VETERINARY MEDICINE

An Illustrated History

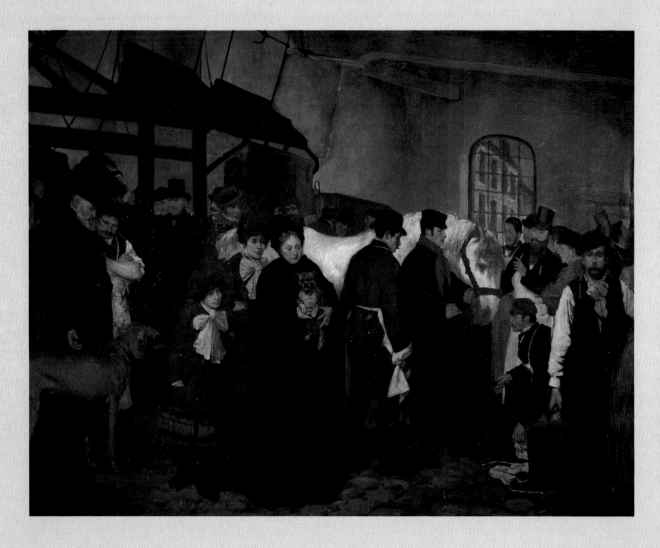

La Clinique Vétérinaire
By Emile Seeldrayers

La Clinique Vétérinaire, an early scene of the veterinary clinic in Brussels, Belgium, was painted in 1884 by Emile Seeldrayers (1847–1933) and is, perhaps, the most intriguing work of art in the history of veterinary medicine. Seeldrayers's painting has been the subject of interpretation for years. It was originally presented to the School of Veterinary Medicine at Cureghem-Brussels in 1961 by the Commune of Anderlecht, in honor of the school's 125th anniversary. It had been purchased in 1893 for 4500 Belgian francs. Tradition, although somewhat ambiguous, identifies several prominent figures from Anderlecht who had been connected with the Cureghem school in its early years in the painting. For example, the figure on the right, wearing a top hat and extending his forefinger, is thought to represent Professor Lambert Hendrickx (1859–1936), lecturing to his students. The figure on the left in his fine overcoat with a fur collar is thought to portray Georges Moreau, the Mayor of Anderlecht. His wife, with their two daughters, is thought to be in the center, holding her small dog. Jean Dupuis (1864–1919), who was to become professor and dean of the school, is also believed to be in the painting.

In reality, Hendrickx was a young teaching assistant in 1884. Dupuis would have been twenty years old. And would Georges Moreau, about forty years old at the time of the painting, have a full white beard?

Whether any identification of subjects in the painting is valid is secondary to the realism of the scene Seeldrayers captured. He followed the Flemish tradition with its legendary attention to precise detail. *La Clinique Vétérinaire*, with its richness of detail, especially in the clothing of the people and the rendering of the animals, provides us with an authentic glimpse of the practice of veterinary medicine at the end of the nineteenth century. The painting now hangs in the Faculty Conference Room of the Faculty of Veterinary Medicine, University of Liège. *(Courtesy of the Faculté de Médecine Vétérinaire, Université de Liège. Mahaux Photography, Liège.)*

VETERINARY MEDICINE

An Illustrated History

Robert H. Dunlop

Cert. Agr., D.V.M., Ph.D., FAAVPT, MRCVS, MACVSc., Ll.D. (hon)

Professor
Department of Clinical and Population Sciences
College of Veterinary Medicine
University of Minnesota
St. Paul, Minnesota

David J. Williams

M.A., FAMI, MMAA

Director and Associate Professor
Medical Illustration and Communications
School of Veterinary Medicine
Purdue University
West Lafayette, Indiana

With 529 illustrations, including 265 in full color

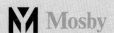 Mosby

St. Louis Baltimore Boston Carlsbad Chicago Naples New York Philadelphia Portland
London Madrid Mexico City Singapore Sydney Tokyo Toronto Wiesbaden

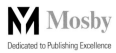
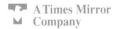

Publisher: *Don Ladig*
Editor: *Linda Duncan*
Developmental Editors: *Kimberly Washington, Carolyn Malik, Jo Salway*
Project Manager: *Patricia Tannian*
Senior Production Editor: *Ann E. Rogers*
Manuscript Editor: *Mary McAuley*
Book Design: *Jeanne Wolfgeher*
Design Coordinator: *Gail Morey Hudson*
Cover Design: *Jeanne Wolfgeher*
Manufacturing Manager: *Theresa Fuchs*
Maps: *Maryland Cartography and University of Minnesota Geography Department Cartography Laboratory*

Printed in the United States of America.
Composition by Graphic World, Inc.
Printing/binding by R.R. Donnelley & Sons Company.

Mosby–Year Book, Inc.
11830 Westline Industrial Drive
St. Louis, Missouri 63146

Library of Congress Cataloging in Publication Data
Dunlop, Robert H.
      Veterinary medicine: an illustrated history / Robert H. Dunlop,
  David J. Williams.
        p.   cm.
      Includes bibliographical references and index.
      ISBN 0-8016-3209-9
      1. Veterinary medicine–History. 2. Veterinary medicine–History–Pictorial works.
  I. Williams, David J. II. Title.
  SF615.D86 1996
  636.089' 09–dc20   95-5238
                                                CIP

95 96 97 98 99 / 9 8 7 6 5 4 3 2 1

Dedicated to

- the goal of strengthening the human-animal bond in all human relationships with the sentient animal world,
- the inspiring leaders and educators who showed the way for the profession,
- the brilliant researchers who advanced understanding or control of animal and human disease,
- the body of the veterinary profession in all its branches which through motivation, learned skills, dedication, and integrity has proven worthy of the high level of public trust it has attained,
- the commitment needed to help the developing world catch up to the current standard of professional ability,
- the goal of restoring and protecting the ecosystems of the world and the animal species they contain.

Dedicated to my wife Josephine Dunlop, who sacrificed countless hours of companionship to sustain my commitment to the production of this opus, and to our six wonderful children, who all contributed in their individual ways, including our beloved youngest son Pytt, who had a special way with animals but whose planned career dedicated to the conservation of wildlife was cut short prematurely.

Robert H. Dunlop

Dedicated to my wife, Andrea, and our children, Lisa, Sara, Anna, and Matthew, who enrich my life in so many ways; to the memory of my parents, Donald and Arlene Williams, who provided me with so much; and to the many individuals by whom I have had the extraordinary good fortune to be influenced and inspired.

David J. Williams

F O R E W O R D

In a classification of thinkers and artists, Isaiah Berlin borrowed a fragment of a poem by Archilocus of Paros: "The fox knows many things, but the hedgehog knows one big thing." According to Peruvian journalist Gustavo Gorriti, this can be taken to mean that foxes have a diverse vision of life, while hedgehogs have a central, systematic one.

To write the book you are now reading, Robert H. Dunlop had to be part fox, part hedgehog, and part encyclopedia. David J. Williams's expertise in the history of art in medicine can be seen vividly in the procurement, presentation, and interpretation of many of the unique pieces of art found in this book. *Veterinary Medicine: An Illustrated History* is a truly monumental work. The history of this most altruistic of healing professions embraces most of human history, as well as the histories of zoology, agriculture, and medicine.

What is now called veterinary medicine began with the earliest people who lived with animals. Then, as now, both utility and compassion surely drove the caring, healing impulse. And these dual motivations continue to drive the profession and those who seek its service.

Michael Ondaarje recently wrote:

The Gurkhas in Malaya
cut the tongues of mules
so they were silent beasts
 of burden
in enemy territories
after such cruelty what
could they speak of anyway . . .

Veterinarians regularly deal with their difficult roles as animals' friends in a world where some animals' other "friends" raise them from infancy to be killed and then eaten.

Animal health remains the primary *raison d'être* for veterinary medicine. And the successes have been stunning: contagious bovine pleuropneumonia, anthrax, tuberculosis, and rabies, to name but a handful.

Not that these animal (and human) scourges have all been conquered, but veterinary medicine now knows how to accomplish that, were there the will to do so around the world.

The study of animal diseases not only underpins the integrity of our meat, eggs, milk, wool, leather, and other animal products; it also sheds light on human diseases. Pasteur, Bernard, Koch, Galvani, and Harvey found animal health and physiology crucial to their breakthrough work, as have, more recently, Carrell, Banting, and Salk.

From the pastoral herders of the Middle East and Africa to the proprietors of "factory farms" in Europe and North America, people and livestock have benefitted from the development of vaccines, treatments, and diagnostic tests. But it was toward dogs and horses, as humankind's first companions, that the earliest healing attentions were directed. These species, along with cats, remain our most important urban contacts with animal life.

The early peoples in Africa and Asia, the early Greeks, the Romans, the Egyptians, and all human cultures so far studied interacted with animals. Animals served as beasts of burden, sources of food or protection, instruments of war, and steadfast companions. They were subjects of scientific study, symbols in art and literature, and objects of religious veneration.

Robert H. Dunlop and David J. Williams's descriptions and anecdotes, throughout both text and legends, portray the sweep and scope of animals and their caregivers, from tribal healers to farriers to today's doctors of veterinary medicine and veterinary medical scientists. Necessarily an overview, this book is historically accurate, cogently written, and enriched with paintings, drawings, and photographs.

This book is to be read, enjoyed, reread, and enjoyed yet again. It is a whale of an achievement.

Franklin M. Loew, D.V.M., Ph.D.
Dean, Tufts University School of Medicine
Member, Institute of Medicine of the
  U.S. National Academy of Sciences

April, 1995

P R E F A C E

Being invited to write *Veterinary Medicine: An Illustrated History* was an honor and provided a unique opportunity to address two goals. The first is to inform the veterinary profession and all its formative groups, including children and students as well as those who might guide their career selection. These people need to become aware of the historical roots, ethos, and achievements of veterinary medicine. The second goal is to educate the rest of the public at large, that is, almost everyone else who might be interested in the topic. Clearly those who own or care for animals would have a special interest. However, there is a much wider audience who find entertainment or fascination in the nature of animals or are intrigued by their roles in the history of science and culture. This book has been developed keeping both of these broad groups in mind, and we hope it will be of interest to both.

The book's theme begins by tracing the regional cultural roots that led eventually to a necessity for a veterinary profession. These began with a growing fascination with and reverence for animals in nature that led to the first artistic expression in caves. The appetite for animal flesh and the use of animal fiber for protection progressed to taming and herding, then to traction and full domestication including dairying, the cultural focus coming on the species that accepted human domination and interaction. The special contribution of the early civilizing cultures of Africa and Asia to medical ideas and to animal health care is examined. The thematic approach then shifts to the great intellectual threshold achieved by the ancient Greeks who laid the foundations for scientific and medical thought. This became the platform that was extended and applied through the Roman and Byzantine cultures and gave birth to the rational and investigational approaches needed for biology and the health professions. The *Hippiatrika* recorded early veterinary highlights, but the trail then petered out into a period of anarchy until it was retrieved by Arab scholars through translation of classic works and their application. It crossed back into southern Europe via the Moors in Spain and the scholarly monastery at Monte Cassino.

From these sites the seeding of the medical schools at Salerno and Montpelier occurred. The enlightened Sicilian King, and later Emperor, Frederic II brought rigor into medical studies and commissioned Ruffus to write all that was known of equine medicine. Progress slowed again in the Middle Ages but was sparked by a few high points for veterinary activities such as the equine medical reporting of Juan Alvarez de Salamiellas in Spain and that of Gaston Phébus in France on the glories of the hunt and the care of hunting dogs. The Italian Renaissance led to a great new surge of rational endeavor built on the classical translations, with the addition of comparative anatomy. However, the need for practical servicing of horses in particular led to concurrent emergence of leaders such as the horse marshals and trades including farriers, grooms, and horse doctors. High points came from the marriage of practical skills and rational thought such as Ruini's equine anatomy and Paré's surgery, which included equine wound treatment. Unfortunately, a great stream of quackery and literary deception developed to capitalize on the burgeoning demand for veterinary care of horses and other animals.

It became evident that an educational program was required to train professionals to provide the medical care needed by animals, and the era of the veterinary schools began at Lyon, on a shaky foundation. However, the examples of a few outstanding individuals set the stage for progress, and the disabling inheritance of intolerance was gradually surmounted. We note how the adoption of a scientific approach in many emerging disciplines played an important role. The discovery of anesthesia and disinfection made possible tremendous advances in surgery. We also show how the adoption of the germ theory and its applications allowed most of the animal plagues and parasites to be controlled. This led to breed diversification and intensification of livestock production while bringing credibility to the veterinary profession as it moved into the modern age of immunology and epidemiology, followed by chemotherapy. The rest of the story encompasses the development of a strong veterinary research arm over the last hundred and fifty years that extended its application from animal health to promotion of public and ecosystem health. The practitioners gradually acquired the satisfaction of competence in diagnosis, therapy, and prevention, while the increasing demand for animal companionship led to the incredible growth of pet animal medicine and the ever-increasing value placed on animals in culture and ecology.

After the early veterinary colleges were established, improved international communication in the more advanced regions led to more homogeneous development of the profession. Therefore, the organizational structure of the book after Chapter 21 changes to focus on the newer traditions of academic disciplines conjoint with the biomedical sciences. The emerging veterinary clinical specialties served by the paraclinical subdisciplines under pathology and microbiology formed another area of focus. Other areas of particular importance to the evolution of veterinary science deserving attention were the concepts of evolution and genetics, veterinary contributions to human and wildlife health, and ethical considerations of animal experimentation and clinical practice. Some influential figures appear in several chapters because of their disciplinary breadth and the multiple ramifications of their contributions.

The originality and breadth of conceptual material required searches of the historical literature that went far beyond the normal coverage of veterinary history. The goals could be met only by consulting bibliographic authorities supplemented by focused browsing and reading over very diverse sections of libraries and manuscripts. The result was being submerged in books and papers over many years while trying to distill and synthesize the perspectives we sought and believed to be valid. Even after the chronological focus zeroes in on more strictly veterinary historical matters later in the book, bibliographic sources were inadequate for the need and a great deal of international searching in scarce historical collections was necessary.

Tracking down relevant illustrations was an enormous challenge that required personal contacts with veterinary historians and the staff of museums and veterinary libraries around the world. In addition, a vast amount of searching in illustrated books and articles dealing with veterinary historical topics was required. The broader topics of animals in culture and public health were easier because there is a great deal of art in these fields and much of it is readily accessible. Nevertheless, the most rewarding moments in this study came in the actual presence of the original art of the cave painters of Niaux; of Gaston Phébus and Juan Alvarez de Salamiellas at the Bibliothèque Nationale in Paris; of the anonymous artist who painted the allegory of Felsina (Bologna) praying for salvation from the rinderpest that destroyed the cattle in the archives of the Stato d'Emilia Romagna; of veterinarian Edward Mayhew's watercolors at the Royal College of Veterinary Surgeons; of Seeldrayers's great painting of the old Brussels veterinary clinic in action, now in Liège; of early equine surgery using anesthesia in Copenhagen; of the fine art of the clinical professor teaching at Vienna commissioned by his admiring students; of the many historical illustrations in the archives at the Royal Veterinary College, London; and in the Comben collection in The Science Museum, London.

Another motivation in producing this illustrated history was the perception that the veterinary colleges have seriously underestimated the importance of a historical perspective to the continuing successful adaptation of the profession. The approach taken has been to track the critical accomplishments that led to progress, perhaps at a risk of underplaying the misdirections and frustrations encountered along the way. We hope that this work will encourage curriculum planners to look again at the need for a historical introduction to the campaigns the profession has conducted in the effort to gain mastery over myriad animal diseases.

Although we are sure to be accused of omissions, a huge amount of information and a large number of illustrations have been left out intentionally because of the limitations of space. Sins of commission are more worrying, and every effort has been made to rectify errors, but some are unavoidable because there are prevalent discrepancies in the literature, especially with respect to dates. Also it seemed important to make a start in gaining a perspective of the veterinary contributions made by earlier Afro-Asian cultures. We hope these innovative but vestigial efforts will spur others to refine their history. We have tried hard to flavor the historical narrative with newly uncovered or reinterpreted information and to use many illustrations that are unlikely to have been seen before. We have avoided focusing too heavily on the nuances of American veterinary history because a number of books have already done so.

We hope that our readers will find that this history broadens their understanding and appreciation of the veterinary profession. The story is fascinating because of the central role animals have always played in human culture and because the creatures themselves are so beautiful and interesting and human-animal relationships can be so rewarding and enjoyable. The veterinary profession has a wonderful story to tell, as the tales of James Herriot have so captivatingly recalled for the era of mixed practice around the time of the Second World War. In addition, the profession has emerged from its various metamorphoses as a field with a combination of advanced practical adaptable professional skills and an expanding potential to contribute scientifically and politically. This is the theme that this book has tried to relate.

Robert H. Dunlop
David J. Williams

ACKNOWLEDGMENTS

Robert H. Dunlop

It is hard to know where to start in acknowledging the assistance I have received along the way; there have been so many contacts. I should start with the Mosby players since without them there would have been no book. Frank Loew and I agreed to take on the project in 1986. Frank withdrew in 1992 because of his mounting workload. David Williams joined me later that year to help with the illustrations. However, when it came to getting the project completed, it was editor Linda Duncan whose patience, assistance, and persistence got us through the process of manuscript completion and illustration listing by chapter. We must be eternally grateful to her for her faith in us and her genuine interest in the project. Conversion of the text to its final form was guided skillfully by senior production editor Ann Rogers. Jo Salway oversaw the preparation of the maps. Two were made by Mui Le and Mark Reimeke of the Cartography Laboratory at the University of Minnesota. However it was horsewoman Linda who kept everyone on the ball, providing appropriate stimuli when needed, although her frustrations must have been many. Her able assistant Kimberly Washington had the formidable task of tracking the ever-changing list of more than five hundred illustrations. Jeanne Wolfgeher engineered the attractive and classic appearance of the book.

Without my son Boadie's contribution in Trinidad in 1990-1991 there probably would have been no manuscript created, or perhaps a much inferior one. He had graduated with a degree in political science at Washington University in St. Louis and brought valuable and articulate perspective from the social sciences that was a challenging sounding board for my ideas. He helped bring order to the vast amount of material I shipped to the Caribbean and translated a substantial amount of veterinary historical literature from German. He became interested in Indian culture and assisted greatly with research on the history of attitudes toward animals and the evolution of medicine in classical South Asian, particularly Hindu, culture using the resources available in the University of the West Indies libraries. He prepared on the word processor the first drafts of all my early writings that were sent to Mosby, with accompanying suggestions for illustrations. Almost half the book was written during that year, appropriately covering mainly the period before the modern veterinary profession was established in France in 1762. After my return to St. Paul I was able gradually to locate more specifically veterinary historical information and illustrations for those chapters. Fortunately, my adaptable wife was prepared to take on the major task of word processing the manuscript and its revisions.

Recalling all the knowledgeable people who gave important assistance in subject matter and art for the book is difficult because of their global and interdisciplinary distribution. Some stand out, however. Library staff of the College of Veterinary Medicine at the University of Minnesota were unstinting in their ongoing support: Livija Carlson and Lisa Berg. Lisa in particular was extremely helpful with searching of the international literature and tracking down items that were elusive. Similarly, their counterparts at the Royal Veterinary College in London, Linda Worden and Jane Kingsley, were very generous in their assistance. Jane, in particular, whose job it was to track and procure old British veterinary literature and illustrations for the college's archives, was a tower of strength in this area. Across the city, Donita Horder, librarian for the Royal College of Veterinary Surgeons, who has had the uniquely valuable role of making library materials available to members of the RCVS, was extraordinarily helpful in finding materials I needed and in making available the Mayhew veterinary paintings for Chapter 25.

On the continent of Europe, August Mathijsen at Utrecht stands out as the great master of veterinary library scholarship and bibliographic development and as the current president of the World Association for the History of Veterinary Medicine. His counsel and assistance on many fronts have been priceless and without peer. Also at Utrecht's veterinary school Peter Koolmees was extremely generous with materials to assist me in preparation for the chapter dealing with the veterinary history of food safety. Fred Smithcors, the doyen of American veterinary historians, has read the entire manuscript, making many valuable suggestions for improvement. So many people have helped that I fear that I may have forgotten some of them. If so I apologize. Many are or were from veterinary school libraries, museums, or faculties: **Germany**: Ernst-Heinrich Lochmann (Honorary President of the World Association for the History of Veterinary Medicine), Barinhausen; Angela von den Driesch, Munich; Johann Schäffer, Hannover; Reiner Grimm, Trauenstein; Martin Brumme, Berlin; Anita Seipert, Leipzig; Friedrich-Wilhelm Schmidt, Göttingen; Andreas Menzel, Giessen. **The Netherlands:** August H.H.M. Mathijsen (President WAHVM), Utrecht; Peter Koolmees, Utrecht; Paul Leeflang (Secretary WAHVM), Utrecht; Ingrid Visser, Drachten. **France:** Jean Brousseras, Alfort; the late Yves Ruckebusch, Toulouse; Jacques Bost, Lyon; J. Blancou, Paris. **Scandinavia:** Carl-Heinz Klatt, Finland; Ivan Katic, Copenhagen; Per-Ola Räf, Skara; Nils-Oler Hellgren, Skara; Folke Rasmussen, Copenhagen; Jorgen Genner, Odense; Olav Sandvik, Oslo; Arne Froslie, Oslo. **Belgium and Luxembourg:** Georges Mees, Brussels; Georges Theves, Luxembourg; A. Albert Dewaele, Liège; Pierre Lekeux, Liège; Robert Marsboom, Vesselaar. **Hungary:** Mary Cserey, Budapest; György Horvath, Budapest. **Czech Republic:** Eva Baranyiova, Brno. **Spain:** Marti Pumarola, Barcelona. **Switzerland:** Werner Sackmann, Basel. **Austria:** Peter Knezevic, Vienna. **Italy:** Alba Veggetti, Bologna; Sergio Biavatti, Bologna; Bruno Cozzi, Milan. **United Kingdom:** Norman Comben, Berkhamsted; Pauline Dingley, London; Benita Horder, London; Jane Kingsley, London; Linda Worden, London; Bob Ablett, Animals in Art, London. **Turkey:** Dr. Erk, Ankara; Ferruh Dincer, Ankara. **Pakistan:** Muhamed Nawaz, Islamabad. **India:** V.V. Ranada, Bombay. **China:** Wang, Qinglan, Beijing; Fengqin Chen, St. Paul. **Japan:** Osamu Katsuyama, Tokyo; Yuzo Koketsu, St. Paul. **South Africa:** Antonie Harthoorn, Kruger Park and East Africa. **Egypt:** Ashraf Saber, Assiut. **Kenya:** David Hopcraft, Athi River. **Australia:** Roger Short, Melbourne; John Fisher, Newcastle, NSW; Helen Fairnie, Perth. **New Zealand:** Ashley Robinson, St. Paul; Roger Morris, Palmerston North. **Canada:** C.A.V. Barker, Guelph; N.Ole. Nielsen, Guelph; Julius Frank, Ottawa; Louis-Phillippe Phaneuf, Ste. Hyacinthe, P.Q. **Mexico:** Miguel Marquez, Contreras. **Brazil:** Isaac Moussatche, Rio de Janeiro; Claudia de Rocha Woelz, São Paulo. **United States of America:** Fred Smithcors, Santa Barbara; Frank Loew, Boston; Andrew Rowan, Boston; Allen Packer, Ames, Iowa; Ole Stalheim, Ames; Claire Fox, Doylestown, Pennsylvania; John Blaisdell, Ames; James Steele, Houston; Calvin Schwabe, Davis, California; C. Trenton Boyd, Columbia, Missouri; William W. Laegried, Plum Island, New York; Roger Breeze, Plum Island; Robert Reichard, O.I.E. Paris; the late Howard Kernkamp, St. Paul, Minnesota; Elizabeth Lawrence, Boston; Robert Shomer, Mahwah, New Jersey; Everett Miller, Wheaton, Illinois; William H.H. Clark, Ringgold, Georgia; Ellen Wells, Washington.

In addition to these individuals, several major libraries have been important sources of published information and illustrations relevant to veterinary history: Bibliothèque Nationale, Paris; The British Library and The Science Library, London; Smithsonian Special Collections, Washington, D.C.; The Wellcome Institute Library, London; Bibliotek Communale, Bologna; the many branches of the library system of the University of Minnesota; and the inter-library loan network.

Several authors, past and present, of books and articles on aspects of the history of veterinary medicine merit special mention: J. Clabby, F. Smithcors, I. Pattison, D. Karasszon, A. Calmette, C. Schwabe, F. Smith, R. Froehner, and E. Leclainche; E. Gattinger, N. Comben, A. Mathijsen, L.P. Pugh, A. von den Driesch, C. Merrilat, E. Miller, W. Clark, R. Thompson, J. Schäffer, G. Mees, C.A.V. Barker, and O. Stalheim.

One thing that has sustained me over the past five or six years has been my growing involvement with veterinary historians, an endangered but wonderful group of people. The World Association for the History of Veterinary Medicine stemmed from German leadership, with Lochmann at the Hannover Veterinary College being the dynamic organizing figure who created the international group. Having had the privilege of attending several of their annual scholarly meetings, I was able to acquire a genuine feeling for historical scholarship. The generous support and assistance I received from several members representing various European countries was invaluable. This was the foundation on which I was able to build, with the help of veterinary and institutional libraries and scholars and by many of my initiatives to make site visits to obtain firsthand the views of scholars elsewhere in the world. My individual contacts throughout the veterinary profession have been extremely rewarding, and they have given generously of their information or provided copies of relevant publications.

David J. Williams

I am indebted to people throughout the world who have assisted me with this project, an *illustrated* history of veterinary medicine. Acknowledging each would be a formidable task, and I ask for understanding in failing to credit everyone here. It in no way demeans their contribution, which I will value forever. Hopefully the credit lines accompanying the figures will indicate to the reader the scope and magnitude of all the individuals and institutions involved.

The School of Veterinary Medicine at Purdue University encourages scholarship and creativity, and this environment is nurtured by Dean Hugh Bilson Lewis, whose friendship and unflagging support of my interest in the history of art in medicine have been invaluable to me. Professor Gretchen Stephens, director of the school's library, and her outstanding staff, have been a godsend. I am blessed to be surrounded by colleagues who have generously assisted me with translations, international telephone calls, and interest in my work. I am especially grateful to Drs. Michel Levy, Melvin Stromberg, Sam Jakovljevic, Augustine Peter, Ourania Andrisani, Elke Scholz, Elikplimi Asem, and Eva Baranyiova, and Mr. Andrew Dziubinskj. Several residents, interns, and students were also helpful, especially Drs. Jeorg Steiner and Claudia Hubensack and Ms. Beatrix in der Wiesche. I am grateful to the staff of Medical Illustration and Communications for their support while I was frequently preoccupied with this project.

Veterinary Medicine: An Illustrated History proved to be a labor of love. While anyone who has worked on an "illustrated" book knows the difficulties inherent in obtaining permissions, especially when artwork is being sought worldwide, the sheer joy of identifying, locating, obtaining, and finally interpreting the beautiful artwork this topic permits was exhilarating. At least half a million images were considered before more than six hundred were ultimately identified as desirable. Librarians and curators proved invaluable in my research for these images and information about them. It is safe to observe that the book would not be possible without their assistance. The following is a small representation of the many who have helped me. Laura Rose, Librarian, National Sporting Library, Middleburg, Virginia; Jane Kingsley, Historical Collections, The Royal Veterinary College Library, London; Benita Horder, Librarian, RCVS, London; C. Trenton Boyd, Librarian, University of Missouri College of Veterinary Medicine; Carolyn Kopper, Collection Development Librarian, Carlson Health Sciences Library, University of California, Davis; Lucinda Keister, formerly Prints and Photography Librarian, History of Medicine Division, National Library of Medicine, Bethesda; Ursula Kolmstetter, Director, Indianapolis Museum of Art Library; Peter Berg, Special Collections, Michigan State University Libraries; Moriya Masashi, Assistant Curator, Osaka Municipal Museum of Art; Dr. M. Redknap, Medievalist, National Museum of Wales; Suzanne Bebbe, Curatorial Assistant, Yale Center for British Art; and Suzanne Whitaker, Veterinary Medical Librarian, Flower/Sprecher Library, Cornell University.

Special gratitude is extended to Dr. Janis Audin, Editor, *Journal of the American Veterinary Medical Association,* whose expertise in art history in general, and animal art in particular, is enjoyed by all who view the beautiful covers of *JAVMA,* which always feature a lovely piece of art demonstrating the human-animal bond. Dr. Audin is continuing a tradition begun by her predecessor, Dr. Arthur Freeman, which has served to enrich the profession and provided me an outstanding resource. I am also grateful to Drs. Emily Teeter, Assistant Curator, and John Larson, Museum Archivist, both Egyptologists at the University of Chicago's Oriental Institute. They patiently assisted me in interpreting the art of this fascinating culture and provided the image of the mummified duck, which is among several pieces of art published here for the first time. Ellen Wells, formerly Head, Special Collections Branch, Smithsonian Institution Libraries, and arguably the world's foremost authority on the history of the horse, made invaluable contributions that found their way into several chapters.

The cooperation, interest, and assistance provided by the international veterinary community have been most gratifying. Dean Albert Dewaele and Dr. Pierre Lekeux of the Faculté de Médicine Vétérinaire, Université Liège, are thanked for providing our beautiful cover art, *La Clinique Vétérinaire* by Emile Seeldrayers. Special contributions were also made by o. Prof. Dr. Peter Knezevic, Veterinärmedizinische Universität Wien; Prof. Dr. W. Schulze, Tierärztliche Hochschule Hannover; Dr. C. Degueurce, Ecole Nationale Vétérinaire D'Alfort; Dr. Vibeke Dantzer and Prof. Dr. Folke Rasmussen, Kongelige Veterinær-og Landbohøjskole, København; Univ.-Prof. Dr. Dr. Johann Schäffer, Fachgebiet Geschichte der Veterinärmedizin der Tierärztlichen Hochschule Hannover; and Dr. Peter Koolmees, Department of the Science of Food and Animal Origin, Faculty of Veterinary Medicine, Utrecht Universtiy.

I am grateful to Mosby for staying the course with this project through thick and thin. I am also grateful to Don Ladig, Vice President, who has supported my efforts on this project from the very beginning. There are simply no words to express my gratitude and appreciation to Linda L. Duncan, Executive Editor for Veterinary Medicine. A better editor could not be imagined by this author. Her interest and level of involvement in guiding this book to completion went well beyond the role of an editor. Kimberly D. Washington, Developmental Editor, also helped bring this book to fruition with her diligence and attention to detail. Both have been a true joy to work with and I cannot thank them enough for all they have done.

Ann E. Rogers, Senior Production Editor, cheerfully saw the manuscript and art through production. Her dedication and concern in bringing this work together were remarkable. I am indebted to the artistic talents of Jeanne Wolfgeher for the unique design and attractive layout of this beautiful book.

Last, but by no means least, I wish to thank Jo Ann Brock, my research assistant. Without her I would still be fumbling to turn on my computer. Her knowledge and appreciation of the artwork combined beautifully with her outstanding organizational skills as a diligent researcher. I wish her all the best as she continues her graduate studies at Purdue.

My contribution to *Veterinary Medicine: An Illustrated History* was accomplished through research at galleries, museums, and specialized libraries. However, the so-called information superhighway also played a key role. Computers, fax machines, and ever more sophisticated software programs enabled me to reach out around the world to not only inquire about but actually see and retrieve images stored in various collections. By this means I became acquainted with many people I hope to meet in person in the future. They confirmed my belief in the innate goodness of humankind. I hope this book will provide them a measure of pride for their contributions.

CONTENTS

VETERINARY MEDICINE
An Illustrated History

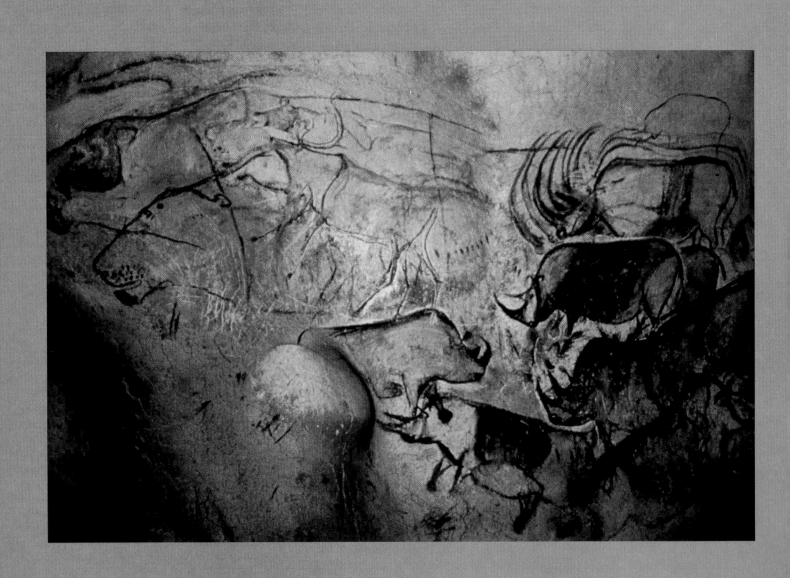

Large Animals Fascinate Paleolithic Artists

PREHISTORIC ANIMAL HUNTERS AND ARTISTS

The publication of Charles Darwin's *The Origin of Species* in 1859 revolutionized biological thought and the way humans viewed their world. At that time Darwin predicted that, ". . . light will be thrown on the origin of man. . ." Indeed the lanterns and flashlights taken into the caves of southwestern Europe that revealed the works of the first *Homo sapiens* artists have illuminated the history and development of humankind and their relationship with animals.

In 1863 the French geologist Edouard Lartet and the English ethnologist Henry Christy began systematic excavations in the Perigord region of southwestern France to establish the sequence of cultural development. From the foundations the scientists laid, the Paleolithic era has subsequently been subdivided based on archaeological evidence, with divisions frequently named after geographical sites at which significant findings were first made.

Hence the Middle Paleolithic period became known as the time of Mousterian culture because of the discoveries in the cave at Le Moustier in the Dordogne region of modern France. This culture, which began about 100,000 years ago and lasted about 65,000 years, is identified with the people known as the Neanderthal, inhabitors of caves and hunters of deer, mammoths, and other mammalian species. The Neanderthal exhibited sentimental behavior in burying their dead with material gifts or relics.

The emergence of the Cro-Magnon race added a new intellectual dimension to what we know of its predecessors. The first part of the more recent Upper Paleolithic period is called Aurignacian because the oldest drawings, paintings, and sculptures were found in the cave at Aurignac in Haute Garonne, also in France. These works are approximately 35,000 years old and appear to be the earliest historical record of artistic achievements made by humans. The crude artistic beginnings of the Aurignacian period were succeeded by the full flowering of animal art in the Magdalenian culture, named for the rock shelter of La Madeleine. The most striking examples of this art are the magnificent animal paintings on the rock walls deep within the limestone caves. In addition to naturalistic animal art, there are examples of symbolic art, including signs thought to depict the external female genitalia. Today three major centers of Magdalenian cave art exist, in the Perigord region, in the central and western Pyrenees, and in Spanish Cantabria; together these centers are known as the Franco-Cantabrian region.

The relics from the Franco-Cantabrian region reveal populations of Cro-Magnon hunter-gatherers who had clearly started to "use their heads" more than 30,000 years ago. Rapid advances occurred in the sophistication of tools. Appropriate materials were selected, and pieces of stone were flaked to yield

1. *Facing page,* One of the many magnificent groups of prehistoric animal paintings in the newly discovered (December 1994) great cavern named Chauvet Cave in a mountainous limestone area near Vallon-Pont d'Arc on the Ardèche tributary of the Rhone river in southern France, northwest of Avignon. Unlike other Franco-Cantabrian art, much of which is hidden away down long dark tunnels, this site consists of a large chamber near the surface. The art has been estimated to be about 20,000 years old, placing it earlier than that of both Cosquer and Lascaux. Another remarkable feature is the wide range of species represented. In addition to a fascination with rhinoceroses, of which about fifty are shown in the cave, and the lions on the left, there were found for the first time a hyena and a leopard or panther, along with bison, elephants, aurochses, deer, horses, bears, and owls. A skull of a cave bear had been positioned on a rock with a backdrop of bear paintings behind it, possibly suggestive of a bear cult. It is considered probable that the enlarged associative and lateral thinking area of the Cro-Magnon brain led to emigration, technological progress, and the creation of symbolic and naturalistic art. Thus the latter may have been an idea whose time had come and spread around the world from its source in Africa. Chauvet's gallery has a greater focus on large and dangerous animals than do the other sites, perhaps implying a sense of awe. *(AFP Photo.)*

2. Map of significant cave locations in Franco-Cantabria and the Spanish Levant where prehistoric animal art has been found.

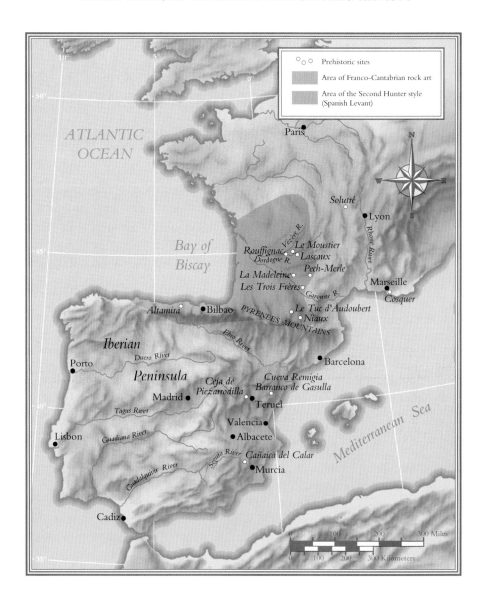

different shapes and degrees of sharpness; these flakes were affixed to spears, which were then enhanced with implements known as spear throwers. Such tools were prerequisites for successful hunting of large animals. Evolving communication skills, particularly the initiation of language and speech, were other essential features that permitted advances in cultural development and hunting strategies.

The cave art of the Upper Paleolithic period in the Franco-Cantabrian region is where recorded history truly begins. The art represents the first attempt by humans to leave a visual record of their times and impressions and thus the first record of the human's relationship with animals. As such, it represents an extraordinary intellectual leap forward in cultural development. The artistry gives us an image of the world of the Upper Paleolithic peoples as one populated by vast numbers of large mammals, as if it were a great game park in which hunting was permitted. In nearly all of the sites, including the famous caves of Lascaux and Niaux, the walls are dominated by precisely painted scenes of large herbivorous mammals. Two classes of animals are predominant numerically in this art: the horses and the ruminants, specifically cattle, bison, deer, and ibex. The supporting cast includes the mammoth, the reindeer, and rarely, the pig. In addition, usually sequestered in a special side chamber, there are images of more dangerous beasts: the bear, large felids, and the rhinoceros. Animals dominated the world view of these artists. Naturally, when these humans felt the urge to create, their art focused on the most impressive animal subjects.

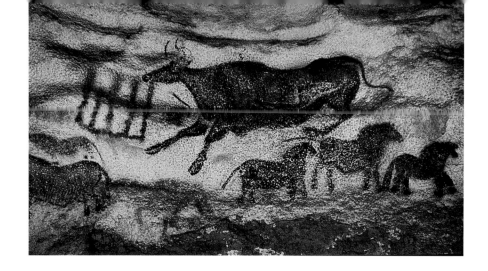

3. Frieze of small horses in the Axial Gallery at Lascaux Cave, Dordogne, France, showing a staggering wild cow that appears to have been speared from the front. The lattice-like structure on the left has been called a trap by some, but it is considered to be a symbolic representation of a hunting magic idea of capturing the spirit of the animal. Early Magdalenian. *(Photo: J. Vertut.)*

4. Mural of second bull and red ox from the Hall of Bulls at Lascaux Cave, Dordogne, France. The scene conveys the mighty power and dangerous horns of the male aurochs, a formidable challenge for the hunters. Early Magdalenian. *(Photo: J. Vertut.)*

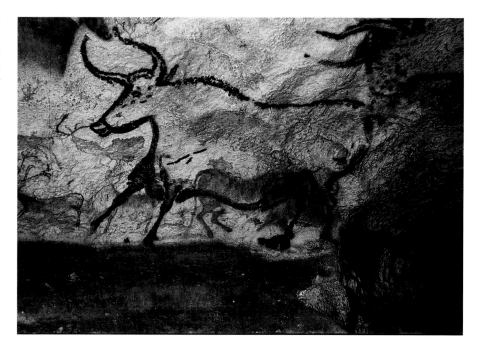

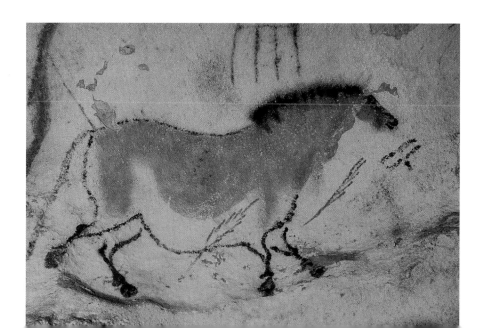

5. Second Chinese horse, so named because of a resemblance to Chinese artists' style of portraying horses as burly ponies with fine bones. The presence of what appear to be flying arrows or spears indicates that this type of animal was a target for the hunt. The image is 140 cm long, from the Axial Gallery at Lascaux Cave, Dordogne, France. Early Magdalenian. *(Photo: J. Vertut.)*

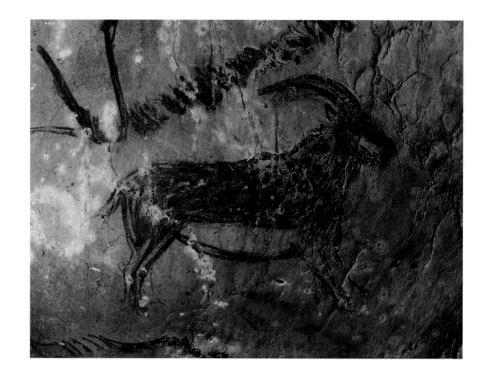

6. Mural of an ibex *(Capra ibex),* the wild goat of the Pyrenees mountains and a favorite but elusive object of the hunt there. From the Niaux Cave, Ariège, France. Middle Magdalenian. *(Photo: J. Vertut.)*

7. Wounded bison from the Niaux Cave, Ariège, France. Middle to Late Magdalenian. *(Photo: J. Vertut.)*

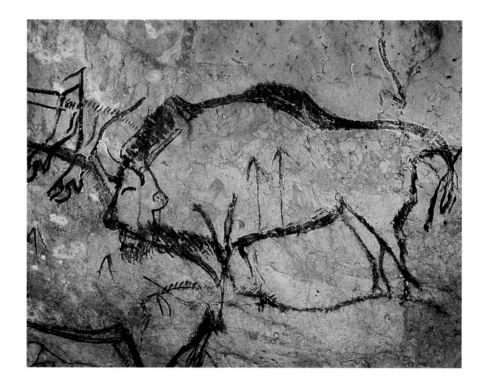

Paleolithic animal art was first rediscovered at Altamira in Cantabria in 1875. The ceiling of the great chamber of that cave is extraordinarily beautiful. One visitor, comparing the cave to Michelangelo's masterpiece in the Vatican, called it the Sistine Chapel of prehistoric art. The dramatic scenes in the Lascaux Cave attracted so many tourists that the art began to deteriorate as a result of biological activity. As a consequence, the cave was closed to the public in 1963, but a complete replica was built nearby for viewing. The simulated art is close in quality to that in the original cave. The cave at Lascaux, among others, is an inspiring attraction for all who are interested in their remote ancestry.

Society owes a great debt not only to the initial discoverers of cave art and archaeologists who worked at the sites, but also to particular scholars such as Abbe Henri Breuil and André Leroi-Gourhan who have made massive efforts to map, draw, classify, and analyze the entire genre of ancient cave art. The latter's *Treasures of Prehistoric Art* and Breuil's *Four Hundred Centuries of Cave Art* are two great classic works in English.

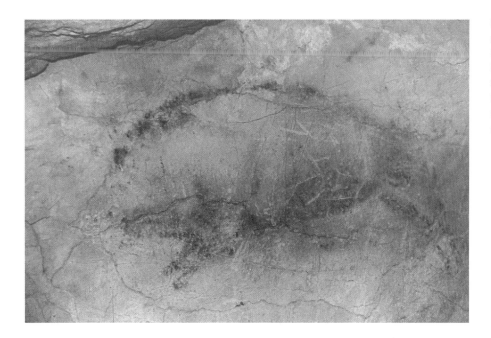

8. Mural of a wild boar, or *Jabali*, found at the Altamira Cave, Santillana del Mar, Cantabria, Spain. The pig is rarely shown in Upper Paleolithic art, and some scholars have recently questioned whether this particular figure is not actually a running bison. Middle to Late Magdalenian. *(Photograph by E. Puig.)*

9. Mural of polychrome large deer, or *gran cierva,* a red deer doe, from the Altamira Cave, Santillana del Mar, Cantabria, Spain. Middle to Late Magdalenian. *(Photograph by E. Puig.)*

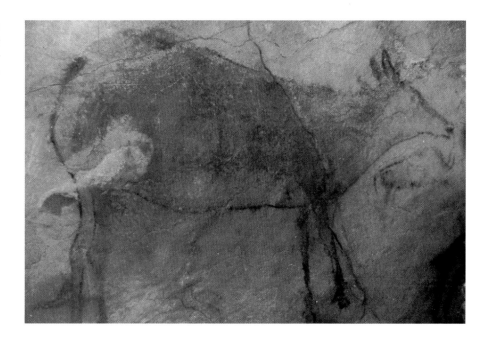

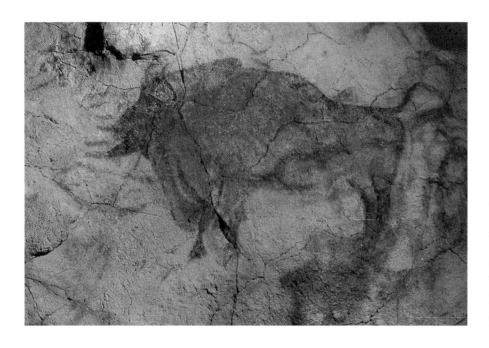

10. The modern discovery of cave art was made in 1879 by the five-year-old daughter of Don Marcelino de Sautuola when she looked up at the ceiling and saw the many magnificent bison painted there. Great standing bison *(Bison priscus),* or what is frequently referred to as *bisonte barbudo* or bearded bison, from the Altamira Cave, Santillana del Mar, Cantabria, Spain. Late Magdalenian. *(Photograph by E. Puig.)*

GREAT AUK IN THE COSQUER CAVE

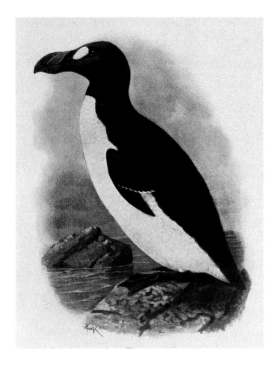

11. The great auk *(Penguinis impennis).* Now extinct, this species once thrived but was eventually destroyed for its flesh, feathers, and fat. The last auk disappeared in 1844. *(Bibliothèque Nationale, Paris.)*

12. Auk, originally mistakenly identified as a penguin. Wall painting from the Cosquer Cave, Cape Morgiou, Marseilles, France. Late Solutrean–Early Magdalenian. *(Photo: F. Broadcast, Gamma Liaison.)*

As recently as July 1991, a great cavern art display was discovered when professional scuba diver Henri Cosquer found access via the cave entrance at Cape Morgiou, more than 120 feet below the current level of the Mediterranean Sea.

The site, 7 miles southeast of Marseilles, includes a narrow entrance to a tunnel that threads 574 feet uphill to the main chamber, which the sea rises to half fill. This perilous underwater passage has already claimed the lives of three divers less experienced than Cosquer who ventured in shortly after the discovery was made. Their deaths led to a decision by the French authorities to close the entrance with concrete once the vital photographs and samples were obtained. The artwork above sea level that has survived includes hand stencils estimated to be 27,000 years old and other symbolic images. More than a hundred engravings and paintings of animals are of more recent vintage, perhaps about 18,000 years old. Thus they are among the oldest of the painted animals of the Ice Age cave period, when the entrance was probably two hundred feet above the sea and well inland.

The repertoire of species represented in the Cosquer Cave is comparable to that of the established Franco-Cantabrian sites of animal cave art; it includes horses, bison, and ibex. However, there are also a few images of sea animals, the most striking being the great auk or garefowl, *Penguinus impennis,* which was seventy-six centimeters long.

The story of the great auk is tragic. The bird could not fly but was an expert swimmer; its medium was the water, except when it came ashore in the spring to reproduce and incubate its eggs. Ungainly on land, it had to find

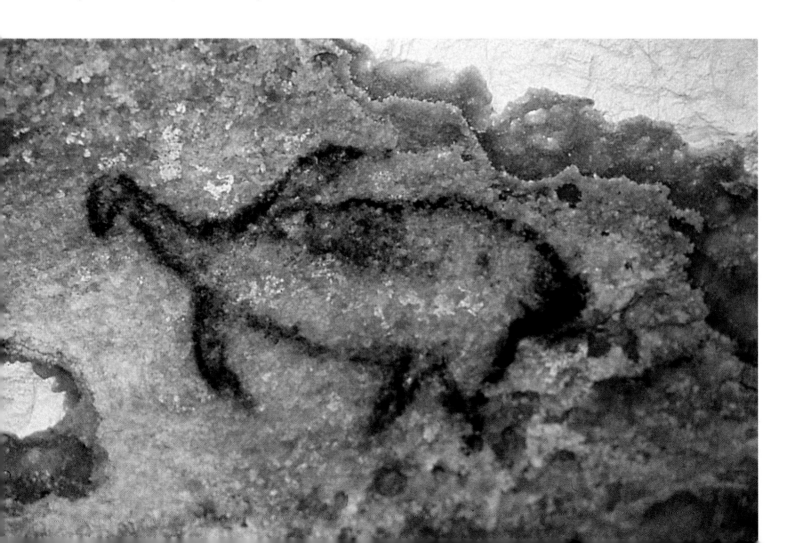

gently sloping rock shelves on which to accomplish these functions. When out of the water, it was uniquely vulnerable to human predators. Until the sixteenth century, when explorers traversed the high latitudes of the North Atlantic Ocean, it was not reported. It became highly prized for meat, hides, feathers, and eggs, and was often carried alive on ships after capture to provide a source of fresh meat. As the oceangoing sailors and fishermen proliferated, the great auk's days were numbered. The last auk was taken in 1844, providing one of the clearest examples of the role of humans in extinction. The visual representation in the Cosquer Cave is thus the oldest record, and confirmation of its ease of capture. Apparently it ranged at that time to southern France and to Spain because of the effect of the Ice Age. The representation of the auk also lends weight to the argument that the animals depicted in the cave art were, at least in part, connected to food harvesting.

LARGE ANIMALS OF THE PALEOLITHIC STEPPE

The animals depicted in prehistoric cave art are nearly all representatives of the class Mammalia. Identifying the individual species has been a controversial exercise for paleontologists and comparative anatomists.

Several types of wild horses were extant after the end of the last glacial era. Some were domesticated and adopted as regional breeds. However, none survived to the twentieth century in the wild state, although some, like the mustang, escaped to exist as feral animals. A wild or feral horse was discovered in Mongolia in 1881 by Nicolay Przewalski. Genetically it is slightly different from the domesticated breeds, having a different number of chromosomes in the cell nucleus. There is evidence that it had been domesticated in ancient times. Today it survives in zoos. Although the horses illustrated by Paleolithic artists show some resemblance to the surviving Przewalsky's horse, they are more lightly built and believed to have been examples of the German loess horse, *Equus germanicus. Loess* refers to a brick-clay geological formation; the fossil bones are found in beds of this material. These horses lived in large herds that spread over the cold steppe of Europe but died out at the end of the last glacial period. Paleopathological studies of the fossil bones have revealed inflammatory exostoses on the metacarpals of some specimens.

Herds of horses presented a serious challenge to the Paleolithic hunters. Their success rate appears to have been low, judging from the fossil bone remains at most cave sites. Only at the early Magdalenian site at Solutré (17,000 BC) on the floodplain in the limestone hills west of the Saone River in east-central France is there evidence of successful large-scale kills of horses. This site shows evidence of the hunters' capacity to plan interceptions of game based on knowledge of the species' behavioral patterns and of the local terrain so that the horses could be driven into a cul-de-sac, where they could be attacked and killed in substantial numbers. The bones from the site show what appear to be butcher marks on both horse and reindeer remains. Sandra Olsen has suggested that the horses passed through the area in bands of six to twelve animals on annual migrations from the winter pastures of the floodplain to the grazing lands of summer in the highlands. The hunters cut them off and steered them into cul-de-sacs blocked by a cliff face, then killed them.

The bison of the cave art is *Bison priscus,* a formidable beast up to six feet high at the withers, with large semicircular, upcurving horns and a prominent mane. A creature of the steppe grasslands, it died out after the adjoining wooded steppe was replaced by forest. *Bison priscus* was supplanted by the European bison or wisent, *Bison bonasus,* a forest inhabitant.

Cattle of the cave pictures are the great aurochs, *Bos primigenius.* Having spread from Asia via damp forests and river valleys, the aurochs took to a grassland steppe habitat but was able to readapt to forest life later, after the last glacial period. It did not become extinct until the seventeenth century, when

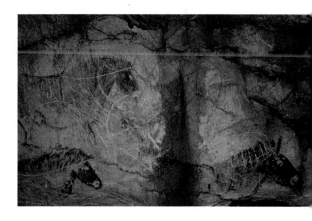

13. The discovery reported by professional diver Henri Cosquer in September 1991 of prehistoric paintings in a cave that opened one hundred and twenty feet below sea level at Cape Morgiou between Marseilles and Cassis revealed a new gallery of the Cro-Magnon artistic representation of animals. Cosquer had to paddle or crawl more than five hundred feet up a narrow sloping tunnel that led to several large, partly submerged chambers to find the art that was still visible above the surface. These three black horses with light muzzles were featured among more than a hundred engravings and paintings. This is the first cave found to portray marine animals other than salmon. At the end of the last Ice Age 10,500 years ago, the sea rose about four hundred feet. Late Solutrean-Early Magdalenian, the art has been dated at about 18,500 years ago. *(Photograph by F. Broadcast/G. Pellisier, Gamma Liaison.)*

14. Location of butcher marks *(1-11)* on reindeer remains found at Solutré, Roche de Solutré, France. Similar signs of meat processing were found on equine skeletal remains. *(Courtsey Sandra L. Olsen.)*

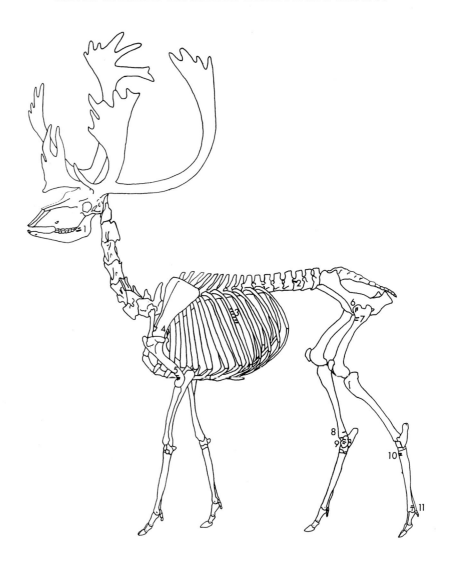

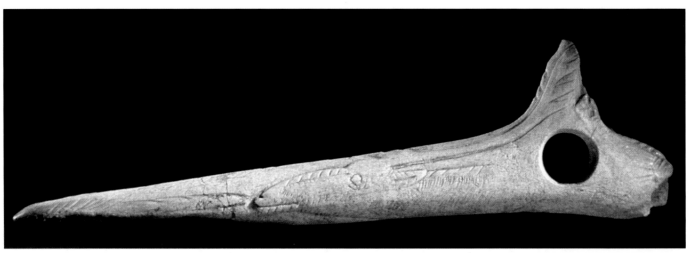

15. The Cro-Magnon's urge for artistic expression extended to carving or engraving animals on everyday objects, such as this perforated staff or spear straightener made from a reindeer antler. The nested signs in front of the animal's head are identical to those found at Lascaux Cave. Found at Laugerie-Basse, Dordogne, France. Middle Magdalenian; 27 cm. *(Photo: J. Oster, Musée de L'Homme, Paris.)*

agriculture and hunting encroached on the wilderness forests. Thus the species survived through the Mesolithic and Neolithic periods into the modern era. The aurochs was a large, dangerous animal with great horns that curved to the side, then swept upward and forward, with an upward twist at the points. Spectacular dynamic examples in cave representations indicate that the aurochs commanded a healthy respect from the hunters. Its remains have been found in peat bogs and old river beds from more recent times.

The reindeer or caribou, *Rangifer tarandus*, although seldom shown in the cave art, was engraved on objects such as antlers and pebbles. This species was a major article of the diet of the Paleolithic hunters, at least at Lascaux. The reindeer were easier prey than the more formidable aurochs and bison or the more fleet horses, ibex, and deer. They abounded in Europe in large herds radiating out from the ice sheets during the last Ice Age. As the Ice Age ended, however, the temperature rose and the forests spread, forcing the reindeer north to Scandinavia and peri–Arctic regions. A migratory species, the young animals may have been particularly vulnerable during migrations, as well as fine fare for the prehistoric kitchen.

Other deer, such as the red deer, *Cervus elaphus,* preferred warmer parkland and wooded country and were more elusive prey for the hunters. These deer made the transition to the forest habitat as the forests advanced at the end of the glacial period. The so-called Irish elk had huge antlers and lived on the steppe but died out at the end of the last glacial age.

The ibex, *Capra ibex,* was a mountain goat of the late Pleistocene period. A prominent feature of some cave paintings, the ibex was admired by the cave artists. It was common in the high plateaus and gorges of the Pyrenees, where a particularly fine representation is found in the art of the Niaux Cave, and in the Alps. Its splendid, divergent, backward-curving ribbed horns were striking. In some areas of high elevation the ibex appears to have been a favorite game species of Paleolithic hunters. It moved down to lower altitudes during cold periods.

The woolly mammoth, *Mammuthus primigenius,* had a thick, hairy coat with an understory, a fat hump, and small ears. These features indicate its adaptation to the cold steppe environment. At the end of the last glacial period the woolly mammoths retreated to Siberia, and their numbers declined rapidly after about 8000 BC, leading to extinction. They appear in cave art

16. Engraving of the "Patriarch," a woolly mammoth *(Mammuthus primigenius),* in the Rouffignac Cave, Dordogne, France. The domed head is clearly demarcated from the powerful humped shoulders, from which the back slopes down steeply to the hindquarters. The massive curved tusks are also portrayed. Middle to Late Magdalenian; 71 cm. *(Photo: J. Vertut.)*

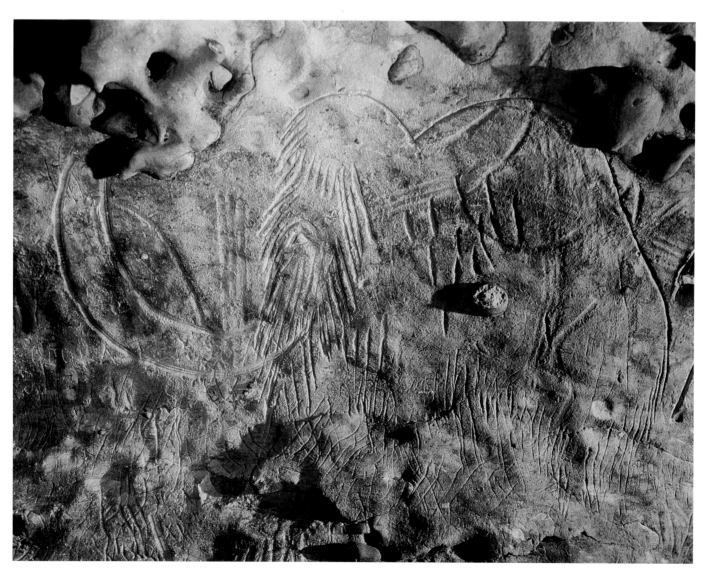

and engravings. Despite their awesome size and great curved tusks, they were hunted successfully by Paleolithic peoples, particularly in eastern Europe and Siberia. The woolly rhinoceros, a grazing species with a furry coat, was adapted to the cold steppe environment but was rarely depicted in the cave art.

The carnivorous species were almost certainly seen as a threat and probably also as competition. The notorious cave bear, *Ursus spelaeus,* did live in caves in the late Pleistocene period, hibernating and giving birth in caves. It was not really a steppe animal, however, and its numbers declined during the last glacial period. Flat molars indicate that the cave bear was mainly a vegetarian. Large and formidable, it had a high, domed forehead. It was replaced by the brown bear, *Ursus arctos,* an omnivorous species with cusped molars that hunted the young of large herbivores. The brown bear is a versatile, adaptable species that can survive in forests and tundra biomes. The cave lion, *Panthera spelaca,* a large, solitary steppe species lacking both a mane and a tail tuft, disappeared at the end of the last glacial period. The cave hyena, *Crocuta spelaca,* was a large, nomadic species of spotted hyena. Its fossils are notable for very large teeth that must have been powered by robust jaw muscles for breaking bones of carcasses. It lived on the open steppe and disappeared at the end of the last glacial period.

The wolf, *Canis lupus,* one of the most adaptable and versatile mammals, was a competitor with humans in the Pleistocene hunt. It can adapt to a wide range of environmental and biological systems. Its dietary needs are met by the expanding population of small rodents in summer and by its hunting of large mammals in winter and spring.

POSSIBLE MOTIVATIONS OF THE ARTISTS

Exactly why the surge of intellectual creativity evident in cave art occurred remains a mystery. There has been no shortage of proffered explanations. An aura of secrecy surrounds the art, with much of it buried deep within dark, nearly inaccessible caverns. Some scholars have inferred from this that the art was part of a magical ritual, possibly conducted by a shaman to ensure success in hunting or some other activity. That the art was simply a narrative and that it served as a way to educate children and facilitate their passage to adulthood are other possible explanations. Some critics have made more crude interpretations of the art, one belittling it as "art for meat's sake," another suggesting that the inaccessible location of the art served as an analogy for the deepest recesses of the female reproductive tract, implying a wish for high fertility rates and burgeoning populations to ensure a steady supply of preferred food and fiber sources. Doodling in the outdoors is a likely explanation for the engravings of reindeer shown on pebbles recovered at the confluence of the Dordogne and Vezere rivers. Coupled with the scene of swimming reindeer painted in one of the caves, the engravings suggest that at this site the deer swam across the river at the start of their migration. Further evidence of some inner creative drive is seen in the exquisite animal shapes carved or engraved on the handles of the spear throwers that date to the Magdalenian period.

The psychological reasons for the Cro-Magnon's artistic explosion will probably never be known for sure, but it is clear that the large herbivores registered as the predominant impression the artists received from their environment, possibly even to the point of becoming an obsession. Maybe just the sight, not to mention the consumption, of these awesome creatures provided the excitement and inspiration for the artistic output of the Cro-Magnon people. Pablo Picasso held the Paleolithic animal art in high esteem. He attributed it to the richness of the faunal environment that saturated the minds of the artists, creating an urge to express the images in pictures, that is, to unload the mind of visions and feelings.

The original artists combined dedicated effort with the unique outpouring of emotion they felt for the objects of their art. Their pictures captured the beauty of form (often in three dimensions) and the dynamism of movement and displayed a powerful feeling for sentience. These creations are all the more remarkable considering that all processes and materials required for their production were invented from scratch. In addition to creating the tools and dyes with which to engrave and color their artwork, the artists made sandstone lamps that burned animal grease to provide a flickering light by which they found their way into the caves and painted. In some caves the artists erected scaffolds so that they could reach the elevated sites, and they used the natural shapes and colors of the rocks to achieve desired effects. The result was the glorious images of animals they created. How fortunate we are to have been left their heritage of art galleries in the caverns of southwestern Europe.

A surprising discovery concerning the relation between the art and the diet of the Cro-Magnon cave dwellers resulted from Jean Bouchud's studies of the distribution by species of the bones found in the Lascaux Cave. The animals depicted apparently were not the main ones used for food. The main animal represented was the reindeer (89% of the fragments); roe deer and wild pigs each contributed 4.5%, and the red deer, 1.5%. Thus the species most commonly depicted in the art (horse, bison, aurochs, and ibex) appear not to have been major items on the Cro-Magnon menu. Considering, however, that the size and weight of the large herbivores would have made transporting them a daunting task, it is possible that larger animals, once killed, were left in the field, with only the hides and large chunks of meat brought back to the hunters' homes. Although this is pure conjecture, it could explain why remains of large herbivores were not found in the caves.

Further studies of the ancient reindeer bones revealed that the phalanges of the reindeer were not fused. Thus they were from young animals taken in the autumn or winter, since reindeer do not easily tolerate temperatures above 55° Fahrenheit (13° Celsius)—partly because of the environmental hazards posed by biting insects, such as mosquitoes and flies, in such warm and moist conditions. In the spring they would have migrated toward higher lands and in a more northerly direction. It seems likely that the choice of subjects by the Paleolithic artists was governed by tastes as much aesthetic as gustatory. Perhaps in this respect they were not so different from many of their successor peoples. Surely the admiration for the horse has not waned, and buffalo, cattle, and other large mammals still hold fascination and awe for most.

More surprising than the lack of connection between the artist's food and art is the absence of interest in representing other things. We find few and mostly feeble representations of people, no vegetation, and only a few birds, fish, and smaller animals. The zoomorphic art of Aurignacian and Magdalenian cultures indicates the enormous importance the people of these periods attached to their relationship with the mammalian world and the surprising humility of their feelings about their own race. The mirror, with its alluring tendency to evoke vanity, had not yet been invented.

There is little doubt that sexuality and fertility were factors in the composition of the pictures. Animals were often shown in pairs, one of each gender, with the male just behind the female in most examples, suggesting an intuitive awareness of the effect of pheromones. Occasional phallic images are indicative of an awareness of the process of fertilization; the many representations of pregnant animals also suggest the artists had some sense of the consequences.

Alexander Marschack of Harvard University's Peabody Museum has published a classic study of symbolism and notation used by the cave artists as an aid to the interpretation of human thought. Marschack's book is aptly named *The Roots of Civilization*. The animals themselves are often symbolic; for example, the ibex is considered a symbol of spring, and bison shown in the molt indicate that summer has arrived. Marschack concluded that the Ice Age artists' cultures were but an instance of the potentially variable human capacity being exploited to achieve adaptation to the opportunities presented by the huge herds that occupied the steppe and tundra biomes of their region at that time. When the climate changed and the herds disappeared, their culture collapsed and the wonderful adaptive capacity of the human brain had to devise new cultural models.

EVIDENCE OF ANIMAL DISEASE FROM PALEOPATHOLOGICAL STUDIES

After an organism dies, there is no opportunity to obtain direct evidence of its behavior or physiology. Once it has decayed, the only direct clues to disease must come mainly from the skeleton and the teeth. Soft-tissue lesions may leave indirect traces of their presence if they caused distortion of hard tissues. The situation is even more difficult in the case of fossils. Remains of extinct species present a special problem because of the lack of extant forms with which to compare them. Although fossilized feces (coprolites) or stomach contents may be difficult to match to the species of origin, they may reveal the presence of fossilized parasites and provide clues to animals' diets.

A remarkable find by archaeologists of the University of Nebraska in 1962 revealed the skeletons of two male mammoths, *Mammuthus colombi,* with their tusks locked in combat. The specimens were estimated to have died about 12,000 years ago. Skeletal injury resulting from physical trauma can leave characteristic visible changes or lesions, particularly fractures and luxations. The cave at Trois Frères in France contained the skeleton of a reindeer that must have fallen into the cave. The deer had shed one antler, indicating that the accident occurred in the autumn. It also had an infected fracture through one side of the mandible. It had had a large abscess with a suppurating sinus and severe osteomyelitis. It appeared that the lesion was at least two months old because a related fracture of the maxilla had started to repair. Some have

17. Illustration of an infected fracture through one side of a reindeer mandible found at the cave at Trois Frères, Ariège, France. The lesions were so severe and of such long standing that the author of the treatise suggested that the animal could not have chewed forage and may have needed human care to survive as long as it did. *(Pales, 1931; de Saint Périer, 1936.)*

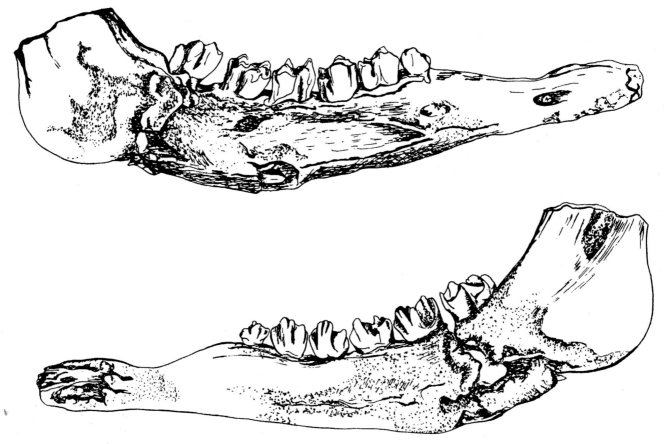

speculated that to survive that long with such a severe disability the animal would have had to receive some nursing care. Another finding, a healed fracture of a reindeer metacarpal, was made at Isturitz.

In many prehistoric skulls and mandibles, dental anomalies have been found. Their incidence became higher after domestication. Equine jaws have revealed teeth that failed to erupt, were turned on their axes, and frequently were overgrown. Such problems are still seen today. Prehistoric dog jaws with a loss of premolars have been found.

Although traumatic and dental injuries are easier to confirm, evidence of degenerative diseases would be of greater interest. If the timing of the prehistoric emergence of diseases in animals could be determined along with information about their paleoepidemiological features, underlying factors that contribute to the genesis of the diseases, the occurrence of cancers, and the causes of extinctions might be revealed. Spread of infectious diseases among species, including zoonoses, would be of particular interest. Recent studies are starting to shed a few promising gleams of light on this area.

During the Wisconsin glacial period in North America, about 72,000 years ago, the Pleistocene lion, *Panthera leo atrox,* and the huge, short-faced bear, *Arctodus simus,* roamed the northern lands. Two specimens of the lion revealed severe disease and congenital abnormalities. An abnormality in both specimens was a lack of incisors, which caused a reduction in overall incisive width. This finding suggests that the northern subspecies carried a genetic factor that caused degeneration of the jaw. The disorder in both cases affected the jaws and teeth. One specimen showed evidence of severe chronic periodontitis and sclerosing osteomyelitis of one side of the mandible, with massive growth of new bone. The other showed loss of a canine tooth with bony overgrowth of the alveolus and a fracture of the other side of the mandible.

Tooth damage and breakages caused by bone crushing are common in large predatory mammals. The lesions in the American lions may indicate a losing battle for successful kills; the lions would have resorted to greater consumption of bone. Other fossil remains of this species have exhibited severe arthritic lesions in the joints of the large bones of the rear limbs.

The skeleton of a short-faced bear, *Arctodus simus,* from about 11,500 years ago was discovered in Indiana and reported in 1987 . The complex bone lesions of periosteal exostoses were thought to be typical of infection caused by organisms of the genus *Treponema,* that is, either syphilis or yaws. This finding, if verified as a diagnosis, raises fascinating questions about the origins of treponemal diseases and the way they may cross the species barrier. Yaws has been found in Eurasian mammals other than humans. There is hope of identifying other diseases that affect the joint tissues, such as brucellosis, in prehistoric specimens.

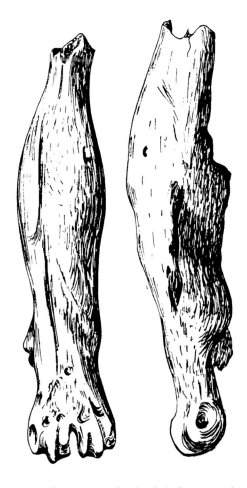

18.   Illustration of a healed fracture of a reindeer metacarpal found at Isturitz, Basses-Pyrénées, France. *(Pales, 1931; de Saint Périer, 1936.)*

UPPER PALEOLITHIC CULTURAL SEQUENCES
FRANCO-CANTABRIA

Years Ago	Cultures	Climate Changes
10,000	Cave art finished	End of glaciation
15,000	Late Magdalenian Middle Magdalenian Early Magdalenian	Warming Cold
20,000	Solutrean	Peak of last glaciation Very cold
25,000	Gravettian	Becoming colder
30,000	Aurignacian	Warmer

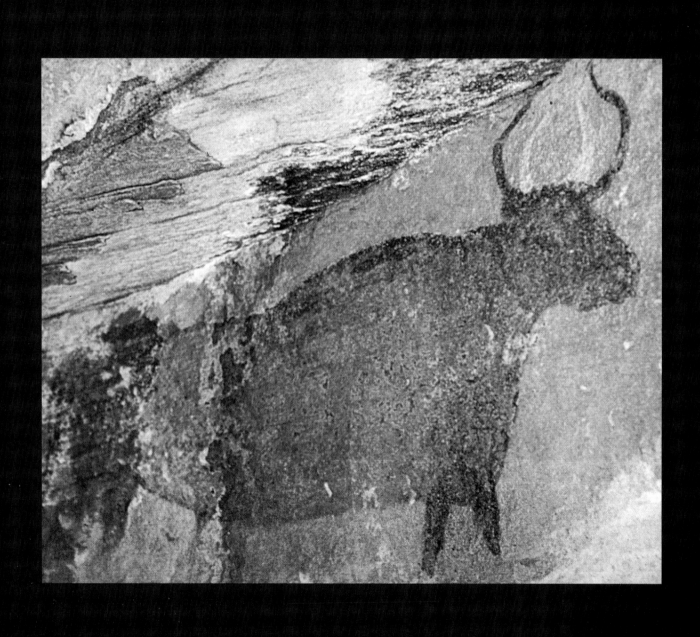

CHAPTER 2

Transition From Hunting to Herding and Farming

~

CHANGING ENVIRONMENTS, MIGRATION, AND CULTURAL EVOLUTION

The period that followed the Paleolithic era, or the Old Stone Age, is called the Mesolithic era, or the Middle Stone Age. The Mesolithic period began as the last Ice Age was ending (about 8300 BC) and evolved into the Neolithic with the spread of agriculture, which was invented roughly 2000 years later. The big thaw was a time of dramatic climatic and environmental change. As the glaciers retreated toward the poles, vast amounts of water were released, causing sea levels to rise throughout the world. The Baltic Sea, English Channel, Irish Sea, and Bering Strait were all formed when the low-lying areas of formerly contiguous land masses were flooded. Air temperatures rose significantly, and with increased precipitation the climate became more humid, particularly at the high latitudes, home of today's temperate zones. These environmental changes led to marked alterations in the biological environment as well. Forests displaced grasslands, spreading northward. Pine and birch, with a hazel substory, predominated at first; however, the deciduous trees, oak, elm, ash, and lime, which took several thousand years to move from southern Europe to southern Scandinavia by 5000 BC, eventually gained the upper hand.

The distribution of animal life changed with that of the plants. Populations of many of the open-terrain species, such as the steppe horse and large bison, declined; others, primarily the reindeer, moved northward with the glaciers. In their place the red deer, roe deer, elk (American moose), aurochs, bear, wolf, and wild pig expanded into the new niches created by the forests.

Human cultures, too, changed considerably during the Mesolithic era. Great geological and chronological variation occurred among societies as people adjusted to changing circumstances. Groups of foragers learned to live by the lakes or the oceans that were rising. The Ertebolle or kitchen-midden culture of Denmark made major use of seafood; the name refers to the middens of discarded shells from oysters, limpets, mussels, and other kitchen waste found beside the camps. The contents of rubbish dumps—skeletal bones of mammals and wild fowl, fish bones, shellfish shells, teeth, hazelnut shells, and spent charcoal—reflect the changes.

The large assortment of Mesolithic cultures makes generalization risky, but some practices were widespread. The bow and arrow, vital to forest hunting, was the most significant new hunting technology developed in that era. Newly flooded coastal shelves provided abundant fish and shellfish, which became a major source of food for coastal communities and spurred the development of harpoons, fish hooks, and fishing nets, as well as rafts, canoes, and boats made of hides, wood, and bark and propelled by wooden paddles. More

19. *Facing page,* The shallow caves and rock faces in eastern Spain along the mountainous borders of the Mediterranean watershed contain a vast, rich artistic record of paintings and rock engravings, which traces the history of the region's earliest inhabitants—hunters and gatherers who eventually became herders. Levantine art, which followed the art of the Paleolithic period, dates from about 8000 to 3000 years ago. It is distinct in its accessibility and the introduction of human figures interacting with animals in the hunt. The black bull shown here, 0.74 m. long, has been carefully painted over a white bull that was drawn earlier. The two bulls are identical except for the horns, which are more pronounced and probably more accurately represented in the latter. This naturalistic bull is the only figure in the cave in which it appears. Ceja de Piezarrodilla, Albarracin (Teruel), Spain. *(Photo: J. Vertut.)*

20. Hunting is frequently depicted in Mesolithic art, as in the scene at right, of hunting wild boar in the Spanish Levant. The original painting is in dark red. Rock shelter of Val del Charco del Agua Amara (Teruel), Spain. *(After Obermaier.)*

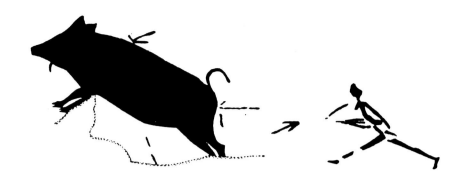

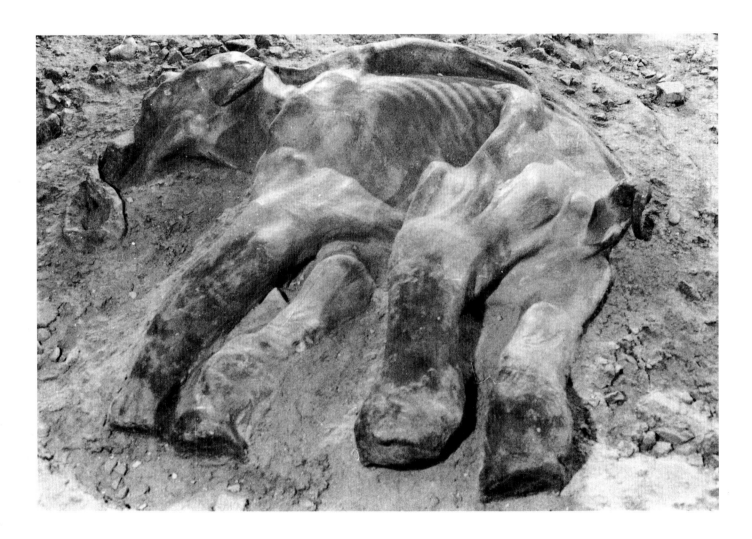

21. "Dima" was discovered alongside the Kirgilyakh River in northeastern Siberia by gold miners working with bulldozers and high-pressure water hoses. The frozen mammoth, 115 cm long and 104 cm high, was estimated to have weighed about 100 kg. It is believed to be about 40,000 years old, and scientists were able to extract DNA from the tissues, but it had undergone considerable chemical degradation. The skin was still intact on the lower portion of the legs. Dima's early death at six to seven months of age reveals the effect of the changes in climate and environment that were brought about by the ending of the last Ice Age. *(Courtesy Biofoto.)*

birds were also consumed. The capacity to develop shelters made of plant materials allowed settlements to become more permanent, since game was no longer as migratory as it had been. In northwestern Europe the Magelmosean culture of the bog people and, further east, the Kunda culture, developed.

The skeleton of an aurochs from about 7000 BC, retrieved intact from the depths of a bog at Vig in Sjaelland in Denmark, had arrowheads embedded in its ribs, and its scapula had been fractured by a spear. Evidently the animal had escaped only to die of its wounds. A set of deer antlers with the frontal bones attached was found at Star Carr in the British Isles. The bones had holes in them, as if to permit tying the antlers onto the hunter's head, perhaps as a decoy or for a ceremonial masquerade. Around 7500 BC, dog skeletons appear in the remains of campsites, suggesting the beginning of domestication of these animals (presumably from species of wolves) for their use as allies in the hunt and perhaps as an early companion species.

The distribution of rock art is remarkably widespread. Examples have been found in the Spanish Levant, the Canary Islands, and over vast regions of Africa from the Maghreb, across the Sahara, through Egypt and the Sudan to Ethiopia, down through central and eastern Africa, to Malawi, Zimbabwe, and South Africa. There are three classes, North African, East African, and the bushmen type of South Africa.

The new hunting cultures that emerged in southern Europe and Africa featured styles of rock art with a focus noticeably different from that of the Paleolithic era. Most of this new art was exhibited in open rock shelters, *abri,* under overhangs in readily visible locations rather than in deep caverns, and the figures themselves are smaller than those of the Paleolithic artists. The hills and gorges of the Levantine region of the Iberian Peninsula between the river Ebro in the northeast and the Seguro river in the southeast, in the eastern part of modern Spain, contain many rock paintings. Most of them were made between 7000 BC and 3000 BC , bridging the Mesolithic and Neolithic eras, although some have been dated to 10,000 BC. Except for these older paintings, in which animals are the focus, the new art is characterized by human figures engaged in daring, vigorous activities such as hunting game (aurochs, deer, ibex, boar, and rabbits) with bows and arrows, fleeing from a wounded bull, and gathering wild honey in trees, suggesting a new militant efficiency.

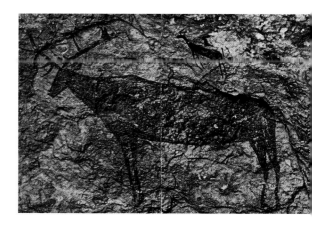

22. The central deer, a stag, from Cañaica del Calar, El Sabinar (Murcia), Spain. *(Photo: J. Vertut.)*

23. The paintings of the Spanish Levant are dominated by scenically grouped hunts, often representing more than one species. The hunter on the left in the rock painting, *below,* is being pursued by a wounded wild ox; the archer on the right has wounded an ibex. Pigs can be seen in the center. Note the stylized human figures in acrobatic dynamic motion. The original painting, in dark red, shows not only the success that is possible in a hunt, but also the ever-present danger. Cave of Remigia, Barranco de la Gasulia, near Ares del Maestre (Castellón), Spain. *(After Porcar.)*

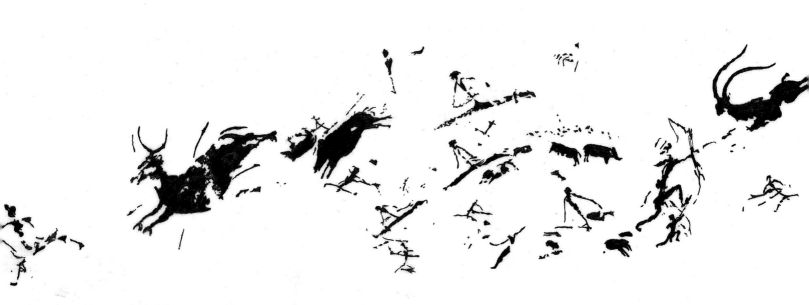

NORTH AFRICAN ANIMAL ROCK ART

Relative dating of the African animal rock art allows four main periods to be identified based on the types of animals depicted. The oldest of these appears to have started about 7000 BC. It is a period of hunting because nearly all the animals are wild species. It is called the *Bubalus* or Hunter Period because the extinct buffalo *Bubalus antiquus* is a common feature along with elephant, rhinoceros, hippopotamus, giraffe, large antelopes, and ostriches. Some domestic animals are portrayed in the transition to the second era, the Cattle or Pastoral Period, which includes a mix of domestic cattle and fat-tailed sheep with a few wild species. This category is thought to go back as far as 4000 BC, at which time the bow had appeared. Third came a Horse Period of three stages, with chariots in the earliest representations about 1200 BC, accompanied by cattle, moufflon, and dogs; these were followed by a Horsemen stage in which riders were shown. After a transitional Horse and Camel stage during the Persian invasions that started in 521 BC, the Camel Period arrived from about 100 BC. It is as if the artists were spectators to a changing tapestry of man's exploitation of animals.

Rock art pervades many parts of the African continent. In the Maghreb region of northwestern Africa the now-extinct long-horned buffalo dominates the art from the oldest period, often accompanied by other large mammal species shown engraved on rock faces. Barbary sheep, especially rams, and

24. Map showing African animal rock art sites. *(Redrawn and modified with permission from Franz Steiner Verlag Stuttgart [formerly Wiesbaden] GmBH.)*

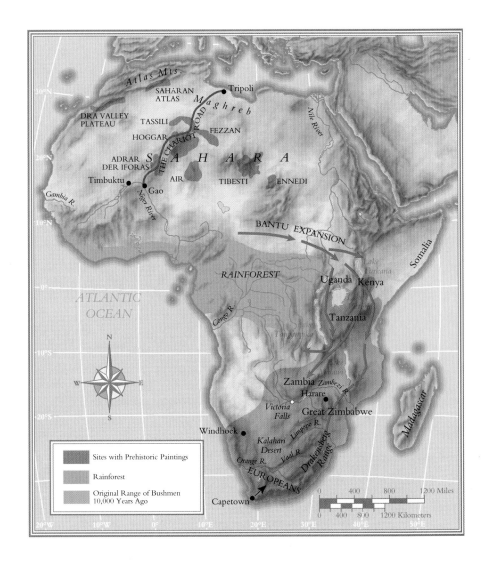

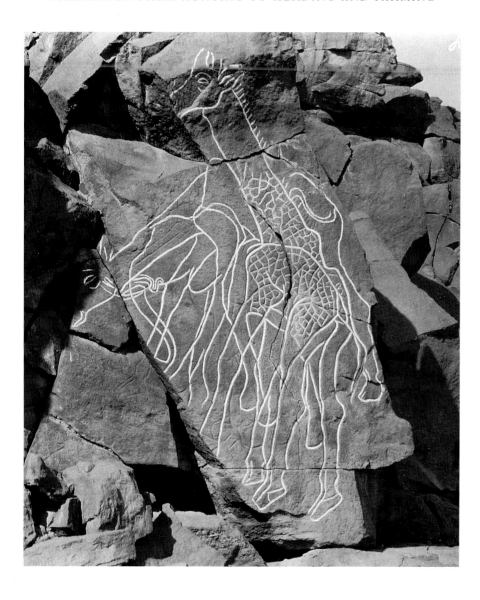

25. The oldest North African art of the *Bubalas* or Hunter Period is distinguished by engravings and paintings of wild species of animals. This Neolithic scene of a giraffe and an elephant was found on a rock formation in Fezzan, North Africa. The chronology of African animal rock art overlaps that of the Spanish Levant but extends beyond it into the modern hunting era, when domesticated animals are represented. *(Photograph by Frobenius-Institut, Frankfurt.)*

ostriches and African large game are also shown. Prolific examples of rock art occur farther east and south at locations called Fezzan, Tassili, and Hoggar. The mentality and motives of the artists parallel those of the Franco-Cantabrian cave artists in their focus on the most dramatic large animals, but the content differs, being supplemented by many human figures. The Sahara then was not the extreme desert it is today. It supported a large human population with various active cultural groups in an arid but habitable environment created by the higher humidity and rainfall that followed glacial melting.

In the central Sahara, the mountainous region including the Hoggar Mountains was a crossroads between the Mediterranean cultures to the north and the Bantu cultures of the Niger River valley to the southwest, as well as a gateway to the Egyptian and Nubian cultures to the east and southeast. The rock faces of the massif attracted artists for several millennia, from the period of hunting societies to that of cattle-herding tribes; their art was seasoned with invaders who had horses and chariots (the sea peoples) and later incursions of camel riders. The artists ranged from buffalo worshippers through bow hunters to members of Bantu cultures. The Bovidian pastoral period around 4000 BC is evident in the art. The equestrian chariots of Cretan invaders from Oea, who crossed the trans-Sahara road as far as Gao on the Niger River in 1200 BC, are depicted, as are Egyptian dynastic influences after 3000 BC and the camel-riders' invasions from Arabia in 100 BC. One of the most artistic representations from the Bovidian period shows a large cattle herd at Tassili Tabbaren and includes a scene of sacrifice. The same style is found in the upper Nile River valley and in surrounding areas of the Libyan-Nubian desert.

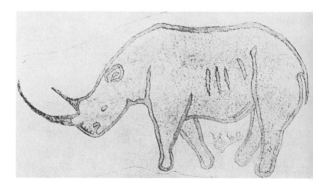

26. Technique and craftsmanship in African rock engravings of animals range from early outline scratchings to more labor-intensive inscriptions that resemble sculpture rather than engraving. Because of such variety, the medium is frequently referred to as *petroglyph*. This engraving of a rhinoceros from the Hunter Period is an accurate representation of the effort and skill that this medium demanded of the artist. *(Courtesy The British Museum, London.)*

BUSHMAN ANIMAL ART OF EASTERN AND SOUTHERN AFRICA

The major artistic culture that emerged in southern and eastern Africa left many engravings and paintings on rock surfaces, under sheltered overhangs, and on fragments of stone. Several artistic styles are represented. One of the artistic groups was the Little People, the *Boismen* (Bushmen) seen by the Dutch explorers. The Khoisan peoples had been the only human inhabitants of a vast area of southern and eastern Africa for 10,000 years until early in the Christian era when the Bantu or Congoid cultures expanded southward and eastward into those regions. At their peak the Khoisan peoples had ranged from the Cape of Good Hope up to Kenya. Two types have been identified among the Khoisan, the Khoikhoi or Hottentots, who were herders who adopted modern life-styles and trained special cattle to guard their kraals, and the smaller San or Bushmen, who remained hunter-gatherers. Around AD 1600 the Sotho crossed the Drakensberg range and were followed by the Shona people. Disaster for the Bushmen resulted from the militant Zulu expansion under Shaka (king from 1818 to 1828) southeastward through Natal, forcing out the other Bantu pastoralists such as the cattle-loving Nguni, who escaped to the north in the 1820s but murdered the Little People as they crossed the Khoisan lands. Eventually they were left with only the inhospitable Kalahari desert. The Bushmen developed a range of arrow poisons made from toxins of animal and plant origin. These included snake venoms (puff-adder and cobra), scorpion and trap-door spider venoms, and a very potent insect toxin from the juice of grubs of certain beetles. The Bushmen used euphorbia juice as a fish poison.

27. The combined scratch-and-punch technique was favored by the early African engraver. *Below,* The eland was carefully cut into dark grey rock (diabase) in western Transvaal. The length of the animal is approximately 40 cm. *(Courtesy Nasionale Kultuurhistoriese Museum, Pretoria.)*

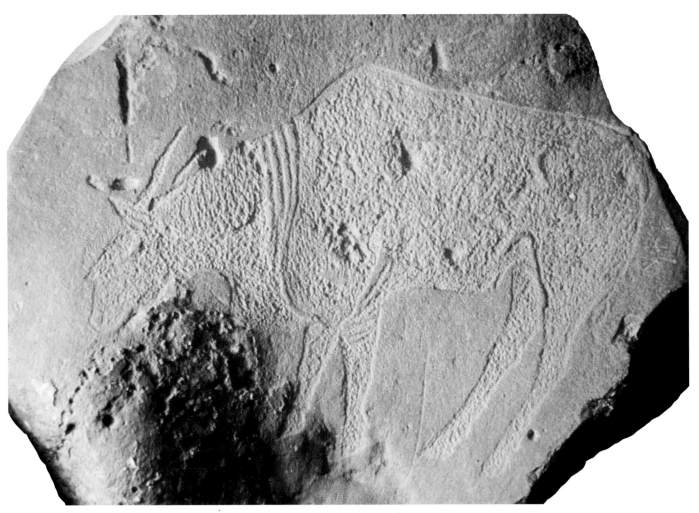

Europeans arrived at the Cape of Good Hope, and the Germans, Dutch, British, and Zulus competed for territory. The Khoisan peoples, having lost their traditional game and sanga cattle to the Bantu invaders, looked to other sources. The adaptive Bushmen became a little too clever as horse thieves and cattle rustlers, probably seeing the European livestock as other fair game but inadvertently bringing the wrath of the new invaders upon themselves. The limited number of survivors of these ingenious hunter-gatherers and their brilliant artists were virtually wiped out by the colonists early in the twentieth century, with only a few pockets of Bushmen remaining in the Kalahari Desert, an area too dry for crops or pastures. Some survived by becoming subservient to the more powerful tribes or colonists. Their art was naturalistic and included people and scenes of daily life.

Many of the Bushmen's rock pictures included animals, often shown alone or being hunted with bows and arrows. Although these pictures vary in quality, some of the representations of animals are striking for their beauty and dynamism, the animal figures always showing an individuality and a personality lacking in most of the human figures. This feature reveals an intimacy with and a focus on the animals' nature. Recognizing their spiritual connection with the animals, the hunters apologized to them after a successful hunt.

Another artistic style, the so-called wedge style, emerged in the area of Great Zimbabwe. Monochromatic paintings in the wedge style represented a broad range of social activities, as well as animals and plants. However, the people who created art in the wedge style did not have the knowledge of animal lore that the Bushmen had.

In 1721 a Portuguese missionary in Mozambique was among the first to report finding Bushman animal rock art. Dutch explorers then found examples of it along the Fish River in the eastern Cape, attributing them to Bushman artists. French explorers found rock art in 1847 in the Maghreb. The German explorer-scholar Heinrich Barth first found the engravings in the Fezzan region in the Libyan Sahara, where paintings were later found, showing abundant fauna that must date back to a much earlier, wetter period.

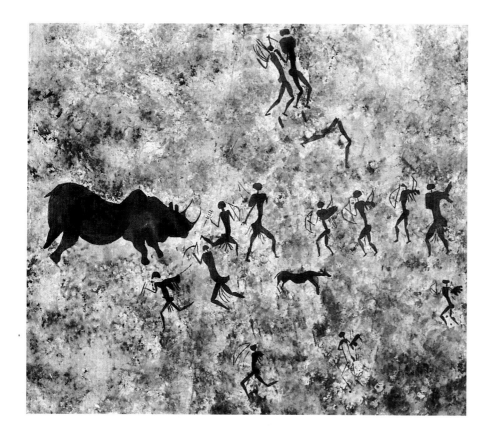

28. Scene of a rhinoceros hunt, including archers and small antelope. Painting on granite. Naukluft, southwestern Africa. *(Copy Weyersberg, Frobenius-Institut, Frankfurt am Main, 1929.)*

George Stow, an English historian with an interest in rocks, recorded the rock art of southern Africa by copying many selections of it. Stow died in 1882; his work was not published until 1930. A major study of Bushman folklore and language was undertaken by another German scholar, Wilhelm Bleck, a close friend of the Stows. A great debt is owed to these two dedicated, painstaking students of Bushman art and culture, because the fascinating Bushmen were to become the target of an extermination campaign by external tribes lacking their aesthetic sensitivity and mastery of their ecological niche as hunter-gatherers.

The capacity of most natural savanna biomes to support fixed human nutritional requirements is estimated at only one to two persons per square mile. Thus as the populations of hunter-gatherer societies grew to exceed this density, their scope was self-limiting. Success in hunting, however, required a cooperative group of sufficient numbers to ensure sufficient kills and protection from predators. When climatic change led to instability of flora and fauna, adaptation to ecological change was necessary. The combination of environmental change and hunting pressure was too much for many vulnerable species such as the mammoth and the ancient buffalo. Humans adapted by restricting maximum group size to be compatible with the carrying capacity of the range. When maximum group size was exceeded, forays were made into new territory. Such forays led to trespassing into other groups' traditional ranges and to competition. Signs of human conflict appeared in rock art.

NEOLITHIC TRANSITION TO PASTORALISM AND AGRICULTURE

Just 12,000 years ago a world in which virtually everyone lived as part of a group of hunter-gatherers was to disappear over the next few millennia and be replaced progressively by a world comprising agriculturalists and herding societies. This change marked the virtual end of human existence as part of natural ecosystems, the end of humans' living within the constraints of those ecosystems. The Neolithic revolution involved mastery over certain life forms (plant and animal) of the planet that could sustain human existence and ensure a dependable food supply. This process, which involved domestication of plants and animals, liberated the human race from the uncertainties of the natural supply of edible nutrients and triggered a population explosion.

The pastoral way of life—travelling over steppes or savannas with herds of ruminant livestock—was a development from hunter-gathering via domestication and early agriculture. Having acquired and expanded domesticated herds of sheep and goats, Neolithic peoples developed patterns of pasturing their herds to exploit the local environments and seasons. Later, when cattle were domesticated, a more aggressive culture emerged, involving longer distance herding on steppe pasturelands that ran from eastern Europe to the Pamir Mountains.

A catalytic step that changed the world followed domestication of the horse in southern Russia: its development as the mode of power for war machines. First chariots provided mobility, then mounted archers and swordsmen brought fighting capacity to a level that had not previously been conceived. The gentle shepherds and cultivators either fled from the horse-powered warriors or were massacred. The use of the horse allowed nomadic barbarian tribes to expand and, buoyed by their success in battle and their dominance over other cultures, they fought among themselves, the winners forcing the losers to move on to stake out fresh territory. The general movement of tribes was from east to west and from north to south across Eurasia. An earlier exception to this trend must have been the movement of the migrants from northeastern Siberia who crossed from west to east and southward to the New World.

In horse-drawn chariots the Hittites took over Anatolia (Asia Minor) around 2000 BC. Other invaders overwhelmed the Hurrians in Syria five hundred years later, and the Aryans surged down into India about the same period. The Scythians, a Eurasian nomadic pastoral tribe that migrated via the Volga River basin to settle on the almost treeless southern Russian steppe north of the Black Sea about 1000 BC, mastered horseback riding for hunting and warfare. They smelted metals for manufacture of weapons and harness parts. Their ferocious bearded warriors were skilled with bow, spear, and sword from their simple padded saddles, even though they lacked stirrups. Their endurance as riders was such that they could spend the entire day in the saddle. They rode only geldings and had learned to castrate. They became undisputed masters of steppe cavalry tactics, enslaved agricultural peoples, and plundered their way to riches. They drank fermented mares' milk and wine and inhaled the smoke from smoldering hemp seed. They loved the exquisite gold ornaments they commissioned from the Greek artisans. Although they stood off the mighty expansionist emperors, Darius of Persia in 514 BC and Alexander of Greece, they became lazy and were supplanted about the third century BC by the Sarmatians, who were unusual in having mounted warrior women as well as men. From the fourth to the sixth century AD the Huns and other nomads overran the Roman Empire and in turn were pushed by others from the east.

Wherever the barbarian peoples went, they maintained a hunting-magical ethos and a belief in shamanism. The animal style of their art reflects their ethos in motifs such as the animal looking backward and the beast of prey at the victim's throat. The so-called x-ray style, which reveals internal structures or patterns of animals and was a speciality of Australian Aboriginal artists in Arnhem Land, and the stag, the favorite animal of the chase, are also hunting-magical features. The stag appears in the art from many regions, but nowhere is it so spectacularly represented as in the Scythian metal works, made in Black Sea settlement towns by Greek goldsmiths.

MIGRATIONS BETWEEN THE NEW WORLD AND EURASIA

Unraveling the contradictory archaeological evidence and subsequent interpretations about human arrival in the New World is a controversial endeavor. There are adherents and detractors for the idea of very early penetration by land to Alaska or of later crossing of the Pacific by ship to establish cultures in Central and South America. There is, however, general agreement on the periods of geological opportunity to make a land crossing via the Bering Strait during the last Ice Age. The massive trapping of water in glaciers lowered the sea level so dramatically that a wide land bridge emerged from the Bering Sea between northeastern Siberia and western Alaska. Thus land animals crossed in both directions: mammoth, mastodon, and steppe bison entered North America very early, long before any humans. On the other hand, the horse and camel traversed westward into Asia and became established there, although their progenitors died out in the New World before 8000 BC. An important argument against early human crossings is the lack of evidence of human settlements on the Asian side above the latitude of 60 degrees north; there were no candidates available to make the trek until late in the time of the land bridges, between 25,000 and 11,000 years ago.

The newcomers arrived near the top of the world in a virgin land that was extremely cold inland from the coastal zone. They probably followed their preferred prey species, which included the large pachyderms and giant bison they had learned to hunt. The people knew how to make protective winter clothing from animal hides and pelts, as well as stone tools for the hunt and fire for heat and cooking. It seems likely that toward the end of the bridge period, some of the newcomers may have brought domestic dogs.

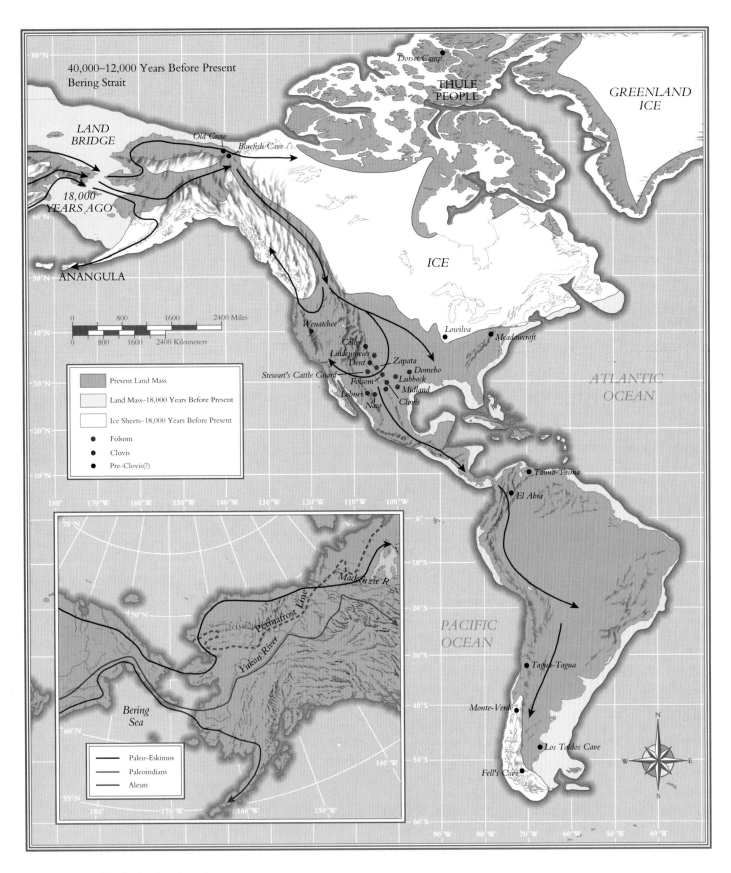

29. Map of Beringia showing the geological opportunity for a land crossing between northeastern Siberia and western Alaska during the last Ice Age. The routes taken by the three main groups who crossed via the Bering land bridge are shown with their subsequent radiation and diversification.

24

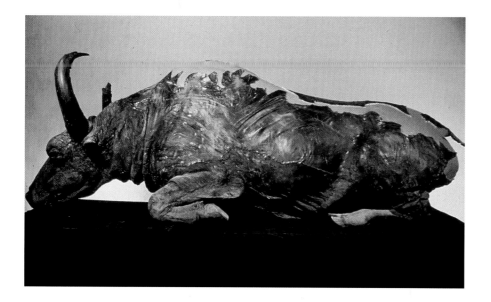

30. "Blue Baby," a bison *(Bison priscus)* that was killed by a lion and frozen in Alaska 36,000 years ago, during the prehominid Pleistocene era. The land crossing via the Bering Strait allowed land animals to cross from both continents, and steppe bison entered North America before any humans did. Taxidermy mount of hide. *(Courtesy The University of Alaska Museum; photo by B. McWayne.)*

Dale Guthrie of the University of Alaska conducted the scientific investigation of the famous Blue Baby, a naturally mummified bison killed by a lion in Alaska 36,000 years ago during the prehominid Pleistocene era. He has described the ecological situation that awaited the immigrants who crossed the Bering Strait. Guthrie traces this fascinating story of progress from the time of the mammoth hunters up to the joint Russian-American research on the DNA of the mammoths of Eurasia mummified in the permafrost.

The last Ice Age allowed land crossings between the New World and Eurasia. It seems that hunting peoples from the Asian continent and maritime Eskimo peoples from the Arctic rim made the crossing to the New World. The former fanned out and occupied the mainland of North America, some proceeding through Central and South America. Many tribes evolved, developing different life-styles, and learning to exploit the native plants and animals. At first the only domestic animal was the dog.

Once on the Alaskan mainland, the people must have ventured into the continent, probably in several waves. Some were hunters destined to become the Paleo-Indians, who headed east, then south and southeast through the Mackenzie River gap to give rise to the diversity of Native American cultures. They advanced throughout the northern continent, then down through the funnel of Mesoamerica to enter the great expanse of the southern continent and a new set of challenges. Other waves were Arctic-adapted maritime people of Aleut-Eskimo type. One of these took the northern route eastward along the Arctic shoreline to become hunters of sea mammals, fish, and caribou. Another group turned back along the Aleutian Island chain. These Paleo-Arctic peoples probably gave rise to the later Aleut and Eskimo cultures.

One ancient site was at Anangula on an islet near Umnak in the eastern Aleutian Islands. Anangula was a major base for boat people who, sealed into their two-person skin kayaks for the hunt, lived off the rich fishing, including salmon and sea mammal ecosystems. Another group that traversed the Arctic shores developed a more diversified life-support system. They headed inland to hunt the caribou and musk-ox and made trips to coastal regions to hunt sea mammals and fish. A third, the Thule people, developed larger boats (umiaks) and the harpoon attached to a line, which would stay in the animal's body and even allowed hunting of whales at sea. It has been estimated that the newcomers to the New World had radiated from the Bering Strait to Greenland within one hundred years of their first entry to North America. Much later they encountered the exploring Norsemen, who reached Greenland and Labrador around AD 1000 and who departed again after two centuries.

The Paleo-Indians had several branches. The Pacific Northwest group moved down the West Coast from Alaska and developed a rich society based on both the excellent fishing, shellfish, and sea mammal resources of the region and the waterfowl, animals, and plant products. The people made wooden houses and large wooden canoes and sculpted wooden totem poles adorned with carved mythic animals and symbols of their ancestors.

The main force of Paleo-Indians who crossed the straits may have been following the woolly mammoth; they are believed to have headed south down the Mackenzie River corridor to penetrate the continent, the various groups then fanning out like prospectors staking their claims to the new land. The distinctive stone tools of the Clovis culture appeared on the Great Plains about 11,500 years ago and spread rapidly. As the glaciers receded to the north, prairie grasslands supported a population explosion of wild game, notably mammoth, mastodon, and bison.

CLOVIS CULTURE AND LARGE MAMMAL AVAILABILITY

The discovery of projectile heads five to thirteen centimeters long, some between the ribs of Ice Age mammoth bones at Clovis, New Mexico, gave the name to the culture and roughly indicated its age. Evidently these ancient hunters thrived on mammoth steaks, their preferred diet, because the culture spread rapidly over the continent. They also hunted a now-extinct form of bison with long horns, *Bison latifrons,* and other species that soon became extinct in North America, such as the tapir, camel, and horse. Although the culture radiated throughout the land from coast to coast, the Clovis people appear to have operated as small, widely scattered bands who hunted at waterholes.

Mammuthus columbi (the Columbia mammoth, not the woolly) was prevalent in the Utah area at the end of the most recent Ice Age, about 10,000 years ago. One specimen was found about 9000 feet above sea level. Skeletal remains showed widespread osteopenia, probably caused by a type of osteoporosis, and arthritis. The condition was described as ankylosing spondylosis deformans, a syndrome found in aging animals, and the estimated age of the specimen at death was sixty-five years.

The Indians who succeeded the Clovis culture used similar methods but developed larger scale operations, specializing in killing bison and some mammoths. The Clovis culture lasted only about five centuries, despite its apparently successful occupation of much of North America. Its extinction coincided with that of several big-game species such as the mammoth, mastodon, camel, and giant sloth. Possible causes included the ecological consequences of climatic change and the hunting pressure of the multiplying new predator, the human being. The Clovis people may have contributed to the demise of the largest mammals, including the mammoth. The Plains Indians that followed, such as the Folsom, specialized in bison hunting, but a significant reduction in numbers of bison did not occur until the invaders arrived from Europe.

Paleontologist Paul S. Martin has calculated that seventeen generations of a band of a hundred hunters would have populated the entire North American continent in 340 years with one person per square mile, assuming doubling every twenty years. He based his estimate on the actual reproductive rate recorded among the mutineers from *H.M.S. Bounty* on Pitcairn Island. Given the slow reproductive rate of mammoths and mastodons and their habitual preference for specific types of environment, it is not hard to envisage a scenario such as Martin has proposed. However, once the breakpoint came and prey density declined, the hunters' population crashed, too. The added factor of droughts in the postglacial era undoubtedly hastened the demise of the large mammals in drier areas, but unanswered questions remain.

BISON HUNTERS

The successors to the Clovis people had to adapt to the changing environment in which several major mammalian prey species had disappeared. The species that dominated the plains, the steppe bison, *Bison priscus,* was well adapted to arid steppe environments in Eurasia before its entry into North America. Other bison species were present, and a new form emerged, *Bison bison,* the one that has survived while all the other species have become extinct. After the Plains Indians emerged, they became proficient in hunting buffalo; it provided most of their necessities of life and became the artistic and spiritual center of their culture. Some tribes exploited the buffaloes' tendency to stampede by driving them over a cliff, or into captivity. The bison and Indians were the main prey-predator system of the Great Plains for more than 9000 years. At an estimated count of fifty to sixty million before the arrival of the white people, however, the buffalo vastly outnumbered the fewer than 300,000 Plains Indians. Thus all the latter could do, before they obtained the horse, was to "nibble 'round the edges" of the great buffalo herds. Agriculture started to develop in Central and South America, and farmers traded with the nomadic hunters to their north.

A great new onslaught was to influence the ecosystems of the Americas with the arrival of Columbus and his ships carrying animals and men with rifles. Thinking erroneously that he had reached his original goal of the opulent East Indies, he named the island natives he encountered *Indians,* and the name stuck. On his second voyage in 1493, Columbus brought the first cattle to reach the Americas, landing them at Santo Domingo. It was 1521 before any reached the mainland at Vera Cruz (Mexico). Subsequently many representatives of Iberian breeds were brought across the Atlantic to become the precursors of the longhorns of the prairie pastures and the criollos of South America. British and French breeds arrived in the 1600s, and the first zebus in the 1800s.

31. Several bison species were introduced into North America, but only one survived extinction, the American *Bison bison.* The first known drawing of the American bison was published by Francisco Lopez de Gomara in *Historia General de las Indias* in Saragossa, Spain (1552-1553). *(Courtesy Bancroft Library, University of California at Berkeley.)*

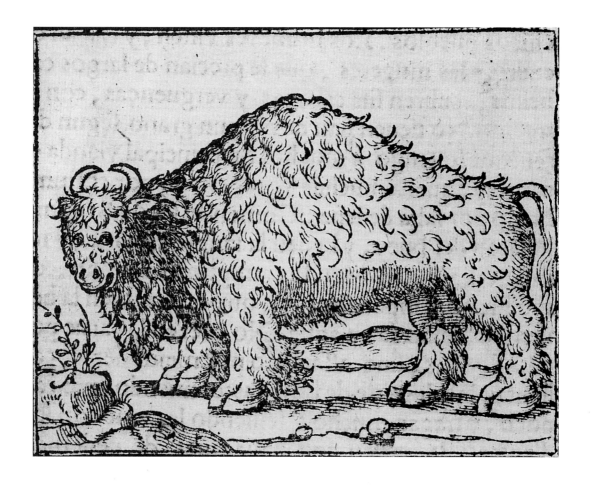

PRE-COLUMBIAN AND POST-COLUMBIAN DOMESTIC DOGS IN THE AMERICAS

Skeletons of domestic dogs that date to 10,500 years ago were found in Jaguar Cave in the Birch Creek valley of Idaho. The short, broad muzzles and crowded premolars confirm that the dogs were a domestic variety, not wolves. They were derived from Eurasian stock resembling remains found at Jericho in the Middle East. Evidently their progenitors had survived a long march with their masters. Stuart Struever's excavations on the Koster farm in the lower Illinois River valley, the Lowilva site of west-central Illinois, revealed skeletons of domesticated dogs dating to more than 8500 years ago. The site is remarkable for its fourteen horizons, indicating occupation throughout the Archaic Indian period, and the Woodland and Mississippi periods (from 7500 BC to AD 1200). The most important animal product for the Lowilva Indians was the white-tailed deer. Many smaller animals, waterfowl, and gamebird species, as well as large amounts of freshwater mussels and several species of fish, were eaten from 6500 to 2000 BC.

Agriculture came late to the area, in about 1200 BC. About five hundred years ago more dogs arrived with Christopher Columbus, some types becoming known as "spaniels," that is, hunting waterdogs from Spain. The conquistadors however, provided other, vicious, larger mastiffs with suits of armor and used them against the Indians in deplorable displays of savagery. The Dogs of the Conquest were used initially in the subjugation and torture of the Arawak Indians of the Caribbean Islands—in "dogging the natives" as it was called—and later against other tribes in Central and South America.

Dogs were popular in Central and South American cultures. They were raised in large numbers and fed on corn to become a dietary delicacy. Some were pets and were buried with their masters. Several types were identified, from minute chihuahuas to much larger breeds. The use of unique, New World species of wild canids in South America as far south as the Falkland Islands was also well known.

ADVANCED CULTURES IN ANCIENT CENTRAL AND SOUTH AMERICA

Amazing developments occurred during the pre-Columbian period in the New World in complete isolation from the civilizations of Eurasia. The Maya of Central America, the Aztecs of Mexico, and the Incas of Peru stand out in their achievements in astronomy, architecture, and culture. Their civilizations, however, were destroyed by the brutal, ruthless ravages of the armed conquistadors on horseback and their fearsome, mastiff-type dogs that were trained to attack people. The military invasions were followed by Catholic clergy who ordered the destruction of all cultural relics of the heathen civilizations, causing incalculable losses of cultural treasures. The less organized "village Indians" of Central and South America, too, were brutalized, enslaved, and murdered.

While the Spanish conquerors were sweeping through the Caribbean and Central and South America, explorers from Portugal laid claim to the land from the Amazon River valley southward on the east side of the continent, the future Brazil. France, Holland, and England made some modest inroads in the Guianas and Belize. The southern cultures' contributions to animal husbandry were only the llamoids, the cavies, the chinchillas, the brush turkey, the Muscovy duck, and the canids. Although Copernicus did not publish his conclusions that the planets revolve around the sun until 1543 at the age of seventy, the Maya had described this celestial phenomenon by AD 1300, which makes it appear that they were the first to show that the planets orbit the sun. The Maya were fascinated by time and calendars; they had complex writing codes and a numerical system.

NORTH AMERICAN TRIBES ACQUIRE THE HORSE FROM SPANISH INVADERS

As the Spanish invaders (de Soto and Coronado) pushed through southeastern and southwestern regions of North America early in the sixteenth century, they encountered Native American tribes. The Indians they met were fascinated and awed by the newly imported animal, the horse, and killed many of the early ones. Much later, the Indians, who had a preference for pintos, gradually obtained horses by theft and possibly by catching strays, some of which became the feral mustang herds. However, the turning point in the Indians' ability to hunt buffalo came after the Pueblo tribe attacked their Spanish oppressors in New Mexico in 1680. After annihilating the Spaniards, the Pueblo captured the colonists' several thousand horses. These dispersed as the nucleus of foundation stock that allowed several Great Plains and intermountain tribes to develop magnificent skills in the saddle as buffalo hunters and warriors within a half century. The inevitable outcome was disaster for the Native American race. This dramatic story, with embellishments, has been told in art and narrative. The relationship between an Indian rider and the horse was a special one involving a combination of athletic and mental domination and intimate affection or bonding. In hunting the buffalo (bison), the Indians developed special skills that included analysis of bison behavior and anatomy to ensure success in the hunt and the kill.

32. With the acquisition of the horse from Spanish invaders, the Native American Indians quickly developed superb riding skills, which greatly increased their ability to hunt buffalo (bison). *Making Medicine, Cheyenne* (c. 1875-1878) illustrates a typical buffalo hunt from the American Indian perspective. *(Private Collection, Native American Painting Reference Library.)*

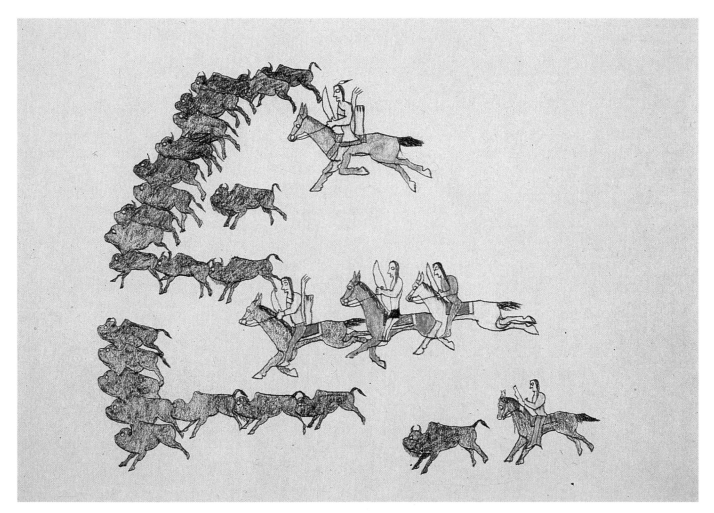

TRIBAL GENIUS IN THE EXPLOITATION OF NATURAL PRODUCTS

A tragic feature of the demise of Indian culture in the Americas is that so much of its heritage was systematically destroyed along with the peoples themselves. Many tribal groups achieved significantly more in their adaptations to the environment than domesticating the dog and mastering the horse. Many crops now used throughout the world for animal and human foods were developed by ancient peoples in the New World, such as corn, cassava, peanuts, potatoes, sweet potatoes, sunflower seeds, and several varieties of beans and tree nuts. Turkeys, waterfowl, clams, various crab and salmon species, lobsters, and other fish of many kinds were all exploited.

Hudson's Bay Company in Canada, founded in 1670, began the North American fur trade after the French traders had ventured up the waterways. Beaver, fox, mink, muskrat, otter, rabbit, wolf, bear, wolverine, ermine, and fur seal provided a remarkable diversity of pelts. South America later yielded chinchilla from the Andes, the Incas ranched rheas to obtain their feathers, and alpacas were ranched for their wool and llamas for pack work. Realization of the importance of fertilizers led to a huge international market for the "mountains" of seabird guano.

A missing link in American development, unlike in Eurasia, was the lack of domestic animals as a source of physical energy: there were no oxen or equids for draft power or for milk. Only the domestic dog was available to help with traction, by means of the travois. Thus Native American agriculture originated in essentially human-powered horticulture supplemented by skillful hunting, trapping, and fishing. Modern agriculture has reaped enormous benefit from these native cultural roots, particularly from the added diversity of exploitable species. Many drugs used for their medicinal and mood-modifying actions have their origins in Native American plant products. The cinchona, or Peruvian bark, gave quinine, a starting point for modern chemical pharmacology. It appears that malaria was brought to the New World by Europeans, and there were plenty of mosquitoes to transmit the *Plasmodium* agent after it arrived. Curare, the "arrow poison," was found to have medical use as a muscle relaxant. Ipecacuanha, or ipecac, was used to treat diarrhea. Cocaine, a drug extracted from leaves of the coca tree, found application as a topical anesthetic in animals and people long before it achieved notoriety as a mood-enhancing drug of abuse.

Some tribes had considerable practical knowledge of anatomy, surgery, and medicinal actions. Castration, suturing, bone setting, trephination, enemas, and treatments for snake bite and fevers were part of the repertoire. A major consequence of the colonization of the Americas was the traffic in alien infectious disease agents between the Old World and the New. The entry of the measles and smallpox agents took a massive toll on Indian life. The impact on animal life was less obvious because there were no large domestic herbivores in North or Central America.

THE FATE OF THE AMERICAN BUFFALO

The American buffalo or bison existed in two subspecies, the plains buffalo, *Bison bison bison,* and the larger, darker woods buffalo, *Bison bison athabascae.* The first post-Columbian invader to see and record a buffalo was Nuñez Cabeza de Vaca in Texas in 1530. At that time the buffalo ranged the grasslands from northern Mexico to northern Canada. Many Native American tribal cultures had become dependent on the buffalo. Courage and cooperation were required to hunt the bison successfully on foot.

The grasslands of the Great Plains were ill-suited to agronomy, and vast numbers of bison, perhaps fifty or sixty million, roamed the prairies and woodlands. Following the emerging grasses in the spring, they made long seasonal migrations of three hundred miles or more, often in huge columns many miles wide. A single herd might consist of several million animals. In the fall they retraced their steps to the southern ranges. As long as the Indian tribes hunted buffalo on foot with bow and spear, their impact on the total buffalo population was minimal. The Indians consumed as much as three pounds of animal tissue per person per day: their first choices were the soft tissues, the tongue, liver, kidneys, bone marrow, testicles, and the brains and blood.

Buffalo intestines were rinsed, packed with blood, and cooked to yield a primitive bloodwurst. Lean meat was dried and stored with herbs between layers of fat in parfleches made of rawhide. Pemmican, the winter staple, consisted of dried meat that was pounded and mixed with fat and berries, then stored in sacks made of the entire skin of buffalo fetuses. It is said that the pasty meconium in a newborn buffalo calf's intestines was a special treat. By-products of the buffalo included clothing and protective coverings made from cured hides, bowstrings made from sinews, diced penis boiled for glue, bile used for decoration, and bone for toolmaking.

After the Spanish came, the natives gradually acquired horses and, later, guns. By the middle of the eighteenth century they had become much more proficient at hunting buffalo. As settlement by Europeans expanded to the west and south, Indians were encouraged to trade buffalo hides for supplies and liquor, then for horses, guns, and ammunition. They also became more dangerous as armed raiders, opposing the trend of settlement on their lands. Despite the incentives of trade and much wasteful killing of the animals, however, the Indians were not the main cause of the population crash of the buffalo that occurred between 1870 and 1890.

The westward expansion of white settlers was at its height between 1870 and 1890. The cavalry was engaged in fighting the Indians to make the territories safe for transport and settlement. Emotions ran high. The tribes were progressively relocated to reservations. Some leaders expressed the view that the only way to make the frontier safe was to exterminate the buffalo and destroy the Indians' horses, a view that became, if not policy, a self-fulfilling prophecy.

A major factor in the decline of the buffalo population became the promotion of buffalo hunting by the new Americans. More powerful rifles were developed to fell the huge beasts: the favorite was probably the Sharps "Big Fifty." Another significant factor was the development of a process for curing buffalo hides that rendered them suitable for fine leather and harness production. This process greatly increased the value of hides and created an incentive for enterprising individuals to develop teams of shooters and skinners.

The coming of the railroads and their advance across the prairies had a devastating impact on the buffalo. The railroads promoted buffalo hunting and sponsored special trips just to shoot the magnificent animals. The carnage was incredible. Putrid carcasses were everywhere. One hunter alone killed 5855 buffalo in two months, keeping five skinners fully occupied. It was not uncommon for one man to shoot one hundred or more from a single stand without moving. When the market for hides became saturated, prices fell again; by 1874 a hide was worth only a dollar or less. It has been estimated that between 1870 and 1875 about 2.5 million bison were killed per year on the North American continent.

After the time of the hunters in the early 1870s, the decimation of the buffalo continued. Some were shot for meat (females were preferred); most were shot just for fun. Huge amounts of buffalo bones littered the plains. Eventually they were hauled away for fertilizer. By 1889, on the entire

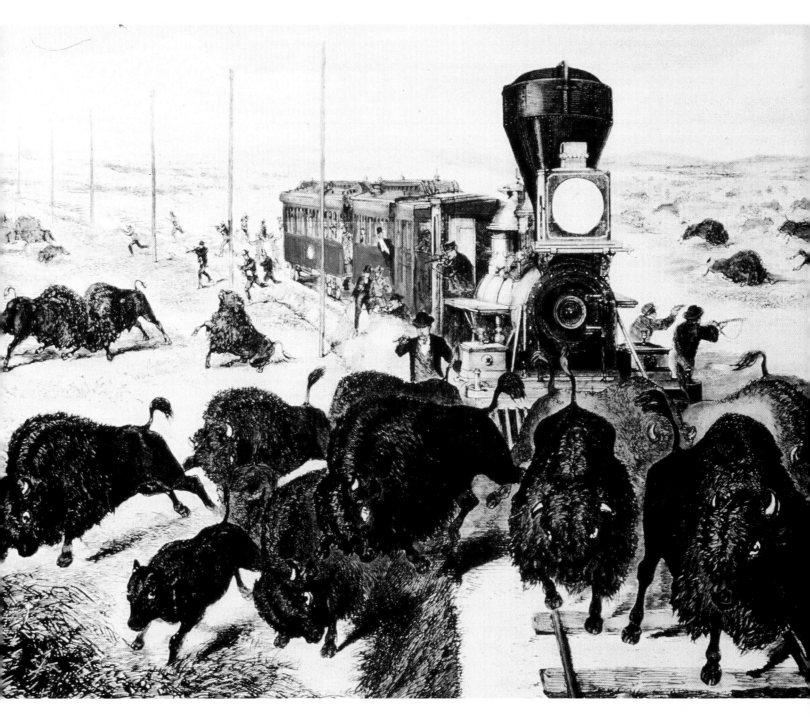

33. *Shooting Buffalo on the Line of the Kansas Pacific Railroad.* Woodcut by Berghaus (1871). The development of the railroads across the prairies contributed markedly to the slaughter of the buffalo, and random killing was encouraged. *(Courtesy The Bettmann Archive, Inc.)*

continent fewer than two thousand buffalo had survived, and the growing numbers of domesticated herbivores had the prairie grasses virtually to themselves. When Native American Chief Seathl of the Duwamish tribe was asked to sell his lands to the government in 1855, he wrote to Franklin Pierce, the President of the United States:

> . . . *I will make one condition. The white man must treat the beasts of this land as his brothers. What is man without the beasts? If all the beasts were gone, man would die from great loneliness of spirit, for whatever happens to beasts also happens to the man. All things are connected. Whatever befalls the earth befalls the sons of the earth.*

Did Americans listen? In the case of the buffalo, certainly not. Twenty-three years after the chief's letter the southern herd had been exterminated, with the smaller northern herd decimated in another five years. From tens of millions to close to zero in twenty-eight years, most of the buffalo were shot for fun or for hides, with the carcasses left to rot. By the 1890s the era of bison hunting was over, and the Native American tribes of the grasslands were reduced to starvation. Anyone who doubts the potential of *Homo sapiens* to endanger the survival of species need only review the story of the buffalo.

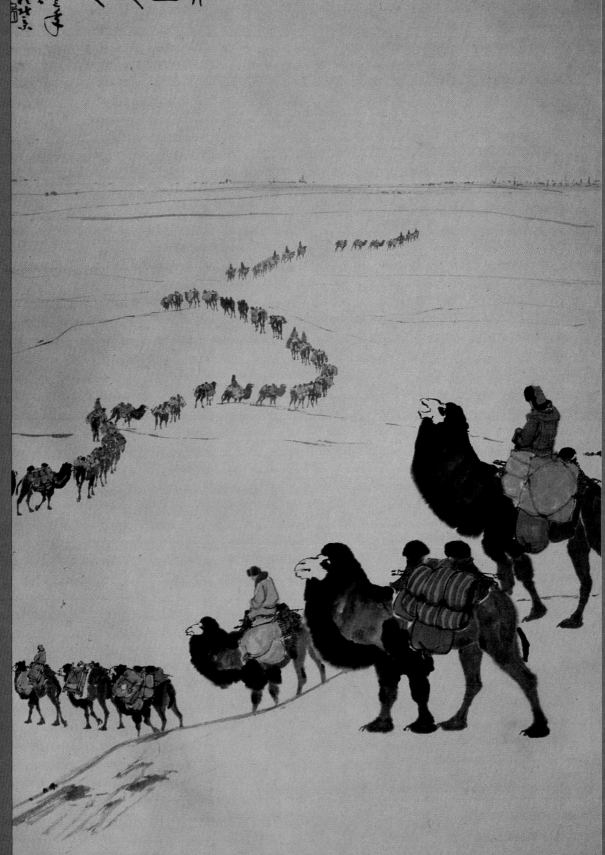

C H A P T E R 3

Domestication of Animals

～

PREHISTORY AND SPECULATION

The idea of gaining mastery over the husbandry of selected plants and animals so that their special attributes could be exploited for human use appears to be only 10,000 to 12,000 years old. Before that great initiative, people had to subsist and meet their needs by hunting and gathering desirable members of the wild species that shared their habitat. Human population densities in habitable regions must have been low enough to allow survival before the Neolithic age. Then the domestication and husbandry of a number of plant and animal species, accompanied by techniques to preserve some of their edible and fibrous products, permitted a revolutionary change in human societies. An unprecedented degree of security of food supply made it possible to establish permanent dwellings and settlements that grew into villages and towns. Nutritional constraints on population growth were lifted, and a progressive increase in population resulted.

There is evidence that many early cultures captured young wild animals, established a human-animal bond by feeding and nursing them, and obtained a relatively tame product. This process can be duplicated today; the classic studies of imprinting of young animals by Konrad Lorenz and others have shown that the human can become recognized as the surrogate parent. Although surrogate parenting may have been one route to animal domestication, it does not of itself constitute domestication. A similar process occurs in animals held captive and cared for in circuses, menageries, and zoological gardens, but few would regard these "prisoners" as domesticated. Some cultures have succeeded in taming and training animals on a large scale, using them to extend human capabilities. For example, the Indian elephant is widely used in South and Southeast Asia, yet seldom bred in captivity. Thus the elephant work force had to be maintained by repeated capture and training. The use of such animals as cheetahs, raptor birds (for example, falcons), and cormorants to assist in hunting or fishing is not classed as domestication. True domestication requires that a subpopulation of a wild species be isolated, bred, and selected to emphasize preferred characteristics and become a dependable supply for human use.

The concept of species today is more plastic than the old idea of a created immutable entity. The current concept entails that the parent wild stock are changing too, so biological species are really moving targets anyway. As Darwin pointed out, artificial selection by breeders of domestic stock is little more than an accelerated version of natural selection in which human agency rather than the environment determines the characteristics that will be favored.

34. *Facing page,* Pack camels, both one- and two-humped, are powerful beasts that can carry several hundred pounds of cargo. Indications of the domestication of the camel are nearly five thousand years old. The Chinese artist, Wu Zuoren (born 1908), trained in Western painting in France and Belgium as a youth but eventually turned to traditional Chinese painting, creating a prodigious number of oil and watercolor paintings, sketches, and calligraphy during a sixty-year career. Many of his paintings are supplemented by poems, which often help to express what the painting, by itself, cannot convey. In *The Burden Is Heavy and the Road Is Long* (1973), Wu has captured the nobility of the camels as they carry their double burden of men and packs across the bleak winter landscape. *(Foreign Languages Press, Beijing.)*

Francis Galton's insightful essay (1865), "The First Steps Towards the Domestication of Animals," spelled out the criteria to be fulfilled for successful animal domestication:

1. The animals should be hardy.
2. They should have an inborn liking for man.
3. They should be comfort loving.
4. They should be useful to the savages.
5. They should breed freely.
6. They should be easy to tend.

Galton stated that failure in only one small particular would condemn a species to wildness and, ultimately, to extinction as civilization extends. The vast majority of animal species fall into the latter category. His list has been amended over time, even by Darwin, who believed that the animals should be of a social habit and that they must receive the human as the "chief" of their "herd." In addition, the species should be compatible with the physical and nutritive environment that can be provided.

The achievement of domestication changed the group dynamics of humans. The possibility evolved of a small group or family or even an individual effort producing a crop or a herd of stock. Although herds (for example, the thorn boma of the Masai) probably required some group activity and attention to security, such as bringing the animals into a fenced compound at night for protection, the individual was able to progressively establish the idea of ownership and attach value to the animals. In many societies domestic animals became the basic currency because they had visible, palpable value and were mobile. Thus they could be swapped alive for tangible possessions, food, or women. As an alternative, an animal could be killed and the meat used to barter for other goods. Special value was attached to breeding stock because the stock could multiply and thus grow in value. Their value created a growing demand for land on which to pasture livestock and grow crops, along with a risk of overstocking and pressure on the water supply.

SPECIES THAT WERE DOMESTICATED

Of the myriad species of animals available in the ecosystems of the world, humans have managed to domesticate only a small number, including about 20 species of mammals. Most of these are in the order Artiodactyla, the even-toed ungulates. These are primarily herding animals of passive disposition; they spend most of their day eating forages or ruminating the ingested roughage, except for the males, which often manifest seasonal aggressiveness, especially during the breeding season. The leading groups among these ungulates are the ruminants. Sheep, goats, cattle (including zebu, yak, and Bali cattle), water buffalo, pigs, camels (dromedary and Bactrian), the Andean camelids (llama and alpaca), and reindeer make up most of the biomass of domestic mammals in the world. Except for the pig, these were all forestomach digesters. Other orders represented are the Perissodactyla (odd-toed ungulates, such as the horse and donkey), the Carnivora (for example, the dog, cat, and ferret), the Rodentia (guinea pig), and the Lagomorpha (rabbit). Species that have been tamed, confined, and used but cannot be considered fully domesticated include the Indian elephant, various species of deer, the eland, animals kept for their pelts, laboratory species used for research and teaching (such as rats, mice, and primates), and exotic pets.

35. *Facing page, above,* Because of their great size and strength, elephants have been prized since early times for heavy labor. However, both qualities present unique problems for actual domestication of the species. Since elephants rarely breed in captivity, it is better to capture the wild beasts and tame them for work. Indian elephants are still frequently caught by the stockade method. Wild animals, attracted by a female decoy, are slowly driven through a long, ever-narrowing stockade until they eventually arrive at a small fenced enclosure from which escape is impossible. Once contained, they can be removed for training. *(From Zeuner, A History of Domesticated Animals, 1963.)*

36. *Facing page, below,* The "pitfall" approach for capturing wild elephants is still used in India. Earthen cavities just large enough to hold the beasts are prepared. Tame females are used to attract the elephants, and they fall into the pits. After a walkway of logs is built, they can be pulled out by tame elephants that are attached to them by rope. *(From Zeuner, 1963.)*

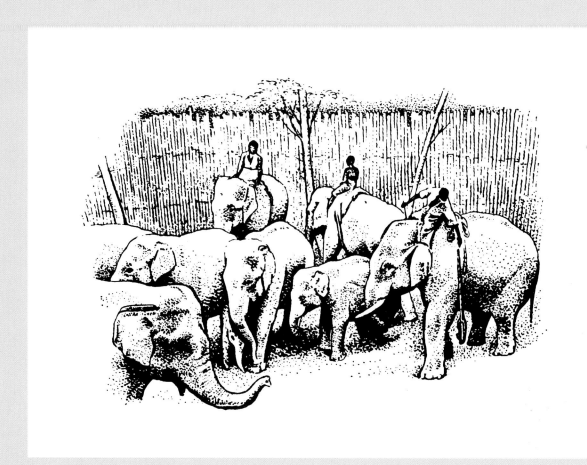

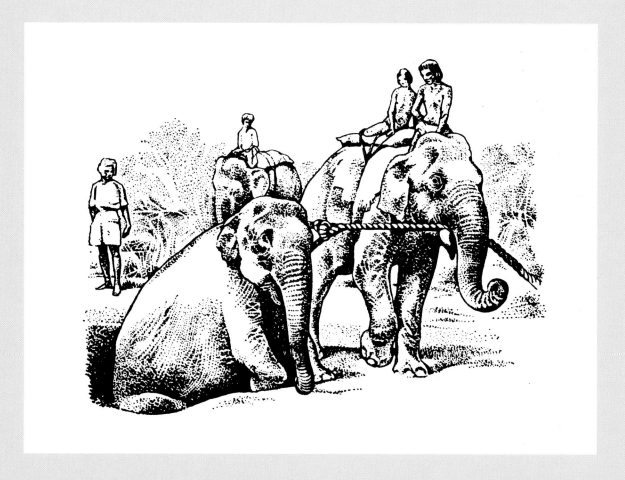

A number of species of birds have been domesticated successfully and play an important role in food production. Many other avian species are kept as companions or ornaments. The fowl or chicken is by far the most important food species (providing meat and eggs), followed by the turkey, some water-fowl (ducks and geese), and some smaller species (such as domesticated game birds, pigeons, and crows). Historically notable among the captive species are the raptors (falcons, hawks, and the like) and the fishing cormorants. Several amphibians and reptilian aquatic species are farmed, including turtles and frogs. The old Chinese development of aquaculture is a rapidly expanding field; many species of fish, mollusks, and shellfish are now being raised for commercial purposes. Among the insects, the silk moth and the honeybee stand out as productive contributors.

37. The order of Carnivora contains several subspecies that were among the first to be domesticated, especially the wolves. *(Redrawn, with permission, after Evans HE:* Miller's Anatomy of the Dog, *1993.)*

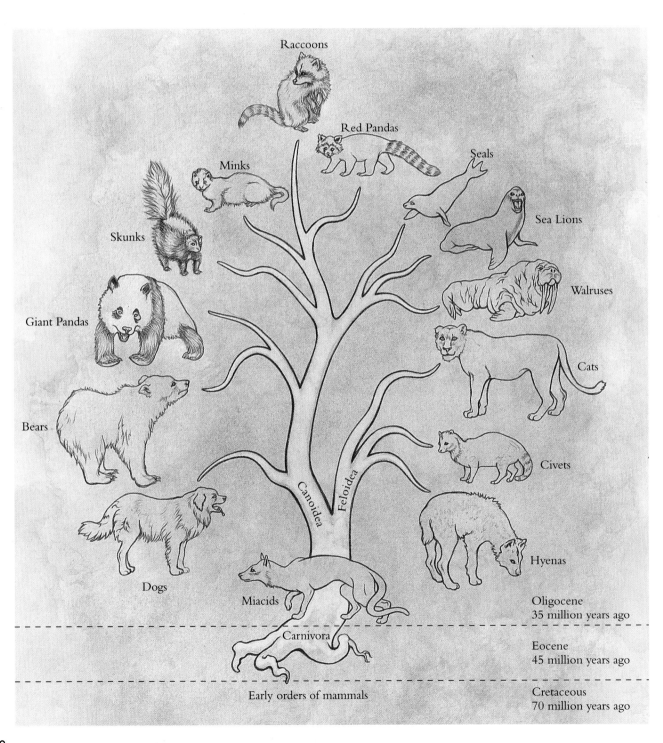

Dogs

Archaeological evidence suggests that the dog may have been the first animal to be domesticated, although the scavenging behavior of the species makes it hard to verify from skeletal remains whether the animals were truly domesticated or just waiting for leftovers. However, when the sites have a disproportionately high ratio of the heavy long bones of the limbs (the ones that dogs cannot crack), the hypothesis that the people cohabited with domesticated canines is strengthened. The dating of remains, too, is nearly always a source of uncertainty. The Palegawra Cave in the foothills of the Zagros Mountains in western Iran was the source of a canid mandible believed to be from a dog dating to about 10,000 BC. Later rock art shows what appear to be dogs assisting humans in the hunt. It seems likely that some kind of link between the human and the dog was established 12,000 years ago, if not earlier.

There is general agreement that the wolf species were the primary progenitors of the dog in all its forms, since they have the same chromosome number, 78. (Chromosomes are the structures containing the genetic material in the cell nucleus.) However, hybrids have been made with other wild canids. It seems that the cooperative, hierarchical pack behavior and socializing propensity of wolves led to their susceptibility to usurpation by humans. If humans adopted pups and got them to imprint on a human instead of a wolf, domestication would have been relatively easy to achieve. This process has

38. Evidence suggests that the dog was the first animal to be domesticated. With 78 chromosomes, the wolf subspecies are considered to be the ancestors of the dog in all its breeds, since they all have this same number of chromosomes. *(Redrawn with permission from Dr. Juliet Clutton-Brock, London; courtesy W.B. Saunders Co., 1993.)*

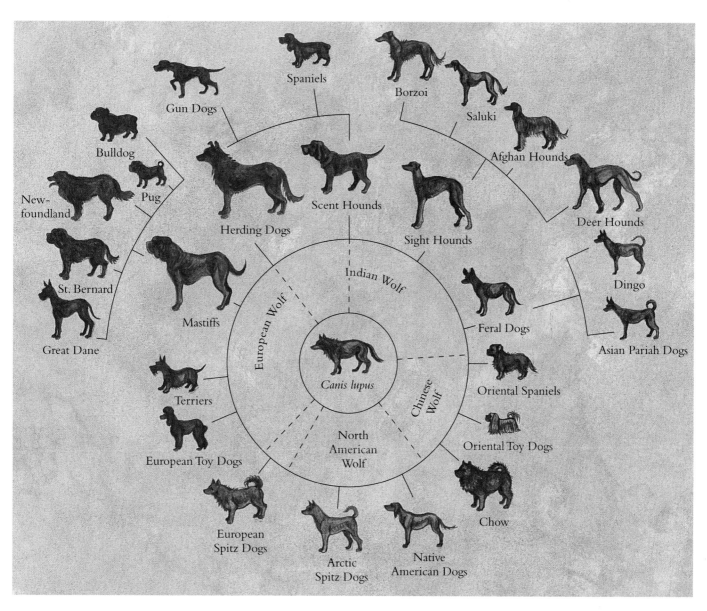

39. Skull of a saluki, dating to at least 3500 BC, found in northern Mesopotamia. Salukis were known to have been used as hunters, running down game by sight rather than smell. This group was bred for speed, stamina, keen eyesight, and powerful jaws. It included greyhounds, afghan hounds, Russian wolfhounds (Borzois) and deerhounds. Such dogs were used for coursing since ancient times, and greyhound racing was developed in the United States in the twentieth century. *(The University Museum, University of Pennsylvania.)*

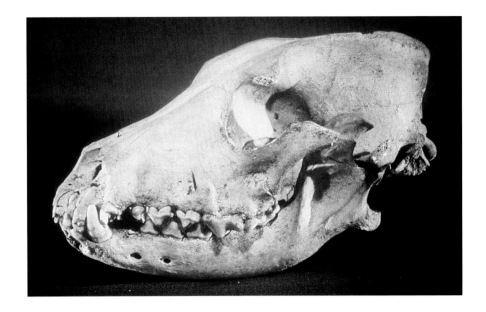

been repeated in modern times. The remarkable feature of the domestic dog, *Canis familiaris*, is the diversity of shapes, varieties, and breeds humans have been able to derive by selection and cross-breeding. Once domesticated, the dog played several roles. It was an assistant in hunting and herding, guarding, and garbage disposal; a companion and playmate; and a source of food. In some cultures puppies were fattened for the pot on a maize or a rice diet (for example, in Mexico and China, respectively).

Small Ruminants

After the dog the next animals to be domesticated were the small ruminant herbivores, sheep and goats. There are several species of wild sheep, but only the Asiatic moufflon of western Asia's Fertile Crescent (the arc of fertile land from the Mediterranean coast around the Syrian Desert to Iraq) has the same chromosome number, 54, as the domestic forms. Sheep were domesticated 10,000 years ago, goats about the same time in the same region. The latter's ancestor appears to have been the Bezoar goat, *Capra aegagrus,* based on the cross-sectional shape of the horns. Although the ibex also breeds with the domestic goat, its horns have a shape that differs from that of the latter's horns.

Herded sheep and goats were the fruits of the pasturelands and browse plants, just as the wild herbivores had been and continued to be. Thus, although crops were the reward for labor on the arable lands, meat and hides were obtained with less effort by herding the land that could not be farmed. In the early centuries of the Neolithic era the combination of crops, domestic stock, and hunting-fishing-gathering skills made possible a new, richer lifestyle than that of the shrinking hunter-gatherer resource that preceded it. The change to habitations and a sedentary existence decreased the hunting contribution and allowed the population to increase more rapidly with the more dependable food supply. Societies were able to trade surplus food and fiber items and develop crafts to display at markets.

With the advent of the wool sheep, reeling of fibers, and weaving, the textile industry was born. The original sheep had colored hair; their coats were useful only for coarse kemp fibers matted into felts. The mutation that led to the origin of the wool sheep was an enormous advance that also brought to an end the spring molt that had caused loss of the kemp. It became necessary, however, to shear the wool to obtain a usable product, a labor-intensive process to this day. The mohair of Angora goats is a fine, high-quality fiber, and cashmere is a product combed from the underwool of goats in molt. Although dating the earliest wool has been difficult, it is unlikely to have appeared much earlier than 4000 or 5000 years ago.

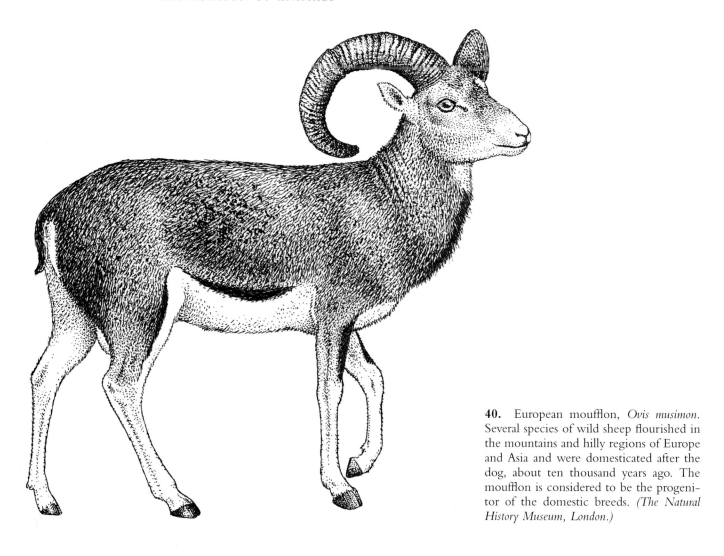

40. European moufflon, *Ovis musimon*. Several species of wild sheep flourished in the mountains and hilly regions of Europe and Asia and were domesticated after the dog, about ten thousand years ago. The moufflon is considered to be the progenitor of the domestic breeds. *(The Natural History Museum, London.)*

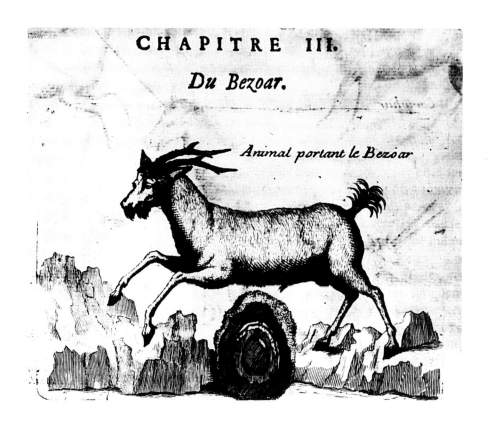

41. Engraving of a bezoar goat, *Capra aegagrus,* against a backdrop of mountains, from Pierre Pomet's *Histoire Generale des Drognes* (Paris, 1694). The bezoar goat is thought to be the ancestor of the domesticated goat. This illustration supposedly depicting a bezoar goat is inaccurate in that the horns should not be branched and should have a more distinctive shape. The picture illustrates the basis for the name bezoar, which is shown as the layered calculus beneath the goat. Such objects were found in the stomach of these goats and were believed to have magical properties to protect against poisons. *(National Library of Medicine, Bethesda, Maryland.)*

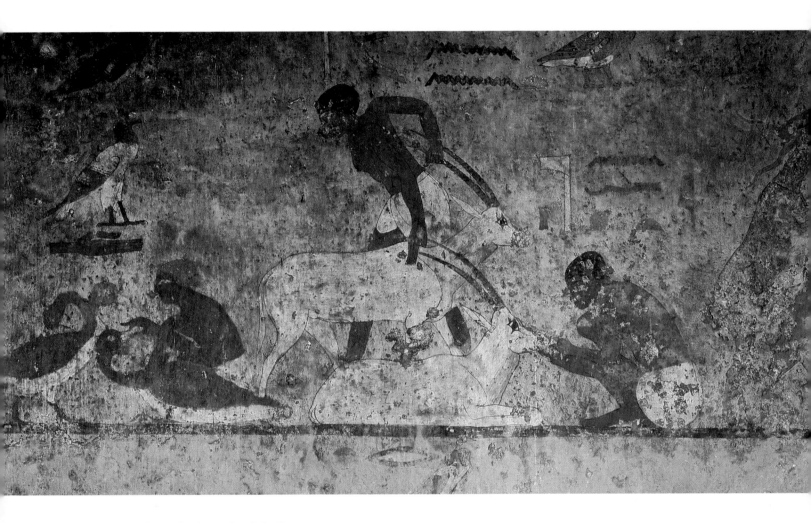

42. Painted mural of men hand feeding oryxes, *Oryx dammah,* from the tomb of Khnumhotep near Beni Hasan, Egypt. Twelfth dynasty (c. 1900 BC). Gazelles, unlike sheep and goats, are not amenable to being controlled by herders over long distances but some species can be tamed and corralled or herded in confined areas. *(Photograph by J. Vertut.)*

Cattle

Cattle *(Bos taurus)* came into the fold later, apparently derived from tamed versions of the great aurochs, *Bos primigenius.* The last aurochs died in AD 1627. The humped cattle, or zebu *(Bos indicus)*, exhibits a small difference in the shape of the Y chromosome from the humpless one. The earliest remains may be from Mesopotamia. A likely progenitor of the zebu, known as *Bos namadicus,* once roamed South Asia but is now extinct.

Cattle were domesticated in Anatolia, now part of Turkey, about 8000 years ago. That site appears to provide the earliest evidence of the domestication of the bovine species. The focal site for the discovery was the remains of the town of Catal Huyuk on the Konya Plain. The town was occupied for approximately 1000 years from the middle of the seventh millennium BC. Other species found to have been present at that time included the moufflon, Asian wild goat, red deer, onager, and dog, although it is estimated that ninety percent of the meat consumed there was beef. Cattle feature prominently in the art found at Catal Huyuk, and there is no doubt that the bovine species has always had special religious significance in many cultures. It has been suggested that the initial drive for domestication of cattle was to meet the demand for sacrificial purposes. Belief that such sacrifice ensured the continuing cycle of prosperity and fertility was widespread. In Assam and parts of Southeast Asia the mithan *(Bos frontalis)*, the domesticated form of the wild gaur cattle, is still controlled solely for ritual slaughter.

The idea developed of using animals to carry loads and, subsequently, to draw wheeled vehicles or sleds. Soon the use of oxen in traction for plowing, cultivating, seeding, and threshing was a logical step. Thus the domestic animals had an enormous impact on the advancement of agriculture and civilization.

43. *Auerochse* (1942) by K.L. Hartig, German. Now extinct, the aurochs, *Bos primigenius,* or Eurasian wild ox, stood six feet tall at the shoulder. It was probably the source of domesticated cattle, *Bos taurus.* Oxen used for plowing, cultivating, and reaping continue to play an important role in some agrarian societies. *(Museum für Naturkunde, Berlin.)*

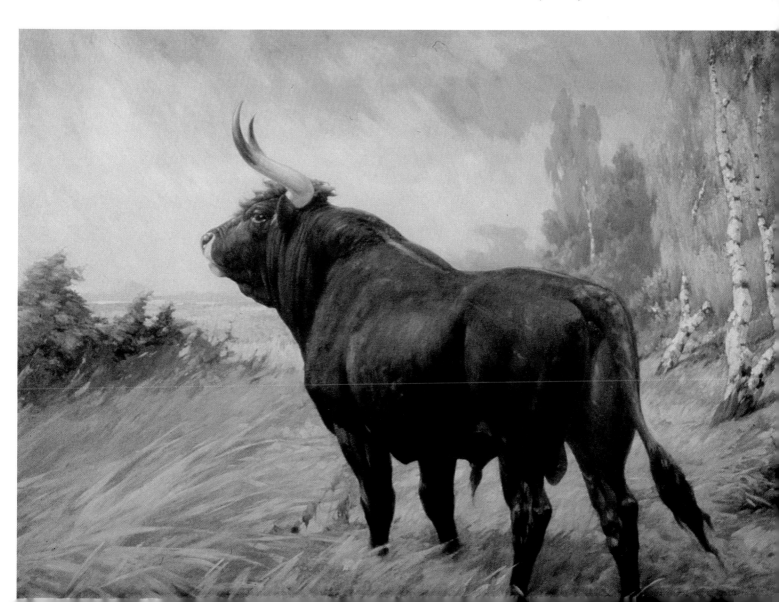

Milk as a product of animal domestication was a later development, since robbing a wild or semiwild mother of her offspring twice a day would have been a challenging undertaking. However, humans suckling animals or vice versa appeared as a theme in ancient mythology; great tales were fabricated around this idea. Some involved a maternal wolf or dog, others the great, universal mother-cow or small ruminants. Still others entailed piglets or puppies raised with the help of human breasts. Presumably ewes and nanny goats would have been the first to be exploited for milk in the real world because of the greater ease in handling the animals and their more submissive natures. Because sheep and goats tended to have short lactations and low yields, however, the benefits were limited. Once the practice was established, cow milking came to dominate the scene. Early strategies would have involved joining in the milking after the calf started to suck, thereby stimulating the let-down reflex that would be blocked by the cow if a direct attempt were made. Progressively over the centuries humans were able to get the cow to dissociate its lactation from the calf's activities after the first few days of nursing. Selection of productive strains led to the development of cows that would yield much more milk than the calf required, and the dairying industry was born.

Although making milk available was an enormous boon for many segments of the global human family, this food did not suit all cultures. The peoples of eastern Asia, in particular, those south of Mongolia, chose to avoid milk. It was considered undesirable because it was believed to give rise to digestive upsets. Lactase deficiency in the intestinal epithelium does occur in a proportion of adults. Not until the 1990s was lactase added to milk to greatly reduce the lactose level, thereby making a commercial product that was safe for such people. Some animals such as sea lions lack the enzyme altogether; to them cow's milk is lethal.

Archaeological evidence suggests that bovine dairying originated more than 4500 years ago in the Middle East and in southeastern Europe. Subsequently other species were milked, notably the river buffalo of Asia, the camel, and the mare. The barbarians of the steppes used mare's milk for nourishment and made koumiss, an alcoholic, fermented form that would keep, to fortify themselves during wide-ranging excursions and battles fought on horseback.

Hides of many species, including the major agricultural ones, were used to produce leather for human footwear, clothing, and accessories, as well as for animal harnesses, furniture, and technology.

Cats

The first evidence of feline domestication was found at Khirokitia in Cyprus, dating to about 9000 years ago. Because there were no wildcats, it must be assumed that the domestic cats were imported to the island, perhaps to control rodents that multiplied on grain stores after cereal husbandry was initiated. The domestic cat is derived from the wild cat, *Felis Sylvestris*. Other early findings of firm evidence of full domestication are much more recent, for example, New Kingdom Egypt, sixteenth century BC.

Swine

The ancestor of the domestic pig had 38 chromosomes and lived in China and Europe twenty-five million years ago. Hallan Cemi, in the foothills of the Taurus Mountains of southeastern Turkey, was a site where preagricultural hunter-gatherers apparently domesticated pigs more than ten thousand years ago. Many bones from male pigs less than one year old with molar teeth of reduced size were found. This unique approach of domestication allowed year-round occupation of stone houses. Subsequently domestication probably occurred in several areas (Europe, Persia, Africa, and China) between 6500 BC and 4000 BC. Evidence for domestication by 2900 BC has been found in China, and a date of 6700 BC has been suggested for Iraq. Despite taboos on the consumption of pig meat in several major cultures, more pig meat is consumed in the world than that of any other mammalian species.

44. *Sus scrofa.* The former subdivision of wild swine into European *(top and left),* Asiatic *(right),* and other types is no longer used; all domestic swine are now regarded as being of the same species. Although the date and site of the domestication of the pig are uncertain, it was probably domesticated between 6500 and 4000 BC. *(From Kloster, 1984.)*

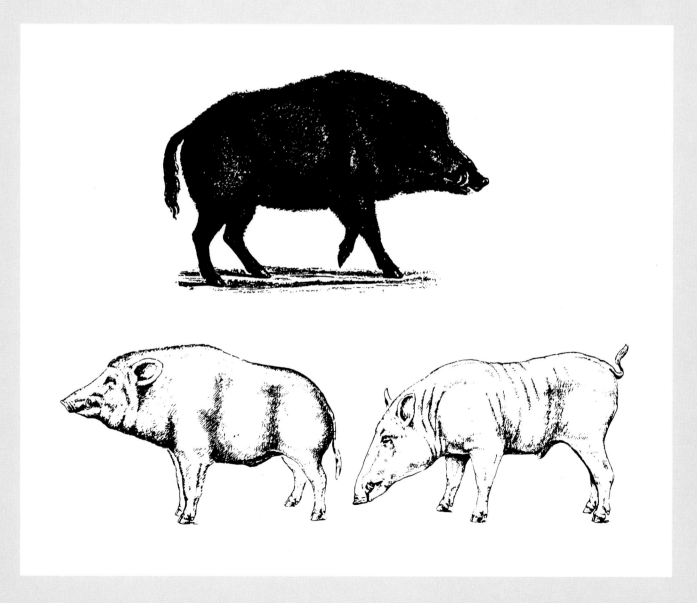

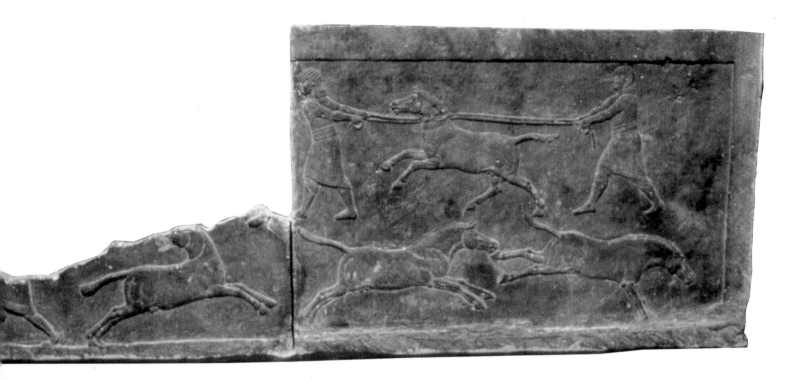

Equids

The equids comprise horses, asses, onagers, and zebras. All breeds of domesticated horses have 64 chromosomes. The only surviving wild species, Przewalski's horse, has 66 chromosomes. Yet both wild and domestic types have 94 "major chromosome arms." It is possible that the domestic forms arose from the now extinct tarpan of southern Russia, but its chromosome number is not known. The horse was domesticated much later than were the ruminant species, probably 5000 years ago.

The Persian onager has 56 chromosomes, and the donkey has 62, yet together with the Mongolian wild ass, all three types have the same number of chromosome "arms." Presumably there were different progenitors.

Camelids

All four camelid species of South America have 74 chromosomes, and they all interbreed. The oldest, thus the likely progenitor, may be the wild guanaco. Another wild form, the vicuña, has a fine coat. The domestic forms are the llama, a beast of burden in the Andes Mountains, and the alpaca, kept for its finer wool. They were domesticated at least 5000 years ago, possibly as early as 7500 years ago. All are members of the genus *Lama*.

The camel comes with one hump (dromedary) or two (Bactrian), each type having 70 chromosomes; the two will interbreed, although male offspring of such a union are usually sterile. The Bactrians are still found in the wild around the Gobi Desert. The earliest archaeological remains indicating domestication of the camel are from Khurasan, Persia, and Turkmenistan and date to 5000 years ago or later. The first-generation hybrid was a powerful beast that could carry nine hundred pounds of freight. It was used on the Silk Road, a trade route connecting the Middle East and China.

All the camelids arose in North America. Early forms moved southward across the Isthmus of Panama and began the line that led to the South American camelids. Others spread to the far northwestern reaches of the continent and crossed the Bering Strait. The camelids in North America died out, but the ones that reached Asia spread westward across the continent, the better-insulated Bactrian staying in the high plateaus and the single-humped variety traveling into western Asia and North Africa, where it became adapted

45. Assyrians capturing wild onagers *(Equus hemionus)* with lassos. Stone relief from Nineveh (c. 645 BC). Although hunted and eaten, onagers were not domesticated but were inbred with horses. Donkeys were induced to breed with horses, the mule being the result of a jackass and mare cross. A stallion and jenny cross yields a hinnie. Male donkey foals to be used for mule production were suckled on mares. *(The British Museum, London.)*

to desert conditions and was the mainstay of desert nomadism and the caravan trade across desolate regions. The dromedary came to serve more diverse functions than its two humped relation: it provided milk, meat, and fiber as well as work, because there were fewer alternative sources in arid regions.

Reindeer

The reindeer occupies a unique position in the history of human exploitation of animals. A major contributor to human subsistence during the Upper Paleolithic era in the late glacial period, it migrated toward northern regions as the planet warmed and the glaciers retreated. After a long period as a preferred target, the species became inaccessible to most hunters when it migrated northward to peri-Arctic regions to stay within its chosen environmental norms. The reindeer, *Rangifer tarandus* or caribou, as it is known in North America, has not escaped human attention. In some areas of northern Scandinavia or "Lapland" it is truly a domesticated species. In North America, however, and in parts of Norway and northern Russia it is still semi-wild or only marginally tolerant of humans. In its ecological setting it is hunted regularly by the wolf. It may be that the behavioral adaptations needed for success in the hunt are similar in the human and the wolf; this may contribute to the relative mutual compatibility that has evolved between these two predatory species.

The reindeer species appears to have been native to the New World, migrating to Asia and Europe via the Bering land bridge like the camel and the horse. The woodland and the tundra reindeer are the two main types. In North America the woodland variety is the Canadian caribou; the tundra reindeer is known as the Barren Grounds deer. The latter type feeds on lichens on the tundra in summer and moves southward to the northern edge of the forests in the winter. During the Würm glaciation (60,000 to 10,000 years ago) the reindeer moved south as far as northern Spain and southern France and eastward across the Riviera to the Alps. The reindeer was present in Britain and in central and eastern Europe and crossed Russia to Siberia. It appears in the cave art of the Magdalenian period, and fossil remains indicate that it was a major dietary component for Cro-Magnon peoples.

Reindeer are essential today to the Eskimo and the Lapland peoples. They are driven, ridden, and used as pack animals. Every part of the animal's carcass is used for food, fiber, or grease; reindeer milk and cheese are used in Scandinavia and northern Asia. In Eurasia the woodland species follows seasonal migrations between the latitudes of 55 degrees north and 65 degrees north; the tundras form at latitudes above 65 degrees north. Certainly the seasonal migrations of reindeer led their hunters to a nomadic hunting life-style and may even have been the origin of nomadic herding pastoralism.

Buffalo

A wild Asian strain of buffalo of Assam, the arnee, is believed to have been the origin of the strains from which domesticated water buffalo were derived. The true buffalo exist as two main species, the intractable and dangerous African buffalo, *Synerus caffer,* and the Asian water buffalo, *Bubalus bubalis.* There are many breeds of the latter in South Asia, the two main types being the river buffalo of drier lands, mainly India, and the swamp buffalo of swampy areas, chiefly south and east of Burma. India has eight or more strains of the river type that are kept mainly for milking (such as the Murrah buffalo) or as pack animals. The swamp buffalo, which are used for draft and for working rice paddies, occur especially in Southeast Asia, eastern Asia, and Sri Lanka and recently have spread beyond Asia to Brazil, Egypt, Italy, northern Australia, southeastern Europe, and Trinidad.

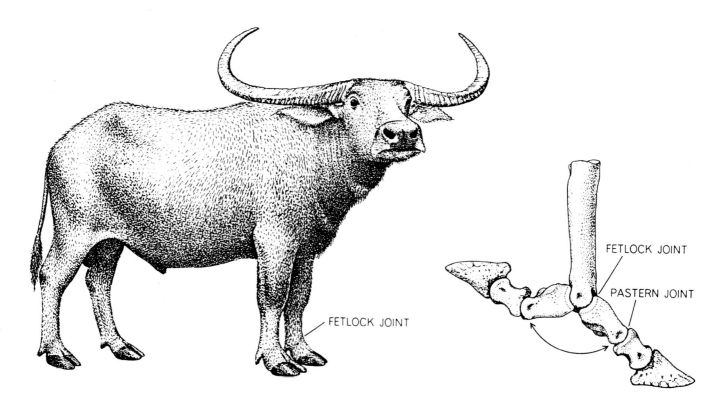

FETLOCK JOINT

FETLOCK JOINT

PASTERN JOINT

46. Swamp buffalo, *Bubalus bubalis.* Varying in size and weight, swamp buffalo have extremely flexible fetlock and pastern joints, making them particularly suitable for working in rice paddies. *(From Cockrill, 1967.)*

The buffalo, although part of the subfamily Bovinae, differ in the number and pattern of their chromosomes (48) from cattle (60) and bison (60) and thus will not interbreed. The bison will cross-breed with cattle to produce the beefalo, but the male progeny are infertile because of differences in the Y chromosome. There are more than 120 million buffalo in the world; eighty percent of these are in the Tropics (the zone from 30 degrees north latitude to 30 degrees south latitude), mostly in India, where they make up about one fourth of the total number of bovids.

The African buffalo never has been domesticated. An extinct long-horned variety, *Synerus antiquus,* was widespread in North Africa, where its skeletal remains have been found, and was frequently depicted in rock art, probably as a cult animal.

Buffalo milk is quite rich, with as much as fifty percent more protein than cow's milk and almost twice the fat content. It is the initial ingredient in mozzarella cheese. The carcass of the buffalo has a greater proportion of lean meat and much less fat than that of beef cattle and is quite palatable.

Ferrets and Rabbits

Ferrets were domesticated from polecats more than 2000 years ago and were used to drive rabbits out of their underground warrens so that they could be caught for food. The ferrets were muzzled for this purpose; otherwise they tended to make a kill underground. Later, they found use in ratting. Ferrets became important when rabbits that had been kept as food animals became a feral pest when they regained their freedom, causing damage to agricultural land and crops. The rabbit was indigenous to the Iberian Peninsula; domesticated and adopted by the Romans, rabbits spread throughout Europe via Italy and France and to the Middle East via North Africa. At some point the albino ferret appeared. It had yellow fur and red eyes and was selected to become the standard form of the domesticated species. In England the ferret became popular with poachers, and ferreting became a sport; a ferreter was appointed to the royal court.

Rodents

Several species of rodents have been domesticated for food and, in modern times, for laboratory work. Outstanding among them is the guinea pig or cavy from the Andes Mountains and surrounding areas. The Incas of Peru made wide use of the guinea pig both as a highly nutritious food and for ceremonial activities, including its mummification. It spread through many of the mountain tribal cultures as a truly domesticated animal, cohabiting with humans. Later it spread throughout the world as a popular pet and a valuable animal for medical diagnosis and research. Most of the rodents that are exploited as laboratory animals today—white rats and mice, guinea pigs and golden hamsters, and the standard laboratory lagomorph, the albino rabbit—were developed to meet the growing needs of medical and scientific research.

In Roman times the fat dormouse, *Glis glis,* was raised as a culinary delicacy. Varro (116-26 BC) described their husbandry in his great work on agriculture. A nocturnal, hibernating, nut-eating species, the rodents were kept for breeding in walled yards with nut trees. The young were provided with acorns, chestnuts, and walnuts and fattened in jars. Today giant rats are hunted for food in West Africa and Southeast Asia, and some efforts have been made to domesticate them in Africa. Their smoked meat finds a ready market.

Avian Species

Nongallinaceous birds, including waterfowl, date to ancient times. The mallard duck and the goose were domesticated in China and Egypt, respectively. These species are popular dietary items but have never attained the productivity of the gallinaceous species. The Muscovy duck, *Cairina moschata,* was domesticated in Mesoamerica and South America. A large black-and-white bird with a bare face and red facial caruncles, it still exists in the wild in parts of Mexico.

Of American domesticates, the most important numerically is undoubtedly the turkey, which was widespread throughout North and Central America and was domesticated long before the arrival of Columbus. The wild form, *Meleagris gallopavo,* was domesticated and has become one of the most efficient producers of high-quality meat among all animal species under modern management systems. However, repeated selection for massive breast musculature has rendered the male incapable of mating, and artificial insemination has become necessary to fertilize the eggs of breeding hen turkeys.

Southern and Southeast Asia are thought to be the homes of the progenitors of the domestic chicken, perhaps the most universally popular source of meat in the world. The red jungle fowl, *Gallus gallus,* has long been considered the progenitor of the domesticated strains. The seals of the Indus Valley civilization portray cocks, and the later Vedic chronicles (Atharva-Veda and Yajur-Veda) praise the cock's courage and his value as a timekeeper for awakening at dawn. Strangely, by about 1000 BC there were strictures against eating chicken meat in India. During the first millennium BC the fowl spread rapidly to Persia and through western Asia into Europe and North Africa. The Greeks bred cockerels for fighting games and adopted the oriental idea that the cock was a divine symbol of light and health. Even Socrates, the great logician, is reputed to have ordered a cock sacrificed to Aesculapius for recovery from illness before taking poison in 399 BC.

The Greeks apparently invented the castration of cockerels to produce capons. The rooster became an erotic symbol and the hen, because of its prolific egg production, a fertility symbol. The breaking of the cycle of an annual clutch of eggs for breeding by selecting birds that would lay as frequently as an egg a day over a long period was undoubtedly the great genetic leap that made the domestic chicken such a desirable species. This capacity also made it possible to multiply the species rapidly when chicken meat came into

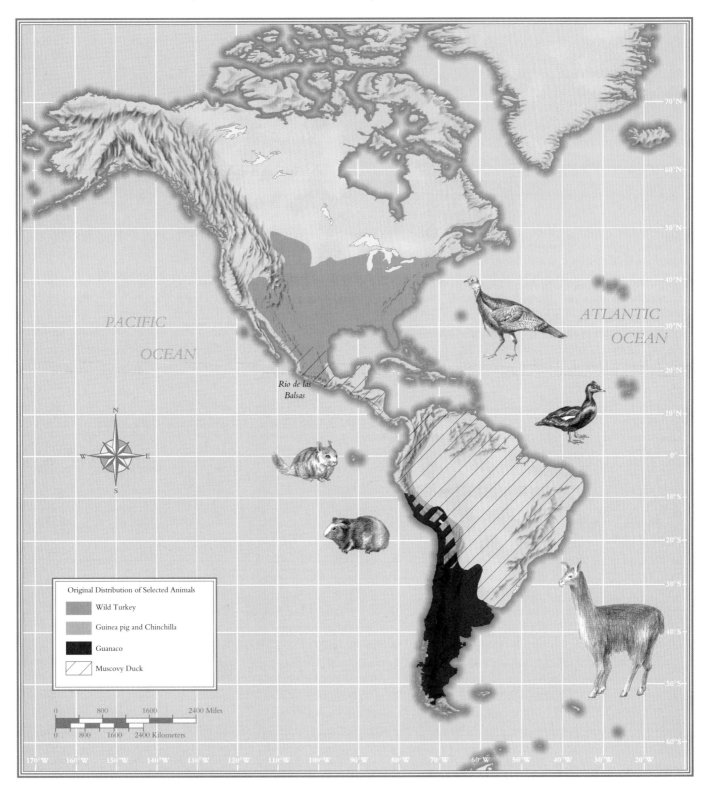

47. Domestication map of the Americas illustrating the original geographic range of the guanaco *(Lama guanicoe),* guinea pig, chinchilla, wild turkey, and Muscovy duck *(Cairina moschata). (Redrawn after Davis, 1987.)*

Original Distribution of Selected Animals

Wild Turkey

Guinea pig and Chinchilla

Guanaco

Muscovy Duck

PACIFIC OCEAN

ATLANTIC OCEAN

Rio de las Balsas

50

vogue. Other gallinaceous species were domesticated, including guinea fowl from Africa and quail, pheasant, and peacocks, but they never attained the productivity and universal exploitation of the chicken and the turkey.

Fur-Bearing Species

Keeping warm in cold climates has always been a major concern of inhabitants of the higher latitudes in the northern hemisphere. Even today at lower latitudes winters are often severe, especially where continental climates prevail. The use of animal skins, pelts, and fibers has been essential to the "hairless" human's survival and adaptation in such environments. The winter coat of reindeer is among the finest insulators available, so techniques for flaying the reindeer and curing the hides played an essential role. Similarly the trappers became popular for their harvest of fur-bearing species, particularly the beaver, fox, mink, muskrat, sable, and ermine, the pelts of which provided warmth as well as objects of high fashion.

Many of the fur-bearing species were placed at risk in the growing demand of the modern era. Silver fox, mink, and muskrat were semidomesticated for mass production. The Eskimos depended on sea mammals for hides and fat as well as for meat. The fur seal, polar bear, and fox were popular. Sea lions, dolphins, and some species of whales (such as the orca) have become attractive entertainers. The annual slaughter of seal pups on the ice floes of the St. Lawrence River recently aroused the indignation of many because of the apparent barbarity. In South America the chinchilla, an attractive rodent, was domesticated and bred for pelts.

Future Prospects

Domestication is not a closed book. Great strides have been made toward domesticating several species of deer (with New Zealand playing a leading role), eland in Africa, bison in North America, moose in Europe, and musk-ox in North America and northern Europe. Several species of gazelle and antelope, including the saiga and blackbuck, although not domesticated, have been controlled in large herds. A few examples of the favorable prospects for aquaculture are salmon farming in Norwegian fjords and elsewhere, trout in many regions, catfish culture in the southern United States, carp in China, tilapia in several regions, and Nile perch in Africa. Shrimp, oysters, and many other crustaceans and mollusks have high potential as mastery of their reproductive biology and health management is attained. The honeybee and the silkworm have been two ancient successes, and opportunities exist for exploitation of other invertebrate species.

One of the remarkable features of "postdomestication" is the tremendous diversity of breeds and strains that have been produced, for example, more than four hundred breeds of dogs. Most of these developments have taken place during the last few centuries and are discussed in Chapters 20 and 31, on animal breeding and companion animals, respectively.

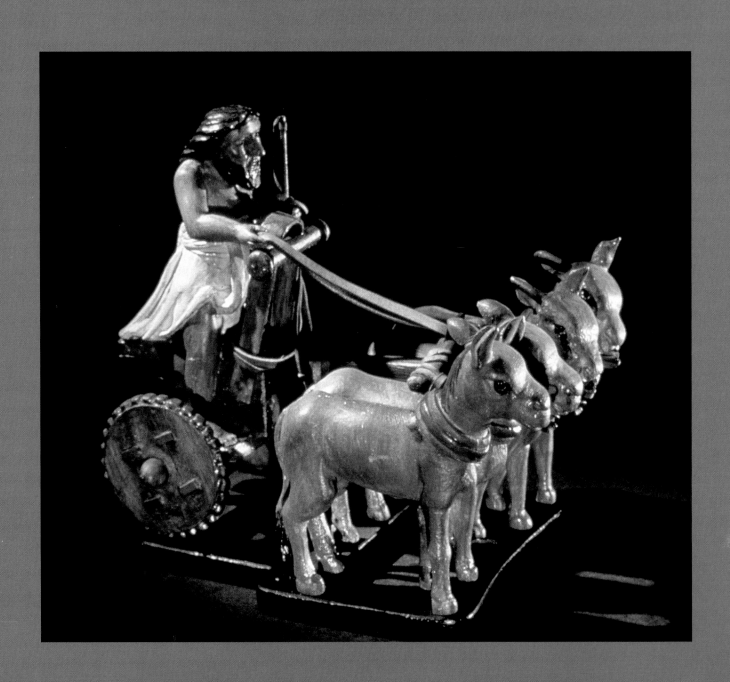

Mesopotamia

First to Depict Animal Doctors

SETTLING THE LAND BETWEEN THE RIVERS

Mesopotamia—the "Land Between the Rivers" Tigris and Euphrates—has been credited with establishing the first urban, literate (based on a cuneiform script) civilization before 3000 BC. The unpredictable precipitation that falls in the form of winter snows in the Anatolian mountains upstream melts in the spring and gives rise to a huge run of water and flooding of the arid areas downstream. The first people known to have settled in the area (more than 6000 years ago) were the Ubaidians, who used irrigation techniques to grow barley and dates along the banks of the Euphrates, a less violent river than the Tigris. Salinization of poorly drained irrigated lands was to become a major ecological problem that constantly threatened agricultural production. These early people formed villages that eventually grew into the first cities in the region: Eridu, Ur, and Uruk.

The centralization of the Ubaidians was caused in part by a rise in sea level stemming from the Flandrian Transgression, which occurred between 5000 BC and 4000 BC. Farming areas were lost to the encroachment of the Persian Gulf. Satellite pictures have revealed that the upper reaches of the Persian Gulf cover lands and rivers that have been submerged, leading some to suggest that this region may have been the site of the Garden of Eden.

ORIGINS OF CATTLE-BASED CULTURES

The Sumerians (origin unknown) began to settle in southern Mesopotamia between 3200 BC and 2800 BC. Most of their cattle were *Bos taurus,* but they also developed the paired zebu team for plowing and had goats and sheep. Cattle were used for draft and yielded milk and dairy products as well as meat and hides. A four-wheeled cart or chariot with solid wheels, drawn by oxen, was developed. These people invented the first written language and created dynasties based on groups of city-states. Around 2300 BC Sargon the Great (2334-2279 BC) overran Sumer and founded the Akkadian Empire, which spanned from the Persian Gulf to Syria, uniting the city-states of southern Mesopotamia. Pigs were bred and castration practiced.

Although Mesopotamians have not been credited with being veterinary trailblazers, an ancient Sumerian-Akkadian script refers to an *azuanshe* and, later, to an *azuguhia* or cattle doctor. Like the Egyptians, they believed in spiritual or mystical demons as the cause of illness, as well as biological aspects that could be handled with physical treatment and medication. Thus a magical role to exorcise the demons, as well as the medical one, was assumed by the complete priest-physician. The supreme god, Marduk, was responsible for genesis of the world, ordering the gods and the cosmology of the universe.

48. *Facing page,* Model of a man driving a copper quadriga pulled by four harnessed equids, perhaps onager-horse hybrids. The original copper war chariot was excavated in the Sahara Temple at Tell Agrab, Iraq, and is thought to date to the Early Second Dynasty (c. 2800 BC). The harness represents the first attempt by humans to control animal power for their purposes. *(The Oriental Institute, The University of Chicago.)*

49. Perhaps the first description of an animal doctor is seen from the impression of this cylinder seal found in the tomb of the Sumerian King Ur-Ningursu of Lagash (c. 2200-2000 BC). The cuneiform script reads

O god Edinmugi, vizier of the god Gir, who attends mother animals when they drop their young!
Urlugaledenna the doctor is your servant.
The script is accompanied by veterinary-like instruments. *(The Louvre, Paris.)*

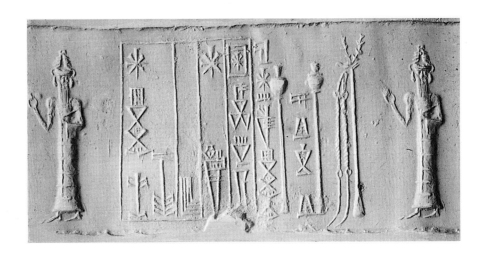

Typically he encountered opposition in the form of Tiamat, his jealous great-grandmother, who created the forces of evil in the form of monsters (one was the Rabid Dog) that were led by the supermonster Kingu. To counter this threat, Marduk attacked the monsters with his bow and a great four-horse chariot, winning the loyalty of his many gods. He created the human race and ordained that they should serve the gods. The earth gods then created a sanctuary for Marduk that they named Babilim (in Greek, Babylon). The next challenge appeared in the form of a great plague known as the evil Namtar. Marduk had to call on his father, Ea, the god of science, glory, and life and the spirit of the waters, for assistance in driving out Namtar.

The general idea of an animal doctor seems to have been described for the first time as a healer, or *azu,* of the herds of ruminant animals. A cylindrical seal from about 2200 BC that was found in the tomb of Sumerian King Ur-Ningursu of Lagash shows this healer, who is identified as Urlugaledenna. He is depicted with veterinary-type instruments and a text in cuneiform script indicating that he performed healing and gave obstetrical and medical assistance to animals.

FIRST BEHAVIORAL STANDARDS FOR HEALTH PROFESSIONALS

The Sumerian Empire of the southern delta region fell into decline and by 2000 BC was once again a disparate group of city-states. Around 1760 BC, King Hammurabi (1792-1750 BC) established the Babylonian Empire in the central part of Mesopotamia; the empire lasted until 1530 BC, when the region came under the control of Kassite tribes, which were followed in turn by Assyrians. Both the Babylonians and the Assyrians were Semitic peoples. Babylon itself fell to the Persians in 539 BC.

During the reign of King Hammurabi the Babylonian achievements in the fields of legislation and public administration were remarkable. The roots of his legal manifesto can be traced to the days of an earlier Sumerian king who collated all laws into a codex, but Hammurabi immortalized his Code of Law revision by engraving it on a diorite stele. Discovered in Susa, Iran in 1902, it is now at the Louvre in Paris. Clearly it was intended to last. Hammurabi's Code provided a legal framework for a moral code that was enforceable and was a great landmark in the emergence of protection of the rights of the individual. Its impact on virtually all subsequent cultures has been immense. All aspects of society were considered, including biology, agricul-

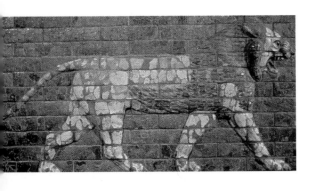

50. This colorful striding lion once decorated a side of the Processional Way, which led out of the city of ancient Babylon through a massive gate named for the Mesopotamian goddess of love and war, Ishtar, whose symbol was the lion. At least one hundred and twenty lions such as this one lined the Processional Way. Molded brick with polychrome glaze. Neo-Babylonian Period. Reign of Nebuchadnezzar II (c. 604-562 BC). *(The Oriental Institute, The University of Chicago.)*

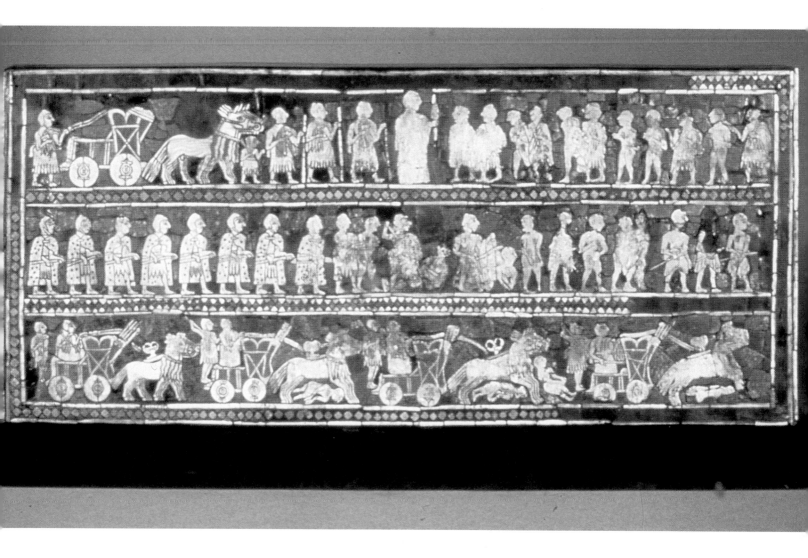

ture, and medicine. The code included rules for veterinary work; overall the medical focus of the code was on surgical interventions:

> 224: *If a "veterinary surgeon" performed a major operation on either an ox or ass and cured it, the owner of the ox or ass shall give to the doctor one sixth of a shekel of silver as his fee.*
>
> 225: *If he performed a major operation on an ox or an ass and has caused its death, he shall give to the owner of the ox or ass one-fourth its value.*

Comparatively speaking, veterinary services were "low on the totem pole" in the class society the code established. Treating a freeman for a broken bone or wound drew a fee of five shekels, but for the son of a plebeian, only three shekels, and for a slave, two. Thus the veterinary doctor got a twelfth of the fee of a doctor of slaves and a thirtieth of the fee of a doctor who treated a freeman. Since ordinary artisans made but a fifth of a shekel per day, veterinary medicine can be assumed to have held an intermediate status.

The code contained severe penalties for errors and failures in medical treatment. When a patient died under the surgeon's knife, the offending hand could be amputated. Those who deliberately injured work animals were punished as criminals. Indeed, the food, fiber, draft power, transport, and military mobility that animals provided made animal husbandry an important skill. The Chaldeans, a Babylonian people who had an elaborate mythology about cosmology and nature, left scripts (at least one dating to 1500 BC) indicating that a broad knowledge of animal husbandry and healing had evolved.

51. Peace and war seem to be represented on this two-sided funeral piece known as *The Standard,* found at the Royal Cemetery at Ur. The lower portion of the "war" side represents an early depiction of using the pulling power of equids. They appear to be controlled by neck collars and nose rings, which, unlike a true harness, would have seriously limited their ability to breathe while pulling. Shell, lapis lazuli, red sandstone, and bitumen. Ur, Iraq (c. 2600–2500 BC). *(The British Museum, London.)*

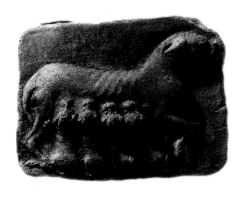

52. Plaque from Old Babylon showing a female dog suckling four puppies. The dog possibly represents the goddess Gula. *(The Oriental Institute, The University of Chicago.)*

SPECIAL RESPECT FOR DOGS AND CONCERNS ABOUT RABIES

Dogs, widely used in hunting, appear to have played an important role in Mesopotamian life. The first mention of rabies occurs in the Eshuna Code of 2300 BC (that is, before the code of Hammurabi). It called for action as soon as rabies was noticed in a dog. The owner was informed at once and had to take preventive action against bites. If the rabid dog bit someone who later died, a heavy fine was exacted.

The Babylonian King Adad-apla-iddina (1068-1047 BC) of the second dynasty of Isin built a temple to the goddess Nin-isina (Lady of Isin), who was represented in art with her holy animal, the dog. Known as Gula, she was worshiped as a healing goddess who protected people from rabies or, if angered by an insult to a dog, would afflict them with the disease through its bites. Many dog burials, often of young dogs, were found in the surrounds of the temple, along with memorial plates. It has been suggested that canine distemper may have been prevalent. A high incidence of healed fractures suggests that abuse was common. Gula was also a healing goddess in a more general sense; it is believed that the dog, by licking wounds or festers and comforting patients, was an assistant in treatment. The dog also served as Gula's mystical symbol to sway the gods in the patient's favor.

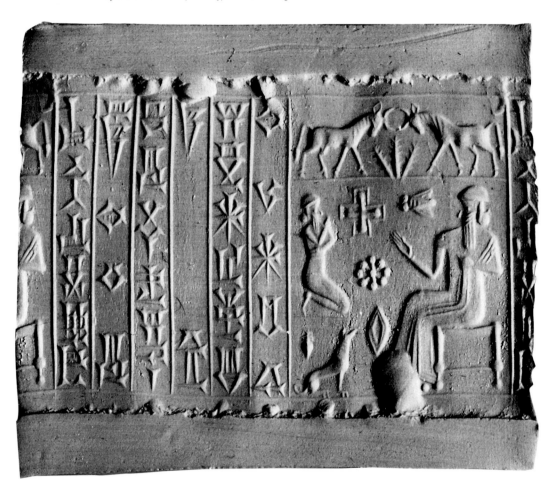

53. Impression of a worship scene from a Kassite cylinder seal showing a dog, the symbol of the healing goddess Gula. She was worshiped in Old Babylon for protecting people from rabies, but if she was angered by an insult to a dog, she could also inflict the dreaded disease. *(Vorderasiatisches Museum, Berlin.)*

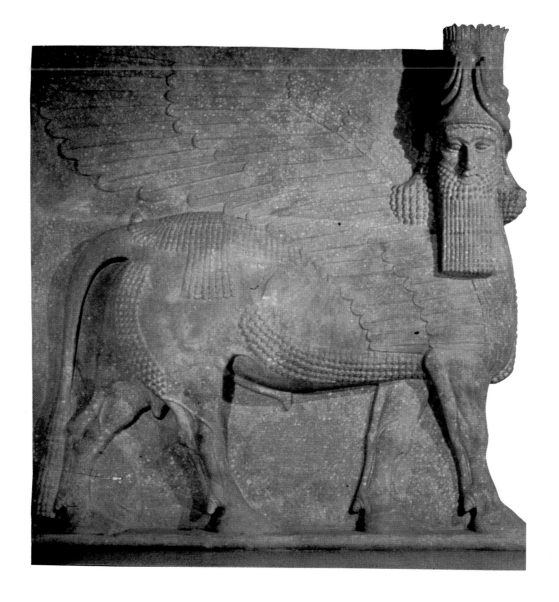

SOCIAL IMPACT OF THE HORSE

Domesticated horses, imported to Mesopotamia from the Anatolian plateau to the north and the Zagros Mountains to the east, first appeared in the area around the end of the third millennium BC but did not become common for another five hundred years. Their relative scarcity early in the second millennium BC may explain why they are not mentioned in Hammurabi's Code. Combined with the invention of the wheel, the horse had an immense impact on militant cultures. Its potential for rapid, effective transport of people and supplies and for chariot warfare was soon realized. Two-wheeled wagons and chariots drawn by two horses were depicted in Mesopotamian reliefs during the second millennium BC.

The Assyrian aristocracy developed a zest for hunting, especially for the hunting of such dangerous predatory adversaries as the lion, which was a threat to livestock. Great feats of courage were recorded on magnificent bas reliefs of Assyrian King Assurbanipal (668-627 BC). Later, lions were purposely bred for the royal hunt in palace menageries. Conclusions about the clinical outcomes of lesions caused by arrows in different organs were derived from observations, for instance, that an arrow through the thorax caused hemorrhage from the mouth and that arrows in the spine could lead to hindlimb paralysis. Elephants, buffalo, wild equids, boars, and the formidable aurochs were hunted, too, with the aid of large mastiff-like dogs. Cheetahs and falcons also were trained to hunt. Sites for the breeding, feeding, and training

54. Human-headed, winged bull from Khorsabad (Dur Sharrukin), palace of Sargon II (722-705 BC). Height, 487 cm; weight 40 tons. *(The Oriental Institute, The University of Chicago.)*

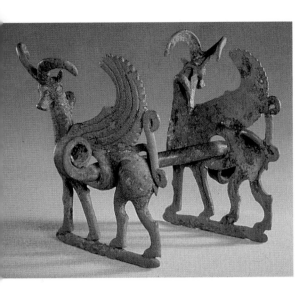

55. Luristan horse bit made of bronze. From Mesopotamia (900–700 BC). With the arrival of the domesticated horse near the end of the third millennium BC, Mesopotamian society realized its effectiveness for military purposes. *(The Oriental Institute, The University of Chicago.)*

56. Stone relief of Assyrian king Assurbanipal hunting wild onagers on horseback with bow and arrow. Nineveh (c. 645 BC). *(The British Museum, London.)*

of horses were established at many locations. The horse became the most valuable animal; those who owned them or managed them assumed special status in the Assyrian kingdoms.

Assyria became the master state in procurement and training of suitable horses. The high priority given to those functions is indicated by the appointment of *musarkisus*, high-level government officers responsible directly to the king, who scoured their provinces collecting horses. King Esarhaddon required daily written "horse reports." A study of a month's worth of these reports showed that horses were acquired at a steady rate of about 100 per day and taken to the royal stables near Nineveh. Of 2911 horses collected in that period, 1840 were classed as yoke or chariot horses, 787 as riding or cavalry mounts, and 27 as stud animals. Two breeds, Kusaean (Nubian) and Mesaean (Iranian), were identified; 136 mules were also obtained.

The first recorded manual on hippiatry dates to the fourteenth century BC and was written by Kikkuli, a Hurrian expert on hippiatry from the province of Mitanni. The manual refers to a central city famed for horse procurement and training, namely Hethiter. Detailed feeding and training procedures are described. About the same time, a treatise on treatment of equine diseases was produced in Ugarit language in Ras-Shamra, Syria, but only fragments have survived. A striking feature was that remedies were always applied via the nasal passages, presumably to be swallowed when they reached the pharynx.

An important achievement of uncertain time and place was the crossbreeding of a male donkey with the mare or female horse to produce the mule. Although the breeders knew the progeny were sterile, they were highly prized for their strength (a trait from the dam) and endurance (a trait from the sire). Although lacking the horse's speed and maneuverability, which were crucial for cavalry charges in chariots, the heat-tolerant mule was ideal for long hauls of wagons and as a pack animal. The onager was cross-bred with the donkey to yield a stronger hybrid.

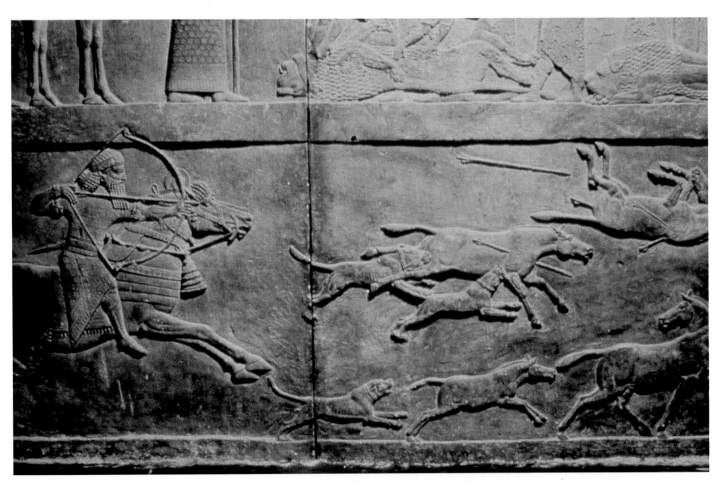

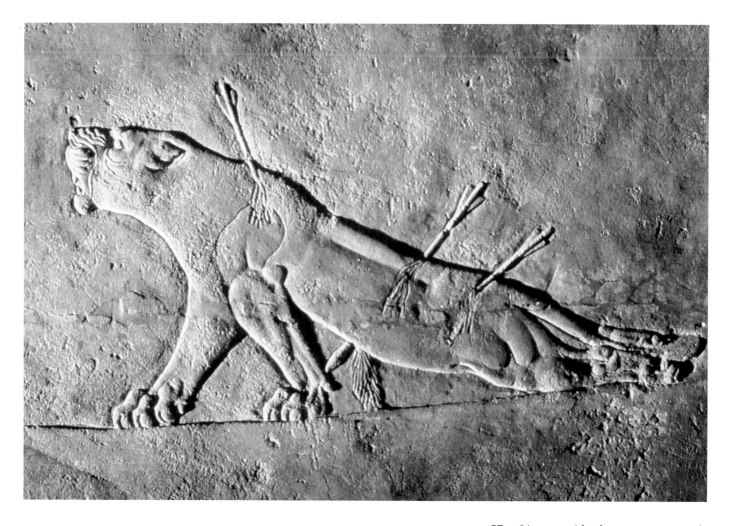

57. Lioness with three arrow wounds that caused injury to the spinal cord and resulted in paralysis of the rear extremities. Detail from *The Great Hunt,* an alabaster relief in the palace of Assurbanipal. Nineveh, seventh century BC. *(The British Museum, London.)*

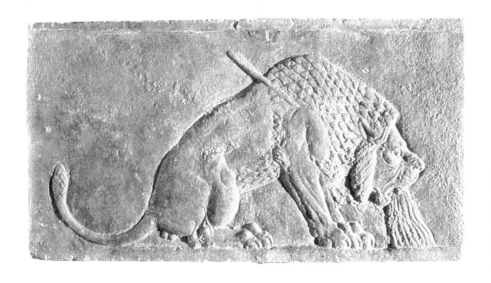

58. The Assyrians hunted lions and later bred them for royal hunts. Observation of arrow wound lesions suffered by the lions led to clinical conclusions represented in Assyrian art. For example, a wound in the lungs brings blood to the mouth. *(The British Museum, London.)*

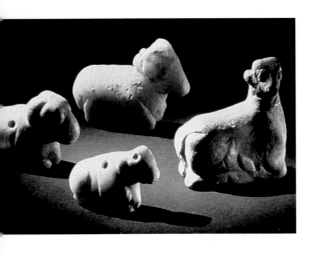

59. Stone amulets in the form of sheep, pierced for suspension, from Iraq. Sometimes such amulets had designs drilled on the bottom and were used as stamp seals. Protoliterate Period (before 2900 BC). *(The Oriental Institute, The University of Chicago.)*

FOCUS ON COSMOBIOLOGY

The history of Babylon is remarkable for its attention to astronomy and cosmology—the sun, the moon, the air (and weather), the planets, and the constellations—and the cyclic changes in these components of the universe that affected the planet. The earliest known representation of the signs of the zodiac was Sumerian and dates to about 2000 BC. The priests were expected to use the cosmic cycles and signs from the gods to forecast the outcome of epidemics affecting humans and animals. Pazuzu, the demon causing fever, was frequently represented as a large fly. Unexpected or inexplicable events and dreams were considered omens and were used in prophecy. The detailed appearance of the organs of sacrificed animals, especially the liver (clay models of the sheep's liver were made) and other viscera, were used by the oracles to divine the course of future events. Ninazu, the snake god, was considered a healing force. His son Ningishida had a rod with two snakes entwined as his emblem in Mesopotamia, an early clue to possible origins of the caduceus. Malformations and abortions received particular scrutiny and recording at Nineveh (in the library of Assurbanipal); they formed yet another basis for prophecy.

Empirical medical and veterinary diagnosis and treatment were also employed at the healing level of the individual case. Clay tablets dated to the sixth century BC indicate that much was known about animal diseases and their medical treatment and surgical intervention. Many remedies of herbal, animal, and mineral origin were known, formulated, and used. Bleeding and the lancing of abscesses were practiced.

HORSE-BASED CULTURES: MEDES AND PERSIANS

After the Assyrian culture went into decline in the eighth century BC, adjacent cultures such as the Medes to the east became free to develop a more creative civilization. The men had become outstanding horsemen and made the horse their main animal of sacrifice. Their priests were called magi and followed Zarathustra (in Greek, Zoroaster), the leader and prophet of the Parsee religion. The Persians followed the Zarathustran philosophy and religion in the sixth century and adopted many features of the Medean culture. Zoroaster's holy book, the Zend Avesta, said its wisdom had come down from the god of joy, Ahura-Mazda. The Parsee was a dualist religion espousing the eternal struggle between the spirits of good and light and evil and darkness. The holy animal was the dog; it was customary to lead a dog to a dying person to ward off the evil spirits. The magi protected the eternal flame, which kept away the evil forces of darkness. The Zend Avesta described animal healing and care in depth. Particular attention was paid to diagnosis and treatment of canine diseases. The soul of a dog-beater would suffer abomination on its passing and would be unwelcome in the next world. The moribund were expected to confess their sins to animals and seek forgiveness before they died.

Domestic animals rated highly in the Persian and Medean world order. The Mithras cult revered an Indo-Persian god and required capture and sacrifice of a bull in the presence of a lion, a snake, and a god. The Medes and Persians were famed for the quality of their horses and the care they gave them. The very word *Persia* was derived from the word for "horseman." Their high-quality horses and the skillful horsemanship of their cavalry formed the basis of Persian power that was to develop into the greatest empire the world had seen under Cyrus (559-529 BC), Darius I, and Xerxes—until Darius III was overthrown by Alexander the Great (in 332 BC).

Persians in the Middle Ages were noted for their exquisite artistry, particularly their miniature paintings depicting legends and complex situations involving people, animals, and the natural environment.

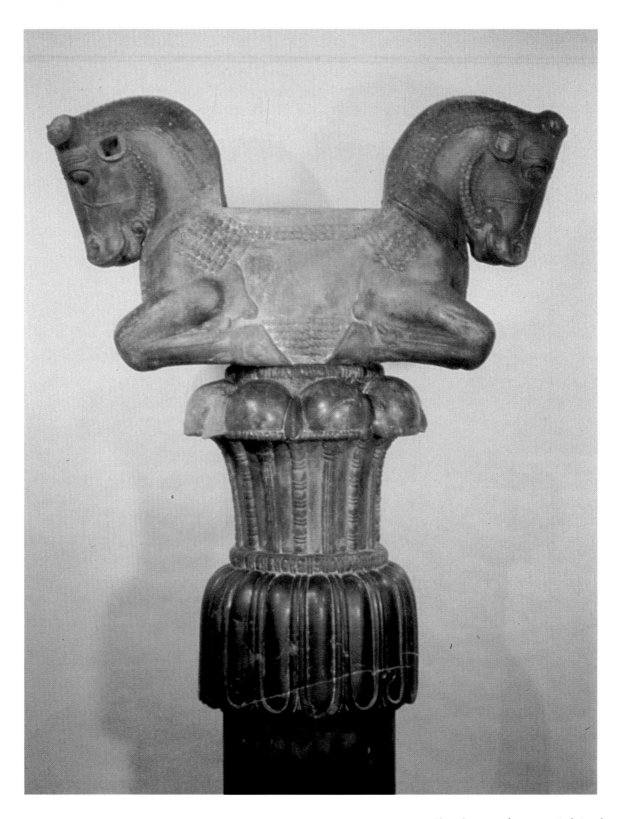

60. Stone column capital in the shape of a double bull. The roof of the Apadana, or audience hall, was supported by thirty-six stone columns, each topped by a pair of bulls placed back to back. The roof beams rested between the bulls almost sixty-five feet above the pavement. Limestone, extensively restored. Iran: Persepolis, Apadana. Achaemenid Period, during the reigns of Darius I and Xerxes (c. 500–480 BC). *(The Oriental Institute, The University of Chicago.)*

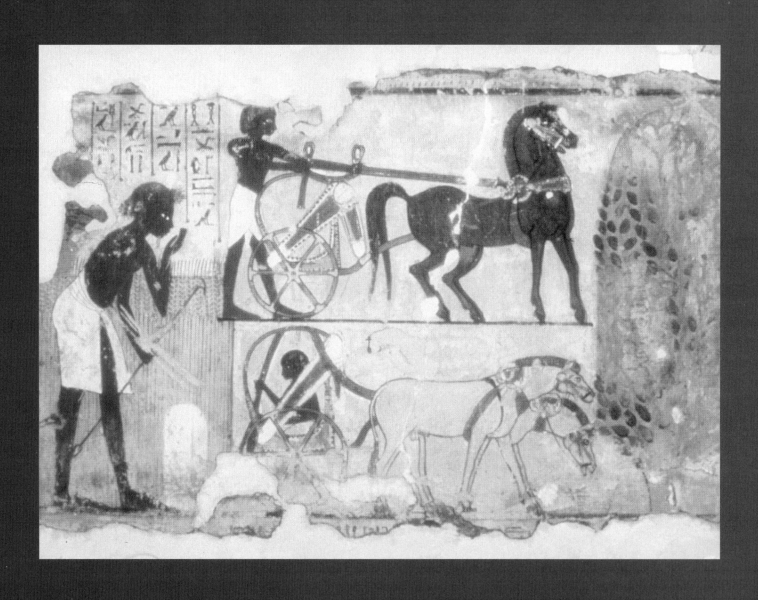

CHAPTER 5

Animal Care in Ancient Egypt

PREDYNASTIC NILE VALLEY CULTURES AND ANIMALS

The Nile River valley of the Old Stone Age received much more rain than it currently does: west of the river a savanna existed where today there is a barren desert. In those days wild game were plentiful, including wild precursors of domestic species such as the aurochs, ass, and wild buffalo. The climate was changing, however, becoming progressively more arid, with desertification advancing as the marshes and water sources were drying up. To the west lay the rocky, mountainous Tibesti Plateau and oases in the land between the Nile valley and the hills. Rock art has been found throughout this region, and remains of large animals have been found in areas north of Khartoum, where they could not survive today.

The hunting peoples of the Paleolithic era were followed by nomadic cattle herders of the Neolithic period. Upriver from Egypt, a transitional culture called the Khartoum Mesolithic evolved between 7000 BC and 4000 BC. These Nile valley hunter-gatherers exploited aquatic species for food, such as fish, turtles, reed rats, and larger mammals. The people used bows and arrows and harpoons, made decorated pottery, and left rock drawings. They may have given rise to the fine-boned Badarian people and the Shaheinab or Khartoum Neolithic culture. The latter became effective hunters of large mammals and domesticated the African pygmy goat. Ample evidence exists of human fascination with animals throughout the predynastic era.

NILE VALLEY CIVILIZATIONS

The great civilization of the Nile valley began about 5000 years ago with the unification of Upper and Lower Egypt under King Menes, who was both a healer and an anatomist. After the unification came the period known as the Old Kingdom or the pyramid age (2686-2160 BC). The question remains: Who were the ancient Egyptians?

Although Egyptian leaders did establish an empire, they did not set out to be a militant regime aimed at the conquest of other lands. Mostly they were prepared to sustain their empire through peaceful coexistence, negotiation, and trade. Indeed, Egypt lacked a standing army until one was created in 1550 BC, at the beginning of the New Kingdom (1580-1085 BC). Before this development, when the *pharaohs* (the Egyptian word for "hereditary monarchical rulers" or "kings") did decide to fight, they used mainly mercenaries hired from other lands. The Egyptians' engineering projects required that timber be imported from Lebanon and Syria, and ores for metalworking from Sinai. Their work with copper and timber was a technical advance from the preceding stone- and bone-based cultures.

One group of cultures often under Egyptian attack was that of the Nubians, who lived farther south in the Nile valley. Toward the end of the

61. *Facing page,* Animals play a prominent role in the art of ancient Egypt, reflecting their lofty status in the culture. This wall painting (c. 1400 BC) from the tomb of Nebamun, a nobleman, shows horses and hinnies harnessed to chariots while a tax collector assesses the crops on Nebamun's estate. The horses in the upper portion are restrained, the hinnies below, submissive. Thebes, eighteenth dynasty (1567-1320 BC). Height, 43 cm. *(The British Museum, London.)*

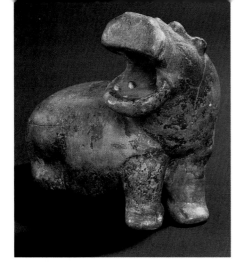

62. Blue-glazed faience of a roaring hippopotamus. The hippopotamus, considered a goddess in ancient Egypt, was especially revered by pregnant women. Middle Kingdom. Height 15.2 cm. *(The British Museum, London.)*

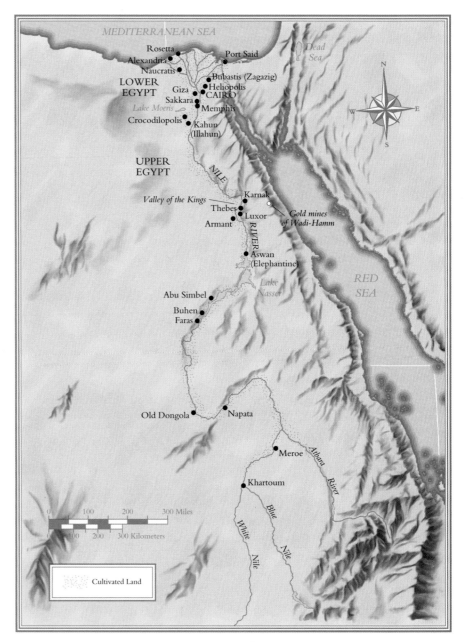

63. *Above right,* General map of Egypt showing the great civilization established along the Nile River valley and most of the sites mentioned in the text.

Old Kingdom, a group now known as the C Group emerged in Nubia. These people were breeders of cattle and makers of high-quality black polished pots; they placed clay figures of cattle on their graves and made rock drawings of cattle. Another culture, the Kerma culture of Kush (in Nubia), made artistic pottery with animal motifs in reddish clay.

ANIMAL WORSHIP AND MYTHOLOGY

Divine association with animals was a major feature of the religion of ancient Egypt. People gained merit by worshipping and caring for animals. Animals represented human spiritual characteristics, and complex rituals were constructed based on these priestly concoctions.

Egypt's regions, counties, and towns coined myths about hundreds of gods. Only a few can be alluded to in this brief discussion of their frequent representation in the form of animals. Perhaps the most widespread central myth was the idea of a creator of the world, Ra or Re (the king of the gods), who was tied to the daily solar cycle. In the beginning Ra was thought to have ruled over his creation, the earth, during the "First Time," when the cycles and rhythms of life were established out of the preceding chaos. Ra's chief enemy was a great serpent, Apep, who tried to block the normal solar cycle

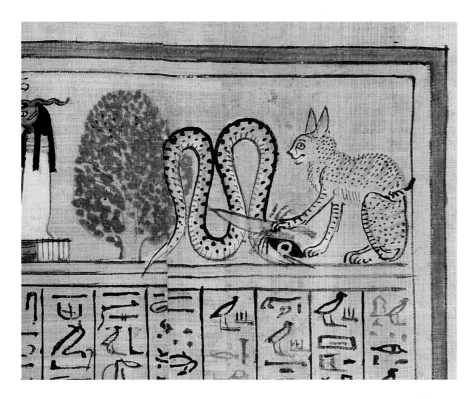

64. Ra, in the form of a cat, beheading the serpent Apep. Ancient Egyptians believed that Ra was the king of the gods and the serpent, his chief enemy, was attempting to block out the sun, which rose each morning above the sacred persea tree, seen behind Apep in this illustration from the *Book of the Dead,* papyrus of the scribe Ani (c. 1250 BC). The demise of Apep preserved light over darkness. Nineteenth dynasty (1320-1200 BC). *(The British Museum, London.)*

of sunrise to sunset. In the papyrus *Book of the Dead* (c. 1250 BC) there is a delightful representation of Ra as a vigilant cat beheading a malignant version of Apep and thereby preserving the daily sunrise over the sacred persea tree. When a solar eclipse occurred, it was feared that Apep had swallowed the vehicle (a barque) that conveyed the sun across the heavens. Ra was most commonly represented as a falcon-headed man because of a complex myth in which Horus the high-flying falcon bore the sun across the sky as his right eye or as a disk on his head. The pharaoh was seen as the living Horus, son of Ra, who became Ra after his death, gaining immortality. Thoth, represented with an ibis's head, was physician to the gods, as well as their scribe of justice.

Apis was the sacred black bull, one of the oldest Nile valley gods, a symbol of procreation and the fertility god of the Nile. Apis was responsible for the Ptah-Seker-Osiris cycle of creation, death, and resurrection. The cat Bast was venerated as a benevolent goddess in many parts of Egypt. Cats were frequently embalmed and buried, for example, at the special cat cemetery at Bubastis. The ram was worshipped, especially the horned head of the ram, often as Amon or Khnum. Anubis the jackal was commonly an object of worship, sometimes along with a dog. Embalmers were represented with Anubis's head, since they arranged for the trip to the next world. The ancient Egyptians were extremely conscious of the importance of birth. The role of the cow was perceived as central to the cosmic rebirth of the sun at dawn.

THE RULING CLASS: PHARAOHS AND THEIR HIGH PRIESTS

During the Old Kingdom the ancient Egyptians had a king, Djoser or Zoser, who is thought to have ruled from 2630 BC to 2611 BC. He had a remarkable adviser, Imhotep, who was renowned for priestly prowess, wisdom, and versatility. Revered as a priest, healer, and architect, Imhotep designed the first pyramid as the royal tomb of Djoser. He also initiated procedures that were to evolve into the practice of preserving the body and soul of the pharaoh in the pyramids. Unlike the mythical Thoth, Imhotep was a real person, although his adulation lived on after his death and he was accorded divine status in 535 BC. Unlike Aesculapius, he is not shown with a symbolic serpent.

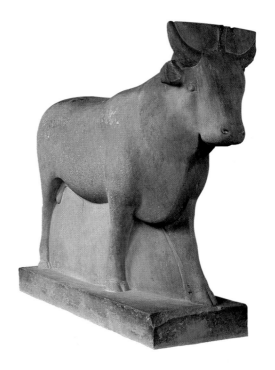

65. A realistic statue of the sacred black bull, Apis, who symbolized procreation and was believed to be responsible for the cycle of creation, death, and resurrection. Granite. Serapeum at Saqqara, near Memphis. Thirtieth dynasty (399-343 BC). *(The Louvre, Paris.)*

66. Detail from the east wall of the sacrifice chamber from the tomb chapel of Hetepherakhti, showing a birthing scene of a goat. The head, neck, and front extremities up to the shoulder are clearly visible. The position of the kid is normal, and the mother appears to have no difficulty with the delivery. Relief from the Mastaba of the high official Hetepherakhti near Saqqara. Middle of fifth dynasty (c. 2420 BC). (*Rijksmuseum van Oudheden, Leiden.*)

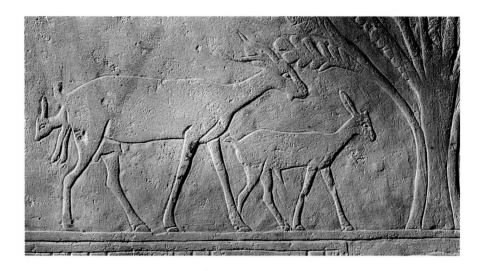

67. Birth of a calf. Group in stuccoed and painted wood. Boy's apron in linen, cow's tail in twine. Middle Kingdom, eleventh to twelfth dynasties. Length of base, 47 cm. (*Royal Ontario Museum, Toronto.*)

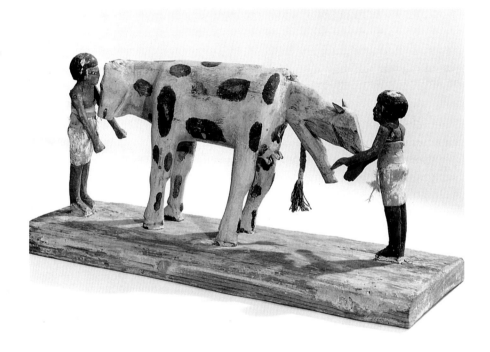

The texts of the papyrus records that were buried with the rulers in the eternal tombs form a bridge from modern times to some of the most distant steps in the cultural and intellectual history of humankind. The lore of the Egyptians became the foundation of and the model for the regional cultures that followed theirs. The wall engravings and painted grave art contain many scenes of animal husbandry, slaughter, and sacrifice, imparting a sense of wonder about the goal of immortality. Many beautiful scenes depicting cows giving birth and receiving assistance indicate considerable knowledge of obstetrics, although the practitioners depicted are believed to be skillful stock handlers rather than animal doctors.

The Egyptian dynasties in their turn inherited the accumulated beliefs, legends, and technology of prehistoric humans. These included many superstitions about the presence of good and evil in events that beset the individual, such as misfortune and disease. The priestly caste had to contend with perceptions of magical powers or genies that were thought to invade the persona of the depraved or sick, and they had to protect the people and animals from the much-feared venomous snakes. Thus their role became that of both priest and physician, the former to deal with the evil spirit and the latter to provide care for the suffering or deranged body and mind. The Egyptian priest-physician, portrayed, for example, as the Nubian clad in a leopard skin, appears to be a much more structured version of and sequel to the shaman or witch doctor. Since disease was considered an invasion by evil spirits coming from the invisible emanations of the curses of the dead or from the angered gods, mystical means involving magic, spells, and prayers were considered necessary to drive them out.

EMERGENCE OF RATIONAL MEDICINE AND HINTS OF VETERINARY CARE

The nonmystical aspect of the priest-physician's role, the palliation of the symptoms of disease, was based on the accumulated lore derived empirically and recorded. A remarkable range of practical measures, which might be classed as nursing care, and of medicinal concoctions, as well as a limited range of surgical approaches and cautery, came into use. Some of these have come to modern attention in the form of documents like the Ebers and Kahun papyri. The Kahun is of particular interest because it mentions a number of animal diseases and is one of the earliest records of a veterinary-type approach to animal treatment. Specific diseases recorded in the papyrus are virtually unrecognizable, although eye problems are specifically mentioned. Egyptian physicians developed specialities based on body systems, such as diseases of the eyes. Of course, the remarkable practices of embalming and mummification have allowed modern pathologists to examine the surviving parts of the body, particularly the skin and bones, for the presence of disease. Mummified cats have been uncovered, and information about their then extant diseases can be gleaned. The ideas of hygiene and preventive medicine were also developed by the Egyptians, who regulated standards of cleanliness for the body, food, clothing, and habitation.

Treatments were focused on controlling putrefaction of wounds. Copper-containing minerals (such as malachite and verdigris) and greasy salves of honey and lint were popular. (In modern times such salves have been shown to be effective bacteriostatics). Use of a hot knife and tapes for closing wounds was described. Bleeding and enemas were widely used. Despite the focus on embalming, the knowledge of anatomy in the health professions appears to have been sketchy.

The oldest veterinary publication is the part of the Kahun papyrus that describes in sacred hieroglyphic script certain cases of animal disease. The town of Kahun of the twelfth dynasty was sited at the Illahun of today, in the Fayoum district. The papyrus, dated at about 1900 BC, has been damaged over the interval of almost 4000 years. Surviving fragments describe three diseases of cattle (two include eye problems) and some snippets about eye diseases of dogs, fish, and birds. The approach is systematic: Title, Symptoms, Admonition, Treatment, Prognosis, Progress, Reinspection, and Further Treatment are typical categories.

The Kahun papyrus, although fragmented and difficult to interpret, illustrates that rational intervention had begun to play a part in animal treatment. Some sense of this shift can be discerned in fragments concerning two cases of disease in cattle. In the first case a bull was "trembling with the worm." It went into rigid extension, fell to the ground, and convulsed. The cow doctor's treatment was, first, to recite the sacred spell to the bull and then to introduce his arm into the bull's rectum. After this, he rubbed the bull's back with the (other?) hand. When the affected site was reached, the cow doctor manually removed all clots and other purulent matter. He washed his hands in a bowl of water after each pass of palpation and evacuation. He could detect that the animal would recover when the pus appeared. This case was the first written record of the use of rectal palpation and evacuation in an animal. The condition appears to have been severe necrotic gastroenteritis.

In the second case a bull appears to have had a high fever and respiratory difficulty. It had dyspnea, and the eyes were running, the cheeks swollen, and the gums inflamed. The first action was to hold its head upright and recite the sacred incantation. Immediately it was to be laid down so that the attendant could cool it with repeated applications of cold water. The aromatic essences of plants or fruits (cucumbers or gourds) were to be applied to the eyes, chest, abdomen, and limbs to "fumigate" the animal. Later, the attendant tried to take the bull to be bathed and immersed in the cold water. If it refused to go to the water, the cycle of cold-water splashing and plant-extract rubbing had to be repeated. As a last resort (perhaps as a partial sacrifice to appease the demon that had possessed it?) the animal was bled from incisions made in the nose and tail. At that point the animal's fate was in the hands of the gods: it lived or died. If it was reluctant to move or was sluggish and the eyes were inflamed, the eyes were wrapped with heated linen in an effort to relieve the lesion. The identity of the disease is uncertain, but malignant catarrhal fever and rinderpest have been proposed as possibilities.

The Bible is a source of information about animal diseases in Egypt. The Book of Exodus describes plagues that caused heavy losses of livestock; the plagues were related chronologically to catastrophic climatic changes that led to floods and droughts. In one of the plagues cattle exhibited clinical signs compatible with the syndrome of anthrax. Some authors have speculated that rinderpest may have been present.

EMBALMING: IMMORTALIZING THROUGH MUMMIFICATION AND DEIFICATION

One of the most extraordinary features of the Egyptian civilization was its attitude toward the embalming and burial of the dead. The viscera were removed and the cavities filled with natron (the natural soda left by the Nile, a mixture of sodium carbonate and sodium bicarbonate); then the body was covered with natron and left to cure in the sun. The final steps were to treat the remains with aromatic resins and to restore the shape with padding.

68. Mummification was an extraordinary feature of ancient Egyptian life. This process was extended to sacred animals as well as to the pharaohs, and radiographic studies of the embalmed species have demonstrated that a variety of skeletal diseases were common. These radiographs show a typical mummified cat and a cat mummy with dislocated cervical vertebrae. *(The Natural History Museum, London.)*

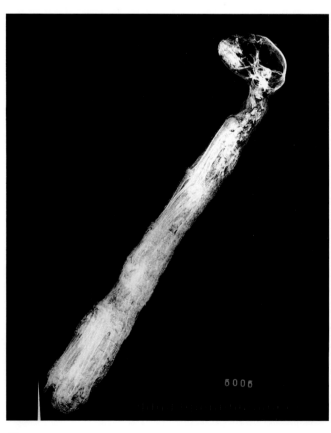

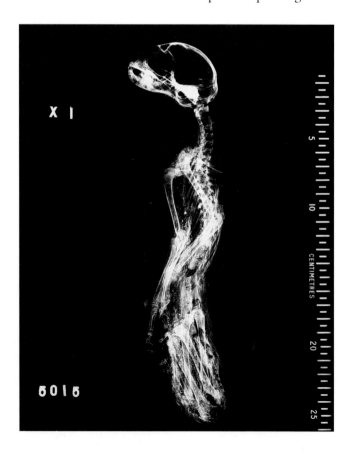

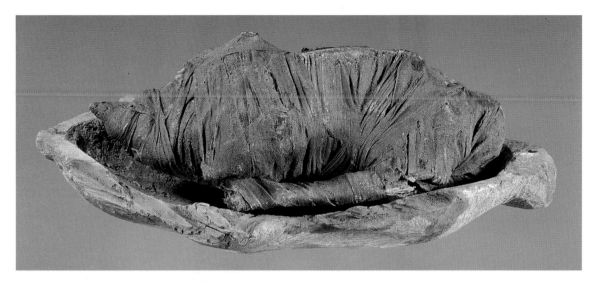

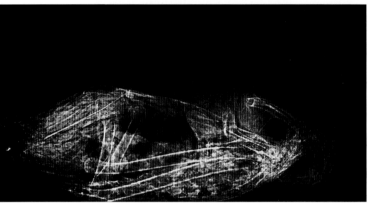 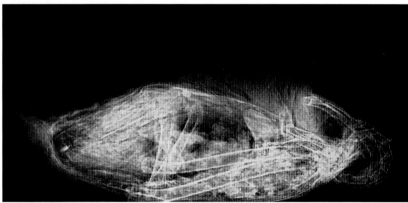

The technique of mummification that preserved the remains of the pharaohs was extended to the most sacred animals as well. Thus Apis, the black bull with sacred markings selected to be the divine representative and worshipped at Memphis, was accorded the fullest treatment, as seen in tombs of bulls in the Serapeum, the temple at Saqqara. The carcass was embalmed and wrapped for sixty days (seventy days of mourning were declared for the pharaoh), and the traditional ceremonial rituals of the priests were performed before it was transferred to the Serapeum. Huge statues of the Apis bulls, twelve feet long and nine feet high and carved from single pieces of granite, were found in the temple. The tombs of sixty-four bulls were discovered by Auguste Mariette in 1851 and 1852. Ptolemy I Soter moved the center of Apis worship to Alexandria. Other bull cults included those of Mnevis at Heliopolis and Buchis of Armant.

Species other than bulls were handled differently. For some, such as baboons, falcons, and ibis, all members of the species were regarded as divine representatives. As a result the baboon galleries at Saqqara contained more than 4000 burials, and those of falcons contained literally hundreds of thousands. The embalming process had to be simpler for these species, and the wrapped animals ended up in pottery jars or relic boxes. The Saqqara animal cemeteries were a vast subterranean necropolis for cattle, falcons, baboons, and ibis. Ram-headed Nile gods known as Khnum were worshipped at Elephantine Island near the first cataract that was considered the source of the river. Dogs and jackals were worshipped at Cynopolis (the "place of Canines") in Middle Egypt. Baboons and ibis were the sacred animals of Thoth, the god of wisdom and writing. Bast's sacred cats were buried at Bubastis. The presence of mummified animals has allowed the study of the incidence of diseases, in particular, skeletal diseases, in ancient Egypt. Study has verified that many modern skeletal diseases such as rickets, arthritis, osteoporosis, and hip dysplasia were present in ancient Egypt.

69. Mummified fowl and its wooden containing case, recovered from a plundered tomb during the Egyptian Expedition at Thebes (1918-1920) by the Metropolitan Museum of Art. Ancient Egyptian tombs contained many objects for the afterlife, including fowl for nourishment. Recent radiographic studies have identified this specimen as a duck, probably from the early eighteenth dynasty (1567-1320 BC). *(The Oriental Institute, The University of Chicago.)*

Most of the animal burials date to the later stages of the classical Egyptian civilization, the late and Ptolemaic periods during which the Egyptians were repeatedly overwhelmed by such invaders as the Persians and the Greeks. Perhaps the priests were calling upon all their spiritual resources to help sustain the traditional culture and to ensure its resurrection.

CULTURAL DEVELOPMENT BASED ON SUSTAINABLE AGRICULTURE

Lake Tana and the Blue Nile make up the conduit for the runoff from the rainy season in Ethiopia, and the White Nile conveys the surplus waters from Lake Victoria and the surrounding regions. The annual increase in flows along the Nile valley began about the end of May; the rising level of the river (measured in "Nilometers") was perceptible by mid-June. The level rose steadily until the beginning of August, when the canals were opened to flood the plains. Animals were removed from the lowest areas, but during a sudden, unusual rise in the flow pasturelands could be inundated and a rescue operation had to be mounted to save the cattle.

The waters of the Nile were the basis of successful crop production in old Egypt. Each year they inundated the lowlands adjacent to the river, and after the waters receded the areas had to be resurveyed to determine ownership. The fertile, friable alluvial soils were worked easily with the aid of teams of oxen drawing primitive plows. The seed was scattered by hand; then goats or pigs were driven across the soil to tread in the seed. The rooting habits of swine were also exploited to clear the land of roots before cultivation. Cattle pulled the plows by means of a simple yoke resting on a pad tied to the withers. Shoulder pieces were slung from the yoke to form a collar. As an alternative, the yoke could be affixed to the horns and to the pole attached to the plow. The Egyptian farmer mastered the art of local irrigation with the aid of an ingenious device called a shadoof, a bucket slung from a long pole with a stone weight on the other end; the pole was attached to a post. The bucket was pulled down to the water level of the river and filled; the weight contributed to the lift back up (or a springy pole could be used to help the lift), and the bucket was swung 'round and its contents dumped into a gulley above the bank that fed into the planted area.

The ideas of agriculture and stock raising (and their adoption) allowed settlements to become permanent or, at least, to have a repetitive, seasonal nomadic pattern. Consequently the Egyptian civilizations left far more substantial physical evidence of their culture than had any previous peoples, and later interpreters, looking back, could obtain a much clearer picture of the setting for the various stages of human progress. After ways were found to communicate ideas, on the one hand, through code words and symbols constructed from hieroglyphs and a basic alphabet and quantities, on the other, through arrangements of numerals, it became possible to leave records that permitted subsequent historians to understand the logic of a culture. Outstanding among these relics was the Rosetta Stone, a large basalt tablet discovered in AD 1799 by Captain Bouchard of Napoleon's invaders at Rashid, or *Rosetta* as the French named it. It contained inscriptions of Ptolemy V's 196 BC Memphis decree in three languages (Egyptian hieroglyphic, Greek, and demotic). The stone was seized by the British, but a copy of it was taken to Paris where Champollion used the comparison to decipher the Egyptian writing in 1822. This achievement allowed the birth of Egyptology based on "the literature" of Ancient Egypt, allowing a great advance in modern understanding of the ancient culture. Many of the original hieroglyphs were based on animals and later were modified and stylized to become letters.

The impact of animal domestication on ancient Egypt was immense. Farmers in the Nile River valley during the times of the pharaohs esteemed oxen above all other possessions. As suggested earlier, oxen imparted to farmers the capacity to work their arable land with much less physical labor, making life bearable and expanding the area that could be tilled. Cattle of both the European type (*Bos taurus*) and the Asiatic or zebu type (*Bos indicus*) were brought in, the zebu later, during the New Kingdom. In the art of the Old Kingdom, long-horned and lyre-horned cattle, as well as short-horned and hornless varieties, were prevalent. Whether these earlier cattle were all imported or some were tamed locally is uncertain. Horned cattle, usually white, brown, black, or spotted, were used as draft oxen. Horn training or deformation, an interesting manipulation, was practiced. Usually one horn was bent down, since that appearance was regarded as a lucky portent of a healthy, productive life. To this day the Dinka and Nuer tribes of southern Sudan perform similar operations on the horns to produce the desired effect. To progressively bend the horn down and forward, the growing horn of a young animal is notched right through to the corium several times at intervals. This painful, bloody operation was performed by a specialist called an atet, who also bled and castrated cattle, provided obstetrical assistance, and treated wounds, dislocations, and fractures. Presumably, similar practices had existed in ancient Egypt. It is clear from the scenes of fattened oxen that castration was practiced widely in ancient Egypt.

Cattle were valuable as a source of milk, which became a staple food. Milking cows are often portrayed as hornless, suggesting that the handlers may have practiced dehorning or had succeeded in selecting for the trait, or both. One sarcophagus shows a cow being milked with a calf tied to its foreleg, a stratagem often employed to initiate milk let-down by allowing the calf an initial short suckle. Fattening of cattle may have been enhanced by castration and restriction of movement. Overgrown hooves are discernible in wall illustrations, and animals are depicted as being hand-fed.

70. The Hathor goddess, in the form of a cow, from the Shrine of Hathor, Deir el-Bahri, Western Thebes. Animals played a major role in the bewildering yet fascinating religion of the ancient Egyptians. Here Hathor is protecting and suckling the young pharaoh, Horus. Deities assumed the form of animals, with Hathor, a sky-deity, taking the shape of the cow-goddess of love and joy. The marks on the cow's hide represent stars from earlier departed pharaohs. *(Egyptian Museum, Cairo.)*

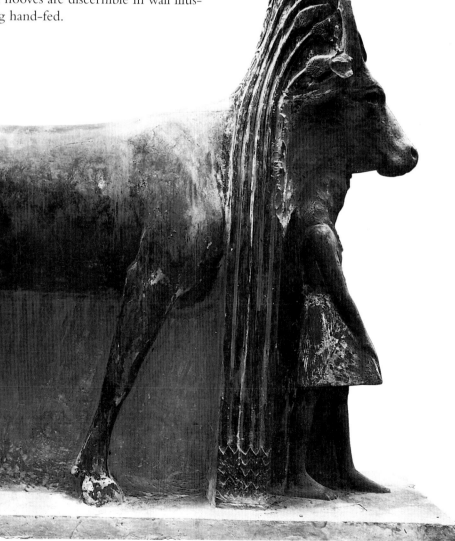

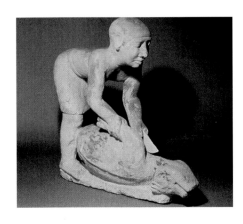

71. Ancient Egypt benefited greatly from animal domestication, and cattle became an important food source. This limestone servant statuette shows a butcher slaughtering a calf. From the tomb of Nykan-inpu. Giza. Fifth to sixth dynasties (c. 2500-2300 BC). (*The Oriental Institute, The University of Chicago.*)

72. Detail of painted geese (c. 2600 BC) from the tomb of Nefermaat and Itet. Fourth dynasty (c. 2613-2494 BC). (*The British Museum, London.*)

Slaughter of cattle involved casting and tying the animal and rolling it onto its back with the neck forced back. Then the throat was cut from ear to ear. Often the blood was collected for cookery: black puddings were popular in old Egypt. Later, both Israelites and Moslems were prohibited from eating blood. The *swnw* (an Egyptian word for "doctor") practiced a primitive type of meat inspection, at least for the sacrificial cattle.

Twisted-horned sheep were popular in the Old Kingdom but were progressively replaced by the more favored fat-tailed sheep during the Middle Kingdom (c. 2040-1786 BC). Goats were common, although given a low value, and donkeys were used as pack animals and ridden, mostly by young boys. The dromedary camel was introduced long after the horse, and even later the Arabs brought in water buffalo as draft animals.

Pigs had been kept in the Nile delta since prehistoric times, thriving wherever moist soils allowed them to root and water holes were available to wallow in for cooling. They were well regarded as food and were sacrificed. One myth tells that in the guise of a black pig the powerful but ambitious god Seth (Set) blinded Horus's eye, with the consequence that Ra reluctantly commanded the people to abhor the swine for Horus's sake, a punishment inflicted on the evil enemy of the gods, Seth, for having injured the eye of heaven. The prohibition may have applied only to the upper classes, since there is evidence that swine, like goats, were kept and eaten in Upper Egypt after it. Herodotus, the Greek historian, reported on the use of squealing pigs and pork baits to trap crocodiles, indicating that pigs were plentiful. However, the Hyskos ("shepherds of the desert") conquerors of Upper Egypt, who are thought to have been a Semitic Bedouin people from Syria, brought a different view. To them swine were "unclean" long before Islam, and prohibitions were imposed on their use, probably based on an arbitrary extrapolation from mythology.

The Nile complex of rivers, lakes, and swamps teemed with fish, and some Egyptian peoples also fished the surrounding seas. A great variety of species were caught, and many were depicted in the art decorating temples and tombs. Waterfowl (ducks and geese) are represented beautifully. The pharaohs were enamored of animals of all kinds, and ornamental fish ponds and waterfowl collections were features of their gardens and art.

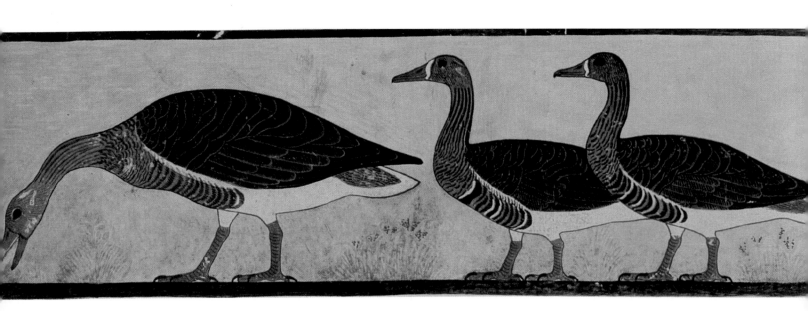

SUSCEPTIBILITY OF STOCK TO INFECTIOUS DISEASES

The narrow strip of well-watered, fertile land along the banks of the Nile River and its delta branches attracted a heavy concentration of livestock. Evidence suggests that this concentration rendered the stock susceptible to recurring plagues of environmental origin, such as anthrax, and to imported plagues arriving with purchased animals or invaders such as the Hyskos. Imported plagues included respiratory and enteric diseases. The concentrated stocking must have led to a high incidence of parasitic diseases. It is likely that the ancient Egyptians had an inkling about vector-borne diseases, since they took precautions to avoid mosquito bites, for instance, by using fine nets in infested areas like the Fayoum basin. The frequent droughts and dust storms must have contributed to the high incidence of eye diseases.

ARRIVAL OF THE HORSE AND ESCALATION OF WARFARE

Because of military threats or ambitious leaders (or both), most of the later cultures placed a higher value on the horse than on the food-and-fiber species. Egypt had the relative luxury of developing its animal agriculture before facing invaders. Egypt did not obtain horses until relatively late, but they became important in the New Kingdom, appearing on monuments for the first time during the eighteenth dynasty, after 1568 BC. Presumably the horses were brought into Egypt from the Eurasian steppes via the lands of the Middle East. The New Kingdom rapidly mastered the new domesticated species and learned to harness and drive them. Instead of shoes, a type of sandal made of matting was used to protect the hooves.

When the Hyksos invaded from Palestine around 1730 BC, they used a new battle technique based on bronze weapons and chariots drawn by swift Arabian horses. The hated Hyksos worshiped the evil god Seth, which heightened the resentment against their imposed dynasty. Not until the Egyptians similarly employed horses were they able to evict the Hyksos in the middle of the sixteenth century BC. Egypt became the leader in breeding

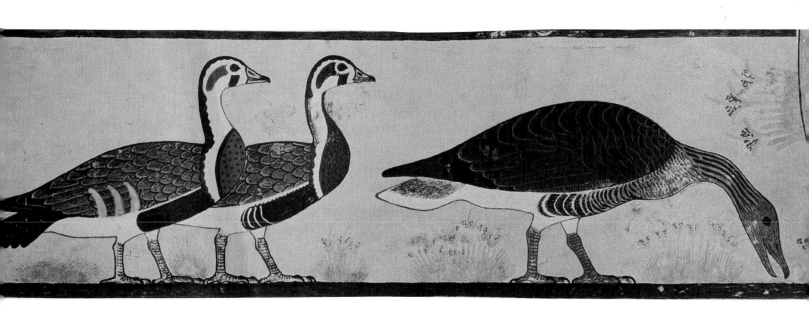

high-quality Arabian horses, and during the New Kingdom these fine beasts were depicted in art. The Egyptian empire subsequently expanded as far as the Euphrates River by using the horse in battle.

Egypt was reunited during the eighteenth dynasty, setting the stage for the Rameses kings from the delta. Later dynasties had to fight the Libyans and the Sea Peoples. The Sea Peoples were great bands of roving invaders from the Aegean region who destabilized the region and laid waste to many states, including Egypt in the time of Rameses III (1187-1156 BC), who defeated them. A general decline set in under the later Rameses kings and their successors. As the glory faded, Egypt became a prize to be fought for, and it suffered many changes of rulers—Libyans, Ethiopians, Assyrians, Saites, and Persians. Alexander incorporated Egypt into his great Grecian empire in 332 BC and established his capital at a magnificent new center called Alexandria, which was destined to carry the torch of intellect in medical and veterinary fields under the Greek-speaking Ptolemies. This change converted Egypt from a unique African state to a Mediterranean state that looked to Europe for its development.

Tomb paintings show pairs of equids that are thought to be hinnies harnessed to chariots. Hinnies are hybrids produced by crossing a donkey jenny with a male horse. The offspring of that match are graceful and tractable but infertile. If the interpretation of the art is accurate, Egypt was unusual in developing this cross and using it for traction and transport. Also controversial is the use of the onager or hemione (half-ass). Although the onager has been considered to have been a domesticated equid in West Asia, it is now believed, because of art reliefs showing the onager being captured in Assyria, that it was used only to cross with donkeys.

ANIMAL SACRIFICE AND SPORT

Vast numbers of cattle and some *Oryx* species (which were semidomesticated) were sacrificed at the temples for the festivals, and various proscriptions applied to several animals. The billy goat was proscribed from use in sacrifice because it was considered the embodiment of Seth, the god Horus's enemy. Nevertheless, evidence suggests that it was sacrificed by the subaristocratic classes. The swineherd, unlike the shepherd, was excluded from religious ceremonies, and in many parts fish were proscribed as food.

Animals played an important part in the Egyptian economy. In the time of the Rameses kings, a bull, depending on its quality, was worth 30 to 120 deben, a donkey about 40 deben, and a goat only 2 deben. (A deben, made of copper, weighed 91 grams and served as an Egyptian medium of exchange.) In addition, the pharaohs imposed a poll tax on livestock, as well as a hide tax. When administration was centralized in the New Kingdom, the pharaoh's overseer of cattle collected the cattle tax throughout the kingdom. Hence animals not only eased the life of the farmer but also served as a source of risk-free wealth for the pharaoh.

Animals were involved in many aspects of Egyptian life. Bullfighting was a sport in Egypt that appears to have involved rivalry between individual bulls, their owners prodding them to dominate their opponents. The ichneumon or mongoose was revered because of its remarkable dexterity in destroying snakes and its appetite for crocodile eggs. Various types of dogs are depicted in Egyptian art. Hunting was a popular means of protecting the flocks from predators such as lions, leopards, hyenas, small wolves, and jackals, although wild animals were also trapped and caught alive. Various weapons were used in the chase: throwing sticks, spears, bows and arrows, and even lassos. Chariots accompanied by packs of dogs were used in some areas. Preserves were maintained for wild animals so that they could be released and hunted later. A great variety of antelopes, gazelles, ibex, and smaller game, including

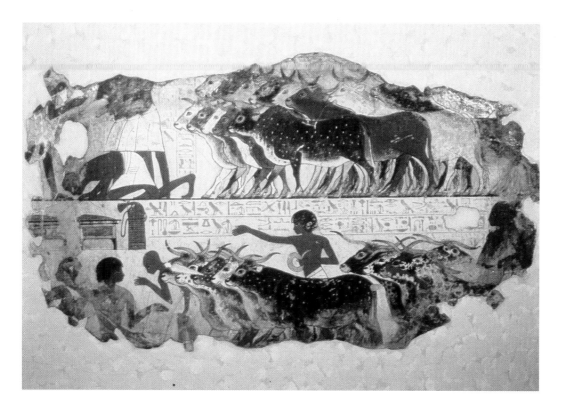

73. Livestock played an important role in the economy of ancient Egypt, with cattle being taxed throughout the New Kingdom. In this wall painting (c. 1400 BC) from the tomb of Nebamun, cattle from his estate are being shown for inspection. Height 58.5 cm. Thebes, eighteenth dynasty (1567-1320 BC). *(The British Museum, London.)*

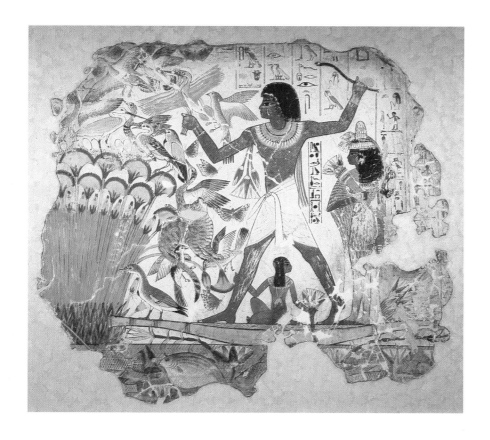

74. The nobleman Nebamun hunting waterfowl in the rich Nile marshes with his wife and daughter. The early Egyptians were great hunters. Here Nebamun is using a throw stick carved like a snake while holding herons in his right hand for camouflage. Wall painting (c. 1400 BC). *(The British Museum, London.)*

75

fowl and fish, were hunted. Birds were plentiful and popular as food, but their numbers declined greatly as the aridity of the region increased and the marshes shrank. They were hunted from small boats in marshy areas like Lake Moeris of the Fayoum Depression. Sometimes live decoy birds were used, and cats were sent to retrieve birds that escaped into the thickets after being felled by a throwing stick.

The origin of Lake Moeris, dating to the thirteenth dynasty, was attributed to pharaoh Amenemhet III, who redirected the Nile through a gap that led it into the Fayoum basin so that it formed the huge lake by controlling inflow and outflow. A huge area of cultivated land was added. The water flowed into the created lake for about half of the year and then out for the other half. Hence the water was returned to the river during the dry season. Aegyptos was the name used in *The Odyssey* for the Nile River. The historian Herodotus stated that Egypt is an acquired land, the gift of the river.

ANIMALS AS COMPANIONS

Evidence of dogs and cats being kept in many homes in ancient Egypt is seen in paintings, figurines, and mummies. The scenes show lively participation in hunting and play; animal caricatures appear in later dynasties. The pets were accorded special names. It seems that most were treated with affection and care, and there seems to have been a preference for cats and miniature dogs. Clearly there must have been some tenacious selection programs to achieve the latter.

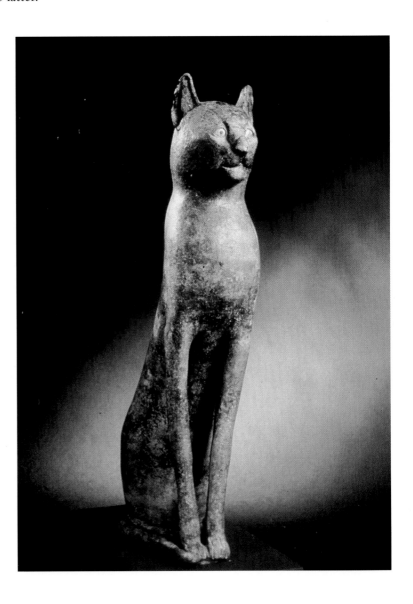

75. Cat figurines from ancient Egypt are common, for cats held special status. They were companion animals in many households and were also used for bird hunting. This bronze figurine is characteristic of the form frequently depicted in works of art. Height, 50.3 cm. Egypt, site unknown. Latter part of first millennium BC. *(The University Museum, University of Pennsylvania.)*

Cats had a special status, especially during the New Kingdom, appearing frequently in works of art. A special form of cat, depicted in statuettes dating to the Ptolemaic period, was lean and superior-looking, almost regal in poise, and had an inscrutable expression that conveyed a slightly sinister aura. Presumably the cat was initially tamed and introduced to the homes to control rodents. The striking scenes of cats participating in bird hunting indicate a high level of communication between humans and cats and the intimacy of companionship.

Large dogs such as greyhounds and wolfhounds were used in the hunt and as guard dogs. Monkeys were imported from lands to the south to serve as amusing pets. Throughout the artwork the image is generated of a people who regarded animals with genuine affection and joy.

76. Wall painting of a cat eating a fish, detail from the scene of Nakht and his wife receiving offerings at the funerary banquet, from the tomb of Nakht. Thebes, Tomb 52. *(The Metropolitan Museum of Art, New York.)*

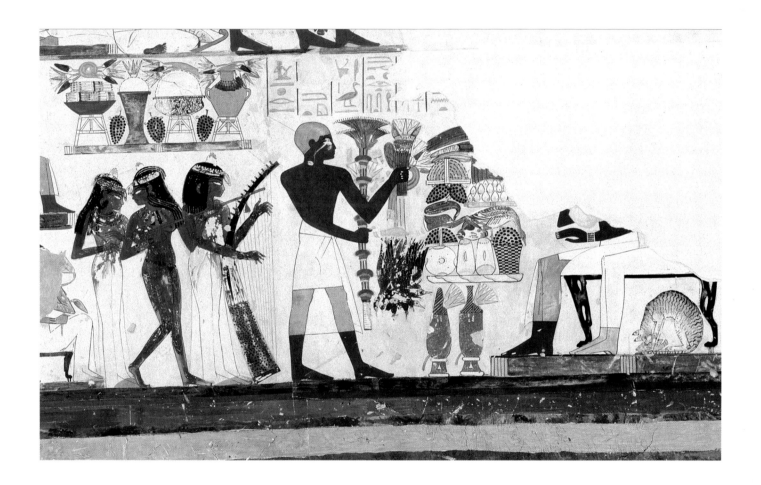

轎車

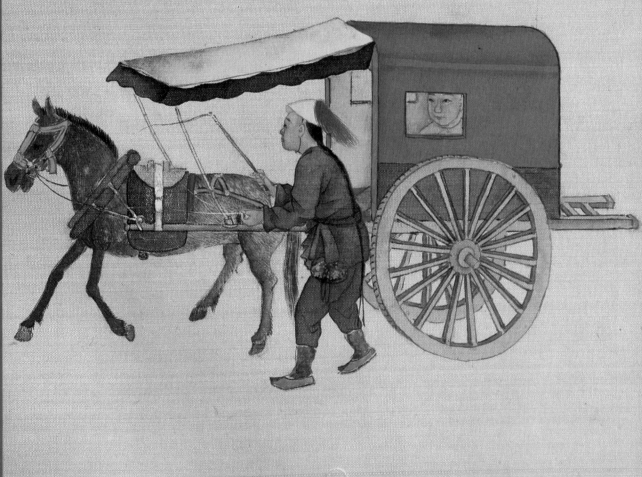

C H A P T E R   6

Roots of Veterinary Medicine in East Asia

GEOGRAPHICAL OVERVIEW

East Asia comprises China as well as Tibet and Taiwan, Mongolia and Siberia in the north, and the Koreas, Japan, and the nations of Southeast Asia. It has had a significant, largely unappreciated impact on the evolution of veterinary medical technology. China's vast population and ancient culture have made it the hub of the region. Domestication of animals and plants began in the middle reaches of the valley of the Yellow River and its great tributary, the Wei, more than 7000 years ago. The semiarid sagebrush steppe's main wild fauna were the burrowing subterranean mole rats or zokors of the *Myospalax* genus that were agricultural pests. Millet and barley farming on dry land was being supplemented with irrigation by the sixth century BC or earlier. China introduced rice and soybeans; the written character for the latter, "sku," may have symbolized perceptively the root nodules containing the nitrogen-fixing *Rhizobium* bacteria as three elongated dots. The soybean has become a major international basis of protein supplementary feeds for livestock. Hemp was grown for fiber, and the mulberry was introduced as food for the voracious silkworm larvae that generated silk.

In southern reaches the 3900-mile-long Yangtze or "Long River" system flows from "the roof of the world" at about 20,000 feet down through the vast grain-producing plains of Szechuan to the East China Sea at Shanghai. Other great river systems flow south to serve the cultures of Southeast Asia and Burma (the Mekong and Salween, respectively). Controlling the vast water resource to prevent flooding, to provide irrigation water, and to make navigable waterways for transport has preoccupied most of China's dynasties. The legendary Yu, a founder of the Xia dynasty (c 2205-1766 BC) allegedly developed a vast complex of dikes on the Yellow-Wei system. "But for Yu," a saying has it, "we should have been fish." The Xia peoples were supplanted by those of the militant Bronze Age Shang dynasty (1766-1027 BC), with their horse-drawn chariots and love of hunting, who invented the character system of writing.

Unlike in the West, where the mythological dragon is a malignant, flame-belching monster, the oriental dragon is always linked to waters. Nor is the dragon always an evil being in the East. Rather it is considered essential, even benign, in the movement of waters, that is, in evaporation, precipitation, and flooding, despite having immense power. The dragon theme is associated with the river valleys on which food production depended.

77. *Facing page,* The collar harness, invented in China by the first century BC, is still the most efficient means for transfer of equid power for traction. Watercolor, dated about 1800. *(Courtesy Board of Trustees of the Victoria & Albert Museum, London.)*

79

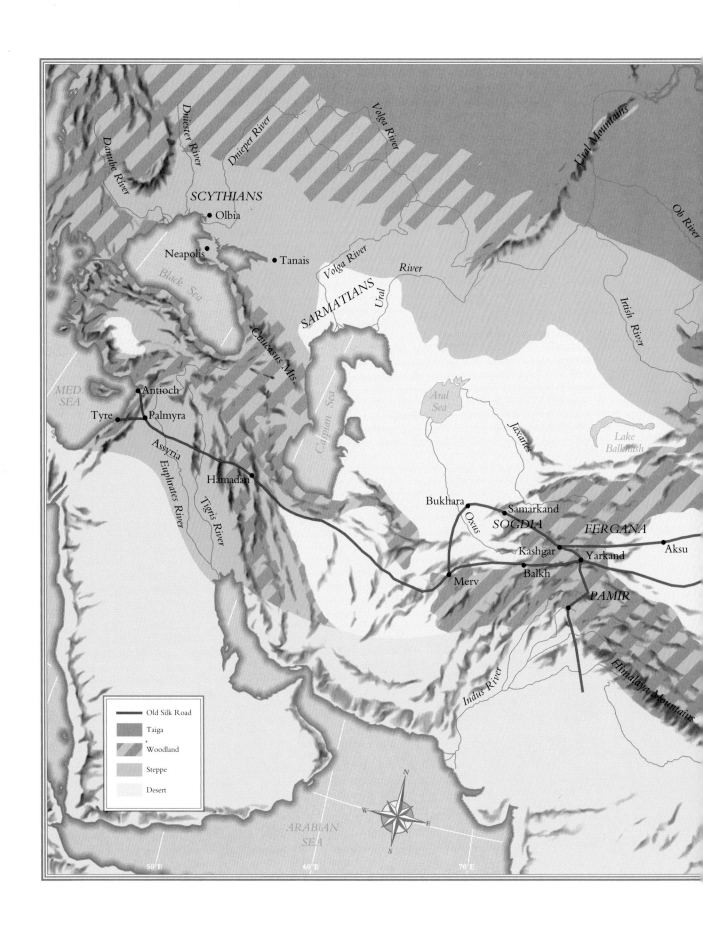

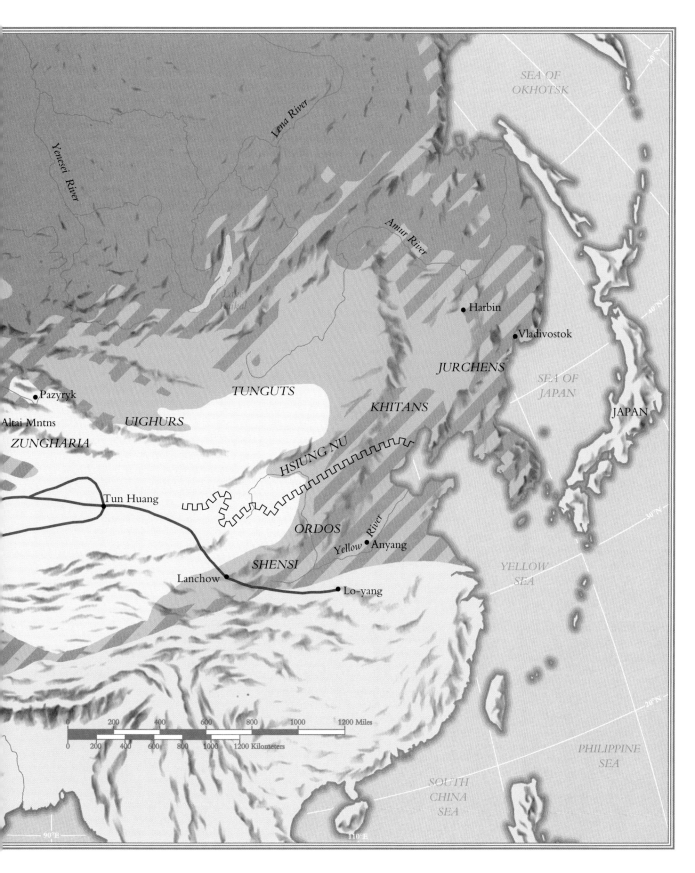

78. Map of Asia and North China showing the Silk Road from Lo-Yang to the Mediterranean Sea, the Great Wall of China, major biomes, geographical features, and tribal regions that are mentioned in the text.

79. The Yangtze River watershed, outlined, showing the only remaining regions within which pockets of giant panda still exist in the wild. These pockets are mainly in special reserves or national parks at high altitudes. The pandas move seasonally, following the growth of different species of bamboo, from 5000- to 8000-foot altitudes in winter to 9000- to 13,000-foot altitudes in summer.

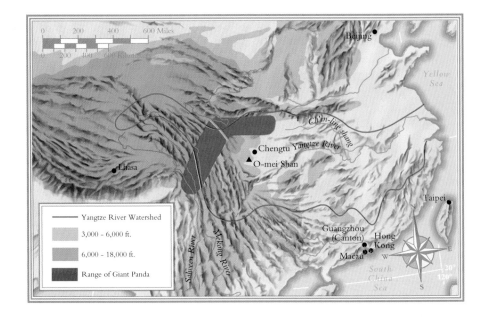

80. The all-inclusive dualist concept of yin and yang underlies the captivating mystical nature of Chinese intellectual inquiry. It is represented by the familiar ideogram of nested shapes of the dark *yin* and the light *yang* forming a circle made of contrasting elements. The scene shows sages meditating upon the symbol in the Qing (Manchu) dynasty. (*The British Museum, London.*)

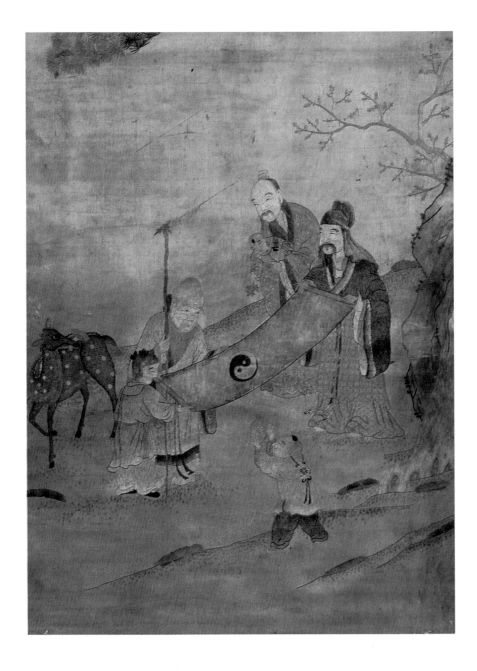

According to Lieh Hsien Chuan in *Lives of the Immortals,* the legendary story of China includes a story about a veterinary surgeon and a dragon. Ma Shih-huang was an expert horse doctor. One day a dragon with drooping ears and gaping mouth came to him for treatment. He punctured its lips and mouth and administered a decoction of liquorice, and the dragon was cured. Thereafter many dragons came to him for medicine, and one day they carried him away, "no one knows where."

The doctrine of the two principles, yin and yang (discussed later in this chapter), from which everything was said to originate, involved a supernatural animal. The symbol of the doctrine, known as the Pa Kua, consists of a circle, representing the infinite void, that contains the two interlocking, curved figures of the yin and yang. The central core is surrounded by eight different combinations of triple lines, some with breaks, and each combination is contained within an octagon. This remarkable symbolic figure was revealed to one Fu Hsi on the back of a dragon-horse that arose from the waters of the Yellow River.

East Asian people had two general life-styles, each conditioned by a particular environment. The first life-style reveals the enormous impact of agriculture on the river valley cultures that developed on the flood plains. Although life was always harsh and occasionally precarious because of catastrophe, the grain-based production of food permitted a population explosion. Food production was accomplished by human manual labor, supplemented in the southern areas with the draft energy of the water buffalo. Today almost ninety percent of the valley land that is usable for agriculture in China is used for crops; only a small proportion is used for pastured stock. Since pigs can be kept on a diet largely composed of crop by-products, they became the major source of animal products, particularly meat. China developed the world's largest populations of swine and Pekin ducks. A consequence of the cultivation of crops has been the extremely high population density in farming areas—now about a billion people—and an unfavorable balance between population and land. As a consequence, the natural environment and the populations of native animals in these crowded core lands of China have largely been displaced or destroyed by the monocultural development of the region.

The second life-style was that of a rim of cultures surrounding the Chinese core that originally were non-Chinese but are gradually becoming integrated. In a rugged terrain of deserts, mountains, and plateaus, these peoples were completely dependent on domestic animals for their survival. Often the peoples were warlike and raided the settled agricultural areas. The arc of cultures, from the northeast to the southwest, included the Man (Manchu), the Mongols, various Turkic tribes, the Tibetans, and others. Collectively the region has sometimes been called Inner Asia. Although the area of land is comparable to that within the ring occupied by a billion Chinese, most of whom claim descent from the Han dynasty (206 BC-AD 220), the total population is only in the tens of millions. Many of these peoples depended on sheep or goats, cattle, and yaks or camels for subsistence, migrating with the seasons for their forage and protection. Once the horse was domesticated, the cultures adopted it for mobility, hunting, and raiding, the latter aided by their mastery of metallurgy. All their needs for food, fiber, shelter, and fuel came from their animals. Many of the tribes (such as the Hsiung-nu) chose their leaders for preeminent ability to succeed in battle rather than by heredity, which was consistent with their warlike tendency. In ancient times they were feared and regarded as barbarians by the Chinese, who built the Great Wall to keep them out. In fact, the Mongol group had conquered China and ruled the land for a span of ninety years, after the fabled Yuan dynasty (AD 1279-1368) was established by Kublai Khan (AD 1215-1294), the Great Khan for East Asia from AD 1260, who ruled all of China from 1279 to 1294. His court was visited by Marco Polo. The jungle hills of Southeast Asia formed a smaller, mostly tropical biome.

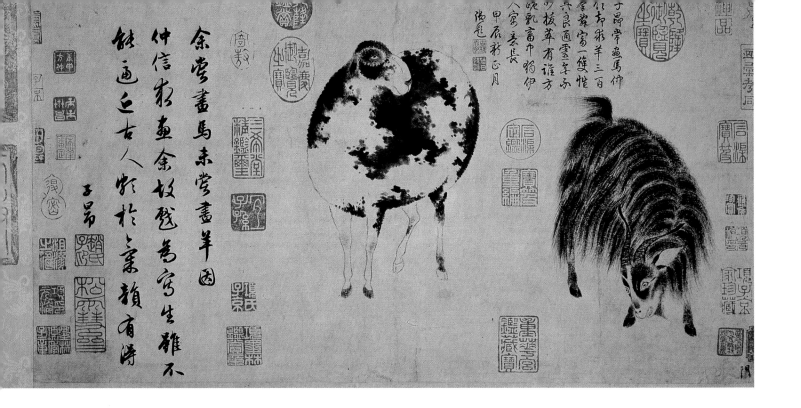

81. *The Sheep and Goat* by Chao Meng-tu (Wu-hsing, 1254-1322). These elegant drawings show the differences between sheep and goats: horn and ear shape, tail position, and texture of the fibrous coat. *(Courtesy Freer Gallery of Art, Smithsonian Institution, Washington, D.C.)*

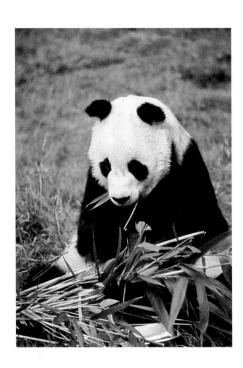

82. China's most famous animal, the giant panda bear. It is now an endangered species surviving in remote bamboo groves in protected highland areas at elevations of up to more than 10,000 feet in central China. Adult pandas weigh about 220 pounds, but the young weigh less than 4 ounces at birth and are very vulnerable. *(Courtesy Black Star.)*

ANIMALS IN PREHISTORIC AND ANCIENT EAST ASIA

The best-known animal species of East Asia is also one of its rarest—the giant panda. Recent efforts to enhance its reproductive success have achieved more publicity than results. As a bear, it is omnivorous and still has a taste for meat in the form of the bamboo rat. Today meat is used as bait to trap pandas so that they can be equipped with electronic collars and monitored by radio; such behavioral studies are aimed at aiding their survival. A few pandas survive in west-central China in three areas with altitudes between 10,000 and 13,000 feet and in groves of its preferred diet, fountain bamboo. Most people would be hard pressed to identify other regional wild species, except, for example, the orangutan and the gibbon in Southeast Asia. Yet North China, Mongolia, and adjacent regions of Siberia are believed to have been the original home range of the tiger, with its preferred diet of wild pigs supplemented by deer. China has many glorious birds, notably the colorful pheasants for which it is the heartland and the spectacular tragopans and cranes. Many of these are on the list of endangered species. Burrowing rodents in the region have been incriminated as vectors of plague.

Domesticated animals such as the Ming-period horses, the yaks of the high mountains, the two-humped camels of the Silk Road caravan route, and the ubiquitous Chinese pig are more familiar than are wild species. Records show that the ancient Chinese nobility were enthusiastic hunters, killing mainly deer and foxes. Later the water buffalo became important in cultivating the rice paddies of the Yangtze basin and South China, and draft oxen were used in the northern and upland areas.

Only bones of pigs and dogs have been found with any regularity in the oldest settlement sites of ancient China, although bones from cattle, sheep, and horses have been found occasionally. Hunting and fishing were important; the bones of water deer are the most common among those of the wild species. From 2700 BC to 2357 BC was an active period for domestication. Later sites yielded more bones of cattle, sheep, and horses, as well as of water buffalo and chickens. Wild fowl were hunted. The credit is given to Dong, Zhongxian (before 2208 BC) for inventing castration by means of a hot iron. Castration of boars was first recorded between 1520 BC and 1030 BC.

Remains from Inner Mongolia reveal a late start on domestication and a great dependence on sheep and cattle. Wild cattle, wild water buffalo, and Mongolian wild horses were present. Goats came later, perhaps arriving via caravans from central Asiatic stock.

CHINESE INVENTION OF AQUACULTURE

The art of aquaculture was invented in China. Evidence of ancient fishermen predates the Shang dynasty, which had metal hooks. The management of natural fish populations began in earnest in the feudal Chou (Zhou) dynasty (1027-256 BC). Fishing for the popular common carp, *Cyprinus carpio,* was regulated by seasonal river closure to conserve stocks. Carp were revered for their strength in ascending the turbulent hurtling waters of the Dragon's Gate rapids in the Yangtze (Ch'ang) River. Knowledge of carp culture for contemplation and pleasure grew after its Chou founder, Wen Wang, built a pond, stocked it with fish, and studied their behavior early in the twelfth century BC while he was confined to his estate by the last Shang emperor.

During the creative "Spring and Autumn" era (722-481 BC) of the early eastern Chou dynasty, Fan Li of Yue recorded available wisdom concerning carp culture in his treatise *Fish Culture Classic* of 460 BC. It included the results of his experimental work on ponds and on the propagation and care of fry. As the purpose of raising fish gradually evolved from enjoyment to food production, the culture of carp was expanded to large bodies of water during the empire of the Han dynasty, then into paddy fields in the era of the Three Kingdoms (AD 220-280) to provide mosquito control. Goldfish and other colored carp were developed in the following Jin era.

A dramatic political change occurred during the Tang dynasty (AD 618-907). An emperor with the same name as the common carp ordered it protected as a royal symbol, and its use was banned. This policy forced the development of other species and led to replacement of the common carp with other species and polyculture systems, including the grass carp (which was used to reclaim land), blackcarp, and bighead carp. Collection and transport of fry were perfected during the Sung (Song) dynasty (AD 960-1279).

Mastery of the intensification of polycultural techniques for freshwater species was perfected during the Ming dynasty (AD 1368-1644). Fish diseases and their control were described in AD 1628. Under the Qing (Ch'ing or Manchu) dynasty (AD 1644-1911), separation of fry species was advanced.

83. Detail from *The Pleasures of Fishes,* painted in 1291 by Chou Tung-ch'ing, a Sung loyalist and native of Lin-Chiang, Kiangi. This breathtakingly beautiful work reveals a remarkable intensity of observation, catching perfectly the carps' freedom of movement in their aquatic medium. The obvious pleasures of the fish in water gave the Sung artists an "indescribable feeling," as they themselves felt like fish out of water under the alien Yuan rule of Kublai Khan (1215-1294). *(From the collection of AW Bahr, Purchase, Fletcher Fund, 1947. [47.18.10.] Photograph by Malcolm Varon. The Metropolitan Museum of Art, New York.)*

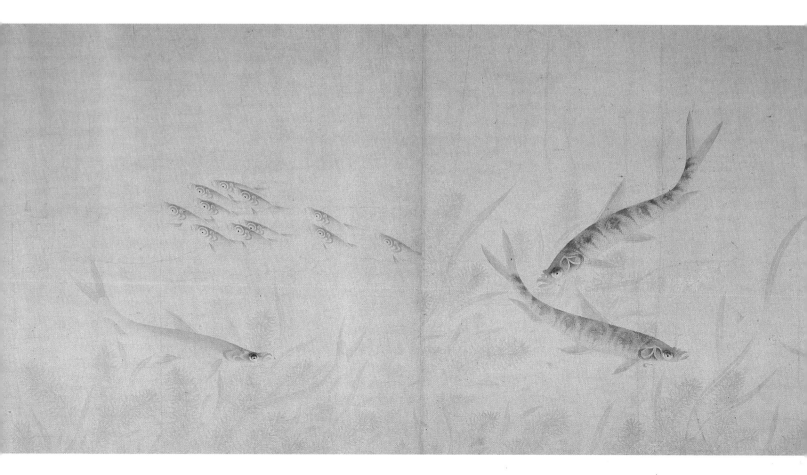

After the stagnation of the twentieth-century warring period, initiatives were undertaken to extend aquaculture to brackish and marine waters. A new thrust in research today has led to better control of epidemic diseases. Integration of aquaculture with livestock and crop systems avoids waste. Ducks, geese, chickens, pigs, small ruminants, and cattle have been used to consume crop products; their excreta provide nutrients for the planktonic algae and zooplankton growth that nourish the fish. Whether these systems may heighten the virulence of human pathogens such as the influenza virus remains to be seen.

MILITARY MIGHT AND THE HORSE IN EAST ASIA

The equine remains in the Bronze Age Shang tombs are of small Mongolian ponies, probably related to the wild horses discovered by Przewalski in 1876. The latter once roamed in great herds over the steppes and semideserts of Kazakstan, Mongolia, Sinkiang, and parts of Siberia at altitudes up to 8000 feet. Sacrificial pits containing nearly a hundred horse skeletons have been dug up at Yin Hsu. Remains of one dog and the meat interred with it were found in the area. Stone statues of animals dating from the Shang period have been found, including a fine likeness of a pig. Individual charioteers were heroes and were buried with their own chariots and two horses. One such burial from the twelfth or eleventh century BC was found at Ta Sau Kung, near Anyang: the ponies were hardy and sturdy and had heavy heads. Much later, during the short, turbulent, dramatic period of the Qin (Chin) dynasty (221-207 BC), China's factions were unified under Shih Hunagdi (259-210 BC), also known as the First Emperor. Cavalry replaced chariots. The emperor's extraordinary burial site included huge underground chambers that contained life-sized terra cotta figurines of a veritable army of horses and men (about 7500 of them). Also, two beautiful heavy bronze carriages were uncovered, to each of which were harnessed four fine horses of the compact Mongolian-pony type. The horses were harnessed as a quadriga, and a weighted pom-pom was suspended from the bridle, Assyrian style.

The quest for larger, faster steeds was pursued during the Han dynasty. Emperor Wu's envoy Chang Chien reported in 115 BC the presence of magnificent horses in Ta-juan (Ferghana, a city-state north of Samarkand). After two envoys who had been sent to negotiate a purchase were slain, Wu sent a vast army and took 3000 horses by force in exchange for gold. He named them the Horses of Heaven. As is often the way with horse trading, not all were magnificent and fewer than fifty of them survived the 2000-mile march home. A spectacular bronze equine tomb sculpture—poised in full run with one hoof on a swallow symbolically bearing it to the heavens—is thought to be of one of these fine horses. The sculpture was discovered at Lei Tai in Kansu province in 1969. The Horses of Heaven are thought to have been a domesticated variety of the plains tarpan that existed in the wild on the steppes of southern Russia and eastward to the Volga River. The tarpan became extinct in the 1880s.

A great equine initiative was developed during the Tang dynasty that envisioned a decisive military role for fast horses ridden by bowmen. Systematic horse breeding and acquisition were undertaken; from about 5000 head at the start of the dynasty, the population increased to 700,000 by the middle of the seventh century AD on the pastures of Shensi and Kansu. Turkish and Tibetan incursions then disorganized the studs, and the numbers fell sharply. The aristocratic passion for horses led to imports of Arabian horses (AD 703), Tibetan ponies, and many other breeds obtained by tribute from other Asian kingdoms. Crossbreeding was practiced to upgrade the small Mongolian steppe horses. The result was a higher, lighter animal than the chunky Mongolian type. The sport of polo was adopted and was popular in Ch'ang-an. Horses

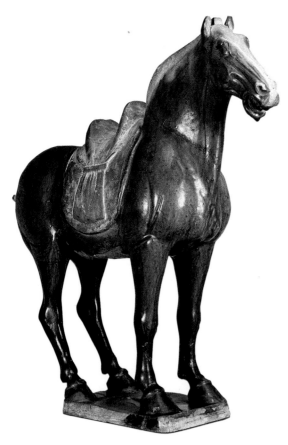

84. Saddled horse. From Tang dynasty, around AD 700. Hardy, muscular, and compact, such horses were the motive power of the Chinese cavalry. *(Museum für Kunsthandwerk, Frankfurt, Germany.)*

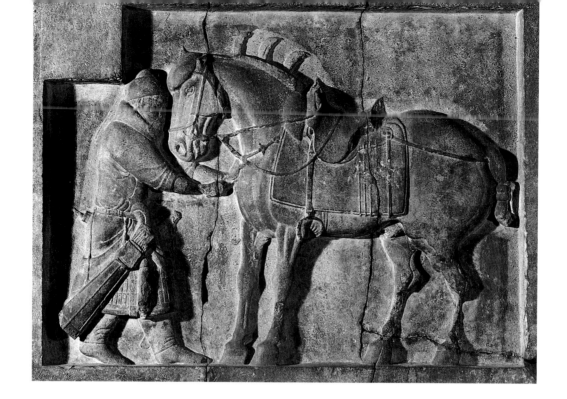

were prominent in the art of the period, which included superb bas-reliefs on the tomb of Tai'-tsung (emperor from AD 626 to 649), funerary figures, sculptures, and paintings (for example, of Han Kan, who lived from AD 720 to 780). However, the Tang forces were unable to keep the nomad and mountain raiders at bay. The Uighurs helped resist the Tibetans and acquired a monopoly over the horse trade, and the Tang had to retreat toward the southeast.

The pony-riding pastoral tribes of Mongolia between the Khinghan Mountains to the east and the Altai and Tianshan Mountains to the west were forged into a single expansionist military nation by Temujin, who became Genghis Khan. He took the Tangut kingdom of Xixia, then crossed the Gobi Desert to attack China, crossing the Great Wall at great cost to human and equine life. By 1215 he had reached the capital, Zhongdu (Beijing today) and destroyed the city. He charged off to the west on the greatest territorial empire-building exercise in history. He left behind a general, Mukali, to govern the conquered lands of China, who was advised by a Mongol mandarin named Yehlu Chutsai. Chutsai advised against converting North China's cultivated fields into livestock pastures and urged Mukali to "milk the productive Chinese cow" instead. He counseled that "the empire was won on horseback but it will not be governed on horseback." The Mongol troops were unbeatable on the battlefield, but Chutsai was able to get Chinese engineers to construct giant catapults so that the fortified cities they came up against could also be made vulnerable. After Genghis Khan's triumphant campaigns to the west, he partook of great celebrations before returning to mop up the rebellious Tunguts in 1227. He died of a fever, but his successors continued the expansion. A remarkable system of courier communication was established, with about 10,000 posts 25 miles apart stabling hundreds of horses. By changing horses, messengers conveyed information across distances of up to 200 miles a day. Kublai Khan, grandson of Genghis Khan, completed the conquest of China but never lost his zest for hunting and hawking. Animals were everywhere in his court—trained lions and leopards, mastiffs, falcons, and eagles, even 5000 elephants. His palaces were carpeted and draped with his trophy furs and hides.

Donkeys and mules have been widely used in China, at least since the Chou dynasty. The crossing of a donkey jack with a Mongolian pony mare produced a hardy mule, the main pack animal. The crossing of a pony stud with a donkey jenny produced the hinny, a rarity in most cultures, which was developed as a thrifty puller of carts.

85. Magnificent stone relief from the tomb of the Tang Emperor T'ai-Tsung, who died in 749, shows a cavalryman removing an arrow from the breast of his powerful charger, which is equipped with stirrups (invented by the third century). *(The University Museum, University of Pennsylvania.)*

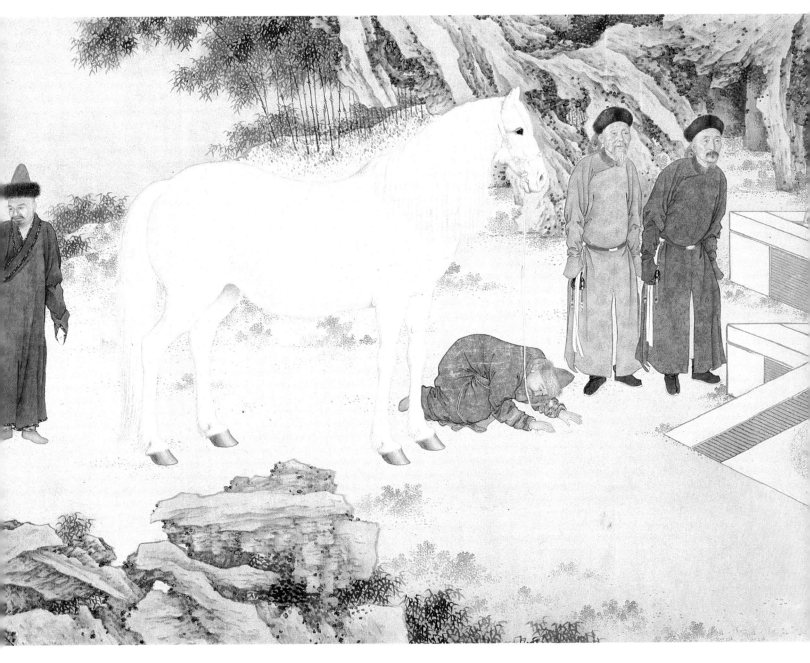

86. Reversal of roles: Ch'ien-lung (1736-1795) receives Kazakh envoys. Before 1644 the Manchus had presented horses as tribute to the Ming emperors. Now, seated upon the throne themselves, they received the same offerings from the tribes that remained beyond the Great Wall. *(Musée Guimet, Paris.)*

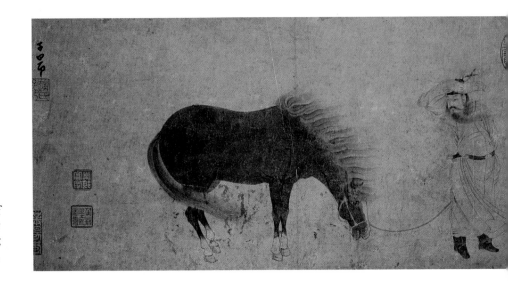

87. A horse and groom feel the bite of North China's winter wind, as depicted by Zhao Mengfu, Kublai Khan's leading painter. *(National Palace Museum, Taipei, Taiwan, Republic of China.)*

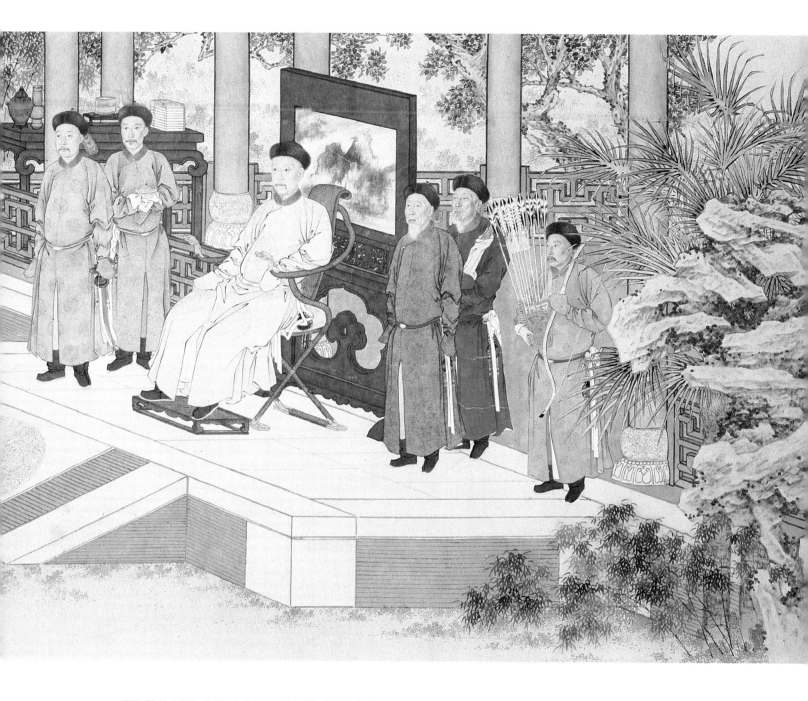

TECHNOLOGY FOR ANIMAL USE

Chinese agriculturists were slow in learning to use and develop dairy products. Avoidance of milk as a food persisted until recent times in large areas of East and Southeast Asia. Perhaps more surprising was the relatively late adoption of draft animals in Chinese agriculture. Although draft horses and cattle were used to pull carts as early as 2000 BC, the simple plow did not appear until the fifth century BC and the ox-drawn one, not until early in the first century BC. At Ur in Mesopotamia, on the other hand, a plow appears on a seal dating to about 3500 BC.

When the Chinese did use animals for physical work, they made better designs for saddlery, harnesses, and farm equipment than did their counterparts elsewhere. By the fourth century BC they had developed the trace harness in which pressure of traction is applied to a band across the front of the horse's chest. In contrast, early Western harnesses used a band across the throat, which compressed the windpipe and neck vessels; this style stayed in use until the eighth century AD. The greatly improved padded horse collar was developed in China before the first century BC, far ahead of its development in Europe and the Mediterranean region. The drawing capacity of a horse with a well-designed collar is more than six times greater than that of a horse with the throat-and-girth collar system. This drawing capacity was one

88. Water buffalo and farmers working in the rice paddies in China. From an ancient print. *(From Zeuner, 1963.)*

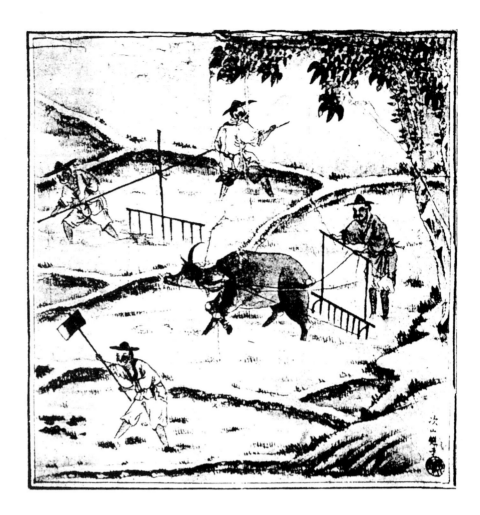

89. A stone relief of the second century AD from Yeng-tzu-shan in Szechuan, shows an ancient plow drawn by an ox. A plowshare and moldboard are already in evidence. Malleable iron plows had been invented in China by the fourth century BC. *(Werner Forman/Art Resource, New York.)*

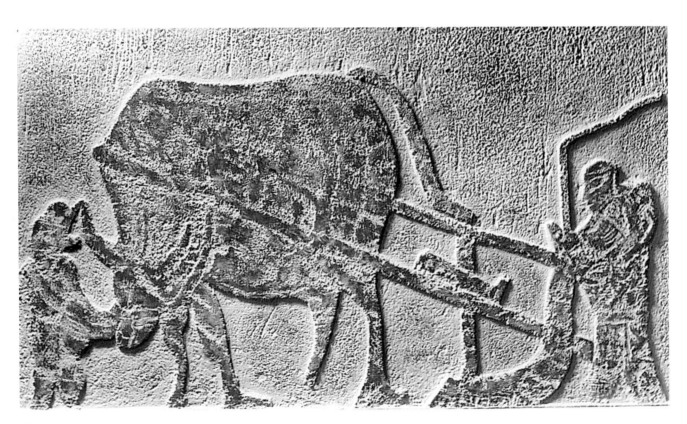

factor in Europe's reliance on ox-drawn transport by means of a yoke and two oxen, which allowed the pressure to be taken against the animal's spinal hump. The Chinese also developed the whiffletree, which made it easier for animals to pull implements or carts, especially when more than one animal was used. Before the Christian era they devised a camel pack-saddle that was kept in place by means of a padded neck support.

China led the world in farm implement design. Ox-drawn ards (plows), first with stone, then with wooden plowshares, were in use for thousands of years elsewhere. The Chinese, however, made the first iron plowshares out of a special, malleable cast iron. They also developed an adjustable fitting that controlled the plowing depth by changing the distance between the beam and the share, as well as a moldboard to turn over the soil. Another major agricultural advance to China's credit was the multirow seed drill, which revolutionized the efficiency of sowing seed crops nearly 2000 years before Europe was able to match this invention.

The enormous military advantage imparted to riders in combat by stirrups was accomplished in China by the third century AD. Chinese expertise with wrought iron made stirrups possible. Adopted in Byzantium and then by the Vikings, the stirrup was slow in reaching the rest of Europe. When it did, it made possible the use of the heavy armor and the great horses of the cumbersome medieval knights by allowing them to stay in the saddle.

A single grave from the Shang period, which began after 1766 BC, is unique in containing the skeletons of an adult male rider, a horse, and a dog. This strange nomad was far ahead of his time because further clear evidence of horseback riding is absent for more than 1000 years. By then nomadic horsemen with bows were common, but the Chinese still preferred chariots. Under Wu Ling, however, soldiers had better bows and learned to ride wearing trousers, which replaced the awkward traditional robe and slippers. They became better marksmen with small, accurate bows probably copied from those of the northern reindeer people. Militant nomads on horseback became such a menace that the state of Ch'in started the Great Wall, as stated earlier, to fence out the Hsiung-nu barbarians.

90. In their days of power the Manchus looked back to their "heroic" age with a certain nostalgia, perpetuating the warrior tradition in their art after it had changed in reality. In this figure an eighteenth-century general, Ma-Ch'ang, is still portrayed in the old epic style as a horseman with bow and arrows. (*National Palace Museum, Taipei, Taiwan, Republic of China.*)

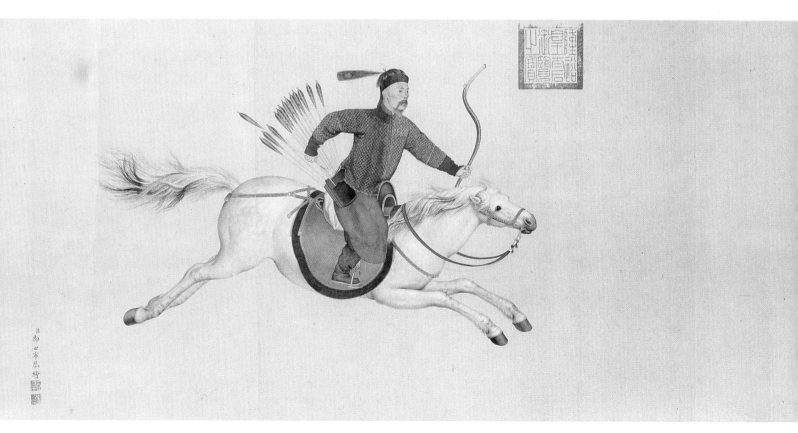

SILK FIBER

Animal life-forms provide fiber as well as food. China acquired wool, felt, leather, and furs from the culture of the raiding Mongol herders. The richest of all the animal fibers, after the fabled pelts of mink and sable, was surely silk. So desirable was this product that a great, hazardous caravan route, the Silk Road, was dedicated to its trade from China by Bactrian camelback around the Gobi Desert to the Middle East and the West during the Han dynasty, since silk was a major luxury item in imperial Rome. The Latin name for China was *Serica,* or "silken." North China's gift to human luxury was the domestication and culture of the moth *Bombyx mori,* which required that the North Chinese master both the management of the moth's breeding cycle and the production of an adequate supply of the special diet of the larvae, the leaves of mulberry bushes.

EARLY EVIDENCE OF VETERINARY MEDICINE

The historians of the Han dynasty, which reunited much of China for more than four hundred years, provided a source of information about preceding cultures in East Asia. Although certainly a mixture of legend and fact, that information is all that remains of the roots of the tradition that set the special nature of China's ethos. Other rulers had deliberately destroyed the classic texts in an attempt to obliterate previous achievements and traditions. Another type of historical evidence is archaeological. The synthesis reveals a cultural tradition deeply rooted in an agricultural environment that oscillated between drought and flood. Awareness of cosmic phenomena was keen, and the people were intuitively adaptable and continuously at risk from aggressive neighboring tribes.

KEY CHINESE DYNASTIES

Before 2357 BC	Neolithic
2357-2208 BC	Neolithic
2205-1766 BC	Xia
1766-1027 BC	Shang
1027-771 BC	Western Chou (Zhou)
771-256 BC	Eastern Chou (Zhou)
722-481 BC	Spring and Autumn
480-222 BC	Warring states
221-207 BC	Qin (Chin)
206 BC – AD 8	Former Han
25-220	Later Han
220-280	Three Kingdoms
285-581	North-South disunion
618-907	Tang
907-960	Five dynasties
960-1279	Sung (Song)
1279-1368	Yuan (Mongol)
1368-1644	Ming
1644-1911	Qing (Ch'ing or Manchu)
1912-1949	Chinese Republic
1949-Present	People's Republic of China

A remarkable feature of oriental (Asiatic) history is the much greater importance given to animals than in other cultures, exemplified in China by the comparative approach to medicine that called for a cadre of animal physicians. As the dynasties came and went, concentrating great central power in one emperor, then fragmenting into multiple warring states before reconsolidation, there was great interest in forecasting the future. The favored method was to use the scapulas of cattle, pigs, and other large animals, which were grooved and scorched to produce fire cracks that were interpreted by fortune-tellers. Huge numbers of cattle were slaughtered to keep up with the demand for scapulas. The breastplate of the tortoise or turtle was used as well.

Priests had held great power in the Shang dynasty of ancient China because they were thought to be able to placate the evil spirits that caused diseases and natural disasters. Animal and human sacrifice was practiced, and there were "horse priests" who could treat animals. Records of thirty-six diseases have been found inscribed on pieces of cattle bone and turtle shell. During the Western Chou dynasty, one emperor's coach driver was a famous horse doctor. He could bleed horses from the neck, for instance, to cure summer fever. He allegedly had this assignment from 947 to 928 BC. A government department of animal medicine existed, and an official title equivalent to "veterinarian" was listed in the government manual *Chon Li* as "one who cared for military horses." The yin-yang hypothesis of balance in nature (discussed later in this chapter) undermined faith in the authority of the priests and enabled the emergence of new health professions based on acupuncture and preventive medicine. Identified cadres of health professionals were the general physicians, the surgeons or wound healers, the dietitians, and the veterinarians.

A great figure in Chinese veterinary history, whose nickname, Bai-le, became a household word throughout China, was Sun, Yang, who lived from 659 to 620 BC in the "Spring and Autumn" period of the Eastern Chou dynasty. He was an aristocrat and a leader in government from the Chin region. Sun acquired a legendary reputation for skill in evaluating horses. He impressed upon his son, who was having difficulty evaluating stamina in horses, the importance of firsthand observation of conformation, performance, and behavior. According to Sun, Yang, one must acquire this expertise not "by the book" but by intense studying of the animal. He had studied anatomy and had rudimentary knowledge of equine physiology and pathology. He became expert at applying the principles of acupuncture to horses and used it to treat all types of equine diseases. Sun is considered the father of veterinary acupuncture in China. *Veterinary Acupuncture* was written not by him but by others who capitalized on his famous name. It listed seventy-seven acupuncture sites on the body surface, eight on the foreleg, and eight on the thigh.

Horse medicine was undoubtedly considered a special career in early times. Those who engaged in it had high social rank and were well respected. The importance of the horse for fighting, transport, and cultivation was recognized. It is said that Shun Yeng, also known as Pao Lo (born c. 480 BC), was the first full-time veterinary practitioner, and he is sometimes considered the "father of Chinese veterinary medicine"; it appears, however, that every major dynasty had such a figure. Castration of food and draft animals, including boars and cocks, was widely employed, and sows were spayed.

About the end of the Chou dynasty the book of odes, *Shih Ching* or *Shijing,* appeared. It described feudal life from the eleventh to the sixth century BC and included a description of the signs of good health in goats. The first named veterinarian was Chao Fu, an expert in animal diseases and a chariot warrior during the reign of Mu Huang (tenth century BC). Han dynasty scholars wrote a history of the Chou dynasty, which transformed China from a pastoral state under Turkish rule to a militant one based on horse and chariot power. During its later period, about 400 BC, government health sciences were organized into five classes, including the Service of Physicians for

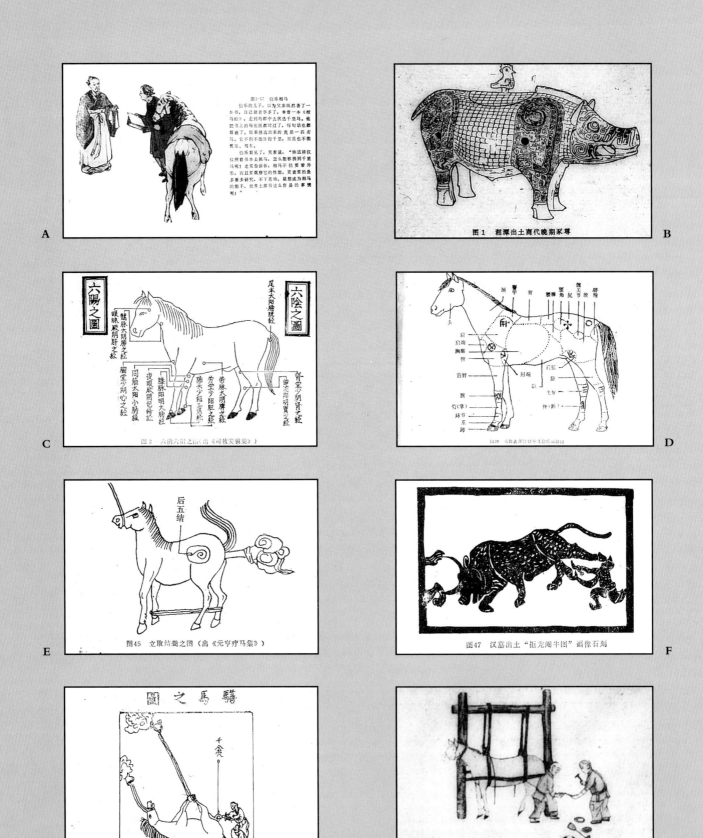

91. **A,** Renowned early horse doctor Bai-le telling his son how to judge a horse. (Seventh century BC, Spring and Autumn dynasty.) **B,** Ancient stone pig from the Shang dynasty. **C,** Horse showing the yin-yang principle. The six front points were considered yang (male), the rear ones, yin (female). **D,** Acupuncture points of a horse. **E,** Removing impacted feces from a standing horse with a severe case of colic. **F,** Castrating an adult bull. Han tomb from Han dynasty. **G,** Castrating a horse. The horse is cast and tied on its back. **H,** Attending to the feet and shoeing a horse that is suspended in the stocks. *(Courtesy Professor Wang Qinglan, Beijing.)*

Animals (the Shou-i, or veterinarians) and the "Shu-ma," or "horse doctor." The role of horse doctors was to heal the diseases of horses. Their duties were to establish a diagnosis by meticulously observing the signs of disease, then to select and administer the appropriate therapy. A sick horse was sprinkled with an infusion of medicinal plants to make it feel comfortable. The horse was made to walk at a moderate pace; then its pulse was examined. This procedure was said to facilitate recognition of the disease. Treatments consisted mainly of herbal drenches. Ulcers must have been prevalent because they received special mention. The importance of good nutrition and nursing care was emphasized. If the patients died, the lost animals were to be counted and the number recorded as part of the veterinarian's merit evaluation; his level of appointment was subject to being raised or lowered depending on the outcome. An animal healer named Cho Li T'ien Kuan has been credited with that proposal. The government also introduced compensation to farmers for losses of animals.

The first book of herbal pharmacy appeared during the Qin and Han dynasties that followed the Chou. Herbs for veterinary use are listed on a wooden slat dated to the Han dynasty. Before the Chinese invention of paper in AD 97 (in the Kansu province in western China), records and texts were preserved on strips of wood or bamboo.

An interesting syndrome was that of the "heavenly horses," whose sweat had a russet hue, probably as a consequence of infection with a filarial blood parasite, *Parafilaria multipapillosa,* which causes seepage of blood from the skin.

UNIQUE FEATURES OF ANCIENT CHINESE HUMAN AND ANIMAL MEDICINE

Acupuncture in the treatment of animals has been used in China for more than 3000 years. Although based on detailed observations and recordings, the technique is empirical and has not received adequate study at the scientific level. Untrammeled by magic or religious doctrine, Chinese scholars were able to develop an original medical philosophy from which many advances were to flow.

The *Classic of Internal Medicine* or *Nei Ching* of the Yellow Emperor (Yu Hsiung), compiled over a long period until the third century BC, included a part called the *Ling Shu* or *Needle Classic,* a book of acupuncture and moxibustion. The combination of these techniques is called *zehenjiu.* Another part called *Su Wen* or *Plain Talk* set out the principles and practice of acupuncture, and these continue to stand virtually unchallenged in Chinese medicine and veterinary medicine. The *Nei Ching* established the meridian theory of acupuncture, the types of needles, the names and sites of acupuncture points, the prescription of each point for diseases, and the distribution of "forbidden points." A similar compendium of medical lore, the *Man Ching,* was later published. These two works became the standard Chinese medical texts.

The underlying principle of acupuncture was the hypothesis of yin-yang balance, which holds that attunement to nature is necessary for health. In Chinese cosmology yin is the feminine principle in nature—dark, passive, and weak; yang is the masculine attribute—bright, active, and strong. In society the yang element of ruler, father, and husband must prevail over the yin element of subject, son, and wife. The combination of yin and yang attributes was said to produce everything that exists, and the hypothesis of yin-yang balance was the basis of the strict moral code of kinship, education, and virtuous behavior that was advocated by Kung Fu-tzu or Confucius (550-479 BC) and his successor, Mencius. Both acupuncture and moxibustion were deployed in restoring the patient's precarious balance when it was deranged. Moxibustion was a method of producing mild blistering by burning the conical parts of mugwort or cotton soaked in an oil on selected skin sites. The Daoism of Lao-tzu, counterpoint to Confucianism, had many followers.

92. O. Kothbauer, in Austria, developed a detailed acupuncture map for cattle. The sites of pain spots or Kothbauer's points on the cow's body and the internal organs to which they relate are shown. Needle therapy has been used in the treatment of reproductive disorders in cattle. *Qi (ch'i)* is a uniquely Chinese concept of the wholeness and viability of an organism, the coordinating factor that accounts for the responses to change that reset the balance among cells and tissues to preserve health and biorhythms. Acupuncture seeks to facilitate that process by influencing specific channels of the body system. *(American Journal of Acupuncture.)*

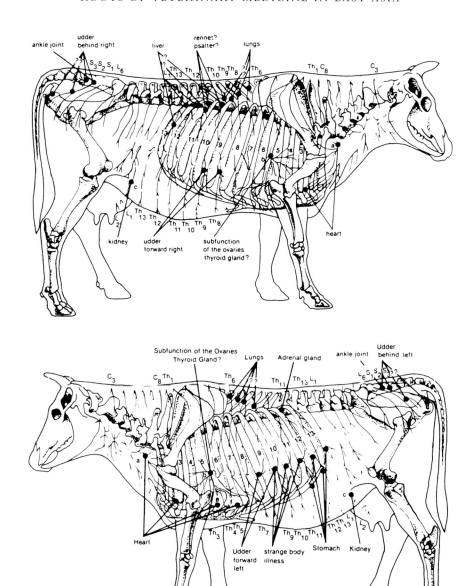

93. Elephant with acupuncture points. *(From the World Health Organization.)*

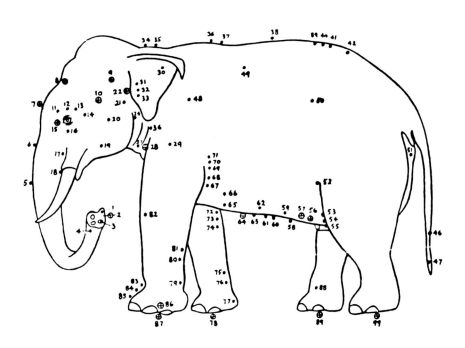

THE RISE OF RATIONAL IDEAS OF COMPARATIVE MEDICINE

Chinese medical knowledge expanded rapidly during the Han dynasty between the second century BC and the third century AD. Elements of Buddhist philosophy combined with rational derivations from the philosophy of Confucius favored the development of the health professions, including veterinary care. Without benefit of dissection, the *Nei Ching* espoused the doctrine of the dual circulation of the blood in the second century BC, long before Harvey. Chinese medicine made a fetish of examining and interpreting the arterial pulse, differentiating twenty-eight patterns while recognizing that the pulse wave originated from the heart. Wang Shu-ho's book *Mo-Ching (Classic of the Pulse)* became a standard text, spreading across Asia and influencing Persian and Arabic medicine and veterinary medicine. The Chinese also conceived of a more mystical second circulation called Ch'i (considered a yang attribute), a form of energy that circulated via invisible tracts. The two circulations, of the Ch'i and the blood, were interdependent, the blood system being regarded as the yin element. This mutual reliance was used as the rationalization of acupuncture. Medical educators even constructed elaborate models of simulated circulation out of bamboo tubes through which liquid was pumped by a bellows. The idea of two interacting systems linking the various organs of the body led to complex concepts of storage organs linked with administrative centers by communicative systems and channels. Chinese thought developed a doctrine of five interactive elements—fire, water, wood, metal, and earth—reminiscent of the Greeks' four elements of air, water, fire, and earth.

The greatest physician of China was Chang Chung-Ching (c. AD 140-220). Regarded as the authority who established the system of differential diagnosis and therapy, he was revered and had the status of a "Chinese Hippocrates." His work was an important contribution to the understanding of disease. He prescribed acupuncture for yang-type diseases and moxibustion for those of the yin type. The concept was that acupuncture should be used when body defenses were at a peak, and when they were on the decline, moxibustion was recommended. In other words, a combination of herbal and needle approaches was used. Massage, cupping, bleeding, and bathing were also used.

During the early empire, Huang-Fu Mi (AD 215-282) wrote the *Treatise of A B C (Chia I Ching),* a great, systematic organization of medical science into categories of physiology, pathology, diagnosis, and treatments, which led to the spread of acupuncture and moxibustion to Japan, Korea, and France. During the Tang dynasty Sun Ssu Miao (AD 590-682) wrote the *Golden Prescriptions (Ching Fang),* which introduced a concept of "tender points." Later, electrical resistance was used to measure changes in diseased organs.

The physician sought to reveal how the patient had violated the Tao (the creative principle that ordered the universe, according to Taoists) so that measures could be taken to restore the balance. The recognition of the interaction between the bodily functions and environmental cycles led Chinese medical thinkers to an awareness of biorhythms and "body clocks" linked to force fields. They described physiological patterns and patterns of disease that followed diurnal ("about a day") rhythms and monthly or seasonal rhythms. The idea of biorhythms was accepted much later in the West. Similar ideas and practices were applied to veterinary problems, especially in the horse. Except for castration of animals to enhance productivity and facilitate handling, there was virtually no emphasis on surgery. The medical focus was on diagnosis and pharmacotherapy, coupled with physical therapy. The first record of a woman doctor was made during the Han dynasty, when Ch'un Yu-yen was called to the palace to treat the queen. Medical education began during the Tang dynasty, when woman doctors were granted recognition after a system of selection, screening by physicians, and examination.

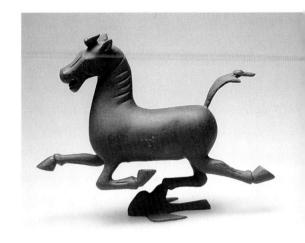

94. This replica of a glorious bronze sculpture of a celestial horse being borne heavenward on a swallow with outstretched wings was discovered in a general's tomb at Wu wei, Gansu. The horse is of the type acquired from Sogdiana or Ferghana during the Eastern Han dynasty, about the second century AD.

PHYSIOLOGY, REPRODUCTIVE BIOLOGY, AND DISEASES OF NUTRITION

Chinese medical scholars accorded endocrinology and sexuality special attention. They isolated gonadotrophins and sexually active steroids in crude form from human urine in the second century BC and recognized that the same could be accomplished in domestic animals. They used products obtained by concentration and crystallization. They even came to recognize that active agents (steroids?) could be purified by sublimation from aqueous solutions in special vessels maintained at moderate temperatures (below 300° C). The technique was applied to volatile herbal medicaments as well. Other chemical techniques were deployed successfully to precipitate biologically active materials. Beans (*Gleditschia* species) that contain saponin (a natural soap) were used to precipitate hormones from urine. The products obtained were used to treat sexual dysfunctions, the idea of bodily regulators for some functions preceding similar Western discoveries by 1000 to 2000 years.

Problems attributed to endocrine agents were important in China. The excessive passing of sweet-tasting urine accompanied by abnormal thirst, or diabetes mellitus, was well known, and three forms of the disease were described. Chinese physicians recognized the value of a strict dietary regimen in treatment. They also prepared thyroid extract from the thyroid glands of gelded rams and used it to treat goiter in human patients before AD 700, providing an early example of veterinary science serving biomedical science. The value of seaweed in treatment of goiter was also recognized in ancient China.

The oldest awareness of deficiency diseases had Chinese origins and allowed understanding of a new concept of animal diseases, specifically, that some were of nutritional origin. Chang had discovered foods that would cure some of these diseases. Han Yu (AD 762-842) showed regional differences in the incidence of beriberi (thiamine deficiency). Hu Ssu-Hui, imperial dietitian from AD 1314 to 1330, in his classic *Principles of Correct Diet* (1330), described wet and dry forms of beriberi and prescribed separate dietary regimens for each. Tooth decay and dental care were addressed. Among ectoparasites, the itch-mite of scabies was well known in ancient China.

CONTAGIOUS DISEASES: SMALLPOX AND THE ECOLOGY OF PLAGUE

A remarkable achievement of ancient Chinese medicine was the development of a strategy to minimize suffering and deaths caused by smallpox (the European name used to distinguish it from the "great pox" or syphilis). Long before Jenner's cowpox vaccine, a technique had been developed in the southwestern province of Szechuan in caves used by Taoist hermits who were reputed to practice "internal alchemy" on the mountain O-Mei Shan. Public recognition of their method was achieved when Prime Minister Wong Tan's (AD 957-1017) son died of the disease. Desperate to avoid further deaths in the family, the prime minister explored all possible avenues, and one of the hermits who had mastered the inoculation method was brought to him.

Apparently the monks recognized two forms of the disease, variola major and a less virulent minor form. They took the pock material from some of the scabs, sometimes from people who had been infected mildly as a result of inoculation, which suggests an awareness of the possibility of attenuation of the infectious agent. The material was stored in a small corked container for twenty or forty days (in summer and winter, respectively). It is now thought that about eighty percent of the virus would have been inactivated. The method of inoculation ("implantation of the germs") was to put the material on a plug of cotton and insert the plug into the nostrils. Thus the virus was to enter via the nasal mucosa. Although the practice was said to be effective and remarkably safe, it did not become widespread in China until the sixteenth century. It spread to central Asia and Turkey, whence the method was conveyed to England and was actively promoted by Lady Mary Wortley Montagu (1689-1762), who had her own family "variolated" in 1718 amidst heated controversy. This method preceded and, later, competed with Jenner's method of using cowpox virus; both were controversial.

The story of progress in controlling plague in China is remarkable. Wu, Lien-Teh was a brilliant "offshore Chinese" scholar in colonial Malaya who went to Cambridge University and matured into an outstanding physician and medical research scientist. He was invited to Manchuria to assist in controlling the devastating plague epidemic of 1910 and 1911 that took 60,000 lives. Chinese confidence in Western medicine was growing because of the success of Jenner's cowpox vaccine against smallpox and the achievements of medical missionaries.

Arriving in Harbin in December 1910, Wu immediately conducted a postmortem examination that revealed classic lesions of plague and isolated *Bacillus pestis* in pure culture. In April 1911 he orchestrated the first international medical conference held in China to develop proposals for a plan of action to control the epidemic. Kitisato of Japan, Zabolotny of Russia, and leading Western experts participated. Transfer of patients to rat-proof isolation hospitals and establishment of a permanent sanitation task force to respond immediately to outbreaks were key features of the plan. At that time it was recognized that the disease was spread by the fleas on rats. Wu's plan was to mobilize support for policies that would break the chains of person-to-person and rat-to-person spread of infection.

Wu initiated a research program to trace the possible origin of plague epidemics in wild species, the "sylvatic" form. He was able to confirm the local view that there was a connection with wild rodents, particularly a marmot called the tarabagan, a hibernating Siberian species. His scientific work soon established that the species was vulnerable to the plague bacillus after experimental exposure. Also, its fleas would attack other mammals, including humans. He negotiated with the Russians for permission to study the disease in nature in Transbaikalia and received solid support from Russian veterinarians. Wu showed that the disease progressed more slowly in hibernating animals and that some of them would survive to initiate an epizootic in the spring.

Wu's conclusion was that the plague organism had been endemic in the marmot populations on the northern Asiatic plateaus since ancient times. Early in the nineteenth century it infected other rodents, then people, via flea transfer. The rodent form in nature was the bubonic, and the pneumonic form arose as a result of it.

The great epidemic of 1910 and 1911 in Manchuria may well have been a result of a fourfold increase in the price of marmot pelts, which triggered a wave of amateur hunters seeking to cash in. The hunters did not know the importance of avoiding contact with animals that were visibly sick, and many became infected. The disease spread along the railway system. When another epidemic occurred in 1920 and 1921, the Manchurian authorities were able to control it with minimal loss of life.

Wu and K. Chimin Wong wrote a valuable *History of Chinese Medicine* in English, which included coverage of veterinary medicine.

BEGINNINGS OF PAIN CONTROL FOR SURGERY

The Chinese, in addition to seeking professional advice to treat their ailments, were enamored of elixirs of immortality, enhancers of life's pleasures such as aphrodisiacs, and relievers of pain and discomfort. Not all their experiments were beneficial. Tonics and elixirs containing heavy metals (such as mercury, arsenic, and lead) were distinctly hazardous; opium obtained from the poppy could perform miracles when properly used but carried the terrible risk of addiction; the "autumn mineral" of sexually active extracts of urine required experience with effects and dosages that were unlikely to be well understood in a period before scientific medical and veterinary experiments; and other herbal drugs such as hemp, hyoscyamine, and ephedrine were a mixed blessing. The quest for surgical analgesia and anesthesia involved the use of hypnotic analgesic drugs, hallucinogens, and acupuncture. Hua Tuo (in the second century AD) concocted an alcoholic drink containing Indian hemp that was said to induce a type of general anesthesia. He was reputed to be the greatest surgeon of his time and to have performed laparotomies and flushed parts of the gastrointestinal tract, but no written records are known. Chiu or alcoholic drinks, including strong, noncarbonated ale, were made by fermenting grains and starchy tubers. Potent distilled grain alcohols were also made, but drunkenness was uncommon. Many medicinal products were prepared as alcoholic tinctures, and similar extracts were used to enhance flavors.

Emperor Kien Lung in 1744 commissioned a comprehensive encyclopedia of medicine and surgery; the result was the forty-volume *Golden Mirror of Medicine.*

EARLY WRITINGS ON VETERINARY MEDICINE IN CHINA

Of nine books listed in bibliographies of veterinary medicine during the pre-Tang period, eight dealt with the horse and one with horses, buffalo, cattle, camels, and donkeys. The Tang government established a department of veterinary medicine and a school of veterinary medicine. The formalization of veterinary practice and veterinary education was first described in AD 618. Li Ssu edited *Collection of Ways to Relieve the Suffering of Horse (Ssu Mu An Ch'i Chi)*. Because it listed seventy-six serious diseases and thirty-six etiologies, it was the first text on differential diagnosis for veterinary medicine. This work was expanded from four to eight volumes during the Sung and Yuan dynasties and included a section entitled *Tested Prescriptions of Nomadic Origin.*

Veterinary works were listed in agricultural rather than medical bibliographies. Wang Yu-hu's catalog of works in Chinese agriculture, which appeared in 1964, revealed the following distribution of works on animal science by species: horses, sixty; silkworms, about forty; cattle, eighteen; fish, twelve; camels, five; swine, two; and ducks, chickens, and geese, one each.

Farm workers were trained to become horse doctors. A military encyclopedia of about AD 1004 described horse diseases and management. It listed the sites on the skin used as major acupuncture points and described the treatment of wounds received in combat. Prescriptions and therapy were provided for many specific diseases, most for digestive disturbances. Impacted feces were removed manually from animals with colic caused by coarse fodder. Mainly herbal remedies were administered in liquid form. A book on pharmacy for animal medicines was produced by the government during the Sung dynasty.

The role of the veterinarian was to master knowledge of animal dysfunctions, to relieve inflammations, and to cure a variety of known diseases. The main route of treatment was to funnel medications as a drench via the mouth. It was also necessary to observe the animal's mood and behavior, to motivate it, and to correct the balance of the deranged yin-yang. For inflammations the animal was dosed with medications to eradicate the causative agent. Food, water, and medications were then provided, along with rest to allow restoration of health.

The *Compendium of Materia Medica (Pen T'sao Kang Mu)* was written by the revered Li Shi-chen, a famous Chinese Ming scholar who lived from AD 1518 to AD 1593. The compendium described mostly herbal medicines tested on himself and was his life's work, filling fifty-two volumes and taking twenty-seven years to complete. It was published posthumously in 1595. The work included comprehensive information about 1871 substances (374 of them new) used in medications; among them, 55 were recommended for veterinary use. The compendium also described methods for collection and manufacture of the folk medicines. Li consulted all 39 previous monographs on materia medica and cited about 1000 references. The opus described 1074 drugs of plant origin; 443 drugs obtained from animals, including 9 kinds of dragons; and 354 from minerals or other sources. Ephedrine, kaolin, and chaulmoogra oil were important items little known in the West until the twentieth century.

During the Yuan (Mongol) dynasty *A Description of the Treatment of Sick Horses,* edited by K'a Kuan Lon, appeared. Further progress was made during the Ming dynasty, when two famous veterinarians, the brothers Yu Pen-Yuan and Yu Pen-Heng, wrote the *Treatise on Horses (Liao-Ma Chi),* a masterful synthesis of the veterinary information of the period. It included an illustration of main acupuncture points. Editions continued to appear until 1957, when the figure of the points was revised. Yang Shih Ch'ao edited *The Book of Horses* and *The Book of Cattle,* and *Prescriptions for Horses* also appeared.

The remarkable drawing of a splendid but pathetically emaciated horse attributed to Sung artist Gong Kai (AD 1222-1307) is thought to express the self-image of the Chinese scholar after the Yuan conquest changed the value structure. They felt condemned to live in a world in which their art was not appreciated. The horse was a traditional symbol of the scholar-official, and the painting was an apt representation of the scholar-official's fate under a dynasty that revered horsemanship rather than scholarship and art.

95. *Emaciated Horse* by Song loyalist Gang Kai (1222-1307) expresses the self-image of scholars during the Yuan dynasty, when their talent was not appreciated. The allegory of a horse of splendid physique deprived of sustenance pointedly conveys the status of the neglected scholars to a conqueror who prided himself on his horsemanship. *(Osaka Municipal Museum of Art, Abe Collection.)*

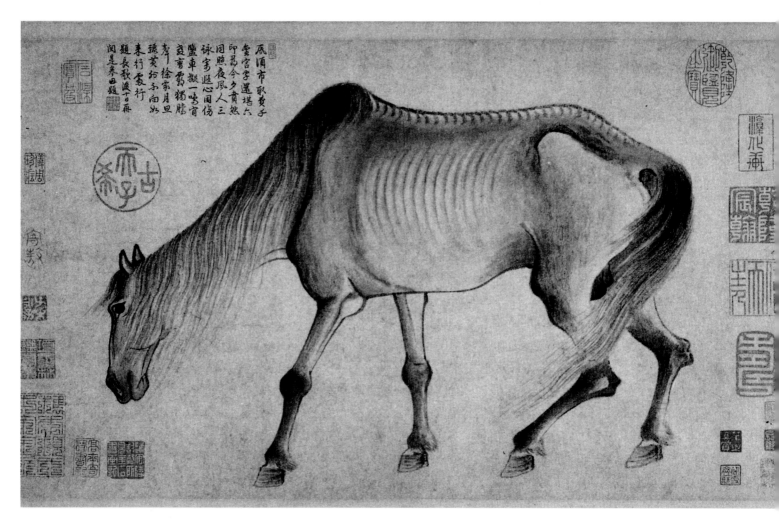

The Qing (Manchu) dynasty provided the *Complete Issue of the Cattle-Classics* about 1680. This work described diseases of cattle and water buffalo, as well as acupuncture points. It identified standard procedures for physical diagnosis. Observation and description of the clinical signs were the keys to decision making. The method required that the practitioner "look, smell, ask, and touch" (take the pulse). The pulse was taken at the base of the tail. Summer bloat in cattle was a recognized condition, and lameness and infertility were common problems.

According to the *Complete Issue of the Cattle-Classics,* first, the general disposition and condition of the animal were evaluated and noted, including its strength or weakness and degree of abdominal fill. Then the position of the head, the bearing of the ears, the temperature of the skin and horns, the moistness or dryness of the muzzle, and the sensitivity of the feet were checked. This detailed examination encompassed the appearance and integrity of the lining of the body's orifices, the nature and odor of secretions and excretions, the composition and intake of the diet, and the texture and condition of the skin. Careful attention was paid to the environment, since diseases were thought to be caused by adverse climatic conditions, spoiled feed or water, or poisons and pests.

A surprising feature was the reluctance of veterinarians to engage in manipulative procedures or surgery. Although they would lance abscesses and castrate, they would not, for example, manually remove a retained placenta. The general tendency was to depend on drug therapy.

The first *Complete Collection of Pig Diseases* by Chu Ching Ta Chi'uan came out in 1900. Diarrhea, rheumatism, and infertility were concerns. Given the enormous numbers of pigs in China, the relative lack of attention to swine medicine was remarkable. Either translations of most of the old Chinese veterinary works are not yet available or the ancient texts have been lost.

APPLICATIONS OF ACUPUNCTURE IN ANIMAL MEDICINE

During the Tang Dynasty, acupuncture was widely used in horses and in small-animal medicine. Wang Tao wrote on diseases of dogs and their treatments, including the use of acupuncture, when sick dogs were receiving little attention in the West. The use of acupuncture in the treatment of elephants was described. French Jesuit missionaries expelled from China brought knowledge of the technique back to Europe, where it was taught in the early veterinary schools in France, Austria, and Germany for several decades. Russia and eastern European nations became aware of the technique. Except in France, it lost favor in Europe in the mid-nineteenth century. Recently, however, growing contacts with China by interested veterinarians have led to a revival of interest in the technique and attempts to extend the more detailed studies of its use in humans to domestic animals.

Jöchle studied Chinese medical philosophy and human acupuncture under Huebotter, one of the first scholars to bring detailed knowledge of these fields to the West (in 1929). In 1958 Jöchle demonstrated a system of lines of enhanced conductance ("meridians") on the body surface of horses, donkeys, dogs, cattle, and pigs. In Austria O. Kothbauer mapped the bovine acupuncture sites, correlating specific points to internal diseases. The technique has been claimed to correct certain reproductive disorders. In China, acupuncture has been advanced by the addition of electrical stimulation of the needles, and prolonged surgical anesthesia with the desirable feature of no recovery period has been accomplished.

VETERINARY MEDICINE IN THE MODERN ERA

Chinese traditional veterinary medicine was abandoned after 1840 and the Opium Wars. The Qing dynasty established a veterinary college specializing in horses. The army's medical and veterinary practices were gradually westernized. After the Republic of China was established in 1912 under Sun, Yat-sen and the modern era began, the first Western-type schools of veterinary medicine were established (after 1917) and informal degrees were awarded. Chairman Mao Ze-dong introduced a new policy in 1944: "We must train rural veterinarians." In 1947 the Northern University School of Agriculture was required to develop Chinese veterinary medicine. In 1956, however, it was estimated that there were about 150,000 untrained practitioners of Chinese veterinary medicine.

The Yu brothers' old book formed the basis of Kim Chung-Tze's *New Treatise on Horses and Cattle* (1955), the first Chinese veterinary book to use modern terminology. In the following year an attempt to organize veterinary medicine began with the publication of research journals such as *The Chinese Journal of Veterinary Medicine* and *Herdsmen and Veterinary Medicine*. The first National Conference on Veterinary Medicine was held in 1958, and the Research Institute of Chinese Veterinary Medicine was founded in Lanchow. The leading veterinary school developed in the capital, Beijing (formerly Peking). A new national initiative in veterinary medicine for companion animals was undertaken in the 1990s.

TIBET: THE HIGH HIMALAYAS

Buddhism began in the foothills of the Himalaya Mountains and evolved as a religion in India. It spread to Ceylon and Southeast Asia on the one hand and to East Asia (including China, Korea, and Japan) on the other. It took root in Nepal and Tibet, and the pagodas of Tibet retained the ancient Sanskrit texts in Tibetan script on wooden blocks. The monks and the lamas (teachers) studied these scripts, which covered Buddhist thought, astronomy, and traditional medicine. Tibetan contacts were made with Mongolia and the Chinese province of Szechuan. The primary intellectual concern was the relationship between the mind and the impurities that surround it. The Tibetan religion included a mythical view of the world as peopled by the Lord of Hell, who must be appeased. The agriculture of this high land made use of the yak for milk, burden, and draft, and donkeys for burden and labor. The Bactrian camel was the hardy vehicle of the desert trade in the north. The product of the Tibetan shawl-wool goats was highly prized by the fashion trade. Flocks of sheep with mounted herders exploited the high pastures.

Tibet was protected by the muddy Yellow River much of the time, but the winter freeze allowed raiders to cross from the north. The vulnerable state strove to preserve its mysteries from invaders, and it was virtually closed to curious visitors, even to scholars. The most revealing cultural discoveries were made in the Cloister of 1000 Buddhas at Tun-Huang, near the western border of China and Mongolia, a former cultural center along the old Silk Road, long since forgotten. The cloister was a fabulous edifice with many grottoes and rooms. The monks evidently had sealed one of the rooms to protect its contents from Chi-Chia invaders in the eleventh century. A Chinese monk found the room to be full of ancient documents, cloths, and statues dating from the fourth or fifth century AD to about 1022 AD, just before it was sealed. International scholars rushed to the site. British, French, and other nationals carried off most of the contents, and many of the materials disappeared en route to Europe.

Enough documents and scrolls from the cloister survived to show that the ancient scribes of Tun-Huang held a significant knowledge of horse doctoring. Not surprisingly, in the rarefied air of those high valleys the main problem was exhaustion, followed by friction injuries resulting from the weight of the rider or burden or from foot diseases. Problems arising from malnutrition were also common. Urethral calculi were encountered, and methods to clear the tube via cauterization or gentle compression of the bladder through the rectum were recommended. Venesection and cauterization or cutting of the skin were used. The Chinese techniques of moxibustion and acupuncture were practiced for lameness and internal disorders. Succinct instructions that could be memorized were set down concerning materia medica and appropriate treatments.

The Tibetan translation of the *Asvayurveda* of Salihotra has been preserved and indicates that Indian hippiatry was well known. There is little available literature on the veterinary care of the other domestic species such as the yaks, asses, goats, and Bactrian camels.

VETERINARY MEDICINE IN JAPAN

In ancient times the Japanese, like other cultures, appealed to mythological figures. Japan identified the need for veterinary skills during the era of rapid expansion of horse stocks for military purposes in East Asia. A veterinary priest-physician was brought to Japan from Korea in AD 598 to train a person of the imperial retinue in the veterinary art. Thus Korean ideas provided the seeds for early Japanese veterinary development. Japan participated in this early version of an arms race in the seventh century AD. During the following century, in 731, the government gave permission for people to become horse doctors, and in AD 804 one of these went to China to learn the current knowledge there. By 877 there were horse doctors in Japan. Military horses were purpose-bred by late in the twelfth century. The civil war of 1467 involved mounted Samurai warriors and triggered a strong demand for horse doctors, so a school was started to train them when Osaka was the capital of Japan. Western concepts of veterinary medicine probably were introduced by Dutch contacts; one Japanese practitioner was trained in their system.

The government of Japan decided to introduce Western ideas and advances in medicine and veterinary medicine about 1880. It was fortunate to locate an excellent and a unique candidate when it approached the Berlin veterinary school with this request. Johannes Ludwig Janson (1849-1914) was born in Baden-Baden and graduated from the Berlin college of Humboldt University in 1869. He spent five years as an Army veterinarian after studying under the famous pathologist Rudolf Virchow for two years. He gained experience of practice at Kroningen in Saxony and in Klefeld, where he was also in the veterinary police. During a year with the army of Napoleon III he learned French and the French style of equine medicine. Back in Germany he spent two years as a veterinary technologist on a farm before returning as Professor Extraordinarius to his alma mater, where he taught anatomy, histology, physiology, and pathology for two years.

Janson was thirty-one years old when he was invited to Japan to establish a veterinary school at Komaba Agricultural College in Tokyo. He developed the academic program and taught ten subjects himself the first year. He was then joined by Karl Troster, who shared the load, and they opened a veterinary hospital so that students could receive practical training. Janson stayed twenty-two years, until 1902, then retired. He was named distinguished professor of Tokyo Imperial University (now Tokyo University), and a statue in his likeness was placed at the front of the veterinary school, an unusual honor for a foreigner in Japan. He taught part-time at other schools and indulged his interest in oriental art and travel. He returned to his native Germany after he

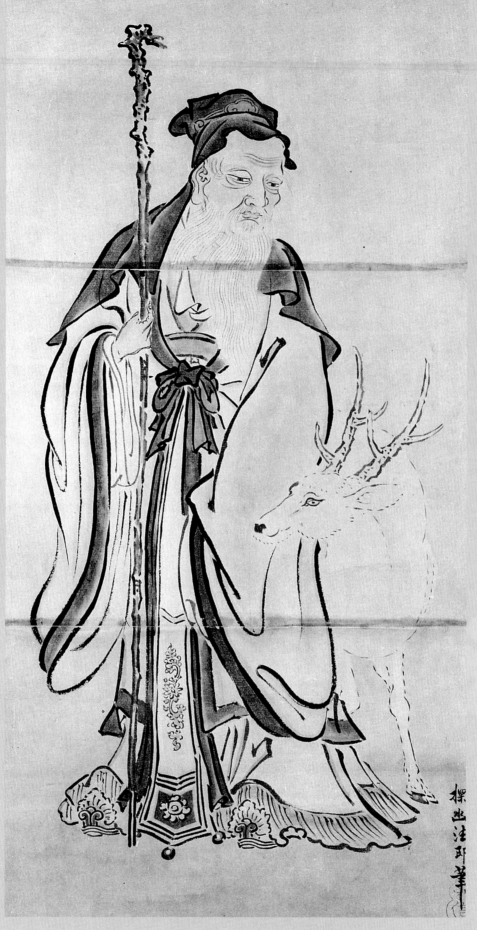

96. *Jurojin, One of the Seven Gods of Luck* (in Japan). He is associated with longevity and is often shown with a crane or, as in this case, a stag. He is usually dressed as a scholar, wearing a headdress. *(Museum für Volkerkunde, Vienna.)*

retired but found that the Orient had stolen his soul, so he returned to Japan and died there on October 28, 1914. His impact in bringing the Japanese veterinary profession into the modern era with high academic standards was significant. Two of his graduates became leaders in the profession in Japan. Sennosuke Katsushima became the first native-born professor of veterinary medicine and attained an international reputation. Yoshiemon Sudo was distinguished in surgery. Janson was a fortunate choice for Japan and left a great legacy. His breadth of knowledge and scholarly interests coupled with his personal commitment and philosophy made him an effective "change agent" for his chosen profession in Japan. He took his unique collection of oriental books on veterinary medicine and animal art back to Berlin.

Before Janson's time Japan had developed its veterinary medicine on the traditional oriental pattern that evolved in China. The Chinese emperor's 1596 book on acupuncture in the horse was introduced. Herbal medical texts described remedies for horses that made use of twenty-five different herbs. They were mixed with honey and administered either to cure the horse or to keep it healthy.

One branch of veterinary medicine has roots that are traceable to the Shogun born in 1685, the Year of the Dog: he decided not to kill dogs and to become a protector of dogs. As early as AD 982 a book was published based on a compilation from Chinese sources on how to treat human disease caused by exposure to rabid dogs. In 1268 a monk made a temple with a hospital for people and animals. Rabies became a major concern in Japan in the second half of the nineteenth century. In one outbreak a rabid wolf bit a number of people, nine of whom died. By 1873 regulations were appearing in Tokyo and Hokkaido prefectures that required the capture of all loose dogs and the killing of those that were rabid, but the disease resurfaced. In 1892 two rabid dogs in the south bit animals of several species, and cows, horses, cats, and poultry died. In the following year during a major campaign in Nagasaki prefecture, 735 dogs were destroyed and 48 of them were reported to have been

97. The oriental genius for drawing and sculpting animals is illustrated in these examples from a Japanese lesson book. They are remarkable for the directness and simplicity with which they display the essence of the animals' forms and natures. *(Gift of William Sturgis Bigelow. Courtesy Museum of Fine Arts, Boston.)*

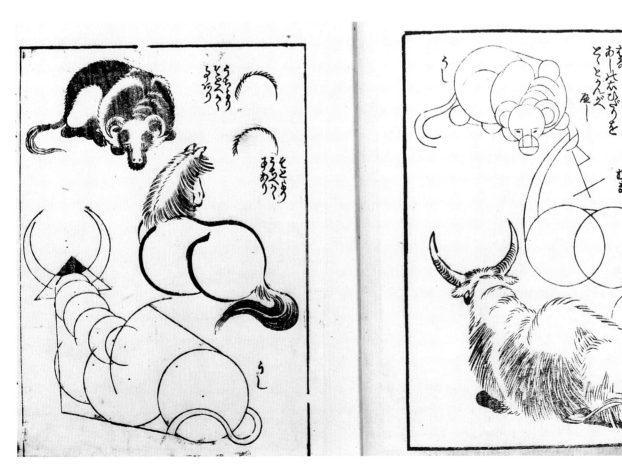

rabid. In 1895 Kuraki Tome made a vaccine, which he called Number 11 Vaccine. He used material from the brain of an infected dog, passaging it via rabbits. It was tested on twenty-five persons who were bitten by a rabid dog, and none got the disease. Later, in 1905, a three-year study reported 4526 cases of dog bites in humans. Forty-nine of the dogs were found to be rabid, and thirty-five people died.

Shibasaburo Kitasato (1852-1931) was an outstanding Japanese scientist whose work had a great impact on microbiology and immunology relevant to veterinary medicine. He was born in Ogunicho, on the southern island of Kyushu, and studied at the new Kojo medical school under C.G. van Mansvelt of Holland. He then studied at Tokyo Medical School before joining the Central Sanitary Bureau to work on infectious diseases. During a cholera epidemic in Nagasaki in 1894 he cultured the cholera bacillus from the feces of patients there. He also isolated *Pasteurella multocida,* the cause of fowl cholera, from dead chickens in Tokyo.

Sent to Germany, Kitasato studied under Robert Koch from 1886 to 1891 at his Hygienisches Institut. Koch had isolated the pathogens of tuberculosis in 1882 and cholera in 1883. During the productive period in Germany, Kitasato published work on the organisms causing cholera, typhoid, and anthrax. The highlight of his stay, however, was his remarkable achievement of the first isolation of *Clostridium tetani,* the spore-forming cause of tetanus, in 1889. He also produced experimental infections in animals and showed that the germ of the infection produced a specific toxin. He then showed that the serum from animals inoculated with the toxin contained an antitoxin. Koch was astonished and overjoyed at his pupil's successes, and Kitasato was given the unusual distinction of a professorship.

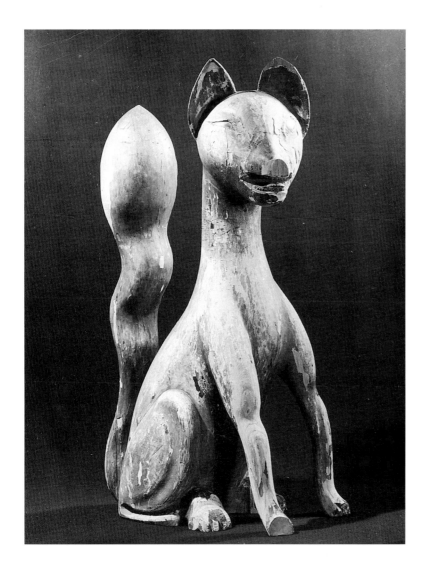

98. A seventeenth-century Japanese wooden carving of a sitting fox. The fox is the messenger of Inari, the god of rice and guardian of the rice crop. But the animal is feared, too, for its malevolence; possession by a fox spirit is sometimes thought to be a cause of insanity, depression, and hysteria. *(Museum für Volkerkunde, Vienna.)*

Emil von Behring repeated Kitasato's approach with the diphtheria organism and published his work jointly with Kitasato in 1890; the publication, *Ueber das Zustandekommen der Diphetherie-Immunität und der Tetanus-Immunität bei Thieren,* is a landmark opus in the initiation of immunology. Returning to Japan in 1892, Kitasato established a private institution that was merged later (in 1905) with the government's Vaccine Lymph Farm and Serum Institute. Kitasato reported in 1904-1906 that native cattle were free from bovine tuberculosis until European breeds were imported in the 1870s. In addition, they were very resistant to the human strain, which was prevalent in Japan. Kitasato went to Hong Kong to study a plague epidemic there in 1904, isolating *Pasteurella pestis* at about the same time that Alexandre Yersin did, then to another outbreak in Manchuria in 1911. He was responsible for building fine research facilities, including a research center for veterinary science at the Kitasato Institute. He became dean of Keio-Gyüka medical college in 1917 and was made a baron in 1924.

The Japanese Veterinary Medical Association was established in 1921. The agricultural ministry expanded and developed specialized subdivisions, including veterinary medicine. The agricultural colleges were associated with veterinary schools. The war with China created new demands for veterinarians. After the war, students trained in veterinary medicine in ten national universities and at the Osaka University of Agriculture and five private veterinary schools. The Japanese Veterinary Medical Association was replaced in 1948 by the Japanese Veterinary Doctors Association. During the American occupation, cultural links were established with the United States. A major initiative was the translation of many veterinary books into Japanese, and educational exchange programs allowed Japanese veterinarians to gain advanced training in America and elsewhere. Research centers were strengthened and became much more productive in the second half of the twentieth century. The Japanese Central Horse Racing Association was established in 1954. The Japanese government assisted veterinary developments overseas, including the establishment of a new veterinary school in Zambia. The 1995 gathering of the World Veterinary Congress in Yokohama, Japan, highlights the profession's progress in Asia.

99. One of the three surviving sections of a famous Japanese handscroll, *Sungyu Ekotoba,* known as *Ten Fast Bulls.* Such powerful bulls were used to pull carriages with passengers. The artist has succeeded in portraying a remarkable sense of virile muscular power. This work is from the militant Kamakura period (about AD 1280) and is of the nationalistic form known as *Yamatoe. (Gift of Mrs. Donald E. Frederick. Photograph by Paul Macapia. Seattle Art Museum.)*

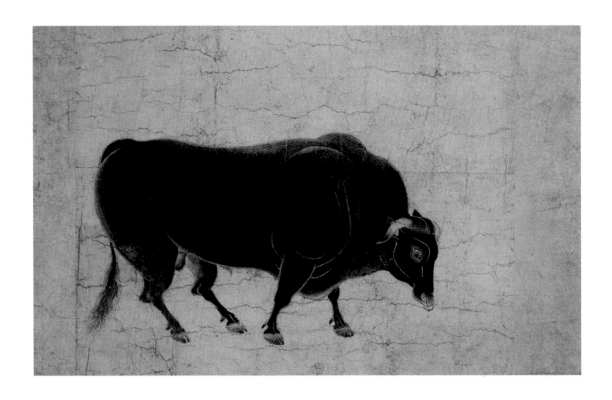

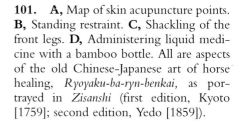

100. Nonomura Sotatsu, who died in 1643, created this deer scroll using a brilliant technique of contrasting gold and silver washes on the simple outlines of the animals. He was a founder of the *Rimpa* or decorative style. The calligraphy was done by Koetsu (1538-1637). *(Gift of Mrs. Donald E. Frederick. Photograph by Paul Macapia. Seattle Art Museum.)*

101. **A,** Map of skin acupuncture points. **B,** Standing restraint. **C,** Shackling of the front legs. **D,** Administering liquid medicine with a bamboo bottle. All are aspects of the old Chinese-Japanese art of horse healing, *Ryoyaku-ba-ryn-benkai,* as portrayed in *Zisanshi* (first edition, Kyoto [1759]; second edition, Yedo [1859]).

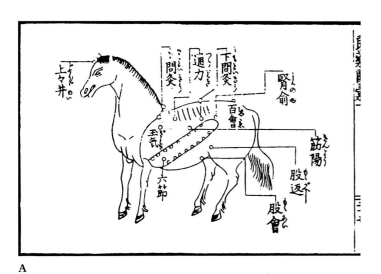

A

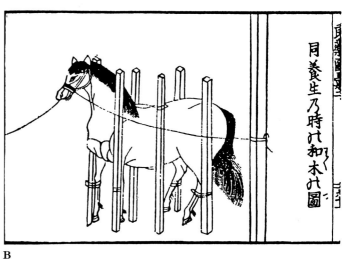

B

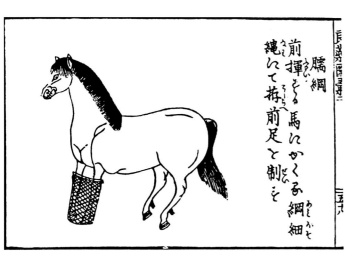

C

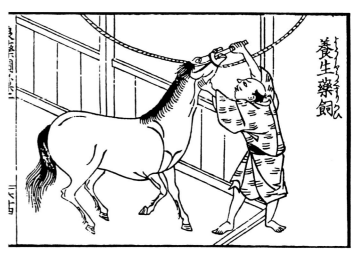

D

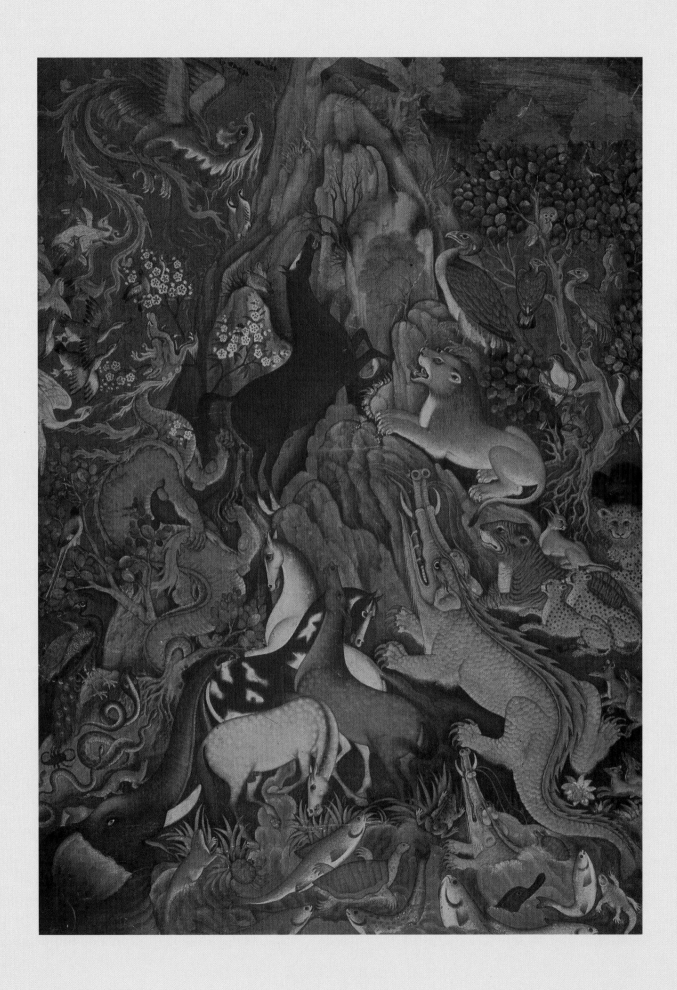

Animal Use and Veterinary Origins in South Asia

ANIMAL ALLEGORIES AND FABLES

Many Western images of India involve animals, perhaps partly because of the adventures depicted in Rudyard Kipling's immortal *Jungle Book,* particularly the nature stories about Mowgli, the child raised by the wolf, and wild-animal characters. Various film images, too, of mahouts with their elephants and snake charmers with their mesmerized hooded cobras have added to the colorful Western conceptions of India. Although not portraying a wholly accurate account of life in India, these entertainments do convey the central role that animals (usually the less exotic ones) have played in Indian history and the remarkable fraternity that has developed between people and animals there over the last twenty-five centuries.

South Asia was an early source of fables, including many short stories in which talking animals exemplified human characteristics and behavioral traits. Pre-Christian examples include the Pali Jatakas or birth stories, in which the Buddhist symbolism conforms to the idea that the Buddha went through several animal stages in his evolution to perfection of spirit. In painted Ajanta caves of the Deccan plateau, a beautiful scene illustrates the altruistic Buddha during a previous incarnation as a white elephant sacrificing his tusks. The most famous collection of Indian fables, the *Panchatantra* of the fourth century, was translated and spread throughout West Asia, the Middle East, and Europe. It included delightful animal tales that encouraged caution and self-interest rather than altruism. The folktales became the model for the *Anwar-e-Suheili* of the Persians and the *Kalila Wa Dimna* of the Arabs, Turks, and Mongols. Each culture developed special artworks to illustrate the fables.

EARLY LIVESTOCK AGRICULTURE OF THE INDUS RIVER VALLEY

Emerging during the third millennium BC was the third of the world's great riverine cultures (after those of the Euphrates-Tigris and the Nile cultures), the Harappan culture of the Indus River valley and the river's tributaries. The ruminants and donkeys helped open the region to grain production. The people who settled in the thousand-mile-long valley are believed to have immigrated from farther west, possibly Sumeria, after 4000 BC. The dependability of the Indus River's water supply was offset by occasional catastrophic flooding. The culture featured two major urban complexes laid out geometrically, one at Mohenjo-Daro, the other at Harappa, several hundred miles upstream. The culture's unique pictographic script, as yet undeciphered, occurs on steatite stamp seals, most of which display animals; long texts have not been

102. *Facing page,* Indian fables, filled with allegorical references to animals, were the precursors of folktales for other cultures in South Asia. The poetry from the Mughal dynasty, in particular, is beautifully illustrated by sixteenth-century Indian artists in a uniquely romantic style. In this album leaf painted by Miskīn (c. 1600), a raven listens to the various animals complain of grievances suffered in their experiences with humans. The theme is from the Ottoman poet Lami'i Celebi (died 1538). Gouache on paper. *(The British Museum, London.)*

103. Steatite stamp seal from the Harappan civilization showing a male zebu and undeciphered script. The Harappan culture had vanished by 1500 BC. Mohenjo-daro, West Pakistan (c. 2500-1900 BC). *(Copyright The British Museum, London.)*

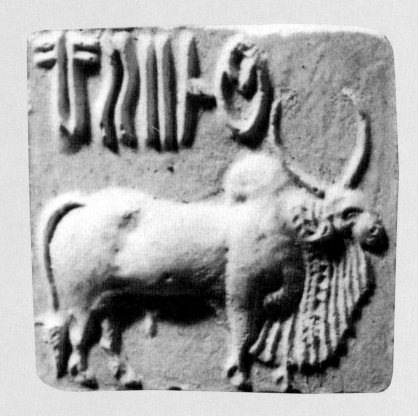

104. *Below,* Cave scene of *Fighting Bulls* from Ajantā, East India. Bulls were popular subjects for Indian artists. Zebu also were frequently depicted in bull-grappling sports. Probably from the Gupta period, fourth to sixth centuries AD. *(British Library, Oriental and India Office Collections, London.)*

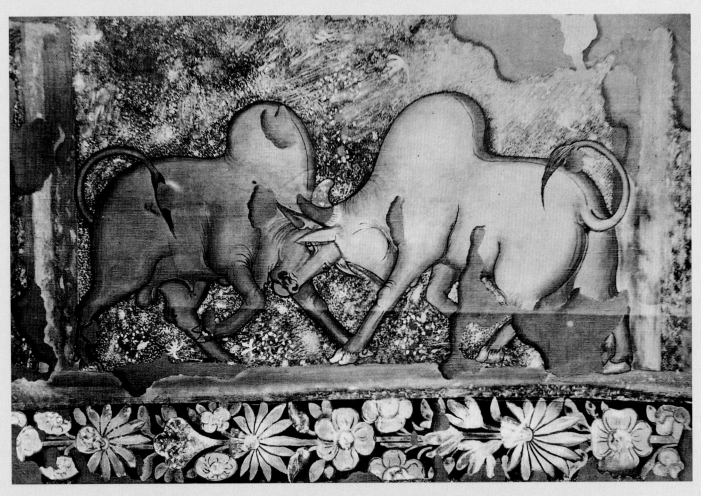

found. The people had both humped (zebu) and humpless cattle, buffalo, sheep, goats, pigs, donkeys, dogs, and fowl. Bulls predominate among their artists' representations and seals and probably had a religious significance as the focus of a fertility cult. Indeed, bull and buffalo sacrifice and bull-grappling sports were practiced. Wild animals are also depicted, including the elephant, tiger, deer, rhinoceros, and monkey. Movable toys were cleverly made in the shapes of monkeys and cattle.

THE ARYAN INVASION AND HINDU CULTURE

The decline of the Harappan civilization around 1900 BC marked the beginning of more than 3000 years of greater and lesser invasions of South Asia by various groups. The first, most historically influential of these invaders, the nomadic warriors of Aryan tribes originating from the steppes of central Asia, may have directly caused the fall of the Indus Valley cultures. These tribes were able to accomplish these challenging translocations in part because of their use of animal power derived from horses and oxen. Without the horse for the charioteers and transport and the livestock (cattle, sheep, and goats) as a continuing source of sustenance, their march through the Kush to Kabul and on through the Khyber and Bolan Passes to the valleys of the Indus would not have been possible. Their self-sufficiency in food on the hoof from the cattle, sheep, and goats that accompanied them allowed a versatility not available to sedentary agriculturalists; furthermore, their mastery of metallurgy permitted construction of light-spoked chariot wheels and effective weapons. These advantages, coupled with an aggressive, confident attitude, permitted the Aryan tribes to defend themselves from attack and to overrun any who resisted. They fanned out gradually through the watersheds of the Indus and, later, the Ganges River and beyond. Most of the tribes eventually settled into agricultural pursuits.

The Aryans had a strict social hierarchy and, although illiterate, did compose hymns that were committed to memory by the Brahmana, or hereditary priests. Later these were to be recalled in the first Indian literature, the optimistic religious hymns and legends of the Rig-Veda, which have been handed down to modern times as traditional utterances telling vaguely of feats of ancient rajas (chiefs). Composed during the second millennium BC and later written down in Sanskrit, the Rig-Veda is full of cattle imagery and the relationship of the species to fertility. *Veda* in Sanskrit means "the knowledge."

The Rig-Veda was followed by the Sama-Veda, the Yojiur-Veda, and the Atharva-Veda, which together compose the Four Books of the Vedas. Prose commentaries of the Vedas, called Brahmanas, describe the role of the Aryan priestly class, the Brahmans, and spell out precisely how sacrifices should be performed. From the names of these works the Aryan religion has become known as Vedism or Brahmanism. In the first millennium BC the religion was challenged by Jainism, Buddhism, and other non-Vedic systems. Hindu philosophy began to emerge from the conflict with the writing of the Upanishads between 600 BC and 200 BC. Although not rejecting the sacred nature of the Vedas, these treatises emphasize the soul of the individual, proclaiming salvation by self-awareness rather than by faith or works.

Hinduism proved to be a diverse, malleable structure over the centuries, adjusting to incorporate the beliefs of other Indian peoples. By this practice a number of different animals found representation in the Hindu pantheon. Brahma, Vishnu, and Shiva are the central gods of Hinduism but are not themselves the highest deities. They are simply aspects of the ultimate divine principle known as Brahman, which is undefinable and incapable of being represented because it contains all possible attributes. Vishnu assimilated many of the gods of the smaller cults and had many animal characteristics. The heroic Krishna, the Divine Cowherd, was recognized by many as an incarna-

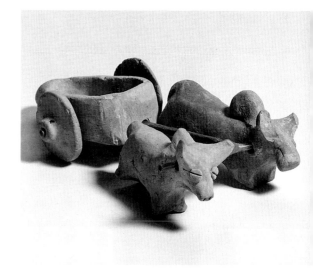

105. Clay toy model of cart and bullocks from Chanchu-daro, Pakistan. Reddish-buff clay (c. 2400–2000 BC). (*Joint Expedition of the American School of Indian and Iranian Studies and MFA. Courtesy Museum of Fine Arts, Boston.*)

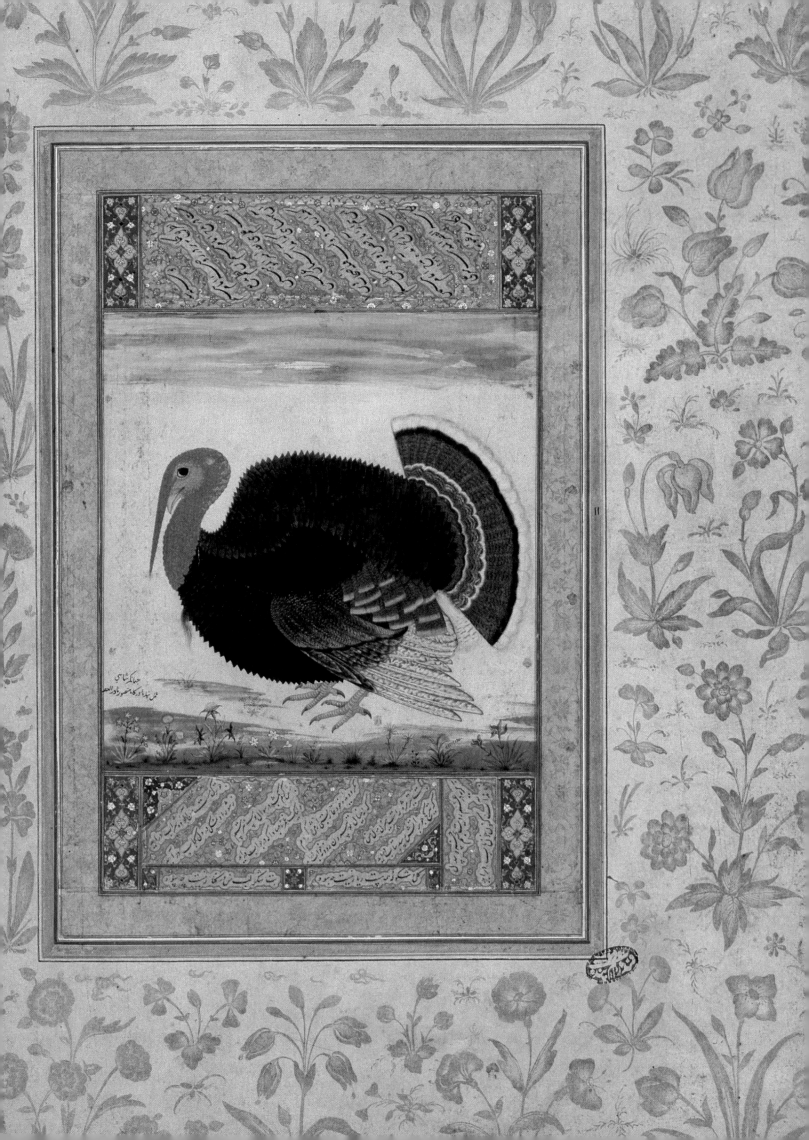

tion of Vishnu, as were other martial heroes. Shiva, the Destroyer, had a bull called Nandi for a mount and was often worshiped as a fertility symbol. Shiva was also the father of Ganesha, a god portrayed with an elephant's head, who removed obstacles from projects to be undertaken.

ANIMAL AGRICULTURE IN ARYAN CULTURE

Cattle were the predominant livestock of the Aryans and in fact served as the currency of the land. The population of zebu *(Bos indicus)* exceeded that of *Bos taurus.* Individually branded, the cattle were often grazed on common grounds and watched by a communal cowherd. Large herds of cattle were maintained under seminomadic conditions by herders in outlying regions. Pairs of oxen were used for burden and traction, particularly for cultivation and transport in dry areas. The draft function was vital to crop agriculture of plowing, irrigation, and harvesting, as well as for pulling the main means of transport, the ox-cart. Muzzled oxen were driven around a post, where cut grain was placed on a packed slab to thresh the seeds from the ears. The manure was important as fertilizer but even more so as a crude plaster for construction and, when dried, for fuel. Milk and curd were important dairy products that balanced the deficiencies of the grain staples of the diet. Ghee (butter oil made from melted butter by skimming off the solid fat) was used universally, since it would keep at high ambient temperatures.

The discovery of iron around 1000 BC enabled a new burst of technology that included metal plows, which facilitated the transition from a pastoral nomadic existence to forest clearing and managing a settled agricultural society. It may have been during this transition that the cow and the draft ox became as important as the mighty bull, which was symbolic of the previous cultures.

The importance of the horse derived from its military function. Horses are mentioned in the Rig-Veda, but they are described as having only seventeen ribs (the modern horse has eighteen). According to the Rig-Veda, the war-horse was used mainly in pairs, to draw a lightweight chariot bearing two warriors, a most formidable cavalry weapon:

> *Rushing to glory to the capture of herds,*
> *swooping down as a hungry falcon . . .*
>
> *And at his deep neigh, like the thunder of heaven,*
> *the foemen tremble in fear,*
> *for he fights against the thousands,*
> *and none can resist him,*
> *so terrible is his charge.*

Evidently cattle rustling was a major activity. Indeed, the Sanskrit word for *war* literally meant "need for more cattle." Although the phrase "not for killing" was applied to milking cows, cattle were not sacred at that time and the high proportion of bones of young animals in archaeological digs is evidence that beef was eaten regularly.

The importance of water buffalo is often underestimated. About 65 million, half the world's population of water buffalo, were present in India alone in 1985. The swamp type has wide, sweeping horns and is widely used in rice-growing areas and river valleys for traction and burden. Male buffalo were used to clear swamps and forests, then to plow the wet land of the rice paddies, which is their continuing role today. The females were the mainstay of local milk production because of the high quality and high fat content of their milk. The main milking breeds, however, are of the river buffalo type, such as the Murrah with tightly curled horns. Goats used for milk and meat were common, and sheep were prevalent, especially in cooler areas. Blankets

106. *Facing page,* Mansūr, one of the Mughal Old Masters, painted this splendid turkey cock for the Wantage Album (c. 1612). The cock was a Portuguese import brought to Jahāngīr from Goa in 1612, the seventh year of Mansūr's reign. The same artist also created superb pictures of a hen and a chicken and of a game duck during the same period. Gouache on paper. *(Courtesy of the Board of Trustees of the Victoria and Albert Museum, London.)*

107. The shawl goats of Tibet depicted in this lithograph by Louard lived in the mountainous regions. The first British veterinary surgeon, William Moorcroft, moved to India as superintendent of the East India Company's horse stud at Pusa in 1808. He made a hazardous six-month journey with his friend Hyden Hearsey to obtain and bring out some of the fabulous fine-wooled goats whose fibers were made into fashionable shawls in Kashmir. *(Courtesy of the Board of Trustees of the Victoria and Albert Museum, London.)*

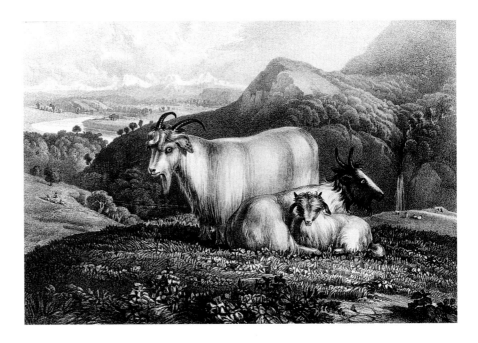

and clothing were made of textiles from the wool of sheep and, in mountainous regions, from the hair of yaks and goats. In some areas pigs were kept, usually in modest numbers.

CASTES AND SACRIFICE

The discrimination of class was an early feature of Aryan society in which an identified nobility was distinguished from the rank-and-file tribesmen. The late Vedic period saw the establishment and concretization of what is today known as the caste system, which hierarchically ordered the members of society on the basis of their occupational niches. Today there are an estimated 3000 castes and 25,000 subcastes in India. Superimposed on this multitude of castes was a far more general grouping of the people into four classes. The priestly upper class of Brahmans claimed precedence over the other classes, including the king and his army, and represented divinity in human form. Their role was to study, teach, and sacrifice. The Kshatriya, or warrior class, ranked next. Its members were expected to protect the people and also to sacrifice and study. The main functions of the Vaishyas were to breed cattle and use them to cultivate the land, and to pursue trade and lend money. The fourth class, the Sudra, served the other three classes. The class distinction also applied to horses, with each human class having its like breed of horse for its use. Thus there were Brahman horses for the priests, a Kehtri for the Kshatriya, a Byes for the Vaishya, and a Seuder for the lowly Sudra.

Sacrificial killings were prevalent under the auspices of the Brahman priestly class. Although buffalo, sheep, goats, and chickens were used, the primary sacrificial animal appears to have been the cow, which the Brahmans sacrificed to propitiate the many gods. The cow was dismembered, and the parts were pointed in the directions of cosmological entities to return the parts to their cosmic origins, allowing the cycle of re-creation to be fulfilled.

One of the most remarkable forms of sacrifice was the royal horse sacrifice or Ashvamedha, in which an ambitious king had a specially consecrated stallion set free to roam for a year and be followed by a selected band of warriors. The chief of every territory the horse entered had to fight or pay homage to the king. If not captured by an enemy, the horse was brought back to the capital at the end of the year and sacrificed in a shocking ceremony in which the king's wife was required to copulate with the dying animal. Despite later rejection of sacrifice, the Ashvamedha continued to be performed on occasion, the last episode being in the ninth century AD.

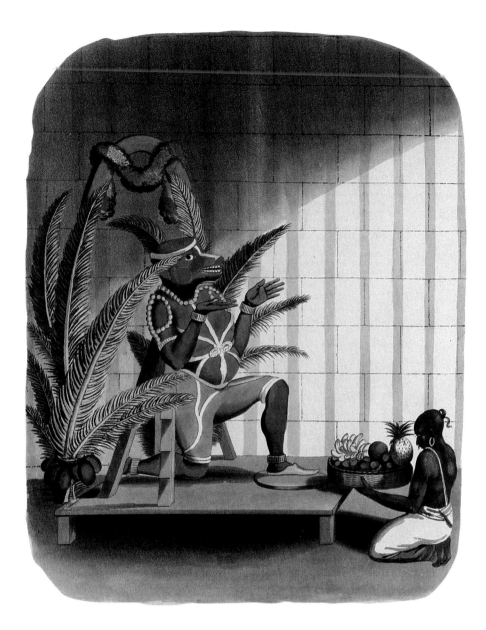

108. A Brahman making an offering of fruits to Hanuman the monkey-god in the temple of Perambur, Madras. Brahmans were part of a complex caste system that afforded power and rights to various strata of society in India. Depending on their level, Brahmans took part in sacrifice of both cows and horses. Colored aquatint by Medland after Charles Gold's oriental drawings of 1806, which were sketched between 1791 and 1798. *(Courtesy of the Board of Trustees of the Victoria and Albert Museum, London.)*

THE GROWTH OF ASCETICISM

During the mid-centuries of the first millennium BC the Indian subcontinent went through a period of tumultuous social change. Tribal affiliations began to decline in importance as the old groups fell apart or were incorporated into more powerful kingdoms. The result was a growth in feelings of insecurity about the future as people found themselves facing the sorrows of hunger, disease, poverty, and death without the old support provided by closely knit groups. United with a yearning for knowledge that could not be gleaned from the Vedas and a dissatisfaction with the pessimistic components of Brahman philosophy, these feelings led to the emergence and growth of asceticism. As asceticism grew, the belief that the functions of the universe depended on sacrifice slowly began to diminish. Instead of atoning for sin through sacrifice, avoiding sin in the first place became paramount.

During the first millennium BC the theories of *samsara,* or transmigration of souls, and *karma,* the idea that actions made in the present or past lives affect one's present and future, came to be widely adopted. These two concepts are crucial to the concept of *ahimsa* (or harmlessness, that is, noninjury to animals and people), and they continue to shape South Asian attitudes toward animals today.

117

BUDDHISM AND JAINISM: AVOIDANCE OF HARM TO ANIMALS

Both Siddartha Gautama, the Buddha or Enlightened One (567-486 BC), and Vardhamana Mahavira, or Great Hero (540-468 BC), were Indian Kshatriyas and aristocrats who left their homes around the age of thirty to lead ascetic life-styles. Both men made ahimsa an important component of their beliefs, although Mahavira carried the concept to the extreme. Unlike the Buddha, who eventually modified his asceticism, Mahavira remained an ascetic all his life. He is generally considered the founder of modern Jainism, which continues to exist and today has more than two million adherents.

Central to the Jain religion is the belief in samsara and the denial of the existence of a supreme being. Jain monks were initiated by having all their hair pulled out by the roots, and they were required to abjure killing, stealing, lying, sexual activity, and possession of property. Ahimsa was paramount. Drinking water was strained to save the animalcula, feather dusters were used to gently clear the path of ants and other insects, and a veil was worn over the mouth to avoid entry and destruction of flying insects. Agriculture was forbidden because plowing and cultivating involved the killing of many plants and soil organisms. Eating meat was proscribed for all Jains. Mahavira himself went naked and said that all things had *jiva* (souls) and to eat them was murder through ingestion. Devout Jains were encouraged to fast unto death, a philosophical goal that was to be adopted as a political weapon against central authority. Predictably a majority of Jain followers took a less challenging path, as Buddha had provided for his believers.

Since the soul could migrate into any animate object, objects were classified into five groups depending on the number of senses they possessed. The highest class had five senses and included gods, humans, and higher animals. The next group was said to lack hearing and included some of the insects. Third came those that allegedly could neither hear nor see, including ants and fleas. Fourth were things that had only taste and touch. The final grouping had only touch and included rocks, plants, earth, fire, and water.

Gautama's discourses were recorded in *sutras*. He strove to define the principles of true reasoning and right judgment. He referred to perception, inference, and comparison, thereby opening the intellectual window to evaluation of traditions and to originality of thought. This effort released a tide of philosophical and scientific energy. The Buddha gave up pure asceticism after many years, seeking instead to lead a life following the Middle Way, a balanced path between the worldly and the ascetic. He gained many followers, teaching his philosophy of transmigration of the soul and the struggle to improve by self-analysis. The Buddha expressed his doctrine as having only one flavor, the emancipation from sorrow, which was derived from cravings for individual satisfaction. Hence the only way to escape the endless, sorrowful round of rebirth was to overcome such cravings.

Buddhist monks developed communities that attracted pilgrims. They developed simple medical care using five basic medicines: butter, ghee, oil, honey, and molasses. These grew into a range of health-promoting foods and a substantial pharmacopoeia as the monks started to serve the laity. From these humble beginnings a new system of medicine began to emerge called *ayurveda* or "the knowledge of longevity."

EMPEROR ASHOKA'S EDICTS AND *PINJRAPOLES*

The nonkilling religions continued to gain followers until the great Mauryan Emperor Ashoka (269-232 BC), grandson of Chandragupta Maurya (whose dynasty was the first to unite the cultures of Gangetic and Indus valleys), adopted Buddhism as the state religion. After a war to conquer Kalinga (now Orissa) that involved massive loss of life, he turned to Buddha's laws. He had edicts carved on stone pillars, one of which specifically prohibited the slaughter of animals. Another edict stated that everywhere provision was to be made for two kinds of medical treatment, treatment for people and for animals. The great impact of Buddhism in India was to turn the Brahmans away from animal sacrifices and toward a new pacifism and humanitarianism.

Ashoka's edicts are the first mention of what are known today as *pinjrapoles* or charitable animal hospitals, although they may have existed before his reign. Which religious sect founded the first pinjrapoles is unknown, but it seems likely to have been the Jains, since they run the pinjrapoles in India today. They are most common in Gujarat, the region with the greatest population of Jains. All kinds of injured and sick animals were and still are to be found in these hospitals, receiving food, shelter, and treatment for their sufferings. True veterinarians seem not to have been employed at pinjrapoles, but the individuals who treated the animals must have become quite skilled at treating fractured limbs and other common health problems. This remarkable idea of animal shelters providing health care preceded human hospital development in most parts of the world.

COW WORSHIP

Hinduism holds the cow to be a sacred animal and bans Hindus from killing cows or eating their flesh. The origin of this reverence for the cow is still debated. Traditionally the sanctity of the cow has been seen to derive from the role of the animal in Vedic ritual and literature and from the concept of ahimsa. Other theories suggest that the cow was used to achieve the economic and political goals of historical Indian states or to combat the influence of Buddhism and Islam.

Belief in the sacred nature of the cow has resulted today in one third (237 million) of the world's cattle being compressed into three percent of the Earth's surface. To Western eyes this situation has seemed odd and irrational; the cows have been seen as competing with humans for resources in a hungry society. In 1966, however, Marvin Harris proposed an ecological basis for the origin of cow veneration. He suggested that cattle and people exist symbiotically in India, the cow and the ox providing crucial services to the rural people. The bullocks give farmers a cheap, reliable source of traction; cows provide dairy products; and both produce much-needed dung for use as fuel, shelter, and fertilizer. Even when the cattle die, they are not wasted, since *harijans* (outcastes) skin and eat the animals. These arguments explain why the tradition has managed to survive over the centuries, but they are difficult to accept as an explanation for the origin of the belief. Certainly, Buddhism's strong opposition to animal sacrifice had a great influence on Brahman practices, bringing an end to cattle sacrifice by the fourth century AD, but it was not an easy battle. In the first millennium BC one Brahman addressed the argument that cattle should not be eaten because the gods had endowed them with cosmic power by replying, "That may very well be, but I shall eat of it nevertheless if the flesh is tender."

The *goshala* is an animal shelter that provides refuge for old, useless, unwanted cattle. Unlike the pinjrapole, a Jain tradition, the goshala is a Hindu institution designed solely to preserve and protect cows. The first goshalas

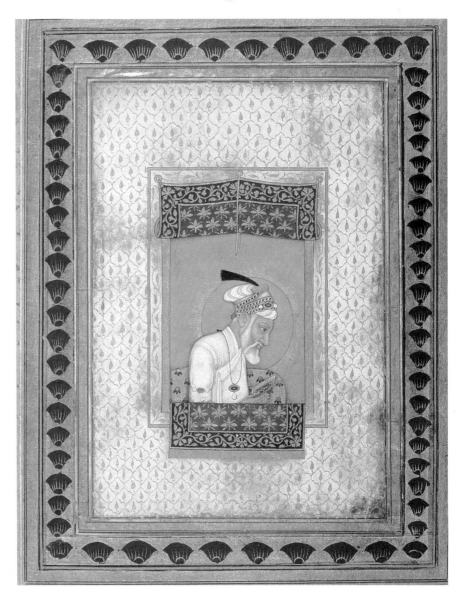

109. Aurangzeb (1659-1707), Akbar's great-grandson, reading from the Koran. *(Oriental and India Office Collections, The British Library, London.)*

110. *Facing page,* Akbar (1555-1606), first of the four great Mughal emperors, shown hunting with cheetahs. Akbar was eventually influenced by Jain monks to prohibit the killing of animals. *(Courtesy of the Board of Trustees of the Victoria and Albert Museum, London.)*

may have been created out of reverence for Krishna, one of the most popular Hindu gods, but today most of them have a secondary role, serving as small dairies. Nevertheless, they are subsidized by charitable donations as part of Hindu commitment to the ideals of *dharma* (righteousness) and ahimsa.

It is probably no accident that the first recorded references to goshalas occur in the twelfth century AD. The rule of Muslim conquerors, whose extensive incursions into India began in the eleventh century, helped make the sanctity of the cow absolute. The Islamic practices of eating beef and sacrificing cattle at the festival of Bakr Id were a source of great tension between Hindus and Muslims. Some Islamic leaders made efforts to soothe Hindu anxiety and create an atmosphere of peaceful coexistence. Babar (1526-1530) is believed to have issued a decree forbidding the killing of cattle, and Akbar (1555-1606), the first of the four great Moghul emperors, was influenced by Jain monks to declare slaughter of animals illegal.

Akbar's great-grandson Aurangzeb (1659-1707) attacked the tolerant policies of his predecessors, and conflict between Hindus and Muslims intensified. The main opposition came from Shivaji (1627-1680), who claimed that his duty was to save the cow and the Brahman from the Muslim. The cow thus became a symbol of Hindu power. The sanctity of the cow again served as an important standard for Hindus in their struggle to gain freedom from the British in the nineteenth and twentieth centuries. Mahatma Gandhi, who played a crucial role in achieving Indian independence, explained the importance of the cow thus:

> The real essence of Hinduism lies in the protection of the cow, the embodiment of the pre-human world, the giver of riches, the basis of agriculture, the mother of the people.

120

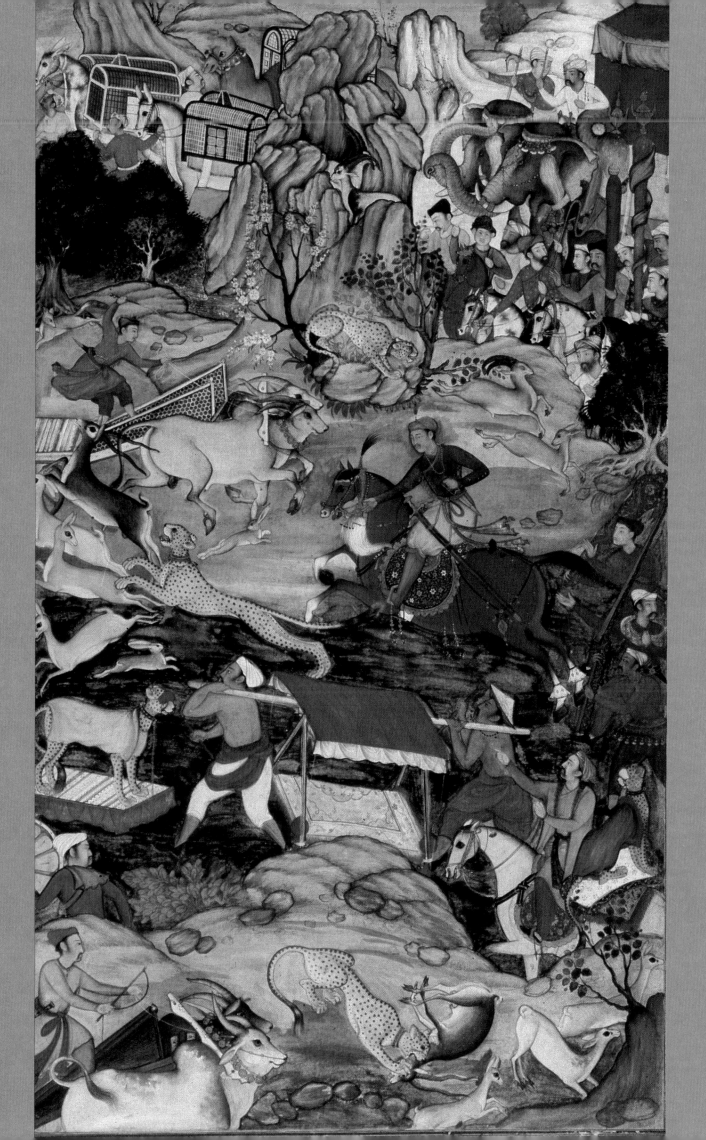

111. The importance of the horse in South Asia developed from its military use. Three of Shah Jahan's sons, Shuja, Aurangzeb, and Murad, are shown on horseback with spears and swords. *(Courtesy of the Board of Trustees of the Victoria and Albert Museum, London.)*

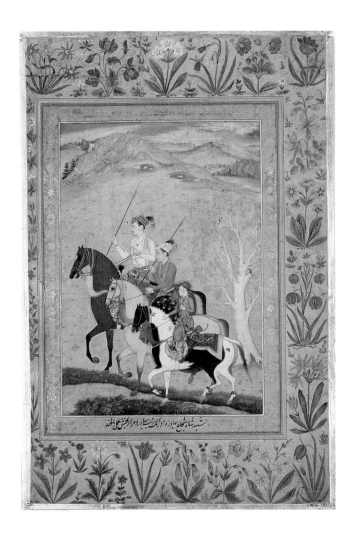

PRELITERATE ROOTS OF INDIAN MEDICINE

The evolution of veterinary medicine in the Indian cultures was influenced greatly by the emergence of medicine as a scholarly field. The ancient mythology invoked other-worldly powers to explain events beyond human control. Belief in demons as causes of sickness and deranged behavior was widespread. The Atharva Veda shows that the priestly class influenced the management of disease in humans and animals through prayers, incantations, spells, potions, and exorcisms. In the Rig-Veda the term *bhisaj* referred to a healer of disease. Later, the traditional doctor became known as a *vaidya.* Yoga was practiced in an effort to gain total mastery over both body and mind via a virtual self-hypnosis; this practice served as an excellent medical preventative. Among the recognized diseases were *takman,* the fever that appeared with the onset of the monsoon, presumably malaria, and *yaksma,* which was consumption or tuberculosis.

Indian approaches to care of the sick included herbal and mineral preparations as treatments. Garlic was thought to promote health. The *Rauwolfia serpentina* plant (Indian snakeroot) was used to treat psychiatric disorders and hypertension; today an extract yields the tranquilizer reserpine, which has been used to avoid panic crowding and hypertension in turkeys. Hemp was used to induce an anesthesia-like trance in people and animals before surgery. *Berberis aristata* was used to check diarrhea. Its active ingredient, berberine, has been shown to reduce fluid loss caused by cholera or toxicogenic *Escherichia coli* infection. Ethnomedicine is largely botanical and applies to veterinary as well as medical applications. P.O. Boddings, in 1927, was the first to collate the aboriginal medicinal plant lore in English, complete with symptoms of diseases for which the herbs were used. The subject has reached vast proportions: more than two thousand herbs are mentioned in the literature.

THE CLASSICAL PERIOD OF HINDU MEDICAL SCHOLARSHIP

Building on the folklore concerning medical matters and the Vedic mythology and scholarship of the priestly class, a cadre of physician-scholars began to emerge. The Vedas allude to the surgeons of the gods, the Asvinkumara twins born of a god in the form of a mare, in a myth remarkably similar to the Greek tale of Chiron. Another legend had it that the god Indra imparted knowledge of life and surgery to the miraculous horse Dhanvantari, to whom the invention of the ayurvedic approach to medicine and health is attributed. Greek ideas may have been incorporated after Alexander the Great's conquest of the Indus valley region in the fourth century BC. Indian medical thought devised a system of three humors, reminiscent of the four Greek humors. The words used, *vata, pitta,* and *kapha* (for wind, bile, and phlegm, respectively), must not be taken literally. They are abstract terms. When all three are in harmonic balance, the human or animal is healthy. When they are not, pathophysiologic activity brings about imbalances among the seven body constituents (chyle, blood, flesh, fat, bone, marrow, and semen), which lead to signs of disease. A remedy must be selected that will bring the humors back into balance, reset the balance of the elements, and restore health.

The legacy of the Indian medical origins was brought together in a great landmark *samhita* or treatise written in Sanskrit by the legendary Caraka, who may have been connected with the great scholarly center at Taxila (Taksasila) about the first century AD, the beginning of the classical period of Indian medical synthesis. He may have lived much earlier, as some claim, and the story may have been written down at that time. His ideas evolved in part from roots that go back to the Buddhist *sangha,* or community. Caraka is also listed as author of a text in verse on animal healing. His acclaimed samhita is probing and philosophical, a comprehensive compendium on matters medical. It is remarkable for the similarity of its eight branches to the modern medical curriculum, except for the notable omission of surgery: Principles of Medicine, Pathology, Diagnostics, Physiology and Anatomy, Prognosis, Therapeutics, Pharmaceutics, and Means of Assuring Success in Treatment. He focused on eight major categories of disease: diarrhea, fever, dropsy, consumption, tumor, abscess, leprosy, and skin diseases.

Caraka's materia medica includes hundreds of herbal products, many mineral prescriptions, and 177 products of animal origin. The latter list tends to jeopardize its credibility to Western readers but illustrates a different attitude toward animal wastes. It includes for external or internal use snake dung; fumes of burnt snake; eggs of various birds and reptiles; blood, excrement, and urine of all domesticated herbivores, as well as their milk, flesh, and fat; and beeswax and honey. Caraka also noted that becoming a *vaidya* or physician was a process of spiritual rebirth and required an ethical oath of initiation.

India attained a high reputation in surgery after the legendary Susruta from Benares on the Ganges River supposedly wrote his compendium while court physician, probably in the time of the Gupta kings in the fourth century AD, although there are no records that allow establishment of exact dates. It may have been much earlier, or at least may have drawn on ancient sources. Susruta's treatise was the first to cover surgery in detail. It lists more than 120 instruments and many surgical procedures. Amputations, lithotomy, and abdominal invasions had become commonplace, along with a wide range of techniques to probe, drain, extract, or suture. Susruta cited the use of certain ants' pincers to close wounds, the bodies of the ants then being pinched off. He described the setting of compound fractures and cesarean sections. He performed cataract operations and provided detailed coverage of ophthalmology. The samhita became famous for its original coverage of plastic surgery. Susruta was said to have pioneered an effective technique for skin flap trans-

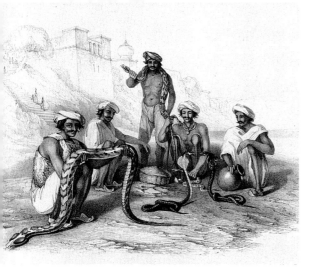

112. In Hinduism the cobra is believed to be a god—Nagar Amman. Both cobras and pythons are used by snake charmers in performing their celebrated feats. The skills of snake catchers are required for the capture of snakes found in the home, since they are not to be harmed. In *Itinerant Snake Catchers,* these unique animal handlers exhibit a supply of pythons and cobras for sale to snake charmers. Drawn from nature on stone by Major Luard in about 1833. *(Courtesy of the Board of Trustees of the Victoria and Albert Museum, London.)*

plants and was the authority on rhinoplasty (after punishment for adultery), reattaching and restoring the natural appearance of noses, ears, and digits that had been severed. Many approaches to bandaging tailored to specific organs were described. Susruta differentiated genetic and dietary forms of diabetes. He described malaria, which was attributed to mosquitoes; plague, which was known to be accompanied by deaths in rats; and smallpox. He mentioned 760 medicinal plants and described external medications.

Strengths of Indian medicine included wound treatment, particularly the removal of arrows and arrowheads, which caused the predominant injury in an age of archery and chariot warfare. Many horses must have sustained this type of wounding and required such treatment. Snakebite was a dreaded eventuality in the land of cobras, and logical therapy was developed, including using a tourniquet, cutting the wound and sucking it, then applying a red-hot coal to the wound. Prayers *(mantras)* were said to consecrate the procedure and invoke the assistance of the gods. More than 10,000 people and untold numbers of livestock may still die of snakebite in South Asia every year.

The Indian medical leadership of the classical era of Caraka and Susruta applied scholarship and intuitive genius to idealistic goals. The depth of understanding of the effects of the physical and psychological environment of the individual was impressive. Considering that there was a taboo on physical contact with human corpses, the Indian achievements are all the more remarkable. Their commitment to dietetics and preventive medicine, to efficacy in treatment, and to the maintenance of health is as valid today as it was 2000 years ago. It applies equally to animals and humans. The two classic compendia form the foundation pillars on which the framework of ayurvedic medicine was constructed.

South Asian medical scholarship went into stagnation and decline around AD 500, when the region experienced the tumult of repeated invasions by aggressive pillagers and conquerors. A bright spot appeared in the seventeenth century, however, when Anandaraya wrote *Jivananda,* a great allegorical tale in which King Jiva (life) suffers many personified diseases in his body fortress.

113. The remarkable range of surgical instruments depicted in this ancient Tibetan medical scroll is comparable to that developed by the famous Indian surgeon, Susruta. His *samhita* (treatise) listed 101 blunt and 20 sharp instruments. The sharps included lancets and knives of various shapes, bistouries, scissors, saws, drills, trocars, and needles. Among the blunts were various forceps, pincers, hooks, loops, tubes, catheters, and sounds or probes. Splints and sutures were employed, and skin grafting for plastic surgery was a specialty. Alcohol was used to suppress sensitivity, and inhalant dispensers were made. Cauterization and boiling fluids were used, suggesting an awareness of the idea of wound contamination. Lithotomy was practiced for stone. *(Courtesy The East Asian Library, University of California, Berkeley.)*

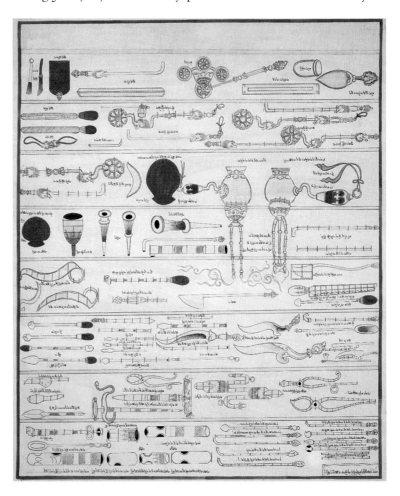

After many mighty battles the enemies are repulsed by the joint efforts of medicine, religion, and yoga. This medical drama characterizes the historical sweep of Indian medicine from its mystical beginnings, its professional scholarship, and its ascetic beliefs. It could be regarded as a framework of thinking for the field of geriatrics. Most Hindus still use some form of ayurvedic medicine today. Starting from a holistic approach to the patient, the practice is based solely on observations and conclusions; that is, treatment is based on inference—experiments are of no purpose. In the words of Caraka, "There is very little that can be obtained from direct proof. The province beyond direct experimental evidence is vast."

Inoculation of people for smallpox was practiced widely in Bengal in the eighteenth century. Although the disease was recognized in ayurvedic texts, there is no word about its prevention by inoculation. Islamic medicine, based on the Canon of Avicenna, *Al-Qanun fi't-Tibb,* came to India after the Afghan invasions in the eleventh century. The Indian name for it is *Yunani Tibb,* an interesting derivation from Greek (Ionian) and Persian. The Yunani physician or *hakim* treats Muslim patients, and ayurvedic physicians treat Hindus.

ANIMALS IN BATTLE

The fighting that marked the decline of medical scholarship paradoxically increased the demand for competent veterinarians. Elephants, horses, and, to a lesser extent, dogs formed important parts of the fighting forces and consequently often suffered battle wounds. In addition, contagions resulted from the congregation of large groups of animals and the various stresses to which they were subjected.

Elephants trained for war duties appear first in the Buddhist texts. The elephant had been tamed before 500 BC but was seldom bred in captivity, primarily because of a phenomenon known as *musth,* the Urdu word for "intoxicated." Musth occurs periodically but irregularly in male elephants and is characterized by various physiological and behavioral changes that cause the animal to become more irascible and dangerous. Plasma testosterone levels climb by as much as fifty-fold, and a profuse, sticky, odoriferous secretion that can be seen running from the temporal glands is rubbed on foliage as a marker. Frequent dribbling of urine occurs, and the elephant displays a characteristic walk with the head held high, often swinging its head in a figure-of-eight motion. Aggressive use of tusks may be seen. Several times each hour the bull emits a deep, low-frequency rumbling sound that carries far. The sounds and associated behavior may arouse the females. In the tamed situation, however, a bull in musth may go berserk and have to be chained to a tree.

114. A Rajasthan miniature depicts a group of armed mahouts trying to restrain a bull in musth that has snapped its holding chains and is running amok. *(Explorer Archives, Paris.)*

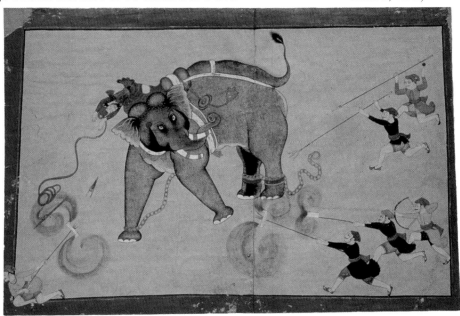

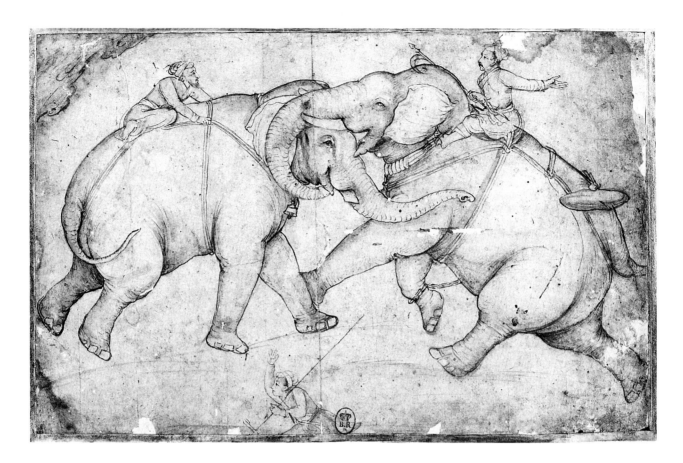

115. Elephant fighting was once a popular sport in some parts. The great beasts were goaded by their mahouts and sometimes were provoked by spectators who waved rods with firecrackers attached. *(Bibliothèque Nationale, Paris.)*

Because elephants were seldom bred in captivity, a continuing demand existed for tracking, hunting, herding, and taming the forest herds. The practical knowledge of elephant handling arose in the non-Aryan aboriginal forest tribes. Capture of wild elephants was accomplished by putting tame females in a stockade to attract their wild conspecifics into it. Koonkies or trained elephants were used to contact the wild ones and calm them during the final roping and training steps. Temperament and health were evaluated under the guidance of the elephant doctor in the selection of animals suitable for domestication. The *Arthashastra,* essentially a detailed government manual used from 300 BC to AD 300, included rules for land use and forest preservation as they pertained to elephant production. It also laid out the procedures for catching, training, and classifying elephants and for their military training, nutrition, management, and stabling.

Elephants were a threat to agricultural crops, and ownership was restricted to ruling families, whom they served as symbols of prestige and ceremony. In battle, elephants were used like a modern tank corps, breaking down fortifications while making openings in troop formations for the soldiers to exploit. They helped move armies through mountainous areas or across shallow rivers and swamps. They were protected with leather armor but could be panicked by fire, and it was a common error to be overly reliant on them. Alexander the Great memorialized in coins his victory in 326 BC over King Porus of Lahore and his army of more than one hundred elephants. Alexander's tactics were to allow the pachyderms to penetrate his lines, then to direct his men to attack their extremities with ax and sword, turning them against their own troops. As the elephants charged back, Alexander's men jabbed them from behind and they trampled the soldiers of Porus, creating panic.

Cavalry, a separate division of the army, was never perfected to the degree attained by many of India's invaders. The two-man fighting chariot was the major military vehicle from the Vedic period through the Mauryan empires (324-187 BC). Horses were bred mainly in the northwestern regions and in Sind or imported from Arabia and Persia, then distributed to the warrior class for military and sporting activities.

Despite having animal brigades, the South Asian forces suffered many defeats in confronting the aggressive forays of the Turkic tribes from the steppes of central Asia, which began in the sixth century AD. These tribes later adopted Islam to varying degrees and formed a loosely knit realm of autonomous groups under military leaders called *khans.* They were nomadic pastoralists and hunters on tough little Mongolian horses, herding sheep over a vast range from the north of China to the Black Sea. A remarkable example of domination and interdependence between humans and animals, they became as one with their horses, managing to control their steeds while shooting rapidly in any direction with their double-curved bows. No other force of their period could compete with their maneuverability and devastating effectiveness. Some of the tribes invaded with the aim of capturing territory, but looting was the usual motive.

The Turkic tribes used camels as well as horses to great effect. After conquering the Indus Valley peoples, Mahmud (leader of the Ghaznavid tribe) crossed the Thar desert in 1024 with a massive caravan of 30,000 camels to attack the sacred Hindu temple of Somnath on the shores of Gujarat. The tribe's sturdy desert horses were far superior to those of the Indians, who lacked the talent and environment favorable for horse breeding. The Ghaznavids were supplanted by the Seljuk Turks or Ghurs, who were led by sultans into India after 1206.

In 1398 Timur the Lame (Tamerlane), a later Mongol conqueror, led a force of Muslims from Samarkand into India through Afghanistan. He marched toward Delhi, where the sultanate was in decline and disintegrating into fiefdoms, and took on the sultan's forces, which included a large number of war elephants. Tamerlane countered the challenge by driving a squadron of

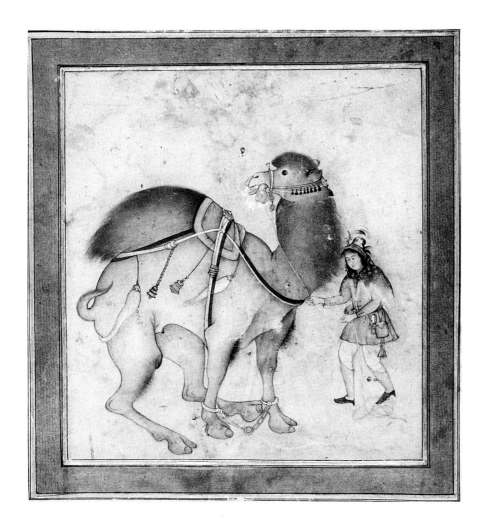

116.   In addition to horses and elephants, the camel was used for military purposes in South Asia with great success, especially by the Turkic tribes. The scene of a camel and its driver was a favorite subject of the Mughal painter Safavid and of the Ottoman genre. This piece dates back to the artist Bihzad in late fifteenth century Herat. Album leaf (c. 1600). *(The British Museum, London.)*

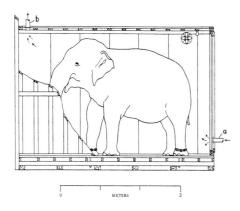

117. Side view of a respiration chamber with pipes to introduce and remove gases, whose volumes could be measured and gaseous composition analyzed to study metabolism. *(From Benedict, 1936.)*

camels laden with bales of straw ahead of his army, then firing the straw as the camels reached the pachyderms and driving the blazing fleet of "desert ships" straight at them. The elephants were terrified and turned to flee through the ranks of their own troops, who fled as well. When the rout was complete, Tamerlane ordered the sack of the city, which yielded him yet another mighty harvest of skulls and slaves.

A final invasion came when Babar, a Mongol, led his warriors into India in the 1520s. He defeated the elephant defenses by using guns and archery to shoot the mahouts. His grandson, Akbar, built the great Mughal empire on a basis of tolerance of diverse religious beliefs. This wise leader had a tremendous knowledge of elephants and was considered an excellent elephant driver.

VETERINARY MEDICINE: PALAKAPYA'S ELEPHANTOLOGY

The heavy dependence on elephants and horses in warfare caused the veterinarian's role to be held in high esteem. There were specific horse doctors, and a detailed text on venesection in the horse was produced. A remarkably large armamentarium of natural products was available to be used in therapy.

A number of animal healers over the centuries are mentioned in the literature surviving today. Some of the Buddhist Jatakas describe elephant doctors as an identifiable professional cadre. Palakapya, a legendary figure of the Epic period, is said to have been the author of the *Hastyayurveda* (derived from *hastin,* the Sanskrit word for "having a hand"—a reference to the elephant's trunk—and *ayur* or "long life"). The treatise was dedicated to the god Ganesha and began with Vedic prayers. The text describes the knowledge of elephant life and health but has not appeared in full in translation. It stated that elephants in the wild seldom get sick but that the captive elephants had many health problems.

The treatise covered diseases in four categories: introduction and major diseases, lesser ailments and poisons, surgery and obstetrics, and therapeutics. Of elephant diseases, 315 are described as attributable to winds, spleen, mucus, or blood or their various combinations, a classification that exhibits some similarity to the Greek concept of the four humors. The Greek connection also appears in a description of the ideal elephant veterinarian, which is remarkably similar to the Hippocratic ideal of a physician. One severe fever called *rakala* was said to be specific for elephants. *Raja yakshma* or tuberculosis received special attention. It was attributed to overwork and working during excessive exposure to sun and heat. A wide range of signs was observed, and the prognosis was unfavorable. The section on surgery included discussions of wound treatment and suturing, as well as the daunting task of restraining the massive patient for surgical intervention. Restraint was particularly challenging because the elephant was not a fully domesticated animal; principles of acupuncture were used to identify sites useful in controlling elephants.

The most common ailments of tamed, captive elephants included skin sores, cracked feet, indigestion, pneumonia, tuberculosis, and inflamed eyes. Two forms of tuberculosis, one a wasting disease and the other a pulmonary form, were described in a 2000-year-old Hindu text. Working elephants tended to be overworked and fed unsuitable diets, which led to exhaustion and colic. War elephants suffered from wounds, embedded arrows, or fractures and subsequent infections. They were frequently given alcoholic draughts with a view to making them more aggressive.

Dental problems occurred in elephants, and age was estimated by examining the color and physical structure of the teeth. If a tusk, which is a modified incisor, was broken short enough to expose the pulp, infection could enter and cause excruciating pain. Similarly, abscesses of the roots of molars

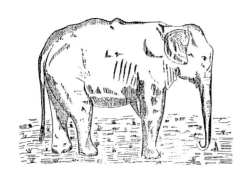

118. Working elephants suffered from a variety of maladies, including soreback, which resulted from the loss of some spinal processes. *(From Evans, 1910.)*

could occur, and overgrowths could lead to malocclusion. To compensate for the tremendous wear on their teeth, elephants replace their teeth five times. When the sixth set of teeth has completed its cycle of wear, the toothless old elephant dies of starvation, usually by the age of sixty-five years.

In Ceylon (now Sri Lanka) King Buddhadasa (AD 362-409) was both a devout Buddhist and a trained practitioner of ayurvedic medicine. He would treat any patient he encountered on his travels who needed help, human or animal, without discrimination. He appointed horse and elephant doctors, establishing a strong tradition for animal care in Ceylon.

Observing the elephant's habit of consuming the soil of salt flats when it has colic is said to have led to the use of salts in the treatment of human indigestion. Sukumara Barkath wrote the *Hastividyarnava* in the eighteenth century, which contained many details about types and individual behaviors of elephants, described diseases, and provided an extensive materia medica. Surgery, however, had been dropped from the repertoire of treatments.

Today forage deficiency and environmental stress resulting from climatic changes are major factors causing losses in the wild. Poaching for ivory is an added risk, particularly for the African elephant but also for the Asian species. Modern studies of infectious and parasitic diseases have shown that the elephant is susceptible to a number of serious viral and bacterial infections and endoparasitic and ectoparasitic infestations.

119. The circus career of Anno, the first Indian elephant to be brought to Germany, began in Frankfurt am Main in 1629. Engraving by Wenzel Hollar. *(Staatliche Graphische Sammlung, Munich.)*

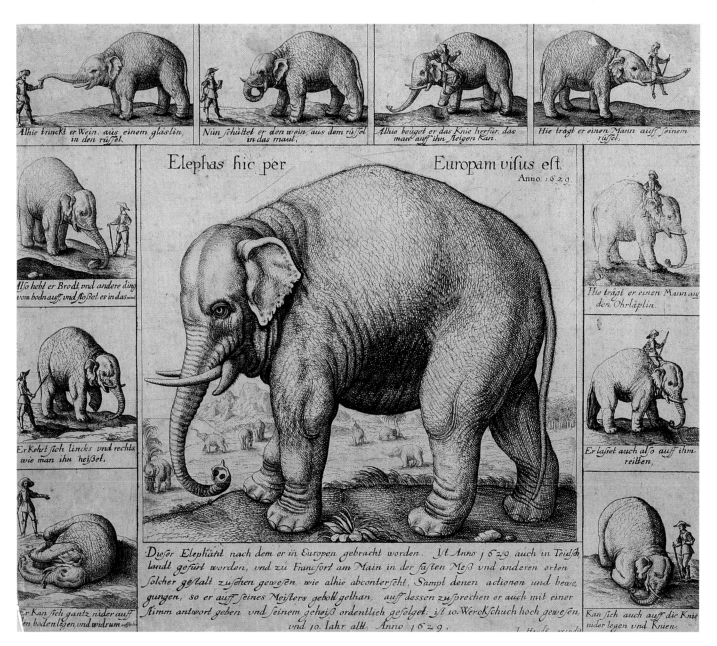

EQUINE VETERINARY MEDICINE: SALIHOTRA

Salihotra of Salutar, near Kandahar, was the first Indian horse-healer of whom records exist. His name is associated with everything dealing with horse care. Veterinarians became known as *Salihotriya,* from which the modern name *salutri* was derived. The Sanskrit term *salihotrasastra* implied veterinary medicine. The *Asvayurveda Siddhayoga Samgraha* of Salihotra dates to the fourth century AD, and his name was invoked again in later texts. Vagbhata, a Buddhist physician famous for his revision of the classic medical texts, was also listed as author of a veterinary text on horse medicine. Drugs were administered by nasogastric tube and via balls (boluses), drenches, and clysters. The traditions of castration, bleeding, blistering, firing, and cautery were practiced. Hooves received special attention, and the eye was examined to confirm the judgment of prognosis.

The Imperial Council of Agricultural Research in 1937 authorized an investigation into the collection of information about an uncharted field, indigenous veterinary medicine, under the direction of Krishnaswamy of the Civil Veterinary Department in Madras. He published a series of articles over the next eight years on animal husbandry and veterinary science in ancient India. He noted that the best source of his information had been the Sarasvati Mahal Library in Tanjore in southern India.

The highlight of Krishnaswamy's findings was that during the reign of Shahjahan a voluminous work on horses and veterinary science, written in Sanskrit by Salihotra, was obtained from Chittur near Madras in southern India. The emperor had ordered that it be translated into Arabic, and it became the *Kitab-ul-Vitrat.* This version was translated into English, and a copy exists in the British Museum. A part of the original work in Sanskrit, thought to be lost, was found in the Tanjore library with material on veterinary science. Other parts may exist in other Indian sites, as well as in Nepal and Tibet.

The *Asva Vaidyaka* in Jayadatta, another ancient work of the Epic period, reviewed earlier works, including that of Salihotra. Topics included equine breeding, feeding, management, diseases, and treatments. It provided, in considerable detail, names for the parts of the body of the horse and measurements based on a unit of a finger's width or *angula.* Of particular interest is the term *marma* or *vidu,* which was defined as the vital point—eleven and one-half centimeters downward from the root of the ear—used to shoot horses for instant killing. Also identified were the *ksirika* or the part inside the cheeks where the pulse is felt and the *asrupata* or site of the angular vein below the eye, which was a preferred vessel for bleeding in certain diseases.

Ancient books gave detailed recommendations on horse management, feeding, rules for training, temperament, gaits, longevity, and determination of age by patterns and colors of the teeth, as well as expectations of the rider. Serious blemishes in horses were considered omens of trouble in the offing. These included monstrosities and disabling deformities as well as obvious abnormalities such as being born with three ears, divided hooves, or only one testicle. Enormously detailed attention was given to animals' colors, the sounds of their vocalizations, and their dimensions and shapes.

CATTLE HUSBANDRY AND DISEASE

Although it is obvious from much of India's ancient literature that cattle were considered essential and valuable to society and were for centuries the basic unit of currency in trading, there is almost no extant literature on cattle diseases and veterinary work. Only a description engraved on the leaves of a fan palm from the Tamil people of the south has survived. Translated into English late in the nineteenth century, it includes illustrations and a materia medica.

Epidemic diseases such as rinderpest, anthrax, and tick fever are identifiable. It must be remembered that cattle were cared for by the peasant-trader class and did not receive the priority status given to the animals of the warrior class, the horse and the elephant. The Salihotriya could be penalized up to the value of the animal for negligence or ineffective treatment.

Many recipes for treatment of common and serious diseases of cattle were developed in ancient India. Even animals afflicted with the plague epidemics of rinderpest and foot-and-mouth disease were treated by the indigenous peoples. Hirachandra reported in 1925 that he had tried such remedies, and he claimed considerable success. The erosive oral and digestive tract lesions of rinderpest were treated with vinegar rinses and drenches. The *bael* fruit was widely used to control the diarrhea seen in rinderpest cases. For foot-and-mouth disease the mouth was rinsed with a decoction made from *babul* bark *(Acacia arabica),* and ulcers were dressed with astringent *neem* oil (oil of *Margosa indica*) mixed with camphor. Dysentery in cattle was treated with the bark of *Hollarrhena antidysenterica,* which contains conessine. Because there was no numerical reporting on survivorship, the efficacy of these early folk remedies remains uncertain. Other bovine epizootics included anthrax, piroplasmosis (tick fever), and hemorrhagic septicemia.

Although rabies was treated, the claims of success are almost certainly exaggerated. Treatment was to be started immediately after the animal victim was bitten by an animal suspected of being rabid. The bite wound was treated with a herbal paste and ghee. Presumably depending on the species, herbal emetics and purgatives were administered. If clinical signs of rabies developed, the body was cooled with water and cooling drinks were given with curd. It was said that this regimen would calm the animal and lead to its cure.

Bloat or tympanitis of cattle was apparently a fairly common occurrence. One village remedy was concocted from ginger root, peppercorns, salt, asafetida, and bark from the drumstick tree. These were pounded together to extract a liquid, which was shaken up in a bottle of warm water and used as a drench. Asafetida, from a species of *Ferula* root, has a powerful odor. Like garlic, it was widely used as an antiseptic to treat wounds and ringworm. Blue stone (copper sulfate?) and petroleum products, after they became available, were popular treatments for foot lesions and for killing maggots. Certain plant extracts were used for their anthelmintic action in calves. A renowned ancient remedy for snakebite in India was *Kuri Mooti Ka,* which consisted of ground *hariali* grass; it was claimed to be quite effective.

Because cattle in India are unique in that they are allowed to complete their natural life span, they tend to manifest degenerative diseases seldom encountered in cattle in other parts of the world. Calvin Schwabe has pointed out that they could be an invaluable resource population for studies of the pathobiologic characteristics of aging.

The indigenous remedy for worms in dogs was powdered areca nut, a purgative and vermifuge. Ipecacuanha root was used in canines as an emetic, an expectorant, and a treatment for severe diarrhea, including that sometimes seen in virus distemper.

The indigenous products used for specific diseases varied greatly by district: more than 2000 have been recorded. This variety suggests that in many cases, clearly effective prescriptions had not been found. There is great potential, however, for finding valuable substances. Today many indigenous plants are being tested for antibacterial, antifungal, anthelmintic, and antiviral properties, as well as for effectiveness in suppression of cancer cell function.

MOORCROFT: AN INDIAN ROLE FOR BRITAIN'S FIRST VETERINARY SURGEON

European contact with India did not occur until the Portuguese explorer Vasco da Gama reached the spice-trading port of Calicut in AD 1498. His countryman Afonso Albuquerque established a settlement at Goa, founding a trading empire on good relations with the native people. The Dutch also had operations in India, but in the latter part of the eighteenth century the British government gradually assumed a dominant role in the subcontinent. Because the cavalry was crucial to maintaining order in the country, farriers became a high priority. Great difficulties were encountered in obtaining suitable horses in India, breeding them in sufficient numbers to meet the army's needs, and keeping them healthy.

The Bengal stud had been established in 1796 at Pusa by the East India Company to breed its own cavalry horses. After initial failures to acquire suitable breeding stock large enough to carry a dragoon and his equipment (252 pounds), the company sought the services of a competent member of the newly established veterinary profession who was a horse specialist to help identify suitable breeding stock for shipment to India in 1800. The person selected was William Moorcroft, the first English-speaking veterinary surgeon, who had graduated in 1791 from the oldest veterinary school in Europe, in Lyon, France, just before England had established its first such school. He served in this consultant role until 1808, when he was appointed superintendent and veterinary surgeon of the company's stud at Pusa and traveled to India to take up his duties.

In London Moorcroft had a large veterinary practice specializing in horses. He had invented a machine to manufacture seated horseshoes that, although well-conceived, was a commercial failure. A truly remarkable man who deserves to be remembered as one of the great role models of the new profession, he was notable for the global compass of his interests and abilities. He was a trained human surgeon and an experienced agriculturist before becoming a veterinarian. A man of vision and curiosity, he combined an adventurous spirit with the incisive ability to take appropriate action that characterizes a skillful surgeon. His passion for horses was matched by a competence that made him the leading veterinary surgeon of his day. Sixteen years after he qualified, he went to India, where he worked for seventeen years until his premature death in 1825.

In India Moorcroft became a legend. He poured his prodigious energies into reforming the mismanaged stud and learning enough about the horse stocks of southern and central Asia to plan a course of action that would allow the company's goals for the stud to be met. His approach was to travel and see for himself the complex network of horse breeders, traders, and users throughout the region. Along the way he visited every British cavalry regiment, horse stud, and horse fair, freely offering his unique skills in management and medical care for animals and humans alike, while accumulating any information that might be of value to the East India Company or the British enterprise in India.

Moorcroft undertook three massive journeys in pursuit of his goals. The first, in 1811, took him more than fifteen hundred miles across India in search of the larger breeding horses he realized would be essential to the stud's success. Although he obtained some animals having better conformation than those at Pusa, he learned that he would have to range farther afield, even beyond India, to locate the class of animal he needed.

On his return Moorcroft made major reforms. He abolished the existing practice of *zamindara* in which many of the stud's stallions were put out with local breeders in the surrounding area on contract for the foals. The concept had potential but had been corrupted by neglect and mismanagement, resulting in inferior progeny, debilitated breeding stock, and compromised quality of the nucleus herd at Pusa because it was stripped of many of its stallions. Another scheme, called *nisfi* (Arabic for "half"), put mares from the stud out with local breeders, who had to bring them back to be bred, the stud guaranteeing purchase of the foal. Half the arbitrated price went to the breeder, the other half to covering the costs of the operation. This was another good idea defeated by the purchase of unsuitable mares, mismanagement and neglect on the farms, and high rates of foal mortality. Moorcroft poured his energies into improving the property and premises of the stud, the quality of breeding stock, and the management and health care of the stock.

Moorcroft's remarkable second journey took him north to Nepal and into Tibet; crossing the Himalaya and Zaskar Ranges he became one of only a few Europeans to reach Lake Manasarowar, at 15,000 feet above sea level. Although he found little to help solve the problems of the stud, he did manage to bring some prized Tibetan shawl-wool goats back with him.

In addition to his personal excursions and consultations, Moorcroft had sent agents to other parts to seek information on procurement of suitable breeders. The solution was identified as the large-boned Turcoman horses of central Asia, which would have to be brought to Pusa from Bokhara across Afghanistan. Thus it became necessary to make a dangerous journey to the northwest to find the sources and negotiate the horses' purchase and transport. Triumph came in 1819 in the form of authorization to make the great journey to the northwestern frontier of India, then across Afghanistan and into the central Asian republics as far as Bokhara. This tremendous undertaking was to command all of Moorcroft's energies for the next six years and to cost him his life.

Although Moorcroft had purchased a few moderately good horses to the east of Bokhara, his journey was scarcely a success as a horse-procuring exercise. His plan was to make a detour from Balkh back to Andkhoi a hundred miles to the west on the way home, having heard that excellent horses might be obtained there. Leaving his main party at Balkh, he rode to Andkhoi and was never seen again. He is believed to have died there of a fever, but mystery surrounds his passing.

On reviewing the Indian phase of Moorcroft's career, it can be stated with assurance that both India and Britain were well served by his presence there. England's first veterinary surgeon and the finest of his times, he brought to his professional role in India the highest available standard of veterinary science and ethics with an enduring commitment to the advancement of knowledge. He was, in a word, unforgettable.

120. British veterinary surgeon Moorcroft and his colleague Captain Hyden Hearsey riding yaks on their perilous mission into Tibet to procure shawl-wool goats. Hearsey had many contacts that facilitated the journey, and he painted this unique picture of the pair en route through the passes of the Himalayas into Tibet. Moorcroft made two other marathon trips in search of better horses for the Pusa stud. The last one was to Central Asia, where he died under mysterious circumstances in 1825. *(The British Library, London.)*

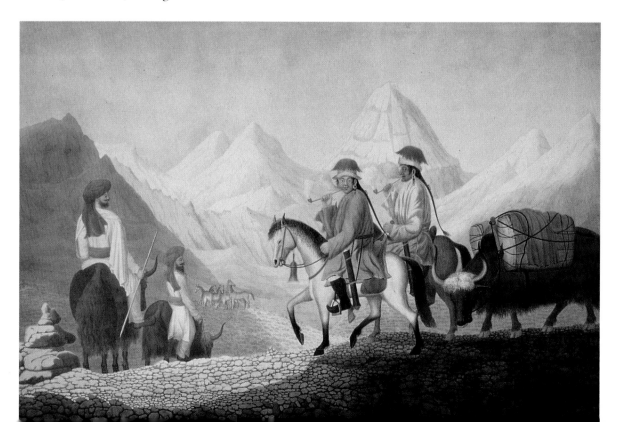

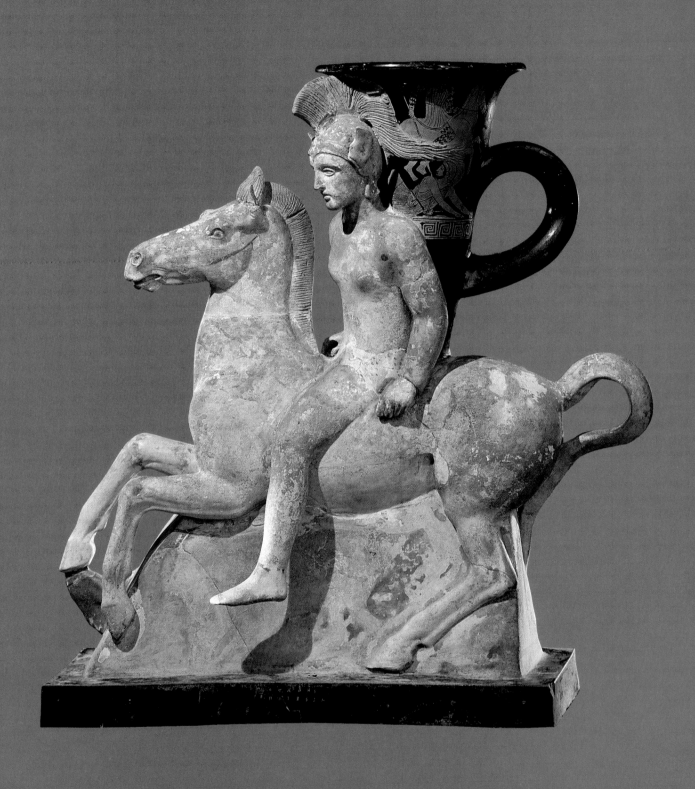

Ancient Greeks

Intellectual Founders of the Health Professions

Ancient Greek civilization stands out from all other civilizations in the course of human history because of its extraordinary commitment to the search for new intellectual truths while casting off the shackles of its rich, often poetic mythology. Yet it is astonishing that this intellectual thrust often was not balanced by a comparable drive to exploit the new knowledge in a practical sense. Also remarkable was the abysmal failure of subsequent cultures to adopt the Grecian achievements and advance them further. Had some of the Greek records not been rescued and translated by Arab scholars, they might well have been lost. Apart from the later flurry of the Renaissance, when serious attempts were made to consolidate what was already known and to take up the intellectual challenge again and make further progress, little intelligent scholarship was accomplished until the second half of the seventeenth century.

The ancient Greeks developed a complex mythology to express the unfathomable aspects of the world they occupied. Their pagan polytheism assigned animal natures to each of their gods. Their mythology comprised many adventurous tales and legends in which animals played prominent roles. Some of the myths were derived from those of the Nile River Valley cultures.

The "roots of the ancient world" for the Greeks meant "Admirers of Mother Earth." Largely an inhospitable, rocky land with many offshore islands, the Greek peninsula and islands spawned rugged seafaring peoples who fished and traded in the Mediterranean Sea. The terrain led to the development of isolated tribal groups with different levels of cultural achievement. The first civilizations were of Achaean people, who shaped the Bronze Age culture of the Balkan Peninsula, its associated islands, and Crete. The old Minoan civilization of Crete became wealthy and developed its own alphabets and written script. The snake, representing the underworld, had to be appealed to as the god of healing before there could be medical intervention for the sick.

Minoan Crete was remarkable for its evidence of a bull cult, presumably based on domesticated cattle brought to the island. The well-known artistic representation of bull-leaping sports in the palace of Minos in Knossos and, later, in Mycenaean Greece shows one of the most daring and acrobatic feats: grabbing the horns while the bull was on the run and somersaulting back over the bull's body.

Mycenae was overrun by Dorians from the north about 1200 BC. Greeks sailed across the Aegean Sea to establish settlements on the shores of Asia Minor that grew into city-states with multicultural trading ports free from traditional patterns of hierarchy.

121. *Facing page,* A bronze rhyton, an ancient Greek drinking horn. An Amazon on horseback makes up the base. In classical Greek mythology Amazons were a race of female warriors believed to live near the Black Sea. Animals figure prominently in Greek mythology, frequently assuming god-like status. From Meroe by Sotades, fifth century BC. *(Harvard and MFA Expedition. Courtesy Museum of Fine Arts, Boston.)*

122. Minoan Crete was renowned for its bull cult. Bull's-head rhyton, found at Knossos, the capital of the ancient Minoan civilization. *(Hirmer Verlag GmbH, München.)*

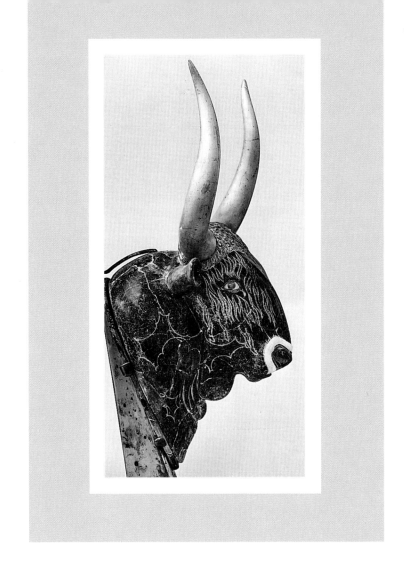

123. Sites of the Greek diaspora of the Classical period and later.

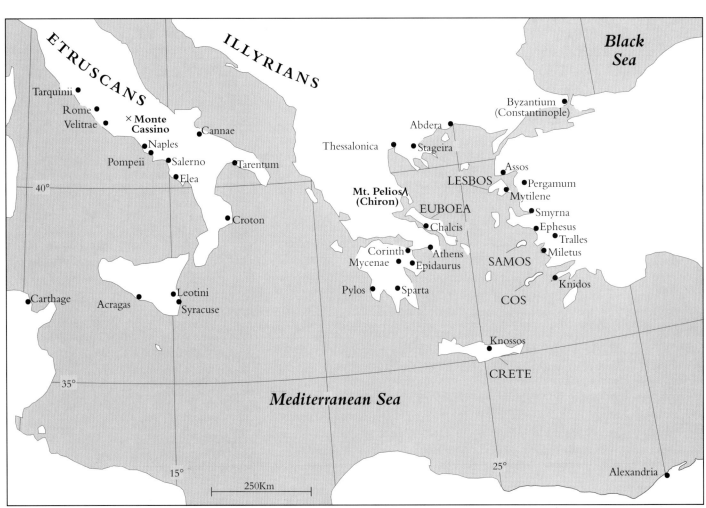

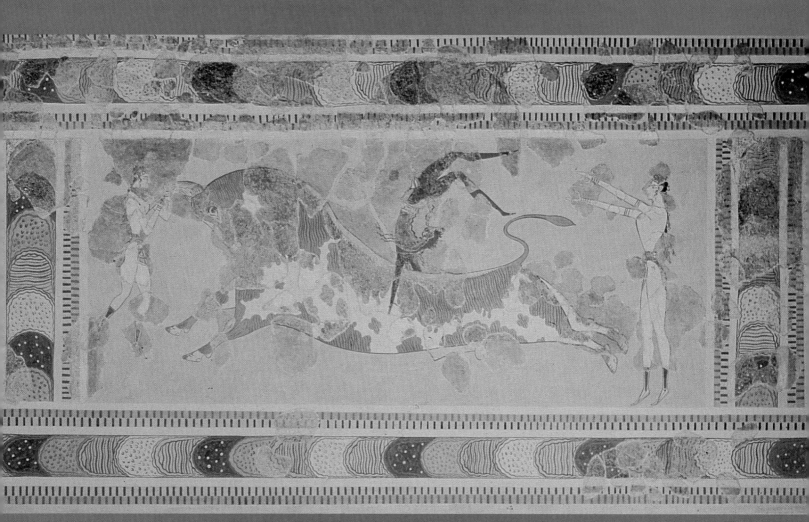

124. The bull-leaping fresco from the palace of Minos in Knossos represents what must have been a risky sport of grabbing the bull's horns and somersaulting over its back. The bull symbolized fertility and power; strength combined with agility would have been needed for such an activity. *(Hirmer Verlag GmbH, München.)*

AGRICULTURAL BASIS OF GREEK CIVILIZATION

Farming and pastoralism provided the livelihood and sustenance for most ancient Greeks, imposing discipline on them and forming the basis of pagan sacrificial religion. A wooden ard drawn by oxen was used to break the ground without turning it. Agriculture, cooking, and sacrifice were the activities that distinguished humans from their wild ancestors and the beasts. Control of the environment was considered essential to farming and to sacrifice, both of which required fire. Provision of animals for sacrifice placed the farmer at the center of civilized existence. The distinction between "wild" and "domestic" was considered essential to an orderly life and extended to personal behavior. Later, sophisticated use of large, yoked teams of oxen was developed to haul the huge stones used for temple construction.

Although some areas such as Epiros, which was noted for its large cattle, had good lowland meadows for every season, Greece was a mountainous region, and pastoral animal production was a significant component of agriculture. The right to pasture animals was restricted to those to whom a grant was made, usually male citizens. Long-distance transhumance of sheep, moving the flocks between winter and summer grazing areas, was common, usually under the aegis of a single city. Occasionally there was cooperation between two city-states. For example, in the second century BC the agreement between Myania and Hypnia was tied to the time of dipping the sheep and the period during which they could graze, but the makeup of the dip was not stated. The movement of sheep was clearly a source of friction and could become an issue of geographical sovereignty. Pasturing fines were extracted for exceeding the allowed number of animals or the agreed period. Fines were higher for pigs than for sheep. Dumping manure was also an offense for which fines could be levied. Special regulations applied to sacred ground; animals allowed to graze there had to be unblemished, but provision was made for the animals of visitors to the festivals, usually asses. Sacrifices and festivals involved cattle (Bouphonia or ox-slaying), sheep, goats, and pigs. Sheep and goats were the usual subjects. Cattle were more commonly sacrificed in earlier, archaic times.

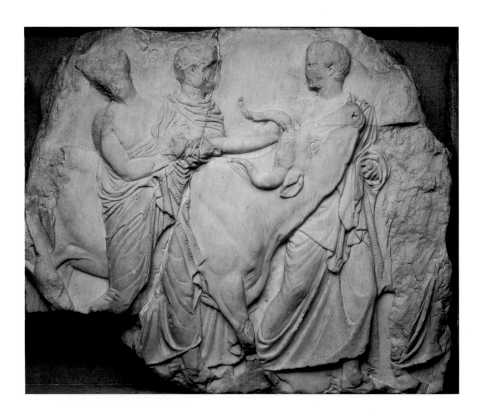

125. At the center of Athenian cult activity was animal sacrifice. A section of the frieze of the Parthenon displays a procession of Athenians and a group of cattle being led to slaughter. Fifth century BC. *(The British Museum, London.)*

PRERATIONAL MEDICAL MYTHS AND LEGENDS

The health professions in ancient Greece, as elsewhere, had their roots in mythology and magic. The gods had to have a doctor, too, and Paian was the first one assigned to dress their wounds and prescribe their herbal medicines. In a tribute to Egyptian prowess in medicine the Greek poet Homer referred to Egyptians as the "race of Paian." Paian was superseded by the legendary centaur Chiron, who became the dominant image in founding comparative medicine; that is, Chiron was both human and animal. A centaur was an imaginary creature with the body and four legs of a horse plus the torso, arms, and head of a man. It has been suggested that militant barbaric cattle raiders from the tribes of Thrace attacking on horseback for the first time (about 1400-1300 BC) may have been the source of the centaur myth. Unlike other centaurs, which were feared and loathed, Chiron was said to combine the basic instinctive knowledge of the natural world (he was a great hunter) derived from his "horsiness," with the higher intellectual traits of a wise man, including sagacity, love of music, and knowledge of the healing arts. Thessaly was a part of Greece that became famous for its horses.

It was said that Chiron was assigned responsibility for educating many exceptional youths, including Asklepios (*Aesculapius* in Latin) and Melampus. He was often regarded as having been a real person who lived in a cave in the Pelion Mountains. A cave that fits the description of Chiron's Cave and Shrine has recently been discovered in eastern Thessaly. Guilds of priest-healers, *Chironidae,* claimed to be descended from Chiron. Aristaios, another pupil of Chiron, became an animal healer. When Chiron died, he became the heavenly constellation Sagittarius. Melampus was said to have learned from Chiron and to have had a unique capacity to communicate with and treat animals. He was said to have been born in 1380 BC and to have lived in Pylos in Messery. He was famous as a shepherd who healed sick sheep. The centaur, symbol of Chiron, was adopted by veterinary groups such as the British Veterinary Association as their distinctive emblem. The United States Veterinary Medicine Association (1863-1898) adopted the symbol as its seal.

Apollo was the mythical god of sickness and healing. The legend has it that his son Asklepios was delivered by cesarean section after his mother was killed, and he was given to Chiron to be educated. Asklepios, Prince of Trikke, became a famous herbal healer and surgeon around whom a cult developed that was based initially on Epidaurus. It was written that he healed humankind and all animals. Roman coins show him treating cattle. Aclianus reported that Asklepios restored the damaged foot of a cock. Dogs, serpents, and birds were kept and were sacred to Asklepios and his daughter Hygeia. Eventually many Asklepions or cult shrines were established, and sick people and animals were brought to them seeking cures. Some became health spas; others evolved into medical schools.

The origin and significance of the emblem of Asklepios, a single snake wound around a stick, is an interesting question, since it has become an international symbol of the medical and veterinary professions. Even the name *Asklepios* was derived from the Thracian words for "snake" *(as)* and "roll" *(klepio).* The sacred snake of Asklepios was a long, nonpoisonous, tree-climbing constrictor species. It is the basis of one explanation put forward as the origin of an alternative symbol of medicine, a rod with two entwined snakes, the caduceus. It seems appropriate to ask why Asklepios had the serpent as his symbol.

A legend was created that the serpent was the real agent of the "dream cure" of the temple of sleep. Entering the innermost depths of the patient's being, the snake accomplished the cure. The healer in human form was excluded from the mysteries of the processes involved. Since this concept was imported to Greece from Egypt, the true healer was the serpent-god

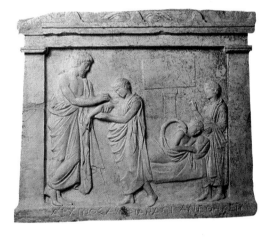

126. According to legend, Asklepios, the son of Apollo, was a great herbal healer and surgeon. Cult shrines were common, and people brought their families and animals for treatment. The staff and snake were symbols of Asklepios; legend determined that the serpent was the source of the cure. In a relief from Attica, Asklepios is shown healing the ailing shoulder of the spirit-form of a boy while the serpent-god Amphiaraos heals the dreaming invalid by taking the injured part in its mouth. This mythology could be the origin of the serpent and staff as the symbols for healing. Fourth century BC. *(National Archaeological Museum, Athens. Archaeological Receipts Fund.)*

Amphiaraos. The idea of the dream cure was vividly expressed in a votive tablet from Attica dating to the fourth century BC, now in the National Archaeological Museum in Athens. The human invalid lies on a couch, dreaming. His spirit-form emerges and moves to the human healer, who then holds his ailing shoulder. Meanwhile, the snake emerges from the dreamer and takes the injured part in its mouth. The cure is effected by the snake for the healer. Perhaps from this complex mythology the idea arose that Asklepios depended on the snake for his healing magic. Thus it could have come about that the single serpent coiled around his staff was considered the logical symbol for the healer and, in turn, for the medical profession.

A design resembling the caduceus appeared on a libation cup of King Gudea of Lagash in Sumeria (in Mesopotamia) dating to before 2000 BC. This was the serpent-god Ningishzida. The legendary Mesopotamian hero Gilgamesh lost the herb of healing to a serpent. In the Gilgamesh epic the hero, having lost his dearest friend to death, seeks to discover the secret of immortality known only to the gods. In a dreaming sleep he learns that death is inexorable and that he should strive to leave a tangible memorial by doing good works.

Later, the Egyptian god Thoth evolved into the Greek god Hermes (adopted by the Romans as Mercury), who was depicted with the caduceus. Hermes was the messenger of the gods but also the god of merchants, whose values were suspect. The wise Thoth was the god who weighed the dead soul's value (representations show the heart) after it reached the underworld. Thoth, however, had no caduceus. Thus the caduceus has hazy links to Sumerian, Egyptian, Greek, and Roman mythology, few of them related to healing. Nevertheless, the caduceus was adopted to represent many medical activities, particularly in publications and by pharmaceutical companies. The premise for such use was tenuous, and many formal medical professional organizations have tended to be more rigorous and insist on the symbol of Asklepios.

After the United States Army Medical Department adopted the caduceus as its insignia in 1902, its use expanded. With a "V" superimposed on the caduceus it became the symbol of the American veterinary profession and the Army Veterinary Corps.

Yet another proposal for the origin of the symbol, attractive but less likely, is that it may have originated from the ancient treatment, still in use, for the presence of an extraordinary filarial parasite, the Guinea (or Medina) worm. The larva of the worm enters via the gut after the host drinks water infected by the crayfish *Cyclops,* the intermediate host. The larva migrates in the body and usually matures into a worm about 1 meter long that locates as a knot in the ankle region. When the afflicted person steps into the water a year later, the mature female perforates the skin and disgorges its larvae into the water to infect new crayfish and sustain the cycle. Wandering native healers had learned that the affliction could be treated by penetrating the developing ankle ulcer carefully and seizing the worm by the head, then winding it gently onto a small stick. The healer turned the stick just a little every day, gradually withdrawing the worm while avoiding the unpleasant consequence of having it void its larvae into the subcutaneous tissues. This healing craft was believed to be the true symbolic intent, that is, of a parasitic worm, not a snake. Other legends involve the special connection between the snake and the underworld and the human need to be on good terms with both.

It should be recognized that the first two of the former suggestions for the origin of the caduceus are, like the centaur, mythological. The biology of the third one is accurate but unlikely to be linked to the legendary origins. Whether the legends of Chiron and Asklepios can be attributed to enlargement upon the skills of real persons or were pure invention we cannot know with certainty. Evidence from folklore indicates that people assuming those names did exist; nonetheless, the truth is obscured by a proliferation of tales.

127. *Facing page,* The frontispiece of David Coster's *Pharmacopoea Hagana* (1738) shows Asklepios paying homage to his father, Apollo, in his chariot in the heavens, and his teacher, Chiron the Centaur. In his left hand Asklepios holds a staff with an entwined serpent, and in his right, in honor of his teacher, an herb. *(The Wellcome Institute Library, London.)*

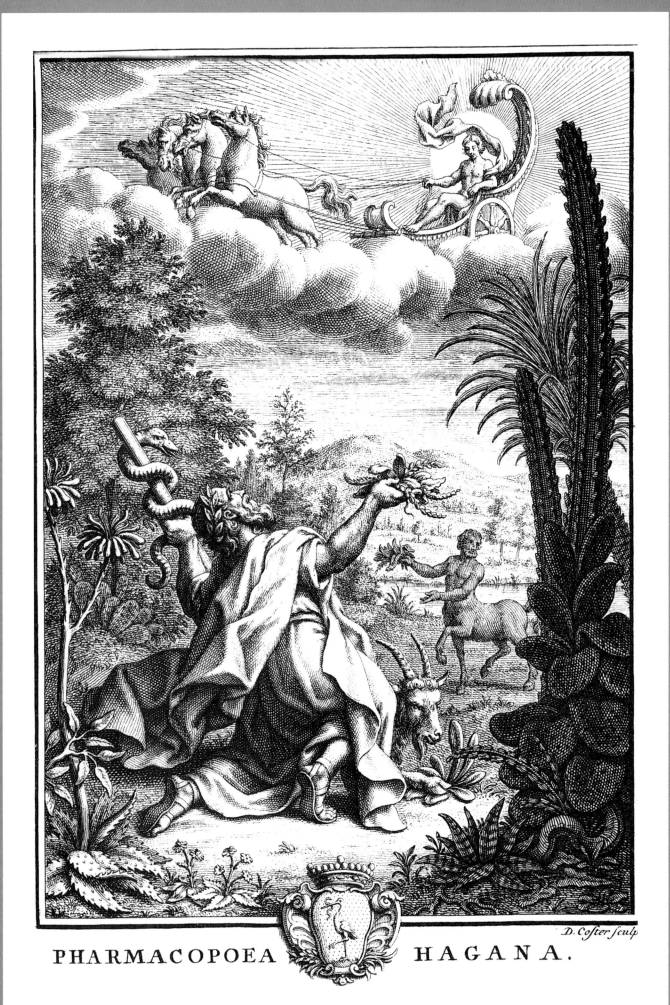

D. Coster sculp

PHARMACOPOEA HAGANA.

SEMINAL GREEK PHILOSOPHER-SCIENTISTS

A surge of intellectual awakening occurred in the Greek port towns of Asia Minor and nearby islands. Tragically, little firsthand evidence remains, but Aristotle (in *Metaphysics*) attributed the start of a great era of philosophy to Thales (640-546 BC) of Miletus, a Greek colony on a peninsula of Caria (now part of Turkey). The new direction was to study nature in a rigorous, rational way, seeking explanations for the changing events free from ordained preconceptions and supernatural speculations or dogmas. This was the creative germ of scientific philosophy. Its proponents have been called natural scientists or philosopher scientists.

Foremost among the philosopher-scientists was the mathematician Thales, who had traveled to Crete, Phoenicia, Babylon, and Egypt and learned about their astronomy, mathematics, and land measurement ("geometry"). He developed an abstract method for calculating areas of any shape and applied it to astronomy. As a result he showed that the Earth orbited the sun and that the other planets, too, followed predictable paths. In 585 BC he also explained a solar eclipse. Thales sought fundamental building blocks for living things and suggested that water must be the elemental material because, for example, the germination of seeds required it. He contributed much, including political theory, to many facets of society and is remembered as the founder of the Ionian school of philosophy and inquiry.

Followers of Thales continued the quest for basic properties. Anaximander (611-547 BC), one of his pupils, speculated that there must be a substance even more elemental than water. He proposed that the spontaneous origin of life took place in the primordial mud and air, concluding that land animals evolved from fish and that human life had arisen from other organisms whose young were more self-reliant. He is also given credit for proposing an experimental approach involving the use of measurements. Anaximenes (585-528 BC) opted for air as the key ingredient because when cooled, it forms water, and heated, it generates fire. Thus it accounted for three of the four elements. He purported that breathing was the basis of life.

The new approach to philosophy addressed the problem of origins and explanations in a heady atmosphere of theoretical speculation (hypothesis) followed by critical reappraisal and revision in a climate of continuous inquiry. The magnitude of this change from its predecessors was and is staggering. It remains as a legacy for all intellectual inquiry, to which the modern era has added the idea of testing hypotheses experimentally. The unpalatability of the philosophy to the traditionalist was manifested when Anaxagoras went to Athens and espoused it. He was prosecuted and banished on a charge of impiety, perhaps partly to discredit his famous pupil Pericles, who matured into the enlightened political leader who led Athens in its golden age.

The idea of fundamental building blocks from which all matter was assembled continued to intrigue the Ionian philosophers. Leucippus of Miletus conceived of the concept of indivisible atoms ("atomon"), and his versatile, brilliant protégé, Democritus of Abdera (470-361 BC), who preceded Socrates, developed a detailed atomic theory based on the premise that the universe consists solely of atoms and the void. He explained air pressure and winds as attributable to their atomic composition. He is credited with introducing the idea of microcosm and macrocosm, the concept that "the living creature is a world order in miniature." He also proposed the theory that the seed is drawn from every part of the body and contains each of its substances.

Democritus's "assembly-kits" version of atomic theory lent itself to physiological reasoning; for example, food could be broken down to simpler components that were absorbed and reconstituted into body tissues. The endless options for atomic assembly could explain the variety of sensations and functions. He also dissected animals to understand the nature of diseases. This area

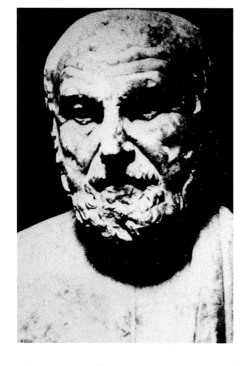

128. Bronze bust believed to be of Democritus of Abdera (470-361 BC), who is credited with the development of the concepts of microcosm and macrocosm. Although his work in veterinary dissection has been lost, his studies have been chronicled in the works of Aristotle. Roman copy of the original of around 250 BC. *(Soprintendenza Archeologica della Province di Napoli e Caserta, Napoli.)*

of his work is of the greatest interest to veterinary history. Because the body of Democritus's work is lost, Aristotle is the source of information on his works. It seems that Democritus demonstrated fatal pulpy kidney disease of sheep and contributed to anatomy and physiology in his seminal works. According to the Roman historian Marcellinus, his studies of diseases led to the prophecy that dissectors who examined the entrails of animals would indicate the measures needed in the future to cure their diseases.

Another Ionian, Heraclitus of Ephesus, is famous for stating that "everything passes," a thought admired by Nietzsche, who modified it by stating that "the only constant in the world is change." Heraclitus considered the basic principle to be fire as the agent of change and believed that tensions between opposing forces are necessary for life and for cycles of the universe.

PYTHAGORAS: VALUES-ORIENTED SCHOLAR AND MYSTIC

The seafaring Greeks spread around the Mediterranean, establishing cultural and trading centers such as at Naucratis on a branch of the Nile delta. Other sites led upward toward the Black Sea via the Bosporus Strait and westward to Italy and Sicily and beyond. Another great strand of Greek philosophical incubation and creativity developed in Elea in southern Italy and Sicily. The important Eleatic branch of Greek philosophy derived in part from Pythagoras, a strange combination of genius and mystic. Born in 582 BC on the island of Samos, thirty miles northwest of Miletus, he became a noted scholar and athlete. He then traveled through Egypt and Chaldea (Babylonia) seeking the insights of the priests and cultivating an awareness of the ancient traditions, including the idea, which he adopted, of the immortality of the soul and its transmigration to other creatures. Xenophanes made fun of this idea in a poem that tells of Pythagoras' admonishing a man for beating a dog by saying, "Stop, do not beat him. It is the soul of a friend—I recognize his voice." This conviction had its roots in the legends about the god Orpheus, who was alleged to have founded a mystic cult in which initiates entered an underworld where they were punished; once their souls were purified and freed from the body, the souls could return to enter the body of another creature. Orpheus was acclaimed as a great musician who would charm wild beasts with his lute. Some claimed he was a real person who lived in Thrace around 1300 BC.

After his travels Pythagoras returned to Samos, only to be appalled at the tyranny of the ambitious Polycrates; he departed, going first to Olympus, then to Croton in South Italy. There he established a philosophical academy that became the Pythagorean Order; the academy incorporated his chimerical belief in both rational knowledge and ascetic religion and accepted both men and women. It had wide appeal based on its reputation in mathematics, music, astronomy, medicine, and religious belief. Pythagoras was the first to assert that the Earth is a sphere and developed the idea that the solar system comprises planets making elliptical orbits around the sun, a concept rejected by a majority of his successors until the sixteenth century. He perceived in the human mind propensities shared with the brute creatures but also nobler seeds of virtue leading to moral and intellectual endeavor. He expected his followers to commit to a life of labor, study, exercise, self-evaluation, and rest, believing that many things, especially love, were best learned late in life.

Pythagoras opposed shedding blood and forbade his pupils to eat flesh or beans or to wear clothing made from animal products. However, one of his pupils (Alcmaeon, the founder of the Croton Medical School) was the first to dissect animal bodies as models of the human frame, describing arteries and veins, the Eustachian tube, the optic nerve, and the brain, which he said was the seat of the intellect. In Pythagoras's philosophy of medicine, surgical pro-

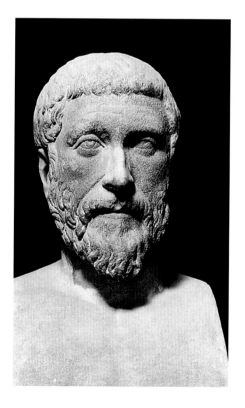

129. Pythagoras of Samos (c. 582-497 BC), a scholar and mystic, was the first to suggest that the earth was a sphere; he also refined Thales' concept of a solar system comprising planets orbiting the sun. His philosophical academy, which became the Pythagorean Order, produced at least one student, Alcmaeon, who had a major impact on early medicine. Roman copy of a Greek bust thought, arguably, to be a general likeness. *(Museo Capitolino, Rome.)*

cedures were forbidden lest they interfere with the soul. He was an elitist who advocated aristocratic rule. After an initial phase of popularity, his doctrines fell out of favor and he was forced to leave Croton; he moved northeastward to Metopontion on the Gulf of Tarento, where he is thought to have died about 497 BC. Subsequently, when a democratic revolution swept through the Greek city-states of southern Italy, the Pythagorean Order was attacked and its facilities were destroyed.

EMPEDOCLES: ELEMENTS, PROPERTIES, HUMORS, AND EVOLUTION

The influence of Pythagoras reached Empedocles (fifth century BC) of Acragas in Sicily, yet another versatile genius and original thinker. He was a philosopher-scientist and physician who followed the ideas of Pythagoras, Parmenides, and Anaximander. Like Parmenides, Empedocles expressed his rigorous thinking in poetry. He emphasized the value of experimentation, using it to demonstrate that air is a substance; he named the substance *aether* and called it one of the four elements. Like the Hindus, Empedocles was a firm believer in the transmigration of the spirit across species lines, even to plants, and he held views on evolution that anticipated some of the ideas of Charles Darwin. He argued that there had been a much greater variety of living organisms in earlier times but that many must have been unable to adapt and multiply, eventually becoming extinct. This was a first grasp of the idea of a possible fossil record of evolution.

Empedocles recognized that light takes time to travel and that the moon's light is reflected. He was attracted to the idea of the fundamental properties or "roots" of all things and was the first to propose the theory of the four elements—earth, water, air, and fire. With the benefit of hindsight one can discern a logical perspective in the struggle to arrive at this concept. These four elements correspond with a modern version of the states of matter as solid, liquid, and gas linked by energy. Empedocles conceived of his four elements interacting with four fundamental properties, namely, hot, dry, moist, and cold. A further link, in the case of the animal body, was to the four juices (body fluids) or humors—blood, yellow bile, black bile, and phlegm.

The theory of the four elements was adopted by the Hippocratic writers and by Aristotle and Galen. Empedocles also believed that health required a balance among opposing forces. He ventured into psychology, perceiving two great currents, love and strife, that ebbed and flowed, influencing the humors to create harmony or disharmony depending on which current was paramount at the moment (shades, perhaps, of China's concepts of yin and yang).

Empedocles used music to redress the imbalance in the insane. He seemed to evince a greater desire than most Greek thinkers to move from ideas to actions. He organized the drainage of a swamp to contain an epidemic of malaria in Selinus, just to the west of Acragas. To use the modern idiom, this project was a rare example of "technology transfer." Because Acragus was destroyed by the Carthaginians about 400 BC, most of the record of Empedocles' remarkable career has been lost.

THE ARRIVAL OF RATIONAL MEDICAL SCHOLARSHIP

A transition occurred away from the many temples to Asklepios and toward new centers of rational medical learning, for example, at places like Cnidus and Cos. On the promontory of Cnidus Euryphon started a trend toward a purely rational medicine based on facts, using animal dissections and post-mortem examinations to gain an understanding of the body and of diseases of animals and humans. Because of this adherence to facts alone, the Cnidian

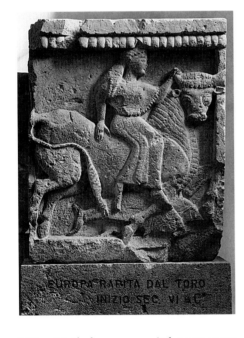

130. Mythology was a vital component of ancient Greek culture, and one popular story was of Europa, who was deceived by Zeus when he changed himself into a bull and carried her on his back across the water to Crete, where she became the mother of Rhadamanthus, Minos, and Sarpedon. An ancient Greek relief shows Europa holding the swimming bull (Zeus) by a horn; a dolphin symbolizes the sea. Metope relief from the Temple of Hera. Mid-sixth century BC. *(Hirmer Verlag GmbH, München.)*

doctors were called "Empiricists." Alcmaeon in Crotonia, Italy, was pursuing a similar approach, but his was intermingled with pythagorean mysticism. The school of Cnidus was a rival of the school of Cos, which attained preeminence in medical history under the leadership of Hippocrates. The Cnidian physicians were accurate observers and stressed the needs of practice. They were weak, however, in the areas of theory and analysis and did not relish debates. They wrote treatises on internal medicine that gave lucid, striking descriptions of symptoms. For example, a patient having difficulty breathing "opens his nostrils like a running horse; his tongue hangs out like that of a dog who feels scorched by the heat in summer." The noble saying that "the nature of the body is the starting point of medical reasoning" was attributed to them. An outstanding treatise by Philiston of Syracuse in Sicily, *Of the Heart,* had Cnidian roots. This remarkably accurate description of the structure of the human heart and its major vessels could have been accomplished only if a real heart had been dissected. Philiston, however, did not advance in understanding from the anatomical to the physiological level.

The vast collation of medical literature known as the Hippocratic collection or corpus compiled in Alexandria under the edict of the Greek pharaoh Ptolemy came from many sources. Three streams or groups of writings are represented: that of the medical theorists, who were speculative philosophers with literary skills, and two other streams, those of the Cnidian and Cos schools. The followers of the latter were the true founders of an all-encompassing rational medicine based on science, experience, and clinical wisdom. They started from observation and proceeded through interpretation and analysis to a rational course of action and prognosis based on the goal of safety for and survival of the patient. So solidly was the foundation of the new medicine set in place by the Cos school that, thanks to its lusty offspring, Galen, it survived the stagnation of the Roman era and the religious quackery and proscriptions of the Middle Ages. Paradoxically, blind faith in Galen's authority had the negative effect of stemming further challenges and progress.

HIPPOCRATES AND THE LEGACY OF THE COS SCHOOL

A contemporary of Socrates (470-399 BC) and Plato (427-347 BC), Hippocrates was born on the island of Cos in 460 BC and died in Thessaly in 367 BC. He studied philosophy and surgery in Athens and traveled widely. Truly the king of medical thought and ethics, Hippocrates has been immortalized by the veterinary profession, which perpetuates his memory as the ultimate role model by requiring graduates in many veterinary schools to take a veterinarian's form of the Hippocratic Oath on graduation. His admonition *primum non nocere,* "above all, do no harm," gives pause to the zealous professional keen to try unproven new ideas and methods. The oath has served as a guide to behavioral values and a reminder of the duties of the health professional for human or animal well-being while protecting the profession's image. The elements of Hippocratic medicine were as follows:

1. Clinical evaluation using all senses and problem-oriented diagnosis
2. Cosmological and ecological factors, hygiene, and expected time course
3. Recording of data and commitment to advance the knowledge of disease
4. Moral commitment to and humanistic concern for the patient
5. Mastery of medicine, which required apprenticeship and study with a master
6. Avoidance of recourse to mysticism while providing psychological support

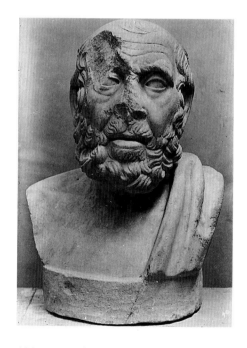

131. Found in a physician's tomb in the necropolis of Isola Sacra near ancient Ostia in 1940, a Roman copy of a Greek bust bears undoubted resemblance to a bust found on a Coan coin marked *Hippocrates.* The influence of Hippocrates on human medicine is profound, and veterinary medicine has immortalized the memory of Hippocrates with its own form of the Hippocratic Oath. His dictum, *primum non nocere (above all, do no harm),* is equally applicable to veterinarians and physicians. *(Courtesy Soprintendenza Archeologica di Ostia, Museo Ostiense, Rome.)*

The genius of the Hippocratic approach derived from an evolving scientific perspective; a base of accumulated and redistilled knowledge of the course, treatment, and outcome of clinical cases; rigorous examination and data gathering; and analysis and decision making leading to intervention for the safety and comfort of the patient. A unique feature was that the frame of reference for each case always encompassed environmental and chronological considerations. The focus was always on seeking outcomes that were favorable. Hippocrates noted that diseases such as epilepsy ("the sacred disease") were held to be of divine origin because they were not understood. *Iatros,* the Greek word for "healer," forms the root of the modern term "iatrogenic" or doctor-induced disease.

The Hippocratic corpus of writings included works by many authors. Treatises covered environmental health *(Airs, Waters, and Places)*, prognosis *(Prognostics)*, contagions and plagues with situational histories *(Epidemics)*, and comparative studies of fractures and luxations in cattle and people (*On Fractures* and *On Dislocations*). In *Aphorisms* the famous aphorism, "Art is long, life is short, the occasion fleeting, experience fallacious, and judgment difficult," encapsulates the challenges of medical and veterinary work.

The Hippocratic school espoused the idea that disharmony among the four humors was the basis for many diseases and could be evaluated by the symptoms. The treatments were directed at correcting the imbalance and restoring a healthy coordination among body functions, but Hippocrates cautioned, "We must not disturb the work of nature." Although prepared to intervene when he judged intervention to be essential, he clearly recognized that many diseases would be corrected without medical intervention. His goal was to bring to bear all his continuously maturing mastery of his profession to understand what was happening in the body of the patient and its causes, while judging what the likely course would be and how he could improve the chances of recovery. The phenomenal erudition of Hippocrates, his common sense and practical skills, his insistence on a code of conduct, his zeal for advancing the competence of his profession, and his cautions against reckless speculations combine to warrant his enduring image as a model for the professions of human and veterinary medicine. He vanquished the ideology of the ancient traditions and myths that called for superstitious acceptance on faith without justification or analysis.

The progress of medicine as a great clinical profession has depended on two ancient philosophical roots. One of these was the medical school at Cos that developed from the intellectual genius of Hippocrates. The other was the idea of advancing basic knowledge by means of scientific research, which would be known today as comparative biomedical science. It was to fall to one who was but seventeen years old when Hippocrates died to assume the mantle of guiding this philosophical branch.

ARISTOTLE'S NATURAL HISTORY AND EXPERIMENTAL BIOSCIENCE

Aristotle, born at Stagira in northern Greece in 384 BC, was brought up in the court of Philip of Macedon; his father was the court physician. The medical craft was handed from parent to offspring. Thus Aristotle became well grounded in the ways and knowledge of the physicians. However, he also developed a keen interest in natural history. In his youth he roamed the valleys, mountains, and shores of Macedonia, making biological observations and collecting specimens and information. When he was eighteen years old he went to Athens (366 BC) to study in the Academy under the renowned Plato, who was then sixty years old. Aristotle stayed with the aging master until Plato died in 347 BC, nearly twenty years later. Plato was the supreme intellectual and elitist. He condemned the senses, revering only the purity of thought un-

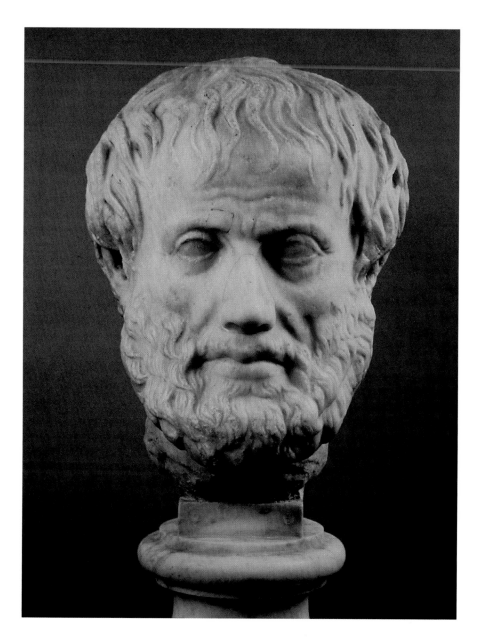

132. Marble bust of Aristotle (384–322 BC). After studying for nearly twenty years with Plato, Aristotle set out to satisfy his interest in zoology by classifying the animal kingdom. His studies resulted in several publications that had a profound effect on comparative biology and veterinary medicine. Copy of Late Classical original, first century AD. *(Kunsthistorisches Museum, Vienna.)*

trammeled by any sensory distractions. Plato denied animals a soul, thereby restricting immortality to the human species and holding the speculative concepts of transmigration of souls and a blissful afterlife in heaven for the worthy. Although an admirer of Plato, Aristotle differed from him in these and many other views. His own standard was to revere the truth above all else. When he was not selected to succeed Plato at the Academy, he left and went to Assos on the Ionian coast. There he married his niece Pythias, who died in childbirth. He moved to Mytilene on Lesbos, where he studied natural history on the coasts, feeding his passionate interest in marine biology.

In 342 BC Aristotle was invited by King Philip II to become tutor to his son Alexandros, destined to become Alexander the Great. Aristotle's three years in that role had a profound effect and won him a wealthy benefactor for his later scientific research. His biological collections were to become expanded on a grand scale. He was disgraced in Macedon when a relative engaged in a political plot, and he returned to Athens. There in 335 BC he developed the Lyceum as his school of philosophy, and his prodigious intellect attained its full productive power. After thirteen years of mature scholarship he encountered political trouble again when Macedonians were purged after Alexander's death; he had to leave Athens and died of a stomach disorder in 322 BC in Chalcis, where he owned property on the island of Euboea. His work at the Lyceum was continued by his trusted friend and colleague Theophrastus, an authority on plants.

During his fruitful years at the Lyceum Aristotle put many of his thoughts into written form, producing a vast corpus on many subjects ranging from the liberal arts to the basic sciences and the learned professions. Because zoology was a major interest, he set out to classify the animal kingdom and study the diversity of form and function among animals. *Parts of Animals* and *Generation of Animals* are two of his famous biological works. He recognized that a species is first defined by the interfertility of its members and can then be studied in an ecological and a behavioral context. One doctrine on generation—that the male provides the form and the female the matter of the offspring—would be rebuffed today on both scientific and political grounds. Aristotle noted that interspecific couplings are rare but do occur, especially around desert watering holes where thirst draws diverse species together. Although Aristotle gravely underestimated the mother's role in genetic transfer, he did foreshadow the science of genetics by identifying the sperm as a carrier of genetic inheritance.

ARISTOTLE'S INITIATION OF COMPARATIVE MEDICINE

Aristotle considered studying common characteristics among species—the body systems approach—preferable to studying all the species individually and exhaustively because the huge scale of the latter project would involve enormous numbers of boring repetitions. Nonetheless, his *Historia Animalium (Story of Animals)* provides information on almost five hundred species; of these he had dissected about fifty. He determined, for instance, that the horse lacks a gallbladder. The disciplines of anatomy and physiology felt his touch. *Parts of Animals* is a four-volume comparative anatomy of animals that also explains the functions of the organs. In *The Gait of Animals* he describes quadruped locomotion and explains why limb sequence is diagonal. Aristotle was determined to classify every living thing. He liked great challenges and carried them out well. On a canvas so vast a few errors were inevitable. Some of these errors may have been made because he quoted reports by others who were less careful than himself, but this is speculation. Considering that Aristotle was exploring virgin territory in most of his many forays into bioscience, the amount of information and analysis he was able to generate remains nothing short of phenomenal.

Aristotle believed that animals have states of mind that are rudimentary forms of those of humans. In comparing the psychic qualities of animals with those of humans, he used the analogy of early childhood, when one can observe traces of a maturing psyche although the general level of mental activity is not markedly different from that of animals. The most surprising among his errors was his siting of the intellect in the heart rather than the brain, even though the writings of Hippocrates were available to him for reference.

Aristotle's *Pathology* revealed a keen interest in animal diseases; he reported on maladies of horses, asses, cattle, sheep, swine, fish, bees, elephants, and dogs. He was well aware of the Hippocratic method of medicine and applied it to veterinary diseases. The most interesting interpretation was of a condition of sheep that Aristotle credited Democritus with explaining. In Leontini in Sicily the animals died suddenly, and the kidneys were found to be encased in fat and degenerated (a condition known today as pulpy kidney disease or ovine enterotoxemia). Aristotle attributed the condition to overeating and recommended the local tactic of reducing the feed intake by keeping the sheep off pasture until evening, an early approach to preventive veterinary medicine. He wrote on two methods of castration (either crushing or removal of the testicles) and its effect on growth if performed on young animals; cas-

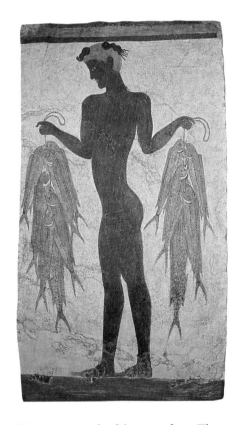

133. Fresco of a fisherman from Thera. Aristotle's *Pathology* included diseases of fish. *(National Archaeological Museum, Athens. Archaeological Receipts Fund.)*

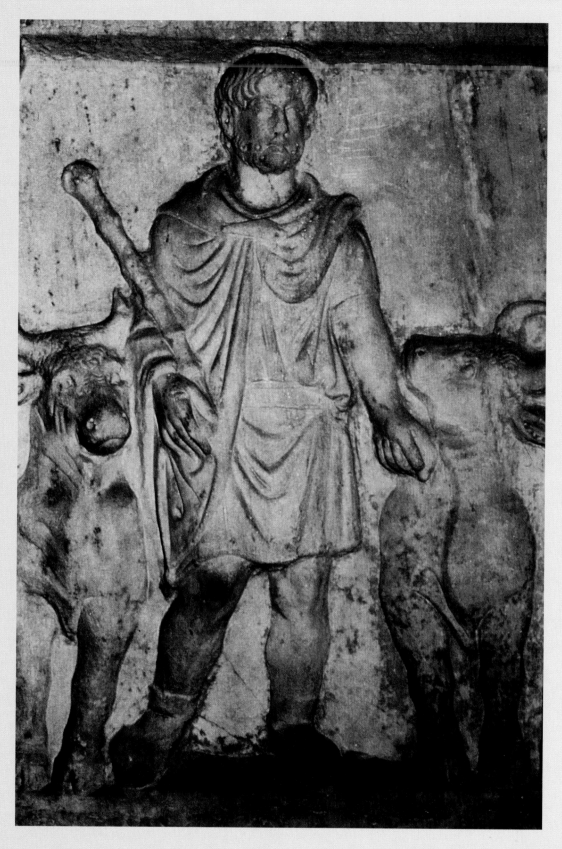

134. Tombstone of Aphtonetos, a Greek cattleman. Greek cattlemen benefited from the teaching and writing of Aristotle on diseases of cattle that were probably contagious—pleuropneumonia and possibly foot-and-mouth disease. First or second century AD. *(National Archaeological Museum, Athens. Archaeological Receipts Fund.)*

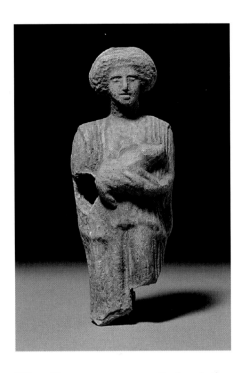

135. Terracotta statuette of a female fig
ure, probably the goddess Demeter, holding a pig. Tegea, fourth century BC. *(The
British Museum London.)*

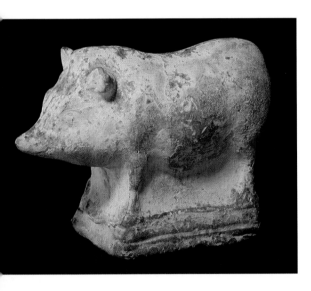

136. Terracotta pig rattle from the sanctuary of Demeter at Eleusis (c. 400 BC).
Votive pigs can often be found at sanctuar-
ies of the goddess Demeter. Aristotle was
probably the first to write on diseases of
the pig, including such conditions as anthrax, high fever, and diarrhea, and described measled swine with a condition
caused by larval tapeworms encysted in the
tongue. *(Fitzwilliam Museum, Cambridge.)*

tration was practiced on fasting sows and female camels via an incision ahead
of the pubis; also, cocks were caponized. His famous work on embryology
was based on meticulous observation of the developing chicken embryo, including insightful views about circulation of the blood.

The eighth book in Aristotle's *Historia Animalium* dealt with illness in animals. He was probably the first to write on diseases of the pig. One lethal disease was supposed to be anthrax; another featured high fevers, diarrhea, and
loss of condition. Measled swine with a condition now known to be caused
by larval tapeworms encysted in the tongue were clearly described; he observed that too much of a favored diet of acorns caused sows and ewes to
abort, and noted that dermal pustules and pimples were observed only in pigs.

Aristotle reported that dogs were susceptible to three major diseases: lyssa
or rabies, which produced lethal madness and the behavior of biting at everything, thereby infecting the bitten subjects; cynanche or quinsey, a strangles-
like condition with throat inflammation and abcsessation that was usually fatal; and podagra or severe lesions of the feet, from which few recovered. Two
epidemic herd conditions in cattle could cause heavy losses. One was a fatal
wasting after pulmonary infection characterized by anorexia, drooping ears,
and hot, rapid breathing, the lungs being decayed on necropsy (this was probably contagious pleuropneumonia); the other involved lesions of the feet (possibly foot-and-mouth disease).

Aristotle stated that horses at pasture were largely free from diseases but
that foot conditions could cause loss of their hooves. Oddly, he supported the
strange idea that the bite of the "shrew mouse" could account for sudden
deaths at pasture. Since the deaths are suspected of being attributable to anthrax, one wonders what evidence could have given rise to this concept.
Unlike pastured horses, stabled horses suffered from many diseases, among
them one recognizable as tetanus. Another was an acute febrile condition; yet
another, known as "barley disease," was surely laminitis. A further observation
was the occurrence of blisters that inhibited or prevented urination. A horse
could suffer "heartache" with excessive movement of the flanks; this condition may have been heaves.

According to Aristotle, an important disease of housed horses was ileus,
an extremely severe form of colicky pain that probably involved invagination
of the intestine and volvulus. This condition may have resulted from inguinal
hernia, and castration was prescribed as a remedy. "Melis," an acute disease of
donkeys, started in the head and resulted in bloody, purulent discharge from
the nostrils. Mortality was high; the disease must have been glanders.

Aristotle described surgical interventions for umbilical hernia, anal atre-
sia, rectovaginal fistula, and ascites. Cautery was used for hemorrhage,
wounds, and damaged tendons. Swabbing and suturing were also reported.

Aristotle's work on animal diseases included dissection-based inquiry, an
early foray into pathology, but it consisted mainly of gathering and classifying
information about diseases. He did not restrict his attention to the horse but
encompassed all the domestic species and several exotic ones, including elephants, camels, birds, fish, and insects. Most ancient Grecian literature relating to veterinary matters during the centuries before and after Aristotle,
almost to Byzantine times, has not survived. Thus written history moves to
the era of Constantine the Great and the brilliant horse doctor Apsyrtos
(c. AD 330) or depends on Roman authors·for their commentaries.

Roman authors such as Varro generally recognized that the Greek horse
doctors or Hippiatroi were indisputably superior to their Roman counterparts. The adoption by the Hippiatroi of the Greek medical system and analytical approach must have contributed to this perception. Some veterinary
historians consider Aristotle the parental intellect of comparative biology and
veterinary medicine.

GREEK HORSEMANSHIP AND HUNTING

Greek horses were probably ponies at first; larger strains were introduced later. Near Eleusinon in Athens, Simon dedicated a bronze horse with his exploits engraved on the pedestal. Only fragments of Simon's writings survive, but Xenophon recalled some of his views. That he was a humanitarian is evident in the following dictum:

> What a horse does under compulsion he does blindly . . . . The horse should of his own accord exhibit the finest airs and paces at set signals . . . the majesty of men themselves is best discovered in the graceful handling of such animals.

Xenophon or Anabasis (430-355 BC), the famous Athenian cavalry general and historian, wrote brilliantly on the management, breeding, riding, and training of military horses, draft horses, and hunting dogs in *Hippiarchos* and *Cynogeneticus*. His writings, which did not include animal healing, have survived to inform historians. Clearly he was above all else a master of equitation.

Xenophon was a Spartan. Because the small horses of his day had to be ridden bareback and were not castrated, the stallions were high spirited. He advocated the use of snaffle cavesson bits with traumatic attachments to aid control until the horse was trained; then gentler, smoother gear would suffice. He taught cavalrymen to ride with straight legs so that, despite the lack of stirrups, they could better grip the horse and use weapons. Horses were trained to lead with the left foreleg when at the canter or gallop because Greek race courses ran counterclockwise and because the right-handed cavalryman could more easily hold his spear in his right hand.

Xenophon used rewards and punishments in training, for example, in teaching the horse to jump obstacles, but emphasized the importance of being calm, patient, and gentle to familiarize the animal with the rider's intentions and win trust, especially of a spirited horse. He made quite a study of the mind of the horse and treated each horse individually in obtaining its cooperation and responsiveness. He said that vocal sounds may be used as specific signals to arouse or quiet a horse but that one must avoid confusing it. He advised the master to instruct the grooms in all aspects of horse management and to watch for signs of exhaustion or sickness such as when the horse does not eat well. It appears likely that there were horse doctors to turn to for advice, but he does not refer to them. He emphasized the importance of good conformation in selecting an animal that would remain sound.

Xenophon was a great advocate of hunting as a way to develop a healthy mind and body and strengthen character. He mentions two breeds of sporting dogs, the Castorian and the fox-like. He kept harriers and followed the dogs on foot. He noted that both types had a large proportion of defective individuals that were undersized, disproportioned, stiff or weak, or unsound of foot; they had poor coats of hair and were inferior in vision or "nose" (scenting ability for tracking).

Perhaps reflecting Plato's attitude toward animals, the Greeks did not consider animals companions, leaving pets to their gods, although some Greeks established strong bonds with their working animals, horses, and dogs. They seemed to like the sounds made by cicadas and often kept them in cages.

SCIENCE AND MEDICINE IN ALEXANDRIA

Alexander the Great, who trained under Aristotle, expanded the Greek empire in a campaign that swept through the Mediterranean, western Asia, Arabia, Africa, and South Asia to the Indus valley, bringing Greek culture and

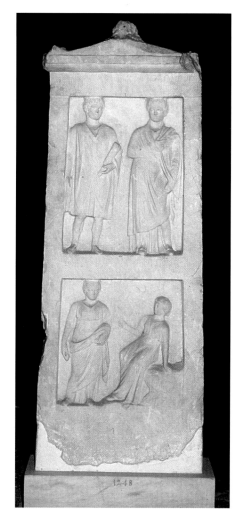

137. Greek horse doctors or Hippiatroi were clearly recognized as superior by their Roman counterparts. Roman monument of the Greek horse doctor Eutychos *(upper left)*, his wife, and two daughters. He is holding castration pincers in his right hand and a large knife in his left. *(National Archaeological Museum, Athens. Archaeological Receipts Fund.)*

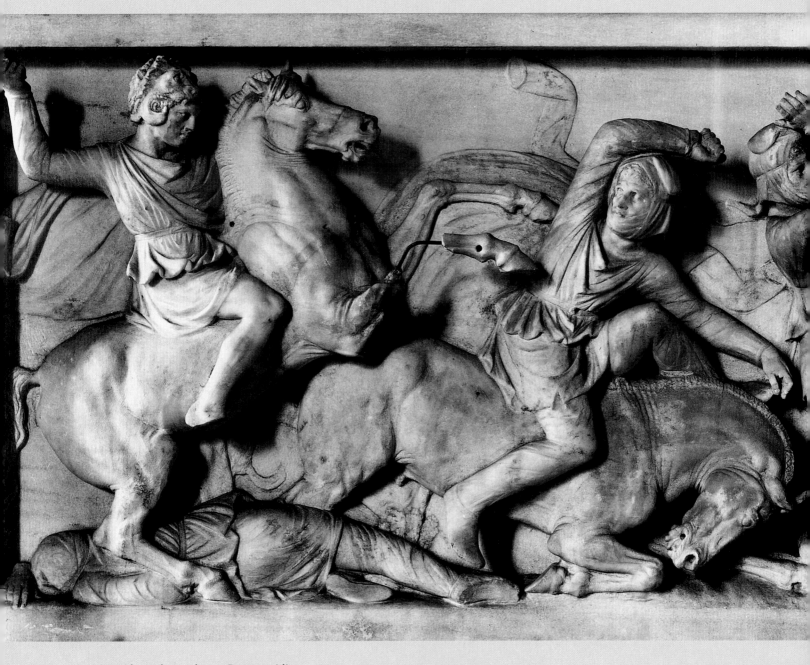

138. Alexander the Great riding Bucephalus while attacking Persian horsemen. Bucephalus, a magnificent black stallion, was said to have been unmanageable by anyone other than Alexander. The horse, given to him when he was a twelve-year-old boy by his father, Philip of Macedon, was his favorite for seventeen years. During the Alexandrian period of learning, anatomical dissection was permitted and early studies of comparative medicine were undertaken. Alexander sarcophagus, Syria. *(Hirmer Verlag GmbH, München.)*

Aristotelian logic to the regions. He founded a fantastic new city that was to be named after him (Alexandria) at one of the mouths of the Nile River. The influence of Aristotle in this venture can be perceived, as no effort was spared in making the new city into a great center for learning and science under the Ptolemys. The core was an enormous library, the Museion, which came to house 700,000 scrolls. A giant observatory enhanced a focus on cosmology and mathematics, and laboratories were established to advance science and medicine on many fronts.

Alexander had a special relationship with his glorious horse Bucephalus, a black stallion said to be unmanageable by anyone else. A Poseidon temple was built by the sea as a focal point for a horse cult.

The Alexandrian center of learning held periodic sway over the intellectual ferment of the world from about 300 BC to AD 500; the first three centuries were its golden age. Religious constraints on dissection and experimentation were discarded. Comparative anatomy was advanced by means of dissections of animals and humans, and physiology was said to have been enriched by experiments in vivisection. The result was great progress in basic medical science. Two great physician-scientists took the lead. Herophilus made detailed studies of the structure of the brain, eyes, nerves, and blood vessels. He speculated on the functions of the brain and made a detailed investigation of the arterial pulse. Erasistratus, a physician from Chios and grandson of Aristotle, studied the upper airway and cardiovascular system, including hemorrhage.

Before Alexandria's initiation of the study of anatomy, it was largely a speculative field because dissection was disallowed. Protovivisection was permitted in some cases, at least in studies made immediately after execution of criminals, although the practice was condemned by Tertullian. Herophilus, the founder of scientific anatomy and originator of its terminology, was able to correct many errors, including Aristotle's error concerning the seat of the intellect (in the brain, not the heart). Herophilus wrote a handbook to help midwives improve their procedures. He clearly differentiated nerves from tendons, showed the vascular system of the brain, and demonstrated that the optic nerve is the visual pathway inward from the eye. He showed for the first time that both arteries and veins carry the blood.

Erasistratus was the founder of experimental physiology and broached pathology. He described the complex form of the throat and the function of the throat in both breathing and swallowing. He distinguished between motor and sensory nerves, conducted excellent experiments, and agreed that the brain was the seat of the intellect.

The great intellectual leaps made by the physician-scientists were too much for the skeptics, empiricists of the worst kind, who held that "everything should be tried without any previous consideration." The skeptics claimed that the causes and essence of disease cannot be found by thinking; they favored intervention, including surgical techniques, which were sometimes skillfully carried out. Treatments then in vogue, such as coprotherapy, are today rejected without question.

Alexandria was the base of the genius Archimedes (287-212 BC) of Syracuse, a mathematician and physicist who died in the Roman siege of that city, and of Hero, a mechanical engineer.

After the learning centers were overrun by the Saracens and concordant with a general decline in the intellectual spirit, religious heretics and mobs attacked the centers. When the Caliph Omar ordered the vast international library burned to the ground in AD 642, countless unique scrolls were destroyed and a devastating scar was inflicted on human intellectual and cultural progress.

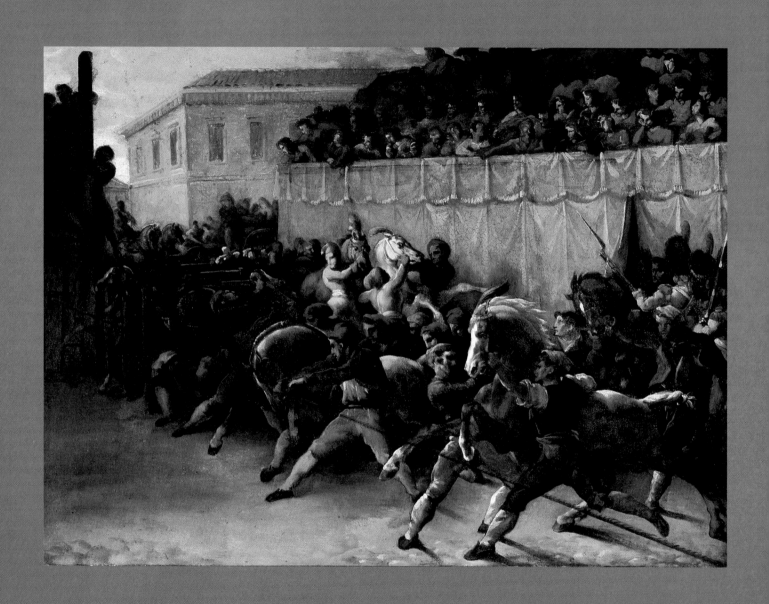

Animal Doctors in Ancient Rome

CONTRIBUTIONS OF THE ANIMAL-LOVING ETRUSCANS

The cultural roots of the Roman veterinary art are traceable to the Etruscans, who loved horses and cattle. The remains of their art in tombs at Tarquinia and elsewhere show fine, long-legged horses suitable for riding and racing, as well as bulls. This art shows connections to that of Greece and its Mediterranean diaspora from about 700 BC to 300 BC. The Etruscans developed divination (foretelling) to the level of an aristocratic calling. Two approaches were used. "Augury" was carried out by individuals who based their predictions on the flight and cries of birds, and "haruspicy" required examination of the entrails of sacrificed animals with special focus on the appearance of the liver. Thus a "haruspex" was an authority on animal diseases and their significance as harbingers of future events, that is, the haruspex was an oracle. Around 200 BC Cato condemned the practice of divination.

The early Romans were people of Aryan pastoral origin who first established villages, then a city-state in Latium on the Tiber River. The forested area was in a volcanic arc. They grazed their cattle and sheep on common pastures and grew grain and figs, and their hogs foraged in the forests. By coalescing several villages, Rome was created, only to be taken over by the Etruscans about 600 BC. Skilled in masonry and metallurgy, they brought an alphabet and artistry. They gave Rome its *cloaca maxima,* the draining sewer that has survived for almost 2500 years, and a famous bronze statue of a mother wolf that was to become the city's symbol. During the Renaissance in the fifteenth century AD the twins Romulus and Remus, who were alleged to have been suckled by a she-wolf and to have founded the city, were added to the statue. Mounted Celtic Gauls from the north overran the Etruscans, who then withdrew from Rome. Later (300 BC), the Celts sacked Rome itself but were repulsed.

POSSIBLE ROMAN ORIGINS OF THE NAME *VETERINARIUS*

The Romans followed many of the Etruscan customs. Animals were esteemed. The very name "Italy" is derived from *Italus,* the name of a bull chased from Sicily by Hercules. *Pecus,* the word for "money," was from the same root as the word for "cattle." Animal and human (until banned by the Senate) sacrifices were practiced. Every year a horse was sacrificed to Mars, the god of war. A special form of sacrifice, given the composite name *suove-taurilia,* involved a pig *(sus),* a sheep *(ovis),* and a bull *(taurus)* and took place in the Campus Martius, particularly after glorious victories.

139. *Facing page,* Spectator sports, especially those involving animals, were performed in circuses and large amphitheaters and were an integral and dramatic part of Roman culture. Horse racing was particularly popular, as seen in *Race of the Riderless Horses in Rome,* a powerful painting done by Jean-Louis Théodore Géricault (1791-1824) in 1817. The Cappadocian, North African, Spanish, and Italian strains were favored by racehorse breeders. The best horses competed until they were twenty years old. *(Walters Art Gallery, Baltimore, Maryland.)*

The animal caretakers were called *souvetaurinarii,* from which the word *veterinarius* may have later been derived. However, the Roman word for "pack animals" was *veterina,* another possible derivation of the term. A *veterinarium* was the compound set aside for the pack animals at a Roman military encampment. The term *medicus veterinarius* was also used on some inscriptions. The scholar Columella, a leading author on agricultural and veterinary matters, used the term *veterinarius* for caretakers of pigs, sheep, and cattle and *mulomedicus* for horse doctors. The latter term was also applied to a slave who had regained his freedom. The term *medicus equarius* also appears in reference to a type of horse doctor who had been demobilized from the Roman army. When Tarrentunus, a Pretorian prefect during the reign of Commodus (AD 180-192), formalized the military regulations, the term *veterinarii* appeared: the *veterinarii* were ranked as "immune subjects" because of their competence in an important speciality. Until then the term *mulomedici* had been used to refer to the special personnel (slaves) who were required to care for the chariot and cavalry horses, pack horses, mules, and draft cattle at each *cursus* or post along the network of roads.

CHALLENGE TO ROME: CARTHAGE AND THE PHOENICIANS

A threat to Rome came from the Phoenicians, whose homeland in Canaan had been overwhelmed by Cyrus. These brilliant seafaring traders and farmers had established a center at Carthage (in today's Tunisia). Having a fine navy and a strong, albeit largely mercenary, army, they blocked Grecian expansion to the west. They developed an advanced agricultural system based on grain and cattle that fueled the Punic commodity trade. The intellectual force behind this system was Mago (550-500 BC), the father of Mediterranean agronomy and animal husbandry and author of a twenty-eight–volume encyclopedia on agriculture. This work was translated by Dionysius of Utica into Greek in 88 BC; the Roman Senate ordered the Greek version translated into Latin. Sadly, all three versions have been lost, and only a few citations by other ancient authors remain. Mago provided details of castration of horses and bulls and wrote on diseases of livestock. Baked clay tablets found at Ugarit (now Ras Shamra in Syria) dating to the period from 1500 to 1300 BC recorded veterinary practices in Canaan before the arrival of the Phoenicians, including the administration of herbal treatments via the nostrils.

Phoenician expansion provoked the ambitious Roman state, leading to the protracted Punic Wars. Rome was forced to develop its navy and expand its highly disciplined army to prevail. Carthage, however, expanded along the North African shore to Spain, where it developed a harbor at New Carthage. From the Spanish base the brilliant general Hannibal, an admirer of Alexander, led a large army of infantry and cavalry with thirty-seven elephants up the Iberian Peninsula, across the Rhone River, and through the Alpine passes at over 5400 feet, to descend on the Po Valley, where he defeated the Roman legions. The elephants are believed to have been mainly of a small North African subspecies, but at least one was from Syria and almost certainly of the Asiatic type. They were a symbol of power, but it is thought that their effect on the outcomes was more psychological than physical. Continuing down the Italian peninsula to its heel, Hannibal was confronted at Cannae by a massive Roman army in 216 BC and annihilated it.

It took the Romans more than a decade to recover. Then, led by Scipio and with an adequate military force, more animals, and reformed tactics, they overcame the Carthaginians in Spain and invaded the heartland of Carthage. Too late, Hannibal was recalled from his long stay in Latium, where he had orchestrated support and resources throughout much of the area south of Rome. In 202 BC a mighty battle was fought at Zama, seventy-five miles from

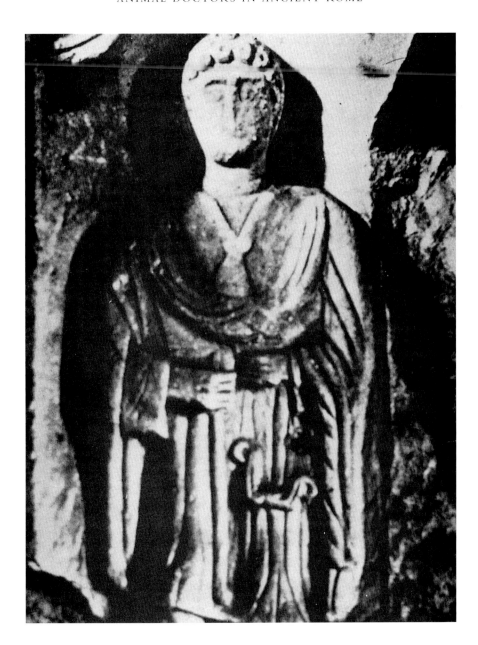

140. Funerary statue of a *mulomedicus* from the Gallo-Roman era. There is some confusion over the use of this term; it was used to describe both horse doctors and slaves who had regained their freedom. *(Lorrain Historical Museum of Nancy, France.)*

Carthage, and Scipio (to be dubbed Africanus) triumphed, thereby establishing the Roman Empire in the former Punic lands west of the Mediterranean. One consequence was a great harvest of slaves who were dispatched to Rome, where their proportion progressively swelled to forty percent of the population. The productive functions of the state became dependent on their labor. Because the ruling class of patricians had less for the plebeians to do, they adopted a policy of "free bread and circuses" to distract them.

ROMAN DEPENDENCE ON THE HORSE

The growing role of cavalry in the Roman armies rendered horse breeding an important function in the Roman Empire. Small landowners with horses supplied mounted sons (equites) for the Roman cavalry. By Julius Caesar's time cavalry was used to overwhelm the regions he conquered and to impress the populace with his power. Horse-borne troops were used for reconnaissance, foraged for supplies for his army while mopping up the enemies' own foragers, and were deployed in coordination with infantry in actual battles. The earliest cavalry wore helmets, carried shields, and fought with lances and javelins. Later, under Flavius, mounted archers were added. The horses were trained in a gyrus or training ring to turn quickly in either direction; trainers

141. The use of the horse in warfare contributed greatly to Rome's domination of weaker foes. *Horseman and Fallen Enemy,* a pen and bistre drawing by Antonio Pollaiolo (Florence, 1426; Rome, 1498), shows an armored Roman warrior riding over his fallen enemy. *(Staatliche Graphische Sammlung, München.)*

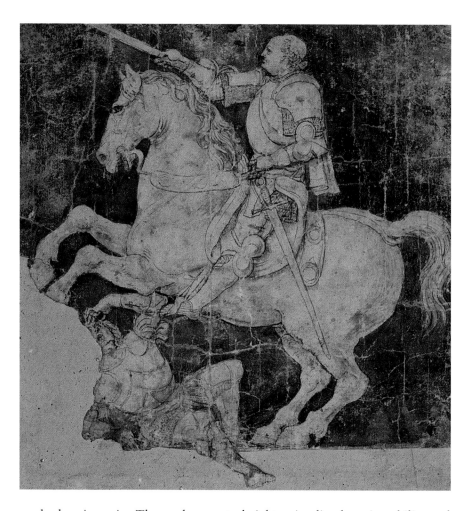

used a lunging rein. The goals were to heighten javelin-throwing ability and to avoid injury to the horses by training them to veer off quickly. This technique was much more effective than the direct charge, with only a spear or lance, into massed infantry, "all-or-nothing" style, which had been used previously by other armies. In the fourth century AD armor was added to the horse, enabling it to survive armed assault or retaliation (war horses did not tolerate wounds well). The armor, however, was added weight and prevented evaporative cooling of the skin, leading to excessive sweating while reducing stamina.

Mule breeding and training were important in the ancient Roman Empire. Reate was an area renowned for the large size and high quality of its mules. A large donkey jack was crossed with a good breeding mare to produce such a mulus. The female offspring are normally sterile because the chromosome count of sire and dam, when added together and divided by two, usually yields an odd number. Rarely, an exception allows an even number and fertility can result. Mules were important for traction and endurance; good specimens were highly prized. Seldom did the donkeys come in for praise, yet they were expected to carry riders and heavy burdens without complaint, despite inferior forage. The donkey was regarded as a lowly creature throughout the Mediterranean region and its health care did not receive much attention. Nonetheless, it was an important adjunct to transport and business activity. Strong bonds formed between boys and their donkeys.

GROWTH OF THE ROMAN EMPIRE

Lacking the innate intellectual curiosity of the Greeks, the Romans excelled in organization and implementation. They learned quickly to adopt to their advantage the advances made elsewhere. The spoils of war brought great wealth to the aristocracy and labor in the form of slaves. The empire grew to

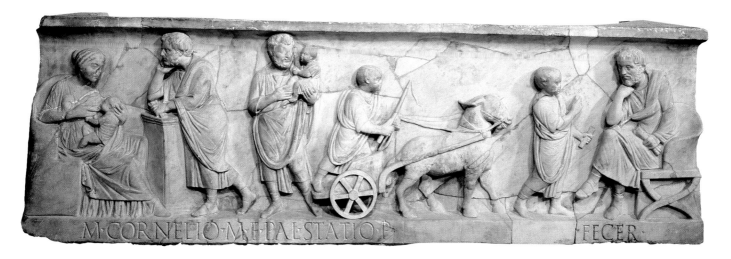

M·CORNELIO·M·F·PAL·STATIO·P· ·FECER·

142. Sarcophagus relief of a boy driving a goat cart. Strong bonds developed between children and their animals in Roman life. *(The Louvre, Paris.)*

the east with the invasions of Illyria and Macedonia. The childless king of the glorious Hellenistic city-state of Pergamon in Asia Minor bequeathed his kingdom, famous for its stock breeding, as well as its culture and architecture, to the Romans, who promptly plundered it.

Julius Caesar brought to submission cis-Alpine and trans-Alpine Gaul, drove the aggressive German tribes back beyond the Rhine, and entered Britain. The Gauls had fine horses and excellent sheep, and the peoples along the northern plains and the Helvetii of the Alpine valleys specialized in cattle, further enriching the Romans' herds and flocks. Despite Caesar's military successes, he was not trusted. At one point (49 BC) the Senate ordered him to return to Rome. Fearing for his life, he audaciously slipped out of Ravenna in a borrowed carriage drawn by mules to reach the Rubicon River, the line between Roman Italy and the area of his command, cis-Alpine Gaul. To cross the Rubicon with troops would be treason. He elected to do so, having sent his legionnaires ahead with this in mind. He marched on Rome and staged a successful coup. Caesar was made dictator of the empire and ruled for ten years, ending its traditional republic status.

Caesar took as a mistress the last Egyptian Ptolemy, Cleopatra, and fathered one of her children. By placing her on the throne, he brought Egypt into a close alliance with Rome. After his return he consulted Egyptian astronomers to reform the calendar, which had become two months out of synchrony with seasonal events, thereby creating the Julian calendar. He poured his prodigious energy into restoring and reforming the corrupted Roman state until he was assassinated in 44 BC.

A struggle for succession ensued. The emperor who was arguably "the greatest," Octavian of Velitrae (63 BC-AD 14), came from the ranks of an equestrian family of modest means. His father's wife, Atia, was sister to Julius Caesar; thus Octavian was the dictator's great-nephew. Caesar, lacking a legitimate son, made Octavian his adopted son to keep alive his name. Octavian was one of the triumvirate appointed to guide the empire after Caesar's death. After the deaths of Lepidus and Marcus Antonius, Octavian came to power in his own right. He was named emperor in 27 BC and given the name Augustus. During his reign, the golden age of the empire, the government was stabilized and the arts flourished. His death in AD 14 was followed by decline and disaster interspersed with a few valiant efforts to restore credibility. Notable reigns were those of Vespasian (AD 69-79), who restored fiscal responsibility, and Hadrian (AD 117-138), who built a wall to keep the Scottish barbarians to the north of it and a 200-mile-long line of forts from the Rhine to the Danube to protect the empire from the Germans. He restored respect and a degree of trust to the empire.

DECLINE OF THE ROMAN EMPIRE

During the watch of Marcus Aurelius (161–180) an epidemic plague arrived from the east. Increased barbarian raiding forced the transfer of forces with medical and veterinary services to the periphery of the empire. The decline of the Roman Empire put increasing pressure on professional services through retrenchment. Diocletian (284–306) passed edicts to control prices that included rules to cap fees for veterinary services, even for such trivial matters as trimming the mane or feet. Bleeding to remove bad blood was recognized to be more specialized and was allowed a three-fold fee increase.

After Diocletian, who in 250 had ordered destruction of all Christian writings and places of worship, Constantine became the emperor from 306 to 337. His reign was a high point in the history of the empire. In 313 he terminated the persecution of the Christians, put the sign of the cross on his battle standard, and declared Christianity the official state religion. In 325 he convened a great church council of more than 220 bishops in Nicaea to attain an unchallenged, official creed that brought church and state together, making the emperor all-powerful on earth. He erected gigantic statues of himself to make the point. He reunited the two halves of the empire (that Diocletian had divided) and became sole emperor by 324. He moved the eastern capital from Nicomedia to Byzantium (Constantinople) on the Bosporus Strait, the strategic waterway to the Black Sea. During his reign the vicious gladiatorial contests were terminated. Near the end of his life he was baptized.

Later, Justinian's reign faced disaster from barbarian invasions and epidemics. The result was massive migrations from the affected regions. Severe economies were implemented, including the closure of all public entertainment, which slashed the need for mulomedici. A law in 370 denied them payment, allowing them only clothing and subsistence. The western empire fell in 476, when Romulus Augustus was forced to abdicate and his army was dissolved. The *Hippiatrika* of the tenth century makes no mention of veterinarians after 488. Theodorus the Great (378–395) had divided the empire again into east and west, and the eastern Empire survived for a thousand years.

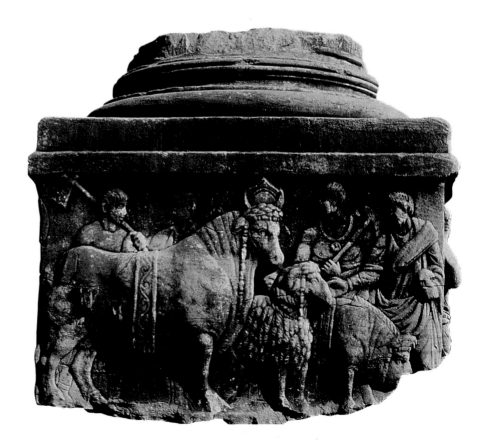

143. Base of the Decennial Monument (AD 303) celebrating ten years of the reign of Diocletian (AD 284–306) shows a state sacrifice of a pig *(sus)*, a sheep *(ovis),* and a bull *(taurus)*. This special form of sacrifice was given the composite name *Suovetaurilia*. The entrails were used for haruspicy. Animal caretakers were *suovetaurinarii*, the possible origin of *veterinarius*. *(Courtesy C.M. Dixon, Canterbury.)*

AN EMPIRICAL ART IN THE SERVICE OF THE ARMY AND AGRICULTURE

In the Roman Empire medical and veterinary work did not lead to high social status and was seen as an empirical, practical art. Treatment of visible, intelligible problems on which intervention could have a discernible effect, such as trauma and wound therapy, bleeding, and obstetrics, required manipulative or surgical boldness and dexterity; it became the forte of the veterinarians. The causes of disease were classified as "communitates." Recognized surgical conditions included penetrating foreign bodies, fractures and dislocations, abscesses and tissue swellings, and developmental deformities. Medical practice was also interventional and empirical and not based on scientific understanding. Medical "science" was primarily an intellectual exercise that was read about. Progress in understanding and effectively treating problems of internal medicine in humans and animals was slow.

Because Roman medical scholarship lagged far behind that of the Greeks, it had to borrow knowledge from them. Although the Romans distrusted the Greeks, they reluctantly had to import some of the skilled Greek doctors. Most of the early Roman writers were encyclopedist generalists who consolidated ideas and practices obtained from a variety of sources. Cato's (234-139 BC) *De Agricultura,* for example, covered many aspects of animal husbandry, such as beekeeping for honey and wax.

Cato distrusted the Greek doctors and their medicines. He extolled the virtues of cabbage, cabbage broth, and herbal concoctions as curative or preventive for most human ailments. He ventured into the realm of animal remedies, stating that a fasting man should prepare the herbal remedy and give the dose to a fasting ox as part of the doctrine of purification. Draft oxen were the backbone of Roman agriculture and transport, so they received a high priority. The bottoms of their hooves were smeared with protective pitch before they pulled loads along roads. If an ox became sick while working, Cato's recommendation was to give it promptly a raw hen's egg, to be swallowed whole.

The farms were worked by oxen and asses. The latter had to stoically turn the mill and carry out manure from the stables to the compost heap in bags tied to the pack saddle. Snakebite of an ox was treated by injecting a decoction of fennel and old wine into the nostrils, and plasters of pig dung were applied to the bite.

Cato recognized the importance of ectoparasitic mites and ticks. He prescribed a preventive lotion of olive oil dregs with lupin extract and wine to be smeared all over the animal after shearing for sheep scab. Two or three days later the sheep was to be washed in the sea. An alternative (for those far from the sea) was to rub the sheep well with salt. Cato was regarded as a callous person who saw most things from a business angle. He urged the farmers to sell their worn-out draft oxen and their blemished sheep and cattle. It is clear that the need for draft animals was reduced by the presence of large numbers of slaves and because the farm equipment for draft animals had not yet been well designed.

Rome was beset by epidemics of human and animal disease. Plagues and pestilence engendered enormous concern and fear in the populace, and the Roman poets immortalized the situation in their vivid descriptions. Describing cattle plague, Virgil (70 BC-AD 19) in his *Georgica* evokes horrific images of the suffering, the losses of animal life, and the stench and devastation that resulted. The mortality rates must have been phenomenally high. To verify the identities of the diseases is difficult, but surely one of the great plagues must have been anthrax.

Virgil observed the practices used to control the devastating "filthy scab" of sheep. Either they were drenched in streams and pools or smeared after shearing with bitter lees of oil and black bitumen. The scabs had to be lanced with steel to allow the inflammation to escape. Another practice for extreme cases was to bleed the sheep from the veins between the underparts of the feet. According to Virgil, if a sheep failed to stay with the flock and lay down, it should be killed to check the spread of the contagion throughout the flock. This dreadful plague was not sheep scab but anthrax. Virgil knew that horses and cattle, too, were affected and that the consequences were lethal: the animals died groaning, with blackened blood gushing from the nostrils or mouth.

When plagues visited Rome, the first in 293 BC, the people lost confidence in their gods and sent emissaries to seek help from the temple at Epidaurus in Greece. They returned with a sacred snake of Asklepios given them there. The snake swam to an island in the River Tiber, where a temple was built to the god of healing, and the plague abated. Greek physicians brought to Rome included Asclepiades of Bithynia (124–50 BC), who became quite popular. Adopting the Epicurean philosophy, he captivated the Romans and gained their trust. He prescribed few medicines. He developed the school of methodics, healing with simple dietetic and mechanical measures such as hot and cold bathing, bloodletting and leeching, laxatives and enemas, liberal use of wine internally and externally, massaging, and exercising. The school of methodics was a forerunner of the health spas that were much later to become so popular in Europe.

The "methodic" approach was developed by a pupil of Asclepiades, Themison of Laodicea, and was well suited to the activities of the early Roman veterinarians and the citizens. The simple, direct mechanical approach allowed the practitioners to be seen as decisive, practical persons of action. However, little intellectual progress in the study of animal diseases was made while this phase of empiricism held sway.

EARLY ROMAN WRITERS ON VETERINARY AND HUMAN MEDICINE

Marcus Terentius Varro

After an unsuccessful military career, Marcus Terentius Varro (116–27 BC) became head of the public library in Rome and dedicated his life to scholarly writing on many subjects, producing hundreds of works, many of which were lost. In his *Rerum Rusticarum* ("Concerning Agriculture") the third book covered agricultural topics, including animal breeding and husbandry. His veterinary comments show that he regarded epidemic diseases as contagious and attributable to invisible organisms that may come with the wind as a miasma from affected areas such as swamps. He attributed many dysfunctions to environmental stresses and management errors such as overwork or feeding too soon after work.

Observing that the medicine of horses was as complex as that of humans, Varro explained that, "on this account in Greece the veterinarians are most frequently called *hippiatroi* or horse-doctors." He divided veterinary care into two categories, one requiring a trained surgeon, the other capable of being mastered by a skillful shepherd. He was conscious of such environmental stresses as the temperature being too high or too low, the workload of draft animals being excessive or too limited to maintain health, and whether food and water intake after work was controlled. He gave special importance to the effects of hyperthermia or overwork: the consequences would be a gaping mouth; heavy, humid breath; and a feverish body. Bathing the animal, rubbing it with warm oil and wine, and covering it with a blanket were measures used to prevent chilling in such cases. If the response was not reassuring, bleeding from the head was called for.

Varro is most impressive in his comments on the idea of contagious diseases. He observed that one sick animal can be a threat to an entire herd. When there was evidence of a sickness spreading, he proposed segregating small groups of the herd "because a pestilence quickly takes possession of a large herd and sweeps it to destruction."

Varro stated that the Roman people sprang from a race of shepherds. Hence penalties were assessed in terms of numbers of animals. He pointed out that sheep were the first animals to be domesticated because of their docility and utility: milk, cheese, skins, and wool were cited, but not meat. He noted that the Latin word for pig, *sus*, is derived from a Greek word meaning "to offer as a sacrifice." He stated too, that "the most important persons of antiquity were all keepers of livestock . . ." The cattle were the foundation of all wealth, and Roman coins bore effigies of domestic animals. The high priority of oxen for draft work, especially the heavy grind of plowing, led to laws against killing working oxen. They could be fattened for slaughter and meat only when they were no longer able to work effectively. Bull calves were castrated at two years of age because recovery was said to be delayed if castration was done earlier. If done later, on the other hand, the animals were apt to become stubborn and useless.

Varro was concerned about the health of bees because honey, the only sweetening agent available in ancient Rome, was highly prized.

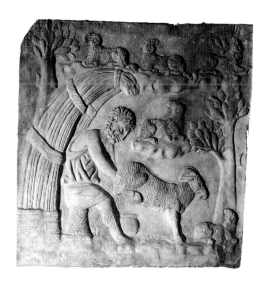

144. Shepherd milking a goat. Relief from Roman sarcophagus. *(Alinari/Art Resource, New York.)*

Cornelius Celsus

Cornelius Celsus (25 BC-AD 50) was a prolific Roman medical writer who, like Varro, recorded a broad spectrum of information. His works indicate that he was a gifted, well-educated man who enhanced the image of the medical professions among the better-educated Romans. Because his primary impact was at the practical level and was written in Latin rather than Greek, he did not receive the recognition he deserved until the Renaissance, when his eight-volume work *De Medicina* was "republished" to wide acclaim in 1478, and he was perceived to have been a "Latin Hippocrates." He stressed the importance of the physician's becoming familiar with the appearance and position of body organs, as were the physicians in the Alexandrian school, where criminals were subjected to laparotomy while still alive. He felt, however, that there were enough clinical cases among soldiers and gladiators to avoid the need to perform such deliberate vivisections. He favored the study of anatomy on cadavers, but this practice was proscribed in Rome in his day. Celsus identified three parts of "medicine"—diet, drugs, and surgery. He was attracted to the last because its impact was visible and obvious. Vitally important to Roman legions and horses was a tool to extract arrows, the Greek-designed Spoon of Diokles, which encircled and neutralized the barbs, allowing relatively nontraumatic withdrawal. Threaded dilators were used as speculums.

Celsus was the first to describe the general phenomenon of acute inflammation: *rubor et tumor cum calore et dolore* (redness and swelling with heat and pain). In addition, he recorded successful transplantation of tissue between human subjects. He described human rabies as a most wretched disease in which the patient is tormented by thirst but is afraid of water. Celsus recommended throwing the patient into a pool of water and holding the head under until the patient was forced to swallow, as well as amputation of the bitten limb and laying on of a hair from the rabid dog (the origin of the popular hangover remedy?).

Celsus recommended burning the base of the scalp with a cautery at two sites in cases of the "sacred disease" (epilepsy), to drain away the noxious humor. According to the famed Greek treatise on this topic (by the Hippocratic school), horses showing signs of nervous system disorders were found to have cysts in the brain on postmortem examination. Ocular discharges were common problems in humans and animals in the lands around the Mediterranean Sea. Celsus recommended the North African approach to treatment: apply the cautery to the crown of the head and burn it down to the bone. Apparently the expectation was that slow scarring of the resulting ulcer would

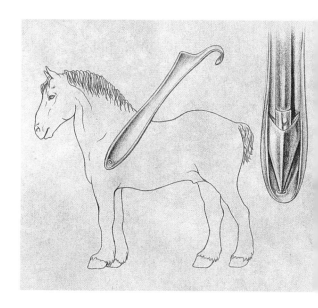

145. The Greek designed spoon of Diokles, somewhat enlarged relative to the horse. The hollow spoon was inserted alongside the embedded arrow; the arrow point was maneuvered into the small hole and the barbs into the wider end of the spoon. Holding the arrow in position, the entire spoon, along with the arrow, could be withdrawn without tearing the tissues. *(Redrawn from Meyer-Steineg, 1914.)*

contract and dry out the tissues, stopping the fluid discharges. Later Roman authors followed this tradition of *purgatio capitus* for cephalic diseases. They recommended it for conditions such as frenzy, rabies, vascular congestion, and circling disease. A guiding principle was that "bad blood" caused disease, and the treatments usually included bleeding from the jugular vein and the palate as well as purging the bowels.

Gaius Plinius Secundus

Pliny (Gaius Plinius Secundus, AD c. 23-79) was born in Comum. He served in many regions of the empire. An inveterate, inquisitive traveler, he wrote *Natural History,* a vast, thirty-seven–volume encyclopedia with 20,000 entries. The work contained an incredible mixture of fact and fable and included many exotic, revolting, and absurd recommendations for medical treatments. He perpetuated the myth that rabies in dogs is due to a worm under the tongue. A few of his claims had some merit, among them the ideas that fern removes intestinal worms, that a plant called ephedron arrests hemorrhage and improves difficult breathing while suppressing cough, and that infant diarrhea is suppressed by rennet. He attributed the discovery of the value of bloodletting to the river-horse (hippopotamus) which, when it has overeaten, finds sharppointed canes on which to press its body and cause bleeding, which cures it.

Pliny made a number of recommendations for treating sick animals. Skin disorders such as farcy and mange were to be treated with a liniment containing an extract of narcissus root. Similarly, the juice of the root of a certain lily (*Ixias* species) would kill mange organisms and ticks of several species and with boiled lupins will cure diseases in sheep and young cattle. He also said that butter was good for horses affected with farcins (farcy) or sallanders and mallenders, chronic eczematous conditions of the legs. Pliny seemed to have a fascination with dubious, revolting remedies such as donkey's urine (sick persons should drink it hot), goat's gall, dung of various species, and fresh, warm blood. Some were to be taken internally, others applied to the skin or to lesions. This damaging tradition later spread throughout Europe. No doubt it was hard to discard the traditional remedies, but they must have reflected poorly on the users, at least among caring, thoughtful people.

One can only conclude that Pliny was a collector of trivia without analytical judgment who delighted in promoting voodoo-like superstitions. In retrospect, Pliny can be credited with one significant toxicological observation: that water carried in clay pipes was much more wholesome than that conveyed via lead ones. He recognized that white lead was harmful to the human system. He noted that inhalation of the deadly vapor of a lead furnace was "hurtful to dogs with special rapidity." When the eruption of Vesuvius buried Pompeii in AD 79, Pliny was nearby and went ashore to investigate, only to die of the poisonous fumes.

Dioscorides

Dioscorides, who lived in the first century AD, (c. 40-90), was a Greek born in Cilicia (now in Turkey). A surgeon in the Roman army, he had a personal passion for collection, identification, and evaluation of healing herbs, extracts, and minerals. He used distillation. He wrote a careful five-volume work, *De Materia Medica,* or *Hylica,* about AD 64-77, which has stood the test of time. The *Hylica* was used by Galen and continued to be used through the Arabian period and the Renaissance for medical and veterinary reference.

Columella

Columella was born in Gades (Cadiz), the former Punic colony in Spain, and later moved to Syria and then to Rome. He lived in the first century AD on a farm far from the city. He was steeped in knowledge of practical agriculture and insisted that farmers should acquire medical experience for the well-being of their stock. An eloquent writer, he produced at least twelve volumes of writings between AD 42 and AD 68. These contained detailed information about breeding, feeding, husbandry, and health of livestock. He predicted that "wild animals once obtained for their fine taste or for sport will one day be acquired and used for gain." He was a keen, thoughtful observer and offered many clear descriptions of animal diseases and medical interventions. He understood parasitism and contagion and was experienced in veterinary techniques, including castration. His writing on veterinary medicine became the veterinarians' bible in many lands and languages, persisting throughout the Middle Ages. He stressed the need for hygiene in buildings and separation of sick animals from healthy ones, as well as isolation of pregnant animals from the herd. In Columella's *De re rustica (On Husbandry),* the volume on animal medical care (book twelve) represented a new pathway for the modernization of veterinary service. He stands above all other Roman authors in the fields of animal husbandry and veterinary science because of his unique combination of scholarship and practical field experience.

Columella provided a valuable record of Roman methods of castration, which was not performed on cavalry horses or racehorses. Compression by a band of cut fennel was used to crush the spermatic cords in the scrotums of young calves. This technique, inherited from Mago's Carthaginian practice, was undoubtedly developed to avoid hemorrhage and infection, as were the strong rubber rings in use today. Presumably the band would be tightened once or twice as it took its effect *paulatim* ("little by little"). Animals destined to become draft oxen were not castrated until two years of age. The animal was restrained, and a special narrow, wooden, forceps-like clamp was applied across the scrotum above the testicles. The scrotal sac was incised, and the testicles were squeezed out and cut off at their attachments to the cords. Part of the epididymides remained attached to the cords, leaving a residue of hormonal production so that the animal retained some masculine features, including greater strength. Evidently the practitioners of castration were aware of the physical and behavioral effects of the male generative organs, since

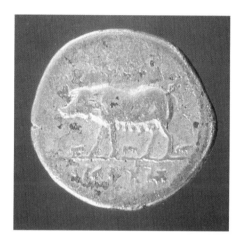

146. Denarius of Vespasian, a Roman coin showing a sow with twelve teats but only three piglets. Vespasian's reign (AD 69-79) was notable for restoring fiscal responsibility to a corrupt state after the assassination of Julius Caesar in 44 BC. *(Courtesy Dr. Rainer Grimm, Traunstein.)*

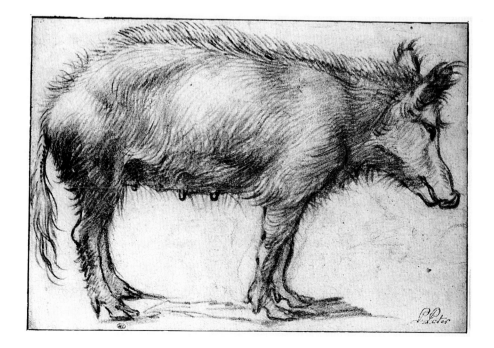

147. *Study of a Sow* by Paulus Potter (1625-1654). This sketch of a tall-standing primitive country pig with long legs, snout, and hairy body is strikingly similar to the sow found on the denarius of Vespasian (Plate 146). *(Armeria Reale, Italy.)*

some of the factors responsible for them survived the technique. The wound was smeared with wood ash and thin leaves of silver. After a few days pitch was applied to deter flies.

Two methods were given for neutering piglets. In the first, two incisions were made quickly through the scrotal wall and the testicular fascia and the testes were squeezed out and cut off. The second method involved making a single incision to cut the median barrier, then reaching in with crooked fingers to pull out the testes.

Serious dystocias in ewes were handled by embryotomy, the deformed or lodged fetuses severed into removable pieces in utero and then withdrawn.

PHLEBOTOMY AND HIPPOSANDALS

Because the Roman veterinarians came to depend on phlebotomy (bloodletting) as their unique skill and as a cornerstone of veterinary therapy, it deserved special attention. The practice can be traced from Egypt's Kahun papyrus through the works of Greek scholars to Roman times. In the Roman Empire, however, it was raised to an "art form" of veterinary therapy. Columella, for example, advised bleeding the entire herd of goats when the first few cases of disease appeared in a herd. He did appear to have some reservations about its efficacy, however, because he advised if the treatment appeared to be of no avail, the animals must be sold or slaughtered and their flesh salted. Even healthy horses were bled seasonally: phlebotomy was used as a spring tonic to remove the old, corrupted blood, a dependable resource generator for the practitioner. The blind faith in bloodletting was a consequence of the prevailing humoral theory of disease.

The technique for bleeding horses involved the use of a special cutting instrument, the sagitta, a sharp-pointed metal device shaped, as the name implies, like an arrowhead. When circumstances allowed, the preparation for bleeding started the night before, with only a light feed being allowed. A rope was tightened around the base of the neck to obstruct venous return and thereby "raise the vein." The horse was sponged with a little water to plaster the hair down, and the contours of the jugular vein stood out clearly. The thumb of one hand was used to stabilize the vein while the other hand, holding the tip of the sagitta in position between thumb and forefinger, drove the point into the vein about a hand's breadth below its bifurcation at the angle of the jaw. The blood streamed forth and was collected in a container. After the desired volume had been extracted, the wound was dressed and the horse was put in a dark, comfortable stall or stable and not moved for two hours. It was common practice to bleed the horses again a week later, this time from the rich venous plexus of the palate. Despite blind faith in the efficacy of the practice, it was common for a rest period of a month or more to be prescribed for work animals after bleeding.

Transportation was enormously important in the Roman Empire. Care of the hooves was a major concern of those who were responsible for working animals such as horses, mules, and draft oxen. Traction, pack burdens, and riders imposed additional heavy stresses on the feet. These frequently were exacerbated by rough or treacherous road or track surface conditions. The Romans studied the maximum weights of loads to which animals could be subjected without damage. They also knew how long animals could be worked in a day and spaced their maintenance posts with this in mind. Cavalry horses were especially susceptible to injury when they were required to gallop over rough terrain. It was recognized that horses were prone to hoof problems when they were put into heavy work after a period of inactivity, and that stall hygiene, that is, preventing the horses from standing in manure or wet areas, was necessary to avoid softening of the hoof. Special hardening preparations and growth stimulators for the outer layer of horn were used.

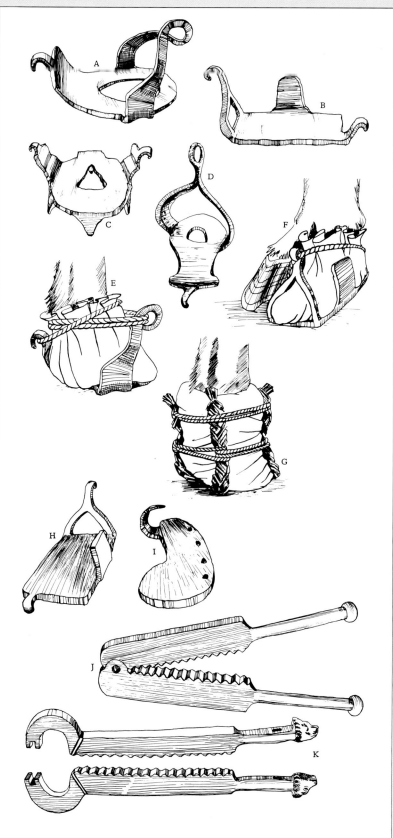

A - "Solea ferrea" (therapeutic shoeing)
Note that support of the sole is possible thanks to the space contrived in the shoeing.
B - "Demi-solea ferrea" (therapeutic shoeing for cattle).
C - "Solea ferrea" (therapeutic shoeing for the treatment of lameness).
D - "Solea ferrea."
E - Dressing protected and fastened by the "solea ferrea."
F - Dressing protected and fastened by the "demi-solea" in the ox.
G - Fleming's shoeing (1907), probably comparable to what the Roman "solea spartea" was.
H and I - Transformation of the "demi-solea" of the Romans (H)
                into the ox shoeing of the Dark Ages (I).
J and K - Comparison between castration pincers ensuring hemostasis.
Model K is a sketch inspired by the piece found in the British Museum in London, and by the one found in the Granet Museum of Aix-en-Provence, with a castration pincers of the XIXth century (J).
To demonstrate the similarity between the Roman instrument and that utilized in the XIXth century, we have eliminated the decoration of the device. It will be noted that the hinge is unfortunately missing on the Roman model.

148. The Romans made significant advances in protecting horses' hooves from wear and injury. Protective cushions or "hipposandals" were tied onto the hooves to hold medications in place and keep the hooves clean. A metal plate with wings and hooks, a *solea ferrea,* was eventually developed; it allowed the hipposandal to be better secured to the hoof. These devices could be individually tailored. (*From Walker,* Ars Veterinaria, *Kenilworth, New Jersey, 1991, Schering-Plough Animal Health.*)

Although the Romans made progress in protecting the hooves from excessive wear and injury, they do not appear to have taken the crucial step to nailed-on, iron horseshoes. Instead, they tied on protective cushions made of Spanish broom, a braided plant material, in the form of "hipposandals." These wrappings were used to hold medications in place for treatment of injuries while keeping out dirt.

Hooves were trimmed by paring. A ridger, a special knife shaped with upturned edges, was used to trim the horn at the angles of the sole and the frog. Incisions were made in the sole to relieve abscesses. The resulting lesion called for a hipposandal containing medication to be applied until healing occurred. A significant advance was the development of a *solea ferrea,* a metal plate with wings and hooks that allowed the hipposandal to be tied securely onto the hoof. These were tailored to match the shapes of the hooves of horses and cattle.

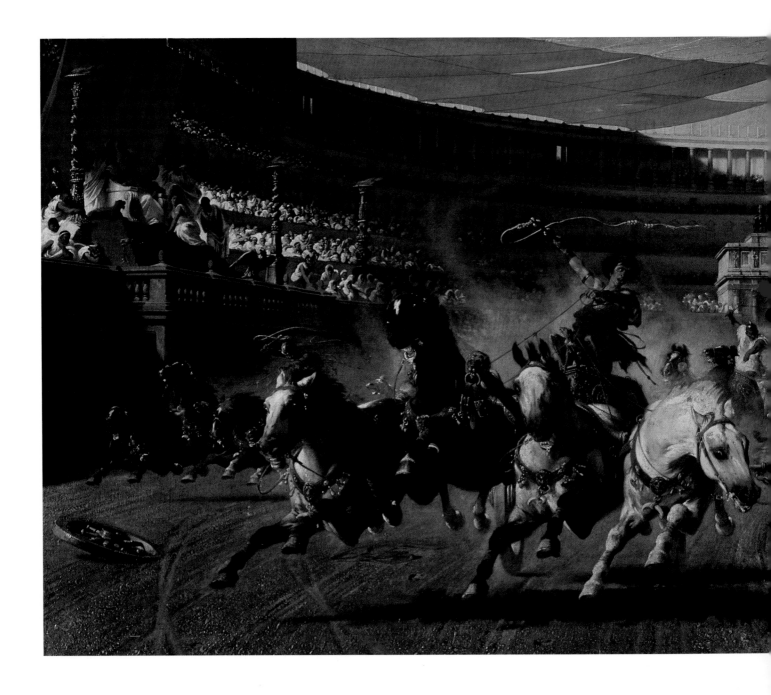

ANIMAL ABUSE FOR ENTERTAINMENT

The Roman culture made an enormous commitment to spectator sports performed in circuses and amphitheaters. Chariot races were held in the Circus Maximus, which held 250,000 people, and horse racing was popular. Evidence of fights between gladiators, between men (usually slaves) and animals, and among groups of animals portrays a progressively more depraved and sadistic society. A large hunting industry developed to trap and transport the wild animals needed to sustain the brutal exhibitions.

Bison were used for spectacular fights in the amphitheater and were regarded as untameable. So, too, was the now extinct wild ox (aurochs or urus), a massive, ferocious beast that had to be trapped in a pit. Julius Caesar had initiated bullfighting on horseback as practiced in Thessaly, the rider galloping beside the bull, seizing it by the horns, and killing it by twisting its neck.

149. *The Chariot Race* by Alexander Wagner depicts the use of animals for sporting entertainment, a key aspect of Roman culture. Chariot races contested in the Circus Maximus in Rome were frequently observed by 250,000 people. *(Manchester City Art Gallery, England.)*

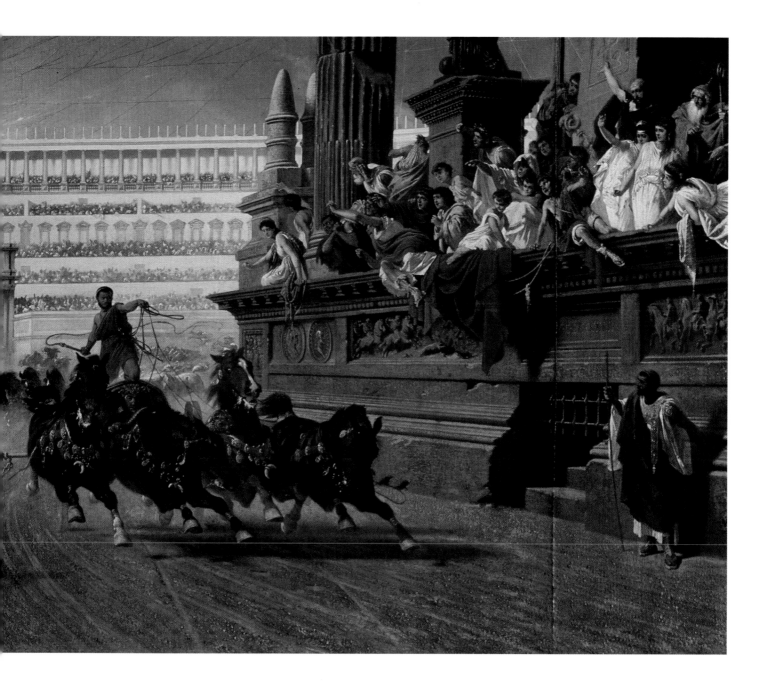

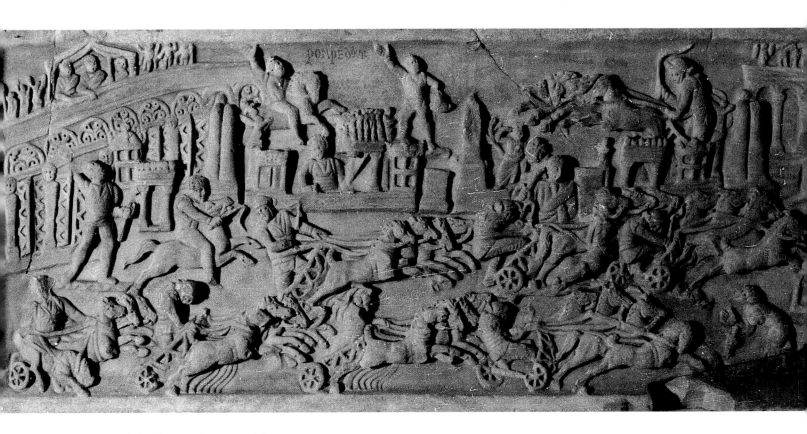

150. While the Greeks enjoyed horse-back racing, the Romans favored chariot races in the Circus. Both four-horse and two-horse chariots were common. A typical race was seven laps or approximately three miles long. The competitiveness of chariot racing took a heavy toll on the horses, and various types of trauma were commonplace. *(Relief from Pinacoteca Communale, Museo Archeologico, Foligno.)*

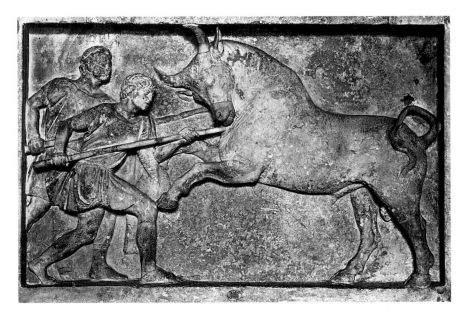

151. As the Roman Empire declined, the nature of the sporting events became more sadistic and depraved. Evidence such as on this stone relief, *Two Roman Gladiators Fighting a Bull,* shows fighting between men and animals. Obtaining wild animals for these brutal spectacles became a major industry. *(Mansell Collection, London.)*

PELAGONIUS: PROMINENT RACETRACK VETERINARIAN

The popularity of chariot racing in Rome was phenomenal. Pelagonius of Illyria, a prominent equine practitioner in the fourth century AD who wrote in Latin, specialized in tending the horses used in the chariot races at the Circus Maximus in Rome. He stressed the importance of good conformation—wide nostrils and chest, powerful musculature with strong quarters, straight legs with a long stride, and black hooves. Horses were selected for behavioral characteristics, too, including a confident, active attitude and a responsive temperament. Many breeds were known by their region of origin throughout the empire and to the east, in Armenia and Persia. Each had characteristics and reputations for performance in war, hunting, or racing. Size was important for the war horse. Racing was followed with such zeal that the performers, both the horses and the charioteers, were studied individually; audiences became obsessed with the complexities of the sport. The finest racehorses were said to come from Cappadocia (now part of Turkey); the best of them were retired to a good life after a productive career at the track, some competing until they were twenty years old.

A continuous search was conducted to locate horses of good quality. Hannibal had developed the North African Arab types as fine cavalry horses. These became known to Romans as Libyan or Numidian horses. Julius Caesar was enamored of Spanish horses because of their speed. He also used the large Gallic horses for cavalry and draught. The larger Parthian horses, with impressive musculature and proud bearing, were considered the bravest in the lion hunt. The closely related Armenian, Cappadocian, and Persian (Nicaean and Medean) types were almost certainly interbred with the Parthians.

The Greek horses were considered inferior, perhaps because those from Thessaly were small and may have been inbred. The "greys" from Mycenae, however, were considered fine racers, probably having been enriched with Persian bloodlines. The breeders of racehorses favored the Cappadocian, North African, Spanish, and Italian strains.

Pelagonius stressed the importance of dry floors in stables kept free of dung. He said that racehorses could be broken at two years of age. After the age of two years, training for racing began, but normally horses were not raced in the stampede-like atmosphere of the circus until they were five years old. The Greeks favored races on horseback, but the Romans much preferred the chariot races of the Circus. Four-horse chariot races were the favorites, but two-horse events were also common. Roman racing had much in common with modern harness racing in North America, complete with starting gates that were wide enough to accommodate the quadriga. Each race was normally seven laps long, requiring about three miles of racing. The actual race was wilder in Rome than in modern racing; collisions and injuries were commonplace. The eyes were particularly vulnerable to blows and to sand thrown up by flailing hooves. Many horses became entangled in chariots or loose wheels and were thrown, with serious damage to chariot, charioteer, and horses a likely outcome. Tendon and muscle strains, trauma to the lower legs and hooves, concussion of the hoof with laminae breaking down or joint injury and hemorrhages, shoulder damage, and tongues cut by the bit were all frequent occurrences. Since no iron shoes were available, hoof wear and abrasion were major problems.

Pelagonius compiled a book in Latin, *Ars Veterinaria (The Veterinary Art)*, in the second half of the fourth century AD. He was a strong advocate of bleeding, relating the site to be bled to the part that was affected. He often recommended that the horse be given the blood to drink after other medications were added to it, or that the blood be made into a salve and smeared on the horse's body. Although he "borrowed" a great deal from other authors, including Columella and Apsyrtos, he failed to adopt some of the latter's insights.

Pelagonius's recommendations are most questionable in the areas of the management and treatment of conditions once they were diagnosed. He gives no evidence of awareness of the contagious nature of epidemic diseases such as strangles, since there is no call for isolation of cases. He addresses this condition under the general caption "Head Ailments." In an era long before the discovery of antibiotics it was difficult to manage conditions caused by bacteria, in this case microorganisms of the genus *Streptococcus*. Pelagonius recommends only hot plasters of resin and grease. For fevers he provides little guidance toward either diagnosis or treatment. He dismisses any value of pulse taking, either for evaluation of heart rate or for the character of the pressure wave. Respiratory problems are lumped in the category "broken wind," and drenches of purgative herbal preparations with oil and wine coupled with application of a hot, caustic salve over the abdomen are recommended. Swollen fetlocks were treated by standing the horse in cold water, bleeding, applying blisters (irritating poultices), or firing with a hot iron to create inflammation.

The narrow range of techniques and medications employed leads one to a conclusion that any claims of efficacy contained more bluff than substance. This explains why mastery of the technique of bleeding was so important. If one could establish the idea that bad blood caused all or part of the problem, efficient removal of blood from the affected region by deft deployment of the sagitta would seem a convincing, positive intervention.

GALEN: FOUNDER OF THE EXPERIMENTAL BASIS OF COMPARATIVE MEDICINE

One figure towers over the medical scene in Roman times. Galen (AD c. 130–c. 200), born in Pergamon, Greece (Roman since 130 BC; now Bergama in Turkey), had studied philosophy and medicine by nineteen years of age. He then traveled for nine years to expand his knowledge, in Smyrna studying the muscles, in Corinth more anatomy, in Palestine pharmacology, and for several years in Alexandria observing dissection and experimental physiology, always recording his consultations. Returning to Pergamon, he became a surgeon to the gladiator school for several years, which provided a unique opportunity for him to pursue his zest for the advancement of knowledge by treating wounded gladiators and dissecting animals killed in the ring. In AD 162, at thirty-two years of age, he departed to chance his arm in Rome and stayed there for twenty-four years. He quickly gained recognition as an influential physician and gave public lecture-demonstrations involving dissection of the animal body, usually pigs, Barbary apes, or goats. He acquired a reputation for wound treatment. He also performed vivisections to show physiological principles and became the intellectual leader of the medical profession. He was asked to tutor the son of Marcus Aurelius. His reputation as a prescriber of effective medications followed his use of mixtures of exotic substances that today are still erroneously called "galenicals." One concoction he made was designed to be a universal prophylactic to protect the emperor from all poisonings and other diseases. Its most potent ingredient was opium. A man of prodigious energy, Galen produced more than four hundred treatises before he died in Pergamon between AD 200 and 210.

Twenty-two of Galen's treatises, about 2.5 million words from his pen, have survived, exceeding in volume Aristotle's works and constituting more than three fourths of all surviving medical works of antiquity. These works are but a fraction of his total output. His hometown of Pergamon was the site of the first use of animal-skin parchment for writing and also claimed the finest library after Alexandria's. Among his many works, the most interesting are *De User Partium* ("On the Useful Parts of the Body"), *De Anatomicis Administrationibus* ("On Anatomical Procedures"), *De Facultatibus Naturalibus* ("On the Natural Functions"), and *De Locis Affectis* ("On the Diseased Parts").

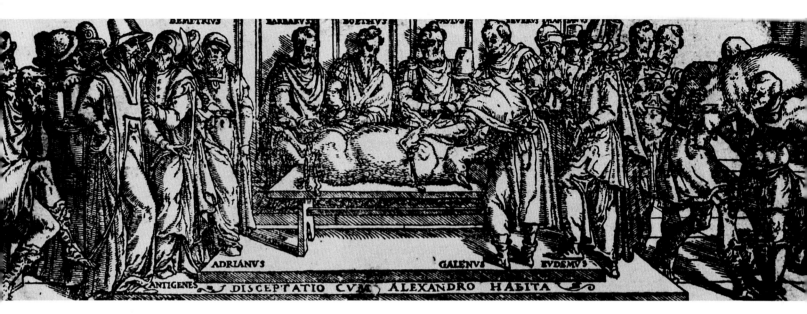

ADRIÁNVS   GALENVS   EVDEMVS

ANTIGENES   DISCEPTATIO CVM ALEXANDRO HABITA

Despite his extraordinary energy, ego, and intellectual dominance of the medical field, Galen was a loner and failed to establish an immediate scientific legacy of scholars to carry on his work. Thus his works were the last in a line of eight hundred incredible years of major Greek scientific and medical illuminations of human thought. For him, every clinical case raised questions to be pursued and ideas to be studied and recorded.

It is astonishing that Galen's writings, so admired in Greece and Rome, remained unknown elsewhere in Europe until the thirteenth century, when they were translated into Latin by Arabic scholars and "galenism" became a medical philosophy in its own right. Galen's contributions to medical progress were legion. His legacy to veterinary thought was an anatomical and physiological perspective based on his animal dissections and functional interpretations.

Despite the enormous respect the world of learning had for the Greek genius Aristotle, not even Aristotle was perfect. He made serious errors that impeded progress because of the tendency to accept his writings as "gospel." It seems peculiar that Aristotle made his biggest mistake about the very organ that he had exploited so effectively, the human brain. He thought that the brain did not fill the cranial vault but left a space for air, the function of which was to cool the heart, which he considered to be the seat of intellect. The error is astonishing, since the Hippocratic (400–377 BC) corpus of works must have been available to Aristotle and the section "On the Sacred Disease" states that

> men ought to know that from the brain, and from the brain only, arise our pleasures, joys, laughter, and jests, as well as our sorrows, pains, griefs, and tears. Through it in particular, we think, see, hear, and distinguish the ugly and the beautiful, the bad from the good, the pleasant from the unpleasant . . .

Galen, on the other hand, was a true disciple of Hippocrates and wrote in depth about his works.

Evidently Aristotle thought he knew better, and uncritical adulators believed his views rather than those of the medical writers. Later, in the newer cultural center of Alexandria, as part of the legacy of Aristotle's pupil Alexander, Herophilus and Erasistratus (about 300–250 BC) studied the nervous system more scientifically. The latter described motor and sensory nerves

152. Woodcut showing Galen (c. AD 130–200) performing vivisection on a pig during an anatomical demonstration. One of the few positive contributions to come out of the Roman bloodsports was Galen's use of the Circus to study anatomy and perform dissections. *(National Library of Medicine, Bethesda, Maryland.)*

and traced them all back to the central nervous system and ultimately to the brain itself. Galen did not go to Alexandria until much later, during the second century AD, but evidently he learned of the medical advances made there and was impressed by them.

Galen's most important contribution to biology was to correct Aristotle's colossal error on the function of the brain, writing, "Aristotle! What a thing for you to say!" Galen was convinced that sensation, movement, and thought all began in the brain. He studied the cranial nerves, the recurrent nerves to the larynx, the systemic and autonomic nervous systems, and the physiological and geometrical aspects of vision, using Euclid's principles to study the latter. Perhaps the most distinguished of Galen's discoveries was the role of the recurrent laryngeal branch of the vagus nerve. Severing this nerve in the pig abolished the pig's ability to squeal. He showed that the same effect on the function of the vocal cords occurred in other species.

Galen performed dissections and physiological investigations on many types of animals, preferring to study pigs, apes, oxen, and goats and extrapolating the results to human function. He held strong convictions of a teleological basis for the design and functions of the body. Also, he was inclined to speculate wildly at times, without benefit of effective methods to test his ideas. Many of these proved erroneous, for example, his doctrine that the arteries actively dilate to fill with blood but do not pulsate. His productive career in medical studies, as might be expected of an active trailblazer, is a vast tapestry of accurate findings and erroneous interpretations.

It is perhaps appropriate that Galen himself made some major misinterpretations of function. Galen's teleology was based on the idea that every structure was designed perfectly for a purpose, nature being the infallible Creator that does nothing in vain. Unlike the revolutionary biology of the nineteenth century, this view aligned Galen, himself a pagan, with religious doctrines of all kinds because it allowed the Creationist view of the infallibility and wonder of creation to be preserved and extolled without threat.

Although Galen derived major discoveries about human function and disease from his comparative studies of animals, occasionally the differences in anatomy and physiology led him astray. His use of vivisections would be unacceptable today on humanitarian grounds, but in his time it did not seem to become a major issue, perhaps because brutality toward humans and animals alike was rampant, even *demanded* as entertainment. This Greek who worked in Rome was the first experimental applied comparative physiologist, the first physician to base clinical investigation on anatomical and physiological studies, and an experimental neurologist whose ideas about medical science, although subjected to many attacks, usually carried the day and held center stage for 1500 years.

VETERINARY MEDICINE DURING THE DECLINE OF THE ROMAN EMPIRE

The period after Galen was a difficult time in the Roman Empire. There was greater recourse to mythology and more acceptance of Greek traditions, including their gods. Horse breeding and health continued to have the highest priority for veterinary duties, but livestock production was also important. Paladius (third century AD) carried on Columella's tradition and had a special interest in avian medicine for farm poultry.

Roman authors after Galen who wrote in Latin on veterinary medicine had the advantage of access to some of the Byzantine Greek works. Although they could be expected to have been more advanced in the principles of internal medicine, this was not always the case. The most important of these Latin authors was undoubtedly Vegetius. His contribution is discussed in Chapter 10. Although the Roman contribution was less than might have been expected, the Roman achievements were practical and were applied on a grand scale. In that sense, as a profession of "doers," veterinary medicine suited the Roman temperament. The Romans established the veterinary profession and gave it the high status of "immunes" in the military units. Warfare, transportation, and plowing were the top priorities. The Roman profession derived its medical acumen from agricultural experience, unlike the Greek profession, which had stronger ties to medicine. Pliny noted that "the horse suffers from the same maladies as man" and that animals have the ability to lead humans to cures useful for themselves.

ΙΕΡΟΚΛΕΟΥΣ ΠΕΡΙ ΠΝΕΥΜΟΝΟΣ ΣΚΕΨ(...)

Ἐὰν ποτὲ τὸν πνεύμονα ... πῶς ἀλγήσῃ. τὸ μὲν
ποιεῖ τὸ σ ... πολυχρέμιον· καὶ πῆ τὸ βαρὺ μάλιστα
ἀστὴρ φ· ὁ ἡμέραλέ· συμπίπτῃ τὸ σῶμα· καὶ
ὑπ' αὐτῆς, ὡς ὁ δοκεῖ ὁ τάριον κατὰ τὸ ... κθραι
μέζας τε ἁμαρᾷ καὶ ... καὶ τὸ μὲν τῶ μ ... καὶ
τὴν τροφὴν πρὸς ... ζλι τῷ· θερα ποιεῖ ἀ ...
τούτου. κρόκου· σμύρνης· κασίας· κινναμ ...
μώμου· ταῦτα πάντα τρίψας καὶ ... δὸ ...
ἅμα μῖξαι τι· καὶ ὅμοιον ... ἀρχὴ μά τι ...
ἀναγκαῖον δὲ προλαμβάνειν τὴν τῆς θερα ...
τε ... ἐὰν γὰρ ... θ ... ὅτην αἱ ὁ πνεύμονα
τύπου. τῷ βυτῷ·

Λ ΤΙΒΕΡΙΟΥ ΕΙΣ ΤΟ ΑΥΤΟ

Λαμπρὸν μὲν καὶ τὸ ... καὶ πρόχειρον ... ταύτην

CHAPTER 10

The Byzantine Empire
A Veterinary High Point

CULTURAL CURRENTS

The Roman Empire was divided administratively into western and eastern branches in the third century AD and recombined later by Constantine. Communication between the branches declined, however, and Theodosius divided the two parts again in AD 395. The Latin west progressively lost its contact with the more creative Greek east and soon succumbed to the barbarians; the east survived for another millennium. The lack of a driving force for natural philosophy in the west allowed it to become relegated to the status of a hobby whose boundaries were prescribed by the church. On the one hand, monastic orders and church schools provided the foundation of education; on the other, they did not tolerate any departure from faith in the Creator-God. Thus Christianity could live with Plato's monotheistic "demiurge" but not with Aristotle's natural philosophy of rational explanations for everything. Christianity was not prepared to grant autonomy to the emerging scientific philosophy. Christian monasticism emerged in fourth-century Italy and spread throughout Europe. The monasteries were places of retreat for those who wished to pursue lives of piety and biblical study. Strict rules were imposed, and secular studies were allowable only if they were directed toward sacred purposes, that is, they had the status of a handmaiden to theology. Nonetheless, the monasteries were the preservers of literacy and scholarship during the Dark Ages.

A Greek colonizer named Byzas had established a settlement called Byzantium, destined to grow into the mighty city of Constantinople (Istanbul today) after Constantine the Great selected it as the strategic site for his capital of the eastern or Byzantine Empire. Because this part of the Roman Empire had been transplanted onto Greek culture, the Greek language and classical tradition survived there long after they withered in the west. The site for the capital was well chosen by the emperor. It was surrounded by water on three sides, and once its fortifications were developed and adequately guarded, it was almost impregnable and hard to blockade. Raided from all directions, the city withstood all assaults—there were many between AD 616 and AD 914, including at least seven by the Arabs—and served repeatedly as the base for conquests and restoration of the surrounding Byzantine Empire. The turning point came in 1071 when, in the battle of Manzikert (Malasgard in Armenia) against Turkish forces led by the Seljuk Sultan Alp Arslan, Emperor Romanus IV was captured and most of his army was destroyed.

Constantine's domination, which had restored the empire's branches, had been obtained at a cost. He had forced the Western and Byzantine churches to accept a single church creed. After he died, bitter theological disputes resurfaced. In one such dispute Nestorios, patriarch of Constantinople, insisted on Christ's humanity and refused to accept Mary as Mother of God,

153. *Facing page,* Veterinary medicine is prominently featured in Byzantine manuscript illumination of the *Hippiatrika.* Commissioned by Constantine Porphyrogenitus, the work is a collection of writings by seventeen authors about the treatment of ailing horses. This folio is from the earliest known copy of the *Hippiatrika,* a decorative edition that is missing its illustrations. Later copies do contain artwork. The writing is by Hierokles and is about diseases of the lungs. Hierokles made one hundred and seven contributions to the *Hippiatrika.* (*Ms. Phill. 1538, fol. 29ʳ. Staatsbibliothek zu Berlin, Preußischer Kulturbesitz.*)

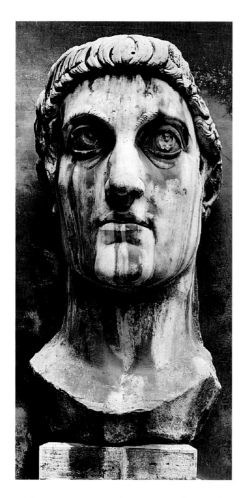

154. Constantine the Great, who established the capital of the eastern or Byzantine Empire at Constantinople. Fragment from a large marble statue. Early fourth century. (*Archivio Fotografico, Musei Capitolini, V.U.O., Rome.*)

whereas the Monophysites gave priority to Christ's divinity. Nestorios was exiled, but his followers, known as Nestorians, developed a school at Edessa in Syria. The emperor closed the school in AD 489, forcing the Nestorians to flee to Nisibis in Persia. One faction then sought protection from King Khusraw in the Persian capital, Jundishapur. A tolerant multicultural university with a medical school flourished there and survived the Arabian conquest in AD 636. The Nestorians undertook the huge challenge of translating the record of Greek culture into Syriac, starting with the works of Hippocrates and Galen. The Syriac versions at Jundishapur were later translated into Arabic and became the link that transmitted Greek scholarship to Islam and eventually to the West.

As for Constantinople, its forces and its will shattered by the Turks, it fell in 1204 to Frank Crusaders who imposed the Roman church. Grassroots ecclesiastical opposition fermented and led to the restoration of the city to the empire fifty years later. No longer able to draw sufficient military resources from its domains, however, the great city, once the vibrant center of the world stage, finally succumbed to the Turks in 1453.

BASIL I: FROM GROOM TO EMPEROR

Byzantine Emperor Michael III, a moody drunkard with an addiction to horse racing, was attracted by a highly spirited but unmanageable horse that no one could ride or handle. A nobleman told the emperor that he had a strong young groom named Basil who was remarkably gifted with horses. Basil was invited to try to control the rearing beast. Grasping the bridle firmly with one hand and pulling the horse's ear down with the other, he murmured into it in a low voice (or did he blow into it?). The horse, as if by magic, became a docile servant. The ecstatic emperor drafted Basil, a young Macedonian of lowly origin who was born in Adrianople in AD 836. Michael left the running of the empire to his uncle, Bardas, who founded a fine university and encouraged the export of religious and scholarly ideas—such as the missionary expedition of Cyril and Methodius, two monks of Thessalonika, to illiterate slavic Moravia. The monks invented a script to allow translation of the scriptures and services, which evolved into the Cyrillic alphabet used by the Slavic church.

After acquiring high status in the court, Basil became co-Emperor and arranged the murders, first of Bardas, then of Michael in 868. The peasant with the gift of horse mastery guided the empire to its golden years, despite the turmoil of competing cultures, and is remembered as the greatest of the later rulers. After his Macedonian clan was replaced, the empire declined until the Ottomans took the city in 1453.

PRIORITY OF CAVALRY VETERINARIANS

The need to maintain powerful, mobile defense forces made the cavalry paramount and gave veterinary medicine an essential role in society: to sustain horse breeding and the health of cavalry steeds.

Horse and chariot racing became major spectacles in stadiums known as hippodromes. During the reign of Justinus I the population was divided into two groups depending on which group of horses (identifiable by colors and flags) they supported. A bizarre civil war resulted in which tens of thousands were killed. The cavalry adopted the tactics of the successful barbarians (Huns or Avars, Magyars or Turks).

Veterinary history is recorded in some of the twenty books of the *Geoponica* ("agriculture"). Based on the Greek works of Democritus and Xenophon and the writings of the Alexandrian poet Nicander, the *Geoponica* was a compilation of works prepared by Cassianus Bassus and issued anew by Emperor Constantinus Porphyrogenitus. Books sixteen through nineteen discussed the husbandry and diseases of livestock. These works commanded respect until the eighteenth century. It seems that even when they were written there were disparities between the agricultural and the medical views about animal diseases. The *Geoponica* contained many superstitious and erroneous statements. The physician Demetrius of Constantinople wrote a fine treatise on falcons and their treatment, which indicates the high priority given to the sport of falconry.

The major focus of veterinary art in the Byzantine era was assembled in the *Corpus Hippiatricorum Graecorum* or *Hippiatrika,* a compilation of knowledge specifically about horse medicine (the editor's name was not recorded). Original works by seventeen authors were lost, but copies giving their identity survived. The *Hippiatrika* was published in the ninth or tenth century AD, although the writings date to the fourth century. The *Hippiatrika* constitutes one of the classics of the veterinary art and a superb piece of literature. It

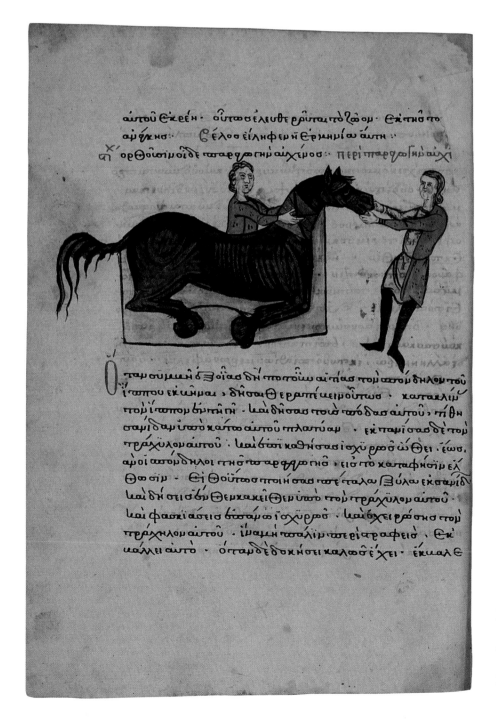

155. Richly illustrated versions of the *Hippiatrika* that have survived all help to clarify the various forms of horse medicine found in the text. This portion of a folio from a fourteenth-century manuscript shows a horse being restrained while its teeth are examined to determine its age. Apsyrtos (c. AD 300–360), a Greek military veterinarian for Emperor Constantine, contributed one hundred and twenty-one writings to the *Hippiatrika;* his description of the dentition of the horse is the oldest known. (*Cod. gr. 2244, fol. 54ʳ. Bibliothèque Nationale, Paris.*)

156. Hierocles, a philosopher and jurist, made one hundred and seven written contributions to the *Hippiatrika*. He is seen as a lecturer in this Byzantine illustration from the *Corpus Hippiatricorum Graecorum*. *(Cod. gr. 2244. Bibliothèque Nationale, Paris.)*

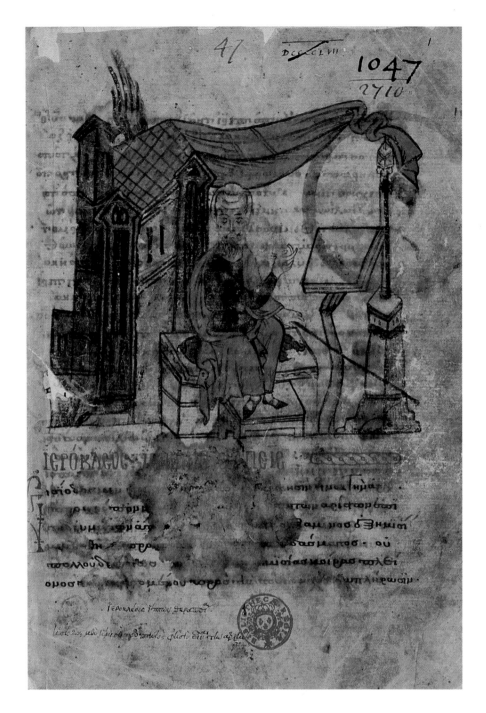

contains writings by Apsyrtos, Hierocles, and fifteen others. Hierocles was a philosopher who recalled much from Greek works on equine care and described foot-and-mouth disease. The hippiatric writings of Grecian veterinarians in the Byzantine Empire during the fourth century reveal that they were trailblazers who succeeded in raising veterinary clinical competence to a high level, especially in equine medicine. They created a focus on veterinary diagnostic, therapeutic, and preventive medicine with a moderate and rational basis.

Although the veterinarians knew the works of Galen and the classical Greek scholars, they were not restricted by the reasoning of the philosophers or the speculations of the agricultural writers. They focused on the highest veterinary priorities, including the treatment of the traumatized horse injured in battle; the importance of care of the locomotor systems, especially the lower parts of the limbs and the hooves, when the horse was carrying loads over rough terrain and sustaining further stresses because of galloping and wheeling in combat; the need to manage nutrition and digestive disorders, especially when high-quality feed could not be obtained; awareness of the contagious nature of certain diseases; and the practical management of reproduc-

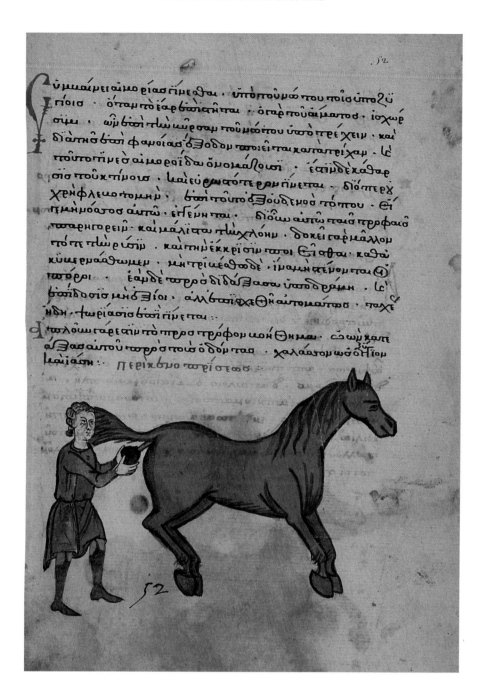

157. An illustration from a fourteenth-century *Hippiatrika* manuscript showing the treatment of distention in a horse. Much of the information on horse care found in the *Hippiatrika* came from the Greeks, and the use of oil and wine for medicinal purposes is frequently prescribed. Here a clyster of wine, oil, soda salt, and the sap from wild cucumber roots is being administered to relieve the distention. *(Cod. gr. 2244. Bibliothèque Nationale, Paris.)*

tion and breeding disorders, including infertility, dystocia, and abortion. They stressed moderation in therapeutic measures, and their most revolutionary conception was the identification of their highest goal as preventive medicine.

APSYRTOS: GRECIAN GENIUS OF EARLY EQUINE MEDICINE

Apsyrtos (c. AD 300–360), a Greek born in Clazomena, was the chief military veterinarian in the Byzantine army of Constantine the Great. He maintained the cavalry horses in the campaigns against the Sarmatians and the Goths in the Danube River valley. The standards of thought and the clarity of his writings were far in advance of their epoch. He provided outstanding clinical descriptions of the main digestive problems in the horse, including specific causes of colic such as overeating, volvulus, acute distention of the intestines, and rupture of the stomach. The descriptions were presented so clearly that the differential diagnosis is readily made in each case. Laminitis was attributed to overeating and handled by dietary restriction, gentle exercise, and mild bleeding, although cooling of the extremities was not mentioned.

Throughout his writings Apsyrtos recommended treatments that exude moderation, simplicity, and common sense enhanced by the authority of thoughtful analysis and experience. He used drenches and ointments. He advised against the common practices of periodic phlebotomy of sound horses and excessive bleeding of sick ones. Apsyrtos wrote the most detailed account of the dentition of the horse that has survived from antiquity. He described the timing of the appearance, shedding, and replacement of the teeth, which allowed the veterinarian to determine the age of a horse simply by examining its teeth.

Apsyrtos recognized anthrax as a specific disease and knew that it would not respond to available treatments. He realized that tetanus was usually a result of puncture wounds or pelvic infections. The clinical signs were described with exceptional clarity and accuracy. Unlike many of the farriers and horse doctors of his day, he differentiated glanders (four forms) from strangles and stated that they could spread from horse to horse.

Apsyrtos practiced surgery, starving the horse before operation. Ligation and cautery were used in castration. Drainage of wounds involved the use of wool setons saturated with pitch or oil. Fractures below the carpus or tarsus were splinted and wrapped, usually with favorable outcomes. Those above the knee or hock and those of the neck were considered incurable and grounds for euthanasia. He advocated sensible surgical techniques and approaches, with attention to sanitation, and knew that some conditions were hereditary. He was contemptuous of all superstitious quackery, divinations, and incantations.

Apsyrtos was an authority on breeding disorders of horses. He observed the gestation period of the mare to be eleven months and ten days. Foals born prematurely could be raised successfully with special individual care, provided the pregnancy held for at least nine months and twenty days. Shorter pregnancies made survival of the foal unlikely. Management of the pregnant mare to prevent abortions and premature births was stressed. Recognizing that some horses are predisposed to attacks of colic and that this condition carries a high risk of interruption of pregnancy, Apsyrtos claimed that such animals must be accorded special attention to diet, avoidance of stress, and use of volatile herbal oils (often by enema) to relax the bowel and assist the passage of feces and gas. Cases of prolonged pregnancy were addressed by blocking the mare's nostrils to induce abdominal presses, supplemented with medications designed to stimulate contractions. Rather more barbaric was the approach to unwanted pregnancies (for example, after a mating with an inferior stallion or when in preparation for racing), which involved manual destruction of the fetus.

It is evident from the following quotation that Apsyrtos was aware of and was a follower of Hippocrates' School of Medicine at Cos. Apsyrtos, too, wrote in the tone of master to pupil and was almost certainly a trainer of other veterinarians:

> Now since we see the most illustrious and trustworthy doctors of humans predict certain symptoms by which each malady might be recognized, so also in veterinary medicine we think it necessary to adopt this mode of forecasting. In men there is an inborn faculty of speech by which they can express what is troubling them, nevertheless, those skilled in the healing art in humans consider the observation of symptoms necessary. How much more needful then, must it be in veterinary practice to observe those symptoms of disease recognizable as such by our traditional art in animals which are dumb by nature.

Apsyrtos's approach to diagnosis and treatment included review of the body systems (digestive, circulatory, respiratory, urinary, genital, and nervous) and was adopted by progressive colleagues, but it seems to have been forgotten again in many parts. If the veterinary profession had moved forward from the high point he brought it to, it would have become a much more effective and valuable intellectual and practical force in society. As a cultured Greek in the Roman Empire, Apsyrtos stood tall intellectually and was accorded high rank by the emperor. It was to be a long, disheartening time, indeed, before veterinary medicine as a profession could stand as tall again.

CHIRON THE VETERINARIAN

Chiron (not the centaur of legend) was a Greco-Roman veterinarian. The name "Chiron" may in fact have been a pseudonym for Hierocles, some of whose writings are also recorded in the *Hippiatrika,* who worked about AD 350. Chiron wrote ten books on veterinary medicine organized by body systems, the *Mulomedicina Chironis.* The book on the nervous system described *purgatio capitis,* the complex routine used to treat most diseases of the head. These included circling disease, frenzy, rabies, fainting, and swelling or tumor of the head. The sequence included fasting from grain, bleeding, sweating, a large dose of the purgative wild cucumber root, rest, bleeding from the palate, and purgation of the head with artemisia (wormwood) or wild radish roots, following which the head was tied down to the lower forelegs for drainage; then mustard poultices and metal cauteries were applied to the parts perceived to be diseased. Chiron's writings manifest a professional standard usually well below that of Apsyrtos, yet he worked during the same period. He acknowledged Apsyrtos as the master.

One topic of particular interest was the method recommended for handling uterine prolapse in the mare. Chiron attributed the method to Apsyrtos. The mare was laid down with her head inclined and turned above her back. Warm water was poured over the uterus to clean it of debris; then it was plastered with a mixture of oil and wine to protect the tissue as it was manually reinserted and repositioned. A bladder freshly taken from an animal was introduced into the lumen of the uterus and inflated, then tied off to seal it. The vaginal opening was closed with three sutures to retain the uterus and its bladder while allowing the escape of urine and any discharges. A concoction of burned laurel leaves and herbal extracts in red wine was poured into the uterine lumen. Twelve days later the sutures were removed and the bladder pierced to release the air and allow its withdrawal. Then, with rest and good feed, a prompt recovery was anticipated.

VEGETIUS AND THE INTRODUCTION OF BYZANTINE VETERINARY PROGRESS TO ROME

Publius Vegetius Renatus, known as Vegetius, wrote the four-part *Artis Veterinariae, Sive Mulomedicinae* in the fifth century AD. Some sixteenth century scholars and publishers believed that he was the same person as Flavius Vegetius Renatus, who wrote on the art of war. Current scholarly opinion favors this view. Vegetius also wrote *On the Distemper of Horses.* He was a layman intensely interested in veterinary medicine. His writings were not original; in fact, the inconsistencies in style suggest multiple authors. Nevertheless, they provided a bridge of information from Byzantium, where active, original veterinary work was going on, to Rome, where nothing had been written since Columella, in the first century AD. Vegetius did add medical ideas to these veterinary writings, such as humoral medical theory, particularly methodics, which was popular in Rome. It is arguable, however, that the ideas of Byzantine veterinarians (particularly Apsyrtos) were more advanced than those of Roman doctors, with the exception of Galen, who was from the eastern Greek culture.

Flauij Vegetij Renati Ain
Büchlein / vonn rechter vnnd warhaffter
kunst der Artzney/Allerlay kranckheyten / ynnwendigen vnd auffwen-
digen aller Thyer/So etwas zyehen oder Tragen mügen /Als pferd/Esel /Maul-
thyer/Ochsen/vnd anderer/Auch wie man allerlay kranckhayten art vñ gepresten
erkesten soll/die mit geerencken/Salbungen/pressungen/Lassen/vnd ander Artz-
neyen etc.zůuertreyßen/Vormals durch Vegetiũ Renatiũ in Latein beschriben/
yetzunder/inn Teütsche sprach verwendt/Allen vich ärtzten/Marstallern/
Schmiden/Reyttern/Burgern vnnd pawren/Auch allen denen die
mit gemeltem vich vmbgeend/gantz nutzlich vnd not-
wendig zů geprauchen.

M. D. XXXII.

158. Title page from the first German edition (1532) attributed to Flavius Vegetius Renatus's *Artis Veterinariae (Veterinary Art)*, c. fifth century AD. Vegetius's writings provided a link for original veterinary work from Byzantium to Rome. *(The Wellcome Institute Library, London.)*

Vegetius had a broad perspective of hygiene reminiscent of Varro's, recommending raised, dry wooden floors to keep the hooves of horses hard and in good condition and well-ventilated buildings that should be fumigated to control infection. He also recommended segregation of animals with contagious diseases lest they infect the others, closing facilities and water supplies that had housed the sick, and burial of the dead. His theme was to prevent disease wherever possible and initiate treatment promptly for the afflicted. He described several forms of malleus (glanders), the plague that knocked horses down as if struck with a hammer, including farcy. He noted that farcy was infectious, and that it and another condition, which he called the "dry disease," should never be treated by phlebotomy. Instead, bleeding and sweating should be reserved for moist diseases. He was an advocate of firing, at least as a last resort, claiming that it cleared up cankered sores, allowing drainage. He noted that the skill of the horse doctor is evaluated by how well he accomplishes curing with the cautery while avoiding deformation. He described laminitis but attributed it to overwork and fatigue. He advocated slinging for treatment of fractures of the limbs, splinting supports for jaw fractures, and incision to drain abscesses.

Vegetius did address diseases of cattle, although the quality of writing is poor and the anatomical information is misleading. He noted that farmers deplored the lack of information about how to handle their cattle. Among the conditions he described, anthrax, rinderpest, foot-and-mouth disease, tetanus, and tuberculosis are recognizable.

Vegetius detailed the woes of the veterinary profession and made a strong plea for society to make a more enlightened commitment to it. He tried to provide that perspective by describing the best practices known at the time. He noted that in Rome the field was unattractive because of its lowly status and poor fees compared with those for the practice of human medicine. Hence the veterinary art became the province of men of lower competence and character. He urged that the profession be restored to the higher esteem it was accorded in ancient Greek culture. His recommendations went unheeded, and the practice of veterinary medicine was relegated to farriers untrained in the corpus of medical knowledge. After Vegetius the decline and virtual disappearance of veterinary scholarship became dramatic. Like the writings of Celsus, the *Mulomedicina* was republished during the Renaissance.

PUBLICATION OF THE *HIPPIATRIKA*

Early in the tenth century AD Emperor Constantine Porphyrogenitus ordered the compilation of all knowledge written in Greek of the veterinary art applied to horses. The result was the *Corpus Hippiatricorum Graecorum* or *Hippiatrika (Equine Medicine),* a collection of writings by Byzantine veterinarians on the practices they employed. It formed the base of recorded knowledge in the field. The identity of the compiler remains a mystery. It was not printed until 1530 in France, in a Latin translation from the Greek by J. Rueil (Ruellius), dean of the medical faculty of Paris. There appears to be no English version readily accessible, a serious deficiency for English-speaking historians. There were seventeen major contributors, with Apsyrtos making one hundred and twenty-one contributions and Hierocles, one hundred and seven. Chiron, Hippocrates (the veterinarian), Pelagonius, and Theomnestos were also contributors. It appears that Apsyrtos had compiled the material initially; most of it dates to his period in the fourth century. The quality ranges from outstanding in Apsyrtos's works to empirical and inferior in the works of Pelagonius. The practice of emptying the rectum manually for digestive disturbances was advocated by Apsyrtos. Hierocles concurred and, unlike the master, had great faith in copious bleeding with his sagitta. The strange practice of treating rabies by surgical removal of the "worm under the tongue"— actually the *lyssa,* as it was called, which was merely a fibrous attachment— seems an extraordinarily dangerous and erroneous technique to have become perpetuated. Theomnestos claimed to cure rabies by dosing with hellebore. Thus the Byzantine veterinary understanding and the insights of Apsyrtos, superior to those of many physicians of his time, were offset by those of other horse doctors whose remedies were anachronistic, even dangerous, yet were pursued unchallenged, with blind faith.

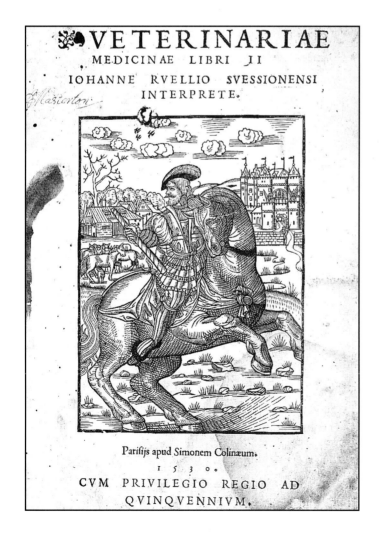

159. Woodcut from the title page of *Veterinariae Medicinae* by J. Rueil (1530), an early Latin translation of the *Hippiatrika*. It was published in Paris, where the French physician served as dean of the medical faculty. *(The Wellcome Institute Library, London.)*

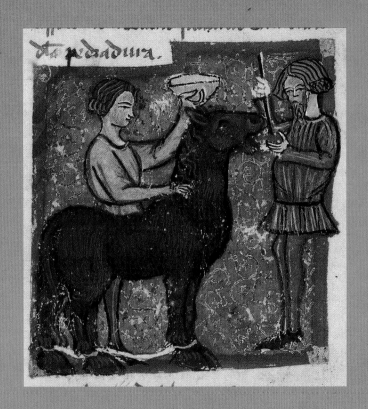

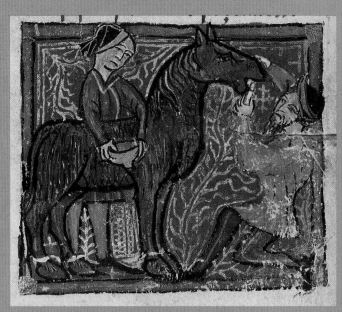

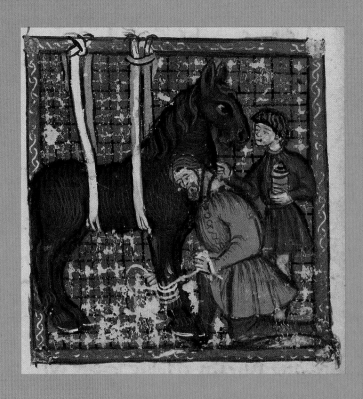

Arabian Medical and Veterinary Progress

ADAPTATIONS TO NOMADIC LIFE IN THE DESERT

The roots of Arab civilization extend back to the original desert nomads. Their harsh physical environment required mobility and a dependence on livestock and crops that could survive the arid conditions. Their endurance, stoicism, and fatalistic outlook may have derived from these ecological challenges. They also had to be ever ready to defend their territorial niche against raiding neighboring tribes. Regular, almost ritual skirmishes were the rule, as if to "keep in shape" for the unexpected. Unencumbered by the trappings and distractions of urban society, the nomads developed superlative memories based on an oral tradition and wonderful gifts of romantic storytelling and poetry.

RELIGIOUS INFLUENCES, ISLAMIC EXPANSION, AND CULTURAL EVOLUTION

The Arab people worshiped at the Ka'abah in Mecca, a cubical building said to have been built by Abraham. Many gods, idols, and icons were permitted there until the time of Muhammad (around AD 570-632), who claimed to be the messenger of Allah, the one true God. He and his successors had to flee by night on camels to Medina, two hundred miles to the north, in AD 622. Seven years later he returned to Mecca in triumph. He purged the Ka'abah of all idols and banned all images of natural things, including animals, thereby giving rise to a special type of symbolic, abstract art and the representation of fantastic forms such as animals with human heads. The Prophet had eleven wives but failed to produce an heir.

Although the Arabs conquered Alexandria in AD 642, the Greek university survived until about 719. The Arabs took over what was left of the Greek writings. After the fanatical stage of conquest during which a vast Islamic empire was built in about a century, the Abbasid caliphs, who around 750 followed the Umayyad caliphs, encouraged the "hellenization" of Islam. The human intellect was prized as one of Allah's gifts, so the Abbasid caliphs allowed reason to probe even the depths of religious faith and established a great center for scholarship in their capital, Baghdad. The forward-looking caliph al-Mamun (813-833) created an academy in which translation was encouraged, and the great Greek writings were conveyed into Syriac and Arabic. The Syrian region had been hellenized earlier, and its language was to form an important bridge between Greek and Arabic. The Nestorian Christians of Jundishapur had made a significant contribution to the earlier Syriac translations. Standing out among the scholars who undertook the academy's work were Hunayn ibn-Is'haq (809-873) and his team. In a remarkable endeavour

160. *Facing page,* Juan Alvares de Salamiellas's *Libro de Menescalcia de Albeiteria et Fisica de las Bestias* was one of the first books written for the veterinarian *(albeytar)* in Spain. This beautifully illustrated mid-fourteenth-century work is truly remarkable for its small, delicate illustrations that provide a view of the life of a medieval horse doctor. The two-part manuscript is profusely illustrated with a variety of scenes of horse care, including the external appearance of horses and the surgical and medical treatment of their maladies. Animal restraint is commonly seen, including the use of hobbles, in various medical procedures. A variety of instruments and their uses are shown. Scenes of oral dosing, examining the mouth with attention to the teeth, and bandaging of limbs are among the many illustrations. Wrapping a fracture of the metacarpus with hemp while the horse hangs from a suspensory harness so that its hooves bear no weight is also illustrated. *(Ms. espagnol 214, Kap. 11. Bibliothèque Nationale, Paris.)*

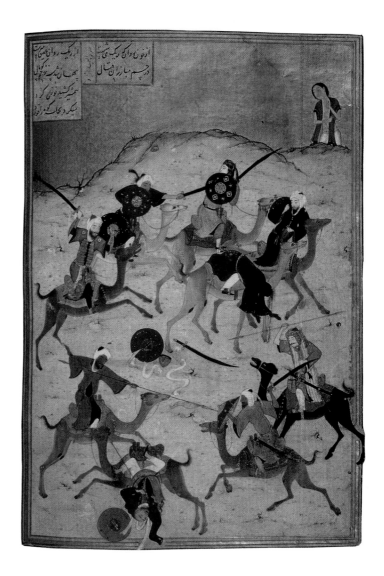

161. *The Battle of the Clans,* a miniature by Bihzad from a Khamsa of Nizami (c. 1490). The scene shows two tribes fighting on camelback. The camels are gnashing their teeth, and their eyes, embellished with gold, seem to show rage. The forlorn figure watching the battle from the hilltop is Majnun. The tribes are fighting an epic battle because of his love for Layla. According to the legend, he lost her to another man, but later, when they finally met, she swooned and he fainted. After her death, he visited her grave and died there. The story is one of the great tragedies in Arab-Persian-Turkoman literature. *(Add. 25900, folio 121ᵛ, The British Library, London.)*

he succeeded in expanding the vocabulary and scope of the Arabic language so that it became a medium capable of expressing complex scientific ideas.

EARLY ISLAMIC MEDICAL SCHOLARS

The Koran, written before the Arabs obtained the works of the classical Greeks, gives no instruction or advice on medical matters, perhaps reflecting the level of ignorance of such things in Arabia in the seventh century AD. Dissection was not permitted under Islam. Diseases and wounds were treated with folk remedies ("bedouin medicine"), and incantations were invoked for serious conditions. Yet illnesses were a prominent feature of everyday experience because of the difficult environment and lack of informed hygiene or medical services. Traditional or folk healers treated the symptoms rather than the underlying disease. Herbal products predominated and were supplemented by animal products, some of them repulsive. Modern chemical science has revealed many pharmacologically active agents in plants that were known to the Arabs.

The 129 translations of Greek medical works cited by Hunayn focused primarily on the bounty that stemmed from Galen's fertile mind. The translations of Galen led to his ideas becoming dominant throughout Islamic medicine. Hippocrates was revered for his ethics, and a version of his oath was required of the Arabic human and animal doctors. The Hippocratic medical writings did not receive the same acclaim that Galen's did, and many were not translated. A selection of multiauthored writings of Galen's era later was translated and compiled as the *Corpus Hippocraticum.* Thus it appears that the transmission of much of Hippocrates' thought was attributable to Galen's commentaries rather than to the direct translation of the works of his great predecessor.

Hunayn was born into an Arab Christian family in Iraq. His apothecary father sent him to the capital for private medical education. He developed an insatiable appetite for written knowledge of the healing art, which fostered his desire to master the Greek language. His precocious genius was recognized, and when he was about twenty-one years old, al-Mamun appointed him to head his academy, the Bayt al-Hikmah. His work was patronized by the subsequent caliphs through the caliphate of al-Mutawakkil, who reinstated him after subjecting him to a period in prison. In addition to translations, Hunayn wrote ten treatises on ophthalmology, which had a profound impact on that specialty for centuries and were built upon by ibn al-Haytham (Alhazen), the greatest of Arab physicists, and others. Hunayn's translations encompassed, in addition to the works of the medical authors, the works of Aristotle and Dioscorides (AD 40-80), a Greek in the service of Rome. The latter's *Materia Medica* became a classic in Arabic versions and an indispensable aid to the health professions. Hunayn also translated the veterinary works of Theomnestus. The life sciences, particularly the medical professions, are indebted to Hunayn, a towering scholar who laid the foundation for subsequent achievements of Islamic scholars and also set the ethical standard for medical and veterinary behavior.

A contemporary of Hunayn, al-Kindi (801–873), was the first Arab philosopher and the first to wrestle with the harmonization of philosophical reasoning with the theological dogma of Islam, a predictable intellectual battleground. He championed the truth as the basis for accord between religion and philosophy. He suggested that the holy texts be interpreted as allegories to guide intellectual endeavour. The philosophers could use their thinking to study the words of revelation that the masses would accept in faith. Al-Kindi, who also served as court physician, had sound advice for his medical colleagues:

> *Take no risks, bearing in mind that for health there is no substitute. To the extent to which a physician likes to be mentioned as the restorer of a patient's health, he should guard against being cited as its destroyer and the cause of his death.*

Ar-Razi (865–925), who became known as Rhazes in the West, was a dedicated Persian physician who went to the great hospital in Baghdad to gain experience, then returned to ar-Rayy (near the site of Tehran) to direct a hospital. He became the most famous of the practitioner-educators and medical authorities of the Islamic sphere of influence. He adopted the mystical doctrine of Pythagoras and Plato that the soul should strive to attain a philosophical ideal, pending which it was fated to go through a series of transmigrations. This doctrine disputed the Islamic conception of divine revelation and brought him into conflict with theologians. Ar-Razi's competence and compass as a doctor were unchallenged, and he contributed to many branches of medicine and pharmacology. His leadership led to care being extended to the tragically disabled such as lepers and the blind. His thinking guided educated animal doctors as well. He had a remarkable intuitive sensitivity for human nature and was an advocate of psychotherapy for the ills of the spirit. He wrote a comprehensive manual of the healing art that won him wide acclaim and provided the first accurate descriptions of smallpox and measles, thereby allowing these two scourges to be differentiated clearly for the first time. He berated quacks and charlatans while espousing collaboration, consultation, and trust between physicians. He was an enthusiast for the idea of continuity of medical care provided by the family doctor and believed in the need for experiments to test the efficacy and safety of treatments. He assembled materials for a vast encyclopedia of medicine, the *Kitab al-Hawi,* but died before it was completed. His students completed it, and it became known as the *Continens* after it was translated into Latin by Farragut in 1279. In 1486 it was printed in the West.

Al-Majusi, a tenth-century Persian from at-Ahwaz, wrote a classic, all-embracing medical text, essentially a synopsis of Galen's works that included his schema of the heart and circulation.

AVICENNA'S *CANON OF MEDICINE*

162. A page, written in Hebrew, from a fifteenth-century Italian copy of the *Kitab al-Qanun* or *Canon of Medicine,* the great encyclopedic opus on medical knowledge compiled by the Persian genius Ibn Sina, or Avicenna (980-1037), as he became known in the West. The *Canon* contained all that was known of medicine at the time. Avicenna also wrote about animal diseases, especially of the horse, and mentioned diseases of the dog and the elephant, despite having no experience with either species. The section on horses was translated into Latin during the reign of Frederick II. *(Ms. 2197, cod. 492r. Foto Roncaglia, Italy.)*

Another Persian genius, Ibn Sina, known to the West as Avicenna, was to make an enormous contribution to medical scholarship in his short life. He was born in Khorasan (Afshana), near Bokhara (part of Uzbekistan), in 980 and died in 1037 in Hamadhan (Ecbatana). A remarkable child prodigy who was practicing medicine by sixteen years of age, he appears to have retained his extraordinary aptitude for scholarship into adulthood: he became one of the most productive intellectuals of all time. Because he was arrogant and his views were controversial, he found it necessary to move often. He settled longest in Jurjan, where he began his great encyclopedic opus on medical knowledge, the *Kitab al-Qanun* or the *Canon of Medicine,* which he completed in Hamadhan. The work opens with a profound definition:

> *Medicine is the science by which the dispositions of the human body are known so that whatever is necessary is removed or healed by it, in order that health should be preserved or, if absent, restored.*

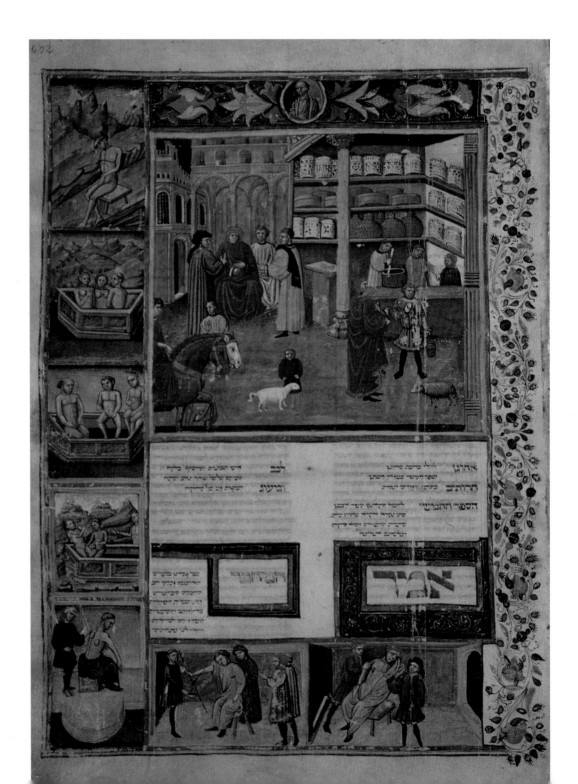

Avicenna, having lost the notes of his own clinical experiences, provided instead a work that is primarily a great, brilliantly systematized conceptual framework for all that was known of medicine. It was translated into Latin within a hundred years of his death and became the standard reference text of the health sciences for many centuries. He listed and evaluated every facet of medicine, recognized that some diseases were contagious, understood dietary and environmental effects on health, urged early and complete excision of cancerous tissue, and recommended testing new drugs by experimentation on animals before testing them in humans. He developed a neo-Platonic philosophy in accordance with the ideas of al-Farabi, which conflicted with Koranic doctrine. Veterinary authors adopted many of his medical concepts. Avicenna wrote about animal diseases in the treatise on science, but this part was not translated into Latin until the time of Frederick II in the thirteenth century. The main veterinary topic was the horse, and Avicenna's views were considered an improvement over those of Aristotle. He followed Aristotle in mentioning diseases of the dog and the elephant but had no firsthand experiences of these species.

When the political power of the Abbasids decayed, there was a swing back to the view of traditional Muslim theologians, who condemned the adulteration of the Islamic dogma that resulted from unfettered philosophical reasoning. They stressed that the intellectual endeavour must always be under the control of revelation. As a consequence, scholars emigrated from Baghdad to the new centers that sponsored intellect, Cordova in the West and Bokhara in the East. An attractive center for scholarship was later founded in Cairo.

ALBUCASIS: MASTER-SURGEON OF THE WESTERN CALIPHATE

In the western caliphate in the Iberian Peninsula great medical schools were established at Seville, Toledo, and Cordova. Al-Zahrawa or Albucasis (c. 936-1013), the court physician in the royal city of az-Zahra, near Cordova, was a brilliant surgeon and author of the encyclopedic *Medical Vade Mecum.* The section on surgery was an extension of the work of Paul of Aegina, an Alexandrian Greek of the seventh century who wrote a book on surgery largely derived from the Hippocratic collection. Albucasis added much material on cautery. His organization and emphasis were strikingly original; in addition, he described more than two hundred instruments. The work was translated into Latin in the twelfth century in Spain and had a significant impact on European surgery. Albucasis was an authority on sutures and antiseptics, the treatment of fractures and wounds, abdominal conditions, and the full range of obstetrical and pediatric problems. He brought status and respectability to the field of surgery. His work placed the Iberian Peninsula at the forefront of surgical technique, including veterinary matters and experimental surgery, for a century.

The Hispano-Arab intellectual thrust came into full flower during the reign of the Muwahhid caliph Yaqoob al-Mansoor (1184-1199). His student, Averroes (Ibn Rushd) (1126-1198), had been appointed Qadi of Seville by al-Mansoor's father and ordered to write a commentary on the works of Aristotle. Born in Cordova in 1126, Averroes was a jurist and physician who became the greatest interpreter of Aristotle and by necessity a brilliant philosopher in his own right. His rebuttal of the devastating attack on the philosophers, *Incoherence of Philosophers,* by the powerful mystic theologian al-Ghazali (1058-1109), was entitled *Incoherence of the Incoherence* and was aimed at defending Aristotle. His translated writings are credited with providing the West with its introduction to Hellenistic philosophy. Ever a humble man, Averroes said, "I believe the soul is immortal but I cannot prove it."

163. *Medical Vade Mecum* was written by the brilliant surgeon Al-Zahrawa, or Albucasis (c. 936-1013). It included a section on surgery in which he described more than two hundred instruments. In a page from an early fourteenth-century Latin copy of the work some of the instruments are used for decorative illumination. In addition to his work in human medicine, Albucasis addressed veterinary care. *(Ms. 28, cod. Fritz Paneth, p. 559. Courtesy Historical Library, Cushing-Whitney Medical Library, Yale University, New Haven, Connecticut.)*

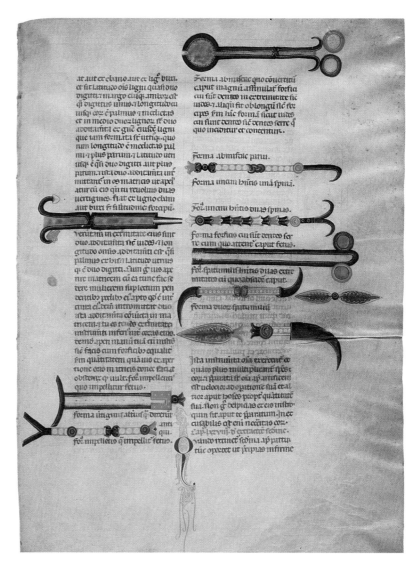

Avenzoar (1113-1162) or ibn Zuhr, a brilliant diagnostician, surgeon, and therapist, addressed difficult thoracic conditions such as pericarditis and mediastinal abscesses. He introduced tracheotomy into medicine, performing the first experiment on a goat. He was also the first to describe the itch-mite, initiating the discipline of parasitology in the Arab world, an advance destined to have major implications for veterinary progress.

Maimonides (1135-1204), also known as Moshe ben Maimon or ibn-Maymun, was physician of Cordova and a distinguished Arabic-speaking Hebrew philosopher who codified the Jewish religion. He was forced by the religious fanaticism of the Almohades to leave in 1148 and settled in Fez, Morocco, then moved to Cairo in 1165. He became internationally renowned as a philosopher and physician for his magnificent introduction to philosophy, *The Guide for the Perplexed*. He was overburdened with medical demands in Cairo; his health suffered and he died and was buried in Tiberias, Palestine. He followed Galen closely in medical matters but criticized several of his philosophical positions. Maimonides regarded the saliva of the rabid dog to be the most dangerous of all "poisons." He also recognized tuberculosis in necropsied and slaughtered animals, and deserves acknowledgement as the founder of veterinary public health.

Ibn Khaldun (1332-1406) described the cyclical rise and fall of societies and observed that urban life and prosperity corrupt human nature. He idealized the desert nomads and their camels and stated that the ideal model for Islam was a holy city with a nomadic surround: the city would provide the base for learning and meditation while the hinterland generated fresh young intellects unspoiled by urban culture.

Ibn Battutah of Tangier (b. 1304) was an inveterate traveler, having covered 75,000 miles using only horse and camel power. He recorded impressions of the world from the Mandingo kingdom (Mali) to Sumatra in Southeast Asia and throughout the Muslim world in the fourteenth century.

REVERENCE FOR HORSES AND CAMELS AND THE EMERGENCE OF BAYTARS

Al-Jahiz, who lived in the ninth century, wrote *al-Hayawan,* the first comprehensive zoology text in Arabic, which described animal life, behavior, and disease in the Mesopotamian region. Much later, in the fourteenth century, the Egyptian ad-Damiri wrote *The Life of Animals,* a comprehensive study.

The golden age of Arab culture addressed the need to advance the fields of agriculture and animal husbandry. One widely used manual was a translation of a Greek text, another was translated from Aramaic (Nabatean). Both the eastern and western caliphates generated original Arabic texts on agriculture. Two that appeared in Andalusia were eventually translated into Spanish.

An old Saharan verse indicates perceptions of the roles of the three major species of large domesticated animals:

> *Horses for a quarrel,*
> *Camels for the desert,*
> *And oxen for poverty.*

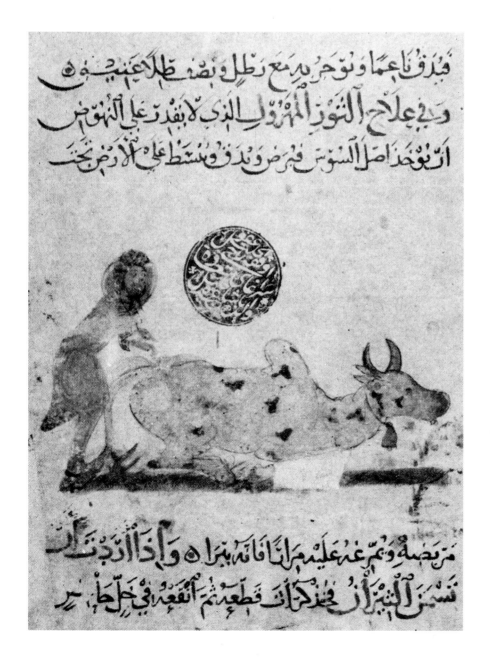

164. A jewel in early Arabic veterinary medical art is the manuscript, *al-Kitâb al-Baytârah (Book on Veterinary Medicine)* of Ahmed ibn Hasan ibn al-Ahnaf from 1209. The text from this illustration states the emaciated zebu is unable to stand by itself and that a litter of chopped liquorice root should be strewn underneath for it to roll on. The round seal is the stamp of the Cairo University Library. *(Egyptian National Library, Cairo.)*

193

165. An illustration of a dromedary suffering from the skin disease *tajja qatta* or "curly leaf disease" (wrinkled dry skin). The prescribed treatment is to administer savin (a medicinal juniper) and millet cooked in lard or cow butter, followed with a half cup of fresh garlic juice. From the 1209 Arabic manuscript, *al-Kitâb al-Baytârah* by Ahmed ibn Hasan ibn al-Ahnaf. *(Egyptian National Library, Cairo.)*

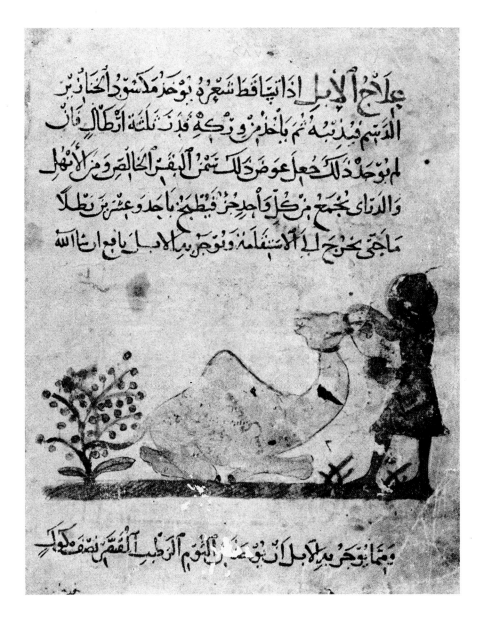

Several Arab writers on veterinary matters addressed the special problems of camel management and diseases. The importance to the desert people of the domestication of the dromedary cannot be overestimated. The remarkable design and physiology of these animals allowed them to travel and live in arid regions where no other domestic animal could thrive. Their unique metabolic system allowed them to withstand the enormous thermal stresses of the desert and long periods without water and food; the anatomy of their feet permitted effective travel over sand while carrying people and loads or pulling carts. Lactating females gave rich milk for a long time, having a variable gestation period of up to thirteen months. Wool, dung, and ultimately meat were other products of the "ship of the desert." Nonetheless, camels required thoughtful management so that overexertion, abscesses, and saddle sores could be avoided. They were susceptible to mange, vector-borne hemoprotozoal diseases, meningitis, and other bacterial infections. Special care had to be taken to regulate food and water intake after long trips such as the journeys made along the major caravan routes from the Persian Gulf to the Red Sea and northward to the Mediterranean. Much of this knowledge was identified by the camel drivers and doctors of Arabia.

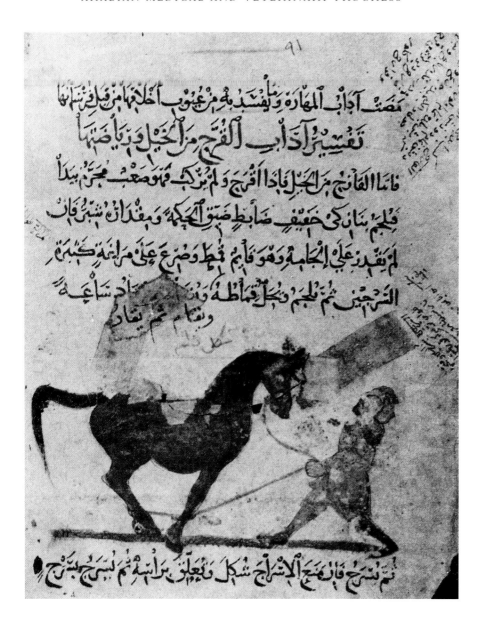

ل

166. This five-year old horse was unmanageable and could not be saddled or harnessed, so its legs were tied together and it was cast down onto a pile of manure. Later it was allowed to rise, the ropes were loosened, and it was led around and untied before saddling. From the 1209 Arabic manuscript, *al-Kitâb al-Baytârah* of Ahmed ibn Hasan ibn al-Ahnaf. *(Egyptian National Library, Cairo.)*

The horse had entered the Middle East and the North African region by the second millennium BC but was not common in the Arabic world until the first century AD. With the coming of Islam, horsemanship, military training, and horse-breeding became important occupations on the political scale. The skill of the cavalry, the high quality of their horses, and the inspiration of their leaders carried the flag of Islam in a single century to the far reaches of an enormous empire. The momentum of the Arab advance was unchecked until the decisive battle with barbarian Franks in armored mail south of Tours in 732.

Ibn Jakoub, son of the "master of horse" and veterinarian to the caliph al-Motadhed, was inspired by Greek, Syrian, Persian, and Hindu veterinarians and drew on these sources to write a book on hippiatry in 695. The first major work on horsemanship and the farrier's art to review the characteristics, behavior, and diseases of horses was written by Akhi Hizam, al-Furusiyah wa al-Khayl, around 860. Many similar, often beautifully illustrated books followed. An extremely high priority was placed on health care for horses because to the Arab warriors their horses were cult animals. As a result, the field of veterinary care for horses was given a special status above that of the care of animals used in agricultural pursuits. Special hospital stables were built, and the name given to those who treated the horses was *baytar*.

In the English idiom a baytar might have been a groom, but in the Arab world it seems that he was a combination of stableman and horse doctor. Baytars were expected to have expertise in mating, obstetrics, foal-raising, training, riding, nutrition, and veterinary care.

Near the end of the twelfth century Abou Zakaria ibn el Awwam of Seville wrote *Kitab el Felahah,* a large, scholarly agricultural book that included discussions of animal husbandry and health care. The hygiene and diseases of cattle, sheep, goats, horses, donkeys, mules, and camels were described. Lameness in horses was a major focus, and the importance of thorough diagnostic investigation was emphasized. The author also provided a detailed introduction to equine dental care and gave methods for correction of defects and injuries. He drew on many sources—classical, Arabic, and oriental—and categorized more than a hundred diseases of the horse by regions or organs of the body, as well as a comprehensive range of therapeutics. Bleeding from various sites, purging, firing, and acupuncture were included. Casting for surgery and shoeing were covered, and surgical removal of osseous tumors was described. Abou Zakaria stands out as the broadest ranging and most able of Muslim veterinary writers.

Abu Bakr ibn el-Bedr al Baytar (1309-1340) of Cairo, horsemaster veterinarian to the sultan of Egypt and son of a veterinarian, wrote a distinguished medieval work in Arab veterinary medicine, the *Kamil as Sina'atayn* or the *al-Nasiri,* as it was called in honor of his master, el Nasser. A copy exists in the National Library in Paris, but the quality of the translation is questionable. The work encompasses all facets of animal husbandry: the care of wild and domestic animals, including birds domesticated in Egypt and Syria; breeding, horsemanship, and knighthood; and animal diseases, drugs, and treatments. The treatise, however, was largely derived from earlier Greek scholars of Byzantium and the compilation of Vegetius.

Abu Bakr's most original and interesting equine contributions related to the conformation and appearance of the horse, dressage, gaits, harnessing, shoeing, determining age and weight, the tricks of the horse dealers, the nature of behavioral problems, training, identifying marks and defects, selection of breeding stock, and the history of famous individual specimens. Abu Bakr observed that the horse was so important to an Arab man that he believed it would be reunited with him and his wives in paradise. The only other animals to accompany him would be his camel and his birds. The horse races and the fights on horseback, along with the love of women, were the celestial treasures promised to the faithful.

The veterinary aspects of the *Kamil as Sina'atayn* display a rich, diverse materia medica. The treatment of vices was given priority, along with wounds and diseases of the skin. The body systems approach to diagnosis was followed, starting with the head. A lengthy discussion of castration condemned the practice in principle. The testicles were removed surgically in rams but were destroyed by crushing in the bull. Damaged hooves were pared with a diamond-shaped Arab knife and a rasp. Iron shoes were applied; padded hoof dressings and leather soles were used. Fractures and dislocations were treated with splints and suspension; wounds were inflated and drained. The fluid of ascites was drained via a copper tube inserted at the level of the umbilicus; the same method was used to relieve gaseous distention.

Sterility in the mare was treated by cervical dilation when appropriate. Embryotomy was practiced in some cases of dystocia; hooks were used in the orbits and elsewhere to give purchase for traction in obstetrics. Prolapsed vagina was corrected by applying pressure using plates attached to the limbs. The disease dourine was characterized as venereal. Signs included pruritus and discoloration of the vulva or swelling and ulceration of the penis.

The most valuable Arabic contributions to veterinary medicine were in physical therapy of the locomotor system, in surgery and wound treatment, in ophthalmology, and in the development of a wide range of pharmacologic

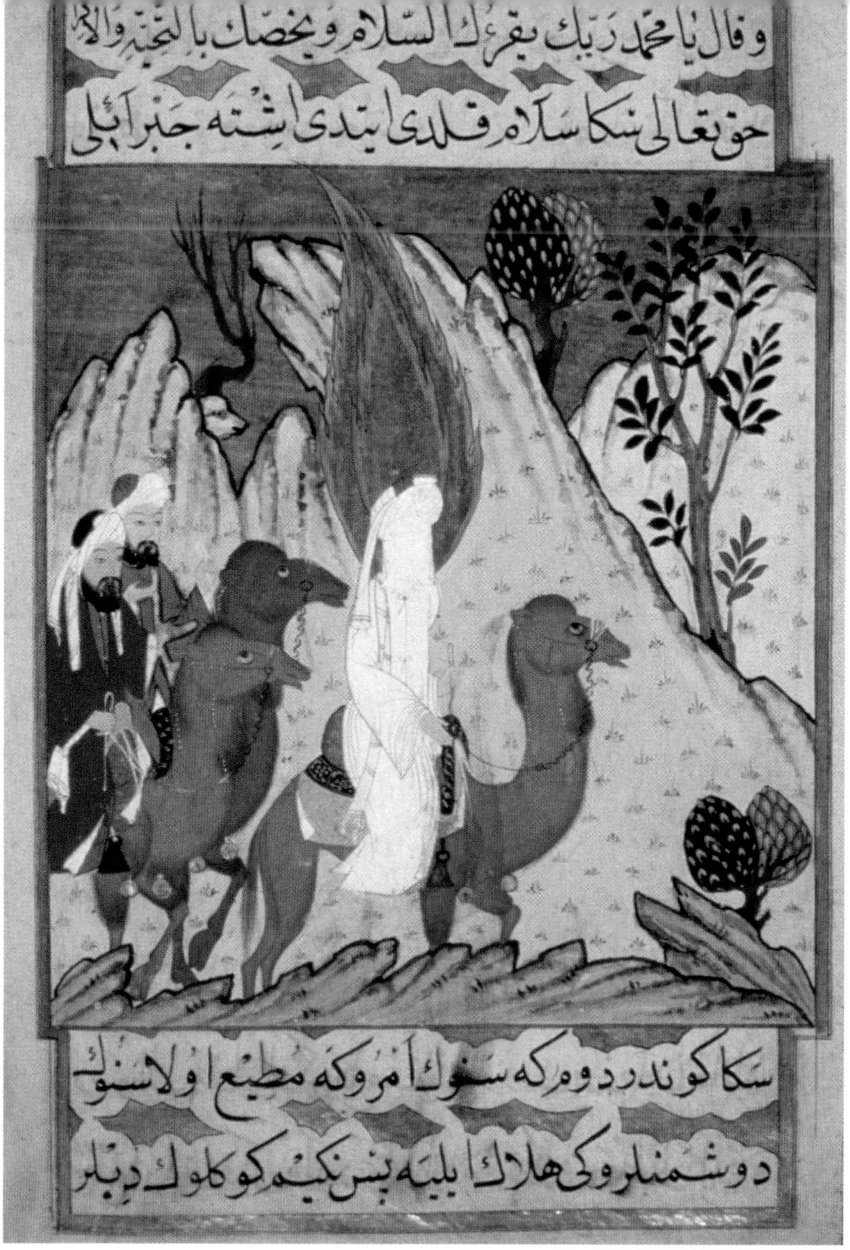

167. Abu Bakr (1309-1340), the son of a veterinarian, wrote an important medieval work on Arab veterinary medicine entitled, familiarly, the *al Nasiri*. In it he described all facets of animal husbandry. In a painting from a life of Muhammad, the faceless Prophet is on his way to Mecca with Ali and Abu-Bakr. In the Ottoman court style (1594). *(Spencer Collection, New York Public Library, Astor, Lenox, and Tilden Foundations.)*

agents composed of natural products. These accomplishments were based on the Greek works of Dioscorides but were considerably amplified. Little progress was made, however, in the knowledge of internal medicine and pathology over that of the Byzantine Greek veterinarians. The diseases of species other than the horse and the camel received little attention. It is claimed that an Arab horse breeder may have achieved the first artificial insemination of a domesticated animal, the horse, in 1332. The view appears to be warranted that the focus of Arab veterinary medicine was toward finding practical solutions for dysfunctions rather than toward advancing the conceptual understanding of the processes of disease.

The Islamic cultures were renowned for their knowledge and use of herbal medications, and veterinary prescribers were no exception. A wide range of aromatic herbs and pharmacologically active plant extracts were dispensed as the tools of the baytar's trade. Those who provided veterinary care were accorded high esteem in most Muslim cultures. Plants that fed the prosperous spice trade grew in the southern coastal region of the Arabian peninsula and on lands facing it on the Horn of Africa (part of Ethiopia and Somalia). Frankincense, a fragrant gum resin from trees, was the source of the incense that was taken north to Gaza on camelback via the incense trade route. Myrrh was prized as a mainstay of treatment for wounds sustained in combat. Other spices and medications were brought from the Orient and transshipped from ports in the area that is now Yemen and Oman. Pleasant smelling extracts were also important in offsetting the vile smells of death and infected wounds.

CONQUESTS BY ARAB WARRIORS ON HORSEBACK

The Arab conquest was made possible by the wonderful horses the Arabs had developed and by their mastery of horsemanship and practical veterinary care. From the Atlantic to the Indian Oceans the Islamic creed was carried on the backs of the Arabian and Barb horses. The prophet Muhammad gave the Arabian horse a major place in the Islamic religion. After his death in 632 his successors led inspired cavalry into a century of conquest that swept through Syria, Palestine, Mesopotamia, Armenia, North Africa, the Mediterranean islands, Persia, central Asia, Afghanistan, and northern India. In 711 they crossed the Strait of Gibraltar.

The Moors marched into the Iberian Peninsula and with the help of oppressed citizens defeated Roderick, the last of the hated Visigoth kings. They continued their drive around the eastern end of the Pyrenees Mountains and surged into Gaul (France), which failed to fight back effectively and was weakened. However, the first minister of the Frankish king, Charles Martel, created a new force of heavily mail-armored knights on horseback, who received land grants for their military service. In 732 a decisive battle was fought at Poitiers, near Tours, a hundred years after the Prophet's death. Protected against arrows and the sword by the sheer weight of their armor, the cavalry on powerful steeds halted the attacks of the lighter Muslim warriors on their agile Arab horses. After frustrating the attacks, the knights charged and drove the enemy from the field of battle. The Arabs did not return but settled in Spain and married there. Charlemagne used armored cavalry to push the Moors back from northern Spain. The Christian knight and the idea of chivalry became symbols of the age. Much later, Alphonso VII (1065-1109) launched the Spanish Reconquista. A popular folk hero, the adventurer Rodrigo Diaz or El Cid, took Valencia in 1094. His famed gray Andalusian war-horse, Babieca, outlived his master by two years and died at the age of forty in 1107.

168. After the death of the Prophet Muhammad in 632 the ferocious Moorish horsemen on their agile Arabian horses began a cavalry campaign that led them, after crossing the Strait of Gibraltar in 711, to eventually settle in Spain. Segment from *Trajan's Column,* second century. *(Peter Newark's Historical Pictures.)*

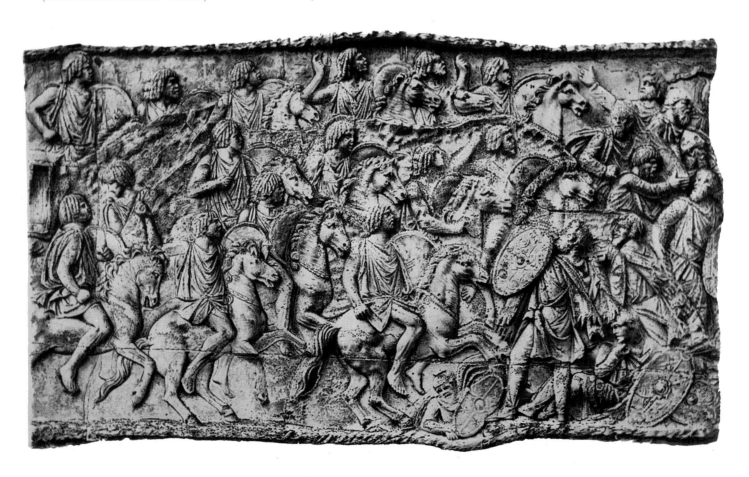

The Arab Empire crumbled during the thirteenth and fourteenth centuries. After earlier clashes with Berbers, Crusaders, Byzantine warriors, and Charlemagne's forces, it was dominated in different times and regions by Berbers, Mamlooks, Mongols, Sarmatians, and Turks. The pattern of interminable internal tribal feuding deflected the leaders' efforts on behalf of the greater empire. The devastation wrought by the plague (Black Death) and other epidemics led to a drastic decline in trade and a severe economic depression. These difficulties led the zealots to launch waves of religious persecution. A Berber tribe rebelled in the Maghreb and in 1269 captured Marrakesh to end the Muwahhid caliphate.

A great equestrian force had emerged from the eastern steppe, the pagan Mongol horde led by Genghis Khan. The Mongols took Bokhara and Samarkand in 1220, then eastern Persia. During later expansion under Hulagu, Baghdad and Aleppo were conquered. Meanwhile, the Mamlooks, descendents of enslaved Turkish soldiers, seized Cairo and gained control of Egypt. They defeated the Mongols at Ain Jalut and took Syria, the Crusader states, and western Arabia early in the fourteenth century. Tamerlane, however, built a new empire through devastation until his death in 1405. The Turkic mantle passed to the Ottomans, who steadily consolidated their gains and took Constantinople in 1453, replacing the Byzantine era with the Ottoman Empire that held sway until 1917.

The Arab state had fluctuated between periods of strong, wise leadership and interregnums of strife and virtual chaos. The splits affected the bitterly disputed selection of the leaders of Islam itself and their doctrines. Two camps emerged, the Sunnis and the Shiites, who differed on who the rightful successors of the Prophet were. These problems have remained insurmountable since the first two or three centuries of the Arab Empire. Arabic medical and veterinary knowledge continued to spread into Europe via Spain, South Italy, and the Ottoman Empire after the Arab Empire crumbled.

EUROPEAN ACQUISITION OF VETERINARY KNOWLEDGE FROM THE MOORS

The Arabian focus on cavalry led to advances in equine management, medicine, and surgery that Spain acquired from the Moors and carried forward to the rest of Europe. The Arabic word for veterinarian, "al-Baitar," was adopted into Spanish as "albeytar."

Juan Alvares de Salamiellas, who lived in Gascony but wrote in Spanish in the mid-fourteenth century, prepared a remarkable book, *Libro de Menescalcia e de Albeiteria et Fisica de las Bestias*. It described and depicted diseases of the horse and their surgical and medicinal "cures." The manuscript is illustrated with many hand-painted miniatures in color depicting scenes of veterinary treatments; only a few copies have survived.

The treatise of Alvares contained two parts, one describing the external appearance of horses, the other dealing with their management and treatment. The arrangement of the ninety-six chapters is somewhat disorderly; a particular condition sometimes is the subject of several chapters. All the horses appear robust, with large necks and chests, sloping pasterns, and large hooves. Many illustrations contain scenes of animal restraint and various veterinary procedures. The latter include oral dosing; attention to the teeth; examination of the limbs; the use of setons in fistulas; work on hooves and shoeing, splinting, or bandaging limbs; rugging; the use of cautery; bleeding; castration; treatment for laminitis; administration of a clyster (enema); blowing medication up the nose; application of salves or blisters; and treatment for urethral stone. Restraint scenes include the use of stocks, nose clamp or twitch, and casting with the feet tied. The *Libro de Menescalcia* is a most valuable document bearing witness to the life of a medieval horse doctor.

In the Arabic tradition Alvares's book illustrated a wide range of surgical instruments, a diverse formulary of medications, and an advanced approach to ophthalmology. Compared with its European counterparts north of the Pyrenees, the Spanish veterinary medicine derived from the Moors was much more advanced. Alvares noted a type of traumatic equine injury to the abdominal wall resulting from the too violent use of spurs. The resulting swelling on the flank ("torondo") might even have been a hernia; the procedure for repair included incision, careful replacement of the bowels, suture of peritoneum with a thread left hanging out so that it could be withdrawn later, and closure.

King Alphonse V of Spain, "Alphonse the Generous," was a patron of science and of veterinary medicine. He required Marshal Don Manuel Diaz to compile the veterinary information obtained in a military expedition to Naples. Diaz completed the assignment in 1443, and his work established the standard for equine management and veterinary medicine, *Libro de Albeyteria por lo Noble Mossen Manuel Diaz (The Book of the Veterinary Art by Manuel Diaz).*

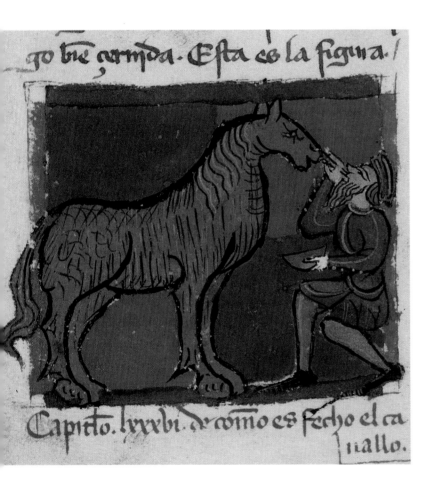

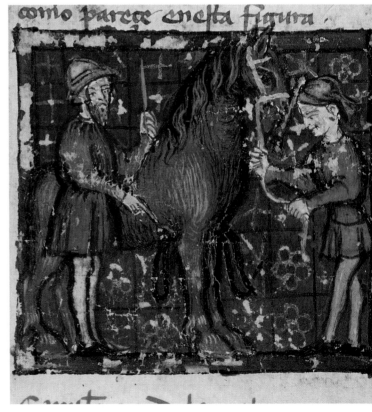

169. *Left,* A miniature showing the administration of medicine through the nose of a horse from Juan Alvares de Salamiellas's *Libro de Menescalcia,* a mid-fourteenth century manuscript containing various illustration of horse care. Alvares's work was one of the first written for the veterinarian (albeytar) in Spain. *(Add. Ms. 15097, fol. 62ᵛ. Bibliothèque Nationale, Paris.)*

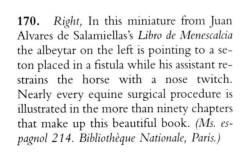

170. *Right,* In this miniature from Juan Alvares de Salamiellas's *Libro de Menescalcia* the albeytar on the left is pointing to a seton placed in a fistula while his assistant restrains the horse with a nose twitch. Nearly every equine surgical procedure is illustrated in the more than ninety chapters that make up this beautiful book. *(Ms. espagnol 214. Bibliothèque Nationale, Paris.)*

The system of albeytars (horse doctors) in Spain originated from Moorish antecedents. The earliest writings about them arose from the Spanish monasteries: the twelfth century *Liber Artis Medicinae* at Ripoll and Frey Teodorico in Valencia covered equine diseases. The Portuguese monk Bernardo wrote *The Seven Books of Albeitary and Science* late in the fourteenth century.

When Isabella, the Catholic heir of Castile, married Prince Ferdinand of Aragon and both attained their thrones (1474 and 1479, respectively), a new Spain was born. They set about creating a church-state throughout Spain by oppressing the large Moslem and Jewish minorities. The Inquisition of 1480 began by examining the sincerity of the *marranos,* Jewish converts to Catholicism. War was declared on the Spanish Moors and they were forced to surrender by 1492 and later to accept baptism, acquiring the label *moriscos.* The Jews were evicted; later under King Philip III, the entire *morisco* population was slaughtered or expelled between 1609 and 1611. In 1500 a law was created that formally established a system of standard-setters and examiners called protoalbeytars, for the new albeytars or horse doctors. This system was to stay in place for more than three hundred years. It did not provide for education because training was by apprenticeship.

The reign of Isabella and Ferdinand was a turning point that marked the end of the Middle Ages and the start of the Renaissance in Spain, with consolidation of monarchial power. In 1492 they occupied the red palace of the Moorish Kings, saw Spaniard Alexander Borgia elected Pope, expelled the Jews, established the Castilian Grammar as the leading language, and sponsored the voyages of Columbus (Colon) and the conquistadors that led to the discovery and conquest of the New World. The system of albeytars evidently travelled with them to the Americas because Don Juan Suárez de Peralta (c. 1536-1590), who was born to a noble Spanish family in Mexico, wrote *Tratado de Albeyteria* between 1575 and 1580. This was the first treatise on horse doctoring written in the New World, and the manuscript survives in the National Library in Madrid.

Back in Spain, after three and a half centuries the Tribunal of protoalbeytars ended in 1847, along with the titles *herrador* and *albeytar,* having coexisted with the veterinary schools for its last forty-three years. The last of the old examinations was administered in 1854.

After the Bourbon (French family) kings came to Spain, the Mesta was ended because it blocked the agricultural and highway developments sought by King Charles III (1759-1788). Two students were sent to Alfort for veterinary education in 1784: Sigismundo Malats y Codina (c. 1756-1826) and Hipolito Estevez. They were charged to develop plans for veterinary schools in Madrid and Cordoba. Under Charles IV and his influential minister, Manuel Godoy, the plan for Madrid a school was approved in 1792, with Malats as the founder and first director. He had been an outstanding student at Alfort and had also studied in Germany, Denmark, and Great Britain. He led the school until 1809, when Napoleon invaded Spain in the Peninsular War. Just before the demise of Napoleon at Waterloo, Malats returned to lead the veterinary school again under Ferdinand VII. Other schools were planned at Cordoba and Saragossa in 1847 and began when the albeytars ended. The Madrid school became part of the University in 1857. The first center of veterinary education in the Americas was founded in Mexico in 1853, a decade before Canada's Ontario Veterinary College in 1862.

Veterinary education in Brazil did not begin until 1913 in Rio de Janeiro, with the first graduates in 1917. Another school was started in 1914 in Rio de Janeiro by the Brazilian Army; to train military veterinarians, with the first group graduating in 1917 as well. A short-lived school began in Pernambuco before 1918. In 1919 São Paulo established a veterinary school that was incorporated into the University of São Paulo in 1935. By 1992 there were thirty-four schools of veterinary medicine operating in Brazil, accompanied by rapid growth of the profession to about 30,000 veterinarians.

INIERPREIATOQUALITER
YNAECCLESIICUSEPIE
DICNTVRAPERISSIME
EPERARCNOEDCLRT

ea dixit dūr ṣodue ṃ ampur
tromum hominū lumuana
tracine qui ẹplerate tẹrra
mulicatorum ẹteece dispdotor
et anum omnam · Faelaut̃ aibi
urcum de lignis quidruat
ridor et ridor pruet
tabicauminubir
tum

AROR
1108

Suaue tracut faubricum pṃuaum
lutcut homo noṣ maupra quam mūdi
monia euūore eiliquancum ea
tollicitau animud uegtione uelim
lnrpicore · procul dubio muant
rucruinamicum ẹpeliter graqu lnlpur
maitrurt eucon lune gomib lnue
nint are disporicum · Sicaumṣa
fucio urcum ericanateri cubicor
longa audinān et quinquaginta
cubicoru luucaudinam collṣemē
fucie urcum etlncubiao
conraminubir tum ẹcrupo
etorouū fucio deliuaur
tabicumouati ta urea
moriaum puciet au
ẹ reliqu ·

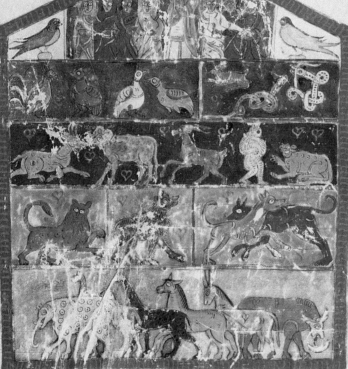
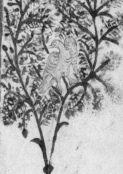

Animals in the Dark Ages

Europe's Gestation Period

～

ROMAN VULNERABILITY IN BRITAIN: BOADICEA'S REVENGE

By the end of the first century AD the entire Mediterranean Sea (Rome's Lake) was encircled by the Roman Empire. Its famous network of straight roads allowed transport by vast numbers of horses, mules, oxen, and donkeys to provide defense and services throughout the empire. Four-wheel carriages were drawn by eight- or ten-mule teams, depending on the terrain and the season, and teams of three were used for two-wheelers. Strict rules were developed to protect the unshod animals from overwork and excessive hoof wear. The capacity of the native Romans, whose population was declining, to staff and govern the realm was exceeded by the vast area and the great distances to be traveled. As a consequence, the armies of colonial provinces recruited more and more of their troops locally or hired mercenaries, and the provinces began to assume greater autonomy. Simultaneously, political intrigues destabilized the central government. The strains increased during the extravagant, decadent reign of Emperor Nero (AD 37-68), who ruled from AD 54 until his death, one sign being a damaging and costly uprising in Britain.

Britain had been settled by successive waves of Celtic tribes arriving from the Continent for a millennium before the first Romans came. They had brought wooden ox plows, farm animals, and capability in bronze metallurgy. Later, tribes such as the Belgae came with their iron technology and metal plows pulled by eight-oxen teams, which could turn the heavy clay soils of river valleys. They also had fine horses. When Julius Caesar invaded in 55 BC, the Celtic forces gave him stiff opposition. He fared better when he returned the following year with two thousand Gaulish cavalry, but the Romans did not prevail over lowland England until Claudius sent a large army in AD 43. Even then the Celts in the mountains of Wales and Scotland were not romanized; the Romans had to deploy their legions mainly in the west and north.

In AD 50 the Roman governor decided to protect his rear guard by disarming the people his legions had already overrun in the lowlands, who had been cooperating with the invaders. One tribe that had fine swords and horses, the Iceni of Norfolk, rebelled and were put down by force. Ten years later, when their king, Prasutagus, died during Nero's reign, the Romans plundered the king's household, flogged his wife Boadicea (Budicca), raped their daughters, and appropriated their hereditary lands on the grounds that there was no male heir. The tribe plotted revenge, and Boadicea led a great rebellion in AD 60 and 61. The Iceni, who were joined by other tribes, sacked and burned the Roman towns of Colchester, St. Albans, and London, butchering any Romans they caught. They chased the Romans up Watling

171. *Facing page,* Animals are prominently featured in many of the illustrated manuscripts produced during the Dark Ages. *Noah's Ark* from *Commentary on the Apocalypse,* written by the Asturian monk Beatus of Liebana in 776, is an outstanding example of how early Christian monasticism viewed God's creatures. In general, these manuscripts portray animals as soulless and estranged from humankind. Some could be eaten, many could be worked, but none could share in the Heavenly Kingdom reserved for humans. Care of the animals was left in the hands of healing saints. *(Ms. 644, fol. 79. The Pierpont Morgan Library, New York.)*

172. Statue of Boadicea by Thomas Thornycroft on the Embankment in London. Boadicea (died AD 62) as queen of the Iceni led an unsuccessful revolt against the Romans in Britain. The Romans continued to face trouble in Britain for more than three hundred years, entirely withdrawing from the island early in the fifth century. *(Hulton Deutch Collection Limited, London.)*

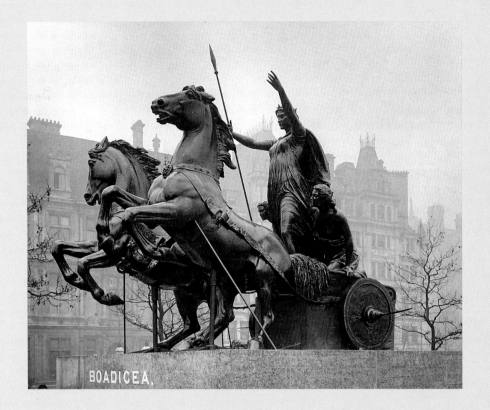

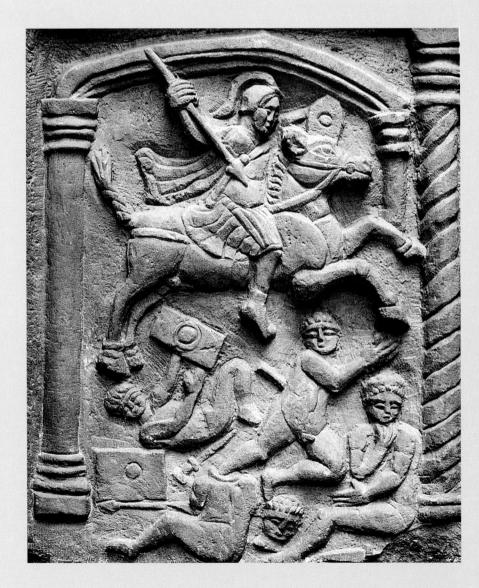

173. Detail of a second-century dedication slab from the eastern end of the Antoine Wall where it meets the Firth of Forth shows a Roman horseman overcoming northern British warriors during the Roman occupation of Britain. *(The Trustees of The National Museums of Scotland, Edinburgh.)*

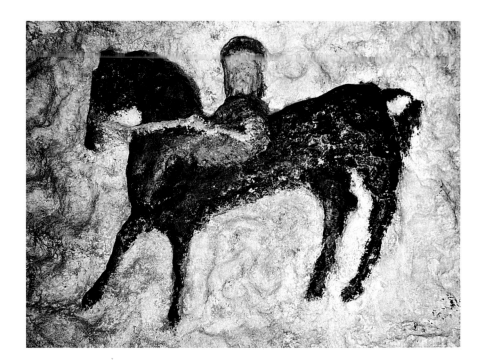

174. Welsh horseman at the base of the Cross of Irbic. The Romans did not dominate lowland England until AD 43, and the Welsh proved particularly resistant to being romanized. *(Peter Newark's Historical Pictures, England.)*

Street to the northwest, but the experienced Roman leader Suetonius set a trap, possibly at Mancetter. The Romans trounced the rebels, and terrible revenge was exacted on the Iceni. A great statue of Boadicea, complete with rearing horses and chariot, stands on the embankment in London in commemoration of the rebellion.

The Romans had further trouble in Britain during the fourth century AD. The Celts were a continual irritant, and the Jutes, Angles, and Saxons from Denmark and northern Germany were moving in from the east and south with the tides via the estuaries and coastal swamps. Early in the fifth century Rome withdrew its forces entirely, leaving the island to the mercy of the new invaders. Because there is little documentation of the period from AD 400 to 1000, it has become known as the Dark Ages. Despite the name, the Dark Ages should be regarded as a time of escape from provincial status and the beginning of the great challenge of nation building. The development of Britain was a particularly difficult process because the indigenous population had to come to terms with the aggressive new arrivals at the same time. The cleric Gildas wrote *On the Ruin and Conquest of Britain* in the 540s. Seven Anglo-Saxon kingdoms emerged: Essex, Sussex, and Wessex (Saxon); Kent (Jute); and East Anglia, Mercia, and Northumberland (Angle). Lowland Britain became the land of the Angles, that is, England; the Celts were pushed back to Wessex, Wales, and Scotland.

THE BARBARIANS' EDGE: MASTERY OF THE HORSE AND BOW

During the fourth century the western empire was no longer able to contain the barbarian migrants and raiders pressing from the east. A chain reaction developed until it seemed that all the tribal peoples of Europe were on the move. Rome's overextended military forces were forced to switch to a defensive posture along natural waterways, notably the Rhine and the Danube.

The Eurasian steppe is a vast belt of grassland stretching from the lower reaches of the river Danube in the west, around the riverine plains that drain southward to form the Black Sea, eastward via the valleys of the Volga and Ural Rivers that feed the Caspian Sea, then across the vastness of southern Siberia to the Altai Mountains. The mountains form an elevated wooded in-

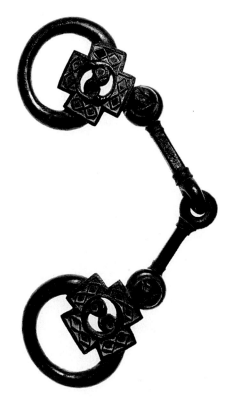

175. The waves of Celtic tribes that preceded the Romans in Britain were skilled horsemen. This flexible Celtic bridle bit found in London demonstrates the excellent cavalry equipment and metallurgy skills of these tribes. *(The British Museum, London.)*

176. The Romans had great difficulty containing barbarian hordes from the east, whose skill in riding and bowmanship proved superior to the Romans' chariots and infantry. Earthenware figure shows a rider and horse clad in cloth or leather armor. Sixth dynasty, seventh century. *(The British Museum, London.)*

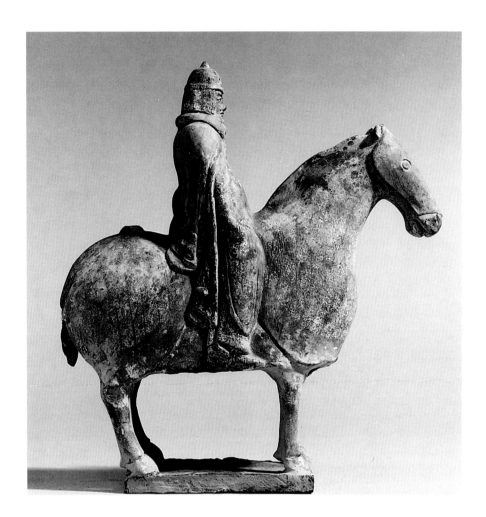

terlude before the grasses continue as a band through Mongolia to Manchuria, where they end at a mountain range just before reaching the Yellow Sea in the Far East. The total span is 4500 miles.

The Altai spawned waves of pastoral mounted tribes, whereas the aggressive Yueh-Chih ("raw-meat eaters") inhabited the more arid lands to their south. Much further east the Hsiung-nu harassed and tyrannized Chinese border areas. Later, during the thirteenth century, the Mongol hordes originated there. The horse gave these tribes the mobility needed to cover vast distances. Their skill in riding and bowmanship, fused to the backs of galloping horses, created a new form of warfare that the legions of more civilized populations were unable to counter with chariots and infantry. The barbarians were more interested in raiding and looting than in settlement. They surged westward and southward, leaving trails of death and destruction. Burial sites dating to about 500 BC, found at Pazyryk and Noin Ula in western Mongolia, suggest that the foothills of the Altai Mountains were the likely site of the seed stock for the expansionist drives. Leaders were buried with their fine Arab-type horses, as well as a few of larger type.

Far to the west the southern part of the area that became the Ukraine had been the home of the Scythians since the first millennium BC. They were famous for the animal style they commissioned in metallic art. They lived in symbiosis with the Ionian maritime settlements along the shore of the Black Sea. The Greeks provided the artistry in brass and gold, as well the wine the fast-living nomads craved. Trading centers grew at the mouths of the great rivers: Olbia commanded the rivers Bug and Dneiper, Tyras the Dneister, and Tanais the Don. On the Crimean peninsula other centers arose, including the colony of Pentacapeum, which developed beside the prosperous Kerch Strait.

Another tribe from the Altai, the Sarmatians, had excellent horses. Because the animals were reputed to be headstrong, only geldings and mares were ridden. As the Sarmatians moved westward across the plains, they encountered the Scythians and displaced them. The Scythians left little for the historical record except recognition by others of their skill in horsemanship and warfare. For example, the Persian Emperor Darius attempted to exterminate them in 514 BC, but he was forced to withdraw by the hit-and-run tactics of the Scythians. The magnificent Greek artistry in metal is the only visible relic of their equestrian exploits.

The Persian-speaking Sarmatians were crowded in their turn by the migratory Ostrogoths (eastern Goths) and moved to the grassy Hungarian plains. The next, even more ferocious Altaic barbarians to arrive were the Huns, who conquered and absorbed the Alans, then ousted the Ostrogoths, whose survivors fled with their herds across the Danube into the Roman Empire. The Gothic cavalry never adopted the "veering bowman" style of fighting used so successfully by the pastoral tribes. Despite their armor, the cavalry could not withstand the Hunnish charges.

Late in the fourth century AD the Huns surged into the Hungarian (Pannonian) plain, where they stayed for fifty years. In 451 Attila mobilized them, and they charged wildly across western Europe before being stopped and defeated southeast of Paris. Even then, they veered south into Italy, ravaging the land as they went. After Attila was killed, the Huns returned to the plains of eastern Europe and were joined by other steppe peoples, the Avars, Bulgars, and Magyars.

The decline of the Roman Empire in Europe was the result of the demoralization of a people rooted, in part, in the oppression and taxation of the peasantry. The barbarian incursions caused a great terror to sweep through the populace; many lives and all valuable possessions were lost, agriculture was disrupted, and there was a loss of confidence in the government. The reproduction rate declined dramatically, and the legions could not be maintained at full strength.

The wandering Gothic tribes, gaining new momentum, marched westward and southward through the empire. The first to mobilize were the Visigoths, who traveled to southern France and made Toulouse their new base, from which they commanded Spain as well. The Vandals took the Maghreb (North Africa); the Ostrogoths conquered Italy itself and replaced the last emperor. The Lombards, too, invaded Italy and made Pavia their capital. Yet another Gothic group, the Franks, spread into Gaul.

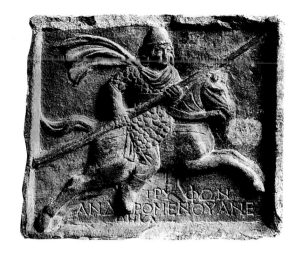

177. Sarmatian horse-warrior. A tribe from the Altai, the Persian-speaking Sarmatians used excellent horses. A headstrong breed, only geldings and mares were ridden. Marble stele found at Tanais in the Ukraine. (*The Hermitage Museum, St. Petersburg.*)

178. The Vandals, a Germanic tribe that sacked Rome in 455, were excellent warriors on horseback. Mosaic from Carthage (c. 500) shows a Vandal horseman roping a stag, an unlikely achievement. The Vandals settled in North Africa, where they ruled the native population. (*The British Museum, London.*)

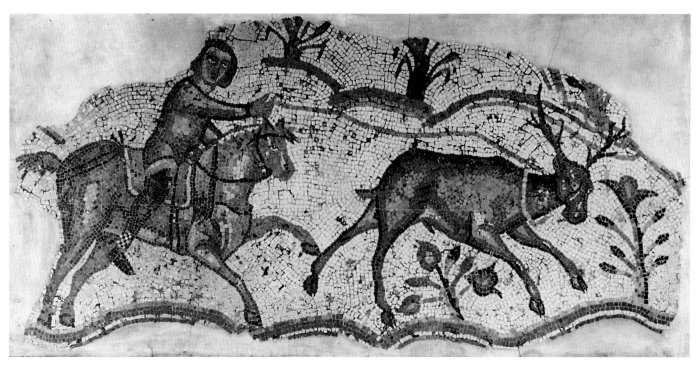

The Goths are thought to have originated in Gotland, Scandinavia, but they became Germanic tribes. From the various factions many of the early kingdoms evolved in the formerly Roman provinces. Some of the groups were absorbed into the more populous regions they dominated; others were later displaced by Byzantines or Muslims. The Franks were the strongest of the Gothic groups. A new form of warfare—armored cavalry on strong horses—was developed by Charles Martel and stopped the Moors at Poitiers in 732, overwhelming the invaders on their light Arab and Barb horses. Martel's son Pepin stopped the Lombards. Then Charles the Great, also known as Charlemagne, became the Frankish king. He set out to unite all the Germanic tribes, destroyed the Avars, and initiated the liberation of northern Spain.

EPIZOOTICS IN THE WAKE OF BARBARIAN MIGRATIONS

Strong evidence indicates that epidemics of animal disease (epizootics) often began in the wake of horse-bound military invasions, especially those from the Asian steppes to the west, in which it was the custom to travel with flocks and herds bringing up the rear. The indigenous stock were particularly vulnerable because they were exposed to virulent infectious agents to which they may have had no previous exposure and thus no immunity. Although the animals of the barbarians, such as the great Hungarian grey cattle, seem to have been resistant to rinderpest, some plagues affected the barbarians' beasts as well. The indigenous people, including the stock owners and the authorities, had no idea how to control the problems. Some outbreaks, presumably of rinderpest, have been estimated to have resulted in mortality rates of ninety-five percent.

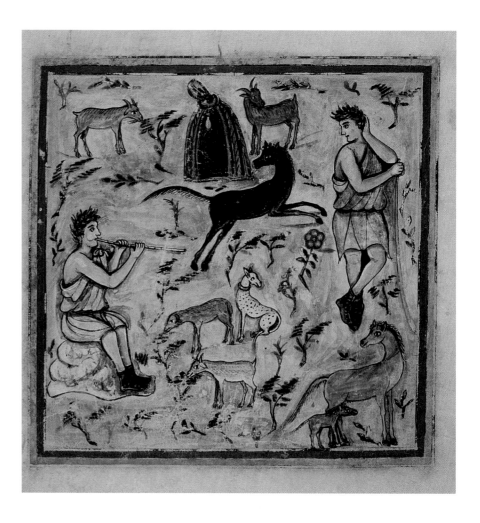

179. *Shepherds Tending Their Flocks,* an illustration in the Roman Vergil (c. sixth century). Evidence suggests that flocks and herds traveling with the horse-bound hordes were susceptible to epizootics, especially the indigenous stock, which had not acquired immunity from previous exposure to the invaders. *(Cod. lat. 3867, fol. 44ᵛ. Foto Biblioteca Vaticana, Rome.)*

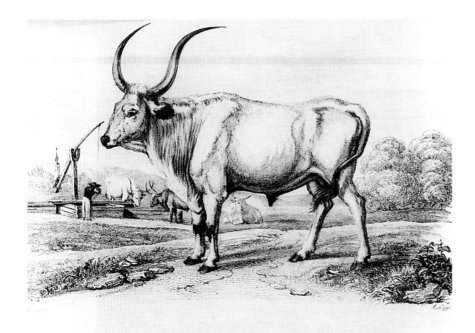

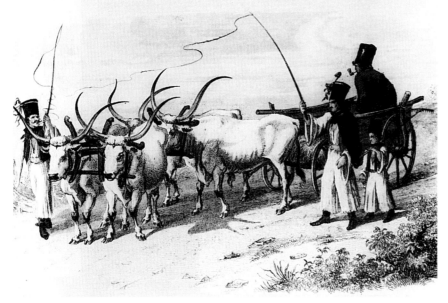

180. Although some plagues did affect the barbarians' livestock, the Hungarian grey cattle of the barbarians were more resistant to rinderpest. *(Courtesy University of Veterinary Science, Budapest.)*

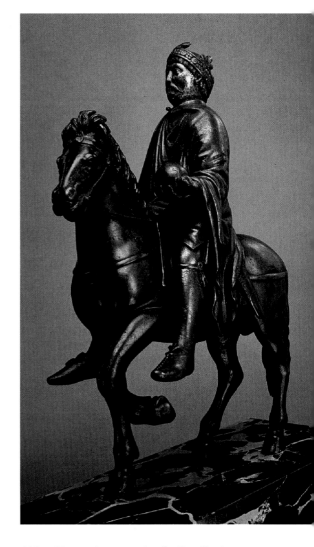

Animal plagues occurred during the first three centuries of the Christian era, but these are poorly documented. It is known that several outbreaks of what must have been rinderpest occurred in the fifth and sixth centuries, after the incursions of the Huns under Attila. Because draft oxen were widely used for cultivation, the entire food production system was threatened. A terrific cost to animal health resulted from exposure to the new, virulent pathogens, the stressful environmental conditions, the lack of forage and feed, and the drafting of able-bodied men into military service. Adding to the misery and suffering, epidemics of rabies occurred on the Continent. The incidence was increased by the custom of some Teutonic tribes to use dogs in war. Cases of rabies appeared in humans as well as in domestic animals.

The "pacification" wars of Charlemagne, like the invasions of Attila, triggered disastrous epizootics of rinderpest. During the first three decades of the ninth century there were massive losses of stock, and recurrent famines were the order of the day from the sixth through the tenth centuries. Not surprisingly, human health also suffered: cannibalism and locust plagues have been reported. Plagues afflicted humans as well as animals, but the medical experts of the day had no answers. The idea of developing a control strategy did not emerge until the Black Death occurred during the fourteenth century. As animals and humans died en masse, the peasants lost faith and turned to mystics and charlatans for advice and therapy.

181. Equestrian portrait of a Carolingian Emperor thought to be Charlemagne. Ruinous epizootics of rinderpest followed the wars of Charlemagne, resulting in huge losses of stock throughout the tenth century. Bronze, ninth century. *(The Louvre, Paris.)*

TENSION BETWEEN SPIRITUAL AND PHYSICAL VIEWS OF HEALING

The monastic movement gained momentum from St. Benedict of Nursia (c. 480–543), who established the monastery at Monte Cassino in southern Italy. He developed the monastic system, which preserved the Christian faith and values during the Dark Ages. His rules governing the lives of monks were widely adopted by monastic orders. One of the Benedictine monks, St. Augustine, was sent to Canterbury by Gregory, the first monk to be made pope, to evangelize the Anglo-Saxons in 597. Augustine was so successful that his parochial system was adopted as the model for the papal administration, and the ecclesiastical organization came to replace the imperial Roman one in the former western empire.

The most dedicated Christians took refuge in the monasteries. The Visigoths, who had entered Spain as allies of a weakened Rome to contain nomadic barbarians, stayed and ruled the peninsula. Bishop Isidore (560–636), who became the archbishop of Seville during Visigoth rule, wrote the famous, encyclopedic *Etymologies,* which covered a vast range of subjects, including medicine. The work was based on the writings of Latin authors and church fathers. The Venerable Bede (673–733), the most significant scholar of eighth-century Europe, generated a great new cultural tradition. His base was the monastery in the Irish tradition at Wearmouth, near Newcastle. Beatus of Liebana, an Asturian monk, wrote a *Commentary on the Apocalypse* (the Book of Revelation) in 776, the outstanding illustrated text of medieval Spain. At

182. St. Benedict of Nursia (c. 480–543) established the Benedictine order at Monte Cassino in southern Italy. In a fresco by Spinello Aretino (c. 1387) St. Benedict is curing a monk. During the monastic movement monks cared for the sick, but the study of medicine was forbidden. Divine intervention alone was required for cures. *(Alinari/Art Resource, New York.)*

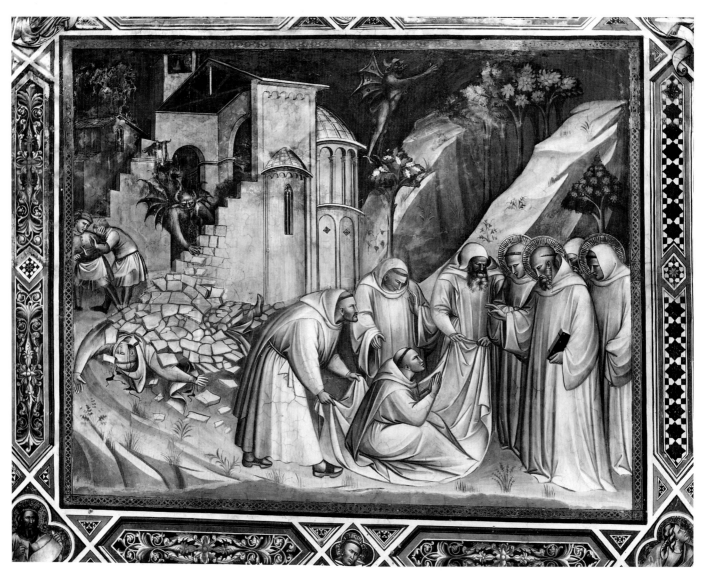

the school and archbishopric of York, Alcuin (730–804), a great scholar, emerged; he was destined to have a great impact on Europe as senior adviser to Charlemagne. John Scotus Eriugena, a brilliant Irishman attached to the same court, wrote *On Nature,* a detailed, well-written natural history of all known created things. Thus the monasteries and church schools provided the few crucial scholars who bridged the intellectual darkness until a royal court gave sponsorship to cultural activity.

The Christian era in Europe aroused a philosophical tension between the Church's supernatural faith in miracles and its conception of diseases (human and animal) as divine punishment for sins and the rational naturalism of the medical philosopher-scientists, who were progressively attributing diseases to explainable natural causes. The rationales for treatment differed, the one spiritual, the other physical. Although religious leaders did not for the most part reject secular medicine, they did object to its being overvalued at the expense of any acknowledgment of the value of spiritual faith and divine intervention. Ordinary laypersons (patients or owners of sick animals) tended to "hedge their bets" by invoking astrological or magical powers in addition to the spiritual prayers and medical interventions. Bede himself recorded many tales of miraculous healing, among other works, as well as a treatise on bloodletting.

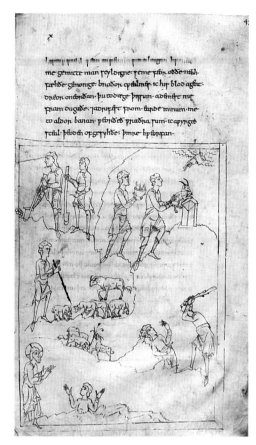

183. *Above,* The rams and goats in this drawing of Cain and Abel from the Caedmon manuscript appear much smaller in scale than the human figures, which suggests that they may be only symbolic. *(Caedmon Ms. Junius XI, p. 49. Eleventh century [first half]. Bodleian Library, Oxford.)*

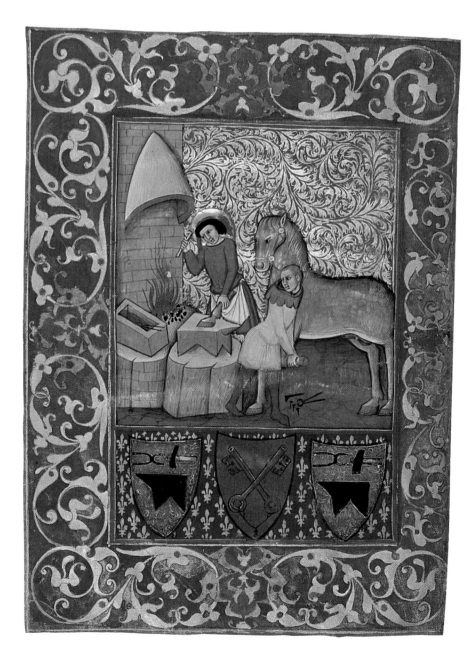

184. Much was made of religious healing of animals, or miracles, during the Middle Ages. One of the most celebrated "cures" is *Il Miracolo di S. Alò.* According to legend, St. Alò, bishop of Noyon, cut off the injured foot of a horse and reattached it completely healed. This miracle was also attributed to St. Giles, who became the patron saint of blacksmiths. An annual pilgrimage of horses in Flanders commemorates a similar miracle of St. Eligius. *(Ms. 4194, cod. 6ᵛ. Biblioteca Universitaria Bologna.)*

211

Shrines that contained saintly relics or were the sites of alleged miracles acquired great magnetism for believers. To this day, many people seeking a share of the mystical, healing power continue to make pilgrimages to the shrines.

As the Roman Church gained confidence, Pope Gregory VII encouraged the Christian reconquest of Spain and considered an offensive against the Muslims in the eastern Mediterranean, a Christian "Crusade." Pope Urban II appealed to the nobility at Clermont, France, in 1095 and gained enthusiastic support from the Frankish lords to deliver the Holy Land from the advancing infidels. The Crusade was begun the very next year with tremendous popular support. Most of Christian western Europe rose to the preachers' call: it was one of the duties of a knight to defend the faith against unbelievers in this world and the next. Several waves of troops were led by mounted noblemen and one, a kind of "People's Crusade," was led by Peter the Hermit on a donkey. Count Emich of Leisingen assembled an army in the Rhineland and threatened the Jews with baptism. As he marched through Germany, he perpetrated a pogrom against any Jews that refused; then Volkmar in Bohemia repeated the action in Prague, as did Gottschalk in Ratisbon.

When the great pilgrimage of 1096 finally arrived at the targeted area, it succeeded in recapturing a 600-mile-long coastal strip of Syria, including Jerusalem, from the Muslims. This great victory was accomplished by a combination of armored knights and disciplined infantry armed with crossbows. The cost in equine and human lives, however, was immense. The gains were eroded, and subsequent Crusades failed to retake the lost areas; instead, during the fourth, final Crusade, the Christian fortress of Constantinople was sacked.

LEECHES: PROVIDERS OF VETERINARY CARE

The term "leech" came to be used for physicians, "horse leech" for horse doctors, and "ox leech" for cattle doctors. The origin of the term has ancient roots. The Greek epic poet, Homer, used the term "leeches" in the Iliad for those said to be skilled in medicine who healed the wounds of the Greek warriors. Two sons of Asklepios were said to be "cunning leeches," heroes who could extract arrows and spread soothing drugs on the wounds, just as Chiron had imparted the cures to their father. It seems that the leech was a surgeon whose work resulted in the drawing of blood. The widespread medical practice of bleeding patients to "adjust their humors" must have given rise to the name, in recognition of the similarity of the practice to that of the blood-sucking invertebrate it connotes. The leech, notably the species *Hirudo medicinalis,* came to be used as an alternative to the fleam in bleeding patients.

The famous martyred twin physicians Cosmas and Damien (third century AD) were born in Cilicia, a Roman province in Asia Minor on the Mediterranean coast south of the Tarsus Mountains (part of Turkey today). They were credited with miraculous cures in humans, including the transplantation of the leg of a dead man to replace a gangrenous leg in a living patient. Their remarkable healing powers were said to apply to actinomycosis of horses. A wave of cattle plagues involving a form of madness, which began in France around 570, took a heavy toll and later spread to deer and sheep. The influence of the tomb of St. Martin was credited with reducing the mortality rate: the oil from the lamp of the shrine was used to dose stock, and the dregs were spread over the pastures. Prevention was said to be achieved by applying the red-hot iron key of the local church to the foreheads of the healthy animals. This superstition persisted almost to modern times. St. Leonhard, who died in 599, is honored in rural Europe as the patron saint of sick animals. A sequence of many plagues of cattle occurred in Ireland in the eighth century and spread to Britain and the continent of Europe. Other quadrupeds were affected in some outbreaks, as were humans.

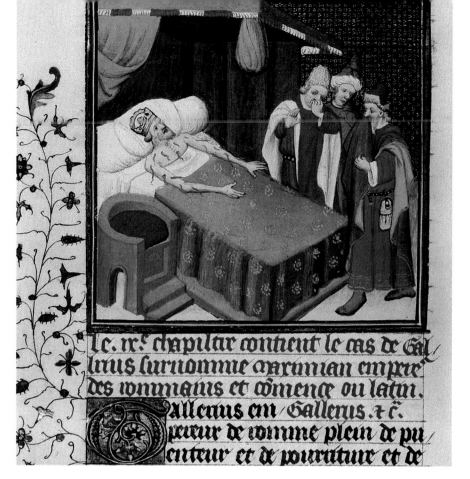

185. The use of leeches *(Hirudo medicinalis)* for bleeding patients lasted well into the nineteenth century. The practice was so widespread that for a time the word *leech* was used to mean *physician*. Eventually the practice spread to animal caregivers. Horse doctors became known as *horse leeches,* and *ox leech* was the euphemism for a cattle doctor. A page from Giovanni Boccaccio's (1313-1375) *Decameron* shows the use of leeches in the Middle Ages. In a rare record of medieval epizootics, the spread of the great plague known as Black Death to swine is also described in this work. *(Jean-Loup Charmet, Paris.)*

Cultural development in Europe after the barbarian invasions had to begin again from peasant roots and priestly leaders. Greek medical literature, corrupted in translation, was filtered through Latin translations to become the main source of knowledge of medical practice in Europe and Anglo-Saxon England. Teutonic tribes had their own mainly magical folk remedies with Mediterranean cultural overtones before they encountered the Roman culture. One persistent superstition was the idea that horned cattle were subject to being "elf shot." Elves were considered small, sometimes terrifying demons empowered with magic. They were alleged to be the cause of certain serious diseases in animals. Perhaps the superstition was just an attempt to explain such then-inexplicable problems as bloat in cattle.

After the general conversion to Christianity the old folk practices tended to be superseded by the prestige of the written word, although the folk magic reasserted itself, for example, in the *Lacnunga,* a poem and a small, commonplace medical book of the eleventh and twelfth centuries. The *Lacnunga* was assembled from several sources. The Anglo-Saxon leech had virtually no original ideas and no understanding of even the rudiments of the science known to classical antiquity.

The Celtic Codes of Wales contained rules defining civil responsibility for animal disease and treatment. A purchased horse that showed any sign of farcy after the sale could be returned to the vendor at any time up to a year after the transaction. Less serious animal diseases had shorter "warranty periods." Also, if someone gave a remedy to an animal, he must be paid for it. If his remedy caused injury to the animal, he had to pay an indemnity. Similar rules had been promulgated earlier in Europe, under Charlemagne.

The earliest surviving Saxon medical manuscript is the *Leechbook of Bald.* It was written in Old English with practical application in mind early in the tenth century, after King Alfred (871-899) had restored cultural activities in the wake of the Danish oppression. The *Leechbook of Bald* drew on Latin works and described charms, incantations, and herbal remedies. Three leechdoms were given against signs of animal diseases: swollen legs, galls, and elf shot (acute bloat). There is no mention of who would have administered the herbal treatments and made the superstitious appeals to God. Useful knowledge was sparse, but the book was an early record of animal care practices.

The leech was both a healer and a priestly figure, the one people turned to in times of trouble. The specialized animal healers—cow leeches and horse leeches—appear to have developed later. *The Anglo-Saxon Leech Book* records that sheep pox was introduced into England by the import of an infected Spanish ewe in 1275. The resulting epizootic lasted twenty-five years. This disease is still endemic in North Africa; it probably reached Spain via the sheep imported by the Moors. •

The Reverend Thomas Oswald Cockayne translated and edited a three-volume collection of *Leechdoms, Wortcunning and Starcraft of Early England* that was published in 1864, 1865, and 1866. He was the leading scholar of Anglo-Saxon folklore, magic, and medicine of humans and animals before the Norman Conquest (1066). A major part of the translations comprised prescriptions of vegetable, animal, and mineral products for the relief of signs of disease in humans and animals. These mainly herbal remedies were combined with magical charms and religious incantations.

Unlike many historians who have sought to record only conceptual progress, Cockayne avoided most latinized texts. His work may reveal a truer picture of the dark, barbaric, almost shamanistic approach to medical matters with cosmological and environmental overtones of the English leeches. Crude links to Pythagorean ideas were evident. More than half of his material was an English version of the *Herbarium of Apuleius Platonicus,* which was derived from pre-Christian, debased Greek sources that had been spread via the monastic system. Hippocrates, Aristotle, and Galen were forgotten. Some of the prescriptions had come down from Dioscorides. Others included disgusting sections from other sources on medicines derived from animals. There is evidence of input from the mythologies of Asklepios, Chiron the Centaur, and the god Apollo. It is thought that Cockayne's three-volume work covers Anglo-Saxon practices from the fall of the western part of the Roman Empire in 476 to the twelfth century. Most of the records date from the time of King Alfred or later.

One section in *Leechdoms, Wortcunning and Starcraft of Early England* is called "Prognostics" and deals with forecasts of outcomes based on dreams and calendar dates. The later part of the collection includes the translation of a text from the medical school at Salerno of about 1100. Differing from the preceding part, the translated text represents a bridge to the new wave of medical thought and avoids reference to supernatural powers.

In Cockayne's work there is one example of a zoonosis related to the treatment of a person bitten by a mad dog: for the bite of a mad dog the wound should be dressed with a mixture of honey, agrimony, and waybroad and the white of an egg. The following examples from Cockayne's collections, which refer specifically to the treatment of animal diseases, indicate the heavy dependence on herbal and mystical charms:

> 78. *If cattle are dying, put into holy water groundsel and springwort and the netherward part of attorlothe and clivers, pour it into the mouth, soon they will be better.*

> 79. *For lung disorder in cattle, pound the wort with . . . waxeth in highways; it is like the wort called hounds mie, on it grow black berries as mickle as other peas, put it in holy water; introduce it into the mouth of the cattle. [This was followed by the instructions to burn several herbs all together so as to make the smoke "reek upon the cattle." Then some crosses made of hassock grass were to be set out around affected cattle and some religious incantations and litanies were to be said. Someone should then] set a value on the cattle and the owner give the tenth penny to the church for God; after that leave them to amend. Do thus thrice.*

> 80. *If sheep be diseased, and for sudden death of them, work to dust black hellebore, lupin, wolfscombe, fennel, stone crop; put into holy water, pour upon the diseased sheep and sprinkle on the others thrice.*

81. *For the pocks and skin eruptions in sheep; lupin and everfern, the nether part of it, the upper part of spearwort, ground, great or horse beans, pound all together very small in honey and in holy water . . ., put one dose into the animal's mouth with a spoon, three doses a day always; for nine times if mickle need be.*

82. *For sudden death of swine, put always into their meat: seethe gladden, give it them to eat; take also lupin, bishopwort, and cassuck grass, tufty thorn, heyriffe, vipers' bugloss; sing over them four masses, drive the swine to the fold, hand the words upon the four sides and upon the door; also burn them adding incense; make the reek steam over the swine and the drink run into every limb.*

If a horse is elf shot, then take the knife of which the haft is horn of a fallow ox, and on which are three brass nails, then write upon the horse's forehead Christ's mark,* and on each of the limbs which thou may feel at: then take the left ear, prick a hole in it in silence . . .; then take a yard strike the horse on the back, then it will be whole. [Then a blessing was to be written on the horn of the knife, because to the elf, this was mighty for him to make amends. This was followed by recipes for the treatment of dysentery and constipation.]

*Christ's mark on the forehead was considered necessary to intimidate the elves and reverse the disease. The elves' shots were not restricted to cattle.

The book *The Medicine of Quadrupeds* appeared in the eleventh century. It developed a largely ineffective system of therapy in which animal extracts were used.

One of the most famous mystical animal healers in medieval Europe was St. Hildegard of Bingen (1099-1179). As a young child she began to have visions, and at fourteen years of age she entered a Benedictine monastery, where she stayed and became abbess by 1136. Her visions continued and intensified; the ecclesiastical authorities accepted their supernatural character and her fame spread and reached the highest authorities. Lacking a scholarly background in medical and veterinary subjects, St. Hildegard's diagnoses and recommendations for treatments of humans and animals may have been derived in part from persons familiar with Aristotle's works. Her ideas on animal diseases were recorded by scribes in two books, *Physica* and *Causae et Curae;* she also wrote in a secret language invented in the convent.

Hildegard's medicaments encompassed natural products, mainly herbs. She also called on religious powers through incantations, blessings, and exorcisms. Stones such as onyx were invoked for the treatment of plagues. She labeled glanders in horses "pest" but thought it was related to strangles. Interestingly, she prescribed a different set of herbal products for each species: for horses and asses, nettle and Levisticum; for cattle, horse-chestnut leaves and marigold for bloat and powder of shell and slag for dropsy; for sheep, spotted pulmonaria; for goats, leaves of ash, oak, or Austrian oak; and for swine, powdered snail shell and dill. For canine rabies the head of a lark was prescribed; bite wounds were treated with honey, egg whites, and achillea, and prevention was achieved by having the animal smell a pungent odor such as acetic ether. Colic or abdominal pain was relieved with lavage, salad, and nettle. Hildegard stood tall in the esteem of the Church and was canonized soon after her death.

The use of leeches to carry out bleeding persisted and became quite popular in the eighteenth and nineteenth centuries. Its greatest exponent was Francois-Joseph-Victor Broussais (1772-1838), who would deploy up to fifty leeches at once on a patient. Leeching became so fashionable that by 1833, forty-one million leeches were imported into France alone. Pierre-Charles-Alexandre Louis (1787-1838), a much more rigorous Frenchman than Broussais and a brilliant medical scholar who founded medical statistics, proved that bloodletting was essentially of no value in pneumonia. Had the practice of leeching survived, there would have been a demand for a veterinary specialty to care for the bloodthirsty little creatures themselves. Marshall Hall (1790-1857), a brilliant Nottingham physician and physiologist who trained in Edinburgh, Paris, and Göttingen, denounced the lancet as a "minute instrument of mighty mischief."

DEFENSE AND AGRICULTURE UNDER FEUDALISM

When the structure afforded by Roman administrative systems collapsed, there was stasis in the rural environment; insecurity and instability reigned during a long, difficult period of agricultural regression and recurrent poverty, plagues, and famine. Gradually tribal factions, villages, and estates became semiautonomous to fill the vacuum in the infrastructure. Provincialism became the prevalent social attitude, complete with dialects, architecture, and all the cultural trappings. Each locale acquired a unique variety and flavor in which it took pride. Incentives for the exchange of information or ideas were absent.

The way was open for the Church to provide a degree of stability by assuming the role of a unifying focus, and to some extent the Roman Church did this. New waves of barbarian raiders, however, such as the Vikings, Slavs, and Magyars, forced the development of a model having military capability. The Muhammadans, too, had become a formidable offensive power. The people turned to strong men to provide security, and the structure that emerged during the seventh and eighth centuries was feudalism. It spread to England via the Normans after the conquest of 1066. The lords or barons who received lands from the king became his vassals and had to swear an oath of fealty to him. Land was also granted in return for military service. Although the manor was the new unit of feudal jurisdiction, the village remained a royal unit for purposes of taxation, administration, and police protection.

In Anglo-Saxon times the village had been the unit of local government, and royal authority was much greater before the Norman Conquest. King Alfred, who defeated the first wave of the Danish invaders and divided the country with them, had imported stallions and built a mounted force of thegns (thanes, or freemen granted land in return for military service). His sons completed the conquest of the Danelaw and established a monarchy over all England with a prototype of a feudal system of local government. The Danes returned under Canute and conquered the land. After Edward regained the land for England, his son Harold died in the Norman Conquest.

Decentralization was a result of the manorial system. The estate was intended to be a single self-sustaining economic entity under a lord selected by the king. The nobleman had a right to a portion of the arable land, his demesne, and each of the manor's tenured peasants had a right to a strip of arable land. Peasants, however, had to provide the master with labor and a portion of the produce they grew. Additional imposts were the heriot, or death duties to be paid whenever a peasant died, and the merchet, a fine to be paid when a daughter married outside the manor and was lost to it.

The restoration of a degree of security and stability allowed the growth of towns, which became pockets of free enterprise in the surrounding countryside, where rural bondage was the rule. Towns developed their own networks, crafts, and markets along with the beginnings of independent literature and art. As the diverse character of Europe began to emerge, the number of new towns grew rapidly and reached a peak in the thirteenth century.

Improvements in agriculture included the three-field system, which was based on a three-year cycle or rotation for the arable land (fall grain, spring grain, and fallow) in open fields, supplemented by grazing for stock. In England sheep were the predominant livestock because of their ability to pick a living off fallow and wasteland in winter. Cattle were kept only where plenty of hay could be made for winter forage or in pasture areas from which they could be driven to market at the end of the grazing season. Transhumance was practiced in mountainous regions such as the Alpine zone, in parts of Scandinavia, and in Spain. Domestic pigs were important only in forested areas; to meet the needs of the family, one or two pigs, fed mainly on wastes and by-products, might be kept for home use.

The importance of animal fibers in the development and economic impact of the European textile industry was huge. The main fiber in western Europe during medieval times was wool. The main sources of fiber were Britain and Spain, and the cloth was woven in Flanders and Italy. England became progressively more involved in the processing and patterning of cloth. Originally the wool was a coarse material; that is, wool fibers were thick. Fine-wool types were imported to Castile, Spain, about 1280. Since the trait for fineness was inherited when Merino rams were crossed with indigenous ewes, Spain became the center of fine-wool production. A feature of the Spanish sheep industry was its custom of long-distance transhumance, the moving of sheep to northern ranges in the summer and to southern pastures in the winter. The gathering place was called a mesta or small commons. A system of sheep walks or canadas was developed; these could be 150 to 350 miles long. Progress was slow through open country, where the sheep could graze, but in enclosed areas the animals could cover distances of 15 to 18 miles a day. In 1273 the king exacted a tax on mesta sheep, which provided a major portion of the crown's revenue. The king forbade the export of sheep, horses, or mules. After the Merinos arrived, demand for Spanish wool expanded rapidly and the mesta organization became powerful. In Castile alone, the sheep population doubled to 2.7 million between 1369 and 1479. Cattle ranching in Andalusia, Alentejo, and Agarve became a major industry in the south. Historical antecedents of bullfighting are evident in cattle-herding techniques used on the open ranges of medieval Castile.

DEFENSE IN THE AGE OF CHIVALRY

The development of nailed-on horseshoes was a major technological step that enhanced the performance of draft and cavalry horses in the Dark Ages. The horseshoe was a Celtic invention from northern Europe; early examples, dating to the first century AD, have been uncovered at Camelodunum (Colchester), England. The Celts were noted for their skill in metalwork. The ingenious idea of shaping a red-hot metal band of iron to fit under the strong rim of a horse's hoof and then nailing it in place revolutionized the usefulness of the horse. The early shoes had six holes for nails. Europeans adopted the use of horseshoes during the Dark Ages, fitting the shoes hot. Calkins were used to reduce skidding. The Muslim world chose light shoes that could be shaped cold; these shoes, without clips or calkins, were thinner at the heel than at the toe, and only two nails were used on each side. To facilitate the task of shoeing, difficult horses were cast.

St. Dunstan (born AD 910), the patron saint of blacksmiths in England, had a forge in his monastery cell, where he made bells and objects for church ceremonies. A legend about him explained why horseshoes were believed to bring good luck. He was visited by the devil, who asked him to shoe his feet. St. Dunstan secured the devil firmly, then inflicted so much pain on him that the devil vowed he would never again enter a place where a horseshoe was displayed. Could that devil have been in the form of a centaur?

The order of knighthood became the strategy used by the nobles to ensure the maintenance of an effective fighting force of cavalry, and the concept of chivalry became codified in the eleventh century. The code of chivalry was instituted to create motivation for aspiring young equestrians to serve the aristocracy in its roles of restraining and defending the people and continuing its own tenure.

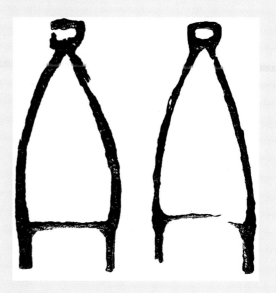

186. Iron stirrups of Viking type found at St. Mary Hill, Glamorgan, South Wales. Probably ninth or early tenth century. The stirrups are one of only two existing pairs of Viking stirrups from Britain and the only stirrups from Wales. From the middle of the ninth century Wales endured Viking raids, but the Vikings eventually settled in Welsh communities and by the eleventh century were fighting for Welsh kings. (National Museum of Wales, Cardiff.)

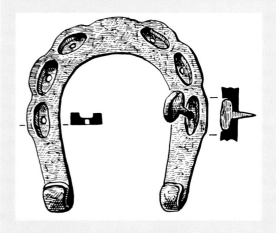

187. Celtic horseshoe. The Celts were noted for their metal work and are credited with the invention of the horseshoe. Shoes of the Celtic type have been found on Roman sites in London. Early Celtic shoes had six oval holes for nails; nail heads were shaped like violin pegs. Shoes were later improved by the use of square nail holes for nails that resembled the letter T. (From Hickman, John and Humphrey, Martin. Hickman's Farriery. London: J.A. Allen & Co., Ltd.)

217

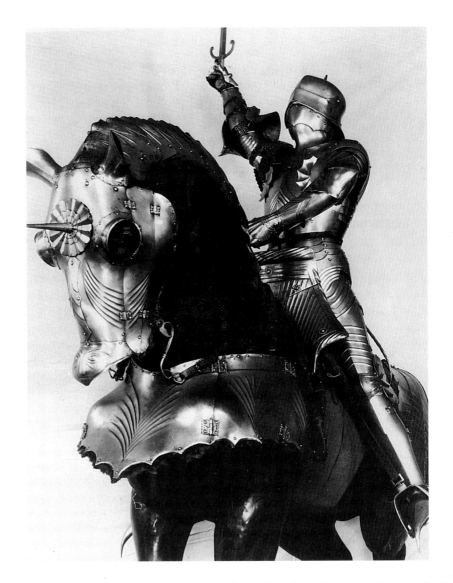

188. Armored knight on an armored horse. In Britain knighthood ensured a fighting cavalry for the nobles. The code of chivalry was created to instill pride in those who served the aristocracy. They not only rode to war but also participated in jousts, evolving into elite mounted soldiers who served a feudal superior. Jousts were an early version of war games designed to keep both knights and horses fit. Jousts were often brutal affairs: King Henry II was a celebrated victim. An armored horse with a rider in full armor would have carried as much as nine hundred pounds of weight. *(Peter Newark's Historical Pictures, England.)*

189. *Facing page, top,* A detail from the Bayeux Tapestry shows Normans and, more important, their horses crossing the English Channel. Wool embroidery on linen (c. 1070-1080). *(Tapisserie de Bayeux, Bayeux.)*

190. *Facing page, bottom,* Detail from the Bayeux Tapestry shows the Norman cavalry using their lances or spears while attacking the English at the Battle of Hastings. The use of stirrups and an improved saddle with supports in front of and behind the Norman riders greatly increased their effectiveness with lances. *(Tapisserie de Bayeux, Bayeux.)*

Recruitment into knighthood was limited to the aristocracy. Ramon Lull reported that only one man in a thousand was chosen to become a knight. The cavalryman needed a good horse and a remount with an attendant, and rituals were followed during a probationary period. Those who were approved developed the common bond of chivalry. Knights were essentially what would be called "officer material" today. They rode to war and participated in jousts. Gradually their status improved, and they evolved into an elite corps of equestrian warriors under a great lord or nobleman.

The Bayeux Tapestry, which dates to about 1080, recorded the way the Norman cavalry rode and used their lances or spears in battle. Some scenes show the tack used on the horse. The introduction of the stirrup had greatly increased the effectiveness of the cavalry. The saddle was designed with supports in front of and behind the rider to allow the rider to stay on board during the impacts. The riders extended their legs forward with the toes up to avoid being thrown forward. The lance could be thrust underarm or overarm or thrown overarm in traditional styles of fighting. In a new method that emerged with the use of better saddles and stirrups for support, a longer lance was held behind its center of gravity and couched firmly under the armpit. The knight was to use the lance as a projectile impelled by the charge of the horse and guided by the rider. The impact could be tremendous, unhorsing an opponent or driving a hole through packed infantry.

The goal of keeping horse and rider fit for fighting and highly motivated between wars led to the development of war games with a romantic touch. The most popular were tournaments or jousts. Separated by a barrier to avoid head-on collisions, the riders were in full armor. The object was for one rider to charge toward the other at full tilt with lance extended and try to unhorse him. A brutal bit with sharp appendages was used to haul the horse back onto its haunches after the encounter, so the reins had to be loose during the

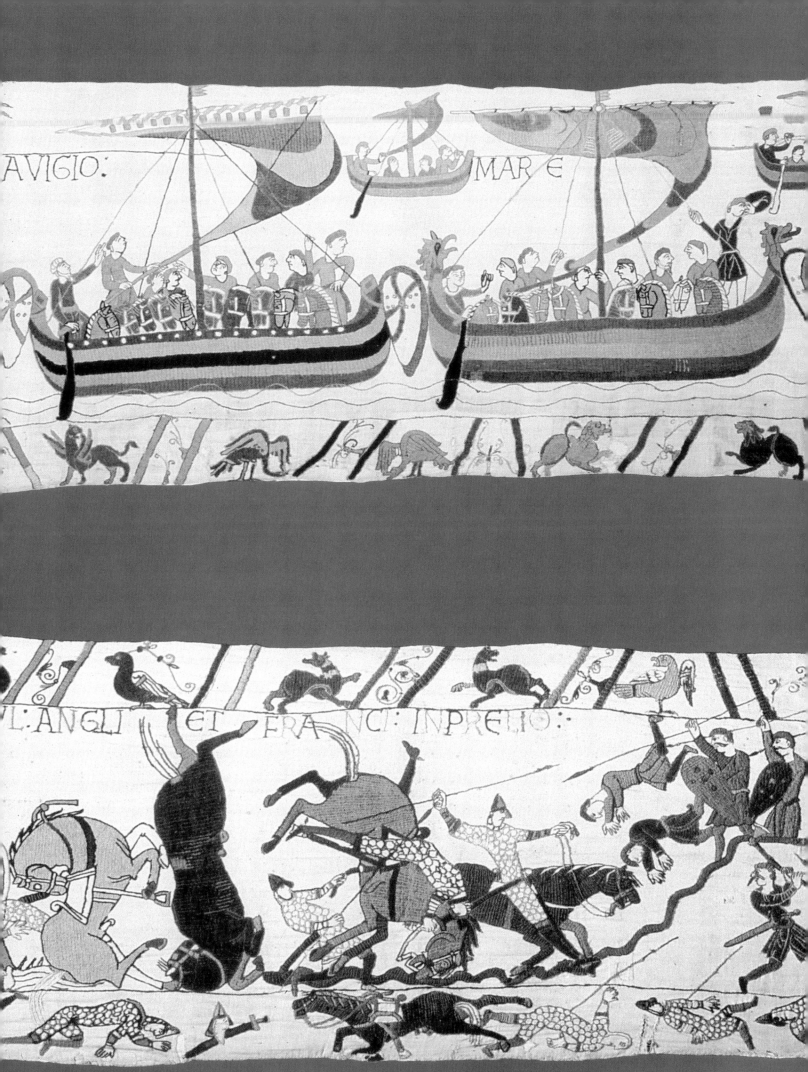

charge or the bit would deter the horse. King Henry II was killed during a joust, when his opponent's lance glanced off his cuirass or breastplate, then lifted his visor and pierced his eye. After the king's death, rules were made to reduce the risks. The weight of armor increased over time; together the weight of a knight and his armor increased from about two hundred and thirty pounds to about four hundred. Later still, when the horse, too, was armored, it had to bear a total weight of as much as nine hundred pounds, and huge horses had to be bred to carry such loads. The invention of gunpowder, however, made these large, slow targets vulnerable, and small, maneuverable horses with little armor were once more in demand for hit-and-run attacks.

THE PIG: A MODEL FOR MEDICAL EDUCATION AT SALERNO

Born at Carthage, Constantinus Africanus (1025-1087) was a polyglot medical and cultural scholar who had traveled to many parts of northern and eastern Africa, the Middle East, and India and had become familiar with various cultural developments and languages. He crossed the Mediterranean to Calabria, on the toe of Italy's "boot," then joined the Benedictine monastery at Monte Cassino, where he translated oriental and Greek works into Latin. He taught at the earliest medical school of the medieval period at Salernum, a spa on the Gulf of Salerno, where the Benedictine order had established a monastery in the seventh century. At that time the region was still Grecian in outlook, and Greek was the spoken language.

The school at Salerno trained doctors in the Hippocratic tradition, drawing on cultural roots of Arab, Greek, Hebrew, and Latin origin. The school was multicultural, nondenominational, and gender neutral. The monks built a hospital adjacent to their monastery, which attracted wounded Crusaders returning from the Holy Land and other patients from diverse regions.

The curriculum was remarkable for its focus on the study of anatomy; dissection of pigs was required, since human dissection was proscribed. Constantinus was a professor of anatomy at Salerno and had translated works of Galen that included studies of the pig. Because the human was considered more like the pig than like other animals, study of the pig became a bridge for the development of comparative medicine. Later, between 1100 and 1150, *The Anatomy of a Sow,* possibly written by Kopho, was published. In one particularly interesting observation the author claimed that "you find two testicles (ovaries) which send sperm into the womb where it joins with the male sperm to form the fetus." This claim was, in effect, flying in the face of Aristotle, who categorically denied the presence of female sperm, saying that the seed came only from the male and that the female's role was to nurture the embryo and fetus. Aristotle's conceptions of physical and biological science were discussed in connection with medical topics.

The Salerno school followed a Hippocratic-Galenic line in stressing a concern for the patient, the importance of moderation in dietetics, rules of good hygiene, thorough physical examination, diagnosis and therapeutics based on experience, and a conservative approach to treatment and pharmacology. Several treatises on aspects of the practice of medicine were produced. The most impressive was a great encyclopedia of internal medicine, the *Tractatus de Aegritudinum Curatione.* Nicolaus Salernitanus's *Antidotarium* was the first formulary and in 1471 was one of the earliest medical books to be printed. The author described the "sponge of sleep," which contained mandrake root, opium, and henbane.

Constantinus's translation of Haly ben Abbas's *Almaleki* as *Pantegni* in 1080 was the main reference to anatomical knowledge. The Persian sage had died in 994, and his comprehensive medical text held sway among the Arabs until Avicenna's *Canon.* Although Constantinus's translations were far from perfect, his most significant contribution was as a "latinizer" of Islamic medical thought. By making Arab medical knowledge available to the West and contributing to the development of comparative anatomy at the Salerno school, his impact on the evolution of medical progress in medieval Europe was substantial. Two surgeons of Salerno, Roger Frugard and his pupil Rolando Capelluti, became famous for their publication *Practica*. Salerno was sacked by Henry VI in 1194 and went into a decline from which it never recovered.

The intellectual flame lit at Salerno was carried forward to Montpelier, Naples, and Bologna. Arnold of Villanova, a Catalan, was the most distinguished medical scholar at Montpelier. Because of its proximity to Spain and the work of Constantinus, the faculty at Montpelier had access to the work of the great Moorish and Arab medical writers and transferred their ideas to Christian Europe. After the popes left Avignon, the authority of Montpelier declined and Paris became the dominant medical center. The flourishing university at Bologna attained a high reputation in surgery after Rolando moved there. Later achievements in that field were underpinned by the anatomical work of Mundinus, whose manuscript of 1316 commanded the field until the time of Vesalius. The work was based on dissections carried out on the cadavers of condemned criminals; legal action was later taken against four overzealous medical students for body snatching in 1319. At the rival school at Padua, Peter of Abano (1250–1315), a brilliant physician and Greek scholar from Lombardy, laid the foundation for the great achievements made there during the Renaissance. His *Conciliator Differentiarum* merged Arab and Grecian views.

The reforming effect of Dominican and Franciscan orders helped restore intellectual approaches to the medical sciences. Albert von Bollstadt (1193–1280) of Cologne or Albertus Magnus, Bishop of Ratisbon (Albert the Great), a Dominican scholar, attempted to reconcile science and theology, in particular, Aristotle's philosophy and Christian doctrine. He read all the available classical literature and subsequent commentaries through those of Avicenna. He taught at Paris, then returned to Cologne. The preeminent naturalist of his time, he wrote *De Animalibus,* a large book on quadrupeds in which he reviewed twenty-five diseases of the horse and other species. His most original statement described the three means by which contagions are spread: entry by bite or injury, contact with a diseased animal or the place where it has been, and the respired air of the sick. Scholars of equine medicine drew from his encyclopedic work from the Middle Ages through the Renaissance. He also wrote *Birds of Prey and Their Diseases.*

PROGRESS DURING THE MEDIEVAL PERIOD

The value of the contributions to cultural progress made during the Dark Ages and the later Middle Ages has been underestimated. The invention of printing alone had a greater impact on human access to learning than any other development since the invention of languages. The establishment of the universities competes with the classical age in Greece in the scale of its impact on human thought. The invention of nailed horseshoes transformed transportation and warfare.

The remarkable developments in science, agriculture, and medicine that began in the later medieval period gradually transformed secular society. Medical education began with a comparative approach in the studies using the pig at Salerno; this approach, coupled with rigorous academic standards, changed the course of the health sciences.

The Christian faith guided by the Catholic Church left a great legacy of administration, architecture, and worship, and the implementation of the political theory of democracy via parliament, law, and representative government was a hard-won accomplishment.

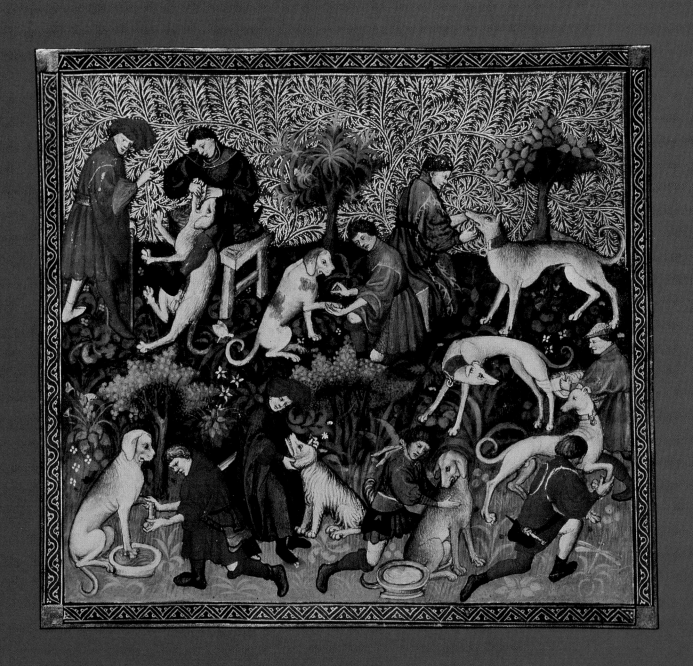

C H A P T E R 1 3

Equine and Canine Medicine in Medieval Europe

~

FREDERICK II: PATRON OF VETERINARY MEDICINE

Frederick II (1194-1250) of the House of Hohenstaufen, who was half Norman and half German, took a special interest in veterinary medicine. He was an extraordinary personality who became the king of Sicily. His kingdom included the southern part of mainland Italy, which contained the medical centers at Salerno and Naples. From 1198 to 1216 the great Pope Innocent III, who declared himself the Vicar of Christ and demanded the allegiance of kings, dominated European politics. He took Frederick II under his protection as a minor, thereby becoming regent of the Sicilian kingdom, and arranged for young Frederick to become kaiser of Germany and, later, to be crowned emperor in Rome. Frederick II negotiated peace with the sultan of Egypt and regained the crown of Jerusalem for Christianity. He was endowed with irrepressible energy, enthusiasm, and curiosity.

Frederick was an enlightened improver of both human and veterinary medicine. After 1221 he required medical practitioners to pass a licensing examination conducted by the masters of Salerno "in order that the king's subjects should not incur danger through the inexperience of their physicians." He issued a decree in 1241 ordering candidates seeking a license to practice as surgeons in his kingdom to study the anatomy of human bodies and attain certification. Presumably dissections were done on animals, notably pigs. He required medical students to have three years of general training in logic, several years of specialized study in medicine and surgery, and a year of practice under the guidance of an experienced physician. The graduates from Salerno were required to take an oath in the Hippocratic tradition and were the first to be called *doctors*.

Frederick II had a general interest in science and, because he was particularly fascinated by animals of all kinds, accumulated a large menagerie of exotic mammals and birds. He had a passionate interest in birds and in that highest of aristocratic sports, falconry. He believed in experimental evidence and established that vultures locate their food by sight. A keen student of the art of falconry, he went to great lengths to learn of the Arabs' experience in the field. They hooded their birds, and he tested and improved their methods, as well as European ones. He composed a treatise on ornithology and falconry, even criticizing Aristotle, who clearly lacked the practical experience that Frederick II had perfected. His six-part book was entitled *De Arte Venandi cum Avibus (The Art of Hunting With Birds)*. It included an introductory section describing falconry as the noblest of the arts. Topics included the habits and structure of birds, the capture and training of birds of prey, types of lures and their uses, the hunting of cranes with gyrfalcons, the hunting of herons with

191. *Facing page, Livre de la Chasse*, a beautifully illustrated practical manual of hunting and animal care published early in the fifteenth century by Gaston Phébus, Count of Foix, signaled a change in equine and canine medicine in medieval Europe. Phébus suggested that instead of the care of these animals being left to the healing hands of saints who were capable of miraculous cures, familiarity and affection for the animals led owners naturally to apply their own methods for caregiving. In this figure from *La Chasse*, great compassion is shown in treating various illnesses and conditions in dogs, Phébus's favorite species. *(Ms. Francais 616, fol. 40ᵛ. Bibliothèque Nationale, Paris.)*

223

192. Kaiser Frederick II of Hohenstaufen (1194-1250), Holy Roman Emperor and King of Sicily and Germany, greatly influenced human and veterinary medicine. His keen interest in birds led him to write *De Arte Venandi cum Avibus* (1247), a richly illuminated six-part manuscript describing the art of hunting with birds. Shown at right is a section of the manuscript depicting the king, with a falcon, addressing some of his falconers. The falconers appear to be paying homage to the king. *(Foto Biblioteca Vaticana, Rome.)*

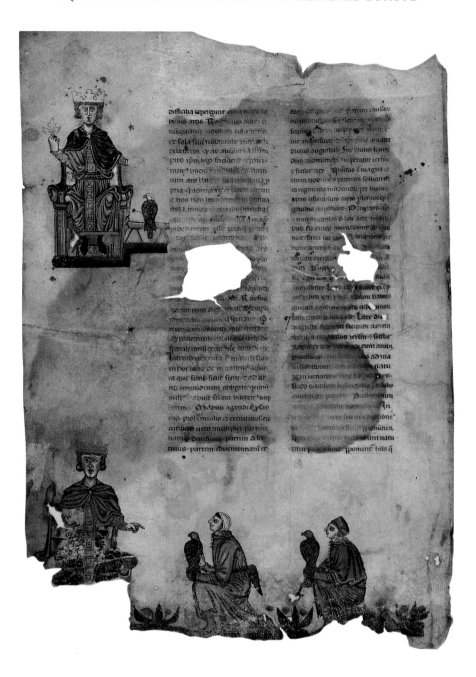

the sacred falcon, the hunting of water birds with the smaller types of falcons, moulting, and the treatment of diseases.

The king's interest in science and medicine extended to animal husbandry, natural history, and veterinary medicine. He had a strong affinity for hunting and required that an excellent stable be maintained for his royal and military roles. In particular, he was aware of the enormous toll in horses sent to the Crusades in the Levant during the twelfth and thirteenth centuries. Thus he perceived the need to develop his equine management, medicine, and surgery to the highest possible level beyond the still-low standards of the Dark Ages. Incorporating all obtainable knowledge from classical, oriental, Islamic, and European sources, he developed a plan of action to address the need.

The emperor, who was dubbed *stupor mundi* ("the wonder of the world"), fell into disfavor with popes after Innocent III. He was excommunicated, found guilty of grave offenses, and deprived of his kingdoms in 1245. Five years later, Frederick II died. Thus ended the career of a great but ruthless innovator, who in knowledge and life-style was something of a bridge between the Muslim and Christian worlds, a premature Renaissance man. Intrigues, power plays, suspicion, and ruthless reprisals characterized his reign. One scholar depicted his behavior as that of a "baptized sultan." He had greater faith in astrology than in theology. He failed to harmonize the new ideas and developments he enthusiastically sought out with the heritage of beliefs and ideals of the Christian faith. Great intellectual gains resulted from his patronage of medicine, science, and the arts in a tumultuous era, but his political legacy was more a blight than a benefit. The kingdom of Sicily went into decline shortly after his death and never recovered. Nonetheless, veterinary medicine in the age of chivalry received a great boost from his sponsorship of improvements in equine medicine and the care of raptor birds.

THE KING'S SPONSORSHIP OF JORDANUS RUFFUS'S *MEDICINA EQUORUM*

To meet the goal of raising the standard of equine medicine, Frederick II appointed Jordanus Ruffus (Giordano Rufo) of Calabria as his chief imperial horse marshal and "mareschallus" or veterinarian. He urged Ruffus to write a book on equine management and medicine. Ruffus undertook this task enthusiastically but did not complete it until shortly after the emperor's death in 1250, when it was published under the title *Medicina Equorum* (*Equine Medicine*).

Ruffus had a military background and was of an applied practical turn of mind. Consequently he regarded the speculative study of the origins of disease and most anatomical studies as expendable. He was content to refer to the old humoral theories and attribute the causes of disease to "bad juices." Like Frederick, Ruffus referred to astrological ideas. He was an empiricist who stressed practical matters like equine eye diseases, lameness, shoeing, and wound treatment. His book was a manual for the user of a horse, written for knights, marshals, veterinarians, farriers, and grooms. He had access to the Arabic literature and through it to Byzantine and Greek sources. Also, Frederick II had in his court the scholar Michael Scotus, who had translated Aristotle's *Historia Animalium*.

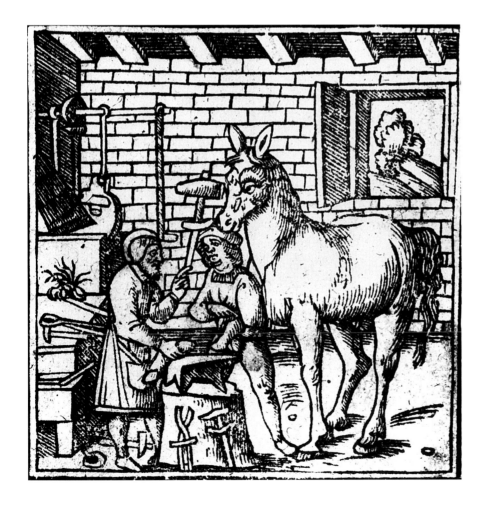

193. Jordanus Ruffus's *Medicina Equorum* was copied many times after its publication in 1250. A woodcut of a farrier (possibly a saint) and his assistant discussing a horse's severed leg makes up the title page of this 1519 Venetian copy, *Libro dela Natura di Cavalli*. This scene is highly reminiscent of the miracle of St. Alò, illustrated in Plate 184. (*National Library of Medicine, Bethesda, Maryland.*)

194. *Right,* Frederick II, who gained considerable veterinary knowledge from the experience of Arabs, appointed Jordanus Ruffus his chief horse marshall. Ruffus published a beautifully illustrated book on equine management and medicine, *Medicina Equorum* (c. 1250). In this folio from an Italian translation, *Libro delle Mariscalcie dei Cavalli,* a horse is being castrated because of damage to its testes. End of thirteenth century. *(Cod. 78 C 15, fol. 14ᵛ. Bildarchiv Preußischer Kulturbesitz, Berlin.)*

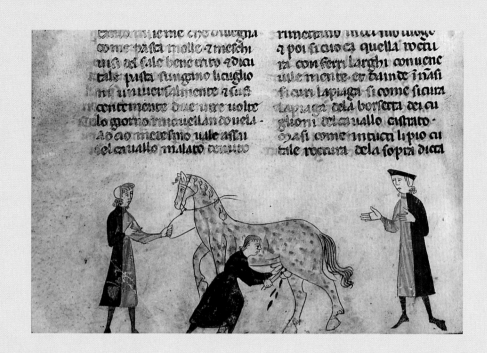

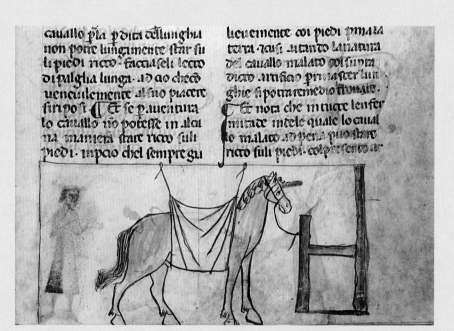

195. *Left,* A primitive hanging apparatus for horses that was used after surgery on hooves. From *Libro delle Mariscalcie dei Cavalli* by Jordanus Ruffus. *(Cod. 78 C 15, fol. 45. Bildarchiv Preußischer Kulturbesitz, Berlin.)*

196. *Right,* Venesection of the jugular vein. From *Libro delle Mariscalcie dei Cavalli* by Jordanus Ruffus. *(Cod. 78 C 15, fol. 9. Bildarchiv Preußischer Kulturbesitz, Berlin.)*

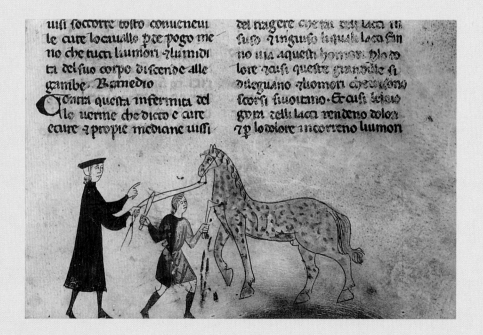

Among his most important contributions, Ruffus paved the way for improved horse management, focusing on the hoof and the mouth. Shoeing of horses with metal shoes can be traced to the late twelfth century in old European and Arabic documents. It was Ruffus, however, who provided detailed descriptions of the foot and of nailed metal shoes. He described innovations in bits and bridles long before those of the great marshals of the sixteenth and seventeenth centuries were introduced, and he wrote about dental care and the filing and extraction of teeth.

Ruffus created the first medieval European system for naming and grouping equine diseases. He latinized names in common use for horse diseases. One large section of *Medicina Equorum* addressed aspects of veterinary hygiene, such as breeding, conformation, breaking, training, daily care, shoeing, bridles, and bits, and differentiated inborn malformations and diseases from those that are acquired. Another major section identified fifty-seven diseases of the horse by name and described the symptoms that give the clue to diagnosis, as well as detailing the recommended treatment. Virtually all the one hundred and fifty or so medications that he listed were products of natural origin—vegetable, animal, or mineral. He recommended measures to gain the trust of the animal. Nevertheless, as was necessary in the days before tranquilizers or anesthetics, he used manhandling and forceful means of restraint involving stocks, ropes and straps, the twitch, and casting as required. Ruffus used surgical instruments and techniques and was among the first to describe the ligation of blood vessels to arrest hemorrhage.

Ruffus's writings contained a wealth of practical information but little to satisfy the intellectual endeavour to address the unknown. Surprisingly, he failed to conduct postmortem examinations to gain insights in the fields of internal medicine and pathology. Even his coverage of malleus, the great scourge of medieval horses, was unsatisfactory. His book achieved great popularity and was translated into many languages. Because of the special interest of the emperor, the importance of the horse, and the comparative component

197. A rather crude but effective method for the reduction of a luxated shoulder. From a northern Italian manuscript illustrating an anonymous and undated list of cures for one hundred and fifty-two ailments suffered by horses. *(Add. Ms. 15097, fol. 94ᵛ. The British Library, London.)*

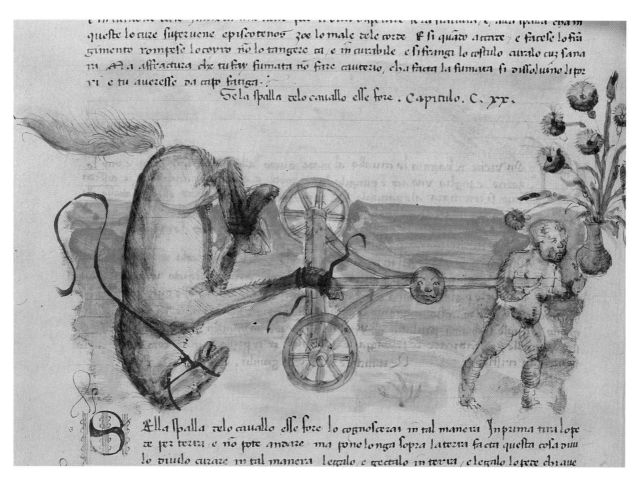

198. Selected sites for the bleeding of a horse. This illustration is at the beginning of an Italian translation by the Dominican Antonio Dapera of a treatise on horse medicine first written by Bonifacio of Calabria during the reign of Charles of Anjou (died 1285), King of Naples. Third quarter of the fifteenth century. *(Add. Ms. 15097, fol. 1ᵛ. The British Library, London.)*

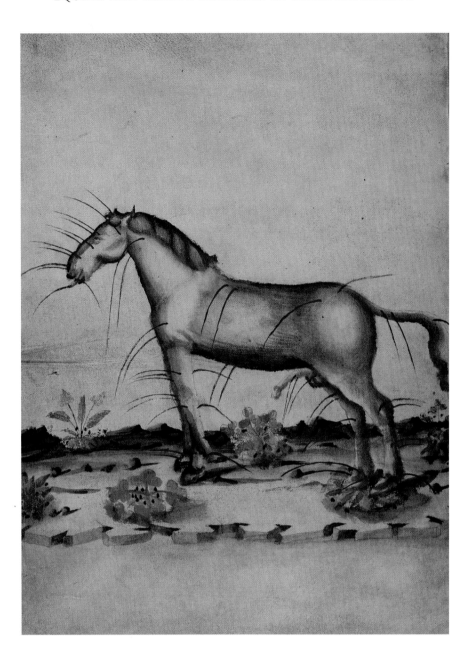

of the developing medical centers at Salerno and Naples, which, as sources of medical renaissance, incorporated Ruffus's work, *Equine Medicine* elevated veterinary medicine to parity with the medicine of the day. Its influence on the veterinary art lasted for five centuries. The appearance of a later translation of Ruffus's *Equine Medicine* under the title *Hippiatria* led to confusion of his book with the Byzantine classic, *Hippiatrika*.

Bishop Theodoric (1205–c. 1296) of Cervia made an interesting contribution to surgery deriving from the veterinary medicine of Ruffus's period. He experimented with applying sponges soaked in hypnotic drugs to the nostrils to induce unconsciousness and analgesia before surgery. Initially he used *Hyoscyamus niger* to calm a horse before surgery, but he continued to try other products such as the opium poppy and mandrake root.

RUSIO'S *HIPPIATRIA SIVE MARESCALCIA*

Lorenzo Rusio (Rusius), who lived from 1288 to 1347, became a marshal and veterinarian in Rome. He compiled the equine knowledge of his day in *La Mascalcia*. He drew heavily on *De Animalibus,* the work of Albertus Magnus, and on that of Jordanus Ruffus (without acknowledgment) and others who preceded him by more than fifty years. Rusio practiced veterinary medicine in Rome, probably from 1320 to 1347. His book was reprinted two centuries after his death as *Hippiatria Sive Marescalcia,* which created further confusion with Ruffus's *Hippiatria* and the earlier *Hippiatrika.*

Rusio focused on the management and hygiene of horses at all stages of life and was systematic in his organization of equine diseases. He noted that violent colic could lead to rupture of the intestine. His discussion of fractures and lameness was detailed. He described the use of a cloth sling to suspend from a beam a horse that was unable to stand or had a damaged hoof. Thus the animal could escape the deterioration of chronic recumbency or protect an injured limb. Rusio applied leeches for inflammation of the legs; his was the first record of their use in veterinary medicine. He also described the brutal practice of removal of the sole for certain diseases of the horse's foot, such as laminitis. Because his *Hippiatria* was popular reading for many generations, it was probably responsible for the later popularity of unsoling, that is, ripping out the sole by brute force, which became a favored technique of farriers. Remarkably, Rusio recognized the likelihood of septic infection of wounds and was the first to show that glanders or farcy could spread from horses to humans, writing of the human form that:

> . . . *the disease arises from the putrid blood which exudes from the veins, and sometimes from a blow or other injury. The disease may also arise from mixing with horses affected with the disease, for farcy is a contagious malady.*

These were the words of a good observer and a sound thinker who was speaking from experience, not "book learning." It is likely that the farriers paid less attention to the risks of infection than to the dramatic operations such as removal of the sole.

JOYS OF THE CHASE AND AFFECTION FOR HOUNDS

The Romans had spectacles, many of them violent or horrific, rather than sporting. The mulomedici served cavalry horses and the veterinarii served agriculture, but neither served the interests of sport other than indirectly, through horse maintenance. The sports of the Middle Ages, on the other hand, arose from the nobles and the warrior class, for whom hunting and hawking formed part of the combat and cultural training of the aristocracy. This perspective emerges from the literature during and after the twelfth century. There were several early medieval writers on falconry, but they mostly described problems and diseases.

The major sports in the fourteenth century were war games and hunting. The art and delights of the chase evoked the following books: the *Livre du Roi Modus et de la Reine Ratio;* William Twice's *Ars de Venerie* (he was master of hunt to Edward II); Gace de la Buigne's *Roman des Deduis;* Gaston Phébus, Count of Foix's magnificent *Livre de la Chasse;* and the great work on falconry by Emperor Frederick II. It should be appreciated that hunting and falconry were privileges largely restricted to royalty and the aristocracy. Special forests were reserved for their use, and ordinary citizens living in the area often had to have their dogs mutilated so that they could not participate in poaching activities. The game included deer, especially stags, wild boar, wolves, and other species such as bear, depending on the region. Cromwell's wars against royalty and the aristocracy led to rapid deforestation of England and a major decline in hunting.

Gaston Phébus was the most eloquent advocate of hunting for pleasure. He extols its joys—finding a great hart, uncoupling the hounds, mounting in haste to keep up with them, observing the behavior of the pack, galloping after them when they are in full cry, and cheering them on. He promises the reader that the activity leaves no place for evil thoughts. Then comes the kill,

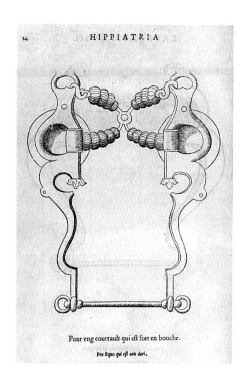

199. Lorenzo Rusio or Laurentius Rusius (1288-1347), a Roman veterinarian, published *La Mascalcia,* a book dealing with horse care that was so popular it was translated into French, German, Italian, and Spanish and republished under different titles, especially *Hippiatria Sive Marescalcia,* not to be confused with the earlier *Hippiatrika.* This picture of a curb bit is from a 1532 edition. *(The Science Museum/ Science & Society Picture Library, London.)*

200. Gaston Phébus's great love and affection for dogs can be seen in the art that illustrates his *Livre de la Chasse*. Phébus believed in the joys of hunting for pleasure and believed in treating the dogs properly after a hunt, as featured in this folio. He wrote that exercise is important for canine health, and sampling a little of the best grass would promote digestion. One dog is being covered with a blanket, and others are being cleaned and checked for ticks. *(Ms. Français 616, fol. 53. Bibliothèque Nationale, Paris.)*

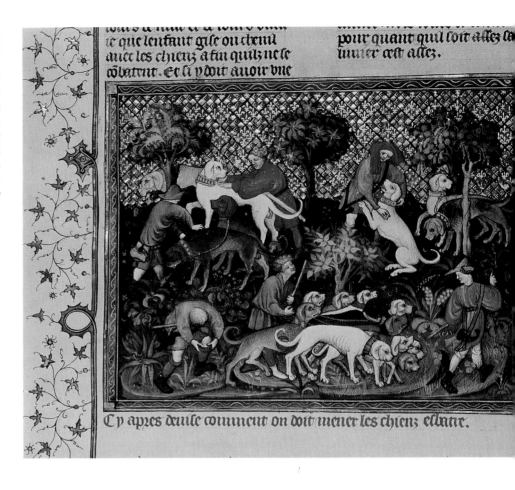

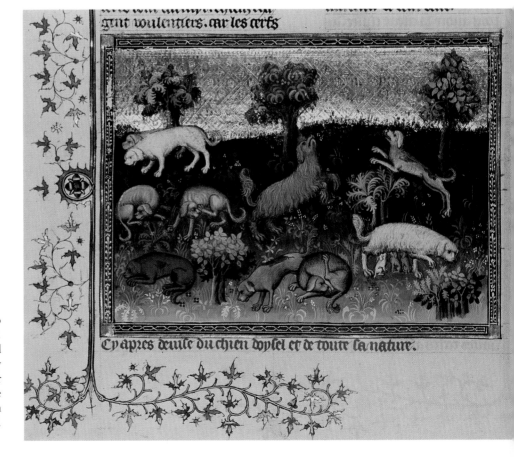

201. The spaniel is featured in this folio from Gaston Phébus's *Livre de la Chasse*. Spaniels were trained to hunt feathered game and were loyal to their masters. They were used to flush the game from its cover so that falcons could capture it. The spaniel and falcon formed a perfect team for this type of hunting. *(Ms. Français 616. Bibliothèque Nationale, Paris.)*

230

the breaking up of the deer, the toast in a good wine, and the ride home, the hunter in a more joyful mood than any other person. He urges all sorts and conditions of men, poor or rich, to participate in some way in hunting or hawking: to live in idleness, without love of sport, is not wise. The Count describes how the freshness of the morning air, the melodious love songs of the birds, and the beauty of the dewdrops at sunrise on the boughs and herbage rejoice the heart and how, finally, after a day spent in exciting and joyous sport, the hunter lies down and enjoys a long, untroubled sleep.

Gaston Phébus's great work stands alone in its remarkable expression of affection for the dog. He devoted ten chapters of *La Chasse* to dogs, mainly to the hounds used as companions in the hunt. He made a study of the behavior of each of his hounds. He recounted stories praising the faithfulness of a dog to its master, even after the master's death. His beautifully illustrated book showed scenes of the chase and of attending to the dogs' needs for medical attention. Phébus died in 1391, passing peacefully after a fine day's hunting in which a boar was killed. His last conversation was with his huntsman; Phébus spoke of how his hounds had performed that day, naming the ones that had run and scented best. His book did not appear in print until 1507.

Anyone who worked with dogs in the hunt had to be wary of the risk of encountering rabid animals. Bartholomew Glanville, an Englishman who studied in Paris in the thirteenth century, wrote an encyclopedic work, *The Properties of Things,* which veterinarians and laypersons alike appreciate for its outstanding description of the behavior of a rabid dog and the effects of its bite:

> *The biting of the rabid hound is deadly and venemous, for it is long hidden and unknown, and increaseth and multiplieth itself . . . cometh to the head and breedeth frenzy.*

> *The rabid hound . . . is always exiled as it were an outlaw, and goeth alone wagging and rolling as a drunken beast, and runneth yawning and his tongue hangeth out, and his mouth drivelleth and foameth, and his eyes be overturned and reared.*

During the Middle Ages, Mandragora or the root of the mandrake plant, described by Dioscorides in his work on herbal remedies in the first century AD, was made into an anesthetic potion or sponge and administered to the patient before surgery or cautery. It induced a deep sleep. Gathering the plant was considered a dangerous undertaking because it was said to utter a shriek upon being uprooted: whoever heard the shriek became insane or died. The solution was to loosen the plant cautiously with the spade, then tie a hungry dog by the neck to the plant and cast meat before the dog but out of reach so that he jerked the root out of the ground, whereupon the dog fell down dead.

PARACELSUS'S IATROCHEMISTRY: CHALLENGE TO SUPERSTITION

Significant advances were made on the scientific front in the thirteenth century. Arnaud de Villeneuve (1235–1315) of Valencia, Spain, traveled to the centers of learning in Barcelona, Salerno, Montpellier, and Paris. He was an alchemist and laboratory chemist of broad interests who showed how alcohol could be used to extract essences from macerated plants. These essences came to be used in pharmacy as "waters of M. Arnaud." Villeneuve became rector of Montpellier University. Roger Bacon (1214–1294), a scholar of Oxford and Paris, urged doctors to escape from inherited dogmas. Although also an alchemist, Bacon was a pioneer in calling for an experimental approach, a precursor of the thinking that led to the Renaissance. Gerard of Cremona went to Toledo in the twelfth century and began translating the Greek classics into Latin.

After the recapture of classical knowledge in the translations from Greek originals in the early Renaissance, physicians lapsed into the hero worship of authorities, notably of Hippocrates and Galen. A confrontation was required to reopen minds to the need for a continuing struggle to advance knowledge, the need to observe, record, test, and rethink phenomena. The challenge came from a freethinker, Theophrastus von Hohenheim (1493–1541), physician of Basel, whose nickname, Paracelsus, was derived from the name of the famous Roman physician and scholar Celsus. Paracelsus frequented the laboratories associated with mines, learning much about mineral chemistry. He was by nature an intellectual revolutionary and an archcritic of the medical establishment and its fixed ideas.

After traveling widely in his youth, Paracelsus acquired a great reputation as a physician, and in 1527 he was appointed to the Chair of Physick at the University of Basel. When the students built a holiday bonfire at the university, Paracelsus marched out with Avicenna's *Canon of Medicine* in his hands and cast it into the fire as a symbolic gesture of breaking the hold of the oracles whose word must not be questioned. He had to flee from Basel within a year of his appointment. Paracelsus was also a student of the occult—of astrology and alchemy. He made predictions about the future in a book entitled *Prognostication*, foreshadowing the famous *Centuries* of Nostradamus, a doctor at Montpellier. Paracelsus, however, provided a bridge between alchemy and true chemistry applied to medicine, particularly that of inorganic compounds. The figurehead of iatrochemistry, he was probably the first to prepare ether, noting that when chickens ingested it, they would sleep for a long time and revive unharmed: he missed a golden opportunity to invent anesthesia. He

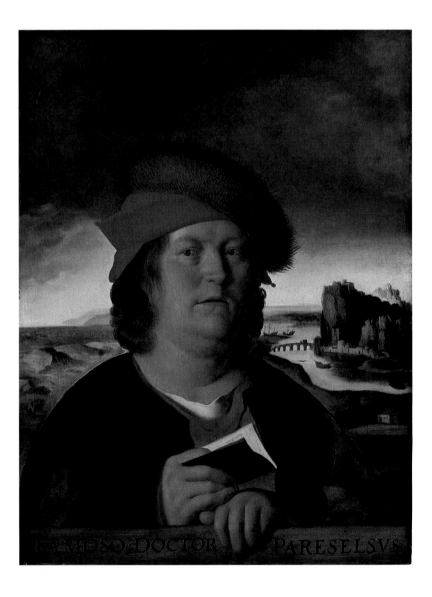

202. *Famoso Doctor Pareselsus* by Jan van Scorel. Paracelsus, formally Philippus Theophrastus Aureolus Bombastus von Hohenheim (1493–1541), was a firm believer in acquiring knowledge from experience, not reading the books and manuscripts of the ancients. This belief was a direct reflection of his understanding of many scientific disciplines, including, among many others, astrology, alchemy, medicine, and pharmacology. His varied experiences were acquired during a lifetime of wandering throughout Europe and into Africa. He treated Danish military horses and published *Die grosse Wundarzney* as a result of this experience. True to his contrary nature, his works were published in low German rather than Latin, making them difficult to translate. *(The Louvre, Paris.)*

was on the track of the role of air in combustion, although he used the term "sulfur," after the Arabs, for the combustible part. He also may have been the first to generate hydrogen gas.

The work of Paracelsus on compounds of heavy metals was the intellectual root of chemotherapy by means of selective toxicity. He treated horses and recommended the use of arsenicals (potassium arsenate and sulfur of arsenic) to treat the dreaded equine disease glanders (malleus), a significant conceptual development in veterinary medicine. He had a great impact on pharmacy, pharmacology, and toxicology. He confronted the old galenical craft of preparing mixtures of herbal products with a new range of chemically prepared medicines (that is, chemically prepared by the spagyrical or alchemical art).

Paracelsus was a man ahead of the science of pharmacology. One of his aphorisms has stood the test of time: "Dose alone makes the poison." He took great pains to determine the correct dosages of his chemical prescriptions, recognizing that in the wrong doses they were poisons. He introduced tincture of opium (laudanum), which became a major remedy in the physician's bag. He was prepared to strive for solutions to the most difficult medical problems, such as syphilis and malleus. One of the most controversial figures in medical history, he became a wandering physician in Germany and died prematurely in Salzburg. His chemical studies were extended by J.B. van Helmont of Brussels, who considered digestion a chemical process.

In 1535 the meticulous Reformation scientist Valerius Cordus in Nuremberg edited the *Dispensatorium Pharmacopolarum,* a great advance in the development of an objective pharmacopoeia of the effects of reputable medicaments. The *Dispensatorium* was a precursor to pharmacology, which emerged as the need for scientific evaluation of drug efficacy and safety became apparent. A range of significant new drugs derived from plants was arriving in Europe from the New World, and gradually the hold of magic potions on the popular mind was being loosened.

SURGERY: A RESPECTABLE PROFESSION

In northern and eastern Europe the Roman church no longer permitted priests to practice surgery on animals. To fill the void, a new cadre of essentially lay surgeons who knew cutting and little else developed from the barbers. They were separated from the physicians or medical practitioners and formed their own guilds. Before the development of anesthetics and a scientific basis for most surgical interventions, it took a callous individual to perform the unpleasant task of cutting open the human body in the face of the screams of agony and the likelihood of postsurgical consequences such as loss of function, disfigurement, infection, and death. The public and academic images of the surgical "profession" never recovered from this early negative image. Traces of it linger today, long after surgery became a legitimate branch of medicine in the nineteenth century.

Only in some Italian and French universities did surgeons receive the rudiments of appropriate education and preparation. The thirteenth century surgeon Guido Lanfranchi was a distinguished scholar who fled to Paris to escape political persecution in Milan. He was listed as author of a book on the surgery of domestic animals, *Practica Avium et Equorum.* The legitimacy of his authorship is suspect, however, since the book was published in 1295, fifteen years after his death. He established an enlightened school in Paris that became preeminent in surgery, thereby restoring surgery's connection with medicine and allowing surgeons to escape the technician label of the barber-surgeons.

The introduction of a thoughtful physiological basis for surgery and the development of effective teaching techniques in Europe has been attributed to Lanfranchi's contemporary, Henri de Mondeville (1260-1320). He stanched hemorrhages with tourniquets, introduced suturing and vascular ligation, and stressed the importance of sanitary practices, including the use of alcohol in wound treatment and in dressing surgical interventions. He also stressed the importance of considerate counseling of the patient and relatives.

Guy de Chauliac (1300-1368), who worked in the great French medical centers and in Bologna, introduced the use of wire in suturing areas under mechanical stress, such as in the closure of a hernial ring, and the use of slings and traction for fractures, thereby developing a great reputation as a bold, innovative surgeon. His surgical text, *Chirurgia Magna,* became a standard for nearly two hundred years.

AMBROISE PARÉ: SURGERY'S REVOLUTIONARY

The Paris school was an island of progressive surgical science in an era when both physicians and society in general relegated the practice of surgery to low-class individuals who were repressed, discriminated against, and despised.

It was, nevertheless, from the lower class that the greatest revolutionary in surgery was to arise. Ambroise Paré (1516-1590) began his career as a barber-surgeon's assistant, trained as a master barber-surgeon, and enlisted in the army, where he developed his dexterity with the knife to a remarkable degree, performing limb amputations in less than three minutes in the time before anesthetics. In the days of the terrifying practice of cautery he adopted the alternative of arterial ligation. The son of an artisan, he knew neither Latin nor Greek, which made it difficult for him to gain acceptance on his return to Paris, but his natural genius, drive, and humanity soon brought him respect. He invented many innovative surgical instruments and designed prostheses, including artificial limbs, teeth, and eyes.

Paré stands as the greatest figure in the history of surgery in the sixteenth century. Of his many books, one, *La Méthode de Traiter les Playes Faites par Hacquebutes* (volume two), dealt with veterinary surgery. The *Harquebus* was a heavy gun. The book is said to deal with restraint of animals and operations, presumably for wound treatment in horses. Paré completely revolutionized the treatment of burns and gunshot and shrapnel wounds, abandoning the standard practice of pouring hot oil into them when supplies ran out during the battle of Turin (1536). He then performed a controlled experiment in which he established that untreated wounds did not show the swelling or cause the "wound fever" typical of those treated with oil. He pronounced that the surgeon dressed wounds but God healed them.

Throughout his career Paré strove to release surgery from false doctrines and dogma. He rejoiced in overcoming the technical challenge that surgical interventions presented but always kept in mind the ultimate goal, the well-being of the patient. Although he had to work with primitive equipment from the medieval period, which was characterized by widespread insensitivity to suffering and much blatant cruelty to humans and animals alike, Paré emerged as surgery's "Renaissance man," who "put it all together." His unusual powers of observation, his remarkable technical prowess, his zeal to relieve suffering, his insistence on evaluation of efficacy in treatment, his intellectual power through a problem-solving approach, and above all, his humanity and concern for the patient, placed him in a class by himself. He vowed in his writings to offer precepts that he would prove by authority, reason, and experience. He wrote many works on a wide range of subjects, among them a major anatomical text published in 1561, just eighteen years after Vesalius' *Fabrica,* as well as a ten-volume set on surgery and a book describing how to tailor autopsy reports to meet requirements of jurisprudence.

Paré's authorities were Hippocrates and Galen; the rest of his wisdom was a product of his personal genius and documented case experience. He was a

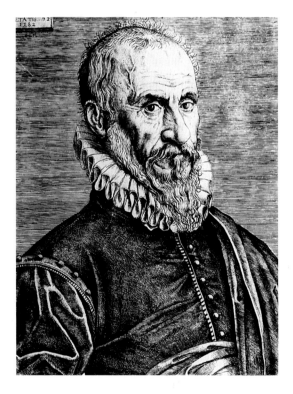

203. Woodcut portrait of Ambroise Paré (1510-1590) at seventy-two years of age. The son of a cabinetmaker, Paré became a leading figure in the development of innovative surgical techniques, which he learned from his experience as a field surgeon. The second volume of his *La Méthode de Traiter les Playes Faites par Hacquebutes* (1545) dealt with veterinary surgery and, more important, established its similarity to human surgery. *(Courtesy The New York Academy of Medicine Library.)*

witness at the scenes of the Italian wars and the wars of religion. He condemned warfare and its evolving technology of ever more infernal weaponry
designed to kill and maim the human and animal bodies. He wrote in collo-
quial French, which made his work readily accessible. Paré's last great work,
Apologie et Treatise, was both a masterpiece of medical scholarship and an autobiography.

THE EVOLVING ROLE OF FARRIERS IN GREAT BRITAIN

Leslie Penrhys Pugh, writing in 1926, summarized the veterinary situation in
the Anglo-Saxon period. After the first horseshoes were invented, the veterinary art was practiced by farriers, who originally were mainly shoers of
horses. Farriery was an "occupation" rather than a profession. Much later it
became a stepping stone to the veterinary art. Even farriers, however, looked
down on cow leeches. Pugh said that "at best, the cow-leeches did nothing
to prevent the recovery of their patients by natural means; at worst, they inflicted unnecessary pain." As individuals started to obtain their own prescription books, "some of the cow-leeches began to rely on incantations, charms
and amulets in order to keep the confidence of their humbler clients." In
some remote parts, especially in the old Celtic regions, such local "wise men"
held their own against the advancing rationalism in animal medicine.

AMULETS BELIEVED TO PREVENT DISEASE

There were incantations to cure red water in Scotland and selected herbs to
protect against sheep pox and sudden death in swine. Urine, salt, and soot
were liberally drenched for supposed therapeutic effect. Witch post amulets of
rowan wood were hung in Yorkshire, and an ornament crafted from the last
sheaf of the season was hung to protect livestock from disease for a year.
Special stones imputed to have magical properties were said to keep the dairy
herd free from mastitis and other diseases for a full year. Most famous of all
was the Lee Penny, a heart-shaped deep red stone of carnelian agate set in an
Edward IV (reigned 1461-1483) silver groat (a four-penny coin) that was put
in a cloven stick and then dipped in the water that was to be given to the cattle to drink. During the Reformation, such amulets became anathema, but
the Lee stone had to be exempted because of the universal faith it commanded.

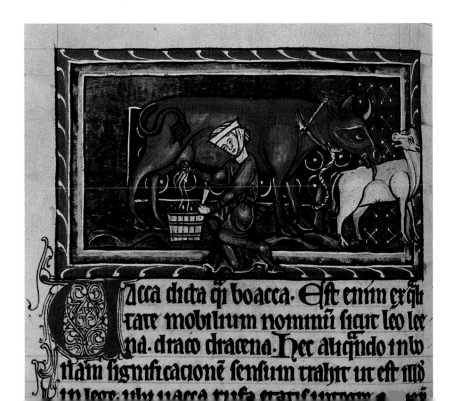

204. Scenes of domestication proliferate
in the manuscripts of the Middle Ages.
Here a cow is being milked while she
cleans her recently born calf. *(Ms. 764.
Bodleian Library, Oxford.)*

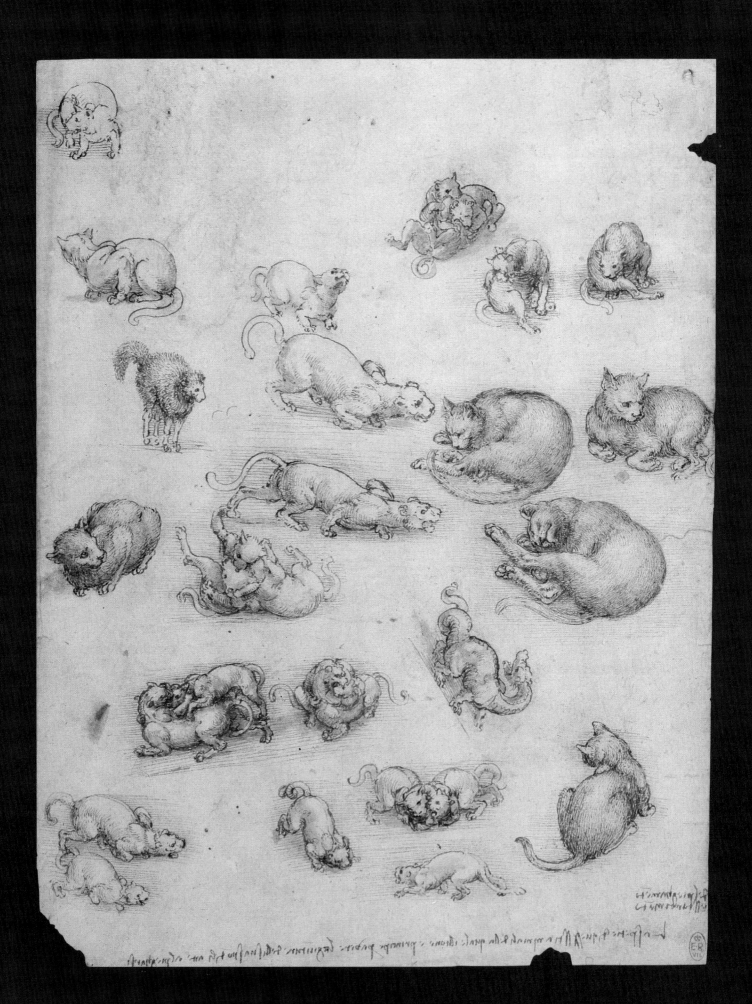

Renaissance in Medical Science

Italian Roots

~

ARTISTIC EXPRESSIONS OF EQUINE ANATOMY

The Renaissance was initially an Italian phenomenon. Towering above other figures early in that period was the great artist and polymath Leonardo da Vinci (1452-1519). Among his works are marvelous drawings of the external anatomical appearances and behavioral characteristics of humans, horses, oxen, and cats. He taught anatomy to medical students in Florence. His insatiable curiosity and artistic drive led him to perfect his anatomical draftsmanship by performing dissections. He used measurements and drawings made with engineering precision in artistic models (for example, in creating the Sforza monument), striving to achieve a perfection of form in the horses he drew or sculpted. This system was later adopted and widely used by artists and students of the relationship between form and function. His biological drawings, which characterized every function—from intimate details of the act of procreation through fetal life to the anatomy of the adult body—have never been equalled.

Leonardo da Vinci studied embryology and obtained specimens from slaughterhouses for work on the bovine embryo. His drawings of horses and cats conveyed dynamic and behavioral images as well as anatomical accuracy and are now enshrined in the royal library at Windsor Castle in England. His anatomical drawings helped others understand the physiology and the behavior of the subject while retaining a sense of the unique, mystical properties of the individual. He captured elements of the human-animal bond and examples of hostility and conflict, yet there is always a sense of interdependence and communication among his subjects and between them and the viewer. He was the real parent of that illegitimate child, the science of anatomy, but of the structures as they are in life, not as cadavers.

Albrecht Dürer (1471-1528) of Nuremberg, da Vinci's contemporary, although more limited in scope as a creative genius, came closest to Leonardo in drawing animals. Dürer had visited the great animal artists of northern Italy who preceded him, particularly Pisanello, who had been the first to draw horses and had made medals bearing equine images with unsurpassed skill and artistry in the early to middle years of the fifteenth century. Dürer made few animal paintings, but his drawings and woodcuts were of superb quality. He had a special flair for animal subjects and even drew pictures of monstrosities such as the pig of Landser, which had eight legs. His symbolic drawings of the medieval plagues of animals and humans convey hints of an appreciation of the idea of contagion.

205. *Facing page,* Perhaps the most influential artist of the Renaissance, Leonardo da Vinci was fascinated with anatomical study, and his drawings of structure and function are among his most masterful works. This particular work, *Studies of Cats* (c. 1506), dynamically captures form and behavior. Like many of his drawings this piece was originally done by Leonardo in black chalk and probably inked in by one of his pupils. *(By permission of Her Majesty Queen Elizabeth II, The Royal Collection, Windsor Castle.)*

206. Drawings frequently identified as being of the brain of an ox but actually showing more human characteristics (c. 1509-1510) by Leonardo da Vinci. The cerebral ventricles in lateral view are at top left; the frontal section is at the upper right; the lower drawing shows the base of the brain and the retiform plexus; the wax cast of the ventricles is set off to the right. The ventricles were injected with wax to preserve their shape. The method of wax injection was his own invention and did not become generally used by anatomists until the seventeenth century. *(By permission of Her Majesty Queen Elizabeth II, The Royal Collection, Windsor Castle.)*

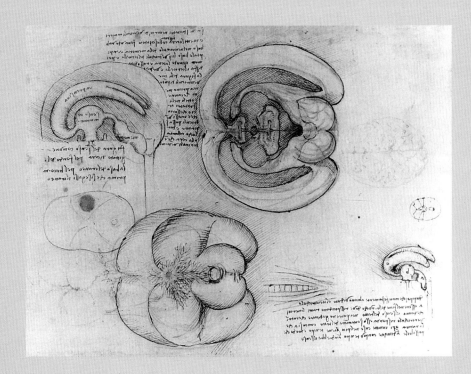

---

207. Drawings based on dissections of the heart of an ox, from Leonardo's latest period. Leonardo drew in remarkable detail the four chambers of the mammalian heart and their valves, which he recognized to be mechanical directors of blood flow and subject to dysfunction. As a consequence, he was puzzled by the then-currently held galenical theory of ebb and flow through the pores in the wall between the ventricles. He drew the coronary vessels and was the first to describe atheromatous lesions with blockage of the arteries in an aged man who died suddenly in Florence. *(By permission of Her Majesty Queen Elizabeth II, The Royal Collection, Windsor Castle.)*

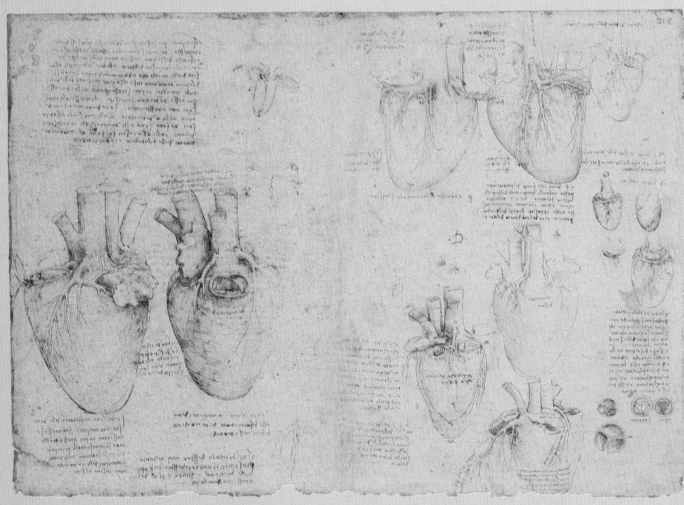

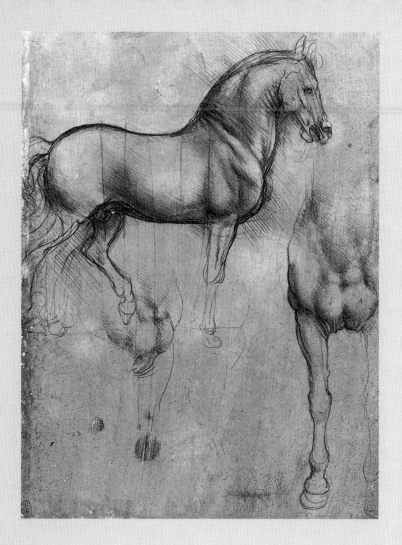

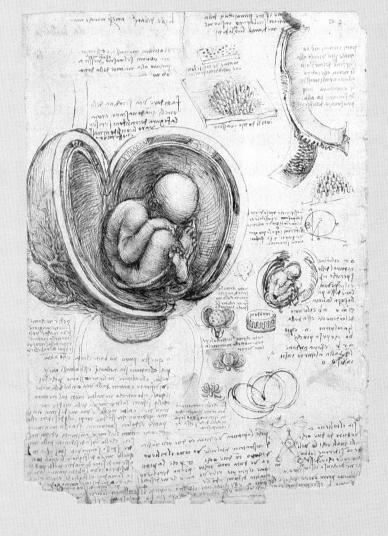

210. Albrecht Dürer, known for his studies of the human figure, was also a keen observer of animals in nature. This watercolor, *The Head of a Stag Killed by an Arrow* (1504), is one of his most dramatic pieces. *(Bibliothèque Nationale, Paris.)*

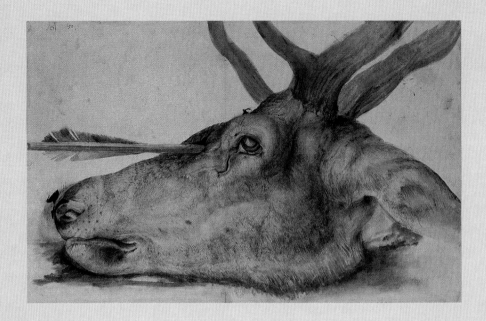

211. This engraving, *The Monstrous Pig of Landser* (c. 1496), shows Dürer's fascination with aberrations of nature. *(Rosenwald Collection, National Gallery of Art, Washington, D.C.)*

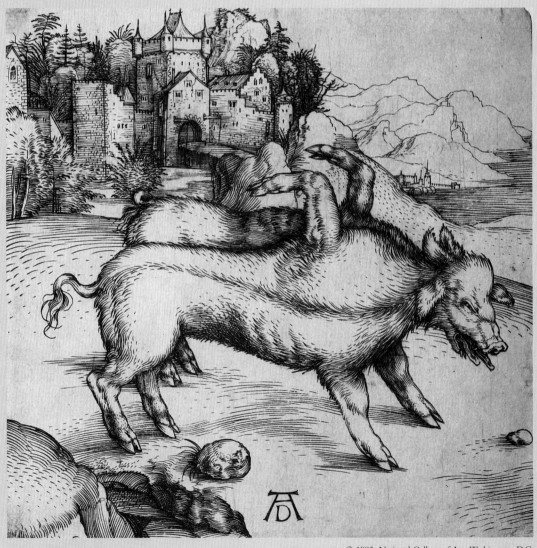

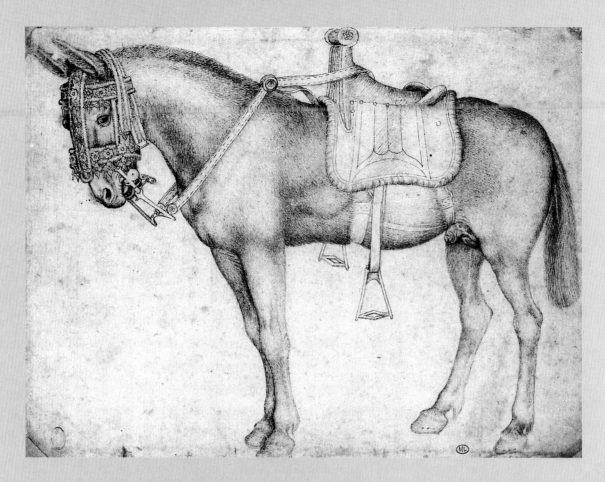

212. *Mule,* by Antonio Pisano Pisanello, Italian (c. 1395–c. 1455). Pisanello's draftmanship illustrates the saddlery of the time in this pen and ink drawing. Although Pisanello's reputation rests largely on his work as a metallist, his drawings and paintings represent the beginning of a new era in which copying traditional forms, which was common during the Middle Ages, gave way to a more delicate, accurate observation of nature. *(The Louvre, Paris.)*

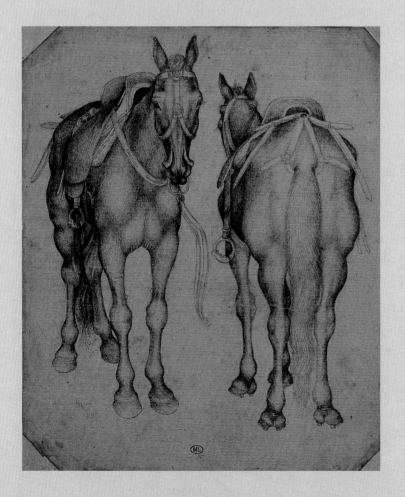

213. *Cavallo (Horse),* by Antonio Pisanello. Pisanello, a superb equine artist, made this study of the same horse directly from the front and rear for his painting, *St. George and the Princess,* in the church of Sant'Anastasia in Verona. Interestingly, the horse is shown with what appear to be surgically slit nostrils, a technique used to increase the animal's respiration and improve its endurance. *(The Louvre, Paris.)*

241

SCIENTIFIC ANATOMY

The development of anatomy as a science in its own right had begun with Galen's dissections of pigs, apes, and other species. His word on morphology was law until the arrival of the brilliant Belgian physician Andreas Witting or Vesalius (1514-1564) who received his medical qualification from Padua in 1537, after studying in Paris as well. Over the centuries the Catholic Church, by banning dissections and any contradiction of the "infallible" Galen, had been a huge impediment to progress in anatomy. Vesalius worked with Sylvius in Paris, then moved to Padua, where he had freedom to dissect. He immersed himself for five years in teaching and mastering human anatomy and produced in 1543, before he was thirty years old, one of the most famous medical books ever written, *De Humani Corporus Fabrica,* a masterpiece with illustrations thought to be by the artist Jan Stefan von Kalkar, who was assistant to Titian. Vesalius had found many errors in Galen's anatomical works (probably because Galen dissected pigs and Barbary apes rather than humans), and his wonderful book triggered a storm of detraction and reprobation—anatomical, medical, and theological—from the old guard. Vesalius was so upset that he burned all his books, critiques, and manuscripts. Anatomy lost its brightest light, its shooting star, because of the same kind of heretical psychology and corrupt bigotry that repeatedly aborted the scientific and scholarly initiatives of the Middle Ages. He became court physician to Charles V and later to his son Philip II of Spain. He died in a shipwreck off the Isle of Zante near Greece. Vesalius had left many able followers, including Fallopius and Eustachius, to carry on his legacy, but they, too, were inhibited. Such was the strength of the conservative, doctrinal establishment of Church and academia that *De Fabrica* languished largely suppressed and unused for a century while the work of the immortal Galen was perpetuated, its flaws ignored.

One of the earliest anatomists to draw from observation of nature and to explore the structure of the brain in detail was Giacomo Berengario da Carpi (1470-1530). He dissected more than a hundred brains and provided clear descriptions of the third ventricle, the basal ganglia, and the pituitary and pineal glands. He developed a test for skull fractures and performed brain surgery.

The Roman Catholic Inquisition, which was reorganized in 1542 (under Pope Paul III) to pursue all deviationists in the attempt to stop the Reformation movement and combat the march of Protestantism, had a deleterious effect on the spread of the new rational science. The Holy Office (that is, the Inquisition) was implacable in its ruthless implementation of torture and terror to obtain confessions of heresy. In fifteenth-century Spain and in Italy during the sixteenth and seventeenth centuries, thousands were burned at the stake, many of them having been tortured on the rack until they confessed. This oppression affected scholars such as Galileo and impeded progress in the professions.

RUINI AND THE BEGINNINGS OF ANATOMY
OF DOMESTIC ANIMALS

Some identify the beginning of the renaissance in veterinary medicine with 1598, the date of publication of the first great textbook on veterinary anatomy, which was designed to be an anatomy of the horse, *Dell Anatomia et dell' Infirmita del Cavallo (On the Anatomy and Diseases of the Horse),* by Carlo Ruini, Jr. (1530-1598). Ruini was born into a prosperous family of Bologna. When he was nine years old, his father was murdered. The son was neither a lawyer nor a jurist, although he did become a senator. He had excellent private tutors; the most influential on his scholarly development was the Aristotelian philosopher Claudio Betti, who developed Carlo's interest in the natural sciences. As a result, Ruini developed a passionate enthusiasm for horses and

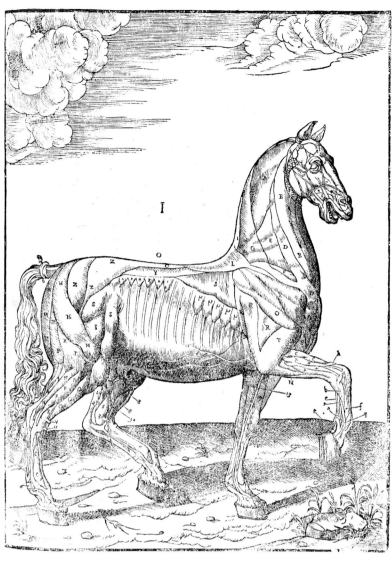

214. Carlo Ruini is credited with the beginning of the Renaissance in veterinary medicine. This side view of a standing horse demonstrates superb superficial musculature and appears in the first great textbook on equine anatomy, his *Dell Anatomia et dell' Infirmita del Cavallo (On the Anatomy and Diseases of the Horse)*, published posthumously in Bologna in 1598. *(National Library of Medicine, Bethesda, Maryland.)*

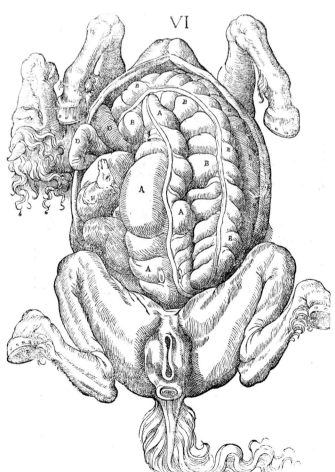

215. Ruini's work demonstrated the exquisite detail of the Italian school of anatomy. This plate from his *Dell Anatomia et dell' Infirmita del Cavallo*, published in Venice (1599), shows the viscera of the horse. *H* in this plate, which appears to be of a foal, is not always present in the earlier editions of this work. *(National Library of Medicine, Bethesda, Maryland.)*

243

equestrian activities, which led him to acquire a great collection of horses of many breeds. Drawing on the great dynamism of the burgeoning scientific and medical culture of sixteenth-century Bologna, he was able to acquire a systematic, experimental approach to the science of the horse. Thus, although lacking membership in the university, Ruini was able to conduct the studies reflected in his early and only masterpiece, which appeared one month after his death, in 1598. This seminal work was republished many times and set a high standard for his successors who were interested in the equine species. It is believed that he made his own drawings, which would have been prepared for printing by the skilled artists and engravers in Bologna. Speculations that Leonardo da Vinci or Titian may have made the illustrations are considered unwarranted. Although the second part of Ruini's book, on equine diseases, consisted of a rehash of the material presented three hundred and fifty years earlier by Giordano Rufo (Ruffus), the anatomical part of the book presents the morphology of the body systems and distribution networks (circulatory and neural). The style of this fine original work, illustrated with magnificent woodcuts, is reminiscent of the work of Vesalius that appeared fifty years earlier.

It is remarkable that a work as specialized as Ruini's was attributed to one who lacked veterinary and medical training and was not a scientist. However, many "amateur" scholars accomplished great works in many fields, especially from the sixteenth century to the mid-twentieth century. The human mind, provided with adequate motivation and access to information, has an innate capacity for self-learning. With tenacity (and, perhaps, a pinch of good fortune), it can attain remarkable scholarly accomplishments.

The quality of Ruini's anatomical descriptions was imperfect and many errors were perpetuated, but the book stood as a marvelous template to be enlarged and refined by its successors. At last a text was worthy to be used in training animal doctors about the complex fabric of their patients' bodies.

216. *Studies of Dogs* by Jan Brueghel d. Ä. Jan was the younger of two sons of the reknowned Flemish artist Pieter Brueghel the Elder, the most original and powerful among the Flemish painters of the sixteenth century. Jan Brueghel (1568-1625), referred to as "Velvet Brueghel," carried on a dynasty of artists founded by his father that flourished to the eighteenth century. *(Kunsthistorisches Museum, Vienna.)*

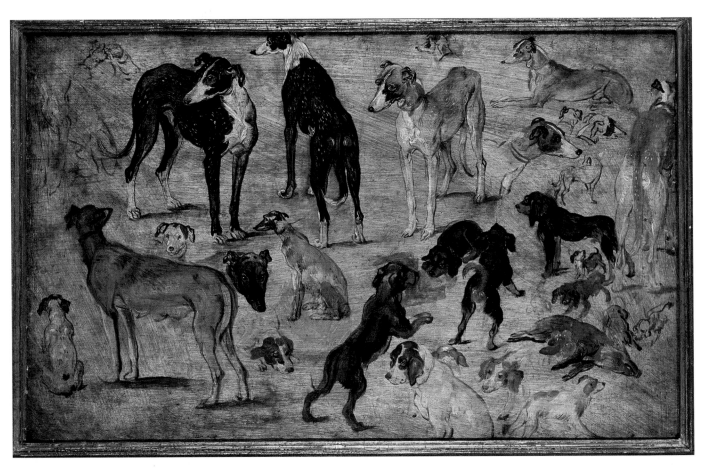

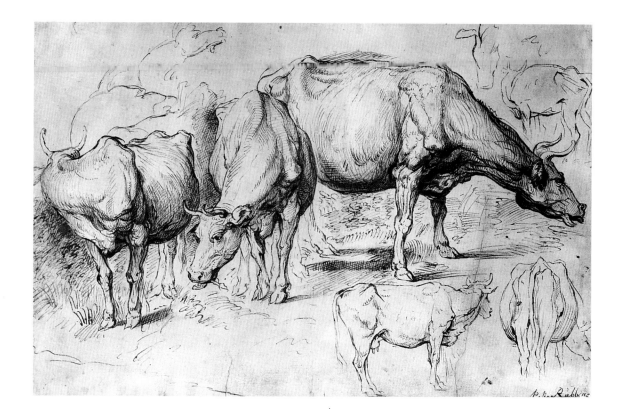

217. The great Flemish painter Peter Paul Rubens applied his academic training of studying the muscular structure of nudes in this rendering, *Studies of Cows* (c. 1618-1620). *(The British Museum, London.)*

Although veterinary anatomy received a new awakening at the beginning of the seventeenth century, no substrate of veterinary academia existed to use Ruini's new book until one hundred and sixty-four years later, when the first veterinary schools were created. Ruini's work, particularly the plates, was plagiarized in the interim, often with the introduction of unpardonable errors, by other authors writing for the large market of horsemen, cavalrymen, marshals, and farriers. Just one year after Ruini's opus appeared, the French physician Heroard published a skeletal anatomy of the horse, *Hippostologie,* in Paris.

Scholars working on the structure and nature of domestic animals other than the horse contributed efforts related to Ruini's. One of the most remarkable was made by Miguel Serveto of Aragon (1511-1553) or Servet, also known as Villanovonus. He studied in Toulouse and was labeled a heretic in Basel for rejecting the doctrine of the Holy Trinity. He moved to Leyden, where he dissected dogs. There he made the remarkable observation that blood cannot pass between the ventricles, refuting Galen's view that blood moved from the right to the left ventricle of the heart through holes in the interventricular septum. Therefore, he reasoned, blood must leave the heart by another outlet, the pulmonary artery. It was left to Colombo and Cesalpino, however, to propose the "second" or pulmonary circulation. On the order of Calvin's Genevan Council, Servet was burned at the stake for his earlier heresies.

Volcher Coiter (1534-1600) of Groningen studied bone development and comparative osteology. He explored the structure of the ear and experimented on decerebrate animals.

Many perils existed for Renaissance scholars as zealous church officials tortured and killed their fellow humans in the self-righteous assumption of collective responsibility to preserve the myths of their versions of "the faith." The unfounded certainty about supernatural direction that had been seeded in the minds of so many in the Middle Ages has lost much of its assurance for modern scholars. None of its advocates ever devised methodologies that could command confidence in directed supernatural phenomena. In its waning centuries, however, its controlling advocates sought to retain their powers and life-styles, turning to means of repression so foul that the last residues of their credibility evaporated.

PADUA'S EXTENSION OF ANATOMY TO EMBRYOLOGY AND REPRODUCTION

Hieronymus Fabricius of Aquapendente, who lived from about 1533 to 1619, carried forward the artistic legacy of Leonardo da Vinci's drawings of embryos. A physician, Fabricius became professor of anatomy at Padua and in about 1600 produced two important embryological treatises, *De Formatione Ovi et Pulli* and *De Formatio Foetu,* although the microscope was not yet available to him. The first book, following Aristotle and Galen, described the development of the chick. The second discussed the domesticated mammalian species as well as the mouse and the shark. Even more significant than these works was the impact Fabricius had on his distinguished pupil, William Harvey (1578-1657) of Folkestone, Kent, a Cambridge scholar who went to the medical center of the Renaissance at the University of Padua to obtain the degree in medicine in 1602. Giulio Casserio (c. 1552-1616), Fabricius's successor, also taught Harvey. Harvey was a pioneer of comparative anatomy. He

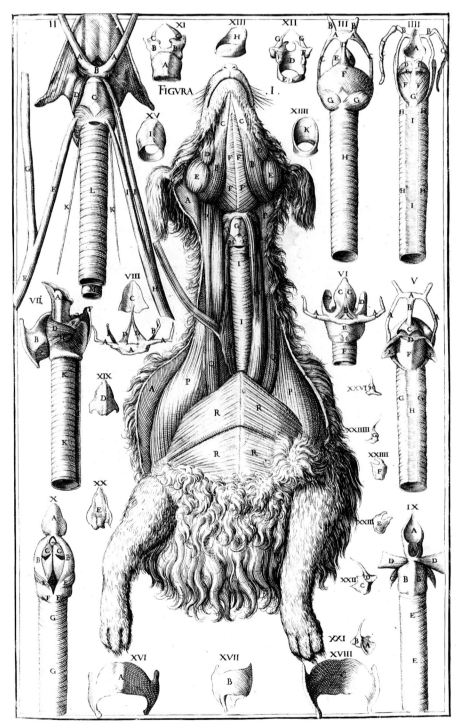

218. Giulio Casserio, or Casserius, of Piacenza was an important figure in the Paduan school of anatomy, succeeding Fabricius as professor in 1604. A teacher of Harvey, Casserius greatly contributed to the knowledge of anatomy, especially of the vocal and auditory organs, as evidenced by the thirty-seven beautiful copperplate engravings found in his *De Vocis Auditusque Organis Historia Anatomica (The Anatomy of the Vocal and Auditory Organs),* Ferrara (1601). Although the artist responsible for the drawings and engravings is not mentioned on the plates, Casserius does cite a German artist, Joseph Maurer, as living in his house to paint his anatomical illustrations. Casserius's work is also important for satisfying the demand at the beginning of the seventeenth century for detailed illustrative anatomical plates that copper engraving made possible at that time. The hyoid, larynx, and musculature of the throat of the dog with various dissections of the laryngeal cartilages are displayed in this plate from *De Vocis Auditusque . . . (National Library of Medicine, Bethesda, Maryland.)*

was famous for combining scientific accuracy with outstanding artistic quality in his *Tabulae Anatomicae* of 1627, prepared by Adrian van Spieghel.

Harvey returned to England and worked as a physician, then became professor of anatomy at the University of London. He began his scientific studies with Fabricius in embryology. Late in life he returned to this subject and wrote *Exercitationes et Generatione Animalium* (1651), in which he corrected important errors made by his mentor about the origin of the blastoderm and about the maturation and subsequent rupture of the blastocyst, findings he achieved with the help of a magnifying glass. He also corrected the collossal speculative error of the "chauvinist" Aristotle that the female contributes only nourishment to the embryo (via menstrual blood), whereas the male provides the effective generating stuff (via the semen). Harvey stated that

> *the egg is to be viewed as a conception proceeding from the male and the female, equally endued with the virtue of either, and constituting a unity from which a single animal is engendered.*

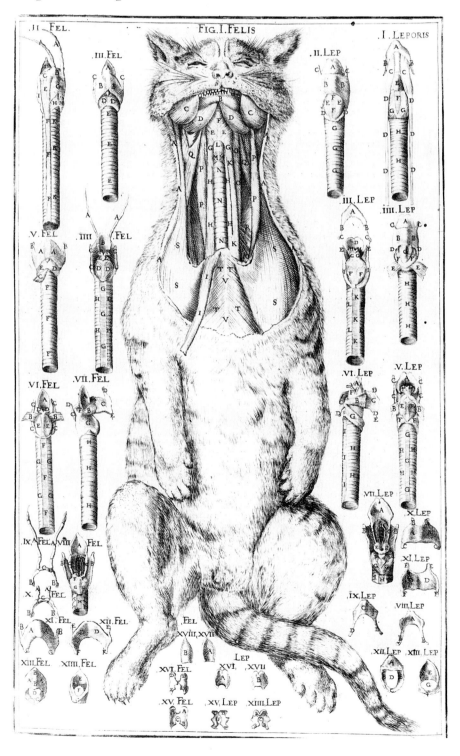

219. The cartilages and musculature of the laryngeal region of the cat and rabbit compared in Casserio's *De Vocis Auditusque . . .*, Ferrara (1601). *(National Library of Medicine, Bethesda, Maryland.)*

Harvey did not answer all the fundamental questions about the generation of life via reproduction or about the process of organ differentiation, but he broke the scholastic stranglehold of blind acceptance of revered authorities.

In the seventeenth century the mammalian ovaries were known as the female testes and were considered organs of unknown function. The Dutch physiologist Regnier de Graaf (1641-1673) of Schoonhoven noticed that some ovaries had spherical structures, which he thought might be the long-sought egg nests. These maturing vesicles came to be called Graafian follicles. A long time later, in 1827, an Estonian biologist named Karl Ernest von Baer (1792-1876) conducted classic studies in his quest for evidence of the real nature of the mammalian egg or ova. He studied many species and showed that the real egg was a "fetal egg within the maternal egg," the latter being the Graafian follicle (named by Haller), the remainder of which, he showed, stayed in the ovary and became the corpus luteum.

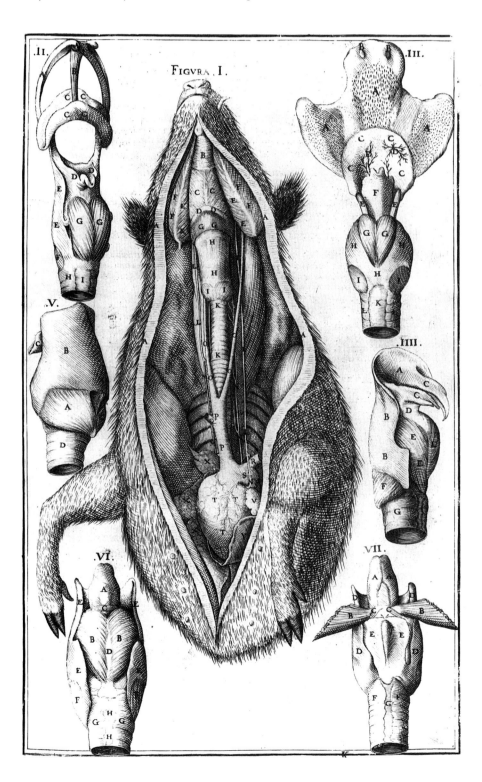

220. The larynx and hyoid structures involved in vocalization of the pig from Casserio's *De Vocis Auditusque . . .*, Ferrara (1601). *(National Library of Medicine, Bethesda, Maryland.)*

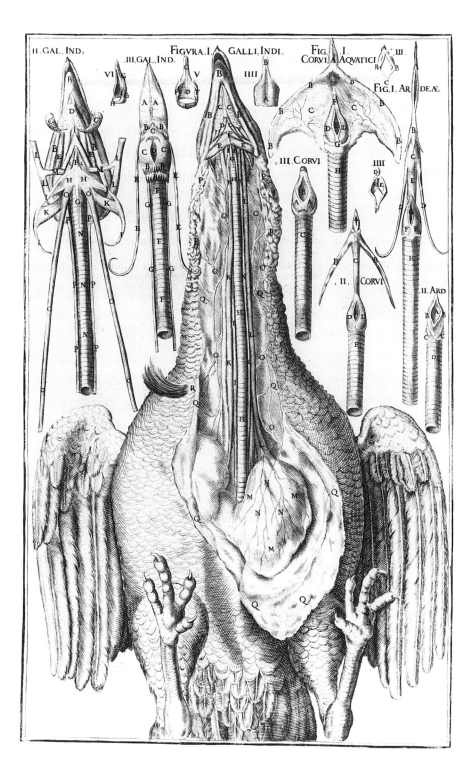

221. The hyoid and larynx of the turkey and other birds illustrating that they lack the epiglottis seen in mammals. Casserio failed to note the syrinx, or posterior layrnx, however. From Casserio's *De Vocis Auditusque . . .*, Ferrara (1601). *(National Library of Medicine, Bethesda, Maryland.)*

222. The anatomical features that control the position and movement of the pinna, or external ear, of the bovine species from Casserio's *De Vocis Auditusque . . .*, Ferrara (1601). *(National Library of Medicine, Bethesda, Maryland.)*

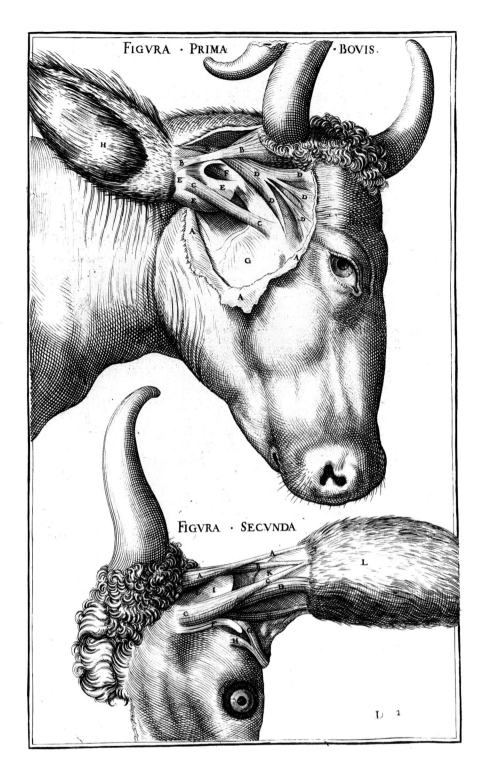

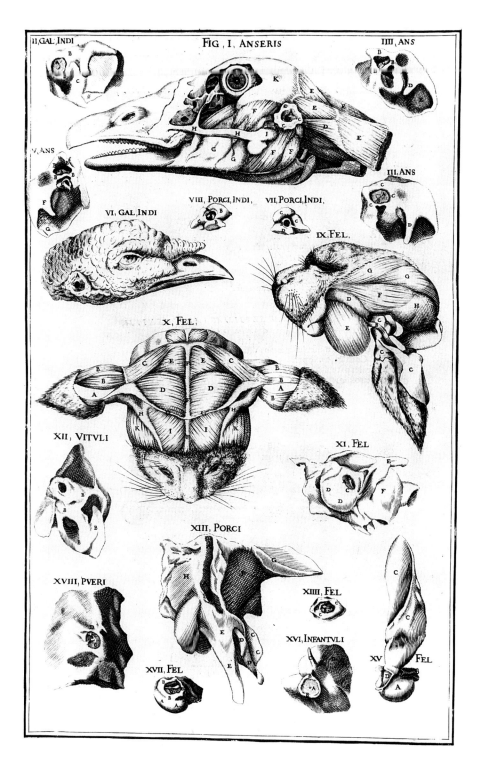

223. Comparison of the muscles of the external ear of the goose, turkey, cat, pig, and human infant, from Casserio's *De Vocis Auditusque . . .*, Ferrara (1601). *(National Library of Medicine, Bethesda, Maryland.)*

224. Jacob Jordaens (1593-1678) was born in Antwerp, where he studied under Adam van Noort. Jordaens was a prolific artist, working mostly in oil and watercolor. His work is classically Flemish in character, with warm color, a tendency to exaggerate form, and an inclination to humor. These characteristics are evident in this study of a goat in red, black, and yellow chalk. *(Yale University Art Gallery, New Haven, Connecticut. University Purchase, Everett V. Meeks, B.A. 1901, Fund.)*

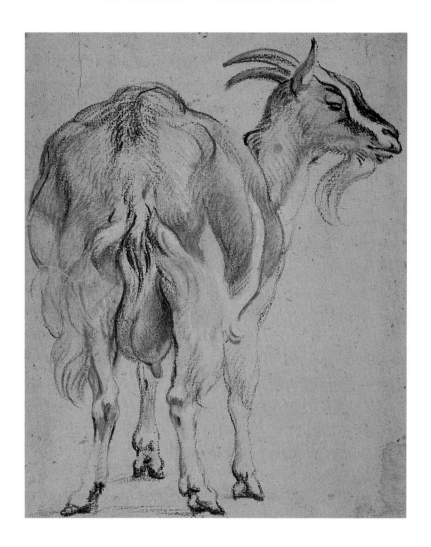

HARVEY'S EXPLANATION OF THE PUMPING AND CIRCULATION OF THE BLOOD

Harvey, one of the great scholars of biological and medical science, was able to make the creative leap from structure to function, thereby providing the foundation for a new scientific discipline based on experimental philosophy, namely physiology. He had acquired familiarity with a vast range of historical writings. He was appointed Lumleian Lecturer to the Royal College of Physicians in 1616, an office he was to hold for forty years, and on April 17, 1617, in his second lecture, for the first time he publicly proposed that the blood circulates in the body. Not until 1628 did he publish *Exercitatio Anatomica de Motu Cordis et Circulatione Sanguinis in Animalibus (Anatomical Treatise on the Movement of the Heart and the Circulation of the Blood in Animals)*, a modest little volume in comparison with Vesalius's glorious *De Fabrica*.

Harvey's work owed a debt to his mentor Fabricius because the latter was the first to provide a detailed description of the valves in the veins, which he christened "ostia" ("little doors") in *De Venarum Osteolis* in 1603. Harvey's mind seized on the role of these "little doors" as one-way valves governing the direction of blood flow. Study of the living heart is extraordinarily difficult, but Harvey wrestled with such work in his vivisections. He worked with several species (the deer was one of his favorites) in the effort to overcome ignorance of the complexities and dynamism of the organ. He established that the mammalian heart was a two-chambered pump (that is, it had two ventricles with valves) whose muscular walls contracted (became harder and smaller)

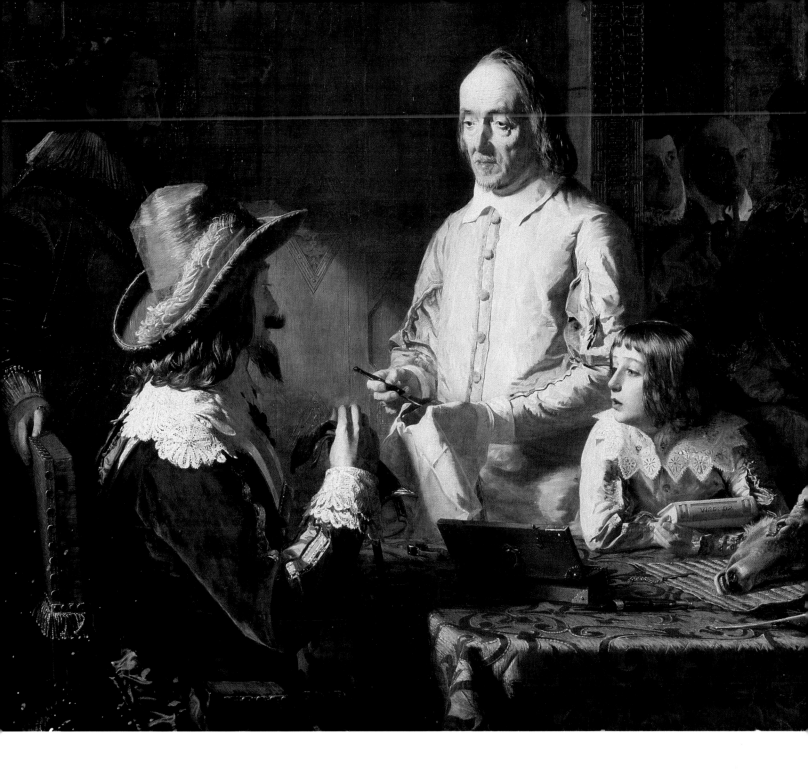

at each beat, forcing the blood out into the arteries of the systemic and pulmonary circulations (from the left and right ventricles, respectively). He showed that the arteries expanded as the ventricles contracted, giving rise to the pulse wave, and that, if cut, the flow of escaping blood was in the direction away from the heart, that is, from the cut end still attached to the heart. He showed that the blood from the right ventricle passed through the lungs and returned to the left atrium and ventricle. He deduced that there must be tiny, invisible vessels or capillaries in the lung and the other tissues to convey the blood, but having no microscope, he could not see them.

Harvey demonstrated how the venous valves worked to prevent backflow and showed that when veins were cut, their blood flowed from the peripheral end, that is, toward the heart. He noticed that the auricles were the first part of the heart to contract and witnessed right atrial fibrillation when a heart ceased its normal pulsations. By physiological reasoning and by estimating the volume of blood ejected from the heart at each beat and multiplying it by the number of beats per unit of time (he chose the half hour), Harvey calculated

225. William Harvey had a profound influence on the development of human and veterinary medicine and is considered the forerunner of modern physiology. In this painting by Robert Hannah, Harvey demonstrates his experiments on deer to King Charles I and the young prince. *(Reproduced with kind permission of the Royal College of Physicians, London.)*

226. Harvey's masterwork, *Exercitatio Anatomica de Motu Cordis et Circulatione Sanguinis in Animalibus (Anatomical Treatise on the Movement of the Heart and Circulation of the Blood in Animals)* (1651), contains his illustrative proof of the circulation of the blood. *(World Health Organization, Geneva.)*

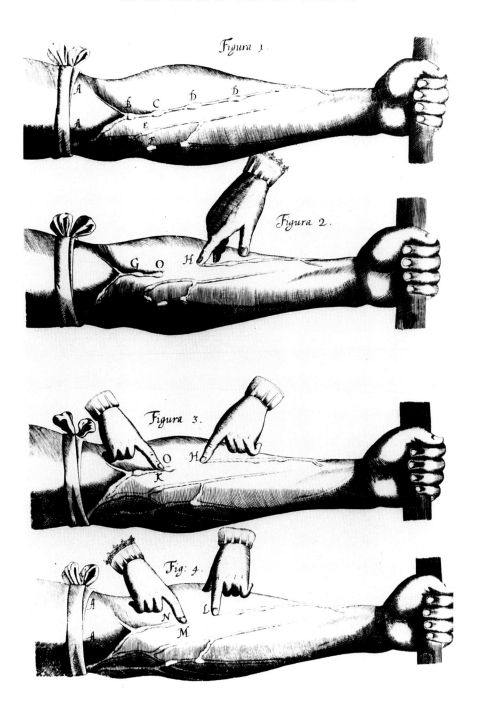

that the entire volume of blood in the body had been ejected in that period. He derived from his calculations the inescapable conclusion that a like volume had circulated and been returned to the heart and hence that the cardiovascular system had an ingenious circulatory mechanism that allowed the blood to be distributed to the tissues to meet their needs and to the lungs, where it was reconditioned by contact with the air.

Harvey's marriage was childless. One year before his death he willed to the Royal College of Physicians his patrimonial estate in Kent to support a librarian, a monthly collation, and an annual feast and oration by a leading figure in the advancement of medicine, thereby establishing the Harveian Oration. These presentations were published as part of the legacy of one of the most influential of all biomedical scientists, a man who was loyal to the quest for progress and truth. His scientific impact was only slowly accepted. The University of Paris, for example, opposed the circulation theory for half a century. Harvey's work was lethal to Galen's theory of an ebb and flow of blood in the vessels. Perhaps more important, the great cornerstone of medicine, the theory of the four humors and all their embellishments, was finally disproved by experimentation and reasoning. Harvey became a role model for investigators in comparative medicine and biomedical science.

Significant details of the architecture of the circulatory system were added by scholars other than Harvey. Gaspari Aselli in 1622 rediscovered the lacteals (known to Erasistratus), and Pecquet in 1647 described the lymphatic system and the return of lymph to the vascular system via the thoracic duct. Just four years after Harvey's death Marcello Malpighi (1628-1694), working as a professor in Pisa, was able to add the missing link to the story of the architecture of the circulatory system by visualizing the capillary vessels with the microscope developed by Leeuwenhoek (1632-1723) and others. Richard Lower (1631-1691) wrote *Tractatus de Corde* in 1669 and showed that exposure to the air in the lungs turned the deep purple venous blood to bright red arterial blood and that the lungs took up some of the air in the process. He also conducted blood transfusions between two dogs and even tried a sheep's-blood transfusion in a man. His fellow Cornishman, John Mayow, explained that the mechanism of the respiratory pump involved an inspiratory effort—created by the contraction of the diaphragm and intercostal muscles—followed by expiration, a largely passive relaxation at rest.

The father of microscopic anatomy or histology, Malpighi described the glomeruli of the kidneys, the structures in the spleen called "Malpighian bodies," and many other previously invisible microstructural features. He made the first drawings and descriptions of the developing chick embryo based on microscopy.

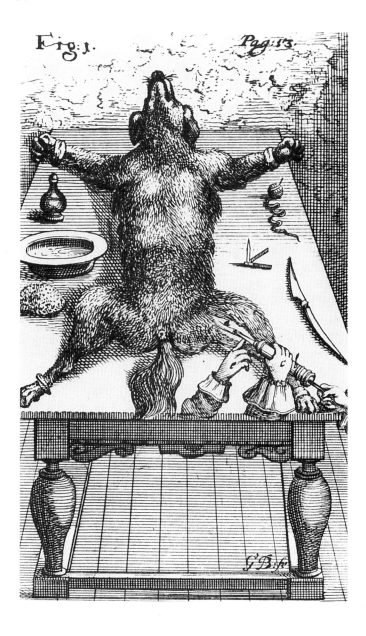

227. Woodcut engraving in Johann Sigismund Elsholtz's *Clysmatica Nova* (1667), showing a dog receiving a venous infusion of medicine in the left rear leg. Elsholtz (1623-1688) was a German physician to the Elector of Brandebourg. He researched and published works on metals, minerals, animals, and vegetables and in 1665 was one of the first to make intravenous injections. *(National Library of Medicine, Bethesda, Maryland.)*

228. Woodcut engraving from Johann Sigismund Elsholtz's *Clysmatica Nova* (1667), demonstrating the techniques of blood transfusion from animal to man and from man to man. *(National Library of Medicine, Bethesda, Maryland.)*

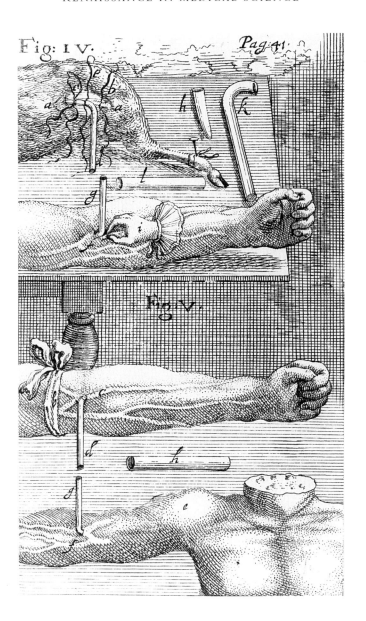

TRAILBLAZERS IN BIOPHYSICAL AND BIOCHEMICAL STUDIES

Harvey's great concept of circulation of the blood was advocated and publicized by the controversial experimentalist and philosopher René Descartes (1596-1650) of Touraine, who worked for twenty productive years in Holland. His stated goal was to reduce the function of the body to a system that could be studied through mathematics, physics, and mechanics. He wrote a challenging theoretical textbook of mechanical philosophy, *De l'Homme* or *De Homine,* in 1662, and held that the body was controlled by the mind, acting through the pineal gland. He conceived of the idea of the reflex arc and the ability of the lens of the eye to focus by changing its form. He created the system of Cartesian coordinates that married algebra to geometry and simplified geometric problems such as vision. He wrote his *Discourse on Method* in Utrecht and published it anonymously in Leyden in 1637.

Galileo (1564-1642), the king of Renaissance physicists, helped Santorio of Capodistria (1561-1636) in his research in physiology. Together they invented a primitive thermometer and a pulsilogue (an adjustable pendulum synchronized with the pulse and read by determining the pulse rate from the length of the pendulum's thread; the pulsilogue was necessary in the days before the invention of watches with second hands). Santorio trained in Padua

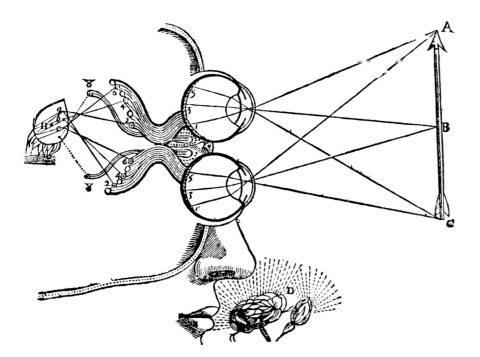

229. René Descartes applied both physical and mathematical principles to the study of physiology. In this illustration from his *L'Homme et un Traitté de la Formation du Foetus . . .* (Paris, 1664) he demonstrates his understanding of the coordination of the sense organs. He conceived of the idea of the reflex arc and the ability of the lens of the eye to focus by changing its form. *(Biblioteca Universitaria, Bologna.)*

and went to Poland, where he worked for twenty-four years as a physician, returning to Padua as professor of theoretical medicine in 1611. He performed dietetic studies on himself for about twenty years, weighing himself before and after every activity, meal, and evacuation. These studies, the earliest chronobiological studies, allowed him to show that he manifested a monthly cycle in weight gain and loss, pulse rate, and temperature. He also proved the loss of weight via insensible water loss. Santorio was truly one of the great pioneers of metabolic physiology, a worthy contemporary of William Harvey.

The chemistry of digestion and metabolism was investigated in Leyden by Francois de la Boe (1614-1672) (also known as Sylvius). He proposed roles for each of the digestive secretions and stressed the central function of the blood. Dysfunctions that could arise because of imbalances between secretions cum digesta and the blood required bloodletting, purging, or sudorific treatments. His was a popular approach that attracted adherents for both human and animal use.

Studies of digestive function in animals were advanced by Johann Conrad Peyer (1653-1712) of Schaffhausen, Switzerland. He was the first to report in depth on the study of ruminant digestion in *De Ruminantibus et Ruminatione,* published in Amsterdam in 1685. He is remembered for his discovery in 1677 of Peyer's patches in the wall of the intestine, which were associated with typhoid fever. Meanwhile, Johan Conrad Brunner (1653-1727) of Dissenhofen, also in Switzerland, was discovering Brunner's glands in the duodenum of dogs, which he considered to secrete a digestive juice. He showed that normal digestion continued after the spleen or the pancreas was excised. In one pancreatectomized dog, however, he noted extreme thirst and polyuria, almost certainly the first case of experimentally induced diabetes mellitus. Regnier de Graaf earlier had studied the exocrine secretions of bile and pancreatic juice.

Robert Boyle (1627-1691), a famous Irish chemist, wrote *The Sceptical Chymist* in 1661. He proved that something in air is essential for animal life. His brilliant studies of blood and gases and his conception of a particulate basis of matter placed him in the front rank of scientists who contributed to animal physiology through experimentation on the blood. In 1667 his assistant Robert Hooke showed that a dog rendered unable to breathe could be kept alive by artificial respiration.

230. The Swiss scientist Johann Conrad Peyer helped advance studies on digestive function in animals. This illustration, from his work on ruminant digestion, depicts the anatomy of the mucosal surface of the forestomachs of the goat. He authored an important book on the compound stomach of ruminants. Peyer's patches in the wall of the intestine were associated with typhoid fever. *(Bayerische Staatsbibliothek, Munich.)*

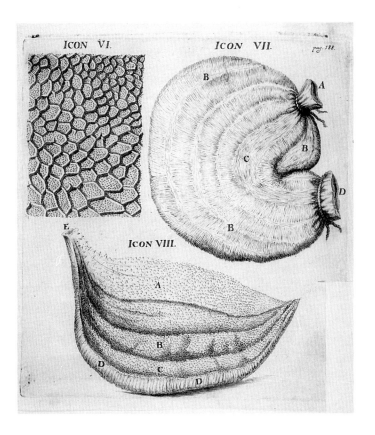

Giovanni Alphonso Borelli (1608-1679) was a friend of Malpighi and a professor of mathematics at Pisa when he began his research on animal movement. Fascinated by the static and mechanical aspects of the human and animal bodies, Borelli applied physical theory to the study of animal terrestrial locomotion and avian flight. He calculated the force of muscle action and recognized that muscles were under nervous control. He attempted to attribute the hardening and tension generated by muscles during contraction to a "succus nervens" transmitted by the nerves to the muscles. He also showed that cardiac muscle, like skeletal muscle, was contractile.

The gigantic strides in anatomical and physiological sciences during the Renaissance, attained before the great advances in instrumentation, are the more remarkable because they were a product of application of the eyes, the brain, and the hands.

A new intellectual revolution was in store, since the new equipment would allow humans to extend the sensory capacities of the body. The simple microscope permitted magnification of visible, that is, macroscopic, organisms and tissues. Early microscopes were small and were limited to 100- to 200-fold magnifications. It was not until the compound (two-lens) microscope was further improved that the body's cells became clearly visible and the pathogenic microorganisms could be visualized at all. Robert Hooke set out the theory in his *Micrographia* in 1665. The Dutch genius Leeuwenhoek attained about 300-fold magnification in 1723 and described the appearance of animalcules (tiny animals) in dental tartar. Lens quality, focusing and capacity, and lighting systems were improved, but Dolland did not develop the oil-immersion lens that made most bacteria visible until 1844. The disciplines of microbiology, parasitology, and pathology could then be developed much more effectively.

Before the physical aspects of physiology and medicine could be studied in greater depth, advances other than the microscope were necessary in physical science and instrumentation. Electrophysiology made it possible to study the function of the nerves and the central nervous system. The kymograph (and its associated equipment) was the forerunner of the force-displacement recording systems, which were vital to the progress of muscular, circulatory, respiratory, and digestive motility studies.

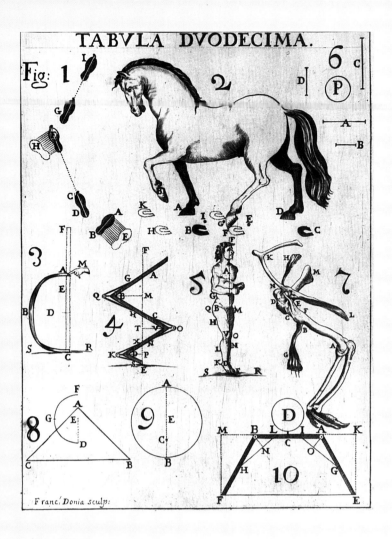

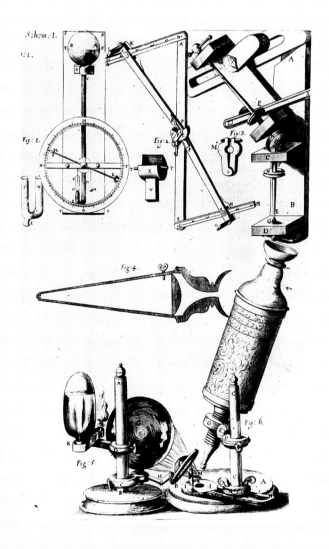

231. A table on the physiology of humans and animals from Giovanni Borelli's *De Motus Animalium . . .* (1680). Borelli, a Pisan professor of mathematics, was drawn to the mechanics of human and animal movement and postulated the relationship between muscle action and nervous control. *(National Library of Medicine, Bethesda, Maryland.)*

232. Robert Hooke's microscope is shown in this engraving from his *Micrographia* (1667). *(National Library of Medicine, Bethesda, Maryland.)*

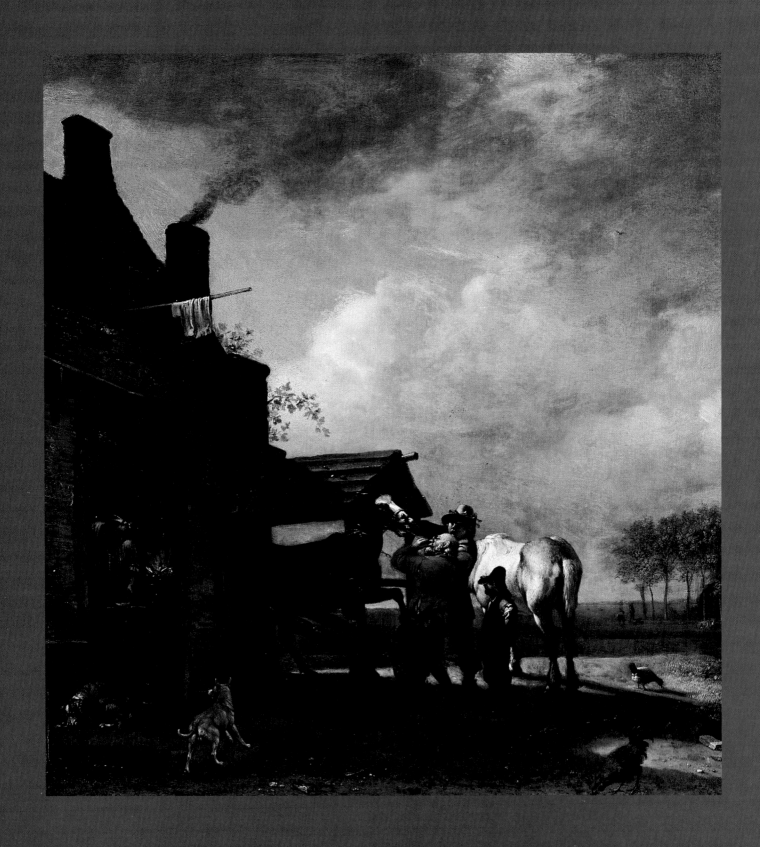

Marshals, Horse Doctors, Cow Leeches, and Authors

SLOW PROGRESS IN ANIMAL DOCTORING ON THE FARM

The *Boke of Husbandry,* an important book with a broad compass of philosophy, agriculture, and general veterinary practice, appeared in 1523 and became quite popular. Its author, John Fitzherbert, has not been fully identified, but he was clearly an outstanding observer and scholar of all things agricultural. He wrote about diseases of horses, cattle, and sheep. Of particular interest in the discussion of horse diseases is his coverage of "morfounde" (founder or laminitis) and its effect on the form of the hoof and the chronicity of the changes.

Fitzherbert gave the first description of the brain surgery required for removal of cerebral hydatid cysts in the "turn" (turning sickness) in cattle. Harward was to perfect this description more than a century later. Fitzherbert described outbreaks of a "murrain" or plague, probably anthrax, and of "long sought," a protracted pulmonary condition similar to contagious bovine pleuropneumonia. Other readily recognizable syndromes included "dewblown" (bloat) and foul in the foot.

In an unusually detailed account of sheep diseases, Fitzherbert's penetrating observational skills and thoughtful, problem-solving approach are evident, particularly in his description of "rot" on flooded lands. He identifies species of grass that were considered bad and makes the profound observation that "white snails be ill for sheep in pastures and in fallows," indicating that he suspected a role for the little white snails that were common in pastures where the rot occurred. He also conducted postmortem examinations of sheep in which he found "little live things like flokes in the liver, full of knots and white blisters." The signs included white conjunctivae with dark streaks; the skin became pale and watery, and the wool loose and easily pulled out. His focus on a likely participation of snails in the syndrome preceded by nearly three hundred and sixty years the scientific confirmation of the snail's serving as an intermediate host in the life cycle of the parasite (liver fluke).

Some of the earliest illustrations of treatment of companion animals appeared in a "book of the chase" by Gaston Phébus in the fourteenth century. In 1576 George Turberville (c. 1540–c. 1610), a sportsman and poet, wrote *The Noble Art of Venerie or Hunting,* a book about the selection, hygiene, and diseases of hunting dogs and the first book of any depth in English that dealt with "cure and medicines for all diseases of hounds." Astrological and astronomical criteria (such as "under the signs of Gemini and Aquarius" and "under a waning moon," respectively) were invoked for breeding to obtain mostly males and to avoid madness. Telegony, the concept that all subsequent offspring of a female will resemble her first

233. *Facing page, A Farrier's Shop* (1648) by Paulus Potter, Flemish (1625-1654). Potter's death at the age of twenty-eight prevented completion of many works, yet he is regarded as one of history's most gifted animal painters. Here Potter shows a horse doctor, wearing a red jacket and leather apron, examining the mouth and teeth of a restrained horse. Inside a grimy blacksmith's house a man is beating a red-hot iron on an anvil. As is common in Dutch seventeenth-century painting, the subject matter looks very real, as if it were done from life. On the doorframe is inscribed *Paulus Potter F. 1648. (Widener Collection, copyright 1993, National Gallery of Art, Washington, D.C.)*

261

successful sire, was believed in absolutely. Faith in the doctrine became set in the public mind because of the outcome of Lord Morton's mating of a mare to a zebra and then to a thoroughbred stud. The first hybrid was striped, but the subsequent foals showed partial striping. The outcome was recorded by artists and received a great deal of publicity. A tragic consequence of the belief was that many good bitches were either spayed or destroyed because of an early mating with a "low-life" dog. Spaying of hounds was evidently a common practice but not before the first litter. It was considered a dangerous procedure for hounds in estrus and in pregnancy; according to Turberville, spaying should be done "as the whelps begin to take shape."

Turberville described six varieties of rabies. The most dangerous was called the "burning madness," in which the dog was running into everything in its path, every animal it bit becoming mad: "They howle a kind of howling in the throats and hoarcely" and live for only three or four days. Turberville considered the "running madness" less deadly because the first animal to be bitten got all the venom and only dogs were attacked. In the "dumme madness" the mouth was open and the beast put its paws in its mouth as if to dislodge a bone in its throat (a dangerous form of rabies because of the temptation for owners or handlers to put their hands in the mouth in an attempt to remove the imaginary obstruction) and the dog also tended to hide. The other forms were the "falling," the "lanke," and the "slavering" madness.

ITALIAN SCHOOLS OF HORSEMANSHIP FOR THE WARRIOR CLASS

After the death of Holy Roman Emperor Frederick II (1250), battles raged for sovereignty of the kingdom of Sicily and Naples. The outstanding quality of Neapolitan horses and their training, a legacy of the great emperor, were often decisive factors in the military successes attained. Fredrick Grisone, who lived during the first half of the sixteenth century, was involved in the establishment of the renowned High School of Horsemanship in Naples, which attracted an international clientele. He is believed to have provided a noted farrier named Hannibal to Henry VIII and did recommend an outstanding horseman to Queen Elizabeth I, Claudio Corte, who stayed in England only six months.

In 1550 Grisone published the *Rules for Riding*, which appeared in many editions; several of these were pirated, embellished by others, and published after his death. Some were translated into French, German, Spanish, and English, the later versions (after 1582) incorporating information on breeding and on diseases and remedies of the horse. Grisone's fame spread widely, and his formal system of riding became extremely popular among European gentry, displacing tournaments and hawking. Riding masters, especially those who were of the upper classes themselves, became influential. The school taught formal, fashionable riding for the aristocracy. No doubt derived from the importance of maneuverability to cavalry training, Grisone's method involved endless twisting and turning in a circle. After the straight-ahead charging of the jousting tournaments during the age of chivalry and with the invention of guns and gunpowder, new tactics and styles were needed.

The deplorable feature of Grisone's method was its basis in fear, which was induced by brutally punishing the horse for any failures to comply. Hitting the horse on the head between the ears was the most commonly deployed insult. Various appalling punitive measures were used, not least of which was the "cure" for running backwards: a live cat suspended from a pole was swung between the rear legs of the horse to claw the scrotum and thighs.

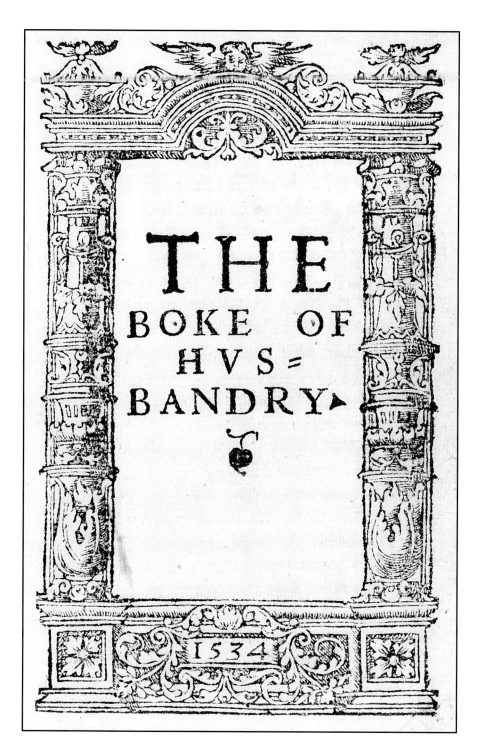

234. Although little is known about the author, John Fitzherbert, *The Boke of Husbandry* (1534) was an important early contribution to the management of diseases of horses, cattle, and sheep. One of the most interesting observations concerned the role of the snail as a host in the life cycle of the liver fluke, which was not confirmed until the late 1800s. *(The Science Museum/Science & Society Picture Library, London.)*

Alternatively, a hedgehog could be used or the gallant rider could jerk a cord tied above the testicles. Although stallions can be headstrong and must be "won over" or dominated, such barbarous methods can only be condemned, not only in the interests of both cat and horse but also to avoid the attitudinal degradation of the horse's trainer. Grisone's countryman Claudio Corte is to be applauded for his rejection of these techniques. Corte's book on the horse trainer, written in 1562, outlined an excellent method to make a horse "handy" without resort to inhumane practices. Grisone's book was translated into English by Thomas Blundeville and published about 1560 without comment on the ruthless practices. Grisone wrote other books on the horse and was said to be more a scholar than a doer.

235. Wood engraving of a horse with its head over a steaming pot, a treatment used to cure respiratory problems such as congestion and bronchitis. From *Trattato di Marescalcia,* Rome (1591), by Scaccho de Tagliocozzo. Numerous books published during the sixteenth century demonstrated a strong interest in hippology, despite their relatively poor scientific value. Tagliocozzo's work passed through four editions, the last in 1618. *(National Library of Medicine, Bethesda, Maryland.)*

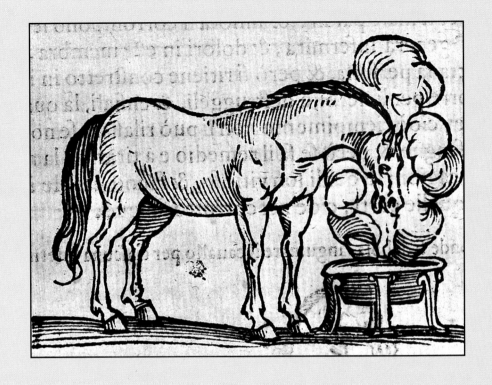

236. The Italian nobleman Cesare Fiaschi founded a school of equitation in Ferrara and was known for his interesting training methods. In 1556 he published what is believed to be the first book specifically dealing with shoeing. He later wrote another book on diseases of the equine foot, although his ideas about shaping the hoof were erroneous. This woodcut, a disease chart of the horse, appears in his *Trattao dell'Imbrigliare, Attegiare e Ferrare Cavalli,* Venice (1603). Many veterinary medical manuscripts and books published from the sixteenth through eighteenth centuries contained so-called disease charts illustrating three general themes. The "blood-letting horse" indicated the best sites for letting blood. The "disease name horse" or "ox" showed areas of disease on the outside of the animal. The "diseased horse" illustrated externally discernible signs of disease. Disease charts were intended to illustratively summarize a book's content and were frequently copied until they eventually lost what little impact they originally provided. They disappeared from the literature with the advent of modern scientific publication at the beginning of the nineteenth century. *(Institute für Paläeoanatomie der Ludwig-Maximilians-Universität, München.)*

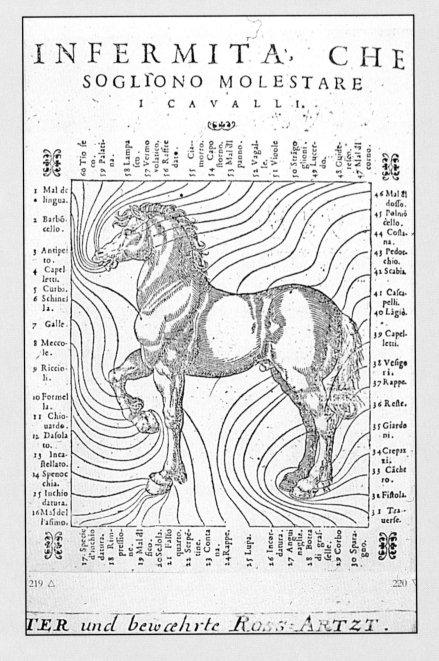

Cesare Fiaschi (1523-1592) was a nobleman of Ferrara, where he founded a school of equitation. A great enthusiast, he strove to accumulate the wisdom of his period in an attractive book, *A Treatise on the Bridle, Menage and Shoeing,* in 1556, probably the first book to specifically address the last topic. The mouth, bits, and bridles are described in detail, and illustrations of complex bits are endless. Fiaschi's approach to training emphasized the expression of vocal commands in modulated and musical tones to communicate the expected movement to the horse. The "shoeing" section contains drawings of types of shoes and a compilation of the advice of farriers, observing that a good one was rare. In the midst of a great amount of useful information an unfortunate error was made that was to be perpetuated by his uncritical successors. Fiaschi stated that the forefeet should be pared at the toe and the hind feet at the heel because the latter were (falsely) said to be thicker there. In 1564 Fiaschi wrote another, less well known book, on diseases of the feet. The Neapolitan teachings were transferred to France by La Broue and by Pluvinal, who trained horses to dance.

Because the cavalry horse had been a decisive factor in medieval warfare, a high priority came to be placed on horse selection and procurement, horse breeding, management and training, harness design and shoeing technique, and horse doctoring. The great "marshals of horse" in turn came to command prestige and began to acquire the status of nobility. England had lagged behind the Continent in the development of cavalry, horse breeding and training, and equine health care. Into this void stepped Thomas Blundeville, a productive, scholarly author of works on the horse, who was neither a practicing farrier or horseman nor a veterinarian.

Thomas Blundeville of Newton Flotman, Norfolk, an Elizabethan scholar of broad interests who wished to see England attain Continental standards of equitation and cavalry training, was the first English author to write about veterinary matters in a systematic way. His birthdate is not known, but he died in 1605. He translated Fredrick Grisone's (Italian) *Rules for Riding* in 1550.

Blundeville wrote on many topics, including astronomy. His most significant work on the horse appeared in 1566: *The Foure Chiefest Offices Belonging to Horsemanship: That Is To Say, the Office of the Breeder, of the Rider, of the Keeper, and of the Ferrer, . . . Painfully Collected out of a Number of Auchtours . . ..* This remarkable undertaking was the first attempt to collate all available written knowledge of horse husbandry, management, riding, and veterinary care in English. In it he assigned to the "Keeper" the role of keeping the horse healthy, especially in dieting, that is, by practicing sound management and preventive medicine, and to the "Ferrer" the role of curing horse diseases. The veterinary section of Blundeville's work is said to be based on information obtained from a farrier named Martin, the court veterinarian of Artois, then part of Pas de Calais, which was occupied by the English until 1558. The book, a valiant attempt to bring order to a vast subject, was tarnished by Blundeville's lack of practical knowledge.

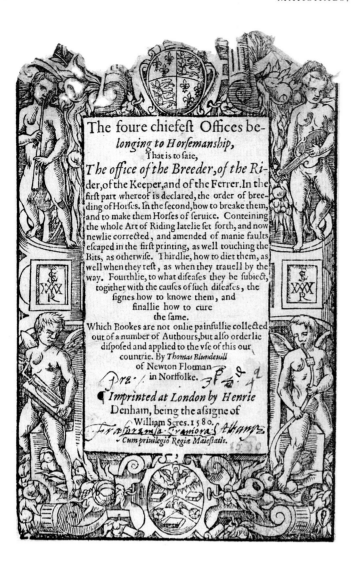

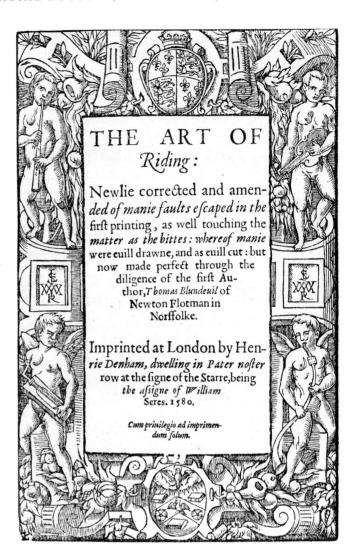

237. Thomas Blundeville's *The Foure Chiefest Offices Belonging to Horsemanship,* London (1580 and 1609) was the first scholarly attempt to amass all available literature on equine breeding and treatment in an English work. Sadly, his work was based on secondhand knowledge. *(The Science Museum/Science & Society Picture Library, London.)*

SELF-STYLED HORSE DOCTORS: ADVERTISING VIA AUTHORSHIP

The most influential writer on veterinary matters in the first half of the seventeenth century was Gervase Markham of Cotham, Nottinghamshire. Markham, the third son of a large family, lived from about 1562 to 1637. He was a commissioned officer in the army of King Charles I and an accomplished scholar of works in Latin and the modern Latin languages, Italian, French, and Spanish. He turned this skill to good advantage by reading extensively and translating selected works into English, publishing the opinions of others under his own name without attribution. In this way he set himself up as an authority, a man well ahead of his time, and fooled many in the process. He approached horsemanship and farriery or horse leeching in the same way.

Markham was a prolific author. Notable among his works were *Cavelarice or the English Horseman* in 1607 and *Markham's Maister-Peece* of 1610, which went through twenty-one editions. The latter essentially contains Blundeville's information on veterinary matters, reproduced and supplemented by Markham's personal contribution, which is nothing more than quackery and includes many disgusting or dangerous items. That those who handled horses succumbed to the braggadocio and false guarantees, to the trickery and the misleading yet effective psychology of the Markham style says something about the peculiar mystique attached to equine matters. His works commanded a loyal following for more than a century after his death; four American editions of *The Citizen and Countryman's Experienced Farrier,* written by "J. Markham, G. Jeffries, and Eiscreet Indians," were published between 1764 and 1839.

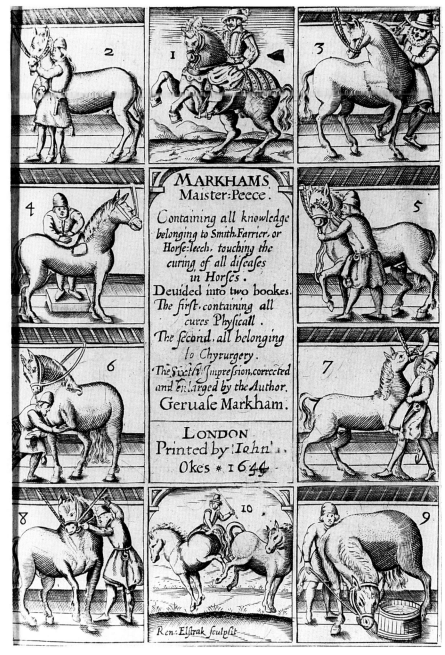

238. Gervase Markham was one of the most prolific writers on veterinary medicine in the first half of the seventeenth century. Unfortunately, many of his works did little more than perpetuate the myths and quackery put forth by his predecessors. This engraving, from his most famous work, *Markham's Maister-Peece,* London (1644), originally published in 1610, shows ten border vignettes depicting various methods of treating and training horses. *(National Library of Medicine, Bethesda, Maryland.)*

Excerpts from Markham's works may convey how ignorant of veterinary remedies the gullible horse owners and grooms were in the seventeenth and eighteenth centuries:

1. *For frenzy, make him sneeze by fuming him with burnt garlic smoke then bleed him in the palate and pierce the skin of the head with a hot iron to release the humors.*
2. *Spurring an exhausted horse to carry on by cutting a slit through one ear and thrusting a sharpened stick through it. Remounted, spur the horse and fret the stick back and fourth through the slit. Alternatively insert three or four pebbles into one ear and sew it to contain them. The noise they make will keep him going.*
3. *For a "sinew strain," take a live cat chop off her head and tail, then cleave her down the chine and clap her upon the strain while still hot.*
4. *For cramp, bury the horse but for his head in a dunghill and sweat him for an hour or two.*
5. *To test for pregnancy, pour water in the mare's ears. If she shake only her head, she is in foal. If she shakes the body too, she is not.*
6. *For sore feet clap two eggs into each sole and crush them, cover with cow's dung and in four hours the horse will recover.*
7. *For a stumbling horse slit the skin from the nose to the upper lip two inches, cut the second skin beneath it, and locate the white sinew beneath it. Take up the sinew with a horn point and twist it round about. This causes him to draw the hind legs forward. Then cut it and the legs will withdraw. The sinew was the cause of the stumbling.*

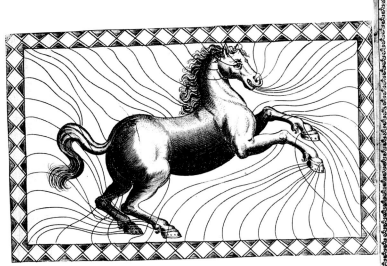

THE
EXPERIENCED FARRIER,
OR,
FarringCompleated.
IN TWO BOOKS
PHYSICAL and CHYRURGICAL
BEING
Pleasure to the Gentleman, and Profit to the
Countreyman.
IN WHICH
You have the Whole Body, Sum and Subhance of
it, in one Entire Volume, in fo Full and Ample Manner, that there
is Little or Nothing more Material to be Added thereto.
For here is Contained
Every thing that belongs to a True HORSE-MAN, GROOM, FARRIER,
or HORSE-LEACH, *Viz.* BREEDING; *The Manner How, The Sea'on
When, The Place Where, The Colours, Marks and Shapes* of all *Stallions
and Mares,* and what are Fit for Generation; *The Feeder, Rider,
Keeper, Ambler* and *Buyer*; As alfo the making of feveral Precious
*Drinks, Suppofitories, Pills, Purgations, Scourings, Ointments, Salves,
Powders, Waters, Charges, Balls, Perfumes,* And Directions how
to ufe them for all Inward and Outward Difafes.
ALSO
The PARING and SHOOING of all manner of HOOFES, and in what Point that
ART doth Confift. The Prices and Vertues of moft of the Principal Drugs, both
Simple and Compound belonging to *Farring,* (and where you may buy them)
VIz. Roots, Barks, Woods, Flowers, Fruits, Seeds, Juices, Gums, Rozins, &c. As
alfo a large Table of the Vertues of moft Simples fet down Alphabetically; And
many Hundreds of Words Placed one after another, for the Cure of all Difeafes; With
many New Receipts of Excellent Ufe and Value, never yet Printed before in any Author.

By E. R. Gent.

LONDON, Printed for Rich. *Northcott* Adjoyning to St. *Peters* Alley in *Cornhill,*
and at the *Marriner and Anchor* upon *New-Fifh* ftreet Hill, near *London*-bridge. 1678.

239. Title page from E.R. Gent's *The Experienced Farrier, or Farring Compleated,* London (1678). Curiously, many of these early books dealing with horsemanship were produced by essentially anonymous authors. It was the tradition to use initials followed by "Gent," to indicate *gentleman.* (*The Science Museum/Science & Society Picture Library, London.*)

A different view of Markham's impact was put forward in 1962 by Poynter, who observed that Markham's writings spanned a wide range of subjects. While recognizing that Markham had been dubbed "a hack" and "insufferably prolific," Poynter concluded that he had been overblamed for what he did ill and underpraised for what he did well. Also, it must be realized that Markham's books were extremely popular when they were written. Poynter felt that Sir Frederick Smith's devastating criticisms of Markham's veterinary writings showed a lack of sense of the historical period, nearly four hundred years ago. Obviously the beliefs at that time cannot be expected to accord with modern ideas, yet that expectation seemed to be the reference point of Smith's conclusions. Veterinary science at that time was nonexistent, and practical animal healing was in a crude and primitive stage. Smith's magnification of the errors became orthodox opinion to be repeated uncritically even by Fussell, the noted agricultural historian, and other authorities.

One of Markham's early books, *Discourse on Horsemanship,* of 1595, included a set of simple cures for horse diseases that generated a strong popular demand. It was this public response that led him to devote an entire volume to diseases of horses, *Markham's Maister-peece,* in 1610. The demand from grooms and horse owners persisted to the nineteenth century, and an abridged version for farriers was put out as late as 1883. Markham's writings on agriculture, especially on country sports, were well regarded. According to Poynter, Markham systematized and popularized a previously dispersed body of "knowledge" obtained from others. This accomplishment prepared the way for the advances in agriculture and animal husbandry that were one of Great Britain's great achievements in the eighteenth century. Nevertheless, the perpetuation of harmful, useless, or unacceptably harsh treatments was a tragedy for the equine patient.

Although the systematic study of anatomy of the horse began after Ruini, equine physiology and medicine were neglected until well into the twentieth century. Perhaps it was typical of the vogue of an unthinking, sometimes brutal approach to equine treatment that a large number of barber-surgeons, especially former military barber-surgeons, were attracted to the field of horse doctoring.

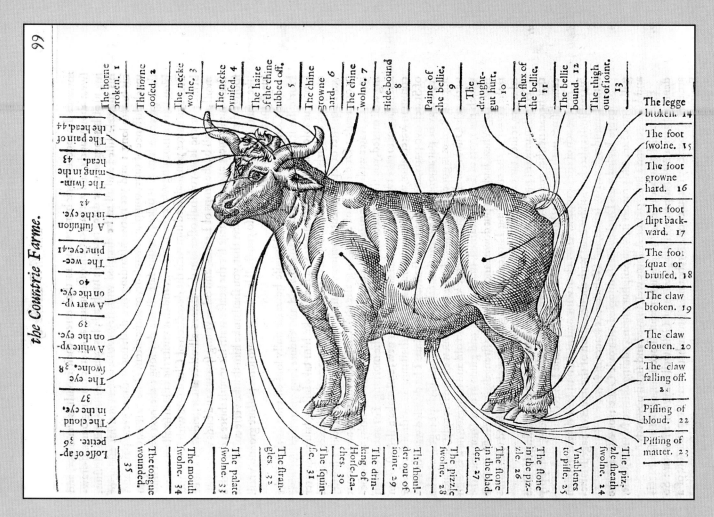

240. *Above,* This disease chart of the bull was originally prepared for Charles Estienne's *L'Agriculture et Maison Rustique,* which was translated into English by Richard Surflet and then modified and published as *The Countrey Farme* by Gervase Markham, London (1616). *(The Science Museum/Science & Society Picture Library, London.).*

241. *Below,* Frontispiece from A.S. Gent's *The Gentleman's Compleat Jockey,* London (1696). *(The Science Museum/ Science & Society Picture Library, London.)*

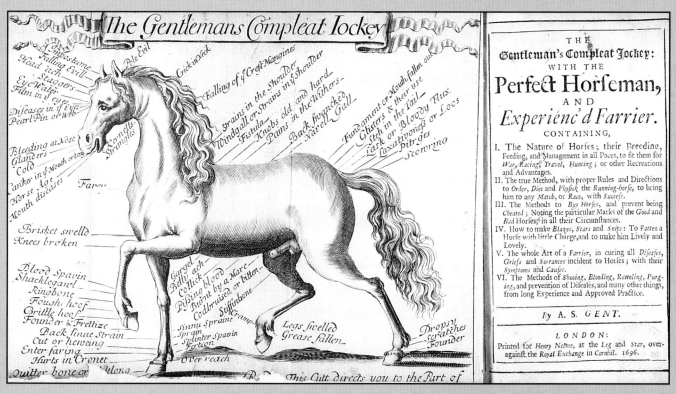

William Gibson (c. 1680-1750) was a military surgeon who turned his hand, with both knife and pen, to equine "curing." After military service he conducted a horse practice in London for thirty years. Like Markham, he drew on the works of others, particularly Solleysel (discussed later in this chapter). Gibson's views were strict in dietary matters but pathetically inadequate in the areas of hoof care and shoeing. He was best known for *A New Treatise on the Diseases of Horses* (1751), completed just before his death in 1750. Its value is little more than that of a small stepping stone in the great stream of ignorance that remained to be crossed. Other English surgeons who exemplified the tendency of their kind to venture into the intellectual void that was seventeenth century veterinary medicine and to publish popular works from a vacuous background included the surgeon John Bartlet, whose most positive contribution was to identify honestly the weaknesses of the medical and veterinary professions of his day.

A somewhat higher plane than usual was reached by a medical scholar who wrote on farriery, Henry Bracken (1687-1764). Bracken was a surgeon's son who apprenticed in that field before continuing with further studies in London, Paris, and finally Leyden, where he studied under Boerhaave, the great medical reformer and educator. Bracken wrote discursively on medical matters, but the veterinary content was limited. He did, however, bring to the field a pinch of the Boerhaave philosophy that for everything there is an explanation and it was the clinician's "bounden duty" to search for it. Bracken translated the senior LaFosse's misleading work on glanders with a critical commentary, and he was well known in horse circles for *Farriery Improved* and *The Traveller's Pocket Farrier* (1742). His contribution to knowledge of horse diseases was limited.

242. A folded frontispiece, a table of diseases showing instruments and utensils, usually bound in the book in a position facing the general title, from William Gibson's *The Farrier's New Guide, Containing, First, the Anatomy of a Horse...*, London (1738). A military surgeon, Gibson established a long-lived horse practice and was best known for his attention to the equine diet. (*National Library of Medicine, Bethesda, Maryland.*)

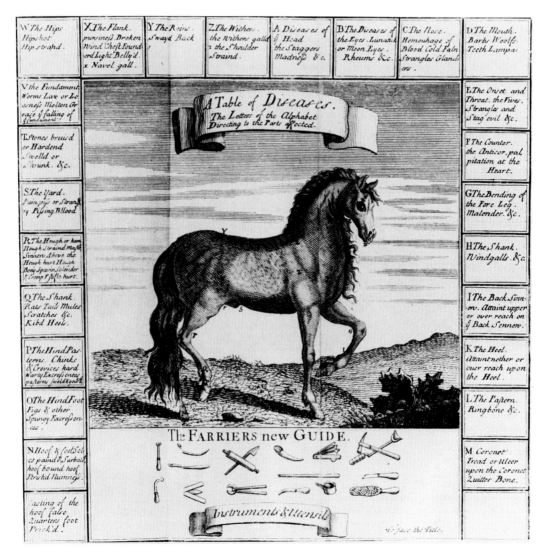

GREAT HORSE MARSHALS OF THE SIXTEENTH AND SEVENTEENTH CENTURIES

William Cavendish (1592-1676), the first duke of Newcastle, was one of the most famous horse trainers of all time, serving royalty and the aristocracy, but was forced to leave for the Continent when Charles I's army was defeated by Cromwell's forces in the civil war of 1642 to 1645. In exile Cavendish developed an outstanding riding school in Antwerp that was considered the best in Europe. He wrote a large-format book that was illustrated with artistic copperplates and published in French in 1658; a different version in English was not produced until 1667. A great judge of horses as well as people, he called the Spanish riding horse the wisest and smartest of all, followed by the Barb as the most resourceful, stoic, and easily trained. The English horse was the most versatile animal.

Cavendish deplored the British lack of attention to improvement through selection of sires. A great advocate of close inbreeding, he was often criticized for this later. Certainly he was one of the great geniuses in getting a horse to bend to his will during training. He was never brutal but insisted on obedience, claiming that "hope of reward and fear of punishment governs this whole world, not only men but horses." Breaking from the tradition of barbarous bits, he used a system of two reins that put pressure on the nose (curb or cavesson). Although he was a strong advocate of purging with aloes, Cavendish's practices and prescriptions were remarkably mild, departing from the dramatic, disgusting, and incompetent measures recommended by most of his peers. He preferred wheat straw over hay as the forage base to avoid the

243. Widely considered one of the most proficient horse trainers in history, William Cavendish, Duke of Newcastle, was exiled from England after Cromwell's defeat of Charles I's army in the Civil War of 1642-1645. Cavendish began a riding school in Antwerp. Symbolic of his supposed ability to train horses to his whim was this scene showing horses kneeling while Cavendish explains to them how to behave. From his book *A New Method, an Extraordinary Invention to Dress Horses: And Work Them According to Nature,* London (1667). *(The Historical Collections, The Royal Veterinary College, London.)*

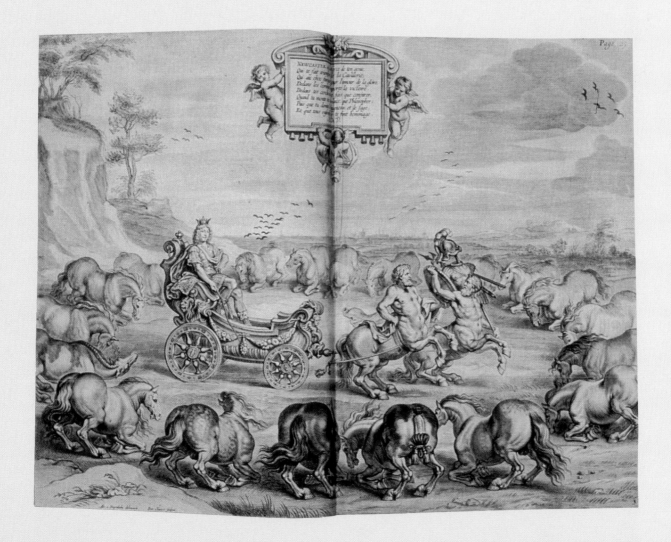

possible association of the latter with heaves or broken wind (emphysema). He was an advocate of shackling both forelegs and one hind leg to reduce the risk of the horse's damaging itself. A trenchant personality, Cavendish did not profess to be a horse doctor, but he condemned Blundeville as a better scholar than horseman and dismissed Markham as being no horseman, merely a copier and lister of medical prescriptions. Likewise, he realized that Thomas de Gray, a contemporary of Markham, was just another plagiarist. Since Blundeville had first copied Grisone, there had been a "chain reaction" perpetuating errors and brutality.

Jacques Labessie de Solleysel (1617-1680) became the dominant figure among the "grand marshals of horse" in the seventeenth century. A person of considerable influence, he traveled to Germany where he worked in Muenster for several years and took note of the well-developed practical veterinary art and gathered as much information as possible about German veterinary methods. He became a riding master in Paris and an admirer of Cavendish, whose systems of schooling he adopted. An extremely able, articulate, and pleasant personality, he brought the latest scientific advances into his erudite thinking. A student himself of all that was known about the horse and its diseases, in 1664 at age forty-seven he produced his famous text, *Le Parfait Maréchal*. This scholarly, well-ordered treatise became hugely popular and was to go through about forty French editions or printings, and others in German. The first English edition was printed in 1696, and was translated by Hope as *The Compleat Horseman*. Solleysel died suddenly at his riding school in 1680 at sixty-two years of age. He was recognized as one of the greatest Frenchmen of his time, thereby elevating the status of horse doctors in society. His well-illustrated book was divided into two parts, the first on all aspects of management of horses and the effect of drugs and the second on equine diseases and their treatment. On management of horses he was a true master, except that he perpetuated the extraordinary error of earlier authors concerning the alleged difference between wall thickness at the toe and heel of the forefeet and hind feet.

On diseases Solleysel brought a fresh perspective but lacked a sound medical grounding. However, he had a clear picture of the contagiousness of dis-

244. The great French marshal Jacques Labessie de Solleysel contributed greatly to the understanding of equine diseases, particularly strangles, colic, glanders, and farcy. His disease chart of the horse, with points of external and internal diseases marked, appears in his classic work, *Le Parfait Maréchal, Qui Enseigne à Connaitre la Beauté, la Bonté et les Défauts des Chevaux…*, Paris (1664). Tremendously popular, the work saw about forty French, two German, and four English editions or printings; it was translated into English by Sir William Hope as *The Compleat Horseman: Discovering the Surest Marks of the Beauty, Goodness, Faults and Imperfections of Horses…*, London (1696). *(National Library of Medicine, Bethesda, Maryland.)*

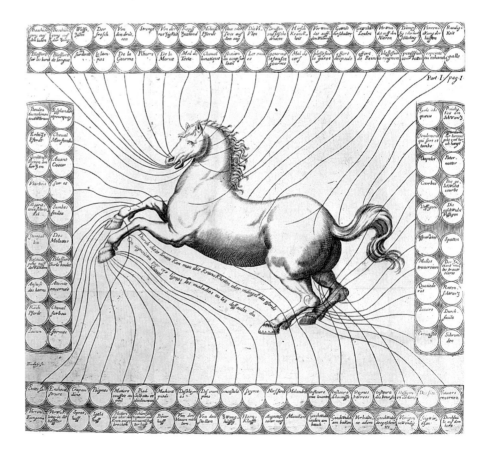

eases such as strangles. He recognized and classified six varieties of colic, including volvulus (twisted bowel), which may arise from gaseous distention or flatulent colic due to wind-sucking; parasitic colics caused by bots and worms; urinary colic; intestinal inflammation; indigestion resulting from overeating, which sometimes led to a ruptured stomach; and excruciatingly painful, violent colic with stasis and putrefaction of the bowels.

Solleysel recognized the close connection between glanders and farcy; he reported these diseases to be unresponsive to available treatments and recommended that therapy not be attempted. His ideas about glanders, a horrible, widespread contagion, were considerably more advanced than those of previous authors. Solleysel actually transmitted glanders from horse to horse, a remarkable experimental advance for the seventeenth century. In his writings he stated that "it communicates its venom . . . and seizes on all horses that are under the same roof with the one that languishes under the disease." He urged the immediate separation and isolation of an infected animal and avoidance of any connection with the others, such as the use of common drinking pails. Despite his forward-looking contribution to scientific progress and living, as he did, in the time of Harvey, Solleysel still retained some of the prevalent superstitious views.

Andrew Snape (born 1644) is the most intriguing of the early farriers, being a kind of bridge between the crude empiricists and the seekers of deeper understanding. Snape came from a family of court farriers, so he had a background of both practical experience and cultural exposure to royal circles. He was sergeant-farrier to King Charles II, who was an enthusiastic patron of medical science. He was appointed warden, and later, master of the company of farriers, being only the second person to hold that position. He had a high regard for education and was considered to have been able to read Latin works. His book, *The Anatomy of an Horse* (1683), was the first on this subject

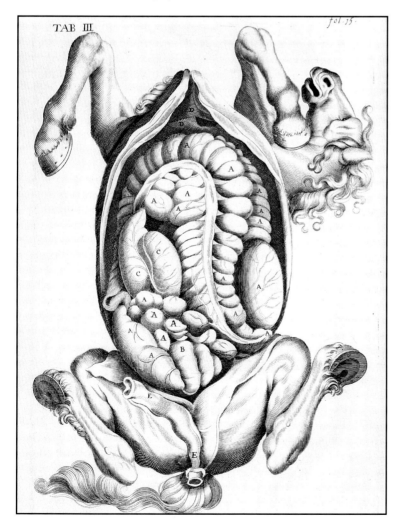

245. The viscera of the horse, from Andrew Snape's *The Anatomy of an Horse: Containing an Exact and Full Description of the Frame, Situation, and Connexion of All His Parts...*, London (1683). Snape's contribution to the understanding of structure and function was regarded as groundbreaking at the time, but it is likely that he plagiarized his anatomical drawings from the great Italian anatomist Carlo Ruini (compare this piece with Plate 215). *(The Science Museum/Science & Society Picture Library, London.)*

in the English language. He is believed to have been a teacher of the farriers, which would explain the use of vulgar terms in his book. Snape copied the plates from a book by Ruini without acknowledgment, and they were erroneously transposed during printing. Thus the plate of the viscera shows their position to be the mirror image of the correct situation. To the horse he ascribed collar bones, which it does not have. Gibson, who wrote the *New Farrier's Guide* in 1720, plagiarized Snape but retransposed Ruini's plates to restore the correct perspective.

The remarkable features of Snape's book are that he strove to explain the function as well as the structure of organs and that he reported the experimental findings of Renaissance scholars. Among these findings he cited the proof of pancreatic exocrine secretion and the controversy over the role of the pituitary gland, which led to the conclusion that it may secrete directly into the bloodstream. Without giving sources, Snape cited research, presumably that of Malpighi, on the internal structure of organs seen with the aid of a magnifying glass or microscope. He described the white nodules of the washed spleen, the presence of kernels in the kidney that may separate the urine from the blood, and the network of microscopic bladders in the lung attached to tiny branches from the pulmonary arteries. He explained the procedure for dissection of the brain and knew of the works of Galen and Willis on the nervous system, his plates resembling those of Willis. The most surprising weakness is his dismissal of the farriers' special area of concern, the equine hoof, by briefly comparing it to the human fingernail.

246. Frontispiece and title page from William Taplin's *Multum in Parvo,* or *Sportsmans Equestrian Monitor,* London (1796). The frontispiece shows a simple view of the method of determining the age (from three to seven years) of horses by the appearance of their teeth. Although his books were widely criticized by his peers for their commercialism, they were popular in both Great Britain and the United States. *(The Science Museum/Science & Society Picture Library, London.)*

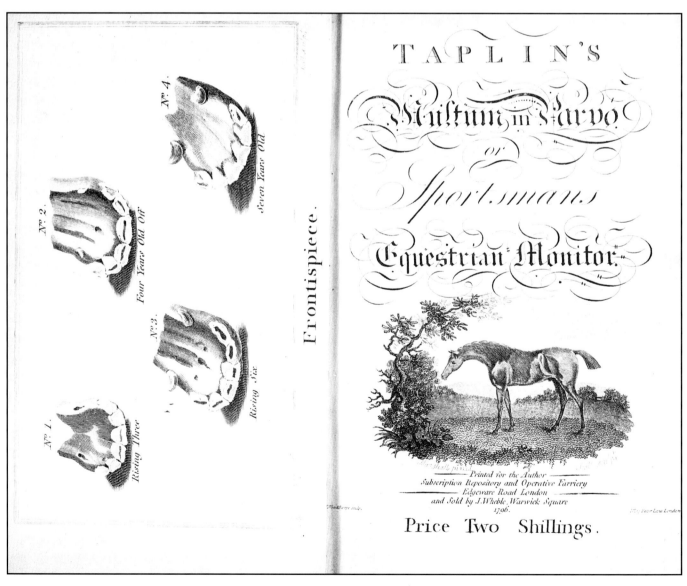

Snape's colleague and the king's physician, Samuel Collins (1618-1710), wrote *A Systeme of Anatomy Treating the Body of Man, Beasts, Birds, Fish, Insects and Plants,* an excellent but little known comparative work that dealt with structures, functions, and diseases.

William Taplin, a surgeon in the last half of the eighteenth century, became a commercially successful practicing veterinarian in Surrey. He wrote several works about diseases in horses and dogs between 1778 and 1803, often in multiple editions. On dogs he wrote of distemper, madness, and rabies; on equine diseases he covered a wide range of topics in a remarkably indifferent way. Considering that he had the works of Clark to draw on and that the first veterinary schools on the Continent had already been in existence for several decades, the professional quality of his work was deplorable. A virulent critic of his competitors, he advertised blatantly; he derived most of his income from drug sales. Although Taplin was widely disliked by his peers, his books were popular in Great Britain and America.

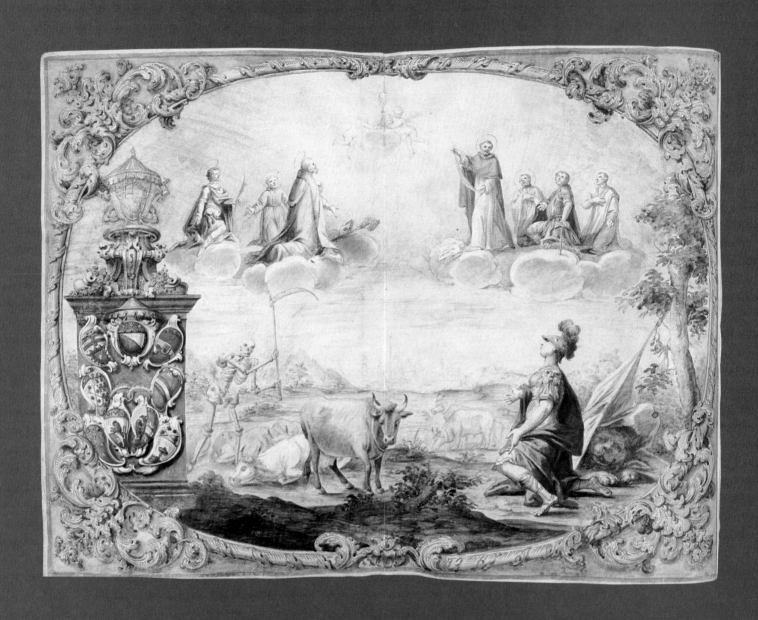

Logic in the Control of Plagues and the Understanding of Diseases

RINDERPEST: MODEL FOR UNDERSTANDING EPIDEMICS

Girolamo Fracastoro or Hieronymus Fracastorius (1483-1553) of Verona studied medicine in Padua when Copernicus and Erasmus were students. He practiced medicine in Verona until 1534, when he retired to devote his life to scientific research, focusing on epidemiology. He developed the concept of "contagium" as the spreading of "seeds of disease," and wrote *De Contagione* in 1546. He made the original description of the lice-borne fever typhus after observing an epidemic in Italy (1533). He was perhaps the first to adopt a genuinely intellectual problem-solving approach to population-based plagues or murrains (epidemics of diseases having high morbidity and, usually, high mortality rates). He applied this intellectual skill in the first instance to a veterinary problem. That beginning was to generate a new discipline that gradually developed the methodologies necessary to address the health management or disease control of livestock and the preventive approach to human epidemics known today as the field of public health.

The initial situation was a spreading epizootic of cattle disease in northeastern Italy. Fracastoro recognized that he was dealing with an outbreak of a contagious disease attributable to an "infectious matter" that could spread from one animal to the next. He envisioned that the disease could be acquired by direct contact with an infected individual, by contact with fomites that the individual had contacted, or via the air that it had exhaled. Whether that first epidemic he confronted was rinderpest or foot-and-mouth disease is unknown, although it was probably the latter, but it should be remembered that nothing was known about viruses and other etiological agents in that period. He had for the first time laid out a template for the understanding of infectious diseases, recognizing that most of them tend to be species-specific. He acquired a great reputation through his early work on syphilis, putting his thoughts into a remarkable poem, "Syphilis. Sive Morbus Gallicus," which captured the imagination of educated individuals and had the effect of christening the disease. A similar poem was written on the diseases of hunting dogs. The lack of an educated veterinary profession meant that there was no intellectual substrate to take the new opportunity to address the strategies for controlling epizootic diseases of animals.

Fracastoro's understanding of infectious disease may have been based on earlier ideas that had similarly been neglected. Lucretius had referred to the idea of contagions, and Albertus Magnus in the thirteenth century had similarly proposed three alternative ways of transmission. After Fracastoro another great lag phase occurred before a reawakening was to appear in the epidemiology of catastrophic plagues. Bernardino Ramazzini (1633-1714), a profes-

247. *Facing page.* This engraving from the twelfth volume of *Insignia Degli Anziani del Commune Dal 1530 al 1796* (Bologna) is an allegorical depiction of the spreading epizootic of cattle disease in the countryside surrounding Bologna in 1713 and 1714. Felsina (the ancient name for Bologna, originally founded by Etruscans) and the heraldic lion next to her are imploring the worshipping saints for protection from Death, seen striking the heads of the cattle. *(Archivio di Stato di Bologna.)*

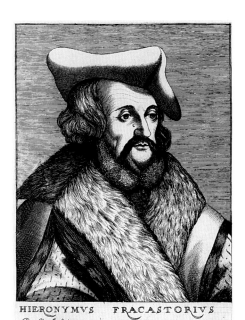

HIERONYMVS FRACASTORIVS

De. Larmassin. scul.

248. Girolamo Fracastoro, or Hieronymus Fracastorius (1483-1553), an important figure who substantiated the spread of disease from animal to animal. In his battle against epizootic disease in cattle, he recognized that many infectious diseases were also species specific. *(The Wellcome Institute Library, London.)*

sor of practical medicine at the University of Padua, wrote a classic text free from unsupportable medieval mystical and astrological rubbish and quackery on the serious new epidemic of a contagious disease of cattle, rinderpest, attributing it to a contagion and environmental factors. Born at Capri, educated by Jesuits, graduate of the University of Padua in philosophy and medicine, and practitioner in Rome, Ramazzini became ill with malaria and went home to Capri to recuperate. He said cinchona (quinine) had done for medicine what gunpowder had done for war. Perhaps the combination of excellent education, experience of practice, and firsthand acquaintance with a major epidemic disease directed his thinking toward a new focus on environmental hazards, epidemics, and occupational diseases.

Ramazzini was appointed to a chair in theoretical medicine in Modena and in a classic work in 1700 described forty occupational diseases. He studied malaria and attained recognition that led to his appointment to the chair of practical medicine at Padua in 1700, where he stayed until his death. He used studies of the pathological features of lesions to refute the prevailing astrological explanations of epidemic diseases such as rinderpest during an outbreak of the disease in 1712. He stressed the importance of detailed study of

249. The term *syphilis* originated from a medical poem, "Syphilis. Sive Morbus Gallicus," penned by Girolamo Fracastoro in 1530. *Syphilis* in Greek means *shameful, hideous,* or *repulsive,* but it is unknown why he chose this title for the disease. *(National Library of Medicine, Bethesda, Maryland.)*

HIERONYMI FRACASTORII
SYPHILIS.
SIVE MORBVS GALLICVS
AD P. BEMBVM.

Vi casus rerum uarij, quæ semi-
 na morbum
q I nsuetum, nec longa ulli per se-
 cula uisum
A ttulerint : nostra qui tempesta-
 te per omnem
E uropam, partim'q; Asia, Libyę'q; per urbes
S æuyt : in Latium uero per tristia bella
G allorum irrupit nomenq; à gente recepit.
N ec non & quæ cura : & opis quid comperit usus,
M agna'q; in angustis hominum sollertia rebus :
E t monstrata Deum auxilia, & data munera cæli,
H inc canere, & longe secretas quærere causas
A ëra per liquidum, & uasti per sydera olympi
I ncipiam, dulci quando nouitatis amore

symptoms and environmental factors and showed how postmortem examination could provide pathognomonic indicators to guide diagnosis. He evaluated all available data to establish that the rinderpest epidemic had been introduced to Europe and that it spread from sick to healthy animals. He reported his detailed findings and his explanation of the nature of the great rinderpest epidemic to the Philosophical College of Padua. At last the message registered in the collective consciousness of the theological, political, and medical leaders, who were faced with devastating losses of cattle throughout western Europe.

Ramazzini tried to protect cattle by applying the principle of variolization that was used for smallpox, puncturing the skin of the brisket in two places and pulling through the subcutaneous tissue a thread soaked in matter from an infected individual. It is unfortunate that there were no veterinary schools, research laboratories, or field epidemiologists to carry forward Ramazzini's magnificent exposition of problem-solving in epidemiology, the discipline of which he must be considered the founder.

The eighteenth century European cattle plague of rinderpest is deservedly described as a "panzootic" after it reappeared in about 1709 from southern Russia, following the path of Swedish and Russian armies. Within five years, 1.5 million vulnerable cattle died, and rinderpest raged from southeast to northwest, crossing the Channel into England. The earliest cases in western Europe were detected in the Italian countryside near Padua on a bishop's estate. Having good connections, the bishop was able to recruit the pope's distinguished court physician, Giovanni Mario Lancisi (1654-1720), to investigate the outbreak. The bishop also asked for assistance from the University of Padua, where Ramazzini took over the investigation in collaboration with Lancisi.

Lancisi had a genuine interest in comparative medicine. He was physician to Spirito Santo Hospital and was appointed professor of anatomy at the Sapienza in Rome in 1684. He had studied febrile diseases in horses and urged physicians to study animal diseases, especially when epidemics occurred. He diagnosed the disease in the bishop's herd to be rinderpest and proposed that strict controls be implemented to check its spread. Like Ramazzini, he described on postmortem examination the lesions that verified the diagnosis. At last a plague with a specific description could be targeted.

Lancisi's investigations during the spreading of the plague revealed that, although city markets had been closed because of the plague, clandestine marketing to evade the restriction was widespread. He deduced that rinderpest must be due to "exceedingly fine and pernicious particles that pass from one body to another." His influence was such that he was able to have his report heard by the College of Cardinals (Collegium Sacrum). He explained that all available remedies had been found to be completely ineffective and advised that every diseased animal should be killed, both to avoid the cost of worthless treatment and to reduce the spread of the contagion.

The cardinals cringed at the thought of a radical policy of slaughter, but eventually Lancisi's views prevailed because they were unarguable. No hard evidence could be brought to bear that would counter them. A papal edict spelled out the draconian measures. It is not clear that slaughter of affected beasts was actually ordained. Any movement of animals from infected areas, however, was prohibited under penalty of death. Dead animals were buried whole in lime. Only inspected and stamped meat could be sold for food. Lancisi had submitted a list of twelve preventive measures to the cardinals. After a further meeting they submitted a set of resolutions to the leading medical fraternities of Europe, and some nations, including France, Switzerland, Germany, and England, paid heed. Because Lancisi's measures were enforced in the region around Rome but not throughout Italy, the Roman region was free of plague within nine months but elsewhere it persisted for several years. It has been estimated that more than two hundred million cattle died in

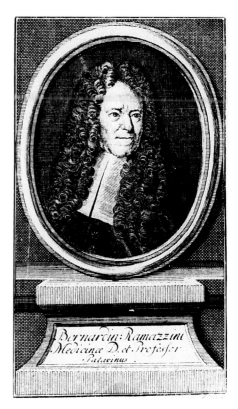

250. Etching of Bernardo Ramazzini (1635-1714). Ramazzini is credited with writing the first text attributing the cause of contagious disease of cattle to environmental factors. As the founder of epidemiological science, his work raised awareness of the biological factors behind the devastating rinderpest. *(New York Academy of Medicine, New York.)*

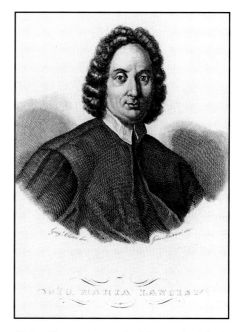

251. Engraving of Giovanni Mario Lancisi (1654-1720) by Marucci, after Cleter. Lancisi's investigation of rinderpest resulted in his recommendation to slaughter all infected animals to reduce the spread of contagion. Had this practice been implemented more widely throughout Europe, a large number of the two hundred million cattle that perished between 1711 and 1779 might have survived. *(The Wellcome Institute Library, London.)*

252. Various scenes of plague in London during the seventeenth century. Although the term *plague* is used for any pestilence of epidemic proportions, it is also used to identify a specific contagious disease of humans that repeatedly threatened civilizations from the sixth to the twentieth century. It occurred in bubonic and pneumonic forms and caused panic among the population. A great medieval pandemic spread to Europe from Asia in the fourteenth century, reaching Britain in 1348, where it gave rise to the Black Death. Another pandemic arrived in 1664 and 1665, some of the consequences of which are shown in these poignant engravings. The roles of rodents, fleas, and bacteria were not discovered until much later. *(Courtesy Master and Fellows, Pepys Collection, Magdalene College, Cambridge.)*

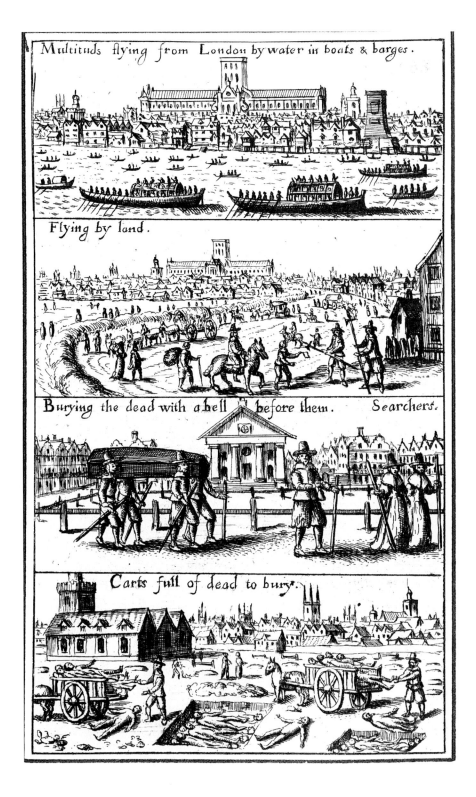

Europe in the sixty-eight years after 1711 as a result of the great epidemic. Clearly Lancisi's visionary guidance was not adopted widely, and the wisdom and resolution to take the necessary measures were absent in influential places. Based on historical evidence, humankind was a slow learner.

In the field of human medicine Lancisi wrote classic descriptions of heart disease as a cause of death and of the epidemiology and control of malaria, noting the role of swamps and mosquitoes and advocating draining of swamps.

In England King George I appointed his surgeon, Thomas Bates, to investigate the epidemic in the face of an outbreak in 1714. He, like Lancisi, was able to define the problem and address it in an effective way with the backing of his royal sponsor. His understanding of the nature of the affliction was much shallower than Lancisi's, but his grasp of what should be done was extremely similar. He had difficulty obtaining information by asking the cow keepers themselves to admit that they actually had the infection on their premises. However, he was able to obtain the desired data from one of the cattlemen and from the cow leeches. He then set up a transmission experiment, housing sick and well animals together in a shed. He was instructed to prepare a written statement of what should be done. His document made six directives and argued for an indemnity of two pounds per sick cow that was burned. Bates started work in July, and by Christmas he had eradicated the disease at a cost of 5418 cattle and a royal indemnity of 6674 pounds. Since Bates appears to have been unaware of the details of Lancisi's work, his achievement is impressive.

PROGRESS IN UNDERSTANDING DISEASES: THE WORK OF MICHAEL HARWARD

Michael Harward of Cheshire, a thoughtful seventeenth century ox leech or animal doctor who later moved to Ireland, made the most significant contribution to veterinary medicine of any Briton of his period. He condemned the widespread superstitious practices and incantations he found among the cattlemen of Ireland, urging that they adopt the way (blessed by God) of a skillful and industrious ox leech, although he saw "very few who bestow any pains on that noble science." His list of prerequisites for a successful cattle surgeon and practitioner is challenging:

Accurate and ready mind
Good memory
Active and nimble hand
Resolution and boldness
Careful and vigilant
Not rash nor hasty

Harward urged the aspiring ox leech to observe butchers at work and study in detail the lay and appearance of the internal organs, including the calf in utero. In 1673 he wrote a short, pithy book, *The Herdsman's Mate,* based on his thirty years of experience in cattle practice. Harward was an accomplished animal doctor who focused on cattle in an age when the horse got most of the attention.

Harward described many infectious diseases, including rabies, and observed the special nature of the poison resulting from the bite of a mad dog. He drew attention to poisonous plants and insects. He knew of bloat and liver fluke ("flouks") and used a cud from a healthy cow to restore the rumen function of a sick one. Harward certainly must have been bold and dexterous as a surgeon, since he gave a detailed account of brain surgery to treat the "giddy" or "sturdy," a turning sickness attributed to hydatid cysts in which the afflicted animal turns to the sound side. He followed Fitzherbert's (1523) description of the surgical method. He was aware that the bladders were situated under the membranes covering the brain. Only if the site was behind the forehead was it operable and then only at the stage when the bone had become soft. After the animal was cast, a large skin flap was peeled up and tied to the horn and the soft spot was located; a circular piece of bone the size of a shilling (or a quarter) was chipped out carefully with the aid of a hammer, and the dura mater was incised cautiously. Careful probing under the dura was used to extract any degenerated yellowish brain tissue so that the parasitic bladder could be located. The animal was then held face down and the nostrils closed manually, causing straining that raised the pressure and forced out the bladder, which could be drawn out the rest of the way. Harward was aware that the bladder contained worms that must not be allowed to escape inside the skull. Harward thus left a record of bovine neurosurgery performed in the middle of the seventeenth century.

253. Title page from Thomas Spackman's treatise on rabies, published in London in 1613. *(The Royal Society of Medicine Library, London.)*

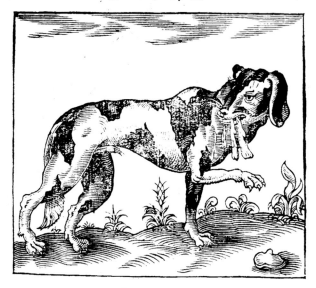

A
DECLARATION
OF SVCH GREIVOVS
accidents as commonly follow
the biting of mad Dogges,
together with the cure
thereof,

BY
THOMAS SPACKMAN
Doctor of Physick.

LONDON
Printed for *Iohn Bill* 1613.

254. Wood engraving showing villagers attempting to slay a rabid dog from *Acerca de la Materia Medicinal . . .* (1565), by the Greek physician Pedanius Dioscorides of Anazarbos. A military surgeon in Hero's army, Dioscorides flourished from AD 40 to 68. His highly regarded work was later translated and published. *(National Library of Medicine, Bethesda, Maryland.)*

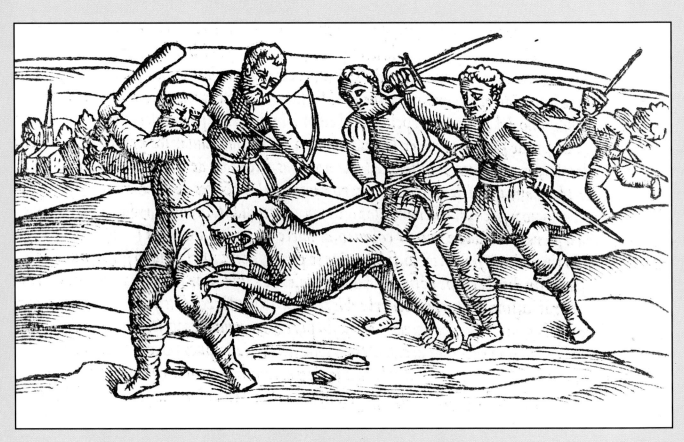

Harward was reputed to have been a superlative obstetrician and was prepared to resort to embryotomy and cesarean section when necessary. He described replacement of the prolapsed uterus and its retention by means of vulval sutures supported by leather strips to avoid tearing. The common problem of removing retained placenta is for the first time addressed; Harward's recommendation was cautious manual removal.

Harward's best-known contribution was to abdominal surgery. Goring injuries received special attention. When they resulted in simple hernias with subcutaneous intestines, they were corrected by waiting ten days, then casting the beast where the feet could be tied vertically to a beam; the skin and sac were cut cautiously and the bowels returned to the abdomen. The inner wound was closed with a continuous suture through the wall muscle and peritoneum; then the skin was closed by interrupted sutures. A supporting canvas roll was applied and sewn into position. In more serious cases, when the abdominal wall was torn and the guts fell out and trailed behind the beast, bolder measures were required. The same approach was used to position and operate on the animal, and the least damaged parts of the bowel were stitched and returned to the cavity. Then followed the innovative procedure. Any pieces of bowel that were too raggedly torn to be suturable or were already black and cold had to be handled as follows:

> First lay the two broken ends that should grow together the one a little over the other in your hand; then cut them both off at once with a pair of scissors, so that the new cut ends may be joined close together, but first cut the two broken ends off close to the midrise and cast them away, then with a fine needle and thread, or silk, stitch the two new cut ends together so that they may gently meet and not be strained. Begin first to stitch at the mid-rise [mesentery] and so round about the gut till you come to the same place again and then make fast your thread . . .

The crucial factor was stated to be the tension on the thread, which should be neither too hard nor too slack. It is clear from the text that in many of these alarming cases the cow survived. Thus it seems that Michael Harward was a pioneer of end-to-end intestinal anastomosis in cattle before it was practiced in humans.

Although some of Harward's ideas and methods had been described in *The Countryman's Instructor,* (1636) by John Crawshey, a cattle and sheep practitioner of Samdall Magna, Yorkshire, Crawshey's work is much narrower in scope than Harward's and the descriptions are rudimentary.

ATTENTION TO VETERINARY PARASITES: THE WORK OF FRANCESCO REDI

English flocks suffered devastating epidemics of sheep scab in the thirteenth century. The "parent of parasitology" was Francesco Redi (1626-1697) of Arezzo and the University of Pisa. He knew of the work of Virgilii Maronis on sheep scab in 1517. Maronis had scraped off the crusts of the scabs, applied ointments, and practiced bloodletting in his treatments. Redi received a letter from Cosimo Bonomo describing the itch-mite *Acarus scabiei* and its eggs as the cause of human scabies (1687). Redi knew the problem of gid, staggers, or coenurosis, and he considered the hydatid cysts in the brain possibly vermicular. Shepherds were aware that the cause was a cystic worm growing in the brain. Treatment for this may have been the origin of animal trephination because the bone over the cysts softens. He published an important work entitled, in English, *Observations on Living Animals Which Are To Be Found Within Other Living Animals.* Redi also did fundamental work on liver fluke. He refuted the theory of spontaneous generation by experimenting with fly eggs and larvae. He always sought the true cause of diseases. His confidence was such that he drank snake venom to prove that it was innocuous unless injected.

EQUINE EMPHYSEMA: THE WORK OF PHYSICIAN JOHN FLOYER

The classic problem of equine respiratory disease, pulmonary emphysema, or heaves, also called "broken wind" because of the characteristic biphasic respiratory pattern requiring a second expiratory effort with each exhalation, had been addressed ineffectually by horsemen, marshals, farriers, and protoveterinarians for millennia. It fell to a brilliant physician, Sir John Floyer (1649-1734) of Litchfield, England, to finally put science on the right track in dealing with this disease. He also developed the physician's pulse watch, which ran for exactly one minute. He made detailed studies of the pulse as a diagnostic technique. In 1698 he published a work on asthma, a disease he had himself. He described the dissection of a broken-winded mare, noting the enlarged lung and the emphysematous air bladders visible on the surface. Observing that the lungs did not manifest the normal elastic recoil after inflation, he concluded that there had been a strain on the lining of the small branches of the airways, leading to some permanent injury to the membranes and trapping of air in the tissues. Floyer's work demonstrates how research in comparative medicine served to benefit knowledge of both animal and human medicine. He had been aware of the physiological experiment of Richard Lower on the effect of severing the phrenic nerves on the respiratory pattern in the dog.

EQUINE LAMENESS: THE WORK OF BRIDGES AND LaFOSSE, SENIOR

Jeremiah Bridges, a practicing London farrier and horse doctor, was among the first to attempt a detailed anatomical description of the horse's foot. He speculated that the weight of the body was borne by the laminae of the four hooves and that the hoof had to be an elastic structure. He noted the springy lateral cartilages that strengthen the heel and restore the shape of the hoof after it is compressed by bearing weight. Aside from mistakenly considering the sensitive laminae to be muscular, probably because of their red color, his anatomical and functional observations were intuitive and enlightening. They provided others with a more accurate basis for further work. His work on the foot was published under the eye-catching title *No Foot, No Horse: An Essay on the Anatomy of the Foot . . .* in 1751.

William Osmer, a mid-eighteenth century surgeon and horse fancier who became a London horse doctor, published several works on diseases and lamenesses of the horse that are mainly derived from the works of Etienne Guillaume LaFosse, Senior. LaFosse, Sr., of Montaterre was the first of a famous Parisian line of horse doctors and veterinarians who made huge contributions to the emergence of equine medicine as a true profession attempting to base its methods on sound knowledge. His book *Observations and Discoveries Made Upon Horses, with a New Method of Shoeing* was published in 1754 and improved in a subsequent edition. He also applied the powder of the common puffball fungus *(Lycoperdon)* to stem hemorrhages, demonstrating its effect in a horse, even in cases of arterial bleeding resulting from limb amputation, before a commission of the Academie des Sciences.

The most important part of LaFosse, Sr.'s work dealt with lameness and shoeing technique. He names the anatomical structures of the foot with the aid of excellent drawings. He described clinical cases of lameness, including fractures of the pedal and navicular bones (embellished with postmortem findings), ruptured tendons, quittor, and puncture wounds.

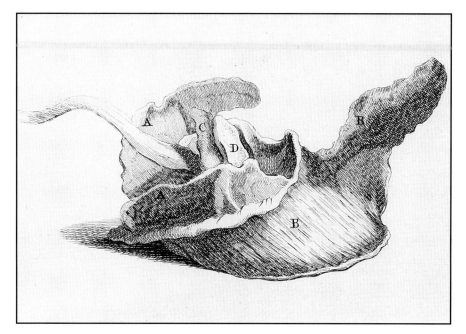

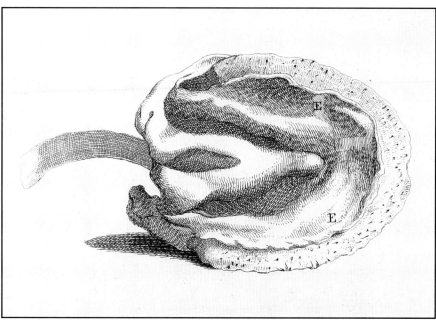

255. *Explanation of the Six Additional Discoveries Made in the Anatomy of the Foot,* one of two plates stitched into the frontispiece of *No Foot, No Horse: An Essay on the Anatomy of the Foot of That Noble and Useful Animal a Horse . . .,* London (1752), by Jeremiah Bridges. In explaining this plate, Bridges wrote:

> *By faithfully following the Knife, and looking into Nature with my own Eyes, I have been enabled to furnish these Additions, which I have not met with in the Perusal of any Authors who have wrote on this subject; neither have I ever seen any of them taken notice of, in any of the Cuts of Anatomy, that have as yet appeared in public.*

(Special Collections, Michigan State University Libraries, East Lansing.)

After introductory remarks in his text on the function of parts of the foot, which, remarkably, neglect the laminae, LaFosse, Sr., illustrated shoeing methods in common use at the time in Europe. He preached reform of the many detrimental farriery practices of the time, particularly the paring out of the supporting sole, the cutting away of the vital cushioning frog, and excessive paring of the wall. He deplored the widespread custom of using long, heavy shoes that put pressure on the sole and distorted the structure and stresses of the hoof by being thicker on the inside branch. He proposed a new method of shoeing aimed at preserving the foot and enhancing the comfort, performance, and durability of the horse. His new shoe became known as the *tip.* His criticisms forced a reconsideration of the principles of shoeing and led others to introduce innovations. LaFosse, Sr., also exposed a long list of errors and atrocities commonly practiced in the treatment of horses. His legacy was carried on by his son Philippe-Etienne LaFosse, known as LaFosse, Jr., who was to become even more renowned than his father in veterinary circles.

JAMES CLARK OF EDINBURGH: VETERINARY PHILOSOPHER-SCIENTIST

One figure stands out from the dismal pack of Englishmen who purported to be animal doctors in the eighteenth century. Many were bold enough to write on veterinary matters, and evidently there was a demand for many of these works. However, aside from the works of a few who, like Michael Harward, were diligent and dedicated rather than commercially oriented and conceited, there is little that could be identified as significant or scientific progress. The exception, who appears to have tried harder than most and with greater result, was James Clark of Edinburgh. Such was his modesty and self-effacement that little is known of him, not even the dates of his time on Earth. Yet he was the role model for Scotland's farriers and became a distinguished veterinary professor. Clark had evolved into the best Edinburgh veterinary surgeon of his day, a man who was prepared to tackle each problem from first principles, unfettered by doctrine and dogma, using his accumulated wisdom, experience, and common sense. He impresses one as having been one of the few truly compassionate veterinarians who sincerely tried to alleviate suffering in his patients and not add to it with the dramatic interventions, which can only be described as atrocities, espoused by many of his contemporaneous colleagues. He had read everything available to him, from the historical writers on matters relevant to veterinary practice such as Xenophon, Columella, and Vegetius, to those of his period, as well as the leading scientific and medical authors (such as Stephen Hales and Boerhaave via van Sweiten's *Commentaries*) and agricultural authors.

Clark brought to bear on his practice knowledge and inspiration from scholars of animal husbandry, physiology, and medicine, as well as his training and apprenticeship in farriery and veterinary practice. He conducted post-mortem examinations to evaluate his diagnoses and treatments. He rejected the traditional doctrine of the imbalance of the humors as the basis of disease. Rather, he insisted on seeking the cause of disease and trying to understand its nature while using the clinical signs to make the diagnosis. Indeed, Clark challenged the whole of medieval medical and veterinary practice and its valueless treatments, including both the universal practice of bleeding to remove the evils and the recipe book of complex formulations of medicinal agents. How refreshing, how extraordinary, how courageous was this man.

Clark's three works were *Observations Upon the Shoeing of Horses,* 1770 (second edition, 1775; and third edition, 1782); *Treatise on the Prevention of Diseases (Incidental to Horses),* 1788 (second edition, 1790; also published in Philadelphia in 1795); and *First Outlines of Veterinary Physiology and Pathology,* 1806 (the preface of volume one advises that volume two is almost ready; alas, since it was never completed, it is lost to posterity). The first of these works used the account of the anatomy of the foot by Bridges and acknowledged earlier publications by LaFosse, Sr. and William Osner. Clark corresponded with the Earl of Pembroke; they had a mutual agreement on many matters relating to shoeing, and the second edition of Clark's work on the shoeing of horses was dedicated to him. Clark called for nothing less than complete reform of shoeing practice, bringing out evidence that many diseases of the horse's feet are a consequence of injudicious shoeing and unnatural treatment—an early allegation of iatrogenic disease.

Clark called for discarding all the usual errors of paring away of frog, bars, and sole, as well as the massive shoes in common use. A narrow piece of iron, flat on the ground surface, hammer-hardened for increased durability, with no more than eight or ten nails in countersunk holes, was all that was required of the farrier's art in tailoring a shoe to the hoof, a shoe that was light in weight, adapted to the size of the foot and the nature of the work, and designed to ensure that the frog could contact the ground. Acceptance of Clark's reforms, as he predicted, came slowly.

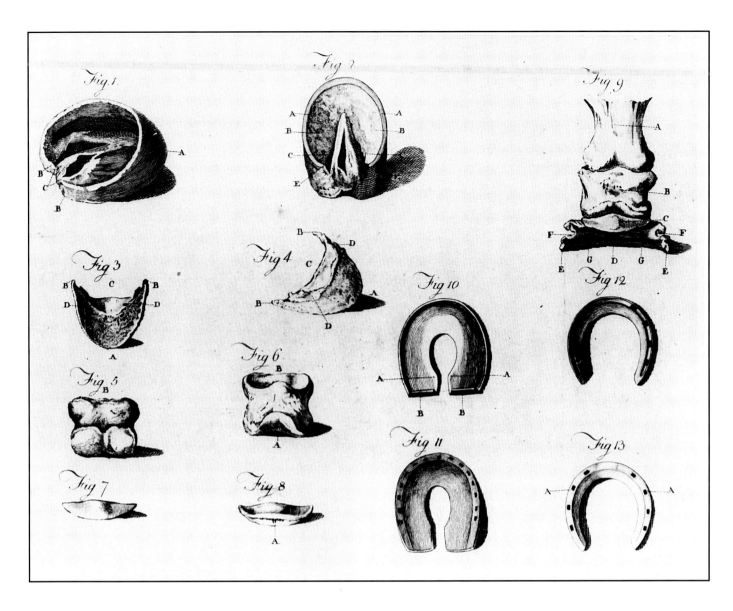

His discourse on diseases of the foot shows a great advance in rational understanding of the pathogenesis and logical approaches to treatment. He divided the conditions into two main groups, accidents and diseases. Considering the lack of antibiotic drugs in his times, he clearly grasped the main principle of wound treatment: to get to the deepest part of a sinus and arrange for drainage from inside out. All oily, tarry, and resinous materials were to be avoided in therapy. He described many diseases well, including laminitis, but was frustrated by the lack of effective therapeutic measures. Nonetheless, he always used conservative approaches and prescribed rest.

Clark's 1788 treatise proposed animal hygiene as a tactic in disease prevention, focusing on the importance of the immediate environment of the horse. Siting and design of stables and the central importance of good ventilation, cleanliness, and comfort were stressed. Nutrition and feeding received detailed attention. Water of good quality and the importance of grooming, regular exercise, and postexercise management were all priorities. The theme of sensible, physiologically sound recommendations pervaded the entire work, including a unique section on nursing of the sick. He emphasized the value of taking the pulse, which had been almost completely ignored in veterinary practice. Also original to Clark was a chapter on kindness to horses. It was too early for him to make sense of the literature on the prevention of contagious diseases such as glanders.

His last book, on physiology and pathology, was intended to become a textbook of lectures he prepared in 1793 and 1794 for the veterinary school the government had assured him would be established in Edinburgh. As such,

256. The Scottish veterinarian James Clark stands out from the farriers of his day for his thoroughness and diligence in scientific endeavors. He also challenged the antiquated and often useless practices of the medieval horse doctors. This engraving, from *Observations Upon the Shoeing of Horses* (1770), one of his three published texts, demonstrates nine hoof problems and four types of horseshoes. *(National Library of Medicine, Bethesda, Maryland.)*

it incorporated advances in physiology and pathology to form a basis for professional education. This assurance led Clark to decline an invitation to replace Sainbel as principal of the London school upon the latter's untimely death caused by glanders. It was disastrous both for the veterinary college and for James Clark when the unstable political situation caused the government to back out of its commitment. For Clark himself it was a shattering disappointment. He had campaigned insistently for the formation of a veterinary school, lamenting the disadvantage of an absence of adequate preparation and training, which left the veterinary art in darkness and obscurity. He noted that such education was already available in France. He urged that a state school be established, and when one finally was established in London in 1791, he pressed for another in Scotland as well. He had been an honorary and corresponding member of the Odiham Society of Agriculture by 1790, when that society was instrumental in founding the London Veterinary College. Clark, although a self-taught veterinary surgeon who had risen from the rank of farrier, had the attitude, interest, and experience that would have made him a better principal for a veterinary school than any other individual in Great Britain. For the Veterinary College in London, Clark's absence proved a catastrophe because one who lacked almost all the essentials, Edward Coleman, was appointed principal; the College became irrelevant as a force in veterinary progress, and the competence of its graduates was questionable for approximately forty years.

OVERVIEW OF THE DEVELOPMENT OF VETERINARY MEDICINE FROM THE MIDDLE AGES TO THE NINETEENTH CENTURY

Just as in France, the best animal doctors in Great Britain were horse specialists in the eighteenth century. Few were qualified to handle the diseases of the other farm animals, pet animals, or wildlife, let alone the basic scientific disciplines, the clinical specialities, or public health. The establishment of veterinary schools would begin to correct that situation and allow the profession to attain respectability.

The overall perception of the evolution of the veterinary art in the Middle Ages is of a time of political fractionalization and repeated warfare on the one hand and of antiscientific theological fundamentalism on the other. These two great authoritarian forces had the effect of suppressing progress in many fields of human endeavor. The human intellect, however, repeatedly exhibited signs of a spontaneous curiosity and drive to learn, with individuals moving to centers of scholarship and cerebral ferment as these were identified. Although these centers were affected by constantly changing political forces as well as repressive church doctrines, the intellectual flame was never extinguished completely and always reappeared elsewhere. Finally, with the Italian Renaissance as the initiating focus, the tide turned, scholarship regained legitimacy, and a long overdue second flowering of the arts, sciences, and professions began. The old dragon of intolerance died slowly, however, because of the attempt to resist the Protestant Reformation that accompanied the other reforms. The overall image is one of the humans' inhumanity to humans and animals alike in the struggle for the human soul.

The narrower view of veterinary medicine's development is one of frustration that a field with such enormous potential for contributing to a value-oriented future was repeatedly prevented from its natural development in society or misdirected by leading figures who sought to manipulate it. The horse had dominated the scene for three thousand years because of its military significance and its sporting attraction to the ruling classes and "landed gentry." Despite the resulting high priority and large investments, horse doctoring never escaped from its own peculiar brand of mysticism throughout the medieval period. The appearance of authority dominated the voice of reason and genuine scholarship in matters equine. No other animal was subject to such atrocities under the banners of training and medical care. Thus, although a larger literature developed on the horse and its management and diseases, the general lack of rigorous scholarship is amazing. The few voices of reason were seldom heard, and the degree of copying and blatant plagiarism that characterized the works of self-styled experts and authors ensured only the perpetuation of errors and resistance to questioning.

The priority accorded the horse meant that the other species got short shrift, a remarkable result in view of the huge losses caused by epidemic diseases of ruminant livestock. The level of ignorance about the plagues was so extreme that there was little grasp of how to address the problem until the scientific method was established. This inability to control disease played into the hands of both the Church and the charlatans. This impotence made it seem that faith was the only hope and that the idea that God was exacting his price for sins was valid. When it was realized, based on the observed results, that that message, too, was false, people turned to the mystics and soothsayers who professed to have charms and magical cures that would protect the animals or save them. All else having failed, the people increasingly turned to witch-hunting, astrology, and prophecy. There were no great philosophical figures in the field of veterinary medicine who could chart a sound course for comparative medicine and articulate it to the authorities. Only Clark had such insight, and he was denied an opportunity to articulate it. Thus the profession was as yet unable to evolve or grow with the advancement of knowledge.

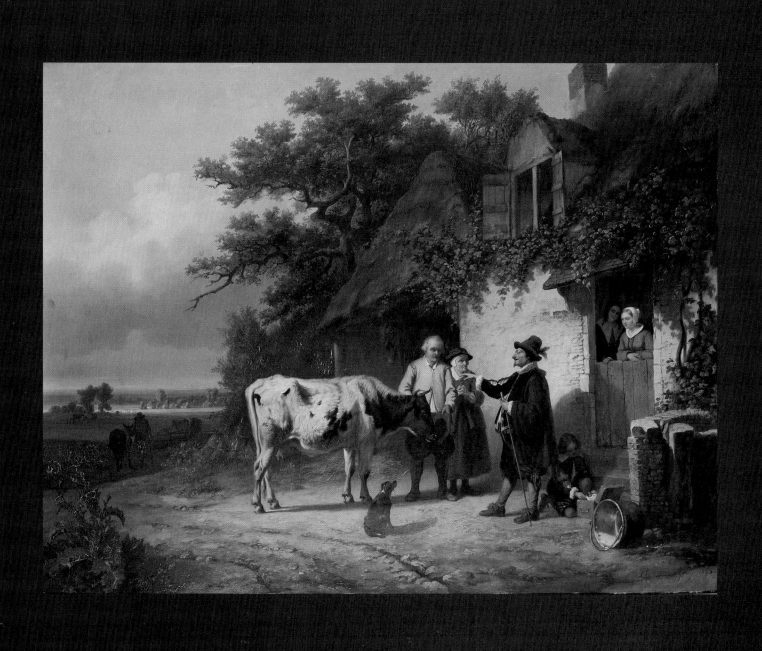

Toward a Scientific Basis for Comparative Medicine

IDENTIFICATION OF A NEED FOR SCIENCE-BASED ANIMAL DOCTORS

Devastating epizootics of contagious diseases of livestock ravaged the herds and flocks of western Europe during the eighteenth century. Foremost among the contagions was cattle plague or rinderpest; massive death rates demoralized the stock owners and destroyed their economy. At last it began to be recognized politically that it was necessary to seriously seek solutions to crises caused by animal diseases. Why did it take such a massive stimulus (millions of dead cattle) to evoke a social response? Leaders of vision were required who recognized the need and had sufficient influence on resources to be able to launch an educational program. The serious contagions of the horse generated concerns similar to those for livestock because in this case the aristocracy was affected directly.

The dilemma was, on the one hand, that the health care of animals was in the hands of individuals who, by and large, had failed to gain the respect of society. The medical needs of the horse had become a kind of mystique in the hands of the equerries or marshals, farriers, and senior grooms. Opportunistic laypersons known as cow leeches were available to treat cattle. The other species seem to have received little attention beyond that of the owner or caretaker. Not surprisingly the type of people engaged in animal doctoring failed to inspire confidence among the educated leaders of society. The other horn of the dilemma was that, although more suitable individuals might be expected to have arisen from the ranks of the medical profession or the zoological scientists, not many deigned to stoop to the level of the farmyard. Among those who did, except for a few notable individuals who had genuine interest and a farming background, medical people were not particularly successful in a veterinary role. So profound was the neglect of the calling that a knowledge base and individuals who were suited to launch it were seriously lacking. Before it would become apparent that a meaningful profession could and should be created, more progress was required.

Progress was to come in the form of great scholars who started to lay the track of disciplined studies that were relevant to a comparative approach to medical sciences. The growing awareness of the idea of the evolution of lifeforms on the planet, particularly from the lower vertebrates to humans, was to become a significant factor in gaining acceptance of the concept that there was an enormous contribution to be made to human medicine through studies of the "lower" animals. It was the vision and scholarship of eighteenth-century biological and medical scientists, however, that were destined to bring about the catalysis: they recognized that there could be a sound scientific footing for the formation of a cadre of people to tackle the problems of animal diseases.

257. *Facing page, L'Empirique* by the Belgian painter Edmond Tschaggeny (1818-1873). Edmond and his older brother Charles (1815-1894) specialized in animal art. Charles was renowned for his paintings of famous horses, whereas Edmond focused on bovine subjects. Edmond frequented the veterinary school at Cureghem, and from his anatomical studies he produced ninety-eight magnificent watercolors of bovine anatomy that were exhibited for their artistic merit at the Paris Expostion in 1864. They were published posthumously in *Atlas d'anatomie de l'espéce bovine* in 1921. In this particular painting, which currently hangs in Buckingham Palace, a smartly dressed individual, probably a cow leech masquerading as an animal doctor, examines a cow in front of a peasant's home as the family looks on. Sadly, this deception was an all too common occurrence before the establishment of a respectable profession based on comparative medicine dedicated to the health of animals. *(By permission of Her Majesty Queen Elizabeth II, The Royal Collection, Windsor Castle.)*

258. Artist's visualization of Stephen Hales (1677-1761), the clergyman of Teddington, and an assistant measuring blood pressure in the horse. The unequal flow of blood within the vessels had been observed by scientists and artists since early times, but it was Hales who developed a classic experiment to measure arterial pressure, the results of which were published in the second volume of his *Statical Essays, Containing Haemastaticks* (1733). *(The Bettman Archive.)*

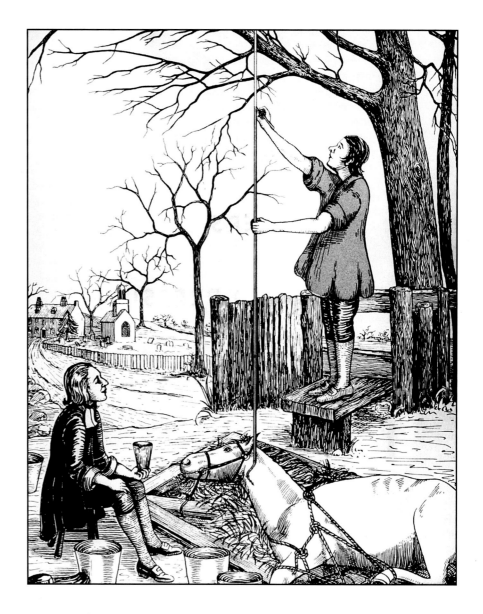

One of the great self-taught entrepreneurs of physiological research was the English cleric Stephen Hales (1677-1761) of Teddington. His greatest biomedical contributions were to the quantitative measurements of arterial blood pressure and hemodynamics. He is renowned for his work on fluid movement in plants and devised ventilation systems for prisons that led to a substantial reduction in death rates among the inmates. His book, *Statical Essays: Containing Haemostaticks* (1733), described the extraordinary experiment of connecting the artery of a recumbent horse via a link of goose trachea to a nine-foot long vertical glass tube and measuring the height to which the blood rose and how much it pulsated with each beat of the heart. More than fifty years later, the brilliant French physician-physiologist Poiseuille repeated Hales' experiment. He used a U-shaped tube containing mercury, which is 13.6 times more dense than blood, to avoid the need for such a long vertical tube. He also found that he could use sodium carbonate solution in the tube to prevent coagulation. With this simple device, he estimated the force of the heartbeat and measured blood pressures.

LAVOISIER'S REVELATION OF THE GASEOUS BASIS OF ANIMAL METABOLISM

Antoine Laurent Lavoisier (1743-1794) decided to apply his intellectual genius to the chemical evaluation of Aristotle's four fundamental elements— earth, water, fire, and air. Lavoisier worked initially in the practical field of geochemistry but made his most important discoveries in studies of air and fire. Robert Boyle had started to characterize the physical properties of gases and to investigate the essential role of the blood in respiration. Steven Hales, who observed that gases could become "fixed" and "collapsed" to a solid or a liquid form, respectively, speaking in 1727 of "air," asked, ". . . may we not with good reason adopt this now volatile Proteus among the chemical principles . . . ?" (Proteus was the Greek god of the sea creatures who had the power to change his shape until firmly held.) Joseph Black in 1755 showed that there was a second kind of "air," fixed air, in substances like chalk, in addition to the atmospheric air. This new gas was carbon dioxide. Joseph Priestley had come close to the discovery of oxygen with his theory of "phlogiston," the inflammable principle of substances.

Lavoisier's insight (1772) was that, instead of something being given off (that is, "losing its phlogiston"), he thought something was being added or taken on. Guyton de Morveau had shown that when some substances were burned, they increased in weight (for example, sulfur and phosphorus). Lavoisier, after his work on saltpeter, which he had shown to be nitrate of potash, showed that it could be made from nitric acid and potash. This led him to study nitric acid and to conclude that it was a compound made of nitrous air and an equal part of common air and a quantity of water. He generalized from this that all acids contain a principle, the purest part of air, that he called "oxigine" (from *oxus*, for "acid" and *geinemai*, meaning "to engender"). Although his generalization about acids was in error (in that hydrochloride does not contain oxygen), the term "oxygen" stuck; its conceptual origin also persists in the German term for "oxygen," *sauerstoff*.

Henry Cavendish had discovered the combustible gas hydrogen and had shown that when it was exploded (burned) in ordinary air, a little dew was formed. When Lavoisier learned of this in 1783, he had already shown that when mercury was heated for several days in a closed volume of air, about one

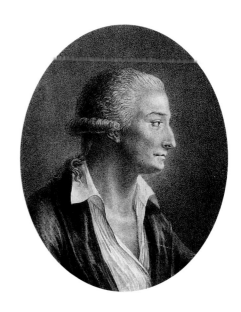

259. Portrait of Antoine Laurent Lavoisier (1743-1794), the French scientist who established the basis of modern chemistry. *(Jean-Loup Charmet.)*

260. Drawing by Lavoisier's wife showing her husband conducting an experiment on respiration while she sits at a table taking notes. *(Eidgenössische Technische Hochschule Bibliothek, Zurich.)*

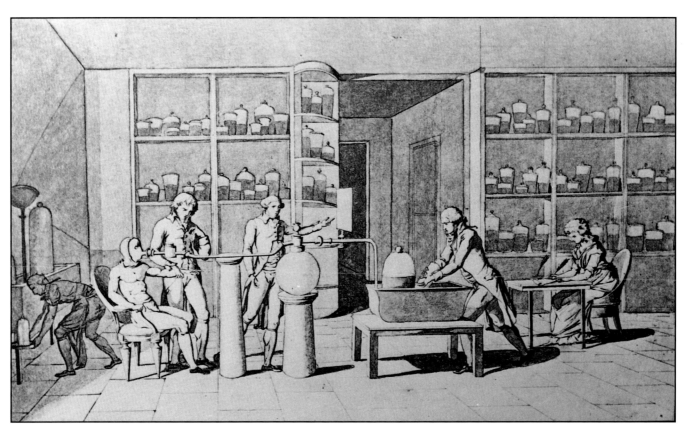

fifth of the air was consumed and a red powder formed on the surface of the metal. A taper would not burn in the residual four fifths of the air. When the red powder was heated, a gas was released in which a taper burned more brightly than in ordinary air.

Lavoisier allowed water to drip down a red-hot gun barrel: the oxygen combined with the metal and the hydrogen was released as a gas. He was now (in 1783) ready to make the momentous proposition that respiration was analogous to combustion. He compared the candle burning in a sealed jar to respiration in a guinea pig: both used up oxygen, both gave out heat, and both yielded carbon dioxide and left a residue of nitrogen. His textbook of chemistry (1789) listed thirty-three "elements," substances that had not yet been broken down into simpler substances. With his distinguished colleagues he also simplified chemical nomenclature to clearly designate the composition of the compounds and by suffixes to indicate the specific forms. This nomenclature led to Berzelius's shorthand system. These efforts set the stage for the atomic theory of John Dalton (1808). Lavoisier is the primary progenitor of the general theory of gases. Veritable master of inorganic chemistry and ingenious developer of experimental equipment, Lavoisier, through his work on gases, formed the basis of respiratory and metabolic physiology. As a "reward" for his much earlier role as a tax inspector, this great revolutionary of the science of chemistry was to have his career foreshortened and lose his head to the guillotine in 1794 in the aftermath of the French Revolution.

LIEBIG'S CHEMISTRY OF DIGESTION AND METABOLISM

Joseph Gay-Lussac (1770-1850) tidied up the master's theory of acidity and proposed a method for analyzing organic compounds that in turn led his famous student, Justus von Liebig (1803-1873), to found a great new school of organic and biochemistry at Giessen, which became the seat of many advances in metabolism.

In 1828 the German chemist Friedrich Wohler synthesized urea, the first organic substance to be synthesized in the laboratory. Justus von Liebig, who was given a personal chair and laboratory at the University of Giessen by King Ludwig I of Bavaria in 1824, carried Lavoisier's flame forward into organic chemistry and its agricultural application. He also continued Lavoisier's tradition of teaching students in the laboratory. A brilliant, inspiring teacher, Liebig left a legacy of research scientists, as well as nearly three hundred scientific papers, two new scientific journals, and a text on organic chemistry. He moved to a chair of chemistry in Munich in 1852. Liebig made several organic chemicals (including tyrosine, chloroform, and chloral) for the first time. He became the parent of metabolic biochemistry by showing that carbohydrates and fats are oxidized in the tissues.

Karl von Voit (1831-1908), the founder of nutrition as a science, was a physician and a student of Liebig who became professor of physiology in Munich in 1863. There he worked with Max Josef von Pettenkofer (1818-1901), who was made professor of hygiene after having held a chair in dietetics and medical chemistry. They studied the metabolic utilization of food, heat production, and respiratory exchange in farm animals. They were able to establish evidence for the law of conservation of energy in living animals. Max Rubner (1854-1932) was a pupil of Voit and continued their metabolic studies. He described the specific dynamic action of feeds and established that metabolism was a function of body surface area rather than weight. He followed Koch in the chair of hygiene in Berlin in 1891. Edward Pfluger (1829-1910) was professor of physiology in Bonn and developed the concept of the respiratory quotient of foodstuffs. Graham Lusk (1866-1932) at the Bellevue Hospital Medical College in New York and Francis Benedict (1870-1957) of the nutrition laboratory of the Carnegie Institution extended these metabolic

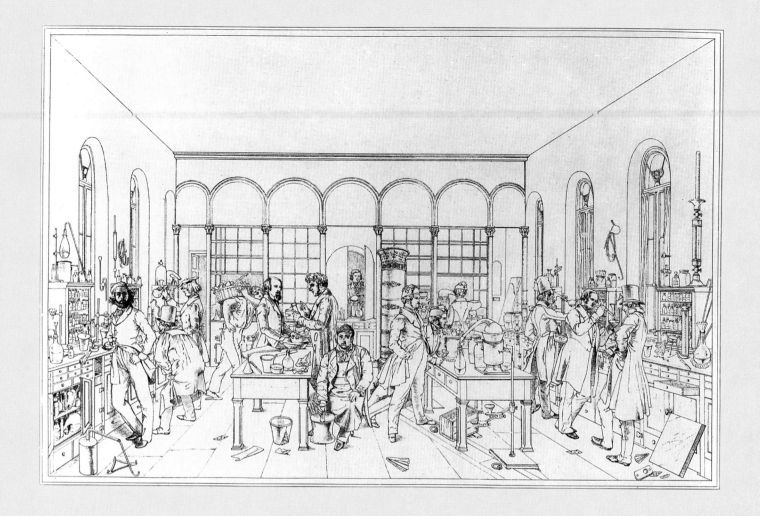

and nutritional concepts derived from animal physiology into the human field. A famous contemporary of theirs was D.D. van Slyke (1883-1971) of the Rockefeller Institute in New York, renowned developer of gasometric methods for blood gases and many other biochemical analyses, including studies of acid-base balance and of urea and the role of glutamine in ammonia excretion. Max Kleiber, author of *The Fire of Life,* brought the German flame to the University of California at Davis, where he was renowned for his ingenious experiments allowing the quantitation of metabolism in animal growth and production.

261. Justus von Liebig's famous chemistry laboratory at Giessen University in 1840. Liebig's reputation attracted students from all over Europe to study with him at this facility. *(Gesellschaft Liebig–Museum, Giessen.)*

EMERGENCE OF BIOMEDICAL DISCIPLINES IN THE EIGHTEENTH CENTURY

During the eighteenth century great scholars and enlightened physicians made the advances that were to form the basis of the new field of comparative medicine. A great arousal of public interest in science and renewed faith in education emerged while unthinking belief in divine ordination was losing its grip. Efforts were made, on the one hand, to "order the world" by classifying all species that could be identified, initiating the broad field of taxonomy based mainly on zoology and botany. On the other hand, particularly in the medical field, the process of reductionism had begun. Medicine was divided into subjects or "disciplines" based on fields of study, usually having characteristic methodologies. The first of these had been anatomy, but now the broader field of comparative anatomy, an essential basis for taxonomic zoology, took hold.

295

The study of living things was a major new field demanding experimentation and hypothesis testing, namely, comparative physiology. The scientific study of disease required an orderly description of changes from the normal condition, starting with postmortem dissection and other studies such as those of microscopic anatomy (histology) to see the changes at the cellular level. Applied to disease, this field became known as pathology. These three great disciplines—comparative physiology, histology, and pathology—led to the basis of a scientific approach to disease in the living patient, again involving the accumulation and codification of a vast amount of detail that could be distilled to guide diagnosis. The art of physical examination to detect pathophysiologic disorders was made more rigorous and formed the basis of clinical medicine. The art of intervention to alter the course of disease required knowledge in the areas of pharmacology and surgery. It was still too early to add the disciplines that would address the etiological agents of infectious disease (microbiology and parasitology) or study disease in a population-based, quantitative way (epidemiology).

STAHL'S MEDICAL THEORY: A COMBINATION OF CHEMICAL AND VITALIST CONCEPTS

During the sixteenth and seventeenth centuries individual scientists had made exciting breakthroughs, but the ideas did not spread as rapidly as might have been expected. Friedrich Hoffman (1660-1742), son of a wealthy physician who died of the plague, studied medicine at Jena. He went to England and met Boyle, returned, and practiced medicine for some time before settling in Halle, where he became a professor at the new university in 1693. He was considered an outstanding clinician and a dedicated teacher who was interested in applying chemistry and physics to medical studies, taking a mechanical view of body functions. He believed in an immortal soul that was not involved in the matter and motion of the body parts. He brought his former student at Jena, Georg Ernst Stahl, to join him as his assistant professor in Halle. He delegated the theoretical aspects of medicine to Stahl.

Stahl (1660-1734), a Protestant from Bavaria, was trained in medicine at Jena and became court physician at Weimar before being called to Halle, where he taught for two decades. Eventually he differed with Hoffman, resigning in 1716 to become physician to the court in Berlin. Stahl was a brilliant chemist who escaped from early indoctrination in alchemy. He proposed the existence of a substance, phlogiston, in metals and combustible substances that was lost when such materials were burned. This idea caught on and held sway until Lavoisier's experiments corrected it by weighing the reactants to determine whether materials were added or subtracted in combustion (oxidation).

Stahl is most renowned for his biomedical theories, which were published in his opus *Theoria Medica Vera,* a general theory of the body and its functions in health and disease focusing on its chemical composition. He ardently believed that an organism was more than a mere mechanism, that it depended on a conscious soul or an anima to keep its complex composition from disintegrating, as it did swiftly after death. Although his chemical discoveries and proposals were but stepping stones to progress, his theory of vitalism (the presence of a life force) was applauded and adopted by many. He considered fever an agent of the anima in combatting disease and thought that bleeding and purging had the beneficial effect of reducing plethora. The physiologist Muller argued that consciousness was separate from the organic creative force, claiming that it created no organic products, only ideas, and was found only in the higher animals.

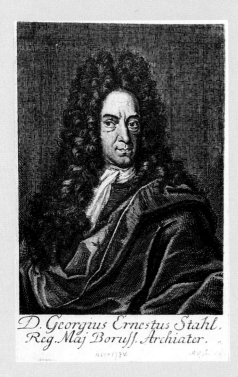

D. Georgius Ernestus Stahl,
Reg. Maj Boruss. Archiater.

262. Portrait of the Bavarian physician Georg Ernst Stahl (1660-1734). He believed in a life force, a conscious soul or anima, that maintained health; his theories on the benefits of fever and bleeding were other important concepts. *(New York Academy of Medicine, New York.)*

BOERHAAVE'S COMPARATIVE APPROACH
TO MEDICINE

The greatest medical thinker of the eighteenth century, who integrated the significant preceding advances and ignited intellectual fires in the minds of the young colleagues he attracted, was undoubtedly Hermann Boerhaave (1688-1738), the Dutch physician who studied philosophy before entering medicine. He was appointed to the first chair of medicine, chemistry, and botany in Leyden and became the leading light of medical progress. He took careful note of the results of Giovanni Borelli's (1608-1679) physical studies on the muscle functions and movements of animals, Marcello Malpighi's (1628-1694) great artistry in microscopic anatomy and embryology, and Frederic Ruysch's (1638-1731) ingenuity in preparing specimens with colored injections that allowed visualization of all the arborizations of the body systems, thereby going beyond the limitations of dissection.

Boerhaave deployed previous advances in developing a new, rigorous basis of theory, effectively building a new framework of medical thought that gained him a reputation as the doyen of physicians and made Leyden the most prestigious medical school in Europe. He became a magnet for the best young minds of his time, and he became mentor to many who were to carry forward the light of learning through the eighteenth century. He applied botany and chemistry to medicine and had a major impact on the adoption of biochemical methods in nutrition. He personally arranged for the posthumous publication of medically trained Jan Swammerdam's (1637-1680) superbly illustrated research on insects, *Bible of Nature,* in 1738.

Boerhaave was a follower of the ideas of Thomas Sydenham (1624-1689), who described all disease as natural history, insisting on the avoidance of philosophical hypothesis and dogma while demanding meticulous observation of actual phenomena. He found that nature unaided often terminated diseases. One of Boerhaave's predecessors at Leyden, Franciscus Sylvius (1614-1672), had been the first to organize modern medical teaching. Boerhaave's genius was contagious; his impact on medical progress was phenomenal and global. Haller, the physiologist at Göttingen; Lancisi in Rome; van Swieten and de Haen in Vienna; John Rutherford at Edinburgh's Royal Infirmiry, followed by Whytt, Cullen, and Brown; and William Saunders at Guy's Hospital in London are impressive examples of medical scholars who made Boerhaave's legacy enduring and built upon it, as he would have wished.

Boerhaave's specific contribution to veterinary medicine, as well as his general impact on medical progress, came about through his protégé van Swieten, whose disciple Pal Adami (1739-1814) was assigned the role of surveying animal diseases throughout the Austro-Hungarian Empire. Baron Gerard van Swieten (1700-1772) was a brilliant, visionary Catholic Dutch doctor and Empress Maria-Theresa's most trusted advisor. She had recruited van Swieten to Vienna to become her chief medical officer for the empire. He rapidly became the great modernizer of medical education in Vienna and the empire, elevating it to its golden-age status, avoiding parochialism, and recruiting the finest medical minds in Europe. He was a strong supporter of veterinary education, but he envisaged it as addressing all animal species and being linked to the medical faculty at the academic standard the latter had newly attained, instead of being merely a form of practical equine medical training at the top of the farrier's art. In preparation for his vision he had encouraged Adami, a highly respected Hungarian medical colleague, in 1765 to study animal diseases in preparation for a leadership role in the new profession.

Van Swieten obtained feedback from early Lyon veterinary school graduates that they were quite unable to develop control measures for the epizootics after their training. Since the Hungarian plain was a major transport

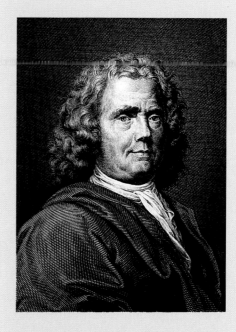

263. Hermann Boerhaave (1688-1738), arguably the greatest medical thinker of the eighteenth century. His status as the principal scientific scholar at Leyden encouraged comparative study among his many students. *(New York Academy of Medicine, New York.)*

route from Asia to Europe, it was particularly vulnerable to the waves of animal diseases, notably rinderpest. Reluctantly van Swieten concluded that it was too early to initiate instruction and that it would be necessary to carry out detailed field studies of the diseases before veterinary education could become fruitful.

The conscientious, brilliant Adami worked untiringly to fulfill van Swieten's vision. He investigated every outbreak of animal disease he could, whether epidemic or sporadic. He conducted clinical and postmortem examinations, accumulating a vast knowledge that allowed him to make a wide range of accurate differential diagnoses. He made the crucial point, overlooked by all other workers on cattle who had focused almost solely on epizootic plagues, that the cumulative toll of the many sporadic diseases surpassed that of the epidemics most of the time and that they deserved a much greater share of the total preventive effort than they had received. He tested treatments rigorously for efficacy. He developed a strict sanitary policy in 1771 for regulation of animal movements wherever contagious epizootics appeared. He wrote a book on cattle plague in 1782. G.F. Sick, who later became professor of the Berlin Veterinary School, accompanied Adami for a period to gain experience.

Maria-Theresa appointed Adami professor of medicine and epizootiology of the University of Vienna in 1775, in keeping with van Swieten's recommendation, although the latter had died three years earlier. When the empress herself died in 1780, however, Adami was dismissed, no doubt as a result of the tug-of-war between military advisors concerned about the real threat to security on the one hand and the empress's societal and rural concerns derived from van Swieten on the other. After Maria-Theresa's son, the Emperor Joseph II, who was influenced more by the military faction, died in 1790, Adami was rehabilitated and in 1804 was made professor of veterinary medicine at a new school at Krakow (now in Poland) whose ancient university had been established in 1364. When Adami retired in 1809, his assistant and interpreter, A.A. Rudnicki, became the first Polish veterinary professor after the annexation of Krakow to the Grand Duchy of Warsaw.

Adami, a remarkable man, was true to the legacy of comparative medicine, advancing veterinary knowledge by deploying the emerging wisdom from studies of human medicine to benefit livestock, exactly as foreseen by van Swieten, and going beyond it through his own investigations to advance understanding. He knew more about the nature of contagious diseases than anyone else of his period, having delved into immunological methods as Ramazzini had long before him. He devised inoculation methods for both foot-and-mouth disease and rinderpest. He implanted threads that had been dipped in saliva obtained from animals with rinderpest and air dried. Thus he demonstrated the loss of pathogenicity on drying (attenuation) and reported successful protection of animals. The authorities in Graz responded with a remarkable decision to ban all further experiments, thereby causing this promising trail to go cold.

THE RISE OF NEW CENTERS OF INTELLECTUAL CHARISMA

The eighteenth century witnessed the rise of new centers of intellectual charisma in the biomedical sciences. After the great launching of anatomical and physiological studies at Padua in Italy in the sixteenth and seventeenth centuries, the pendulum was to swing to Leyden, Holland, and Göttingen, Germany, in the eighteenth.

Bernhard Siegfried Albinus (1697-1770), born in Frankfurt, became professor of anatomy and surgery at Leyden and by the age of twenty-four years produced a classic illustrated work on the human musculoskeletal system. His

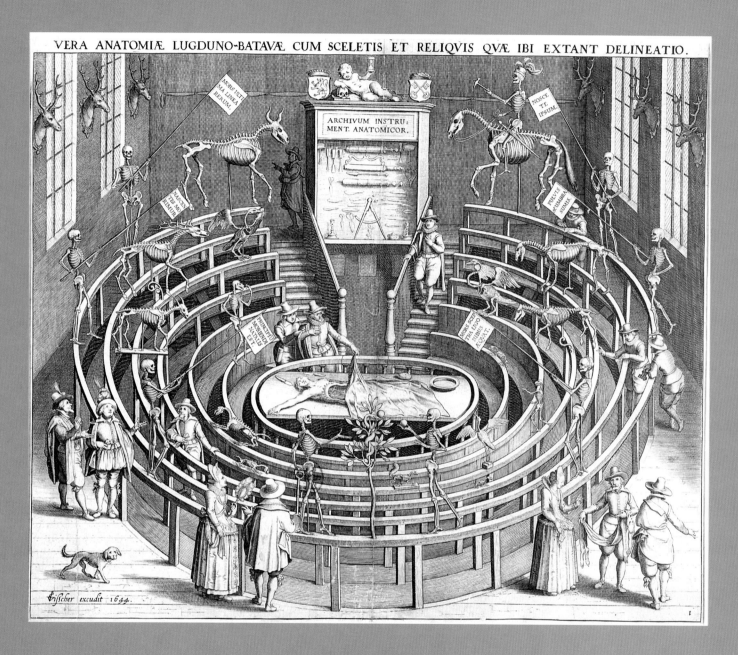

VERA ANATOMIÆ LUGDUNO-BATAVÆ CUM SCELETIS ET RELIQVIS QVÆ IBI EXTANT DELINEATIO.

264. An amusing seventeenth-century engraving of the anatomy theater at Leyden, where Bernhard Siegfried Albinus (1697-1770) lectured on anatomy and surgery. He was the pioneer of a new anatomy in which all investigations were carried out with exacting thoroughness. A close look at this engraving reveals that it manifests the comparative approach and is filled with reminders of death. From the apparent attempt to sell what appears to be a complete human skin to the woman in the lower right-hand corner to the skeletons all around the room, we are forced to confront our own mortality. *(Leiden University Library. Collection Bodel Nÿenhuis.)*

265. Illustrations of the elephant's stomach and cecum by Petrus Camper (1722-1789), a student of Albinus and a peer of John Hunter. *(Artis Bibliotheek, University of Amsterdam.)*

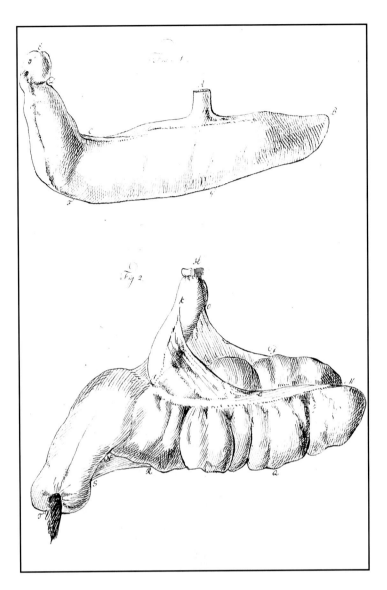

brilliant student Lieberkuhn (1711-1756) described the crypts in the small intestine that are named after him. He made such investigations possible by inventing injection preparations as a technique for microscopic studies. Another of Albinus's pupils, Petrus Camper (1722-1789), had a remarkably broad spectrum of interest, encompassing veterinary surgery and biological illustration. The method of craniology in humans and the great apes is derived from his scientific drawings. He published anatomical studies of exotic animal species such as the rhinoceros, elephant, and reindeer. He extended these studies to a more comparative plane with investigations of the air sacs and air-filled bones of birds and the auditory structures of the widely different aquatic lifeforms of fish, reptiles, and whales, as well as the different effects of air and water media on sound conduction. Camper was a contemporary of the great surgeon and comparative anatomist John Hunter.

HALLER: FOUNDER OF EXPERIMENTAL PHYSIOLOGY

Albrecht von Haller (1707-1777) was born in Berne. An infant prodigy, he knew Greek and Hebrew by the age of ten years, wrote epic poetry by fifteen, and was a doctor of medicine at nineteen. He studied at the University of Tübingen, at Leyden under Boerhaave, and at Paris. He was one of Boerhaave's favorite pupils. Returning to practice medicine at Berne, he became renowned as a botanist and a poet. By 1736, at twenty-nine years of age, he had been appointed Professor of Medicine at the new University of Göttingen, where he did notable work in physiology for seventeen years and influenced many scholars, including the microbiologist Robert Koch. Haller returned to Berne in 1753. Although his extraordinary scientific productivity yielded six hundred and fifty publications, he became troubled about the appropriateness of the suffering caused to animals by the vivisection his work had involved earlier in his career and by the large number of physiological experiments performed before anesthesia was developed.

As a botanist Haller disagreed with Linnaeus's "artificial" system of classification of plants and proposed as an alternative a "natural" system based on the character of the fruit or seed. Although Linnaeus's scheme prevailed, Haller's mind was of a much larger compass. He was a master of many fields, above all, of physiology; essentially, after Harvey's breakthrough on the circulation of the blood, Haller was the founder of the discipline. He produced an immense compendium of his wide-ranging studies in physiology, as well as a brilliant, concise handbook of physiology that became a popular manual. William Cullen (1710-1790), professor of medicine, first in Glasgow, then in Edinburgh, was noted for his system of classifying diseases on the basis of symptoms, that is, based on functional principles being related to structural ones. This nosology was popular with physicians in its day and brought a new order to the understanding of neurological disorders, in particular, affections of sensation and motion. Cullen did a great service by translating Haller's book into English as the two-volume *First Lines of Physiology, By the Celebrated Baron Albertus Haller* in 1786.

The nature of the physiological approach is indicated by the statement attributed to Haller that ". . . more exact divisions of measuring instruments are more important than all of Descartes, all of Aristotle." He adopted the

266. Engraving from Albrecht von Haller's (1707-1777) *Elementa Physiologiae Corporis Humani,* Lausanne (1757). A small dog is lying on its back on a table; scalpels and other surgical instruments are scattered about; an enormous heart is at the left in front of a cherub; and another cherub is holding an anatomical chart. *(National Library of Medicine, Bethesda, Maryland.)*

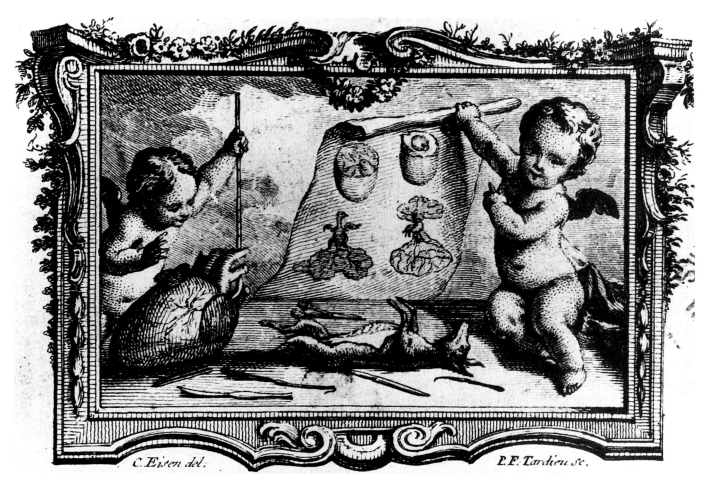

C. Eisen del.   P.F. Tardieu sc.

267. Illustration from Haller's *Mem-oires sur la Nature Sensible et Irritable des Parties des Corps Animals* (1756). A pro-digious researcher, Haller published eight volumes summarizing the major physio-logical discoveries up to the mid-eigh-teenth century. His research included the function of muscles and nerves, and he dissected more than four hundred cadavers during his scientific career at Tübingen, Leyden, and Göttingen. *(National Library of Medicine, Bethesda, Maryland.)*

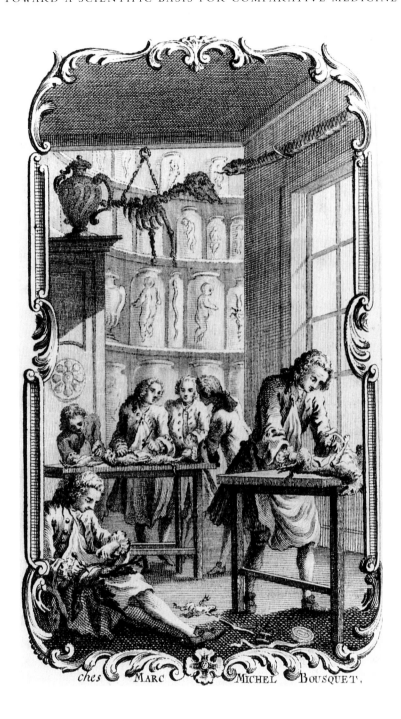

idea of the "physician's pulse watch" with a second hand, developed first by Sir John Floyer, to run for exactly one minute so that physicians could study the pulse rate.

Haller was inspired by Newton's concept of a mechanically ordered world, using it to formulate a new approach to nerve-muscle physiology. Haller identified the distinct roles of the nerve impulse or "sensibility" and of contraction or "irritability." Although obviously not the first to study the functions of the body's parts, he merits the title "founder of the discipline of physiology" because of the enormity of his experimental work on animals, his remarkable erudition, and his international recognition and prestige. He brought his full compass to bear on the issue of developing a comprehensive bibliography of earlier work and became a significant medical historian.

Haller's views on neuromuscular physiology were challenged by Robert Whytt (1714-1766), professor of the theory of medicine at the University of Edinburgh, another former Leyden student. A remarkably astute clinical ob-server, Whytt focused on reflex activity and conducted experiments on frogs, which demonstrated that even a small segment of the spinal cord could sus-tain reflex contractile responses to skin stimuli. He studied the reflex responses of the pupil of the eye to changes in light intensity. He emphasized that there were involuntary as well as voluntary aspects of reflexes, in other words, that there was an unconscious response principle or mechanism that influenced muscle activity. Clinical experience had taught him that tendons, joints, and ligaments were sensitive to the knife and that inflammation of the lining of the thoracic cavity (pleura) and of the membranes covering the brain (dura and pia) was accompanied by severe pain. Haller was so obsessed with his doctrine of irritability that he disputed Whytt's views. Felice Fontana (1730-1805) set out five "laws of irritability" to resolve the disputes and also proposed that nerve conduction was electrical.

BEGINNINGS OF ELECTROPHYSIOLOGY

In Leyden Pieter van Musschenbroek designed a glass vessel coated inside and out with metal that would store a large charge of static electricity. This was the first capacitor and became known as the Leyden Jar. Discharge from several jars wired together was shown to kill animals. By charging such a jar from a kite flying in a thunderstorm in 1750, Benjamin Franklin showed that lightning is static electricity discharging. Luigi Galvani (1737-1798), professor of obstetrics at the University of Pavia, published *Commentarius* and initiated electrophysiology in 1791. (Although translated into German in 1793, the work did not become available in English until American translations were published in 1953.) Beginning with frogs, he claimed to have shown "animal electricity" in several species of vertebrates (frogs, birds, chickens, and sheep) by using nerve-muscle preparations. Galvani's other legacy was the invention of the galvanometer, a delicate device used to measure electrical current, which became an important tool in physiological research.

268. Luigi Galvani (1737-1798) provided the experimental basis that gave birth to the age of electrophysiology. This 1791 illustration demonstrates his idea of animal electricity, which led to the term *galvanism*. The galvanometer, named after him, became an important physiological evaluation device used to measure electrical current. *([RSL]. RRx. 7. Bodleian Library, Oxford.)*

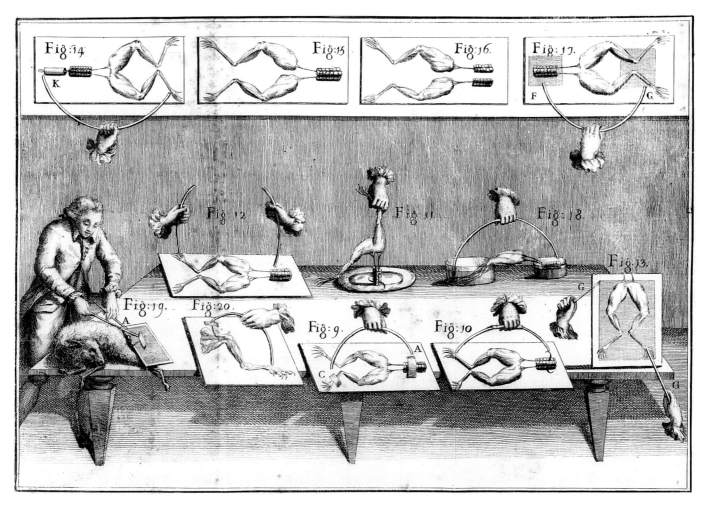

At first Volta (of Bologna) supported Galvani's conclusions that he had obtained evidence of a genuine animal electricity in nearly all animals. Volta changed his opinion in 1799, after he showed that an electrical discharge could stimulate sensory nerves as well as muscle fibers. The device he constructed was a pile of copper and zinc disks separated by damp plasterboard that generated electricity, the first battery and the first device to provide a continuous flow of electricity. The stimulus for this research was his idea that contact of two different metals in a damp environment (brassed iron) could have generated a current that excited the tissues of the animals used in Galvani's experiments.

SPALLANZANI'S ACHIEVEMENT OF ARTIFICIAL INSEMINATION IN A DOG

Lazzaro Spallanzani (1729-1799), a famous eighteenth-century Italian researcher, held professorships at Modeno and Pavia (in philosophy and natural history, respectively). He demonstrated the flaws in the apparatus used by those who claimed to have proven spontaneous generation in 1776. A brilliant physiologist, he studied respiration, including the transfer of gases via the skin; cardiac physiology; and the digestive capacities of saliva and gastric juice. He showed that death resulting from anoxia was caused by changes in the central nervous system. He showed that body parts regenerate in invertebrates and lizards. Of particular interest to veterinary medicine, he was the first scientist to demonstrate that spermatozoa were essential for fertilization of the ovum and to achieve artificial insemination in the dog. He was an ordained priest and became known as Abbe or Abbate Spallanzani.

CLASSIFICATION OF ORGANISMS

Most of the early lists of animals were bestiaries, "collections of animals with human features," the creatures' lives being allegories for human nature and destiny. The authors of fables with moral overtones used the alleged character traits of animal species to convey their message.

The science of "ordering" or classifying the world of living things, at least those visible to "the naked eye," began during the seventeenth century. By 1608 Edward Topsell had produced a tome entitled *The Historie of Foure-Footed Beasts and of Serpents* (second edition, 1658) placing animals in alphabetical order, a meaningless approach from any viewpoint except encyclopedic location. His work was based on the Swiss Konrad Gessner's (1516-1565) *Historia Animalium,* a great five-volume work that was produced from 1551 to 1587 and did not appear in completed form until twenty-two years after his death. Gessner's work is remarkable for its historical compass of animals in ancient literature, not for its taxonomic value. The two authors, consequentially, described many alleged creatures drawn from earlier mythological ideas and writings. Topsell, a clergyman, urged that his book be read on Sunday because knowledge about beasts was "divine"; he drew upon chapters of the Book of Genesis, which stated that the four-footed animals were created immediately before humans. An unusual index in his book listed diseases that could be cured by medicines of animal origin. Pierre Belon (1517-1564), a keen dissector and traveler, made a greater contribution to taxonomy in his works on natural history of aquatic forms, in which he showed that dolphins have mammary glands, and in *The History and Nature of Birds* (1555), in which he made detailed comparisons between the skeletons of birds and humans, a magnificent beginning of comparative anatomy. Another Frenchman, Guillaume Rondelet (1507-1566) of Montpelier, created a great comparative encyclopedic treatise, the Latin text of which appeared in English in 1588 as *The Complete History of Fish.*

Clergyman John Wilkins, one of England's most interesting scholars, became caught in the web of power politics after helping to dispel the constraining webs of an old order. Oxford University had to be purged of Royalist "malignants" after the Civil War. Having been chaplain to one of the leaders in Parliament under the Commonwealth, Wilkins became warden of Wadham College, Oxford, and attracted a remarkable team of scholars, including Boyle, Hooke, and Wren. He married Oliver Cromwell's sister and was appointed to the high office of Master of Trinity College, Cambridge. Unhappily, this was shortly before the restoration of King Charles II to the throne in 1660; hence Cromwell's Royalist predecessor was restored to office and Wilkins lost his job. He became a bishop, however, and ironically was the key figure behind the creation of the Royal Society of London (established 1660), of which he became the first secretary. Thus he played a significant role in establishing high intellectual standards for British science and greatly influenced the aspirations of the health professions.

Wilkins was a remarkable reformer who deplored the departure of the learned world from a common language, Latin, into the use of vernacular languages that resulted from the rise of nation-states and wars between religious groups. He sought a new, universal international language such as the language of mathematical symbols. With the goal of a pictographic language in which the symbols stood for recognizable things, he urged experts in natural history to help prepare the ground. John Ray (1627-1705) was selected for botany, and the marine biologist Francis Willughby for zoology. The result was the book *A Real Character* (1668) by Wilkins. Later books on classification were produced by Ray, who edited Willughby's works, *De Historica Piscium* and *Ornithology,* after his death in 1672, and wrote the synopsis *Methodica,* which contained volumes on mammals and serpents (1693), insects (1710), and birds and fish (1713).

The English medical scholar Sir Thomas Browne (1605-1682) performed a valuable service in writing *Pseudodoxia Epidemica* ("*Vulgar Errors*"), which attacked the allegorical approach to zoology, exposing the credulity of authors who had imparted human qualities and traits to animals. He also distinguished between "common farriers" and "good veterinarians." Browne was a member of the Royal Society. The birth of academic societies in Italy, Britain, and France in the seventeenth century brought new standards and aspirations to the scientific community. Journals appeared, and the "scientific paper" was created as the vehicle for distribution and communication of scholarship.

The dominant personality in zoology during the second half of the eighteenth century was George Leclerc, Comte de Buffon (1707-1788), known as Buffon, keeper of the royal garden in Paris (which became Le Jardin des Plantes) and author of the impressive, encyclopedic *Natural History, General and Particular* in forty-four volumes (1749-1804), the last eight appearing posthumously. His narratives were augmented by Louis Daubenton's (1716-1800) anatomical descriptions. Daubenton thought that all animals should be compared on the basis of their organs. Rather than using the morphological approach taken by Linnaeus in his *System of Nature,* Buffon defined "species" as a population capable of interbreeding, that is, on a basis of interfertility.

Buffon was born in Montbard, Burgundy, in 1707 to a noble family. He traveled in Europe with Lord Kingston, a scholar of natural science, and accompanied him to England, where he studied for a year during the exciting period when Newton, Ray, and Hales were active. On Buffon's return to France he published translations of Newton's *Fluxions* and Hales' *Vegetable Staticks,* two trailblazing works. He was made an associate of the French Academy of Sciences in 1739 and obtained substantial support for his researches from King Louis XV. Eventually he was made a count and a full

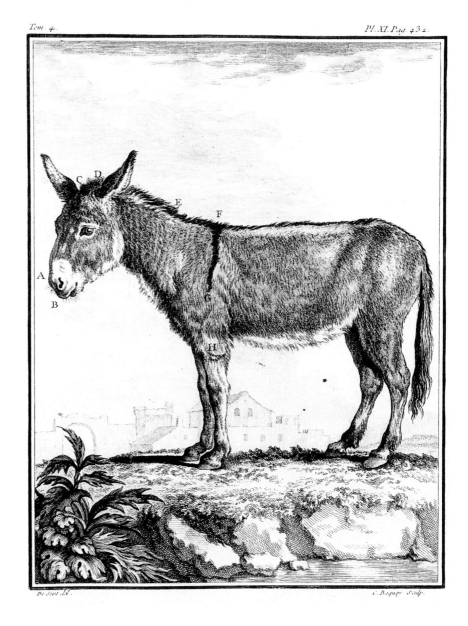

269. *The Ass,* from George Leclerc, Comte de Buffon (1707-1788), *Histoire Naturelle,* Paris (1749-1804). Buffon was a controversial figure in the mid-eighteenth century because of his theories that there were no large animals in America and that the stock was far inferior to European stock. *(Special Collections, Smithsonian Institution Libraries, Washington, D.C.)*

member of the academy. Buffon's work was controversial; he pricked American pride by stating that there were no really large animals there and that their animals had degenerated in comparison with those of Europe. The latter speculation also got him in trouble with theologians because it implied that species had changed since the creation.

Felix Vicq d'Azyr (1748-1794) combined Daubenton's comparative anatomy with Haller's comparative physiology in a penetrating focus on comparative organ structure and function of birds and quadrupeds. A physician who helped found the Royal Society of Medicine (Paris), he was asked to help control epidemic diseases of humans and animals and made several contributions to veterinary science. He drew attention to the adaptations of structure and function in the competition among life-forms. Vicq d'Azyr was among the first to describe the convolutions and sulci of the brain and discovered the lamination of the cortex. He produced an illustrated atlas of the brain, studied the flexor and extensor muscles of animal limbs, and described the vocal cords.

MORGAGNI: FOUNDER OF ANATOMICAL PATHOLOGY

The role of postmortem examination or necropsy in advancing understanding of disease was first addressed systematically by Giovanni Battista Morgagni (1682-1771), professor of theoretical medicine, then of anatomy, at Padua. His seminal work, *De Sedibus et Causis Morborum per Anatomen Indagatis (On the*

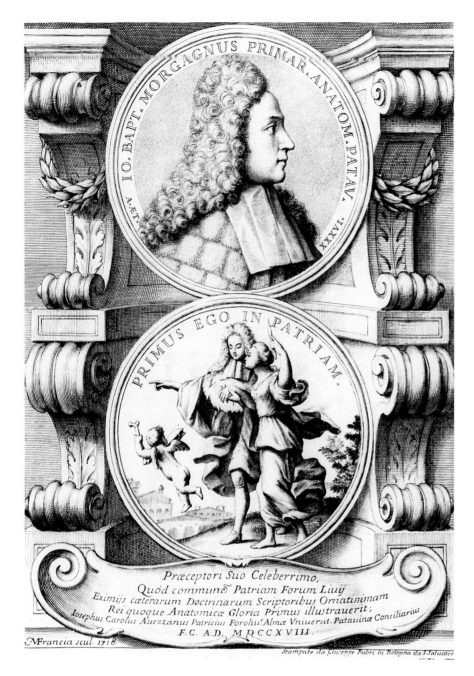

270. Giovanni Battista Morgagni's (1682-1771) monumental *De Sedibus et Causis Morborum per Anatomen Indagatis* (1761) was a collection of seven hundred cases describing patients' medical histories, clinical signs, and necropsy findings. He augmented his theories on pathogenesis with animal experiments. This approach had a tremendous impact on veterinary medicine by providing a systematic way of diagnosing disease before and after death. Morgagni's *Ubi Est Morbus? (Where is the disease?)* prompted research throughout Europe in animal as well as human diseases. *(New York Academy of Medicine, New York.)*

Seats and Causes of Disease Investigated by Anatomy), was published in 1761, a year before the first veterinary school opened. A medical student in Bologna, Morgagni worked with Antonio Valsalva before going into practice in his hometown of Forli. A professor by the age of twenty-nine, he came to occupy at thirty-three years of age the chair made so famous by Vesalius. He communicated his many observations to colleagues by letter. At the age of seventy-nine, he published his great work in five books. Quite remarkable in its almost Socratic style, it is presented as seventy letters describing seven hundred case histories, purportedly written over thirty years in scholarly Latin prose to a young gentleman much given to the study of the sciences and medicine. It was translated into English by Benjamin Alexander in 1769.

The approach in Morgagni's letters was to describe the patient's medical history and clinical signs, then the gross necropsy findings, with great clarity; a clinicopathological correlation followed. Morgagni conducted animal experiments to support his dynamic view of pathogenesis. He was the first to correlate the clinical signs of neurological disease with the anatomical disorders of the brain and the first to describe accurately lesions of the heart valves, syphilitic aneurysm, cirrhosis of the liver, tuberculosis of the meninges and of the kidney, and the Stokes-Adams syndrome. His work led to the nosological approach of systematic pathology, that is, the identification and classification of diseases. The five books were *Diseases of the Head, Diseases of the Thorax, Diseases of the Belly, Surgical and Universal Disorders,* and a supplement with indices. The enormous value of his approach to the progress of veterinary science cannot be overestimated. Specific diagnoses of animal diseases in life and after death became possible, culminating in the superb work by Hutyra and Marek on the clinicopathology of animal diseases in Budapest in the nineteenth century.

Matthew Baillie's (1761-1823) *Morbid Anatomy of Some of the Most Important Parts of the Body* (1794 and 1797), focused on clinicopathological correlation. Baillie married John Hunter's sister and later inherited the Great Windmill Street School, the famous private medical school and London's first medical school (1767) founded by John Hunter's distinguished brother William Hunter. It closed in 1833.

John Abernathy (1764-1831), a pupil of John Hunter who became a charismatic surgeon at St. Bartholomew's Hospital in London, was so popular as a lecturer that a medical school was established at "Bart's." He analyzed "tumors" and separated the swellings resulting from blood, pus, or other fluids from those resulting from true growths of adventitious tissue. He recommended classification of tumors by their anatomical structure and provided an example by listing eight types of sarcoma.

Marie Francois Xavier Bichat (1771-1802) of the Jura, an army surgeon during the French Revolution, was appointed to the famous "Hotel Dieu" in Paris at twenty-eight years of age without a medical degree. A brilliant anatomist, he was the first to use the term "tissues" in the modern sense and insisted that pathological changes affect cellular tissues rather than organs, identifying twenty-one different types. His original approach brought a new logic to the thinking about disease and contributed to the ultimate demise of the theory of four humors. He was a leader in pathophysiological reasoning. His focus on elemental tissues rather than complex organs set the stage for Virchow's later view that the cell was the fundamental unit to be studied. Also, Bichat expressed the view that all tissues have the capacity of independent growth and that cancer is a rebellious overgrowth of a specific tissue that leads to malignancy. He died young of an infection contracted in the dissection room.

LINNAEUS: THE ORDERING OF TAXONOMY

The master of biological classification was the botanist Carolus Linnaeus (1707-1778), or after his entry into the nobility of Sweden, Carl von Linne. He produced three systems of classification—for plants, animals, and minerals. Educated at Lund and Uppsala, he developed a passion for botany and a keen interest in classifying plants on the basis of their sexual organs. He was appointed to develop a flora of Lapland in 1732, a role that required him to travel throughout northern Scandinavia. During his survey he studied animals, too, and showed that reindeer run in fear of a fly that deposits its eggs in the skin; the larvae migrate to the sinuses to complete their life cycle as head grubs before forming the adult fly. He named several other parasites of domestic animals.

Linnaeus trained in medicine at Harderwijk, Holland, before going to the academic mecca of Leyden University, where he spent three extremely productive years, the outcomes including *The Genera of Plants* (1737) and the classic *System of Nature* (1735). The latter set out his proposition for the way to classify natural things in eight large sheets of tables, which he enlarged and improved in later editions. The last (tenth) edition in 1758 had an earthshaking impact. It put forward his two-name system in which a genus name is followed by a species name, for example, *Canis lupus* for the wolf. This idea literally swept the world in its adoption. In his lifetime he classified 5897 species.

271. Carolus Linnaeus (1707-1778), the progenitor of the binomial system of naming plants and animals. *(Universitets-bibliotheket, Uppsala.)*

Linnaeus became professor of botany at Uppsala, where he established a magnificent botanical garden and remained until his death. He was an ardent supporter of the goal of training individuals in animal medicine: one of his protégés was destined to found Sweden's first veterinary school with his active promotion.

ALEXANDER VON HUMBOLDT'S DEFINITION OF BASIC BIOGEOGRAPHY

Exploration of the world by sea, which included scientific objectives, had an enormous impact on the arousal of intellectual curiosity and the development of geological, geographical, and biological knowledge. Joseph Banks (1743-1820), the botanist who accompanied Captain James Cook on his famous voyages to the Pacific and Australasia, became influential as president of the Royal Society for forty years. Georg Foster (1754-1794), the naturalist on one of Cook's voyages, met the young Berliner Alexander von Humboldt (1769-1859) at the University of Göttingen. Foster captivated him with tales of his experiences, took him on a tour of Europe, and introduced him to Banks. Humboldt determined to become a scientific explorer and prepared himself by studying geology at Freiberg in the Academy of Mines, where the director, Abraham Werner, expounded the sedimentary theory of rock formation. (This theory was disputed by James Hutton at Edinburgh University, who insisted that rocks were formed by volcanic heat, as witnessed during the eruption of Vesuvius.) Humboldt was at first indoctrinated in Werner's "Neptunist" views but became more convinced that Hutton's theory had relevance after seeing the landscapes of South America with his own eyes.

Humboldt was destined to mingle with great individuals from all walks of intellectual life. He knew the German poet-scientist Johann von Goethe (1749-1832), having met him for the first time when he was twenty-five years old and Goethe was forty-five. When the French Revolution occurred, Humboldt was twenty years old. He was later sent to Paris and settled there during a difficult time after Napoleon's conquest of Prussia.

Humboldt developed his biological interests. He had published a flora at the age of twenty-four and made four thousand experiments on animal electricity, which were published as *Experiments on the Excited Muscle and Nerve Fiber* in 1797. He also conducted meteorological observations in the Tyrol and geological studies in central Spain. Clearly a great polymath was in the making when Humboldt realized his dream of exploring South America. In 1799 he obtained permission to visit the Spanish colonies there and jumped at the chance. Accompanied by his dearest friend and colleague, the botanist Aimé Bonpland, he embarked on a five-year exploration of Mexico, Cuba, and the northwest quadrant of South America. Well grounded in the earth sciences, botany, and physiology and driven by an insatiable curiosity, Humboldt and this voyage of discovery were to become the model for Charles Darwin's voyage on the *Beagle* from 1831 to 1836. These two men and their feats have had an enormous impact on the advancement of human thought.

The energy Humboldt and Bonpland poured into their scientific expedition was phenomenal. The two men collected 60,000 plant specimens. Humboldt learned from South American Indians how to make their paralytic arrow poison and brought the drug curare to Europe for medical science; he also brought cinchona bark for quinine. The travelers located the Casiquiare Canal, which links the headwaters of the Orinoco and Amazon rivers. They discovered the unique night-flying oilbird, which nests in caves and picks an oily tree fruit in the dark to feed its obese young.

While traveling on the corvette Pizarro, the crew was forced by a typhoid epidemic on the ship to land at Cumana in Venezuela. The scientists went to Caracas, then explored the highlands to the south, crossing over to the valley

272. *Following pages,* Alexander von Humboldt (1769-1859) and his traveling companion, the botanist Aimé Bonpland. During their travels to Mexico, Cuba, and South America they collected tens of thousands of plant specimens and conducted numerous studies. Their achievements in natural history were forerunners for Charles Darwin's later voyage aboard the *Beagle.* *(Berlin-Brandenburgische Akademie der Wissenschaften, Berlin.)*

309

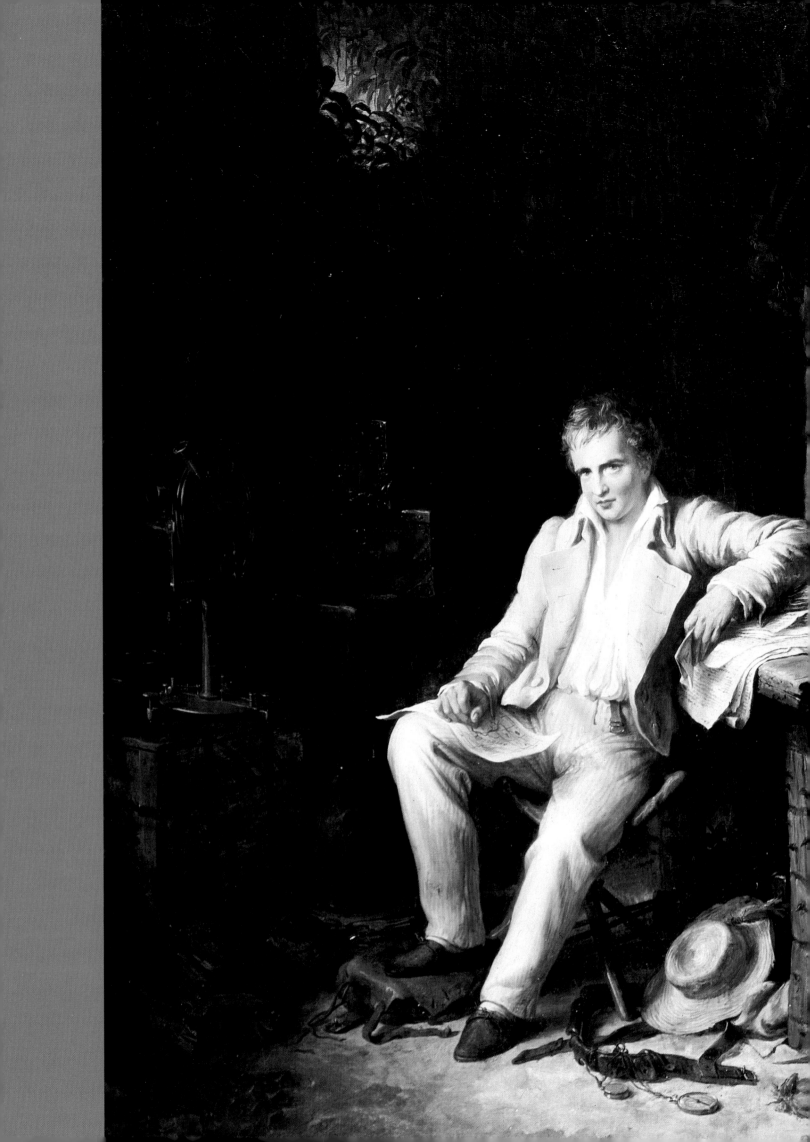

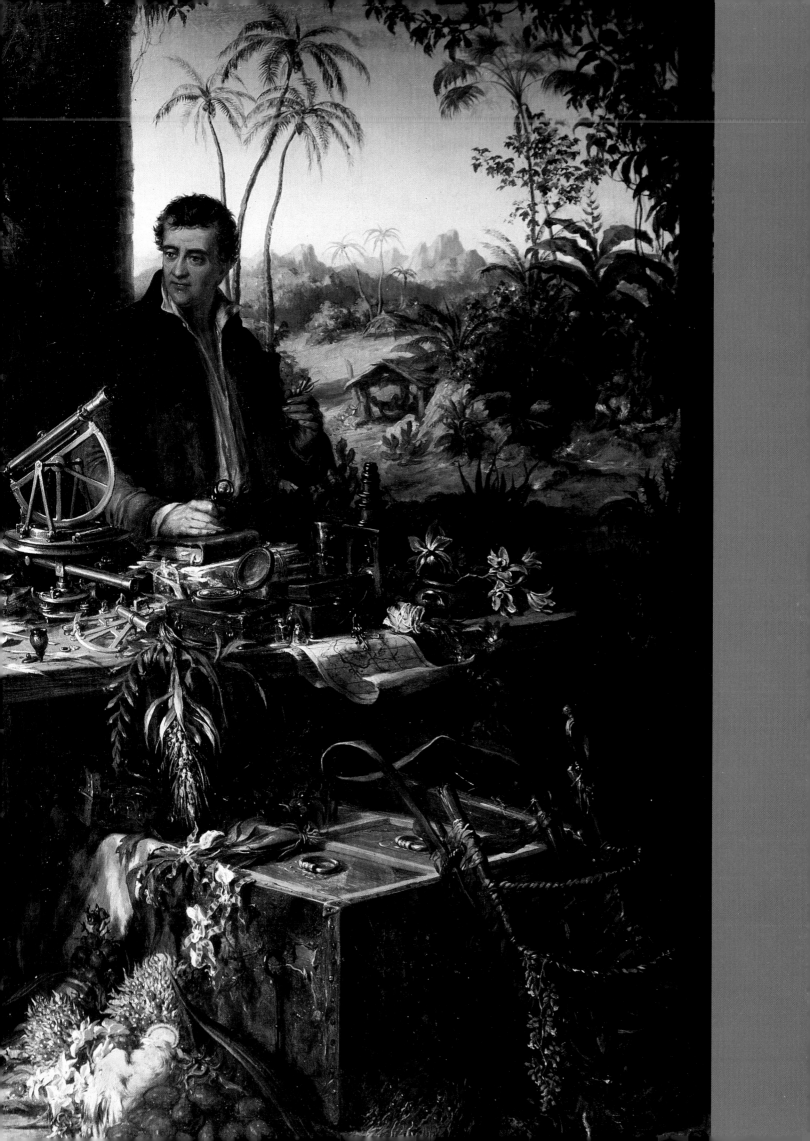

273. Illustration of the oilbird, the "fat bird of Caripe." Discovered by Humboldt in a cave near Caripe, the oilbird is uniquely nocturnal, picking oily tree fruit for its young until they weigh more than one hundred percent of their adult weight. *(Natural History Museum, London.)*

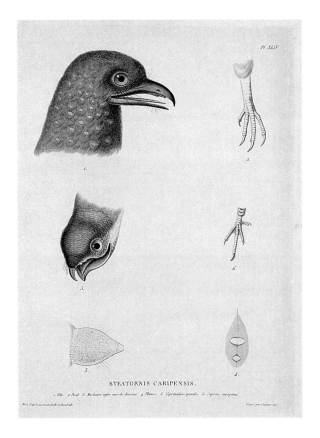

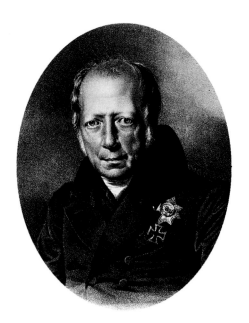

274. Portrait of Wilhelm Humboldt (1767-1835), the eldest brother of Alexander von Humboldt. The leader in reforming German universities after the Napoleonic Wars, Wilhelm was instrumental in establishing the University of Berlin in 1810. He and his brother Alexander had a profound impact on the development of veterinary schools in Germany. *(Bildarchiv Preußischer Kulturbesitz, Berlin.)*

of the Orinoco River. Leaving their Venezuelan collections in Cuba, they sailed to Cartagena, Colombia, and then set out for Bogota, where Bonpland fell ill. After he regained his health, they made their way to Quito, climbing to within 500 meters of the summit of the great Mount Chimborazo (6269 meters). They journeyed on to Lima, where Humboldt collected seabird guano, which proved to be extremely valuable much later, after Liebig had shown the importance of phosphate as a fertilizer. From Lima they set sail for Mexico, where they spent a year exploring before returning to Cuba to pick up the specimens and recrossing the Atlantic to Europe.

Humboldt's observations expanded his overview of nature and led him to examine the basis of biogeography. His ideas were forerunners of the great conceptions of Darwin and A.R. Wallace (1823-1913) about the evolution of living things by natural selection. Both these men were enthusiastic followers of Humboldt and both engaged in biogeographical studies and considerations. Humboldt was an exceptional observer and recorder of the physical environment. His mountaineering exploits allowed him to correlate the effects of altitude and temperature on the distribution of plant species. He also observed the destruction of forests by settlers and forecast long-term climatic consequences of such actions. His oceanic temperature recordings along the Pacific coast allowed him to demonstrate the northwardly flowing Peruvian cold current, known as the Humboldt current. The breadth of his interests made Humboldt the forefather of the science known as ecology.

Humboldt returned to Europe in 1804. En route he received accolades from the American Philosophical Society in Philadelphia and advised President Jefferson in Washington on territorial issues. His native Prussia, however, was in grave crisis. Napoleon invaded and occupied Berlin. Humboldt was sent to Paris as a key member of the Prussian delegation, and he made Paris his home for two decades. He published more than thirty volumes on his South American explorations, including *Personal Narrative*.

Recalled to Berlin, Humboldt lectured to huge crowds on the scientific and integrated understanding of nature and sounded the death knell of Hegel's romantic, antiscientific philosophy. He published his lectures in a five-volume set called *Kosmos*.

Humboldt's only major exploration other than the five-year voyage came when the Russian czar sought his advice on mining the Ural Mountains in 1829. He used his geological knowledge to locate diamonds and converted this opportunity into a massive adventure that took him across Siberia to the Altai Mountains and the Chinese border, returning via a look at the Caspian Sea. He added to his global studies of temperature and magnetism. He was able to persuade many nations to set up global observation stations for gathering geophysical data, to advance understanding of phenomena at the planetary level.

The impact Humboldt had on higher education was profound. He had had the good fortune to attend one of Europe's most enlightened universities, Göttingen, established in 1737 by the Hannoverian royal family that at that time ruled both England and Hannover. An academy of sciences was soon established in the city, and an outstanding academic center resulted. After the devastation of the Napoleonic Wars, German universities underwent reform spearheaded by Alexander von Humboldt's older brother Wilhelm (1767-1835). The model chosen was Göttingen: the primary task of the university should be to develop individual character; rather than follow the tradition of rote learning, professors should explore topics with the students and the focus should be on the search for new knowledge. While minister of education in Prussia, Wilhelm was able to implement these ideas by establishing the University of Berlin in 1810, which soon showed the power of his educational philosophy and was named after the brothers. Science, teaching, and research thrust Germany into the forefront of international academia and graduate training for research to the doctorate level, establishing the model for the modern research university.

Alexander von Humboldt died in the very year that Darwin's *Origin of Species* was published. He would have approved of its author and the great idea of evolution. He was a strong supporter of the establishment of veterinary schools in Germany and used his influence at the highest levels to promote their ideas.

GEORGE STUBBS: ANIMAL ARTIST AND EARLY EQUINE ANATOMIST

George Stubbs (1724-1806), son of a Liverpool currier, had a predilection for art from childhood and worked at it full-time from the age of fifteen years. An independent spirit and largely self-taught, Stubbs painted portraits in northern England for thirteen years. He traveled to Rome when he was thirty years old to evaluate the aesthetic doctrine that nature is inferior to art and returned convinced of its inaccuracy. While living in York (1745-1752), Stubbs worked with a surgeon to study equine anatomy and illustrated a book on midwifery. He moved to an isolated farmhouse in North Lincolnshire (Horkstow) for a year of intense anatomical studies of the horse, a gruesome exercise. He obtained horses, bled them to death, injected them with preservatives, and carried them upstairs to his studio on the second floor, where he dissected them and drew, from nature, the anatomical arrangements. As the bodies rotted, he replaced them. He exhibited his anatomical drawings, which led to commissions. In 1766 the drawings were published in *The Anatomy of the Horse*. His superb anatomical work, depicting the skeleton and its motivating muscles in their dynamic relationship in life, contained eighteen plates. He did not, however, attempt to depict the thoracic and abdominal viscera.

Stubbs' drawings were the most artistic of all those of animal anatomists. With his gifted pencil he was somehow able to convey the life force to his representations of the dead tissues of his dissected specimens. In his paintings of horses, however, he perpetuated errors about the movements of the four limbs in gaits, which were not corrected until the serial photographic studies

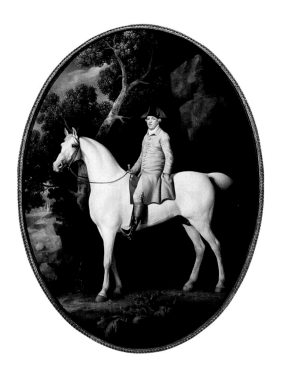

of Muybridge appeared more than a century later. After forty-five years of painting animal and sporting scenes, including some of the greatest paintings of horses and dogs ever made, he returned to a work on comparative anatomy, which he was unable to complete, at the end of his life.

George Stubbs was aware of the new veterinary school at Lyon and wrote:

> *As for Farriers and Horse Doctors, the Veterinary School lately established in France shows what importance this profession is held in that country . . . they have frequent opportunities of dissecting and many of them have considerable skill in anatomy.*

Of his own anatomical work he commented, "If what I have done may in any sort facilitate or promote so necessary a study amongst them I shall think my labour well bestowed."

275. *George Stubbs, Self Portrait on Horseback* (1782). The actual identity of this portrait was not confirmed until 1957, when it became the third known self-portrait of Stubbs. It was originally thought to be of Josiah Wedgewood I, Charles Darwin's maternal grandfather. *(Board of Trustees of the National Museums and Galleries on Merseyside. Lady Lever Art Gallery, Port Sunlight, Cheshire.)*

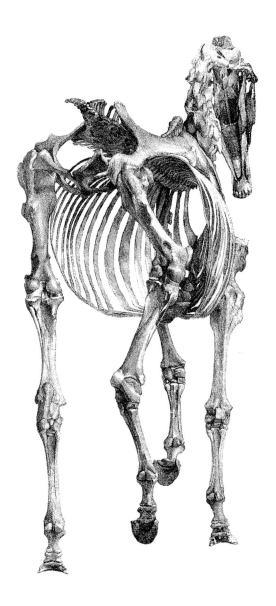

276. George Stubbs (1724-1806) was a superb artistic anatomist. This engraving, *Second Skeleton Plate*, was done by Stubbs himself from his own anatomical studies of the horse and was published in his book, *The Anatomy of the Horse*, London (1766). *(National Library of Medicine, Bethesda, Maryland.)*

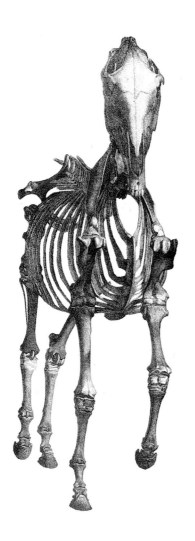

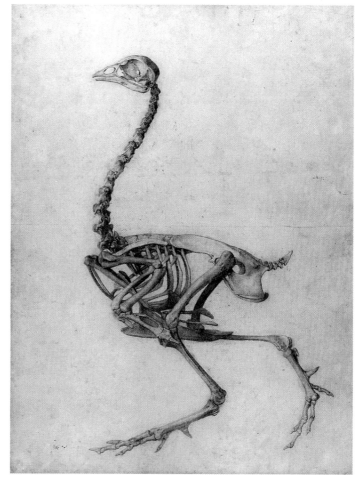

278. *Right, Table V, Fowl Skeleton, Lateral View* from George Stubbs, *A Comparative Anatomical Exposition of the Human Body With That of a Tiger and Common Fowl,* London (1804–1806). Originally the work was to consist of thirty tables, but Stubbs completed only fifteen during his life. The work was published posthumously by Edward Orme in 1817. *(Yale Center for British Art, New Haven, Connecticut.)*

JOHN HUNTER'S DEFINITION OF COMPARATIVE MEDICAL SCIENCE

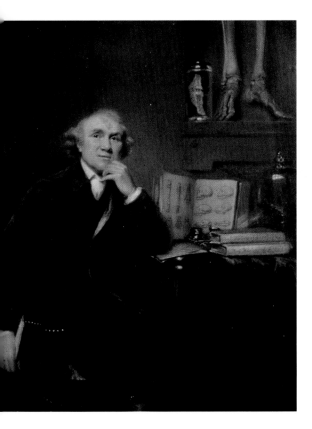

279. *Portrait of John Hunter* by Sir Joshua Reynolds (1786). Hunter (1728-1793), a London surgeon, was the most important visionary of the comparative approach to medical studies. He transformed surgery into an intellectually challenging field based on experimental science, including research on inflammation and wound healing in dogs. *(Royal College of Surgeons of England, London.)*

John Hunter (1728-1793), son of a poor Scottish farmer, orphaned early and lacking good education, went to London at twenty years of age to work with his distinguished elder brother William, a surgeon and anatomist. There John Hunter's inherent intellectual potential took the spark and became a flame that never dimmed. He became London's leading surgeon but never lost his fascination with all things anatomical and physiological. His commitment to curiosity and investigation was total, and he became the leading scholar of comparative anatomy, developing a remarkable museum. His original work on the origin, growth, and diseases of the teeth allowed the then lowly dentists to become scientifically based professionals. After years of dissection and work as house surgeon at St. George's Hospital his health suffered, so in 1760, two months after the French surrendered to the British in North America, he enrolled as an army surgeon in the Seven Years' War for a change of air. He gained experience in military medicine and pursued studies of marine organisms with a passion.

Edward Jenner was John Hunter's favorite pupil and lived in Hunter's house for several years. Hunter urged him to "try the experiment" when Jenner floated his idea about using cowpox matter as a vaccine against smallpox. The medical museum at St. George's has part of the hide of Blossom, the cow from which Jenner's dairymaid Sarah Nelmes contracted cowpox. From Sarah he first obtained the infective material he used in his vaccine.

The framework of thought and the process of scientific inquiry matured in the eighteenth century under outstanding intellectual leaders. The earlier trailblazers such as Harvey and Paré had not found a favorable mental environment and had frequently been blocked by naysayers. In Hunter's time the "neural substrates" were more receptive. He was an unorthodox visionary who became the greatest medical naturalist. He transformed the profession of surgery from one requiring only bold dexterity with little regard for the outcome into an intellectually challenging field rooted in experimental science and concerned about the patient's survival.

Hunter proposed that a predisposition to cancer exists in the surrounding tissues before a tumor appears. Consequently he stressed that the surgeon should remove not only the tumor in its entirety but also some of the surrounding tissues "in which a diseased disproportion may probably have been excited." He loved the outdoors, and his ecological curiosity was insatiable. Driven by an inner need to know, he adored dissection, acquiring every rare specimen he could get and keeping many of them in a den and stables at his home, from bees and silkworms to waterfowl, buffalo, and leopards. When the debate about animal electricity was raging, he was asked to dissect a torpedo ("causes torpor") fish, which has the capacity to deliver electric shocks. He showed that the fish had two electric organs, each several inches long and composed of 470 perpendicular columns supplied by nerves arising from three extraordinarily large trunks that emerge from the rear of the brain.

After rupturing his own Achilles tendon, Hunter conducted experiments in dogs, severing the tendon via a tiny hole in the skin, then demonstrating for the first time that tendons heal by means of a scarring process. He undertook the first serious study of inflammation, concluding that it was not a disease but a salutary response often leading to a cure and that only when unable to effect a cure does it cause mischief. His experiments on gunshot wounds were classic. His inductive approach to experimentation led him to the successful transplantation of tissues: he implanted the spurs of a young cockerel into the comb and its testicles into a body cavity. Even a human tooth grew in a cock's comb after he implanted it there. He performed the first recorded, successful artificial insemination in humans. He was the first to demonstrate the development of collateral circulation after obstruction of the arterial supply, using as the model the antlers of a young stag.

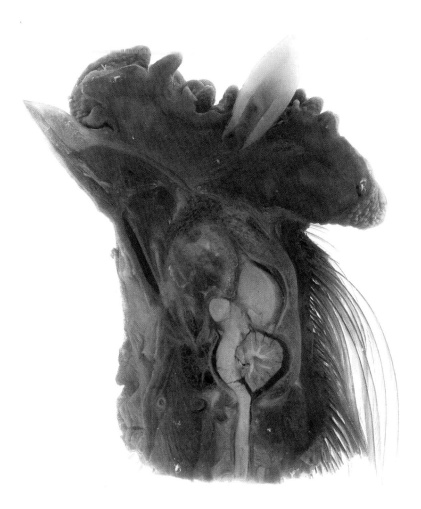

280. Section of the head of a cock into which a freshly extracted tooth was implanted by John Hunter. The cock was killed some months afterward, and the head injected to show the blood vessels of the comb penetrating the tooth. Hunter observed that:

> . . . the external surface of the fang adhered everywhere to the comb by vessels similar to the union of a tooth with the gums and sockets.

(Royal College of Surgeons of England, London.)

Hunter was a great collector, acquiring more than 14,000 animal specimens. Twelve years after he died, his collection was purchased for the nation as a museum of the Royal College of Surgeons. Hunter's museum was designed to serve as a basis for instruction in comparative anatomy, experimental pathology, and surgery, providing real-world examples of the themes he expounded. Tragically, a large part of it was destroyed in German air raids on London in 1941. Hunter's brother-in-law and executor, Sir Everard Home, disgracefully destroyed all Hunter's notebooks and manuscripts in 1823, having published under his own name many of the findings.

Hunter was a prime mover in promoting the goal of a comparative medicine for the treatment of animals. He lent his weight to a plan that resulted in the establishment of Britain's first veterinary school in 1791 and encouraged the young surgeon William Moorcroft to go to France for training. Moorcraft became England's first veterinary surgeon to be trained in a veterinary school.

Benjamin Brodie of Winterslow, one of Hume's pupils, followed Bichat in early studies of autonomic physiology of animals before becoming a skillful surgeon of diseased joints and varicose veins. Brodie studied anatomy under John Abernathy (1764-1831), who was John Hunter's successor and who founded St. Bartholomew's medical school (Bart's). True to the Hunterian legacy, Brodie's interests ranged from anatomy, physiology, and pathology to the quest for understanding any surgical intervention. He took over the surgical practice of Astley Cooper, who chaired the board of the Royal Veterinary College. Brodie became president of the Royal College of Surgeons and of the Royal Society. Also, he was the foundation president of the General Medical Council, which was empowered to control medical practice under the Medical Act of 1858. This recognition of wisdom attests to the importance of John Hunter's broad interests in the evolution of the health professions.

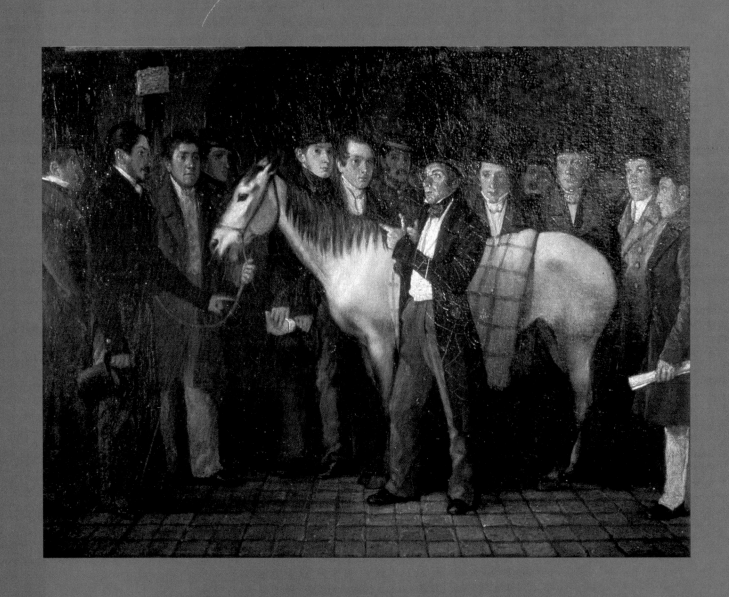

The Launching of European Veterinary Education

RATIONALE FOR A VETERINARY PROFESSION

The study of animal medicine should have accompanied the development of human medicine in Europe from its earliest roots at Salerno. On a few occasions in history individuals such as Apsyrtos in fourth-century Byzantium and Ruffus in the thirteenth century had begun to provide a framework for a veterinary profession, but their efforts were not sustained. These early attempts derived primarily from the authorities' preoccupation with striving for military superiority, which required that their horses be kept healthy or be repaired if they were not. Similar motives were at work in the modern era, when the time finally arrived for the veterinary profession to be reborn. Two were identified repeatedly: the need for better equine medicine and the high costs of repeated agricultural crises created by recurrent epidemics of cattle plague accompanied by high mortality rates. The plethora of less dramatic diseases of livestock received little attention.

The seventeenth-century medical thinker Thomas Sydenham (1624-1689) emphasized the importance of detailed observation in the study of disease. He stated that "all diseases could be described as natural history." Like Hippocrates, he insisted that nature left alone and unimpeded terminates many illnesses without any medicines at all. He was a friend of the influential British philosopher John Locke (1632-1704), who wrote the *Essay Concerning Human Understanding*. Locke was also a physician and was interested in science. He assisted Richard Lower in physiological experiments and studied chemistry, botany, and medicine. He compensated for his lack of clinical knowledge by serving an apprenticeship with Sydenham to "fill the gaps." Locke also worked with Boyle on studies of air and blood. During an extensive tour of Europe (from 1676 to 1679) Locke kept a journal and made numerous notes on all veterinary treatments that he encountered; his journal is now a valuable record of the practices and superstitions of the day. He believed in natural rights and the sovereignty of the people. His philosophy had a profound impact on liberal individualistic thought. He contended that critical reason, modeled on the procedures of natural science, could be applied with benefit to defective social institutions, thereby to diminish the suffering that humanity had imposed on itself by ignorance, sloth, and a lack of intellectual courage. He surmised that ideas arise from sensations and that the mind processes the ideas into abstract forms but that care must be used in expressing them in language, since this step is prone to error. Locke's psychology complemented Newton's (1642-1727) brilliant physics and led to the analysis of Immanuel Kant (1724-1804), who even dared to explain metaphysics. Voltaire spent three years in England and brought to France an overview of the great achievements being made there.

281. *Facing page,* Tzt. Dr. med. Anton Hayne (1786-1853) is lecturing to his students and colleagues at the Veterinär-medizinische Universität Wien in this painting. Founded in 1767 as a school, veterinary medicine achieved university status in 1908 and was granted the same rights and privileges as other Austrian universities in 1920. Professor Hayne was a well-respected member of the Vienna veterinary school, and the veterinary students who had received their diplomas in 1834 wished to present a group picture to their beloved professor as a souvenir. Hayne, an excellent painter in his own right, recommended the painter Anton Neder for the commission. Reminiscent of Dutch and Flemish guild paintings, Neder's composition portrays an appropriate scene in a clinic stall with Hayne, surrounded by students, standing next to a small, thin white horse. He appears to be counting off on his fingers the horse's symptoms in arriving at a clear diagnosis. The nine veterinarians who commissioned the painting can be found in the composition. *(Courtesy o. Univ. Prof. Dr. Peter F. Knezevic, Veterinärmedizinische Universität Wien.)*

CHANGES IN ATTITUDES ABOUT ANIMAL DISEASE: THE NEW RATIONALISM

Locke was in many ways a precursor to the Enlightenment, a movement of thought that rejected the idea of authority as guarantor of truth. Instead, it insisted that the realms of religion, politics, morality, and social life should all be subjected to the scrutiny of reason. Rooted in the scientific "revolution" of the seventeenth century and the new liberal philosophy, the Enlightenment was international but became centered in France in the eighteenth century, where the leaders were the "philosophes," the lettered individuals of Paris. Diderot and d'Alembert had been commissioned to produce a comprehensive encyclopedia in the French language, and a group developed who became known as the Encyclopedists. The group involved 139 authors in this massive task and used the grassroots approach of the Enlightenment, departing from orthodoxy in favor of factual and rational treatises. The work, which required twenty-one years to complete (from 1751 to 1772) and produced seventeen volumes, was extremely controversial and unorthodox, trampling on the toes of established authority on many topics.

The authors included Montesquieu *(Persian Letters* and *Del'Esprit des Lois),* Jean-Jacques Rousseau *(The Social Contract* and *Discourse on the Origins of Inequality),* and Voltaire *(Candide).* The Enlightenment of the Encyclopedists gradually accumulated principles and values with which many people who considered themselves well-informed, progressive, and unprejudiced agreed because they regarded them as self-evident truths. Thus the Enlightenment, as a living, mutable, maturing body of thought that could help point the way ahead, became a major intellectual force in society. It was ended by the French Revolution of 1789, which adopted some of its thinkers as heroes.

Julian Offroy de la Mettrie (1709-1751) studied medicine in Paris and at Leyden with Boerhaave. He translated Boerhaave's works into French and fell into disfavor with the unenlightened Parisian faculty, much as Vesalius and Harvey had at an earlier time. La Mettrie came under attack when his controversial book *The Natural History of the Soul* appeared. He went back to Leyden, where he published *L'Homme Machine* (1748), a satire on the medical profession that got him into trouble even in Holland, where attitudes were hardening as the economy faltered. He moved away to seek the protection of one of his admirers, Frederick II of Prussia, in Berlin. He died young of food poisoning. He had been the most extreme and provocative of the reformers.

Before the Revolution the Enlightenment had an extraordinary impact on literate, thoughtful individuals in society, albeit only a small percentage of the population. It reset the intellectual climate to become one of questioning and expectation of change for the better by the application of reason in solving problems. At the same time there were attitudinal changes. Rousseau contributed a romantic perspective of rural life that raised the standing of agriculture and nature in the public eye. Given the lowly status of most people who worked with animals and the devastation of the repeated epidemics of cattle plague, the time was ripe for an attack on the unsatisfactory status and capability of animal medicine.

ROYAL SPONSORSHIP OF A VETERINARY SCHOOL IN FRANCE

King Louis XV had established a magnificent new military school in the middle of the eighteenth century, which inevitably heightened the emphasis on medical care for horses, including control of the dreaded glanders. Napoleon Bonaparte was a graduate of this school.

THE LAUNCHING OF EUROPEAN VETERINARY EDUCATION

The advance of sciences relevant to comparative medicine was another major preparative factor for a veterinary profession. Buffon, in his zoological description of the horse, had stated his perception of a need for a scientific medicine of animals:

> I cannot end the story of the horse without noting with regret that the health of this useful and precious animal has been up to now surrendered to the care and practice, often blind, of people without knowledge and without qualifications.

Cattle losses in France and Belgium as a result of cattle plague between 1713 and 1786 were estimated to have been about ten million. Rinderpest hit the Lyonnais region hard in 1744. As worry about its ravages mounted, the Academy of Sciences, acting on Buffon's advice, in 1745 named a commission composed of physicians, surgeons, and botanists to study the problem. It became (by decrees of 1748 and 1751) a permanent body, the Academy of Surgery. Thus the epizootics began to preoccupy public opinion and the administrative authorities, and the stage was set for a new approach. Coupled with the enormous losses of horses during the almost continuous wars of the preceding era, the terrifying losses of livestock that the authorities were powerless to check demoralized the countryside.

The rural crisis came at a time when the human death rate was declining rapidly in Europe and the population was expanding. This situation was tied to dramatic progress in agriculture, along with steady industrial and economic progress aided by growing trade between colonial empires and the great powers. The disparity between the progress in human health and the decline in ability to suppress animal epizootics became obvious.

France at the time was a victim of inexorable class laws and lacked the incentives that had developed in Great Britain for the advancement of agriculture and livestock improvement. The French peasants were still very much "the base of the pyramid," and their agriculture was the victim of disincentives and unjust taxation policies. Rousseau's famous comment, "Man is born free but everywhere he is in chains," echoed his view that humans were born good but were corrupted by society.

The king's controller-general, who had special responsibilities for agriculture, was Henri-Leonard-Jean-Baptiste Bertin (born 1719). Bertin had friendly relations with Claude Bourgelat, director of the Academy of Equitation in Lyon, who conceived the great idea of founding a school for the treatment of the diseases of livestock, especially horses. Bertin, who was devoted to the improvement of agriculture and wanted to find ways to attenuate the huge losses of livestock resulting from epidemics, obtained authorization for the world's first veterinary school to be established at Lyon under Bourgelat. Finally a decree of the Royal Council on August 4, 1761, awarded Claude Bourgelat a grant for the operation of a veterinary school at Lyon. The decree was signed by Lamoignon de Malesherbes and the controller-general. The wording of the document left no doubt that the goal of protection of farm livestock was the justification for the decision:

> . . . to open a school where would be taught publicly the principles and the method to cure the diseases of livestock that would procure imperceptibly for the agriculture of the Realm the power to conserve livestock in times where this epidemic desolates the countryside.

Later, in 1764, the school received a royal charter authorizing it to be renamed the Royal Veterinary School. L'Ecole Vétérinaire de Lyon became L'Ecole Royale Vétérinaire de Lyon. After the Revolution, when France became a republic, the "Royale" was dropped and all veterinary schools become L'Ecole Nationale Vétérinaire de . . . (Lyon and Alfort, and later Toulouse, then Nantes).

BOURGELAT: FOUNDER OF THE MODERN VETERINARY PROFESSION AT LYON

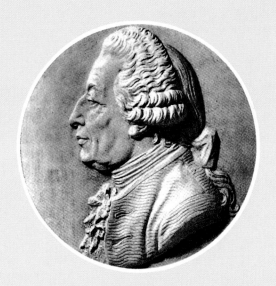

282. Relief profile of Claude Bourgelat (1712-1779), whose Academy of Equitation in Lyon became the world's first veterinary school in 1762. Bourgelat's influence led to the establishment of a second veterinary school at Charenton in 1765, which was soon moved to the Chateau d'Alfort in 1766. *(Edité par la Fondation Mérieux, Lyon.)*

Claude Bourgelat (1712-1779) was born at Lyon, France. His father was nicknamed "La Plume d'Or" ("the Golden Feather"), having been a sheriff in Lyon and a silk trader. Bourgelat was an excellent student under the Jesuits and studied law. He had a turbulent youth, being lazy, playful, and libertine although gifted with a strong intellect. It is said that he left the law when he won a case in which he knew that the client he defended was guilty, which he considered a gross injustice. He joined the army, where his special talent as a horseman capable of riding and breaking horses with the best became evident. He became an equerry. He was certified as officer in charge of l'Academie d'Equitation de Lyon in 1740, soon attaining fame for his cavalry training. Frederick the Great consulted him on the best gait to use in the charge. An ardent follower of the great trainers of horses and riders of the previous era, the Duke of Newcastle and Jacques de Solleysel, Bourgelat updated their works with *Nouveau Newcastle, or a New Treatise on Cavalry . . .* in 1744 and *Elemens d'Hippiatrique* in three volumes (1750-1753). In the latter set he indicated the necessity of creating schools to teach equine medicine. This thought reverberated in the European cultural and scientific establishments.

Bourgelat was active in intellectual affairs and was made a corresponding member of the Academy of Sciences of Paris in 1752 and of the Berlin Academy in 1763. Bourgelat considered all available works on hippiatry inadequate. He said, "It is only by studying the book of nature that we can acquire certain knowledge." Consequently he applied himself to the study of the anatomy of the horse and other domestic animals, then became familiar with the principles of human medicine with the intent of applying them to the study of animal medicine. He was assisted in this goal by two surgeons of Lyon.

Bourgelat was a friend of d'Alembert, who with Diderot was coeditor of the great *Encyclopedie* and had invited Bourgelat to write articles for it in 1755. He was even considered an Encyclopedist. Thus he was a contributor to the reformist movement of the Enlightenment. He tried to explain the functions of the animal body on a mechanical basis and apparently could become tedious in expounding on this theme. It is evident, however, that he was caught up in the stream of liberal scientific thought.

Bourgelat's genius lay in creating the first two European veterinary schools, at Lyon and in Paris at Alfort. Having been struck by the glaring inadequacy of contemporary knowledge about equine diseases and their treatment compared to the rapid development of human medicine, he conceived a project of creating a school to train young men in filling the gap. This task required not only that he have a good reputation with the equestrian community, including influential officers in the army, but also that he could get the ear of the king. Being a royal equerry in good standing, Bourgelat's vital ingredient was his favorable rapport with Bertin, the king's controller-general of finances and a former steward of the Generality of Lyon.

Bertin was attracted by Bourgelat's plan and was able to obtain King Louis XV's support for it. Bertin, however, had an even grander design in mind. He had a deep concern for French agriculture and the heavy losses experienced as a result of diseases of farm livestock, such as the recurrent epidemics of the cattle plague. Thus Bourgelat was able in 1761 to upgrade his Academy of Equitation in Lyon, where he trained young gentlemen mainly in the equestrian skills they needed for military service, to become the world's first veterinary school, L'Ecole Vétérinaire de Lyon, cradle of a new profession, veterinary medicine.

The new school opened on January 1, 1762, in the buildings of the Inn of the Abundance on the main road that became the Rue de la Guillotière. The event of its opening attracted the attention of the executive bodies that advised royalty throughout Europe.

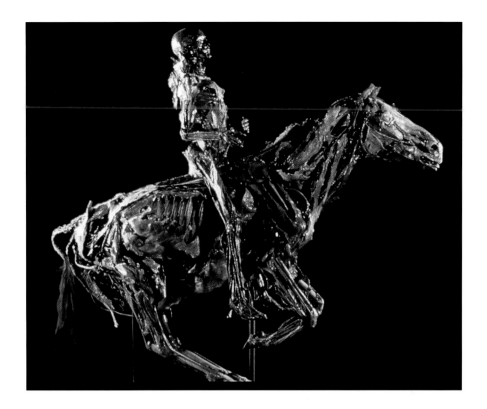

PARISIAN CENTRALITY AND THE
SECOND SCHOOL AT ALFORT

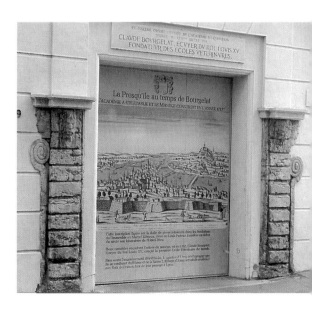

283. *The Flayed Rider* by Honoré Fragonard. A first cousin of the famous painter Jean-Honoré Fragonard, he accepted Bourgelat's offer to become the principal and professor of anatomy at the new Royal Veterinary School at Maisons-Alfort from 1766 to 1771. During these years Fragonard prepared thousands of anatomical models, among which were at least fifty "ecorchés." He improved the well-known methods of wax injection for preserving anatomical dissections, and his subjects, reflecting his eccentricity, were always shown with theatrical flair. The horseman in this particular figure, modeled after Albrecht Dürer's *Horseman of the Apocalypse,* originally held red velvet reins. Fragonard's association with the school ended abruptly when he was fired by Bourgelat, who, in concurrence with many of his colleagues, considered Fragonard a madman. Today only a few of his magnificent models exist. This particular work remains the most spectacular among the exhibits at the Museum of the National Veterinary School of Alfort. *(Photo by Patrick Landmann, Liaison International.)*

Bourgelat knew many of the influential figures of the times, including Lamoignon de Malesherbes and Voltaire. It is necessary to grasp the nature of the upper echelon of French society at that time to appreciate why it was the appropriate seed bed in which to germinate the new veterinary profession. The social and political hub was the king's royal court, a colossal establishment supporting 15,000 people and 5000 horses. This "party of privilege," a hotbed of politicial intrigue that lived by a code of hereditary entitlements, extended its tentacles to the farthest reaches of the French empire.

A "party of reform," as well as the party of privilege, was a force running through the higher intellectual levels of the "philosophes": the genie was let out of the bottle. Although the Enlightenment was an international development, its focal point was in Paris. The population of France was twenty million, but then, as now, all major decisions were made in the capital. At that time the horse was vital for the life-style of the aristocracy, for running the country, and for the maintenance of military power. There were well-established grounds for wanting capable horse doctors to maintain all these functions effectively. The needs of farm livestock received little attention, except when the great plagues struck and devastating losses resulted.

The timing of the establishment of the two veterinary schools at Lyon and Alfort in the 1760s was fortunate. It would not be long before the country became embroiled in the Revolution and the Reign of Terror that followed it. Had the schools been founded fifteen years later, it is unlikely that the idea of veterinary medicine could have come to fruition in France amid the great turbulence.

It soon became clear that Bourgelat saw his breakthrough in achieving the establishment of the Lyon veterinary school as merely a stepping stone to Paris. Thus he lobbied Bertin to allow the transfer of the newborn school to the capital. Minister Bertin, however, committed to a broader view of the role of veterinary medicine, was adamantly opposed to closure of his only school at Lyon. Instead he agreed to the creation of a new school in Paris that might train students of a superior order who could become leaders in a string of provincial schools. His goal was to open more schools to train the new cadre of professionals, not to close the one he had already established.

284. Entrance to the Bourgelat riding academy, which became the world's first veterinary school in 1762. Today it is the headquarters of the Fondation Mérieux, the Institute Mérieux, and Rhône-Mérieux. *(Edité par la Fondation Mérieux, Lyon.)*

285. Skeletal anatomy of the horse from Claude Bourgelat's *Elémens de l'Art Vétérinaire,* Paris (1769). Bourgelat's skills as a superb organizer were apparent in his establishing the schools at Lyon and Alfort, but his publications lacked practical knowledge of medicine and surgery. *(National Library of Medicine, Bethesda, Maryland.)*

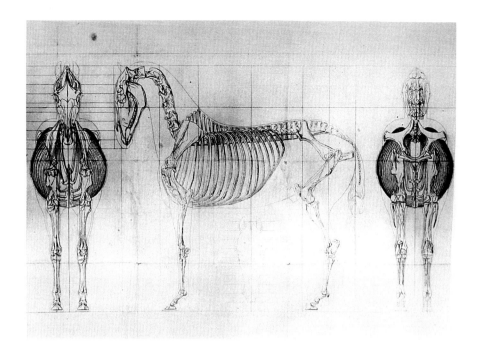

The Parisian school was installed provincially near the Boulevard de la Chapelle in Charenton in 1765. Bourgelat succeeded in his grand design by getting it moved to Maisons Alfort, where it occupied the vast domain of the Chateau d'Alfort, acquired at great expense from the baron of Bormes. It became the Royal Veterinary School of Alfort and remains at this impressive site today as L'Ecole Nationale Vétérinaire d'Alfort. Bertin appointed Bourgelat to a new position that satisfied both the latter's ego and his own vision, that of "Inspector-General of all veterinary schools."

The location in Paris was marvelous because the capital was then the seat of power, the magnet of the world, and the eye of the intellectual storm. Thus the creation of the second veterinary school at Alfort put the new profession firmly on the map, and the profession became caught up in the great movements for change that overturned tradition and threatened hierarchies.

Although Bourgelat had a flair for organization and knew well the corridors of influence from his legal training, he lacked the qualifications and style needed to become a truly effective academic leader. He had made a valiant attempt to acquire knowledge of anatomy and medicine, but he was more the cut of a marshal or an equerry than a veterinarian. He seemed to demonstrate little commitment to the needs of farm livestock, his personal experience and obsessions being tied to the horse. Students sent from abroad to acquire training in the new profession were uniformly disappointed in the lack of studies relevant to animal production and epidemics. The initial curriculum consisted of little more than anatomy, farriery, and equine medicine.

THE REMARKABLE PHILIPPE-ETIENNE LaFOSSE: PARISIAN LEADER IN HIPPIATRY

Bourgelat had a powerful rival who was regarded as the outstanding horse doctor of France, Philippe-Etienne LaFosse. Born in 1738, he was the son of E.G. LaFosse, Sr., the distinguished marshal of the king's equerries noted for his own works on shoeing and glanders. LaFosse, Sr., set his son on the right path by having him train as a groom and as a marshal while also obtaining a good education. Philippe-Etienne attended the flaying yard to study equine anatomy, making necropsies and collecting diseased specimens. He accompanied his father on his visits to sick horses and learned his treatments, operations, and dressings. He was teaching anatomy to the cavalry at Versailles by

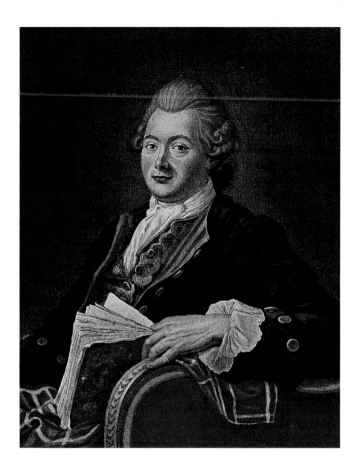

286. Philippe-Etienne LaFosse (1738-1820) was a prominent veterinary figure and is, perhaps, the most famous hippiater of France. He had been provided a strong foundation by his father, Etienne Guillaume LaFosse, an innovative farrier and horse doctor. An equine anatomist, researcher, and clinician, Phillipe-Etienne LaFosse published many works throughout his long career, but his *Cours d'Hippiatrique ou Traité Complet de la Medecine des Chevaux,* a two-volume opus featuring sixty-five beautifully engraved plates, gained him international acclaim. Some editions were hand-tinted in color. It remains one of the most beautiful equine anatomy books ever published. *(Courtesy Loren D. Carlson Health Sciences Library, University of California, Davis.)*

the age of eighteen years and put on a course for marshals in the family home. His scientific bent was soon manifested in a *Memoire on the Bite of a Shrew-Mouse,* which he submitted to the Academy of Sciences, where Buffon was an examiner, in 1757. He showed that the malady attributed to such a bite was none other than a form of anthrax. LaFosse, Jr., was inducted into the army in 1758 to recommend measures to control glanders outbreaks in the cavalry and served in the Seven Years' War. Two years later he registered in the faculty of medicine, producing his *Dissertation on Glanders in Horses* in 1761.

LaFosse, Jr.'s father died the year the Alfort school opened. Despite his obvious superiority in veterinary knowledge, Philippe-Etienne LaFosse was not invited to the faculty. He remained productive, publishing *Guide for Marshals* in 1766. In the following year he opened a course in hippiatry in an amphitheater constructed at his own expense in competition with Alfort, that is, a private veterinary school, but he closed it in 1770 to complete his masterpiece, *Cours d'Hippiatrique (Course of Hippiatry or A Complete Treatise on the Medicine of the Horse).* This magnificent opus appeared in 1772 in two volumes with sixty-five engraved plates; it was said to have cost him 70,000 pounds. His reputation became international overnight. Haller acclaimed him as the most famous of hippiaters. The work was translated into German and Spanish. Two years later he was back in print in French with *Memoire on Epizootic Diseases,* which was followed by his *Study Dictionary of Hippiatry, Cavalry, Horsemanship and Marshalry* in four volumes, and his popular cavalry officer's *Manual of Hippiatry.*

LaFosse, Jr., became an ever more acerbic and embittered critic of Bourgelat and his school. Because of LaFosse, Jr., who considered himself far ahead of Bourgelat and his faculty as an experienced animal doctor, horse marshal, and farrier, the early period of the Alfort School was turbulent. It is evident that he was extremely disturbed by Bourgelat's success in establishing a veterinary school in his "territory" of Paris and obtaining the government's support for it. LaFosse, Jr., embarked on a destructive, vitriolic campaign with the intent of destroying the reputation of Bourgelat and his school.

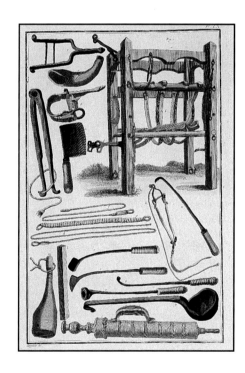

287. *Panche LX, Représentant divers instruments servant à la ferrure aux opérations,* one of many hand-tinted plates from Philippe-Etienne LaFosse's *Cours d'Hippiatrique ou Traité Complet de la Médecine des Chevaux,* published in Paris in 1772. Color editions of this work are rare today. This particular plate illustrates a wide variety of instruments used by farriers of the time. The stock in the upper right is complete with a sling and attachments for the extremities and head. *(Plates 287 through 290 courtesy Loren D. Carlson Health Sciences Library, University of California, Davis.)*

He was incensed at being passed over by Bourgelat for a faculty appointment. He sought to have the Alfort school closed and replaced by one he would lead but was foiled in his many attempts to achieve this end. He had a personal passion for equine medicine and its advancement through scholarly works.

LaFosse, Jr., accepted enthusiastically the idea of liberty, distinguished himself at the taking of the Bastille, and became veterinary inspector-general of remounts. He himself was accused and imprisoned for a year during the chaotic aftermath of the Revolution. In 1790 he published a memoire, *The Royal Veterinary School at Alfort; Reason for the Inutility of That Establishment and Means of Replacing It With Great Economic Saving for the State*. Even after Bourgelat's death in 1779, LaFosse, Jr., having outlived him by more than thirty years, published a final violent, unjust diatribe against the two veterinary schools under the seemingly innocuous title, *New Theory and Practice of Equitation*.

Despite injudicious, inappropriate behavior with respect to the Alfort school and its proprietor, Philippe-Etienne LaFosse has a secure place in history as one of the early masters of hippiatry. As the third generation of a family committed to service of the "equine industry" and the horse itself, he represented the natural evolution of competence from his grandfather, who was among those who attempted to generate empirical equine medicine through experience and application but without benefit of specific professional education. LaFosse, Jr., acquired the cumulative knowledge of two preceding generations, along with a passionate love of his art and sound, competent judgment in practicing it. His genius was in his commitment to the next step, which was to acquire the progressive aspects of the contemporary approach to

288. *Planche XV, Représentant le cheval dont on a enlevé les muscles de la peau,* demonstrates the superficial musculature of the horse in exquisite detail. Like Ruini and other classical anatomists before him, LaFosse showed the anatomy of the horse in stages, beginning with the external features and gradually proceeding to the skeleton.

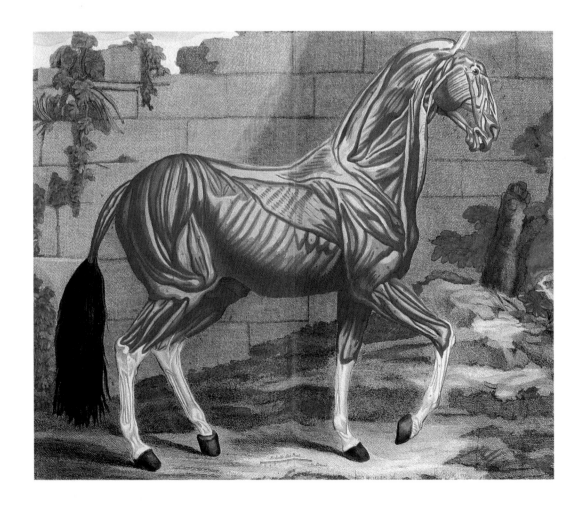

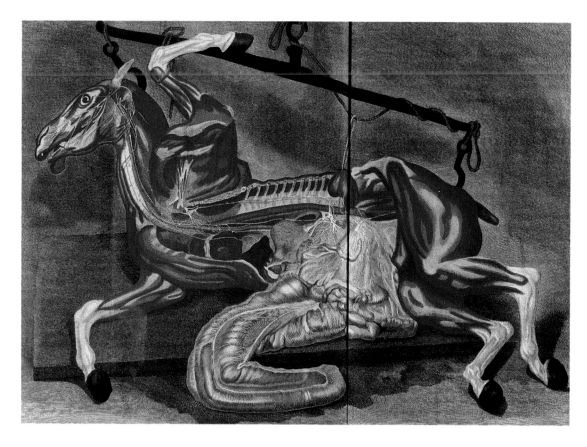

289. The distribution of cranial nerves exiting from the base of the skull are dramatically shown in *Planche XXXIV, Représentant la distribution des dix paires de nerfs sortant de la base du crâne.* LaFosse's work has been criticized for plates showing horses in various stages of dissection hanging from hooks, but in reality large animal dissection rooms resembled slaughterhouses. In this plate the aorta and anterior mesenteric plexus are prominently displayed, with the large colon clearly visible.

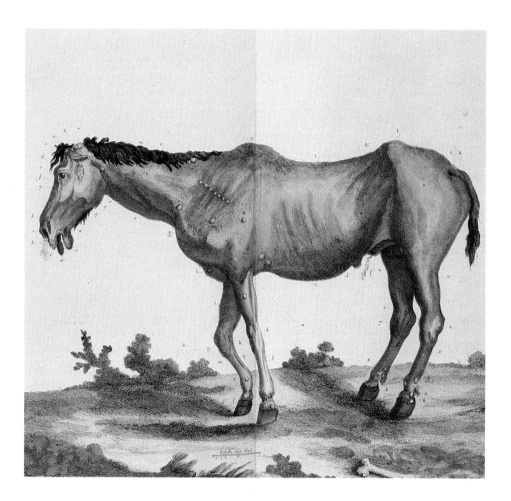

290. A defective horse is seen in *Planche XLIX, Représentant un autre cheval défectueux,* complete with wind puffs, mallenders, or chronic dermatitis in the carpal fold, and wind galls. Wind puffs or wind galls are synovial swellings of joints or tendon sheaths resulting from trauma and are commonly seen in overworked horses. A sebaceous cyst is seen on the horse's chest and eczema is present on the right rear leg. The left hip is higher than the right and looks like a "horn."

science and medicine and apply them to veterinary problems through his research and scholarly writing. His efforts to bring down the Alfort school were in vain, since the faculty was able to defend itself against his destructive tactics, no doubt benefitting from the stimulus of competition along the way.

The Lyon school was beset by financial difficulties after Bourgelat departed, and in 1793, during the Reign of Terror that followed the French Revolution, the school was bombarded during the siege of Lyon. The new director, Louis Bredin, saved it by moving the students, the animals, and the collections to his property at Eailly, several kilometers from Lyon. It was moved in 1796 to a site in the ancient convent of the Dames de Sainte-Elisabeth called the Cloitre des Deux Amants.

VETERINARY SCHOOLS IN THE AUSTRO-HUNGARIAN EMPIRE

The establishment of veterinary education and the new veterinary profession in the Austro-Hungarian Empire of the late eighteenth century was a complicated process. Apparently the leadership was watching closely for new developments among the powerful monarchies of Europe. Maria-Theresa, who became empress of the Austrian Empire (because of the lack of a male heir) and Queen of Hungary, had followed Linnaeus's model for Sweden and sent three students to Bourgelat's veterinary school in Lyon the year after it opened. Among those selected was Ludovico Scotti (1728-1806), the son of an Italian farrier of Cremona. He studied anatomy in Rome and became renowned for his skill in treating cavalry horses. He was from a region of Italy that became part of the Austro-Hungarian Empire after it evicted the French. Recognizing that the Austrian public held animal workers in low esteem and in preparation for the new class of animal doctors, the empress issued a decree in 1765 ordering punishment for anyone who opposed the teachers of the new veterinary profession. Her son and coregent, Joseph II, appointed Scotti to head a hospital and school for horse medicine and surgery in Vienna in 1766, the first in a German-speaking country. This hospital was disbanded in 1777, and a new school was established to replace it.

During a time of tension between the empress and the military, it appears that she was concerned about the health and welfare of all her people and supported genuine scholarship. Joseph II wanted to restore the waning military power of the empire and became a creature of the masculine world of the military, the aristocracy, and the horse. The military leadership recommended that a field surgeon be sent abroad for training in veterinary medicine. It seems that the army leadership wanted to have military men leading the veterinary school to ensure that the new profession gave priority to the horse and the army's need for horse doctors.

Johann Gottlieb Wolstein (1738-1820), a German field surgeon who had battle experience with the Austrian army, had been invited to Vienna to study medicine. He was well regarded and was recommended to Joseph II and his military advisers. They selected Wolstein in 1769 to go to the veterinary school at Alfort for a study program in the new profession. There he studied under Bourgelat, Fragonard, and Chabert but was not satisfied with the program. Thus he also attended the private veterinary school of LaFosse, Jr. Wolstein and LaFosse, Jr., were of the same vintage and saw eye to eye on professional matters; they became firm friends and lifelong colleagues. Wolstein also looked into the devastating epizootic diseases that were plaguing French farmers. He then crossed the Channel and studied the excellent progress being made there in sheep-breeding improvements and horse husbandry. Proceeding to Holland, northern Germany, and Denmark, he obtained an excellent overview of animal husbandry, horse studs, and the state of the veterinary art in northern Europe.

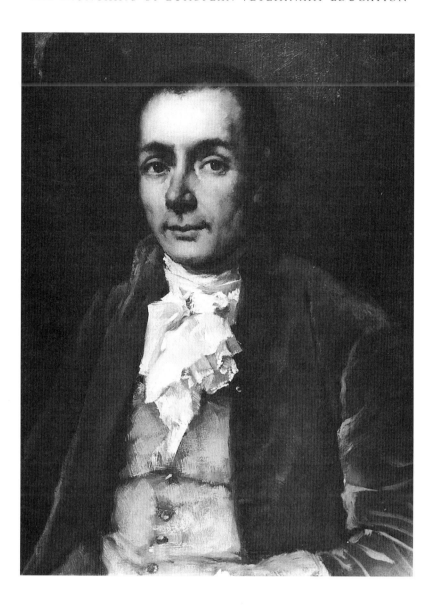

291. Portrait of Johann Gottlieb Wolstein (1738-1820). A student and life-long friend and colleague of Philippe-Etienne LaFosse, Wolstein was asked to improve the existing veterinary school in Vienna. It flourished under his leadership and attracted students from outside Austria. His success in Vienna was followed by an invitation to assist in the establishment of the veterinary school in Budapest in 1787. (Courtesy Der Rektor, Veterinärmedizinische Universität Wien.)

Wolstein went to Jena, where he obtained qualification as a doctor of medicine and surgery in 1775. Upon his return to Vienna he was invited to develop a design for a new, independent veterinary school. The existing school was basically a horse infirmary that had been established by the Lyon-trained Italian veterinarian Scotti to form horse doctors for the army. This arrangement did not meet the expectations about medical standards implanted in the minds of the empress and Joseph II by van Swieten.

During the spring of 1777 Joseph II visited Paris as a guest of his sister Mme. de Pompadour and his brother-in-law King Louis XV. While there, he visited the world's second veterinary school, the Alfort school. It was the principal "repair and maintenance center for the nation's equine force and therefore its main source of agricultural and aggressive energies." Thinking ahead to future wars and the growing Prussian threat from Frederick the Great, the young Emperor foresaw the need for an invincible cavalry on high-quality, well-fed, well-shod steeds free of contagious diseases, their wounds repairable by skillful veterinary surgeons. The director at Alfort assured the emperor that once the school had trained two generations of army veterinarians the French cavalry would be unbeatable.

La Vie Parisienne de Louis XVI described the Alfort school as handsome and spacious, with a natural history collection including many dissected specimens, a fine chemistry laboratory, a full-time apothecary who prepared remedies for sick horses, and a large forge run by excellent blacksmiths. It reported that skillful surgery was performed on the equine patients.

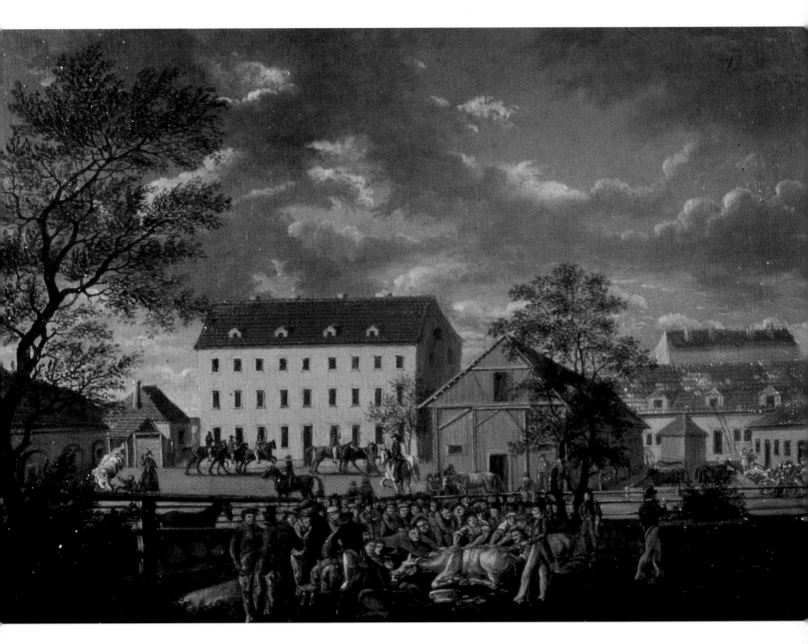

292. A painting of the Veterinär-medizinische Universität Wien in 1783 during Johann Gottlieb Wolstein's tenure as director. A professor, perhaps Wolstein, is lecturing about a cow to a group of students in the foreground. Horses are being exercised in the background. *(Courtesy o. Univ. Prof. Dr. Peter F. Knezevic, Veterinärmedizinische Universität Wien.)*

Initially Wolstein had been given the opportunity to establish a new school elsewhere in the empire, on the outskirts of Budapest, but he declined and insisted he should establish one in Vienna. Wolstein's school developed a good reputation and attracted students from outside Austria. His surgical and medical training coupled with his broad interest and his six-year study tour of western European veterinary medicine prepared him well. He wrote a series of short books on veterinary subjects. He was a strong advocate of raising standards of animal production and veterinary care while overcoming the ignorance of the animal caretakers. Thus his graduates were soundly based in both preventive and therapeutic veterinary medicine.

Wolstein assisted in planning a new veterinary program in Budapest and took the nominated Hungarian professor Sandor Tolnay, a medical graduate, into his school for two years for training. The initial goal was to establish a course in epidemiology and epizootiology for Hungarian veterinarians. Wolstein had a major shortcoming: he was a vitalist who did not believe in contagious diseases, preferring to insist that they were a result of environmental factors. At first, Tolnay had to follow this line of reasoning.

Wolstein's fate, after seventeen successful years of running his Viennese school, was to be arrested in 1794. He was imprisoned in irons for two years and stripped of all his offices and honors. Joseph II had died in 1790. At that time the Austrian Empire was a strict Catholic domain fearful of the contagion of Protestantism with its call for liberty and equality in the aftermath of the French Revolution. Wolstein was a Protestant and was known to be sympathetic to the French Jacobin movement. It is not without relevance that his close friend Philippe-Etienne LaFosse took part in the storming of the Bastille on July 14, 1789, and subsequently took an active leadership role, becoming the veterinary overseer of the remounts.

Joseph II, who had instituted many reforms liberating the empire in his early years, had become reactionary as society became impatient for faster change. His brother, who succeeded him on his death, seems to have been more susceptible to the views of the military and Catholic establishments that feared a slide into anarchy. The month before Wolstein's internment, the members of the Society for Freedom and Equality in Vienna were arrested and seven of its leaders were executed, including the man who had translated from the French Rousseau's *Social Contract* and several other "provocative" works, the Hungarian Szent-Maryam. Thus the Enlightenment was squelched by the Austrian ruling powers.

Wolstein escaped with the help of influential friends, who were appalled at his undeserved treatment. Because he could not return to Austria, he settled at Altona near Hamburg, where he lived for twenty-five years. He reattained a high reputation in Germany but declined offers of appointment at several universities. He died at eighty-three years of age, within days of the death of his esteemed colleague LaFosse, Jr.

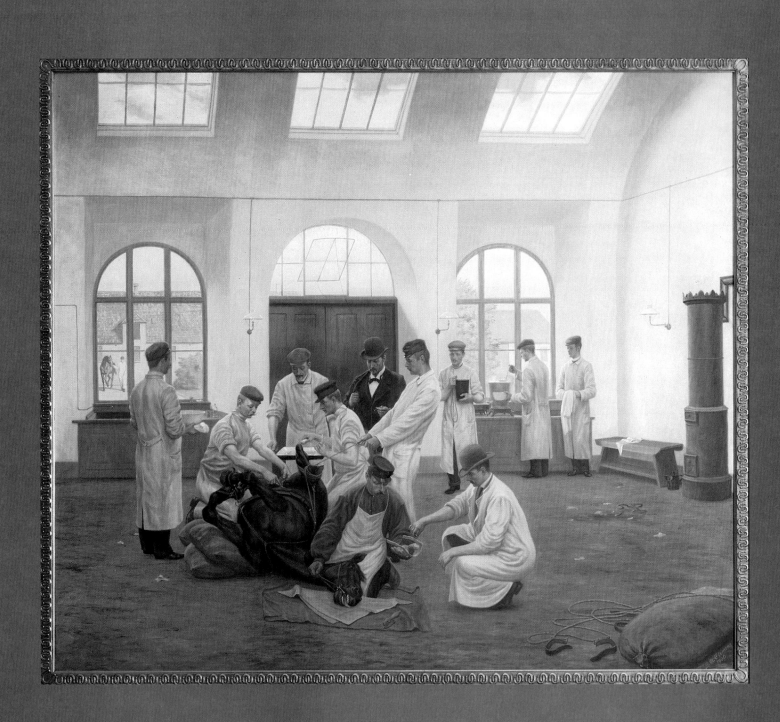

An Increasing Demand for Veterinary Schools

VETERINARY BEGINNINGS IN ITALY

Charles-Emmanuel III, king of Sardinia, sent four students to the Lyon veterinary school in 1762. One of these, Giovanni Brugnone, was named veterinarian of the royal stud; another, Toggia, became chief veterinarian in the army. In 1769 a veterinary school was built in Turin in northwestern Italy under the direction of Brugnone, who designed it. The school was run by the minister of war and was organized along military lines to train veterinarians for the Piedmont army. During the French occupation after 1800 the development of the school was disrupted; it was moved and there were several changes of leadership. In 1834 it was transferred to its present site at Fossano, near the railway station of Turin. Giovanni Battista Ercolani (1817-1883) became the director until he moved to Bologna in 1854.

Venice and Lombardy in northeastern Italy were in the Austrian Empire in the late eighteenth and early nineteenth centuries. The empress agreed to send three students to Lyon to train as veterinarians in 1772. Two others were sent from Milan, one in 1774 and the other in 1776. Two of the Lyon graduates, Volpor and Lucchini, became teachers in a new veterinary school. The scheme was complicated by the idea of a "major veterinary" course for veterinary experts and a "minor" course for farriers. Later, a third stream was added of "communal veterinarian" study for veterinarians who were to work with farm livestock other than the horse. The latter course of study already existed at the Vienna school for students in the Tyrol region.

ORIGIN OF THE FIRST GERMAN VETERINARY SCHOOL AT GÖTTINGEN

Developments in German-speaking states were less susceptible to orchestration than were those of France, the Austro-Hungarian Empire, and Scandinavia. Veterinary science developed more locally because of the greater fragmentation of power into principalities.

Baron J.B. von Sind (1709-1776) of Cologne, a German cavalry officer responsible for horse management and veterinary care, prepared an important manual describing the state of the art in his field. His *Introduction to the Science of the Stallmeister* (Horse Marshal) was published in 1770, during the first decade of the first French veterinary schools. As an analytical critique of the world of the eighteenth-century horse doctor, the book was a transitional landmark. A great advance over the dogmatic style of Solleysel (1617-1680) and others of the seventeenth century, it reflected a growing concern about the inadequacy and outright cruelty of many common practices that had become traditional methods of intervening in equine ailments, including rou-

293. *Facing page, Operation i Kirurgisk Klinik,* an oil painting done around 1898 by G.A. Clemens, shows an operation in clinical surgery at the Royal Veterinary and Agricultural University in Copenhagen. The horse is lying on special moss in the surgery hall, held in position by sacks filled with straw. A student helps by holding a rope attached to one leg. The horse was cast and fixed by the "Abildgaard Casting System" in which manacles were placed around all four pasterns and around the chest; a rope is pulled up and through a ring, bringing the legs together and causing the horse to fall. Abildgaard was the first to design this technique around 1800, and it was modified by Professor Sand in 1890. Interestingly, this harness for restraining is still used for several surgical procedures in horses and is known throughout Europe as the Danish harness for restraining. Professor A.W. Mørkeberg, second from the left, is performing the surgery. Jørgen Hansen, the responsible animal attendant, has placed a cloth under the horse's head to keep the dusty sphagnum moss from entering its eyes and nose. He is also holding Professor Stockfleth's wire net device containing absorbent material, onto which a student is dropping chloroform. Other students are holding a bowl of disinfectant and a tray of boiled instruments. Professor Sand, wearing a dark suit, is observing the whole procedure. Just behind him a student holds a jar of disinfectant fluid ready to flush the surgical site. Note the gas heater, gas lamps, and the old oven for heat and boiling water. *(The Royal Veterinary and Agricultural University, Copenhagen.)*

294. Front of the old building that was occupied by the first veterinary school in Italy before its destruction during the second World War. The *Scuola di Veterinaria* was founded in 1769 by the king of the Sardinia Kingdom, Charles-Emmanuel III, in Venaria Castle, near Turin. Its first director was Giovanni Brugnone (1741-1818), a surgeon who had studied with Claude Bourgelat at Lyon. The school was moved to its present location at Fossano, near the railway station of Turin, in 1834. The facility was rebuilt following the war and remains the school's site. *(Courtesy Dr. Marco Galloni, Università di Torino.)*

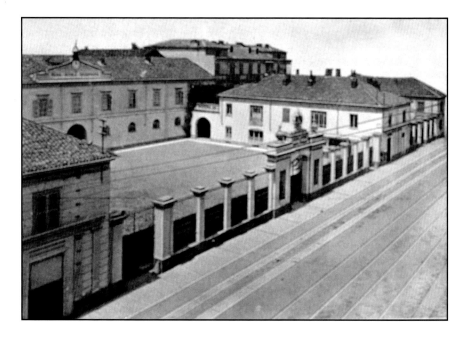

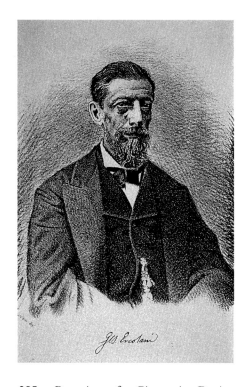

295. Portrait of Giovanni Battista Ercolani (1817-1883). Ercolani became director of the Turin school when it was moved to its current site at Fossano. He later moved to Bologna where, in 1863, he established the Veterinary Pathology and Teratology Museum. Ercolani believed a dynamic knowledge of anatomy was an essential prerequisite for surgery without anesthesia. Today the Ercolani Museum contains 5350 original items. *(Facoltá di Medicina Veterinaria, Universitá Degli Studi di Bologna.)*

tine "preventive" procedures such as bleeding and purging. Farriers in some parts had formed a guild aimed at enshrining their role as sole purveyors of these barbarities. Von Sind labeled them ignorant of both the anatomy and the medical basis of their procedures. He called for a new, scientific approach to horse surgery and made an appeal to humanitarian considerations in treating animals.

Von Sind's descriptions of operations, including treatment of cataracts, nasal polyps, inguinal hernia, and vesicular calculi and trephination of sinuses, called for superior surgical skills based on comparative anatomy and empirical experience. He deplored excessive venesection and inappropriate hoof care.

Von Sind described a significant advance in healing fractures, which was aided by a greatly improved design of suspension devices for horses. Noting the difficulty of immobilizing a fractured limb in a large animal and the enormous pressures it brings to bear in rising from a lying position, he concurred with others' perceptions of a need to protect the splinted parts by supporting the animal in a sling. He observed, however, that slings in use elsewhere, which fully suspended the animal by means of straps, caused severe pressure-trauma followed by inflammation at the sites of the straps and that the trauma could be lethal before the bones healed. Von Sind's new apparatus called for a sheet of cowhide hung from above the sides, which covered the lower thorax and abdomen and provided a large area for weight bearing. The supporting material, however, was pulled up only far enough to allow the horse a choice of standing on its sound legs until it became tired or relaxing onto the support if it got tired, without having to bear weight on or cause pain in the fractured limb or limbs. He described ways of bone setting, fixation of the fractured bones, the necessary follow-up care, and complications. In his publication he claimed success in treating ten fractured limb bones in horses.

Johann Christian Polycarp Erxleben (1744-1777) considered von Sind's work outstanding and overdue; he edited and revised it. Johann was the sixth child of the diakon (deacon) of Quedlingburg. The family was not well off. Johann's mother was unique in the history of medicine and of academic studies in Germany. Dorothea Christiane Erxleben was the first woman to study at a German university (Halle) and the first to graduate as a medical doctor. Born in 1715, she was the daughter of a physician, Christian Polycarp Leporin, who helped her learn by self-study. She gained much experience by assisting him in his practice. Accepted to study medicine at Halle University in 1740, she was unable to take the opportunity because her brother, who was a student there, deserted to avoid being drafted into the army. As a conse-

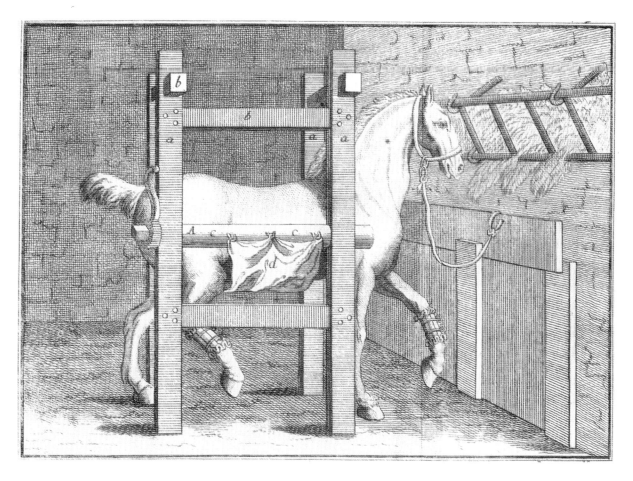

quence, her father was forced to flee from the town, and Dorothea had to stay at home and take care of the entire family. At twenty-seven years of age (in 1742) Dorothea Leporin married Erxleben, a widower with five small children, continued successfully providing medical services, and supported the family. At last, in 1754, she wrote a dissertation and graduated as a medical doctor in Halle, and her detractors had to accept her qualifications to practice. In 1742 she had written a popular paper on the role and possibilities of women studying at universities. She died young, at forty-seven years of age, in 1762, but she had conveyed her unusual talents and drive to her son Johann.

Johann Erxleben had studied medicine but had not completed the examinations. He had obtained a stipend for teaching physics and chemistry. Despite his immature academic background, on October 13, 1768, he wrote a remarkable letter to Freiherr von Munchausen, curator of the flourishing Georgia Augusta University in Göttingen. Erxleben proposed that the introduction of animal medicine as a program at Göttingen's university would be useful. He claimed that for some time he had been dedicated to medicine and had acquired the scientific basis for it and that afterward he had learned animal medicine. He asked the government, therefore, to allow him to teach veterinary medicine and materia medica for six months a year. In the remaining six months he would teach specific diseases of animals and their treatments.

Erxleben's proposal encompassed the following objectives:

1. He would teach people who would like to become farriers.
2. He would treat sick animals himself as a component of the teaching process; that is, he would like to build a small "ecole vétérinaire" (veterinary school).
3. He would perform public necropsies of animals, teaching the makeup of the animal body, knowledge that was necessary to the study of animals.
4. He planned to write a book that would be understandable to uneducated people about the art of treating animals.

296. Plate 5 from Baron J.B. von Sind's *L'Art du manège pris dans vrais principles, suivi d'une nouvelle methode pour l'embouchure des chevaux.* . . . (1772). Von Sind (1709-1776), of Köln, used his experience in horse management and veterinary care as a German cavalry officer to publish a landmark work calling for a new, scientific approach to equine surgery and greater humanitarian care. *(The Royal Veterinary College, London.)*

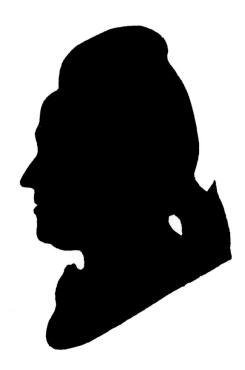

297. A silhouette of Johann Christian Polycarp Erxleben (1744-1777). He was Germany's first veterinary professor and encouraged that animal medicine be taught at the university level. This silhouette is the only known existing portrait of Erxleben. *(Niedersächsische Staats-und Universitätsbibliothek Göttingen.)*

298. The old Viehärznei-Institut, the oldest German veterinary institution. Pen-and-ink quill drawing from a student's family book dated 1801. *(Niedersächsische Staats-und Universitatsbibliothek Göttingen.)*

He expressed the hope and belief that changing the medical approach of the veterinary art in this way would convert the university's losses and lamentations into considerable profits.

When Erxleben set out the preceding vision of veterinary education, he was twenty-four years old. He also asked for modest financial assistance as a teacher of mathematics, physics, natural sciences, and natural history. It was unusual for such a young scholar to make such demands, and his hopes of a professorship were considered unrealistic. At first his proposal was not accepted because it was felt that animal medicine should not be taught at all at the university level, although its importance to agriculture and riding was recognized.

During the eighteenth century, ninety percent of the population was engaged in agriculture. When rinderpest arrived from Asia, it eradicated almost all the cattle and sheep, and serious diseases of horses were widespread. His Royal Highness G.A. von Munchausen, the father of Georgia Augusta University in Göttingen, was eighty years old. A gifted man with great foresight, he drew his own conclusions free of prejudices and decided that the time had come to make animal medicine into a science. Just three days after receiving Erxleben's proposal, he had a letter drafted in reply to him, saying that he thought it would be "very nice" and "interesting" for the new science to start.

Von Munchausen advised Erxleben to conduct a little experiment by producing a book on the art of animal medicine and its teaching. Accepting this advice, Erxleben published a book in 1769, the very next year, called *Introduction to Veterinary Medicine.* It was translated into Dutch the next year.

The book was an encouraging start, but Munchausen was a thoughtful, careful innovator. Because Erxleben was a self-made person in the field, he sent him to study in places where animal medicine was more established, such as Köln (Cologne), where Stallmeister Oberst J.B. von Sind was regarded as one of the finest horse doctors in Europe; Holland, to study rinderpest; and Lyon to the veterinary school.

When Erxleben returned in 1770, he started lecturing in veterinary medicine. He became the first veterinary professor in Germany and the first ever to be a university professor of veterinary medicine. He worked an exhausting schedule to launch his school and was involved continuously with the students in instruction, dissections, and demonstrations in anatomy during the winter. In the summer he switched to the theoretical aspects of veterinary science and animal diseases; also, he treated animals for free two days a week with his students so that they could learn from hands-on practice. Furthermore, he asked the rural priests to spread the word about this service so that animals would be brought in from afar to strengthen the clinical teaching program.

Students were required to be eighteen years of age and had to be able to read, write, count, and understand some Latin and French. Such diligent, able young persons could be turned into good, capable, presentable veterinarians in two years. Erxleben obtained buildings to house the veterinary institute, its teaching programs, and the animals. Thus he was the first in Germany to place veterinary medicine on a scientific basis. Although he remained a member of the philosophy faculty and taught basic subjects as well, veterinary medicine became his main field. In 1775 he was invited to move to the Realschule in Berlin, but Göttingen promoted him to full professor in the philosophy faculty and he decided to stay there. He took over responsibility for an abbatoir in 1776 but died prematurely in the following year, at thirty-four years of age.

After Erxleben's death the school foundered but was maintained by the faculty of medicine and pharmacy. Karl Friedrich Lappe (1787-1854) became director in 1816 and restored the veterinary clinical program. Hannoverian politics, however, had dictated that a new "vetering" school be established at Hannover in 1778, and Göttingen's fine beginning eventually lapsed.

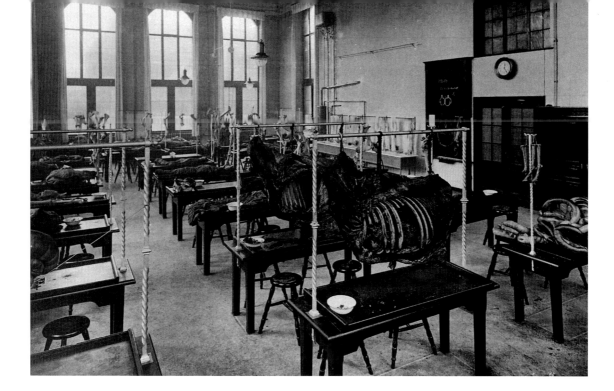

Johannes Kersting, calling for a three-year course, tried to put the Hannover school on a strong scientific path, but his successor, Havemann, changed it back to a duplicated one-year program of mainly practical instruction. These events occurred during the reign of the third Hannoverian king of England, George III (1760-1820), and the American Revolution of 1776. Later, Hannover's veterinary school became quite distinguished.

299. The old dissection room in the Institute of Anatomy at the veterinary school in Hannover, founded in 1778. *(Courtesy Prof. Dr. W. Schulze, Tierärztliche Hochschule Hannover.)*

LINNAEUS'S PROTÉGÉ HERNQUIST: FOUNDER OF SWEDEN'S FIRST SCHOOL AT SKARA

Peter Hernquist (1726-1808), who came from a parish just south of Skara, Sweden, was a pupil whom Linnaeus (the professor of medicine and natural history at Uppsala) personally chose to send to France to study the new field of veterinary medicine at Claude Bourgelat's veterinary school at Lyon and to study with Philippe-Etienne LaFosse in Paris. Hernquist also studied human medicine and surgery in Paris. Upon his return to his homeland he proposed the establishment of a veterinary institute and an animal hospital in Stockholm. His plan was turned down by the authorities. In 1772, however, he moved to the beautiful rural town of Skara to teach mathematics at high school and to start teaching veterinary science in a small way (taking only two students every three years). He persisted in his quest, and three years later, in 1775, a royal proclamation gave him the Brogardenestate in Skara, right in his own hometown, on which to establish a veterinary school. He personally supervised its construction and unearthed an ancient monastery while digging the foundations. He was careful to complete the excavation and record the findings.

Linnaeus selected Peter Hernquist to found the new profession in Sweden because he could best penetrate the most difficult sciences and because he had the gift of writing. When he was sent to Lyon in 1763 to acquire the knowledge and skills needed for the new profession, he was disappointed by the lack of focus on species other than the horse. His home district, after all, was a dairying region. He spent six years in France. He collaborated with Philippe-Etienne LaFosse, the famous hippiatrist, and extended his medical and surgical studies, which included the latest findings on venereal diseases. Hernquist planted three ash trees close together on the Brogardenestate and christened them Bourgelat, LaFosse, and Abildgaard after three heroic founders of the modern veterinary profession. They stand tall to this day as a living monument to the three great trailblazers.

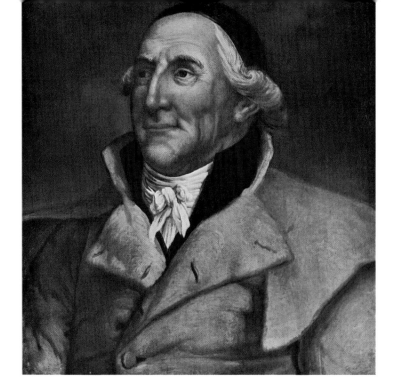

300. Portrait of Peter Hernquist (1726-1808) by Per Krafft, Jr. In 1775 Hernquist founded the veterinary school in his hometown of Skara. He originally studied veterinary medicine at Lyon and with Philippe-Etienne LaFosse in Paris. As with many of the early founders of veterinary programs, Hernquist also studied human medicine and surgery. *(Veterinarhistoriska Muséet, Skara.)*

Hernquist practiced medicine as well as veterinary medicine and established a hospital for the treatment of venereal disease. He was the first to use mercurial salts to treat syphilis in Sweden. He was an outstanding pharmacist because of his training in botany, natural history, and medicine, and his cattle pharmacy has been preserved in Skara's fine veterinary museum. He was a man of extremely broad intellectual compass and interests. He required veterinary students to have a sound constitution and a good singing voice, the latter because the social status of animal owners was low and he felt that it would be unfair for veterinarians, too, to have a low status by association: he linked the school to the church and developed a choir to raise the students' standings in their communities. He ran the school for thirty-three years, until his death in 1808. A marvelous personality, Hernquist left the legacy of a viable, respected model for the profession throughout Scandinavia.

Hernquist's disciple, Sven Adolf Norling, succeeded in establishing a second school in Stockholm. This energetic man commuted between Skara and Stockholm by sleigh and carriage. The Stockholm school was moved to Linnaeus's former base, the University of Agricultural Sciences at Uppsala, in 1976, and the Skara Veterinary Institute became a field station attached to the faculty. Today it has a large veterinary hospital for horses and dogs, gives practical training to veterinary students, guides regional cattle practices, and conducts research on metabolic and nutritional disorders of cattle. Its excellent veterinary museum was inaugurated by the king in 1975 in recognition of the bicentennial of the start of the school in Skara.

ABILDGAARD'S VISION: CREATION OF DENMARK'S FINE COLLEGE IN COPENHAGEN

The Danish envoy to Stockholm, J.O. Stack Rathlou, observed Linnaeus's initiative in getting the Swedish government to send students to Lyon to study at the new veterinary school because of the rinderpest epidemic and recommended to his government that Denmark should follow suit. The medical council supported the proposal, and it was adopted. The outstanding member of the selected group of students was Peter Christian Abildgaard (1740-1801). He arrived in Lyon in 1763, was admitted to the three-year course, and completed it in two and a half years. He was disappointed to find that the critical problem of rinderpest was not addressed, the entire focus being on "hippiatrics." He also found Bourgelat to be extremely proud and vain, provoking "multitudinous annoyances" for the students. No internal medicine was taught at that time, but Abildgaard was able to supplement his studies with courses in human medicine and comparative anatomy. On returning to Denmark he found that the interest in establishing a Danish veterinary service had almost evaporated in the new government formed after the death of King Frederik V. During Christian VII's reign, however, the court physician (Berger) was able to have Abildgaard's stipened extended for two years for the study of rinderpest.

Abildgaard developed a medical practice after obtaining his doctor's degree in medicine based on a thesis in 1768. The political climate changed again three years later, when the prime minister called him to a meeting to discuss plans for establishment of a veterinary school at Frederiksborg Castle. The minister wanted the school to be sited at the royal stud at the castle, but Abildgaard urged that it be in Copenhagen, where it would be easier to recruit teachers and students. After another change of ministers the king finally approved the school in 1773, and Abildgaard was appointed the foundation professor. Although some government support was provided, it was to be a private school. It opened with twenty students and only a single teacher, who took on both an enormous work load and the task of meeting the costs. In 1774 Abildgaard was asked to combat a new wave of rinderpest invasion, and he developed a rigorous control program that progressively eradicated the disease.

By 1776 a proposal was put forward to expand the facilities and seek a royal charter. The king signed a constitution for the school in 1777, making it a state institution rather than a private school. Abildgaard's interests encompassed all of natural history, agriculture, medicine, and veterinary medicine. His personal library contained 2156 volumes in seven languages ranging over all these fields. About ten percent were on veterinary medicine, but it must be appreciated that the new profession had a modest base of literature at that time.

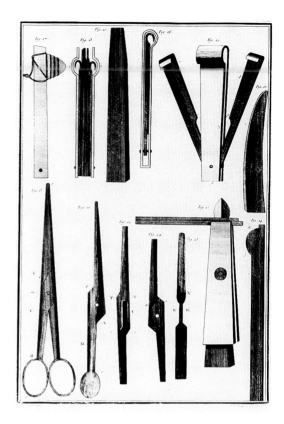

301. Various bloodletting instruments used for the treatment and care of horses. From Jean Jacques Perret (1730-1784), *L'art du coutelier*, Paris (1771-1772). *(National Library of Medicine, Bethesda, Maryland.)*

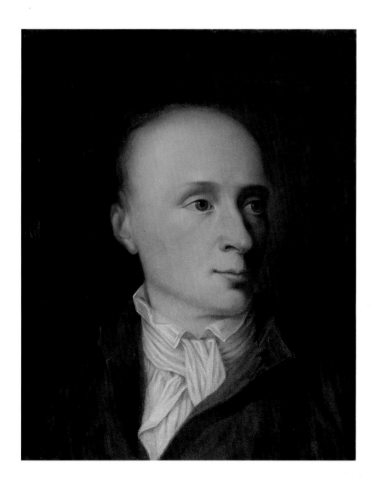

302. Portrait of Peter Christian Abildgaard (1740-1801). A graduate of Lyon, he returned to Denmark to found the first Danish veterinary school in Copenhagen in 1773. It was a private school with twenty students and a single teacher until 1777, when the king made it a state institution. *(The Royal Danish Veterinary and Agricultural University, Copenhagen.)*

Abildgaard was involved, when time permitted, in geology, physics, chemistry, botany, zoology, and natural history, including fossils. He had a special aptitude for and made contributions in parasitology, describing several parasitic species for the first time and wondering whether some of them might have a beneficial or symbiotic effect. In a paper published in 1791 he disputed Troyel's idea that ergot on rye was attributable to a fungus, a rare error on his part, but the paper, nonetheless, was a valuable contribution as a review of fungal diseases of crop plants and their medical significance. He wrote a highly regarded text on physics, and he was later offered the chair in physics at the University of Copenhagen but declined it. His interests included geophysics, magnetism, and electricity. He also constructed a hot-air balloon.

Abildgaard kept abreast of new developments in physiology and attempted in vain to resuscitate the failed heart with electric shocks, an early conception of what has become known as defibrillation. He was both intellectually brilliant and conscientious, demonstrating dedicated commitment to excellence and service. During his stay in France he had mastered the state of the art in horseshoeing, and he incorporated this skill as a requirement for veterinary students. He developed a new horseshoe design that superseded its predecessors and became widely used in Europe. He recruited an outstanding farrier to carry out this phase of the clinical teaching program. Abildgaard also invented the Danish restraining harness, which allowed examinations and surgical procedures to be conducted safely on large animals.

Abildgaard was a leading member of the Royal Agricultural Society, becoming its vice president for four years. He was keen on improving the nation's breeding stock. In 1771 he had written *Information on Horses, Cows, Sheep and Pigs, How These Must Be Tended and Raised; Their Diseases and Their Medicines and Remedies.* This work, written before the veterinary school had been established, reactivated interest in it and led to his being asked to develop a plan for one. He was particularly interested in improving the wool quality of Danish sheep. From 1793 to 1794 he traveled extensively in Germany, Italy, Spain, and Portugal, paying particular attention to the breeding and management of the Spanish Merino sheep. He had been able to import fine-wool Spanish-type sheep from Sweden for breeding studies at the royal sheep breeding station at Gladsakse; after he established contacts in Spain, sheep were imported directly. He and his assistant Erik N. Viborg wrote the excellent *Guide to Improved Sheep Breeding and the Care of Spanish Sheep in Denmark and Norway.*

Abildgaard was considered indispensable to the protection of the impressive (800-head) royal horse stud at Frederiksborg Castle, making regular inspections and being called in when serious diseases were encountered. He became a member of the board of directors and in 1790 was asked to study horse breeding throughout Denmark and the duchies of Schleswig-Holstein. When Edward Jenner published his great work on cowpox vaccination for smallpox in 1798, Abildgaard immediately ordered vaccine from England and conducted the first human vaccinations in Denmark at the veterinary school.

Everything one learns about Peter Abildgaard leaves one with the impression of a man of enormous ability and tenacity coupled with a profound social conscience. He strove to improve the health and well-being of the people, the success of the livestock farmers and the royal stud, the quality of veterinary education and of the new profession, and the advancement of scientific understanding. The only harsh judgment of him came, strangely and irrationally, from Bourgelat, who said of him that "false of heart, hated by his fellow-countrymen, intelligent, he has established a school without having much ability for it." The historical record has established that this statement would have been a more appropriate assessment of its author than of its target. Probably none of the early leaders of the schools had a record as outstanding in its achievements as Abildgaard's. He never lost his zeal for learning and for conveying what he learned to his colleagues and students.

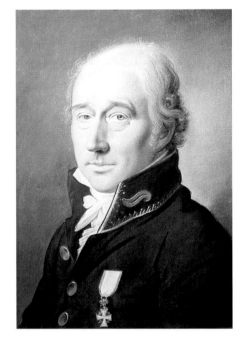

303. Portrait of Erik N. Viborg (1759-1822), an assistant to and successor of Peter Christian Abildgaard as the principal of the Danish veterinary school. In 1807 Viborg founded the world's first veterinary society, Fautores Rei Veterinariae, in Copenhagen. *(The Royal Veterinary and Agricultural University, Copenhagen.)*

Abildgaard chose his staff well. His assistant Erik N. Viborg (1759-1822), a botanist before becoming a veterinarian, was an outstanding scientist. He became a professor in the school in 1796 and succeeded Abildgaard as principal upon his death. They had worked together for eighteen years to bring the school at Christianshavn to the forefront of veterinary education. The veterinary museum at the school has a particularly fine selection of old veterinary instruments and mementos. Viborg developed suitable facilities and an experimental approach to the study of infectious diseases that placed Denmark at the forefront of eradication and prevention of contagions. Thus Viborg was able to make a clear differentiation between glanders and strangles in horses. He also recognized that glanders could take several forms depending on which organs were affected and whether the condition was acute or chronic. His work on glanders reigned until the discovery of the infectious agent. His technique for locating the site at which to introduce the trocar and cannula to the rumen in relieving bloat in cattle became known as Viborg's triangle. In 1807 the forward-looking Viborg founded in Copenhagen the first veterinary society in the world, the Fautores Rei Veterinariae.

During the early period of the veterinary school, Denmark ruled Norway and the duchies. The prevalence of contagious diseases created a recognized need to have veterinarians available in agricultural districts. Abildgaard had developed a recruiting scheme to meet the nation's needs for rural veterinarians that was approved by a royal order in 1792. The scheme called for provincial magistrates to select a literate young man, the son of a farmer or a blacksmith, every third year and send him to the veterinary school. Such students received subsidized education for three years. They agreed to return and settle within the sponsoring dioceses. This plan was accepted enthusiastically, and the first crop of "diocesan veterinarians" were qualified in 1796. The balance of students gradually swung from a predominance of military-sponsored students to equal proportions of military and rural veterinary students. Arrangements were made for the school to provide veterinary services to the members of the distillers' corporation who kept cows in the city; this would ensure a good supply of bovine clinical cases for the students.

304. Illustration of Erik N. Viborg's (1759-1822) trocar *(trommespyd)* from his *Efterretning om Trommesygens Behandling,* Kiøbenhaven (1792). Viborg modeled his trocar after the German style. Its introduction led to wider use of the instrument to release gas from the rumen in cattle. The technique is essentially the same today. *(Den Kongelige Veterinær-og Langbohøjskole, Frederiksberg.)*

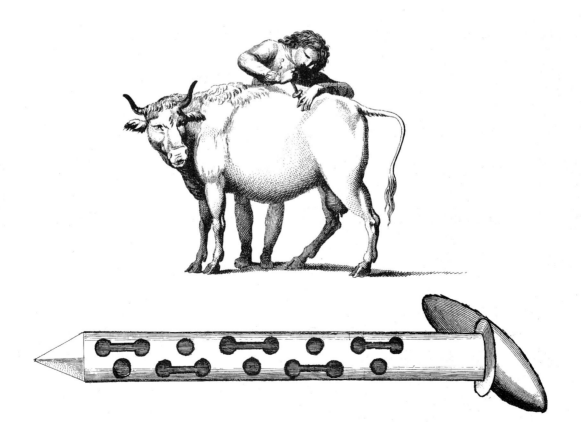

MOORCROFT: THE FIRST ENGLISH-SPEAKING VETERINARIAN

William Moorcroft was one of the most remarkable individuals to enter the veterinary profession. Born illegitimate in Ormskirk in Lancashire in 1767 to the daughter of parents who were pioneers of dairy farming, he was baptized under their name and came to be raised on the estate of his grandfather. His earliest memory was of riding astride the saddle of his grandfather's horse as a young child. Twenty years earlier the Moorcrofts had lost most of their herd to the cattle plague epidemic, a vivid reminder of the need for knowledge of matters veterinary. Thus he obtained his roots in agriculture and animal husbandry and was soon able to indulge a latent thirst for knowledge in his grandfather's fine library, which was later left to the young William.

As one of the forward-looking landowners of the district, Moorcroft's grandfather was a close friend of his distinguished neighbor Thomas Eccleston, one of the keenest promoters of improving agriculture by using new scientific ideas. He undertook initiatives in horse and cattle breeding, along with every advance in drainage, machinery, fertilizing, and cropping. He virtually adopted young William and seeded in him a love of the land and its management that never left him. Eccleston introduced William to England's most famous stock breeder, Robert Bakewell, who in his old age gave William a personal tour of his improved herds and flocks in Leicestershire.

When the time came for young Moorcroft to embark on a career to support himself, he decided on the emerging field of surgery, which was just attaining respectability after a trammeled past as the work of barber-surgeons. Based on their reputations the preferred avenues for his entry into the profession were to attend the elite private school of John Hunter in London; to attend a university medical school, preferably in Scotland; or to apprentice to a surgeon with a good reputation in a large regional hospital. Moorcroft selected the latter option, probably because of his proximity to the high-quality infirmary in the rapidly growing port city of Liverpool, just thirteen miles away. An Ormskirk native, Joseph Brandreth, was on its staff, and Eccleston was a financial supporter of the infirmary. William was granted an apprenticeship under John Lyon, one of the infirmary's leading surgeons, who had trained with the renowned Percival Pott of St. Bartholomew's Hospital in London, the leading surgeon of his day.

Surgery in the "age of agony" before anesthetics and antiseptics had been introduced was, indeed, a grim trade. The pain of the operation itself, followed by the almost certain sequence of infection and complications, deterred all but the most resolute of aspiring surgeons. Moorcroft, however, applied himself with dedication, and by 1786 John Lyon had offered him both a partnership and a hospital appointment.

Chance was to play one of its strange tricks in the form of a devastating attack of cattle plague on the estate of Thomas Eccleston, who begged his medical friends at the infirmary for assistance. They decided to send Moorcroft, because of his background, to discover what could be done to stop the spread of the lethal disease. He tried the best available medical and surgical treatments with the help of the local farrier, to no avail. The best he could do was to insist that all carcasses be buried six feet deep to stop the contagion from spreading.

Eccleston complained that the animal breeders would never get a cure for the dreadful plague because of the ignorance of the cow doctors. What was needed, he said, was a "veterinary school." He noted that other countries already had such schools, there being two in France and one in Copenhagen, and that horse surgery and farriery were much improved as a result.

Human surgeons had finally escaped from their lowly status as barber-surgeons, but animal medicine and surgery were still in the province of the uneducated cow leech or farrier. Moorcroft later recalled how he had come to make a momentous change of career goals from surgery to veterinary medicine. He felt that if he devoted himself to improve a degraded profession intimately connected with agriculture, he might be of much greater value to his country than if he continued in one already cultivated by highly talented men. His master, John Lyon, and his personal friends deplored his decision to forgo his promise in surgery for a career they perceived to be degrading. Nevertheless, he prevailed. As a practical, well-educated person who loved and had grown up with animals, yet had acquired a thorough scientific and medical training, Moorcroft was uniquely and ideally suited for the role he had chosen. Well aware of the outcome of the scientific revolution in agriculture, he was excited by the prospect of what could be achieved in veterinary medicine.

John Lyon persisted in his opposition to Moorcroft's plan and finally persuaded him to travel to London to meet the then pivotal figure of surgery, John Hunter, himself a former student of Percival Pott, for arbitration in the dispute. The visit was made about the end of 1788. Hunter, however, did not succumb to the pressure of the "old boys' network." After hearing Moorcroft's side of the story, he responded, "If I were not so advanced in years, I myself would begin on the following day to study the profession in question." Within a year Hunter was in fact lobbying forcefully for the establishment of a veterinary school in England. With the support of the Odiham Agriculture Society of Hampshire, the London school was founded in 1791, just one year after Moorcroft went to Lyon, France, for training to become the first Briton to receive formal education in veterinary medicine. Before proceeding to Lyon, Moorcroft attended Hunter's lectures in London and was elected to the Society of Arts.

Moorcroft arrived in France in the tumultuous wake of the French Revolution and left before the relatively moderate revolution degenerated into the great terror in 1792. He was disappointed with the standards of the society he found in the city and probably also with the dinginess of the school itself and its cramped, unhygienic site. There were only two faculty members at the time, the director, Louis Bredin, and the professor of comparative anatomy, Jacques-Marie Henon, who conducted research on helminth parasites. Moorcroft's instructors rated him "a model of work and application. Clever, intelligent and well educated, he knows a great deal for his age."

From Bourgelat's ambitious four-year program the course had been shortened to twelve months. The courses were anatomy (with dissection); natural history (actually animal husbandry); medicine (including chemistry, botany, and pharmacy); and pathology (internal and external diseases and their chemical and surgical treatment).

On his way home from France Moorcroft made a detailed, on-site study of horse-breeding practices instituted earlier by Bourgelat and of animal management in Normandy. On his return in 1792, Moorcroft established England's first veterinary horse practice worthy of the name. It was a propitious time for such a venture, since society had become totally dependent on the horse. Transport, agriculture, sport, and the army all used the horse as the source of physical energy. Many auxiliary industries catered to the needs of 150,000 horses and their handlers. Moorcroft wrote a case report of surgery on the brain of a cow at Ormskirk before starting his practice. Also, he worked with an Italian doctor named Vali on animal electricity, translating a text into English and dissecting a horse for him.

TRANSITION FROM FARRIERY TO VETERINARY MEDICINE

The story of the origin of the modern veterinary profession in Great Britain has been told brilliantly by Leslie Pugh in *From Farriery to Veterinary Medicine 1785-1795,* published for the Royal College of Veterinary Surgeons in 1962. According to Pugh, the seed that, after germination, was to lead to the establishment of the Veterinary College of London, was sown by a motion of Thomas Burgess at a meeting of the Odiham Agricultural Society of Hampshire in 1785. Part of this visionary clergyman-farmer's motion bears repeating as a commentary on the state of the art of animal care in Britain:

> . . . that Farriery, as commonly practiced, is conducted without principle of science and greatly to the injury to the noblest and most useful of our animals. That the improvement of Farriery established on a study of the Anatomy, diseases and cure of cattle particularly Horses, Cows and Sheep, will be an essential benefit to Agriculture and will greatly improve some of the most important branches of national commerce, such as Wool and Leather . . .

The Odiham Society included Arthur Young, a noted agricultural observer and writer who was destined to become the president of the board of agriculture. After Burgess's motion had been accepted in principle, two years elapsed during which Young studied the agriculture of France. His visit included a tour of the veterinary school at Charenton, near Paris (it was later moved to Alfort), conducted by the director, M. Chabert. Young was impressed by the facilities and the quality of the professors and the training they provided. He noted that the student body was in excess of a hundred and included students "from every country in Europe except England." The following year the society agreed to send at least two boys to stay there.

James Clark of Edinburgh's book *Prevention of Disease* appeared in print with a preface insisting that veterinary education had become a necessity at a time of rapid improvement of British livestock through selective breeding. Consequently the Odiham Society raised their sights and determined that ". . . the improvement of Farriery would be most effectively promoted by a regular education in that Art on Medical and Anatomical principles." This was a clear call for a veterinary school to be founded on British soil. Britain was well off the pace; the creation of the two French schools had soon been followed by others at Turin, Copenhagen, Vienna, Dresden, Göttingen, and Budapest in the 1780s.

Charles Benoit Vial of St. Bel, a controversial, adventurous French veterinarian and a graduate of the Lyon school, appeared on the scene in England. He had taught at the veterinary school in Paris and at the medical school in Montpellier and was a king's equerry in Lyon. He studied English agriculture and the growing industry of the thoroughbred horse. He also brought a plan for a veterinary school and married an Englishwoman. During a revisit the following year the most famous English thoroughbred stallion, Eclipse, took ill and died. The owner, Philip O'Kelly, hired Vial (who became known as Sainbel in England after he began calling himself Vial de St. Bel) to direct a detailed dissection of the animal and record his vital statistics for posterity. This brought Sainbel's name before the public and the equine industry. In 1789 Granville Penn (grandson of Quaker William Penn of Pennsylvania) met with Sainbel and realized that he could be the missing link between the aspirations of the Odiham Society and its goal of creating a veterinary school, a person with the perspective of the profession and the teaching experience needed to make the school possible.

Penn moved incisively to redraft Sainbel's plan in a style "better adapted to the customs and genius of the nation." He claimed that it was as absurd to continue entrusting the care of sick animals to the shoeing smiths as it would be to entrust human health to a shoemaker, absurd to expect of the shoer of

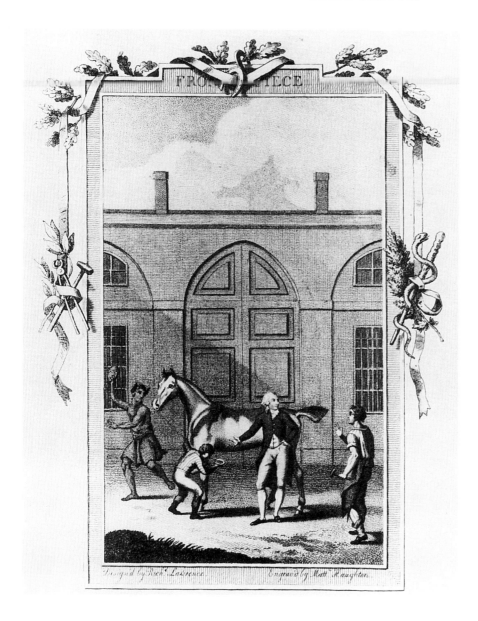

305. Frontispiece from *Elements of the Veterinary Art* by Charles Vial de Sainbel, published in London in 1797. A graduate of the Lyon school, Charles Benoit Vial of St. Bel, a controversial French veterinarian, directed the first English veterinary school, which opened in London in 1792. *(National Library of Medicine, Bethesda, Maryland.)*

a horse qualification for a task that would, if perfectly performed, "demand the united skill of a Harvey, a Boerhaave, a Duhamel, and a Reamur." Penn put together a strategic organizational structure that would enable the plan to acquire the necessary support and legitimization. The Odiham Society appointed a London committee to implement the plan in 1790.

The London committee resolved to break away from the Odiham Society and take the name of "The Veterinary College, London." Also it was resolved that "Mr. Saint Bell" be appointed professor to the college. The council added members, including the Earl of Pembroke, who had made a great commitment to improve the life of the cavalry horse and had focused particularly on improvement in the design of horseshoes. He later supported the policy that every cavalry regiment should have a veterinary surgeon. Most significant of all, John Hunter, the comparative anatomist who transformed surgery, was recruited and elected one of eight vice-presidents in April 1791. He had campaigned for a veterinary school and had encouraged Moorcroft in his ambition to go to France and acquire a veterinary education. Also the president of the Royal Society, Sir Joseph Banks, accepted membership.

According to William Youatt, one of the most distinguished graduates, Hunter became the life and soul of the undertaking after the school was established in 1791. After Sainbel's untimely death, Hunter saved the new school from catastrophe and helped during the difficult transition to new leadership.

ENGLAND'S FIRST VETERINARY COLLEGE: A CHAOTIC START

England's first veterinary school was founded in London in 1791, and the temperamental Charles Vial de Sainbel was to lead it. The school opened in 1792, but its founding professor died suddenly a year and a half later, after contracting glanders from an infected horse. Moorcroft was the logical choice to replace him, but Moorcroft had just begun his London practice in an ideal location on Oxford Street, a main traffic route. He offered his services until such time as the vacancy was filled.

Edward Coleman (1765-1839) was born near Burmarsh in Romney Marsh, Kent. As a young surgeon he began a practice in London and had conducted physiological experiments on asphyxia in dogs and cats, for which he was awarded a medal by the Humane Society. Astley Paston Cooper (1768-1841) was a close friend of Coleman. Cooper was a protégé of John Hunter and became the best-known surgeon in London. He and Coleman had both attended Hunter's lectures. Cooper later became the chairman of the governing body of the veterinary school.

The year after Sainbel's death a compromise was made in the selection of his replacement after a long series of deliberations. The position was offered jointly to Coleman and Moorcroft, both at professorial rank. The latter was reluctant but was finally persuaded to accept an arrangement that allowed him to continue developing his practice. However, after a few weeks he resigned, no doubt finding the shared authority incompatible with his temperment as a challenging innovator and being pulled by the demands of his practice, which allowed him full expression of his ideas. Shortly thereafter Moorcroft hired an assistant, John Field, whom he had known as a student, and together they provided the best possible service in their veterinary practice.

Moorcroft's withdrawal meant that Coleman became the principal of the school. He faced a formidable challenge: to create a viable, effective institution with an inadequate background in the field and inadequate facilities. His critics charged him with lowering the standards both of admission and of professional education, but at that time people who worked with animals were regarded with disdain, and many were illiterate. The school under Sainbel began with high hopes, requiring its students to be fifteen to twenty-two years of age and giving preference to those who had the elements of a good education. Thus the students were a mix of young boys fresh from school and medical students who had served several years of apprenticeship to a surgeon. Under Coleman virtually anyone was admitted who had the necessary tuition fee of twenty guineas, which the principal pocketed. Coleman was reported to have said that a combination of talent and an early knowledge of the horse led to the best veterinarians. In other words, he preferred farriers' sons to surgeons.

It appeared that Coleman reduced the length of training from the original plan of three years to a few months. William Dick obtained his diploma in three months. The first diploma awarded by the college was to Edmund Bond on April 22, 1794, after eighteen months of resident instruction. Of course, Sainbel had been dead for eight months by then, and Moorcroft resigned in the same month. The school also came in for criticism because its sole focus was the horse. The same allegation could be made about several of the early schools in Europe. It would be unjust to praise Bourgelat and condemn Coleman unless one can forgive all shortcomings of the former because he was first. Being first, however, does not make the narrow focus excusable. Great Britain was becoming the greatest center for the development of improved breeds of livestock for the production of food, fiber, and draft power, yet the new school gave no priority to such animals. The school, in the heart of London, was badly situated to attract agricultural animals, but no conception of the broader role emerged and no creative proposals were put forth to meet the need. In those areas Moorcroft would have shone, with his vision and tenacity in pursuit of a goal and his Ormskirk farming background.

The first half-century of the London school seems to have been a golden opportunity lost during a time of great scientific and agricultural awakening in Great Britain. Although Coleman had started his medical career as something of an experimentalist, he did not remain true to the legacy of enquiry he acquired from John Hunter. Because he had charm and eloquence and understood the political establishment and the importance of influential contacts, he stayed in office until he died, forty-eight years after the school opened, after serving for forty-five years as its principal. He considered his chief contribution to have been making the veterinary profession respectable by ensuring that its practitioners were entitled to appointments with

306. The establishment of the Royal Veterinary College (RVC) in London did not meet with everyone's approval, especially the farriers, as evidenced by two hand-colored engravings (Plates 306 and 307) by Francis Jukes (1747-1812) that were published in 1792, the year the RVC opened. In the 1897 publication by James Beart Simonds, *The Foundation of the Royal Veterinary College, 1790-91 with biographical sketches of St. Bel, Edward Coleman, William Sewell, and Charles Spooner, chief professors in succession, 1791-1871,* Jukes' engravings are described as ". . . evidently the work of a severe satirist, whose object would appear to have been the placing of newly-created Veterinary Surgeons, by the establishment of the Veterinary College, on a par with common Farriers." The following introduction precedes the engravings:

"To the Noblemen, Gentlemen, & Others: Patrons, Presidents, & Professors of the Veterinary College; Plates exhibiting the New Methods & Machines chiefly employed for the Reformation & Improvement of Farriery & the treatment of Cattle in General, are most respectfully dedicated by their Obedient Servants, NIck [. . . ?]
Phil [. . . ?]

The first engraving (Plate 306) is identified as "2nd Lecture upon the newly approv'd Method of Casting and Fireing. London. Pubd According to Act of Parliament. March 28, 1792, by F. Juke's." A horse tied with ropes is held by three men outside a blacksmith's shop; to the right, an assistant with bellows works a fire; a small dog stands in the foreground. *(The Royal Veterinary College, London.)*

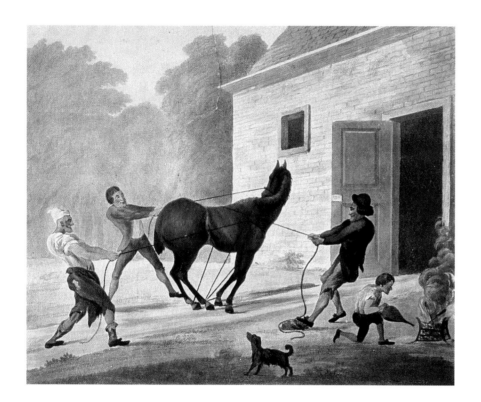

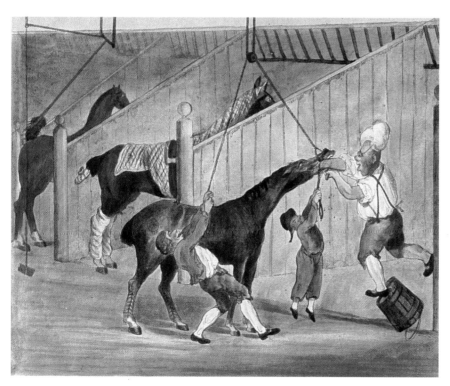

307. "3rd Lecture, Upon the most Novel safe and sure method of Popping a Horse-Ball. London. Pubd May 30, 1792 by F. Jukes, Howland [Housland?] Strt." In a stable two men with ropes that are tied around the jaw of a horse pull in opposite directions to hold the jaw open; another man, falling off an overturned bucket, is attempting, with some difficulty, to put a ball (pill) down the horse's throat. *(The Royal Veterinary College, London.)*

commissions as officers in the cavalry. Although he was an advocate of "proper status" for veterinarians, he accepted that their status should be below that of surgeons and medical practitioners. The indictment of Coleman resides in the comparison of the Edinburgh and London schools as providers of "seed stock" for the New World.

DICK'S EDINBURGH SCHOOL: ACHIEVEMENT OF INTERNATIONAL RECOGNITION

The veterinary college with the greatest impact on veterinary education in North America was established in Edinburgh by William Dick in 1820, the second school to be established in Great Britain. The Highland and Agricultural Society (HAS) of Edinburgh in 1823 hired William Dick to be lecturer in veterinary medicine. Its intentions were modest:

> . . . to get hold of the more intelligent working blacksmith and give him such a training in anatomical and clinical knowledge as would fit him to treat the ailments of animals in a manner less barbarous than then in vogue.

Dick, a farrier's son, was born in Edinburgh. He traveled to London, no doubt by stagecoach, in 1817 and obtained his diploma from Coleman's diploma mill three months later, in 1818. Returning to his hometown, he worked as a farrier and studied anatomy under Barclay, who later helped obtain the patronage of the HAS for a course of veterinary lectures commencing in November 1823. Dick used funds from his practice to found the Edinburgh Veterinary School, arranging for the HAS to issue certificates of competence after approval of an examining board composed mainly of medical professionals and the principal until more veterinarians were available.

The British Army and the East India Company soon began to accept the Edinburgh graduates into their veterinary services. The new faculty achieved a strong international reputation, comparable with the best, by the 1840s. William Dick himself taught hippopathology and directed the clinical work. He was reputed to have been an extraordinarily gifted and subtle diagnostician, frequently diagnosing lameness in horses on the street without leaving his chair. His early colleagues included Thomas Strangeways, Allen Dalzall, and Peter Young. Dick died in 1866, but by then the classes of 1861 and 1862 had produced three great men who carried the Edinburgh tradition across the Atlantic Ocean.

Andrew Smith, founder of the Ontario Veterinary College in Toronto in 1862, graduated in 1861. His classmate James Law was selected by White, the president of Cornell University in Ithaca, New York, to become the first professor of veterinary medicine in the United States in 1868. Law had coauthored (with John Gamgee) two well-illustrated volumes on the anatomy of domestic animals in 1861. He wrote a masterpiece on veterinary medicine in five volumes around 1900, long after he emigrated from Britain to America. Smith and Law were destined to have enormous influence upon the development of the profession in Canada and the Unites States, respectively. The Edinburgh class of 1862 included Duncan McEachran, who went to Canada and founded a private veterinary school in Montreal. He set exceptionally high goals for his school and managed to obtain the assistance of William Osler, who became the greatest medical leader of his day. The son of a veterinarian who trained in Montreal recalled his father commenting frequently on the inspiration he received from Osler as a teacher. Osler's talent took him from McGill University to found the Johns Hopkins School of Medicine in Baltimore and, later, to become Regius Professor of Medicine at Oxford University. Harvey Cushing, in his biography of Osler, credited him with naming McEachran's veterinary school "The Faculty of Comparative Medicine."

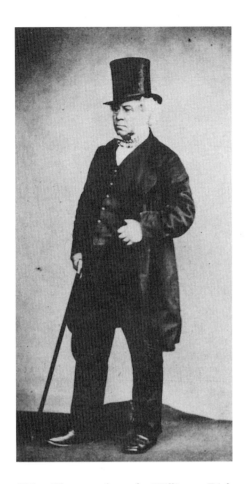

308. Photograph of William Dick (1793-1866), who qualified at the Royal Veterinary College, London, in 1817 and founded his own veterinary school in Edinburgh in 1823. *(British Veterinary Association, London.)*

McEachran's school, however, was too good to be true, too far ahead of its time. He encouraged the development of a veterinary school for those who spoke French, which replaced it. McEachran's vision persisted, however, and in 1880, recognizing the great potential of the developing cattle industry, he went west. He formed a partnership and established the Walrand Ranch, and he was appointed Canada's first inspector of stock. In this capacity he demanded quarantine and inspection facilities for all imported animals. His admonition bears repeating:

> There is some danger that pleuropneumonia may be carried to the unfenced ranges of the far West and it is incumbent upon the Government to take preventative measures to protect the cattle interests of the Canadian NorthWest, if not by prohibition or quarantine at least by rigid inspection before admission to the Dominion.

The Contagious Diseases Act of 1879 allowed preventive measures to be implemented. The first veterinarian in northwestern Canada, John Poett, a veterinary staff sergeant in the Mounted Police based at Fort MacLeod, was appointed in 1884 to inspect 25,000 head of cattle entering from Montana.

ELUSIVE EXPECTATIONS FOR THE FASHIONABLE FIELD OF VETERINARY MEDICINE

After Bourgelat succeeded in creating a veterinary profession in the eighteenth century, it is quite remarkable how rapidly the idea was adopted throughout Europe. The founding of veterinary educational institutions became a veritable fashion trend. Between the beginnings at Lyon in 1762 and the turn of the century, no fewer than nineteen veterinary schools were created. During the same period only six faculties of medicine and two in agriculture were initiated. Along with compelling practical reasons for forming the new professional cadre, such as keeping horses operational and attempting to contain animal plagues, there was also a sudden development of public awareness of the importance of animals. This more subtle perception—that the lives of humans and animals were truly mutually interdependent in a healthy society—seems to have appeared like a revelation to capture the collective imagination.

Expectations, however, ran ahead of realities. The early instructional approach was derived in large part from human medicine, and the early teachers must have had an arduous time "getting up to speed." For the first fifty years or more the field of clinical veterinary medicine was largely empirical. There was no real understanding either of the nature of infectious diseases or of the physiology and pathology of the animal body to allow sound diagnoses and treatments to be developed. The goal of veterinary education was a controversial issue. Should it be to train practical field workers or scientifically based professionals who could solve problems and advance knowledge? The curricula of the various schools oscillated between these extremes, from short, practical training programs to in-depth science-based learning and questioning that required more time.

"Leeches," marshals, farriers, and horse doctors continued to practice animal treatments, but the new veterinary professionals perceived them to be charlatans or "quacks." Consequently moves were made to require licensure and restrict the right to practice to those who were qualified by education, and competition existed in the marketplace. The educational standard for the entering students was too low to achieve the higher goals some institutions strove to attain. Scholars sent to acquire veterinary education elsewhere seem to have had the greatest impact on veterinary education in Great Britain. Excellent students without dogma, bringing an interdisciplinary perspective and becoming aware of deficiencies, they had the vision to create better models in their homelands.

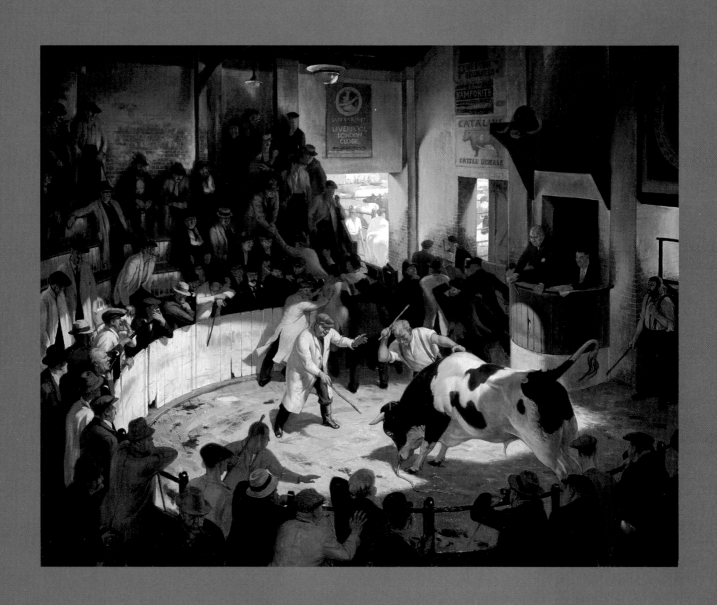

Livestock Improvement by Animal Breeders

BRITISH INITIATIVES TO ADVANCE LIVESTOCK AGRICULTURE

Walter Blith, an English agricultural author of the mid-seventeenth century, was the early master of the fundamentals of agriculture who revolutionized British farming. His *English Improver Improved* of 1652 set out a string of six successful practices that became widely adopted. The list included "drowning" of water meadows (flat riverside pastures); drainage of wet soils and reclaiming of fens; enclosure of land to permit intensification of crop and livestock husbandry and reduction of the spread of animal disease; plowing of old pastures and sowing of deteriorated arable land to grass (the principle that was the forerunner of ley farming); the selection and importance of manures; and the afforestation of land unsuitable for cultivation. Blith conducted field trials of various combinations of fertilizers and manures and was a committed advocate of red clover, although he knew nothing of the legume's root nodule bacteria that fix atmospheric nitrogen.

Establishment of the Royal Society (1662) of which King Charles II became patron fostered the generation of scientific information and recommendation of new crops (such as the potato) and equipment such as the light, streamlined plow. The introduction of root crops, such as that of the turnip by Sir Richard Weston (1645), who integrated it into rotations with clover, made it possible to carry breeding stock through the winter in better condition. Weston's *Discourse of Husbandrie* was published in 1650. Jethro Tull of Howberry, Oxfordshire, invented the seed drill (1701) and the horse hoe, which made possible the low seeding rates and interrow cultivation used in productive row-crop culture. His book *Horse-Houghing Husbandry* (1731) expounded a new perspective of deep cultivation focused on the importance of the complex root structure of crop plants and the use of draft power of oxen or horses. His technique eliminated the need for the wasteful fallow and set the stage for the Norfolk crop rotation of the nineteenth century.

The great advances in animal agriculture in Great Britain, however, derived from the pasturelands. Grasses as the primary nutrient sources for herbivorous domestic animals have been the foundation of milk and meat production since the origin of domestication. Dried forage in the form of hays and straws has been a key factor in getting stock through the winter. Good-quality hay was required to maintain high production, and the improved pastures and leys made possible the increases in quantity and quality.

The British environment, so well suited to grassland and fodder crop production and freed by its aquatic isolation from much of the continuum of wars and animal plagues that spread repeatedly throughout continental Europe and

309. *Facing page, Commotion in the Cattle Ring,* painted by James Bateman in 1935, depicts the busy market in Banbury, Oxfordshire. In response to an unpredictable British Friesian dairy bull, farmers make a rapid exodus from the ring while the two ring handlers distract him and the auctioneer looks on. It was common practice to affix a piece of rope or chain around the horns and run it down through the nose ring to facilitate safe handling of bulls. *(Tate Gallery Publications, London.)*

310. *Herdsman Tending Cattle,* by the famous Dutch animal painter Albert Cuyp (1620-1691). The polders of the lowlands of Holland were the sites of selection and improvement of short-horned cattle for milk production. *(Andrew W. Mellon Collection, copyright 1994, National Gallery of Art, Washington, D.C.)*

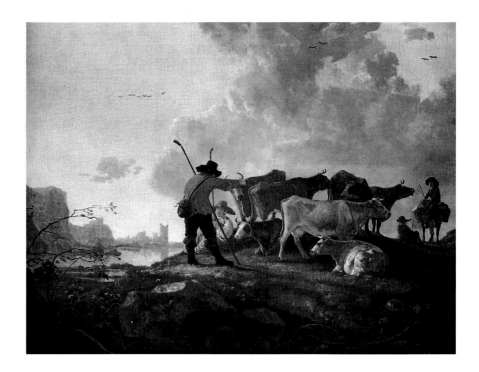

311. *Facing page,* Map of the British Isles showing the regional areas where some of the major breeds of farm livestock originated or were improved. A few of the early breeders who had major impacts on their development are identified. Also shown are the sites of the six veterinary schools and some important centers for research or education to promote livestock health and productivity.

352

devastated flocks and herds, proved to be almost ideal for livestock breeding and production. Other sites in Europe were similarly favored, such as the relatively isolated Alpine valleys and mountain pastures; much of lowland Scandinavia, except where it bordered on the main land mass; the Low Countries with their productive grasslands and mild climate; and the Iberian Peninsula with its great tradition of producing fine-wool sheep and riding horses that arose from strains imported from North Africa and western Asia. The intimate connections among human and animal migrations, geography, and animal health, particularly the epidemiology of infectious diseases, were and are major factors in the development of useful breeds.

Progress in animal breeding through selection and in seasonal nutritional management through enclosure, along with grassland improvement and the exploitation of root crops, gave an enormous boost to British agriculture in the eighteenth and nineteenth centuries.

The great medieval war horses of Europe gave rise to the large breeds of draft horses such as the Flanders and Belgian breeds on the Continent and the Shire in England by the seventeenth century. A feature of British stock farming was its diversity, every region developing localized strains of cattle or sheep. Even after the consolidations of modern times and the disappearance of many local varieties, there are approximately three dozen breeds of sheep, two dozen of cattle, and a dozen or more each of pigs and horses or ponies that originated in Great Britain.

Animal agriculture developed rapidly in Europe in the eighteenth century. Earlier, pastures were being improved and legumes brought into use in them, especially in pastures planted after grain crops on arable land. The old natural pastures such as the Essex marshes carried heavy stocking with sheep, producing wether mutton for the London winter market from Lincoln and Leicester breeds. Lincoln and Norfolk stock grazed the Brecklands, and the incomparably productive Romney marshes fed the renowned Romney Marsh sheep breed. Sheep farmers on the chalk downs of Hampshire, Wiltshire, and Dorset adopted root crops for folding the Hampshire Down sheep, the Dorset breeds, and the Wiltshire horned, a hair sheep. The urine and manure treaded into the soil improved the productivity of subsequent grain crops such as the famous malting barleys used to produce the popular beers and ales.

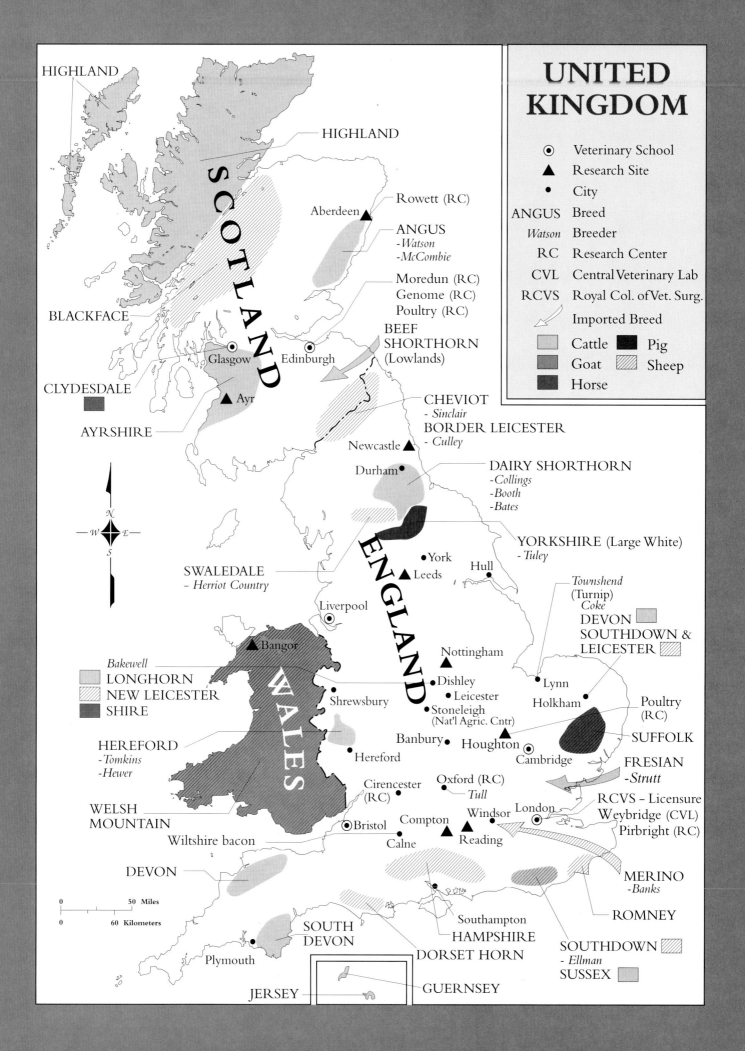

HIGHLAND

SCOTLAND

HIGHLAND

Rowett (RC)

ANGUS
-*Watson*
-*McCombie*

Aberdeen

Moredun (RC)
Genome (RC)
Poultry (RC)

BLACKFACE

BEEF
SHORTHORN
(Lowlands)

Glasgow

Edinburgh

CLYDESDALE

Ayr

AYRSHIRE

CHEVIOT
- *Sinclair*
BORDER LEICESTER
- *Culley*

Newcastle

Durham

DAIRY SHORTHORN
-*Collings*
-*Booth*
-*Bates*

YORKSHIRE (Large White)
- *Tuley*

Townshend
(Turnip)
Coke

DEVON

SOUTHDOWN &
LEICESTER

ENGLAND

SWALEDALE
- *Herriot Country*

York

Leeds

Hull

Liverpool

Nottingham

Lynn

Holkham

Poultry
(RC)

SUFFOLK

Bangor

WALES

Bakewell
LONGHORN
NEW LEICESTER
SHIRE

Dishley

Leicester

Shrewsbury

Stoneleigh
(Nat'l Agric. Cntr)

Banbury

Houghton

Cambridge

FRESIAN
-*Strutt*

HEREFORD
-*Tomkins*
-*Hewer*

Hereford

Cirencester
(RC)

Oxford (RC)
Tull

London

RCVS – Licensure
Weybridge (CVL)
Pirbright (RC)

WELSH
MOUNTAIN

Bristol

Compton

Windsor

Reading

Wiltshire bacon

Calne

MERINO
-*Banks*

DEVON

ROMNEY

Southampton

SOUTH
DEVON

HAMPSHIRE

SOUTHDOWN
- *Ellman*

SUSSEX

Plymouth

DORSET HORN

JERSEY

GUERNSEY

0   50 Miles
0   60 Kilometers

353

HUMPED CATTLE IN DEVELOPING COUNTRIES AND THE TROPICS

The humped cattle, *Bos indicus,* differ strikingly in appearance from the humpless varieties, grouped under the species name *Bos taurus.* There are two general kinds of humped cattle. One has a muscular hump in a cervicothoracic location and is seen in South African Sanga-type cattle and in crossbreds of *B. indicus* and *B. taurus.* The other, the zebu type, has a fattier hump in a thoracic location. Archaeological evidence indicates that the neck-humped kind appeared earlier than the back-humped kind. The two types interbreed without difficulty, which suggests that they were derived from a common ancestral stock that branched into two types of the primitive aurochs. The humped branch, now extinct, has been tentatively named *Bos primigenius namadicus.* The humped varieties were adapted to hot environments and were more resistant to ticks and tick-borne diseases. The humped cattle today are typically part of extensive pastoral systems in developing countries. They make up two thirds of the world's cattle population but produce less than a third of the beef consumed and less than a fourth of the milk. However, they play a major role in draft work in agriculture and transport while providing other essential products such as dung for fuel, shelter, and fertilizer and hides for leather. There are many breeds, particularly in the warmer parts of Asia.

BAKEWELL: ARCHITECT OF BREED IMPROVEMENT BY SELECTIVE MATING

Great Britain became famous for its development of breeds of domestic livestock, particularly sheep, cattle, horses, pigs, and chickens. The development of breeds was largely the result of empirical efforts by farmers who had an ideal type in mind and a good eye for selection of breeding stock. An early proponent of long-horned cattle was Webster of Canley, Warwickshire. His animals provided some of the foundation stock for the most famous of the early improvers, Robert Bakewell (1726-1795), tenant farmer of a 600-acre property at Dishley, Leicestershire. Bakewell showed how a desired type could be developed by locating and purchasing animals having relevant traits and outbreeding from them to determine whether better combinations could be formed. These would then be "fixed" by repeated inbreeding from the finest specimens. His ideal types would not be so today, but there was a valid demand for the goals in his period. His followers were to apply his methods and develop many of the breeds that spread from Great Britain to improve many existing Eurasian breeds and, in pure form, to populate the great virgin pasturelands and intensive systems of the Americas and Australasia.

Bakewell had the eye and mind of a "natural" stock breeder. He was an astute judge of quality, using the senses of sight and touch in evaluating animals. He also looked for a vigorous constitution and a competitive appetite. Britain's stock owed a great deal to Dutch imports in the seventeenth and eighteenth centuries. The previous, simplistic view of the purpose of animal husbandry was that the horse was used for battle and transport, the ox for its labor, the cow for its milk and dairy products, the sheep for its wool, the pig for bacon and ham, and the hen for its eggs. Thus beef came from bony, spent draft oxen and aging dairy cows, mutton from sheep that were often kept for four shearings before slaughter, and veal from calves that tended to fatness. Bakewell perceived the new demand for high-quality beef and tallow (a valuable commodity then), so he selected stock with a propensity for fattening and early maturity. His father remained an active farmer until Robert was in his forties, so he traveled around Europe to observe animal breeding practices on the Continent and in the British Isles. He noticed that a few breeders practiced inbreeding to fix a type, although many were averse to the practice, and he adopted judicious inbreeding as a strategy, concurring with the old adage

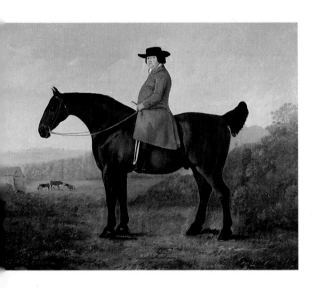

312. Robert Bakewell (1726-1795), perhaps the most significant forerunner of modern livestock breeding, sat for this fine painting by Boultbee (1745-1812) on his estate at Dishley in Leicestershire. *(Leicestershire Museums, Arts and Records Service, England.)*

that "like begets like." However, he was aware of the need to crossbreed first to get a variety of types, some of which would be endowed with the traits he sought.

It is important to keep in mind that Bakewell was active before the science of genetics came into being. He kept specimens of his best animals in pickle to provide evidence of his progress toward fineness of bones, better muscling, and fat thickness. He was the first to apply the concept of progeny testing, deferring wider use of stud males until he saw the results of their early matings and frequently letting out bulls and rams by the season to observe their effects on other herds. He was much more focused on performance for economic efficacy than most breeders, who went after beauty to behold. He insisted on gentle stock-handling methods, and his animals were renowned for their placidity.

Bakewell applied his innovations to all aspects of farming and was an early user of grassland irrigation and concentrate feeding. He weighed his pigs and the food they ate, tracking food conversion. His cattle were known as the improved Longhorn or New Leicester. Hardy, yet fast-growing and efficient, they met the grazier's or beef producer's needs. He did not, however, pursue the goals of increased milk production or fertility. His stock were to be overtaken by the Shorthorn cattle bred by Charles Colling (1751-1836) and his brother Robert of Ketting, Durham. They had studied with Bakewell but set a goal of a dual-purpose animal that would provide milk as well as fatten. Their instincts in the matter appear to have been better than Bakewell's, since their cattle soon became more popular than the Longhorns after Bakewell's death. Nonetheless, the more popular beef breed, the Hereford, grew out of the old Longhorn stock.

313. Painting of the famous Longhorn bull, Shakespeare (c. 1790), bred by Robert Fowler of Little Rollright, Oxfordshire, a contemporary of Bakewell. Such cattle should not be confused with the Longhorns of the American ranges, which were derived from the imported Spanish Criollo stock. *(Courtesy of the University of Reading, Rural History Centre, Berkshire.)*

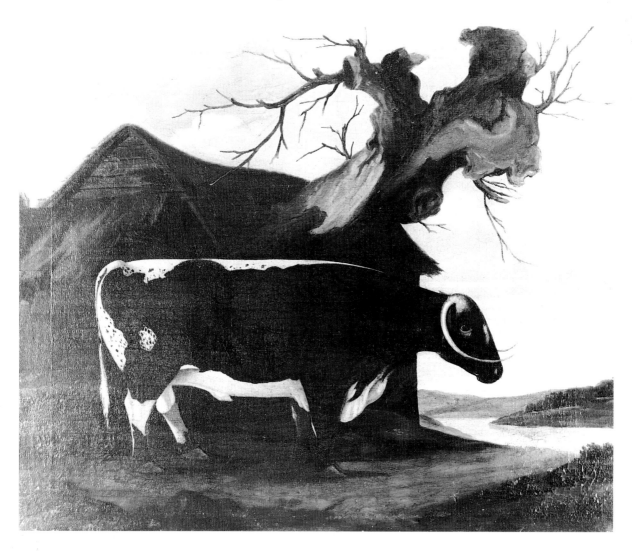

314. *Sir John Palmer of Withcote Hall, Leicestershire, Inspects His New Leicester Sheep, with Shepherd John Green,* painted by John Fernley in 1825. Bakewell developed this breed, also known as Dishley sheep. *(Leicestershire Museums Art Galleries and Records Service, England.)*

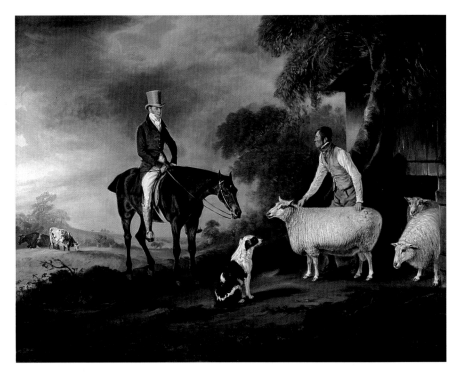

Bakewell's breed of sheep, the Dishley or New Leicester, was outstandingly successful: his finest ram, known as the Two-Pounder, earned eight-hundred pounds in one year for his services, an astonishing amount for its time. Here again, Bakewell was prepared to sacrifice desirable traits to achieve his primary goal of economic meat production, settling for a poor wool clip. This breed had a worldwide impact, and its derivatives such as the Border Leicester are still a major force today in crossbreeding for lamb production. Bakewell bred the large, superior shire horses. He also applied his special talent to the improvement of pigs, but his improved Leicester pig, although it fattened rapidly, was criticized for having leg problems. Joseph Tuley of Keighley, Yorkshire, was the most renowned breeder of Great Britain's most famous breed, the Large White or Yorkshire pig.

SPANISH MERINO VERSUS BAKEWELL'S NEW LEICESTER: WOOL OR LAMB

The Spanish Merino sheep's geographical and genetic precursors are obscure, but great skill must have been applied in their selective breeding for the finest wools. The industry became the preserve of the Mesta, the controlling guild that forbade export of the breed until 1765. A change occurred after the industrial advances in the north permitted mass production of woven cloths so that the Spanish textile manufacturers could not compete. The first Bourbon king of Spain, Felipe V, secured the throne in 1700. He found the Spanish wool trade mainly in the hands of the Dutch, French, and English. In return, Spain had to buy the luxury goods it needed, especially the fine woolen cloths. The Spanish king set out to change this situation by starting to produce finished cloth in royal Spanish factories. The first was in Guadalajara in 1718, and others followed. They had difficulty competing successfully, except for a period after 1740, when Thomas Bevan, a skilled weaver of Melksham, Wiltshire, and his fellow craftsmen supervised production.

The Merino sheep were kept in a transhumant cycle (one of seasonal migration to and from upland pasture) that sent them south to warmer Estremadure for the winter. In May they were moved to Segovia, where they were shorn before being sent to the cold mountains of Leon to graze for the summer. The embargo on the export of live Merinos was broken, first, by a Swedish visionary, Jonas Alstroemer, in 1723, then by the great French scholar

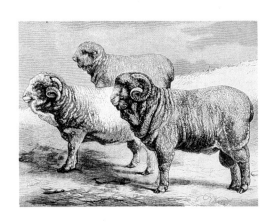

315. Three specimens of Spanish merino sheep fostered at King George III's farm near Windsor by Sir Joseph Banks. He arranged for a shipment to go to Australia with Captain Macarthur, having envisioned their successful adaptation there. They did not thrive in the cool, damp English environment.

Louis-Jean-Marie Daubenton (1716-1799), the distinguished comparative anatomist who had worked with Buffon at the Jardin des Plantes. Daubenton was asked by the government of Louis XV's controller general, Trudaine, in 1766 to "investigate by a series of well-conceived and carefully executed experiments the most favorable natural conditions for the improvement of wool." The concern behind this initiative was the perception of a need for France to develop the capacity to produce its own raw material for cloth manufacture, fine wool, in case the Spanish supply was cut off, as it might be in a war.

A flock was established at Montbard on the Cote d'Or in Burgundy. The achievements of Daubenton in commissioned studies stand as an early, classic effort in animal breeding targeted to improve both the rural economy and a major industry. He was uniquely prepared by his twenty years of research in zoology and comparative anatomy. He obtained parent stock from Roussillon and Flanders as well as from England, Morocco, and even Tibet. The experimental plan called for a ten-year crossbreeding program carefully monitored for the quality and amount of wool produced. Daubenton also included in his protocols all matters affecting the health, feeding, and management of all the strains. He recognized that different factors caused them to vary in the same environment. Exact records were kept of every ewe and lamb and of the ram used in every mating. Deaths were studied by necropsy to find the cause, if possible. Daubenton introduced objective standards for the wool: he used the microscope to determine fiber thickness, creating a scale of seven grades from coarse to fine. He found that he could eliminate coarse, hairy fibers by selection and also select for fineness. Remarkably, he observed that he could produce crosses in which the weight of the lambs' fleece increased as much as threefold from that of their dam's. Also, these factors were modified by their health and nutrition. After ten years of selection he could prove that his finest fleeces were superior to those of Roussillon.

Daubenton's finest wools were just one grade below those of the Escorial flock, reputedly the best in Spain. He reported his results in 1777 to the Academie Royale des Sciences, concluding that it would be possible by selection of the best Roussillon rams to improve the wools from French flocks to the second degree of superfineness. To attain the very highest quality, however, would require the importation of appropriate genetic stock from Spain itself. A new controller-general of finance, Turgot, took the point and authorized such importation. This was accomplished, although the means were not disclosed. Nine years later, Daubenton completed his experiments with the superfine imports and made his final report to the Academie Royale in 1785. He then carried out the ultimate test of having the preeminent clothing firm compare his fleeces with those of the top Spanish firms for cloth manufacture. His were judged to be indistinguishable in fineness, and the Montbard wool was superior in the brilliance of its dyeing. He presented this information to the Academie Royale as an addendum the following year, and it was combined with the report and published.

Daubenton's fine work led to his recruitment to a new chair of rural economy at the Royal Veterinary School at Alfort by Bertier de Sauvigny, who also persuaded him to establish a small breeding flock at the school as a demonstration farm for the Royal Society of Agriculture. Daubenton accepted the professorship and built a small replica of his bergerie at Montbard.

The way was open for France to attain independence in growing fine wools if she wished. The president of Britain's Royal Society, Sir Joseph Banks, obtained a copy of the Academie Royale's publication in 1787. An earlier publication had been based on the first round of experiments at Montbard, *Instructions for Shepherds and Flock-Owners,* in 1782. It went through several editions and continued to be reprinted long after Daubenton's death.

Countries other than Great Britain were on a similar track. Merinos were imported to Saxony (in 1765 and 1778), to Austria (in 1775), again to France (in 1786), and finally, under the prodding of Banks, to England. King Carlos

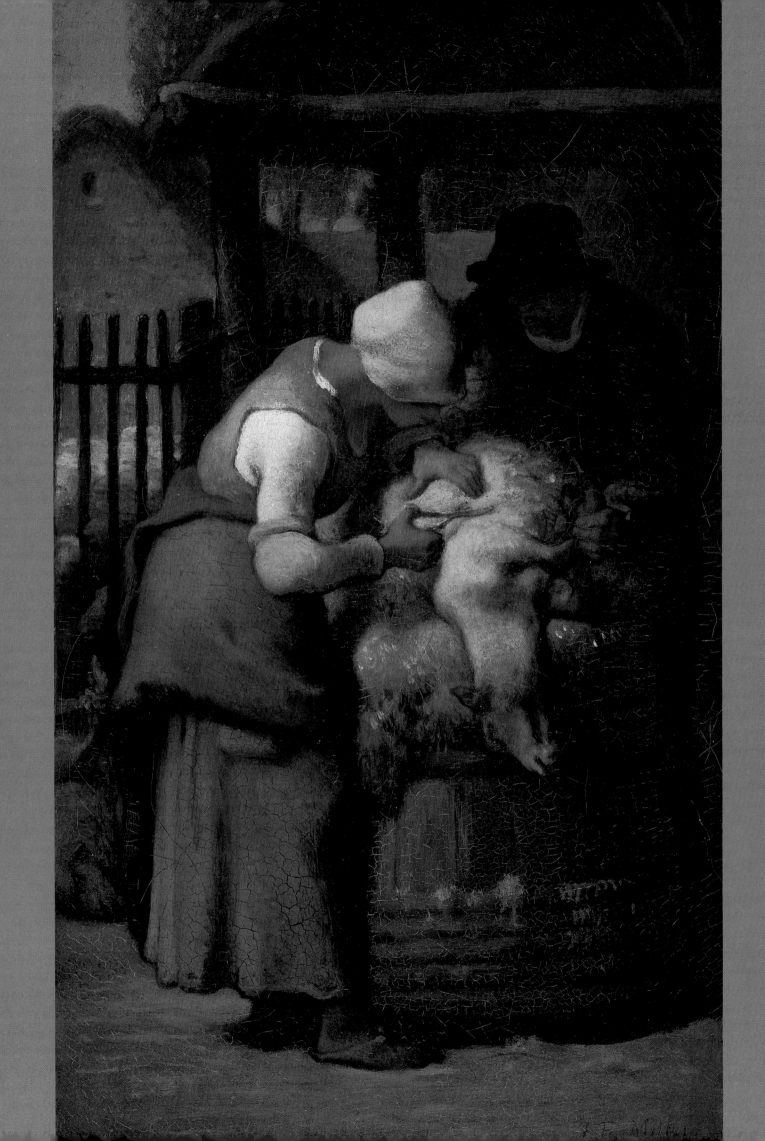

III and his minister Campomanes's reforms included inquiries into the pastoral regime in 1771 and 1779 that were followed by a reduction in the monopolistic powers of the Mesta. It appears that Spain had acquired a purblind mystique that nowhere outside its peninsula could such fine wool be grown. The data for 1667 show that Spain exported about 8 million pounds of fine wool in that year, more than half of it via the port of Bilbao. More than half of the wool went to Holland, Hamburg, and adjacent states; about 1.3 million pounds went to France, around 1 million to England, and 0.6 million to Venice. This supply was harvested from about 4 million sheep, most of them in the transhumant practice of the cabañas.

Bakewell's impact was tremendous. To his agricultural contemporaries he was the inspiration for change and the catalyst of a new synthesis that transformed British farming and livestock husbandry. His development of the New Leicester sheep at Dishley Grange was followed by dissemination of its genes to every sheep-finishing region. The new "fatstock" farming for better-quality meat was adopted rapidly as the land use control provided by the enclosures legislation was implemented. Except for the Spanish Merino fine-wools, wool was the loser in the tug-of-war between meat and wool production. The new sheep were long-wool rather than clothing-wool types. The result was a problem for the fine-wool cloth industry and trade of western England, initiating a controversy that pitted the Spanish Merino against the New Leicester. This skirmish was overridden by the onset of the Napoleonic Wars, which led to the transfer of the arena of competition to the virgin pasture-lands of Australasia. There was legitimate concern about maintaining the supply of fine wools from Spain in the event of war. The realization of the potential for improvement through selection for desired traits and the progress Bakewell had demonstrated led to a great increase in the value of high-quality breeding stock for sale or service, which in turn led to a steady increase in the demand for competent veterinary services.

316. *Facing page, Shearing Sheep,* painted by the superb French artist of rural peasant life at Barbizon, Jean-François Millet (1814–1875) in 1853. At that time wool was the supreme textile fiber in Europe. *(Gift of Quincy Adams Shaw through Quincy A. Shaw, Jr., and Mrs. Marian Shaw Haughton. Courtesy Museum of Fine Arts, Boston.)*

317. *The Shepherd's Return* (1882) by a leading German animal painter, Heinrich von Zügel (1850–1941), the son of a sheep farmer. *(Gift of the René von Schleinitz Foundation. Milwaukee Art Museum.)*

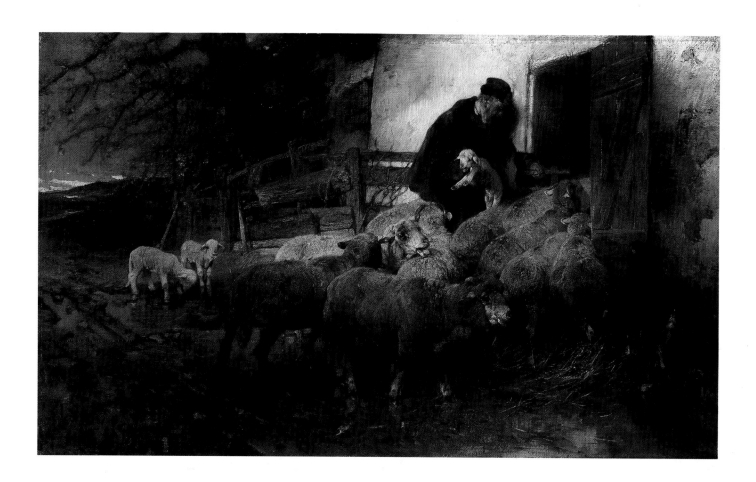

BANKS: SETTING THE STAGE FOR THE AUSTRALIAN WOOL INDUSTRY

Sir Joseph Banks (1743-1820) was one of the greatest figures in the history of scientific culture. Educated in botany at Cambridge, he soon developed an insatiable thirst for knowledge and international perspective, traveling to Newfoundland in 1766 and being selected to fellowship of the Royal Society upon his return. This led to his selection as scientist on Captain James Cook's great voyage of exploration on the Endeavour from 1768 to 1771, during which Banks roomed with the great navigator and greatly expanded the scope of botanical knowledge. In 1778 he was elected president of the Royal Society because of his contributions to botanical science, his wealth and recognized authority, and above all, his good standing with the king. Through his persistence and influence his tenure was marked by the transition in the public image of science and philosophy from one of derision to one of virtually unqualified respect, even admiration. He remained president of the society for forty-two years during this remarkable transformation. By the age of thirty, in 1773, he had been made scientific advisor to the royal gardens at Kew. During his tenure he was largely responsible for adding approximately seven thousand new plants to the collection, obtaining seeds and seed stock with a global reach, and establishing Kew as a testing ground for their potential contribution to the service of humankind.

In 1786 Banks advised the "Heads of a Plan for the Establishment of a Colony" in New South Wales, and he succeeded in obtaining specimens of the wonderful Merino breed of sheep from Spain in the following year. In 1779 he had put forward the proposition that Botany Bay become the site of reception of convicts, since they could no longer be sent to North America. After adoption of the plan he labored hard with his usual persistence to ensure the survival of the faraway settlement and colony in competition with the demands of the Napoleonic Wars. That he succeeded is confirmed by the words of Charles Darwin, who said in 1836 of firsthand impressions after his return from the voyage of the *Beagle*: "Australia is rising . . . into a grand center of civilisation which . . . will rule as Empress of the Southern Hemisphere." The Merino sheep played a major role in the development of Australia.

Banks had kept in touch with the French work with the breed and obtained the king's support for a scheme to import Merino sheep to England. Captain John Macarthur was destined to become the instrument for the selection and importation of Merinos to his Camden property in Australia. Banks never wavered in his support for this enterprise, despite repeated undeserved criticism from the irreverent captain, and Australia became the world's leading supplier of fine wools and, after New Zealand, a leading producer of sheep meat. John Macarthur arrived in Sydney in 1790 as a lieutenant in the New South Wales Corps. In 1797 Captain Henry Waterhouse and William Kent purchased some Merino sheep in South Africa and took them to Sydney. Macarthur bought some of them and started to develop a flock. He envisioned the potential of fine wool production as an exportable product that would carry low labor costs yet have a high value per unit weight, sufficient to recover more than the heavy transport costs from a remote land. Wool had the additional advantage, in the days of sailing ships with no refrigeration, of being nonperishable.

However, in 1801 the governor of the colony had Macathur arrested for challenging the governor's commanding officer to a duel. Sent to England for trial, he wisely took samples of his sheep's fleeces and convinced textile manufacturers there that Australian wool could compete with Spanish fine wools within two decades. With Banks' strong support, he obtained five rams and a ewe from the royal flock of King George III and five thousand acres of prime grazing land from Lord Camden, the colonial minister. The first shipment was

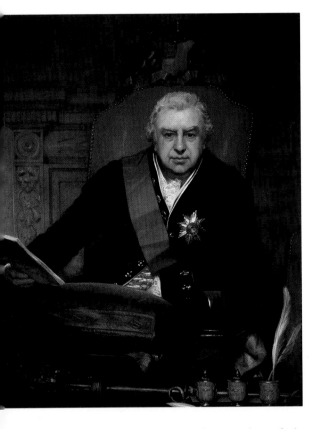

318. *Sir Joseph Banks, President of the Royal Society,* painted by Thomas Phillips. Having travelled as a botanist on the voyages made by Captain Cook to Australasia and the Pacific islands, Banks became influential in science and technology after his return to England. *(By permission of the President and Council of the Royal Society.)*

made in 1807, but Macarthur's optimistic project took thirty-five years to match the level of imports of Spanish Merino wool to Britain. After the Blue Mountains to the west of Sydney were crossed, vast areas of treeless savanna lands were settled by sheep farmers. The only labor required was for shepherding and shearing. Bullock-wagons hauled the wool to the port for shipment to Britain. Thus the animal industry of Merino wool production became a pillar of the Australian economy. Exports of llama, beef, and live sheep were later developments.

IMPROVEMENT OF BEEF CATTLE: ANGUS AND HEREFORD

The breeds of beef cattle that stand out for their wide influence on both the British and the global bovine genome are the Angus and the Hereford. Hornless black cattle were said to have been brought to Britain by Celtic migrants before the Norman Conquest. The polled trait was either conserved or selected for by Scottish breeders. By the sixteenth century they were known in Aberdeenshire as hummels and, later, in the adjacent shire of Angus, as doddies. Cattle trails from this region led to the finishing pasture farms of the Border country. As the black polled cattle became widespread, they became known as Aberdeen-Angus. After the union of England and Scotland in 1707 a great demand developed for prime Scottish beef south of the Border region.

Hugh Watson (1789-1865) of Keillour was the master breeder who laid the foundations for the Angus breed with the great matriarch Old Grannie, who had twenty-nine calves before dying at the ripe old age of thirty-six in a thunderstorm in 1859. No doubt her genes provided the base for the stamina and fecundity that became the hallmark of the Angus breed and ultimately led to its radiation and popularity around the world. Watson's Old Jock was the first bull recorded in the *Herd Book* of pedigrees. William Fullerton's fine herd at Ardovie was tragically decimated by contagious bovine pleuropneumonia in 1859, and Alex Bowie's at Mains of Kelly met a similar fate as a result of rinderpest in 1865, after producing the great sire Cupbearer.

Building on the preceding bloodlines, William McCombie of Tillyfour emerged as the second great architect of the breed, the one who established its international reputation. At first he practiced inbreeding to catch outstanding traits; then he switched to outcrossing to build vigor because he be-

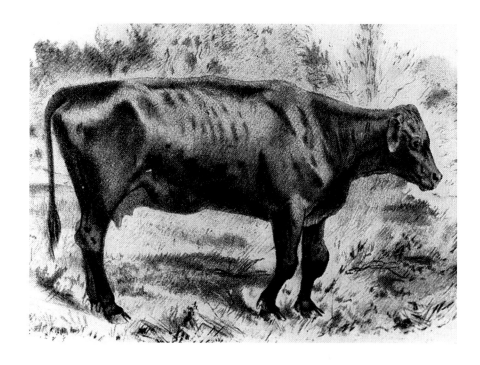

319. Old Grannie, the first recorded Aberdeen-Angus cow. She died at thirty-six years of age after producing twenty-nine calves. This matriarch of the breed, seen here as a "senior citizen," imparted her fecundity and longevity. *(From the Aberdeen-Angus Cattle Society, Perth, Scotland.)*

lieved inbreeding to be "against nature." McCombie's stock triumphed in the show rings at Birmingham and Smithfield in 1767, his steer Black Prince being the first Angus to win. Queen Victoria asked that it be sent to the royal farm at Windsor, and a baron of beef from the carcass was served in Windsor Castle, putting the breed in the spotlight with royal patronage that continues today. Competing from strength to strength, McCombie's entry won the world championship for cattle at the French International Exposition in Paris in 1878; Sir George MacPherson-Grant's won the reserve championship.

In 1873 a Scotsman who had purchased land on the Great Plains between Hays and Russell, Kansas, imported fine Angus bulls to the United States and exhibited them at the Kansas City Livestock Exhibition. Although the Scotsman died the following year, the outstanding dressing percentage of the Angus carcass was recognized and more were imported. The first purebred Angus born in North America was at the Ontario Veterinary College in Guelph, Ontario, in 1880, where Professor George Brown had imported Angus in 1876. Kansas State University played a similar role for the breed in the United States.

The Hereford or white-face type of cattle arose north of the River Wye in far western England, an area protected by the Norman forts of the Welsh border. The *Domesday Book* describes an unique category of villager for Herefordshire—originally a region of great oak forests—the oxman or bovarius, a specialist in plowing who could handle the teams of strong oxen required to break the stiff clay soils of the region. Since eight oxen were necessary for the task of plowing an acre of such soil a day, it is not surprising that a powerful, muscular animal emerged. This area was under monastic leadership until the sixteenth century, when Henry VIII decreed in the Act of Union (1536) that Wales and the Marcher lordships were to be brought into the kingdom and the monasteries closed. Welsh farmers and their stock then moved into the area.

Until 1700 there was a great diversity of cattle types in the region. A yeoman, Richard Tomkins of King's Pyon, then exhibited superior skills as a breeder of working oxen that would put on flesh quickly after being retired from the yoke. He left to his fourth son, six-year-old Benjamin, his finest cow, Silver, and her calf. Ben gradually transformed the breed from a source of

320. The Stocktonbury sale ring in 1884, where Lord Wilton, Thomas Carwardine's famous eleven-year-old bull, was auctioned for one thousand pounds. This bull was extremely influential in the improvement of British Hereford cattle. Another, Anxiety 4th, bred in the same herd, dominates the pedigrees of American Herefords. *(By courtesy of the Hereford Herd Book Society, England.)*

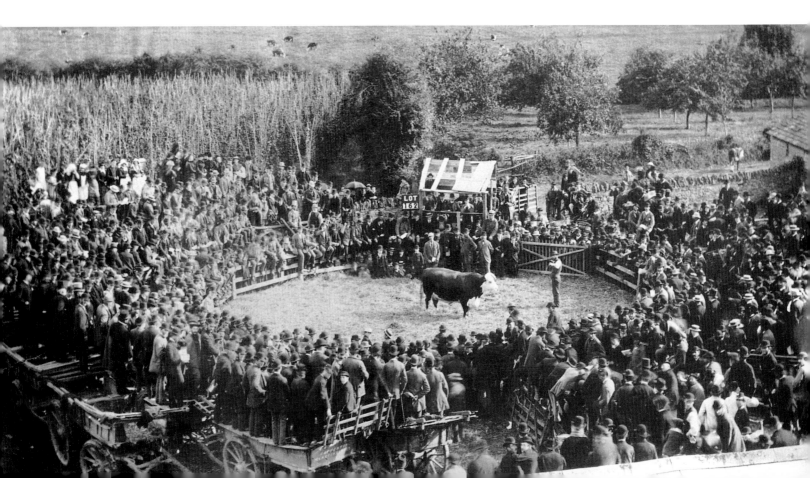

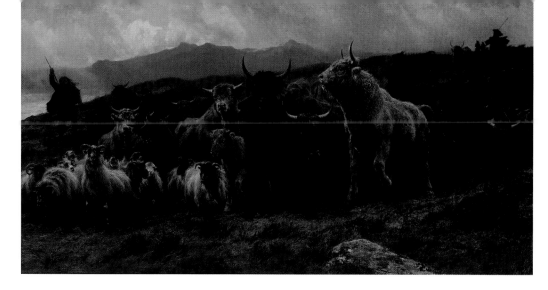

plow oxen into a wonderful beast that met the demands of both grazier and butcher. The man who did more to fix the modern Hereford type than any other was John Hewer, son of William, another great breeder. John Hewer's type had uniform markings, superb quality, and good size and was highly pre-potent. His bulls were widely used, often being leased; consequently his line had a huge impact on the standardization and advancement of the breed.

Although Herefords were imported to North America by Henry Clay of Kentucky as early as 1816, it was not until 1875 that ranchers adopted the breed to upgrade their Spanish Longhorn-derived herds and a strong market developed for export of high-quality bulls. When the American Breeders Association banned registration of British Herefords in 1883, however, South America became the main market for exports. The polled trait was cultivated by the end of the century, and a separate Herd Book was created. This idea was adopted by British breeders, and it was destined to become the dominant form. Exports were stopped because of a severe epidemic of foot-and-mouth disease in the 1920s.

321. *The Highland Raid,* painted in 1869 by one of the greatest animal artists, Rosa Bonheur (1822-1899), who developed her skill in her native France by making anatomical studies at abbatoirs. In this fine Scottish scene two hardy breeds are shown, the slow-growing Highland cattle and the productive Scottish Blackface sheep. *(From the collection of Wallace and Wilhelmina Holladay.)*

DAIRY CATTLE: SHORTHORNS, HOLSTEIN-FRIESIANS, AND JERSEYS

Short-horned cattle were developed in Holland and the surrounding regions and were noted for their high quality. Around the end of the seventeenth century some were imported to the Holderness district in Yorkshire. Their superior quality was recognized and they spread, developing a strong base in the Teeswater area. Later, two of Bakewell's disciples, Charles and Robert Colling, used these short-horned cattle to meet their goal of dual-purpose production of both meat and milk. The Shorthorn breed soon surpassed Bakewell's Longhorns in popular demand. The Colling brothers bought the great three-year-old bull Hubbock and made him the foundation sire of their line of stock. One of his descendants was the famous champion bull Comet, another the acclaimed Durham Ox (1796). The latter was exhibited by John Day for nearly six years until it was injured, dislocating a hip, and had to be slaughtered. Many of the early shorthorns were large and slow-growing but were good milkers. The Colling brothers inbred their best stock to fix a more attractive type that was good for meat and milk production.

A true dairy shorthorn strain was developed by Thomas Bates (1775-1849) to recover the lost yield consequent upon the dual-purpose breeding of the Colling brothers. He purchased Duchess I, the renowned cow sired by Comet, at the Collings's retirement sale in 1810. She soon achieved name recognition for the "Duchess line," and Bates's cattle were exported. They played a major role in the development of the North American Shorthorn, which was used widely to upgrade the hardy range stocks of Spanish Longhorn cattle and produce beef animals of higher quality. Scottish Short-horn breeders specialized in beef production, and the Scottish Shorthorn be-

363

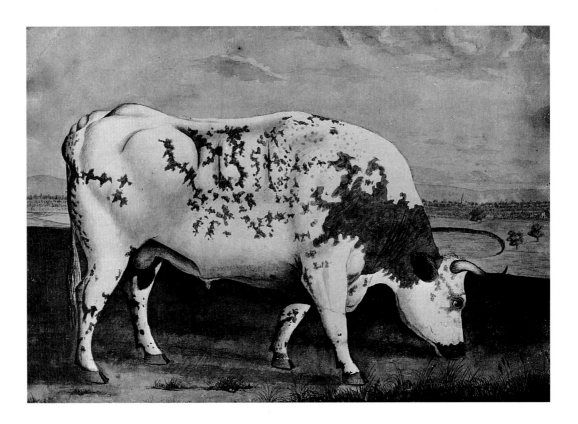

322. The Blackwell Ox, a Shorthorn ox, killed at Darlington in 1779, that was bred and fed by Christopher Hill, at Blackwell, County Durham. This painting was made the year after the ox died, but the print did not appear until 1809. Note the improved form of this fine beef animal with balance between the forequarters and hindquarters. It is an example of the type developed by the Colling brothers and Thomas Booth. Their progress with Shorthorn breeding eclipsed Bakewell's success with Midland Longhorns in the early nineteenth century. *(Courtesy The University of Reading, Rural History Centre, Berkshire.)*

came known as the beef Shorthorn. They have been crossed with the colorful but slow-growing Highland cattle to develop better suckling cows for the poor hill pastures. In modern times the introduction of bulls of Continental beef breeds for crossing has led to the decline of the Scottish strain.

Shorthorn pedigrees were first recorded in *Coates Herd Book* in 1822. The Breed Society was created fifty years later. The Shorthorn breed was dominant in the British cattle population until the Second World War and the advent of artificial insemination. Then dairy breeds became the vogue, and the British Friesian eclipsed the Shorthorn within a few decades.

Fine British dairy breeds other than the Shorthorn made their mark and were exported, including the Ayrshire or Dunlop breed that was derived from crossings between a black strain local to Ayrshire and imported brown-and-white Dutch cattle. It was the custom in Holland for women to do the milking, dairy work being an affair of the household. This resulted in selection for small teats. Also, the Ayrshire cattle did not fatten well when they ended their dairy run. The Ayrshire inherited from its local ancestors sharp, upturned horns and a tendency to kick defensively. The breed became the basis of a strong local butter and cheese industry. After 1945 the farmers moved more rapidly than their counterparts south of the border to become providers of tuberculin-tested cattle. When a national test and slaughter scheme was adopted to eradicate bovine tuberculosis, English dairy farmers imported many tuberculin-tested Ayrshire cattle to accelerate their attainment of tuberculosis-free status. The more productive black-and-whites, however, displaced them within two or three decades. Nevertheless, in Finland the hardier and thriftier Ayrshire breed has maintained pride of place.

Dairy breeds were developed in the Channel Islands, British lands in the English Channel near the French coast. The breeds' histories are uncertain, but they may have included some Asiatic blood among the Breton and Norman stock imported from France. Importations were stopped around the end of the eighteenth century, and this closure led to the fixation of the island breeds. These cattle were known collectively as Alderneys, after the island of that name, until the middle of the nineteenth century, when the Jersey and Guernsey breeds became clearly established in the British Isles. Over time the Jersey became more popular internationally, but both of these were

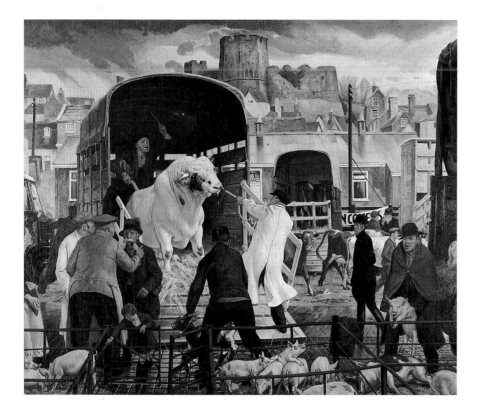

323. *Pulling Shorthorn Bull Off Cart at Lewes Market* (1937) by James Bateman (1893-1959). At that time the dual-purpose Shorthorn breed was the preferred breed; within thirty years the Friesian had displaced it. *(Tate Gallery Publications, London.)*

renowned for their high yields of fat-rich milk. This popularity led to an enormous "gene drain" from these islands to France, the United Kingdom, and North America in the latter part of the nineteenth century, and the Channel Islands had to place restrictions on exports to preserve their nucleus herds. The small Jersey cow has only a little more than half the body mass of the Holstein-Friesian, yet can produce the same weight of butterfat in a lactation. Storage of surplus fat in the more readily mobilizable abdominal deposits is a factor in this remarkable characteristic. Only after the recent decline in the value of butterfat and the growing preference for low-fat milk on health grounds has the Jersey's popularity declined. Today even the large statue of a Jersey cow at the Tillamook cheese plant in Oregon has had to be replaced by a Holstein.

Some Continental breeds such as the brown Swiss and the Simmental have been popular as dairy or dual-purpose breeds, but only the Holstein and Friesian stocks have attained a dominant status internationally.

Early imports of Dutch cattle to southern England included red-and-white as well as black-and-white strains in the first part of the nineteenth century. Many imported cows were destined to a one-lactation sentence in a squalid urban dairy before being fed to slaughter for beef. Before pasteurization was developed, the unsanitary conditions and frequently diseased cattle produced a product that contributed to rather than offset the fearsome levels of infant mortality. Growing concern about the public health hazards associated with such urban dairying coupled with the devastating outbreaks of contagious bovine pleuropneumonia (around 1860) and rinderpest imported from Russia (in 1865) rang the death knell for most of the town milking units. Foot-and-mouth disease was endemic on the continent of Europe. Growth of the railway network allowed milk to be delivered from the rural surrounds. Veterinary concerns that the imported plagues were threats to British native stock led to a ban on live imports except for direct slaughter in 1876. In 1892 all such imports were banned. Thereafter, unmet needs had to be filled by imported chilled or frozen meats.

The Dutch cattle in England went by three names: Friesians, Frieslands, and Holsteins. Their total numbers were low. The Honorable Edward Strutt, inheriting lands near Terling, Essex, that had been abandoned by tenants af-

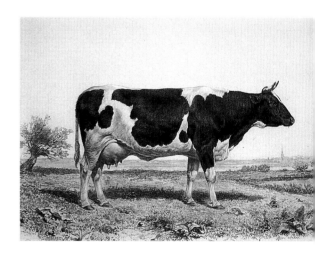

324. The finest Holstein-Friesian cow at the Paris Exposition of 1856. The remarkable potential of this breed for high milk production was already in evidence in this fine specimen. *(Courtesy A. Mathijsen, Utrecht.)*

325. Vriesland-Kleistreen bull from the Netherlands, where the Friesian breed was developed as the leading dairy breed. The Friesian and Holstein breeds have amalgamated as Holstein-Friesian for most national societies, but there are differences in conformation and productivity between them. *(Courtesy A. Mathijsen, Utrecht.)*

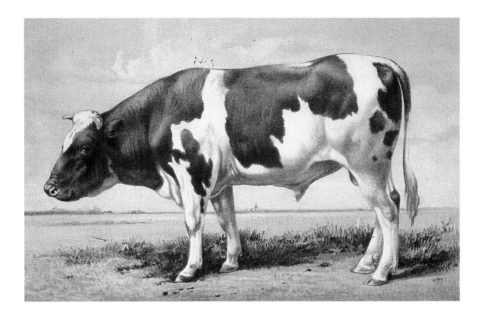

ter the agricultural depression of 1875, brought a scientific turn of mind to the family's dairy operations. His approach was different from that of the early improvers, who had built their stocks' reputations on the basis of pedigreed bloodlines, success in the show ring, and name recognition. Strutt started recording milk production figures in 1896. His results soon showed that the improved Holstein-Friesian breed outperformed all others. Importation of breeding stock, including some Canadian Holsteins, was allowed. The herd book was started as a record of the British Holstein Cattle Society in 1909, but the name of the society was changed to Friesian during World War I. Live imports from the Netherlands were resumed just before the Great War, during a lull in the incidence of foot-and-mouth disease. By 1922 the disease was raging again in Europe, and imports of Dutch stock were made from South Africa.

Compared with the North American Holsteins, the British Friesians are smaller and make a better beef carcass but do not reach quite the same capacity for milk production. The British Friesian soon came to dominate the national dairy herd. Establishment of the Milk Marketing Board in 1933 saved the dairy industry from chaos and possible collapse resulting from oversupply. The Milk Marketing Board has also been a leading organization in advancing the genetic potential for milk production through artificial insemination and progeny testing. Most calves born to dairy stock are derived from artificial insemination.

Although Herman Le Roy and others brought Holsteins to New York in 1820 and 1825, the American Holstein breed was not founded until Gerrit S. Miller of Peterboro, New York, imported the bull Billy Boelyn from West Friesland in 1875. The potential of the breed for high-volume milk production became recognized progressively, and it came to dominate dairy production in the United States.

Since the early 1960s a new search has been under way for genetic improvement in beef cattle in strains from western Europe, Asia, and South America. The main thrust of the effort has been to produce a large, better-quality beef carcass based on the improved Continental beef sires for crossing on the basic beef-cow population or on dairy cows to generate better dairy-beef calves. The first of these to attain the spotlight has been the white Charolais stemming from the Charole region of France. It has been thought that the breed had benefitted from an introduction of beef Shorthorn blood from an imported white bull. The large size of the calves led to a higher incidence of dystocia. Efforts are being made to overcome the problem. Other breeds have followed, including the red French Limousin and the yellowish Simmentals from Germany and Switzerland. The latter have been particularly successful in North America. The "double-muscling" trait has been selected for in the Belgian blue and the Italian Piedmont.

When the Americas were colonized, the first cattle were brought from Spain by the explorers and conquistadors. These criollo cattle were lean and had long horns and came to be known as Texas Longhorns. They learned to survive on poor pastures under harsh conditions but were not productive. Imported beef bulls were used to upgrade these early cattle, but better pastures were required. The French brought their small Normandy cattle when they settled in Quebec after 1608. Dutch settlers in New York brought the first Dutch cattle in 1625, which gave good milk production. The improved strains, however, were not brought in until the middle of the nineteenth century.

In the days before mechanical transport was developed, cattle were driven to market or moved over long distances. This practice carried the serious risk of spreading contagious diseases, although the risk does not seem to have been recognized at the time. The majestic Hungarian Grey Steppe cattle are preserved today only as a rare breed of historical importance. Their origin dates to the fourteenth century, and they have much in common with some Italian breeds. These cattle were alleged to have some resistance to the cattle plague of rinderpest.

American cattle in the southern states were plagued by a deadly disease called Texas fever that was particularly acute when it struck imported stock. It was discovered that the criollo and the zebu breeds were more resistant than most improved *Bos taurus* varieties and were also more tolerant of high temperatures and more resistant to ticks and tick-borne hemoprotozoal diseases like Texas fever. The zebus also have a cervical or thoracic hump. These breeds are thought to have arisen in the Indus River valley or elsewhere in

326. *The Cornell Farm* (1848) by Edward Hicks (1780-1849). An Indian summer view of the farm and stock of James C. Cornell of Northampton, Bucks County, Pennsylvania, which were awarded the Premium title in the Agricultural Society on October 12, 1848. *(Gift of Edgar William and Bernice Chrysler Garbisch, copyright 1994. National Gallery of Art, Washington, D.C.)*

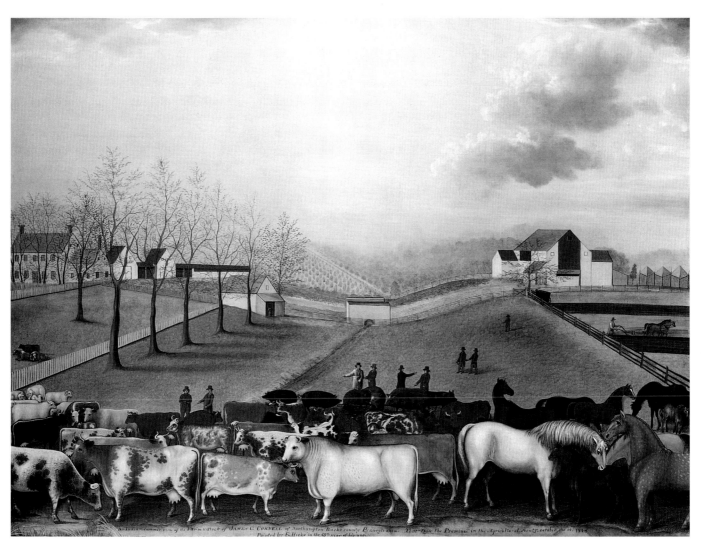

West Asia and to have spread across the Indian subcontinent of South Asia. Crosses between *Bos indicus* and *B. taurus* were developed to be more productive than the former yet more tolerant of heat and disease than were the pure *B. taurus* breeds. Many of the zebus in Asia and Africa are used for draft work for several years or for lactation and calf raising before being used for meat and leather or, as in India, before being pensioned to live off the landscape, contributing only manure for construction, fuel, and fertilizer. The American Brahman was developed as a heat-tolerant beef breed from imported stock.

BORDER LEICESTER AND HILL AND DOWN BREEDS: FORMATION OF AN INDUSTRY

The British sheep industry is remarkable for the way it has developed regional hill breeds such as the blackface, the Swaledale, the Welsh mountain, and the Cheviot for their ability to survive in harsh environments and for splendid mothering qualities. Another feature of the central strategy was the mating of these ewes to rams, typically Border Leicesters or blue-faced Leicesters, that imparted prolificacy and thriftiness to the offspring, a half-bred ewe; the offspring was then mated to a Down breed ram. Initially the improved Southdown was used, then the Suffolk. More recently, some breeders, in a modern move toward "lean" control, have used the Dutch Texel, which was derived by careful selection for meaty carcasses with less fat from Bakewell's Leicester on the island of Texel and comes closest to the modern criteria for his goal of carcass quality. The half-bred ewes produce large numbers of fast-growing lambs of excellent carcass quality. Only New Zealand, with its improved Romneys mated to Down breed rams and its more favorable environment, has been able to outperform the British model economically.

The Southdown rams were developed from the indigenous hornless, speckled-faced sheep that had been kept on the chalk downs of southeastern England for centuries. Although they were small and slow-maturing, they were renowned for the carcass quality of their mutton and for their hardiness, particularly their relative freedom from foot disease or foot rot, that plague of shepherds. This was the substrate that was taken by John Ellman of Glynde, near Lewes, Sussex, who inherited his father's farm in 1780 and converted its line of sheep into one of the most significant improvers of sheep meat by selective breeding. His product was fine of bone and early-maturing, with a carcass that produced a round, short leg of delectable, tender lamb that would catch the buyer's eye. The rams had the capacity to pass on their strengths to their progeny.

Ellman was a leader in animal agriculture who shared his knowledge openly and generously. He was one of the leaders in instituting the Smithfield cattle show. He walked off with most of the prizes for his sheep and also did well with his cattle. His Southdowns were in demand worldwide. The influential Thomas Coke of Holkham, Norfolk, became an ardent promoter of the breed. Jonas Webb (1796-1862) of Babraham, near Cambridge, further improved the breed by selecting for increased size and setting standards. His ewes took all the major prizes at the Royal Agricultural Show in 1840 and held the preeminent position in the show ring for the next twenty years. In 1855 he presented his champion ram at the Universal Exhibition in Paris to Emperor Louis Napoleon. Today a distinguished Agricultural Research Council station for basic research on livestock is sited at Babraham Hall and estate. New Zealand breeders exploited the Southdown breed to the full, using the rams on their Romney ewes to produce top-quality, cheap lamb that appealed to the British taste.

In the first volume of the Suffolk flock book, royal show champion ram (1886 and 1887) Bismark was the model used to establish the breed's scale of points. In particular, the remarkable length of the back, the meatiness of the

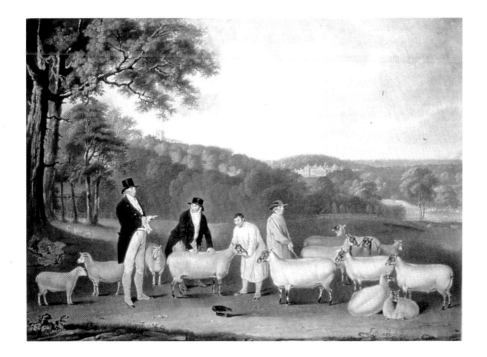

327. *Thomas Coke, a Famous Southdown Breeder, Mr. Walton, and Shepherd with Holkham in the Background,* an engraving taken from a painting by Thomas Weaver (1808). A famous agricultural improver and innovator, Coke was quick to see the quality of the spectacular Southdown breed developed by John Ellman at Glynde, near Lewes, and adopt it. *(Courtesy The Lawes Agricultural Trust, Rothamsted Experimental Station, England.)*

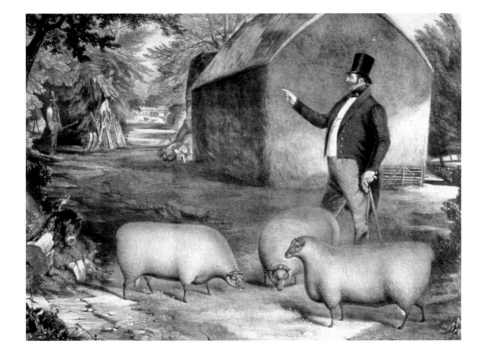

328. *Jonas Webb with Three of His Southdown Sheep.* Lithograph by Hullmandel after J.W. Giles (1842). Webb owned Babraham Hall near Cambridge and became so famous for his Southdowns that he attracted the interest of Napoleon III. The breed's fine reputation led to its international dispersion. Babraham is the site of a distinguished agricultural research station that is focused on science in the service of the livestock industries. *(Courtesy The Lawes Agricultural Trust, Rothamsted Experimental Station, England.)*

animal, and its striking appearance, with a black head free of wool, were noted. It became the most popular breed of rams for crossing as the terminal sire in fine lamb production. This status was not seriously challenged until the Texel arrived from the Netherlands. The Texel's remarkably high carcass quality made it and its crossbred lambs winners at the Smithfield show.

Professor Yvart at Alfort founded the Ile de France sheep breed, involving a New Leicester crossed, probably, with a Rambouillet strain. The goal was to achieve out-of-season breeding and the high-quality carcass for the midwinter lambs demanded by the Ile de Paris market.

Northern Europe has sheep strains of great prolificacy that bear litters of lambs instead of singles or twins, commonly three to five to a litter. Most notable among these is the Finnish Landrace, which has come into prominence in crossbreeding to enhance fecundity in the modern era. Not surprisingly, these sheep do not develop prize-winning gourmet roasts. They are, however, good milkers, as they would have to be. In many parts of the world sheep are milked for whole milk, yogurt, cheese, and in some cases ice cream production. The famous Roquefort cheese from France, for example, is made from sheep's milk. The most productive of the dairy breeds is the East Friesland from Holland and adjacent areas of Germany.

GOATS FOR MILK AND FINE FIBER

Like sheep, goats are milked in many parts of the world. They are a popular species with smallholders, especially in the regions around the Mediterranean. Because they browse more than they graze, they can be damaging to the environment. Goats are popular in tropical and subtropical regions as an adjunct to cattle and sheep. They may be used less seasonally than sheep for an occasional meat meal. Goat meat is widely used in developing countries.

One breed that appealed to British interests was the Anglo-Nubian, derived from stock imported from the Middle East and India. Its long, lopping ears give it a distinctive appearance. Developed as a type to provide milk for long ocean voyages, it yields milk with a high fat content. Most of the other British goats are of Swiss origin, such as the Alpine, Saanen, and Toggenburg, all of which are improved dairy breeds.

Other than milk, a valuable product derived from goats is the fine wool from strains that yield cashmere and angora wools. The Tibetan Kashmir goat is renowned for its ultrafine wool. "Angora" is an old name for "Ankara" and thus represents a wool derived originally from Turkish goats. Some feral goats in Australia have been found to have an undercoat of wool of cashmere quality, and this finding is being exploited.

The use of goats for meat is widespread but has not been developed as systematically and intensively as for sheep.

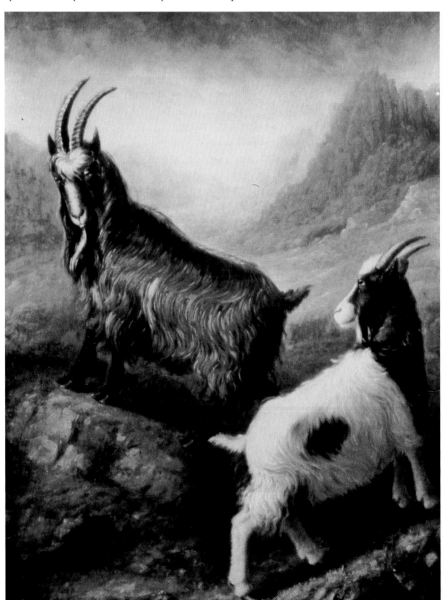

329. *Welsh Goats.* Although the Welsh mountain sheep breed was developed skillfully by breeders, the same cannot be said of the hardy goats of the Welsh hill lands. Goats received little attention from breeders until dairy breeds (Toggenburg, Alpine, and Saanen) from Switzerland and Nubians from the Middle East brought the milking goat a better reputation. This piece was reputed to have been painted by Elizabeth Bradley (c. 1830-1840) but more likely was the work of William Shiels, who was commissioned by Professor David Low of Edinburgh. *(Welsh Folk Museum, Cardiff.)*

TRANSFORMATION OF SWINE STOCKS IN GREAT BRITAIN AND DENMARK

Medieval pigs in Europe were put out to pannage, that is, to roam the forests and forage for their food. These pigs were lean and slow-growing. The British model was a small, sturdy forager and rooter of the soil. Regional varieties evolved and were being improved empirically by the mid-eighteenth century. The dwindling forest ranges were replaced by confining the pigs in sties and feeding them whey and distillery and other food wastes. When Chinese, Siamese, and their derivative Neapolitan strains were imported for crossing with the local stock, the pace of improvement accelerated. Better feed was required, and potatoes became popular as pig food. The new strains were short, docile, and remarkable for their tendency to fatten—ideal for the palate of the times, with its preference for fat pork and bacon. The imported genes transformed the old British breeds. Bakewell tried to develop a large Dishley porker but could not eliminate leg weakness in his heavy strain. The early breeds, like the black Berkshire, were roly-poly and were developed for the fat pork market; they remained the star performers in carcass competitions until the end of the World War. The middle-white pork breed declined dramatically after World War II. The sheeted black-and-white saddleback breeds, the Essex and the Wessex, followed in a wave of popularity, and the Wessex gave rise to the Hampshire in the United States. The early saddlebacks were kept outdoors in areas like the New Forest and later were fed outdoors. Their suitability, like that of the Large Black, has declined with the advent of programmed management for productivity rather than breed purity.

The most important factor that led to changes in the prevalence of different breeds of swine was the change in consumer demand from a preference for fat pork to one for Wiltshire bacon, lean ham, sausages, and lean pork loins, chops, and legs. A longer, leaner, meatier, faster-growing prolific model was required. A British swine breeder, Joseph Tuley of Keighley, Yorkshire, rose to the occasion; a weaver who kept a few Yorkshire pigs in his backyard, Tuley at first was producing the popular, massively overfat model for the fat bacon and showed it at the Royal Show in 1851. However, he was quick to

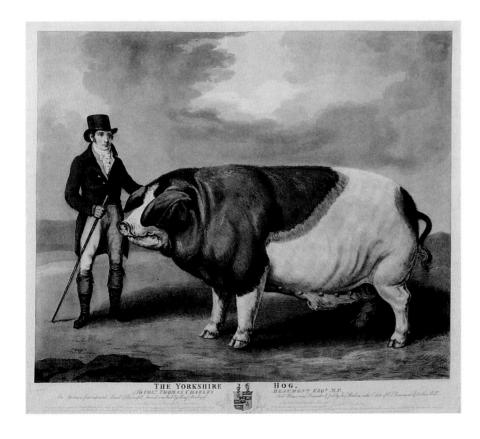

330. *Yorkshire Hog,* painted by an unknown artist and engraved by Pollard (1809). The massive pigs of Yorkshire were precursors of the world's major developmental breed, the Large White, or modern Yorkshire. This stupendous exhibition specimen weighed 1344 pounds at four years of age. *(Courtesy The Lawes Agriculture Trust, Rothamsted Experimental Station, England.)*

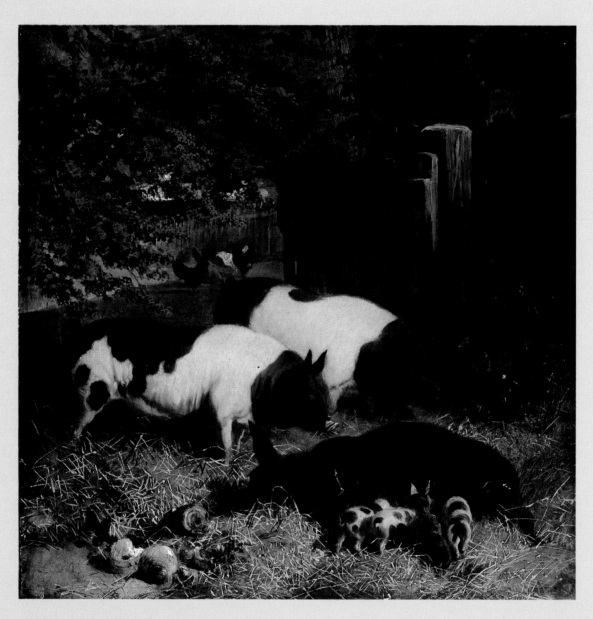

331. *Farmyard Scene* by John F. Herring, Sr. (1795-1865). The artist is famous for detailed work, as is evident here in a typical farm scene of sows and piglets before the age of mass production. *(Courtesy The Sporting Gallery, Inc., Middleburg, Virginia.)*

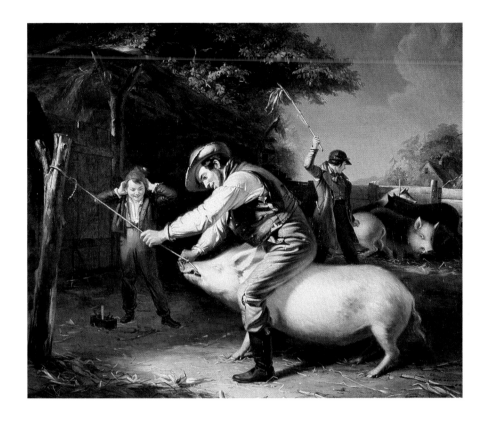

332. *Ringing the Pig* (1842) by William S. Mount (1807-1869). Pigs have a great propensity to root in the ground, with considerable damage to pastures. It was usual to insert copper rings in their noses to prevent this. *(New York State Historical Association, Cooperstown.)*

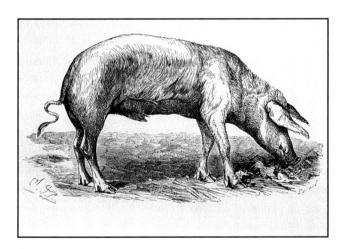

A

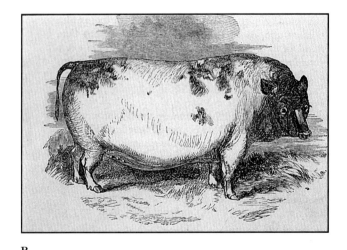

B

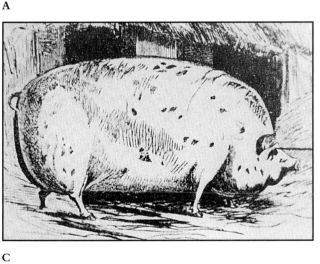

C

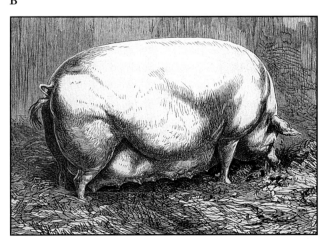

D

333. *Four Breeds of Pigs,* an illustration prepared from old books on the subject. The breeds are *(A)* the common pig of Europe, *(B)* Chinese pig, *(C)* Joseph Tuley's Large White pig, and *(D)* Youatt's Large White pig.

recognize the changes in society. The Wiltshire cure of bacon developed at Calne called for a long body, thin back fat, light shoulder, and heavy hams, with a minimum of offal and low-value parts. Tuley set out to transform his pigs to meet the new goals, and the result was the Large White, which became the most dispersed breed in the world.

Competition came from Denmark, where the cooperative system moved quickly to generate highly competitive products to suit the new consumer demands. Great Britain was the Danish pig farmer's prime customer. The decision was taken to selectively breed the native white Landrace stock. Later, the Danish breeders added selected Large-White genes to meet their goals.

Today a major effort is under way in the use of sophisticated genetic plans to efficiently meet the changing consumer expectations in the twenty-first century. Hardiness is also important because of a new trend in Europe of keeping pigs outdoors.

A GLIMPSE OF POULTRY IMPROVEMENT

The origin of the breeds of domestic poultry is a subject too vast for this text. The ancient terrestrial wild forms such as guinea fowl, peafowl, pheasant, quail, and jungle fowl have all contributed to the gene pool that has given rise to the most commercialized domestic forms today, the chicken and the turkey. Similarly, on the aquatic side a great variety of wild waterfowl share genes with the domestic duck and goose breeds. The Muscovy duck is a separate species that originated in Central and South America and was domesticated there by pre-Columbian Native Americans.

A similar history attaches to the turkey, a small, wild, black American strain that was domesticated in Mexico before the arrival of the conquistadors, who took live specimens to Europe, where the strain became established and spread quickly. The turkey was brought back to North America in the sixteenth century, and wild eastern turkey toms courted and mated with the domestic black hens, imparting genes for the well-known bronze color. The eastern native was never domesticated and imparted its genes without paying the usual price of taming and captivity. The hybrid strains developed into the dominant domestic line; some were shipped back to Europe, the stock becoming known as the American bronze. An English gamekeeper, Jesse Throssel, is credited with the development of the broad-breasted variety there. He emigrated to Canada in 1926, then imported just one tom and two hens of his own stock. He was able to build up a flock from them and exhibited some in the United States, where they triggered a huge demand and transformed the industry.

The domestic chicken's history is much more complex, from its origins in the jungle fowl of Asia to the multitude of breeds that were developed during the "hen craze" of the nineteenth and early twentieth centuries. Charles Darwin listed thirteen "chief" breeds of chickens in 1868, a year after his friend Tegetmeier's *Poultry Book* was published. Local breeds were crossed with Asian strains. Oriental chickens were brought to the Americas and contributed to the dual-purpose breeds developed in the United States.

The most productive of the breeds kept as layers of white-shelled eggs were the Leghorn ("Livorno" in Italian) varieties from Italy. Some were brought to the United States as early as 1830. Some consumers preferred brown eggs, and American poultry farmers complied by using the Plymouth Rock, New Hampshire, Rhode Island Red, and Australorp. The fantastic increase in the hen's capacity for egg production should be noted. In antiquity birds laid only a single clutch of eggs per year. Now they have broken away from seasonal hormonal cycles and constraints and can lay an egg every day.

The extraordinary progress in the broiler-chicken industry is based on selection from the Cornish breed that was developed from Asiatic fighting stock in the United Kingdom and on the white Plymouth Rock, a chance mutant of the standard breed in the United States. Crossings between the Cornish and the white Rock formed the basis for the present generation of broilers. Mass production is required to keep up with demand, and a new generation of genetic improvements is planned.

The domestic ducks are mainly old breeds: Darwin knew half a dozen. The breed that has become preeminent for meat production is the Pekin, which arrived in Great Britain and the United States in 1972 and 1973, respectively. A new twist in France has been the development of duck-breast steaks called *maigret*.

Geese, although they were ancient domesticated animals, have shown less progress toward "industrial" production. They are thought to have African and Chinese roots. Their use is more traditional than commercial, and they have been the subject in major studies of animal behavior, including the phenomenon of maternal imprinting by goslings on the first living object they encounter. Force-feeding of geese to produce that gourmet's delight, paté de foie gras, or fatty liver, dates to ancient times.

VETERINARY IMPLICATIONS OF TRADE IN FOUNDATION STOCK

As the quality and value of domesticated livestock increased and as the level of intensification, nutrition, and management became more exacting, the need for competent veterinary clinical services became greater. Even more important, however, was the imperative to keep out devastating contagious diseases or, if they gained entry, to implement an effective control and eradication program without delay. The British Isles were fortunate, indeed, to have an oceanic barrier between them and the continent of Eurasia that kept out most of the great contagions, except when infected stock were imported. This advantage protected the British breeders from most of the catastrophic plagues that hit their colleagues across the Channel. In the modern era of intensive production systems and rigorous market demands, the pressures to achieve a high-quality, standardized product could be in conflict with the goal of increasing efficiency.

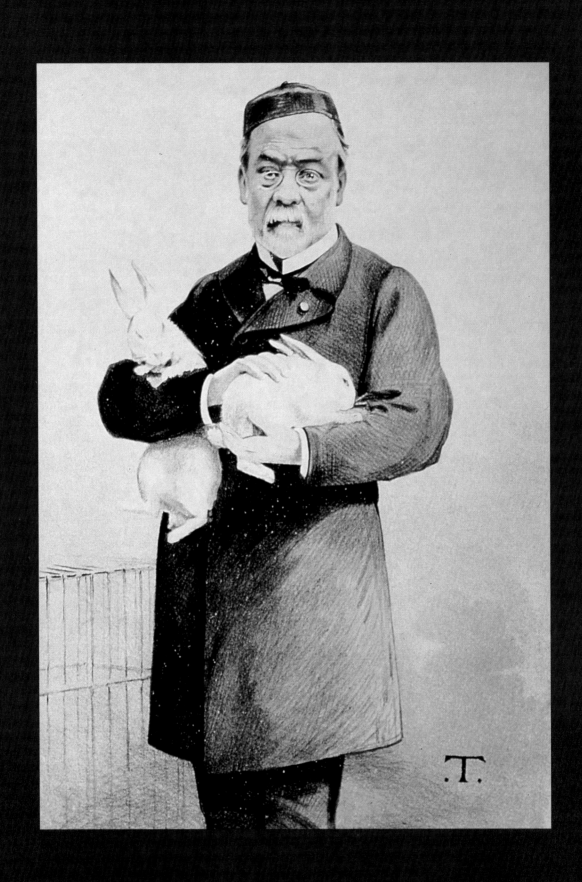

Some Animal Plagues Unmasked

~

THE HISTORICAL SETTING OF CATASTROPHIC EPIZOOTICS

It is hard to imagine the fear that struck people's minds when animals and humans died in droves after contracting epidemic diseases about which no useful knowledge existed. In Rome during the first century BC Virgil described the devastating animal plagues then rampant as ". . . many diseases of cattle, killing not one here and there, but a whole summer pasture." So desperate was the situation that the peasants themselves had to take the place of draft oxen and ". . . tug the creaking wagons over a towering hillside." His descriptions of symptoms are suggestive of anthrax.

Cattle plagues, the most lethal of which was rinderpest, were introduced repeatedly via infected animals brought by raiders from the east. The plagues swept away virtually all the cattle in western Europe. The Russian word for rinderpest, "tchouma," is the same as the one used by the Mongols and the Tartars, suggesting a common origin. The British media in the mid-nineteenth century adapted the term *steppe murrain* for the disease.

There are few dependable records of animal diseases and deaths before the nineteenth century, but crude estimates have been made of the number of deaths resulting from some of the plagues. The great devastation and its recrudescences that began in the early eighteenth century have been calculated to have destroyed about two hundred million head of cattle. Perhaps the very scale of this catastrophe and its social consequences were the stimuli that awakened concerns leading to a new, scientific focus on animal care.

A major epizootic of rinderpest surged westward from Russian Asia across Europe in the 1850s. The rapidly evolving cattle industry of Britain became alarmed, and the professor of bovine pathology at the London veterinary college, J.B. Simonds, was sent to the Continent to investigate the disease. The first cases in Britain were diagnosed in London dairies by Simonds in 1865, and he advised against treatment. He urged control by restrictions on movement of stock. It seems astonishing that many leaders in the medical and veterinary professions, as well as the clergy and the leading analysts of the media, were not yet convinced of the validity of the germ theory of infectious disease. The leading veterinary authority, John Gamgee, was roundly criticized for demanding a policy of trade restriction and slaughter. Even Professor Dick of Edinburgh was an anticontagionist.

It was the British experience with the cattle plague that convinced many of the need to reevaluate the widely held miasma theory of disease causation. John Simon, the medical officer of the Privy Council, focused on the necessity for scientific inquiry, and funds were authorized for research on rinderpest by the Cattle Plague Commission. L.S. Beale, a distinguished microscopist, noted that thoughtful, laborious, and prolonged investigations would

334. *Facing page,* Louis Pasteur (1822-1895), who by thought, investigation, and experiment established that many diseases of animals and people are caused by microscopic organisms. The rabbit was symbolic of his development of rabies vaccine to save human lives by attenuation of an organism that was then still invisible under the microscope. *(National Library of Medicine/Mark Marten.)*

be required. J. Burdon-Sanderson showed that the blood of animals infected with rinderpest contained the poison of the disease and that the serum inoculated into a healthy animal induced the disease. He collaborated with Chauveau at Lyon; the outcome was the Cattle Disease Prevention act of 1866, vaccination having been tried without success. The disease was eradicated from the British Isles after an estimated 400,000 head of cattle had perished. Slaughter of affected animals, with compensation for their owners, was an essential ingredient.

THE ADVENT OF MICROBIOLOGY

Before microbiology could emerge as a field of study, it was necessary to break the hold of Aristotle's idea of spontaneous generation on conventional thought. Francesco Redi (1626-1679) carried out experiments on maggots and the effect of screening meat from flies, establishing that intermediate forms were not created by the decay but rather were the cause of it. Louis Joblot (1645-1723) conducted controlled experiments on boiled plant material in which he protected one part from the air while exposing the other and showed that organisms appeared only in the latter. Abbe Spallanzani (1729-1799) confirmed Redi's work and showed that not even minute life-forms appeared when boiled materials were protected from the atmosphere. He refuted the views of Buffon and of Needham, who claimed to have evidence of spontaneous generation.

Gay Lussac studied composition of the gases in jars used by Nicholas Appert, who recommended in 1795 that heat treatments be used for wine and in 1804 that the treatments be used when meats, fruits, and other plant materials were being preserved in bottles and cans. Lussac concluded in 1810 that anaerobiasis, that is, a lack of oxygen, was the condition necessary for the preservation of animal and vegetable products. In 1802 Erik Viborg in Copenhagen's veterinary school established that equine strangles was a transmissible disease. Thus he established that certain diseases were attributable to invasion by other living organisms.

The mid-nineteenth century saw an intellectual revolution in the health sciences, and veterinary science began to play a leading role in the search for an understanding of infectious diseases of farm animals. Improvements in microscope design had a major technological impact: the macroscopic ectoparasites and endoparasites that had been discovered earlier to be the agents of disease were more visible. Redi made major contributions in the area of microscopy. The compound oil-immersion microscope made it possible to magnify extremely small organisms to the point of visibility. At last the speculations about contagion could be demonstrated. As early as 1823 Eloi Barthelemy, a professor at the Alfort veterinary school, transferred anthrax from an infected sheep to a healthy one and to a horse by inoculation with blood. The first veterinarian to be elected president of the Academy of Medicine in France, he also showed that gangrene could have an infectious origin.

Augustino Bassi (1773-1856) of Milan reported in 1835 that muscardine disease of silkworms was caused by yeasts. He proposed that many diseases of plants and animals may be due to microscopic organisms. Initially the microbiology of plant pathogens proceeded more rapidly than that of animal pathogens because many of the plant diseases studied were caused by fungi such as rusts, smut, and ergot, which are much larger than bacteria. The first demonstration of a microscopic agent in an animal disease was made by Johan Lucas Schonlein, a founder of clinical medicine, who showed that favus, a skin disease of chickens, was caused by a pathogenic fungus (a *Trichophyton* species) in 1839.

Christian Gottfried Ehrenberg (1795-1876), in his seminal work on protozoa, *The Infusoria As Complete Organisms,* in 1838 coined the term "bacterium" and classified bacteria on the basis of morphological features. He also described 533 types of protozoa (more than 300 of these for the first time) and their structural features or organelles. He ascribed a genetic function to the nucleus. He christened the infusoria "polygastria," but they were renamed after von Siebold at the University of Freiburg suggested "protozoa" in 1848. Ehrenberg accompanied two scientific collecting trips to Asia, one of them with the insatiable German geographer-geologist-physiologist-naturalist Alexander von Humboldt.

David Gruby of Hungary trained in medicine in Vienna and moved to Paris, where he founded medical mycology between 1841 and 1845. He inoculated various animals with the favus organism, establishing that it was infectious and describing the organism and the pathological response. He also described the fungus that causes thrush, *Candida albicans,* and the dermatophyte genera that cause ringworm (*Trichophyton* and *Microsporon* organisms). Easy to see with the aid of the microscope, pathogenic fungi proved to be hard to culture in the laboratory. Gruby's fine laboratory work was transferred to the clinic by Raimond Jacques Adrien Sabouraud (1864-1938), the famous French dermatologist and mycologist. Gruby also gave the genus name *Trypanosoma* to flagellated protozoa he observed in the blood of amphibia.

During 1849 and 1850 Aloys Pollender, Pierre Rayer, and Casimir Davaine all observed the agent of anthrax using the microscope. Henri Delafond, the director of the Alfort veterinary school, cultured anthrax rods in vitro in 1860 and guessed that the spore was involved in the origin of the disease. He also showed the extraordinary rate of multiplication of the organism in the blood and tissues of the host after a few drops of infected blood were inoculated into it, which explained the virulence and high mortality rate of the disease. Anginiard in 1859 transmitted equine anemia. Chauveau (1827-1917) at Lyon proved that tuberculosis was infectious in animals in 1868. Edoardo Perroncito, microbiologist and parasitologist at the veterinary school of Turin, actually observed microbes in the blood of chickens infected with fowl cholera in 1878. This observation followed the demonstration by Delafond at Alfort in Paris in 1851 that the disease was transferable between chickens.

Henri Bouley (1814-1885), the son of a veterinarian, graduated from Alfort in 1836 and soon began a distinguished career in academia at the Alfort school. Within two decades he was elected to the French Academy of Medicine and became an active member of a group dedicated to the study of the comparative pathology of infectious diseases. The Parisian medical research environment in the second half of the nineteenth century was at a unique stage: veterinarians debated with medical practitioners on virtually equal footing. Popular topics were anthrax, tuberculosis, glanders, and the use of vaccinia virus for smallpox vaccination. The possible origin of the vaccinia strain from a type of horsepox that had been passed to cows was a controversial issue. Jenner himself believed that the vaccine strain had come from an equine disease called grease. Bouley's experiments on this subject led to the conclusion that there was an entity called horsepox. Although the mystery of the vaccine strain's actual origin was never resolved, Chauveau pursued the question later.

Chauveau at Lyon became involved in microbiology and immunology when he was asked to chair a commission to study vaccinia and variola. His finding was that variola passed through cattle still produced variola in humans. His assistant, Jean-Joseph-Henri Toussaint (1847-1890), a veterinarian with doctorates in science and medicine, isolated the agent of chicken cholera in 1879 and confirmed that microbes observed by Perroncito caused the disease. Toussaint cultured them in vitro in neutralized urine in 1879. He sent the head of one of the dead birds to Pasteur, who isolated in a liquid medium the organism that was to become the first species of the *Pasteurella* genus. Later, the same organism, left to languish forgotten in an incubator, was tested again and was found to have lost its virulence. Nonetheless, it was found that this "attenuated strain" was still able to stimulate the host's defenses, and the great idea of immunizing against infections was born, partly as a result of serendipity. Toussaint was awarded the Barbier Prize of the Academy of Medicine in 1881 for his brilliant discoveries in bacteriology and immunity, which included an earlier anthrax vaccine that preceded Pasteur's.

George Fleming (1831-1901) was veterinary inspector to the British War Office. In 1880 he urged at a conference on animal vaccination that chairs of comparative pathology be established at all British medical schools, as they had been on the Continent. He felt that knowledge of animal diseases would be much more valuable to doctors than their existing curriculum's comparative anatomy and zoology were. Chauveau at Lyon and K.H. Hertwig (1798-1881) at Berlin were notable examples of veterinary scholars in academia who were in the forefront of extending the curriculum and related research to encompass the pathology and microbiology of diseases. In Prussia and France persons interested in combined medical and veterinary studies were actively encouraged. One encouraging factor was the growing use of animal experimentation in infectious disease research, which allowed rapid progress in veterinary knowledge. McFadyean, with training and interests bridging science, medicine, and veterinary science, became the role model for the British scholar. In 1871 Fleming wrote an important book, *Animal Plagues*. He deplored the decision (in about 1835) to open British ports to imports of foreign cattle, since the consequence was that bovine pleuropneumonia, foot-and-mouth disease, and rinderpest all found their way across the Channel.

PASTEUR: INTUITIVE GENIUS OF MICROBIOLOGY

Strangely, it was a veterinary problem, the dreaded disease of anthrax, that drew two of the finest and most focused minds in the history of biomedical science (Pasteur and Koch) into the challenge from which the science of veterinary and medical microbiology was born. "Anthrax" is an ancient word meaning "malignant ulcers" or "carbuncles," which are a common sign of the infection in humans and dogs. The more commonly affected sheep, cattle, and horses may die suddenly or manifest fever, depression, and hemorrhages from body orifices and especially, edematous swellings along the abdomen and thorax and on the perineum and external genitalia. Swelling of the pharynx region in pigs can lead to asphyxia. The blackish-red spleen is the derivation of the German name for the disease, *Milzbrand*. Workers with fleeces and hides were at special risk, hence the name "woolsorter's disease" for a pulmonary form in humans.

Louis Pasteur (1822-1895) was neither a veterinarian nor a physician, yet few in these two health professions have contributed more to the advancement of the well-being of animals and humans than he, through his discoveries in pathogenic bacteriology and immunology. He was a combination of intuitive visionary genius and intense applied scientist. His disciplinary compass knew no bounds because he was above all a problem solver who used or created disciplines as he needed them. Born at Dole, near Dijon, of a long line of tanners, he became fascinated at school in Paris by Biot's discovery that some substances in solution rotate polarized light, as had been previously known of crystals. This fascination led Pasteur to discover optical isomerism and molecular asymmetry in tartaric and lactic acids, thereby creating the field of stereochemistry, which became significant in biochemical research.

Recognition of Pasteur's accomplishment led to a professorship in chemistry at the age of twenty-six (in 1848) in the faculty at Alsace, which grew into the University of Strasbourg. He found that grapes contain dextrotartaric acid but that if they are allowed to ferment, the levorotatory form could be obtained. He concluded that bacteria could use only the dextroisomer. His

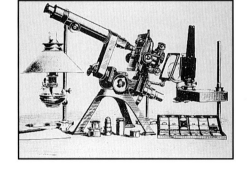

335. Engraving of a very high-resolution optical microscope suitable for bacteriology made by Powell and Leland in the mid-nineteenth century. The lamp, adjustable stage, slide tray, and spare lenses are shown. The genius of Leeuwenhoek had paved the way. *(Dr. Jeremy Burgess/Science Photo Library.)*

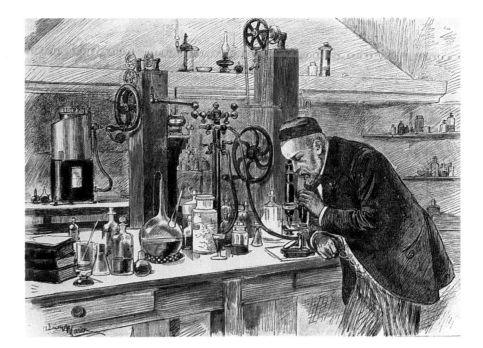

336. Pasteur is shown using a compound microscope to study microorganisms in his laboratory at the Ecole Normale in Paris. *(Mary Evans Picture Library/Photo Researchers, Inc.)*

interests in biology increased, and he moved to Lille in 1854, where he was made dean of the faculty of science. He began to offer courses in fermentation, his new speciality.

The renowned German organic chemist Justus von Liebig held firmly to the view that alcohol was formed from sugar by purely chemical processes. He chose to ignore both that brewers used yeast cells to promote the fermentation of grain and that Theodor Schwann (1810-1882), who discovered animal cells in 1839, had demonstrated that yeast cells divide and grow during fermentation. Pasteur extolled the explanation that fermentation was the biological role of yeast. Liebig was not converted; much later he attacked Pasteur's views in a book that appeared in 1871.

Ever seeking explanations of natural phenomena, Pasteur turned his attention to the souring of milk. He soon showed that a rod-shaped organism was associated with the formation of lactic acid, another optically active substance. Gradually he developed a new branch of science, which he preferred to call "microbiology" (French) rather than "bacteriology" (German). Just three years after moving to Lille, Pasteur was called to Paris to become director of scientific studies at the renowned Ecole Normale, where he had worked with Biot. Ten years later, being perceived as too authoritarian and overpowering, he was required to leave his administrative post and was made director of physiological chemistry until his retirement in 1888. He had to build his laboratory with his own funds.

Pasteur developed the liquid broth technique for bacterial culture. When he found that some species were active only in the presence of air and others only in its absence, he dubbed the former "aerobic" and the latter "anaerobic." This finding led him to the concept that anaerobes may start the process of fermentation or putrefaction, after which their products serve as substrates for the aerobes. These integrated roles showed that microbes have an essential function in recycling detritus. He demonstrated by rigorous experimentation that microbes were necessary for fermentation and that, when present, they used up oxygen and produced carbon dioxide.

When Pasteur came onto the scientific scene, the idea of spontaneous generation of living organisms from decaying organic matter ("heterogenesis") was being espoused forcefully by Felix-Arichimede Pouchet of Rouen in a book published in 1859; he claimed that he had proved it experimentally.

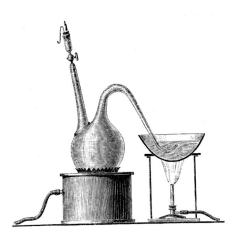

337. The swan-necked flask that prevented the entry of air, which was designed by Pasteur to prove that putrefaction occurred only when air containing organisms was allowed to enter. This experiment was a devastating blow to the then widely held theory of spontaneous generation. *(Ann Ronan Picture Library at Image Select.)*

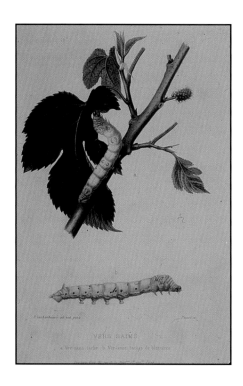

338. Painting of silkworms from Pasteur's 1870 *Etudes sur la Maladie des Vers à Soie,* in which he described two devastating diseases caused by microorganisms. He showed that the diseases could be controlled by examining the worms for the presence of the infectious agents and using for breeding only those in which the agents were absent. *(Institut Pasteur, Paris.)*

Pasteur responded with a series of classic experiments. He heated long-necked flasks with his broth inside, driving out the air, then sealing them. He took some flasks to the countryside and others up a mountain, then opened them for a time before resealing them. After culturing in the laboratory, life-forms developed in forty percent of the "country air" flasks and in only five percent of the "mountain air" flasks. Other scientists joined the fray. An English pathologist, H. Charlton Bastian (1837-1915), presented new arguments for spontaneous generation in *The Beginnings of Life* in 1876. Pasteur knocked his arguments down, but the skirmish shed light on the effect of acidity on sterilization. William Roberts of Manchester showed in *Studies in Biogenesis* (1874) that neutralized cultures were harder to sterilize than acidic ones.

As early as 1865, Pasteur had urged the heat treatment of wines and beers to 55° Celsius before allowing them to cool for storage, to prevent spoilage or souring caused by microbial contaminants in the yeast-fermentation vats. This principle was later applied to the protection of milk both from souring and from infectious agents by heating it to 65° Celcius (149° Fahrenheit) for thirty minutes. This process, known as pasteurization, has been modified slightly over the years but remains a cornerstone of veterinary public health. Pasteurization became imperative toward the end of the nineteenth century, when bottle-feeding of babies became fashionable but led to a substantial rise in rates of infant diarrhea and mortality. Linked to the campaign to eliminate bovine tuberculosis and improve sanitary practices, the adoption of pasteurization had brought about by 1900 a significant reduction in rates of infant mortality and in the incidence of types of human tuberculosis attributable to *Mycobacterium bovis.*

Pasteur, having established his new science of microbiology and converted most of the skeptics with his work on fermentation, putrefaction, pasteurization, and sterilization, turned his attention to the study of the possible roles of microbes in diseases. Ever attacking practical problems and seeking solutions, he accepted the challenge of investigating a disease of silkworms that was threatening the French silk industry.

By 1865 silk production had dropped to less than a sixth of its earlier level. Pasteur went to the center of the industry at Ales and studied the problem. He found a high incidence of unsuccessful, nonproductive cocoons. He labored for five years, showing that there were several distinct diseases, before he came up with the practical solutions he sought. In a disease called pebrine the silkworms carried corpuscular or granular structures. Pasteur's solution was epidemiological. After the females mated, he had the eggs checked by microscopic study. If the eggs contained the corpuscles, they were discarded. The corpuscle-free eggs raised healthy larvae, despite the overall infection of the brood. The second condition was called flacherie (flaccidity), which he attributed to a motile *Vibrio* organism. He showed that this organism produced a form that was extremely resistant to drying and to heat. He proposed that this property was attributable to the highly refractive bodies he observed under the microscope. Using this new knowledge of persistent structures (later known as spores), he devised a control strategy.

One of the most remarkable features of Pasteur's style is that he was able to break through to practical solutions even in the absence of basic understanding. For example, pebrine was later shown to be caused by a protozoan, *Nosema bombycis,* and flacherie by a filterable virus that predisposes the worm to the bacterial agent seen by Pasteur. In both cases he did not have the full picture but he was able to reason his way to an effective solution.

Pasteur's great works had established the principle of chemical asymmetry and the germ theory, and he had addressed practical industrial problems of fermentation (production and preservation of wine, vinegar, and stored foods) and diseases of silkworm stocks. Pasteur suffered a stroke at forty-six years of age, which left him paralyzed on the left side for the rest of his life. At fifty-five he turned to the study of diseases that afflicted the vertebrate animals and might have a microbiological origin. He started with the dreaded *charbon* or anthrax that caused huge losses in the sheep industry and in cattle and other species. Its contagious nature had been recognized in Europe for several decades.

Casimir Davaine (1812-1882), a French physician, demonstrated microscopic rodlike organisms in the blood of cattle affected with anthrax in 1863. The organism was named *Bacillus anthracis.* In the same year Louis Pasteur discovered a nonpathogenic anaerobic bacterium that formed spores, which he named *Bacillus butyricus.* The anthrax organism multiplies rapidly in the body and forms toxins. On exposure to air it forms spores that can persist for centuries in soil and organic matter. Anthrax is unusual among infectious diseases because of its persistence in spore form and its capacity to spread via airborne particles.

Pasteur's approach in 1876 was, first, to capture the suspected culprit microbe and then to "tame" it, that is, get it to multiply in an artificial laboratory environment that he created for it so that it could be studied in depth. He developed a liquid broth medium that sustained the organism's growth. The medium could also be diluted to determine the lowest dose that could produce a lethal infection when inoculated into a susceptible animal. Later he was able to show that the virulence of the culture could be attenuated by repeated cultural passages and environmental stresses.

To create a vaccine in 1880, Toussaint had used heat to attenuate the anthrax organism. The procedure was clearly tricky because the thermal conditions had to be carefully controlled. He used defibrinated blood heated to 55° Celcius for ten minutes. Pasteur, Chamberland, and Roux claimed to have improved on the method in 1881 by using air at a temperature of 42° Celcius to 43° Celcius for attenuation and to avoid spore formation. When Pasteur's original laboratory notebooks were released in 1874, questions were raised about the procedures actually used. Apparently the public report and the notebooks did not agree entirely, and he had used some of Toussaint's procedures. Pasteur's claim of his vaccine's efficacy was challenged by a critic, so he put on a dramatic public trial before a large crowd, including the media, at Pouilly le Fort. Twenty-four sheep were divided into two groups; one group was given a series of inoculations with the vaccine beforehand, the other was left unvaccinated. All the sheep were then given a lethal dose of a culture of anthrax organisms. All the vaccinates survived and all the controls died;

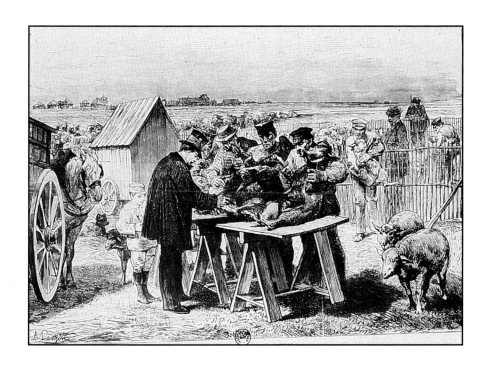

339. An artist's rendition of Pasteur inoculating sheep with his attenuated anthrax vaccine in the famous anthrax immunization experiment at Pouilly le Fort, fifteen miles outside Paris, in 1881. All of the twenty-five vaccinated sheep survived the challenge with a lethal dose of virulent organisms two weeks later, while all twenty-five of the unvaccinated control sheep died. *(Institut Pasteur, Paris.)*

Pasteur's vaccine was vindicated. It is probable, however, that Toussaint's contribution of the first anthrax vaccine did not receive due recognition. Sadly, this creative scholar had a nervous breakdown and died prematurely in 1890.

Pasteur's ability to translate field observations into ingenious ideas for near-conclusive experiments has never been approached by any other investigator over such a broad front. He literally created new subdisciplines to focus on the missing conceptual understanding. Certainly the microbiology of veterinary infectious diseases was one of these. Part of his genius was his tenacity in striving to obtain the crucial pieces of information or experimental results through a combination of field work and laboratory work. Faced with the challenge of determining how animals in the field acquired anthrax without benefit of injection of a living culture, he fed contaminated hay to cows with negative results. Undeterred, he added thistles that were prevalent in the pastures to the fodder, and the disease occurred. He was tested again on the issue of how the disease reappeared on premises where affected animals had been buried. He reported that the busy earthworm recycled the decaying material, including the anthrax spores, and returned them to the surface with its casts.

A veritable "ecologist of disease," Pasteur was also a master of the art of attracting the attention of his clientele to his work. The whole of France monitored his progress; indeed, much of the developed world wanted to keep in touch with his scientific revelations. He developed a vaccine for swine erysipelas in 1882. Then he showed that his bacteria-free filtrates of the *Pasteurella* organism, obtained by means of Chamberland's filter, caused hens to go into a deep sleep. Toussaint had initiated work on microbial toxins in 1878. Pasteur concluded that the organisms had produced a chemical toxin, opening a new avenue of research. By this unique strategy of holding the focus of professional, political, and public attention he was, as if by magic, able both to bring the intellectual climate of his day into a state of readiness to accept his series of discoveries and to block his critics' efforts to discredit his work. His accomplishment was remarkable because, as this modest history of veterinary progress has shown, society and the various cultural establishments were all too often unwilling to accept or take action on great conceptual breakthroughs. Veterinarians and veterinary scientists who have made important discoveries have seldom received due credit.

KOCH'S SYSTEMATIZATION OF PATHOGENIC BACTERIOLOGY

Friedrich Gustav Jacob Henle (1809-1885), anatomist and pathologist, discovered that Henle's loop was a component of the basic architectural unit of the kidney, the nephron. Although not a microbiologist himself, Henle studied Bassi's work on muscardine disease of silkworms and proposed in 1840 that many animal and human diseases may be attributable to invasion of the body by living parasitic organisms. He held several academic chairs; in his chair at Göttingen he had a profound influence on Robert Koch, who became a great enlightener in the understanding of infectious diseases.

Henle proposed that his hypothesis about the possible microbial origin of disease should be tested in every instance by subjecting the disease to four rigorous criteria:

Specific organisms were always present in cases of the disease.

These organisms could be isolated and cultured independently in the laboratory.

Their inoculation into healthy subjects would reproduce exactly the disease symptoms and outcome.

The organisms must be observed in and recovered from the experimentally infected animals.

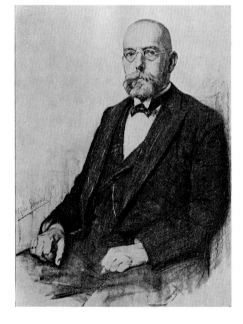

340. Robert Koch (1843-1910), the physician who developed important techniques in microbiology that are still in use today for the isolation of organisms in pure culture. He was the first to demonstrate and culture the agent that causes tuberculosis. His work led to the establishment of laboratories for medical and veterinary microbiology and set the standards that were used to determine whether an agent caused disease. *(Photo: AKG, Berlin.)*

Henle's criteria were to become known as Koch's postulates in recognition of their magnificent deployment by the noted German physician and microbiologist, Heinrich Hermann Robert Koch (1843–1910). He was born in Clausthal in the Harz Mountains, the third born of thirteen children. He was interested in natural history and cared for the family's livestock—a cow, a pig, a horse, and chickens—as well as his own rabbits and guinea pigs. He studied medicine at Georgia-Augusta University of Göttingen, at that time still a rural community. The faculty when Koch graduated in 1862 was remarkably advanced and inspiring. It included Wohler (who accomplished the first synthesis of urea), Krause (who identified sensory nerve endings), Meissner (whose name identifies autonomic nerve plexuses of the gut wall), Hasse (known for his scientific approach to medicine), and Henle (who studied renal architecture and epithelia and established criteria for proof of the bacterial origin of disease).

The students at Göttingen were encouraged to participate in research, an ideal opportunity for the young Koch. Later he credited Henle, Hasse, and especially, Meissner for awakening his interest in research. He won the university prize for a paper on ganglion cells in the nerves of the uterus. Metchnikoff came to work with Henle when Koch graduated, in 1866. Koch worked briefly in Hamburg; during a cholera outbreak he demonstrated wavy, whiplike microbial structures in intestinal contents, his first encounter with the "bug" he was later to identify as *Vibrio cholerae*. He benefitted from the forward-thinking ideas of the pathologist Edwin Klebs (1834–1913) of Königsberg, a persistent advocate of the germ theory of disease and a pioneering microbiologist. Klebs invented the method of obtaining pure cultures by "darwinizing" or using successive dilutions to kill competing organisms.

Koch practiced medicine in rural Rakwitz in Posen; he served in the medical corps in the Franco-Prussian War in 1870, then returned to Rakwitz and soon became the district health officer in nearby Wollstein. He had obtained a microscope and developed a laboratory in his home. Anthrax was rampant in the livestock of the region, and he took up the serious study of the disease. It served as an excellent problem and an opportunity for Koch to establish himself as a new force in the study of infectious diseases and microbiology. It was fortuitous for veterinary medicine that such a trailblazing genius applied himself to an important veterinary problem, thereby setting a standard for subsequent veterinary investigations that ensured rapid, rigorous progress. Koch himself noted the enormous advantage of working on a human disease that was readily transmitted to animals, since the origins of such a disease could be studied and control strategies could be developed in a comparative and experimental way.

The German veterinarian Frederick Brauell (1856) had shown that anthrax was surely a zoonotic disease by transmitting it from humans to sheep and that human deaths resulting from it were common in rural areas. He obtained blood samples from the slaughterhouse and inoculated mice, which died with their blood rich in the little rodlets described earlier by Davaine. Koch then embarked on the problem of in vitro culture. He conceived that the medium should not only sustain the organism but also must be sterilizable, to avoid contamination, as well as solid and preferably somewhat transparent, to allow separation. At first he used potato slices as the medium, then meat extract in gelatin. Koch even used the aqueous humor of bovine eyes as a culture medium for anthrax. He developed a unique system of culture plates, which could be inoculated in sections at angles and permitted intermittent sterilization of the inoculating loop, thereby ensuring sufficient dilution to allow colony selection and subculturing as necessary. The technique was a huge success. Even Pasteur, whose relations with Koch were strained, acknowledged it publicly by declaring "C'est un grand progres." One of Koch's assistants later suggested that he try agar obtained from seaweed in preference to gelatin, and another, Richard Petri, devised the small glass dish with a matched, close-fitting lid—the Petri dish.

Empowered by the new technique, his improved status, and his own remarkable experimental intellectual drive, Koch developed pathogenic bacteriology. Independent of Pasteur's work, he studied spore formation in anthrax. He took his work on anthrax and spores to Ferdinand Cohn and Julius Cohnheim, professors at the University of Breslau, and Cohn arranged for the publication of his paper on anthrax in 1876. Cohnheim was enthralled and is reported to have announced, "This is the greatest discovery ever made in bacteriology." Koch's international reputation blossomed. Koch followed his pioneering work on anthrax with an important study clinching the role of bacterial infections of wounds in 1878. In 1880 he was appointed to the Imperial Health Department in Berlin and was assigned two assistants, Friedrich Löffler and Georg Gaffky, both former Prussian army surgeons. In 1885 he was invited to fill the new chair of hygiene at the University of Berlin. During this phase of his career, when tuberculosis was the preeminent human disease in Europe, accounting for at least one in every seven deaths, he systematized bacteriology and trained future researchers. Koch turned his energy away from the rural scene and focused on the quest for the tubercle bacillus.

When Koch went to Berlin (Reichsgesundheitsamt), he exemplified the combination of personal dedication to rigorous scholarship and focus on the practical problems of disease control. He held his chair in public health until 1891, when a special center was built for him, the Institute for Infectious Diseases. During his time in Berlin his passion was directed toward the conquest of tuberculosis. He discovered and demonstrated the tubercle bacillus, having developed a way to visualize it selectively with his staining technique. He showed that the characteristic nodules (tubercles) had a caseous center made up of dead cells.

He collaborated with Wilhelm Schütz, head of the Pathology Institute of the Berlin veterinary school, and worked closely with a physician on his staff and his own trainee, Friedrich Löffler. A veterinarian, Paul Frosch, was Koch's assistant and Löffler's colleague in research. Carl Jensen, a Danish veterinarian, worked with Koch and later received recognition for his pioneering work on transplanting tumors in mice.

Koch reproduced tuberculosis by inoculation with his pure cultures in guinea pigs, rabbits, cats, and field mice; a progressive infection resulted, with caseous ulceration at the injection site, emaciation, pulmonary disease, and swollen lymph nodes. Pulmonary tubercles were observed.

Tuberculosis ("consumption" [wasting] or "phthisis" [pulmonary tuberculosis and wasting]) is a chronic progressive, contagious-infectious disease of animals and humans characterized by the development of nodules or tubercles that undergo cell proliferation and central necrosis with caseous degeneration. Tuberculosis had been a human disease since the earliest civilizations; the Egyptian mummies bear witness to this fact. Both the Talmud and the works of Hippocrates described a prevalent syndrome that could be none other than "TB," as tuberculosis came to be called. It was present in Italy at the start of the Christian era and spread northwest, even to England, via imported cattle as well as via contact with human cases. The leadership of British farmers in stock breeding led to dissemination of their purebred livestock to all corners of the globe, some delivering tuberculosis as well as better genes. It is believed that the disease became widespread in the human population only after the establishment of town dairies during the Industrial Revolution (from about 1750).

An ancient disease of cattle, known as pearl disease because of the lustrous appearance of the bovine tubercles, was at one stage thought to be a form of syphilis resulting from unnatural unions between humans and animals. Early in the nineteenth century the resemblance between pearl disease and human

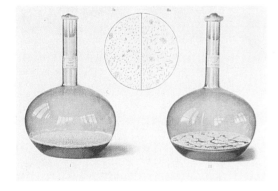

341. An illustration from Calmette's famous book on tuberculosis, published in 1923. Glycerine-broth culture flasks for, *left,* bovine and, *right,* human strains of the causative agent and the microscopic appearance of the tubercle bacilli in each case are shown. *(From Calmette, 1923.)*

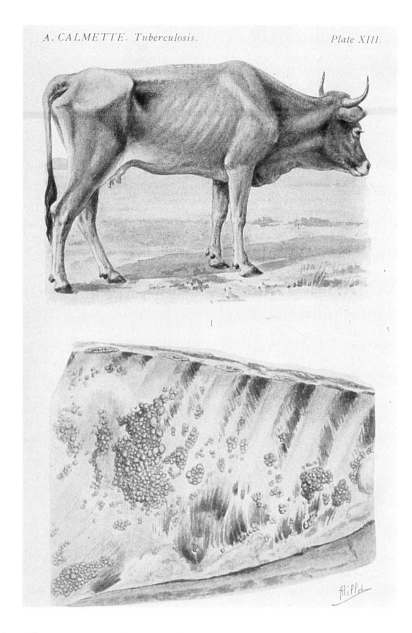

342. Artist's rendition from Calmette (1923) of, *top,* a cow affected with tuberculosis and, *bottom,* the appearance of the pleura after slaughter. Typical pearl-like lesions of vegetative tuberculosis of the pleura are evident. *(From Calmette, 1923.)*

tuberculosis was noted by some but disputed by others, including the influential pathologist Virchow, who categorically denied that tuberculosis occurred in animals. French veterinarian J.B. Huzard proposed in 1790 that tuberculosis was transmitted from animals to humans.

A brilliant specialist in diseases of the chest made the critical steps toward an understanding of tuberculosis. René Laennec, the person destined to make this great service to humankind, was born in Quimper, Brittany, in 1781. Left motherless by the forays of consumption at six years of age, he went to live with an uncle, a noted physician in Nantes who became rector of the faculty there and was an ardent admirer of John Hunter. Young René decided on a medical career. Early in his medical career he invented the stethoscope and used it in describing the clinical signs of diseases of the chest; a book he wrote on the topic of auscultation constituted a great leap forward in physical diagnosis (1819). Thus Laennec gave physicians the tool that has become their insignia and allowed them some familiarity with the functions of the heart and lungs. Laennec, who was himself afflicted with tuberculosis and eventually died of it, laid the foundation for the understanding of the disease. He showed that the several stages of the disease—from translucent granulations to opaque caseous nodules to an apurulent stage—were all part of the same tuberculosis syndrome.

In 1868 Villemin transmitted the disease to rabbits, then between species of animals. During the same year Chauveau at Lyon transmitted the disease by feeding animals tuberculous material from cattle and concluded that Villemin had been correct in his conclusions about the organism's ability to cross the species barrier.

343. The finest early illustration of the lesions in the lung of a cow infected with tuberculosis. From R. Carswell's *Pathological Anatomy, Illustrations of the Elementary Forms of Disease,* London (1838). *a,* Catarrhal mucus in a bronchus. *b,* Fibrous capsule enclosing caseous mass. *c,* Such capsules after caseous contents are removed. The probe shows connection to bronchial branch. *d,* Acinonodular lesions. *(As reproduced in Francis J: Bovine tuberculosis, 1947.)*

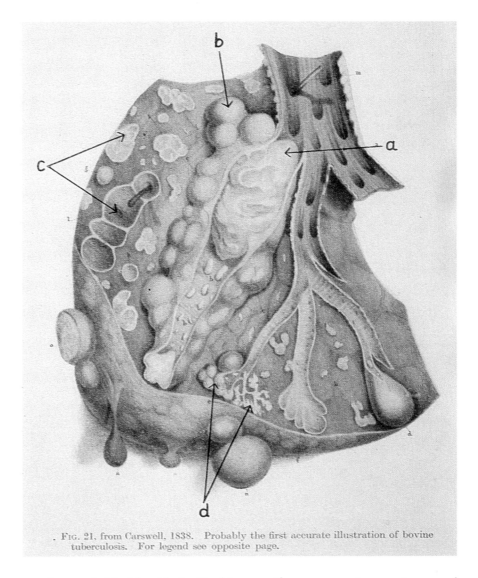

. Fɪɢ. 21, from Carswell, 1838. Probably the first accurate illustration of bovine tuberculosis. For legend see opposite page.

A remarkable blemish in Koch's magnificent career in veterinary and medical research was his adamant refusal to accept that the bovine strain of the bacterium was infective for humans, perhaps out of respect for Virchow's views that tuberculosis did not occur spontaneously in animals and that domestic animals were insignificant in its transmission to humans. Koch was, however, inconsistent on the subject:

> *Tuberculous domestic animals are only of minor etiologic importance. Animals do not discharge sputum and tubercle bacilla are found only rarely in their feces. However, the milk of tuberculous cows can be a source of infection. Except for that, animals can be a source of infection only after death, through ingestion of infected meat. In that case, the infectious agent will invade through the digestive organs and the first evidence of disease will appear there. . . . Regarding milk as a source of infection, organisms are infrequently found in the milk of infected cows. Tubercle bacilli occur in the milk only when the mammary glands are infected, but tubercles do not develop often in the udders.*

It appears that he was referring to the human strain of the organism.

Koch had a burning ambition to find a cure for tuberculosis. At the Institute of Hygiene he worked with Pfeiffer, Kitasato, Behring, Ehrlich, and Uhlenhuth. When he had an opportunity to present his findings at the tenth international medical congress in Berlin in 1890, it was rumored that a momentous announcement would be made. The title of his presentation was *Bacteriological Research.* He stated that after many failures he had found a substance that inhibited the growth of tubercle bacilli both in laboratory cultures in vitro and in live animals. When injected into guinea pigs with advanced tuberculosis, it arrested the disease. He expressed hope that it might be effective

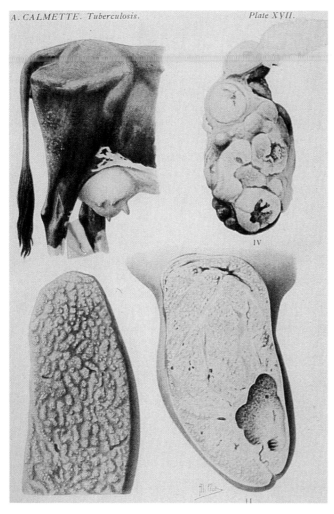

344. Four illustrations from Calmette (1923) of mammary tuberculosis in a cow. *Upper left,* The distortion of the udder. *Upper right,* Section through esophageal lymph glands. *Lower left,* Transverse section above the cavity. *Lower right,* A cavity within the udder. The veterinary contribution was to insist that the bovine strain of the organism was infectious to humans and that infected milk or meat was a risk to public health.

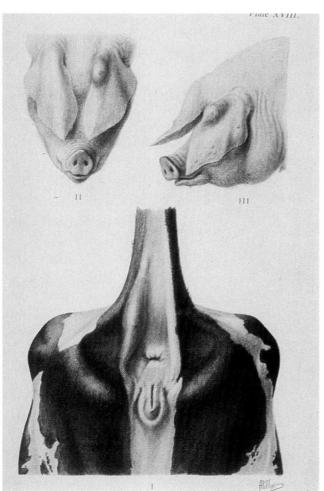

345. Koch's tuberculin was the basis of a diagnostic test when given intradermally to animals, causing a purple swelling in the ear of a pig, *top,* or in the tail fold of a cow, *bottom. (From Calmette, 1923.)*

389

in human therapy. A few months later he published a report indicating that humans, unlike guinea pigs, underwent a severe febrile reaction when given a small, 0.25-ml dose of the substance. The reaction was minimal at a dose of 0.01 ml unless the person was infected, in which case a generalized febrile reaction with malaise set in. In cases of phthisis, the dose had to be lowered to 0.001 ml and repeated daily until no temperature rise occurred. The report stated that in early cases the patients were free of symptoms in four to six weeks and could be considered cured.

The consequence of Koch's report was that the demand for his treatment was overwhelming. There were fatal reactions to the treatment, and public opinion turned against Koch. Although the "tuberculin" was abandoned as a therapeutic agent, its true value as a diagnostic reagent surfaced. Koch received a patent for it, but he was surpassed in immunological research by his former colleague Emil von Behring. The controversy surrounding the importance of bovine infection in public health was finally resolved when Theobald Smith in the United States separated and isolated the human and bovine strains of the tubercle bacillus. An avian strain was also found. Koch was at last convinced that the bovine strain was infective for humans. He accepted Smith's findings and in 1884 incorporated them into public health proposals. Despite these findings, the compulsory pasteurization of milk products that was introduced in 1898 was undertaken to prevent tuberculosis in pigs and calves fed separated milk obtained from large dairies.

Koch's statement that bovine tuberculosis was not transmissible to humans had been challenged by several leading veterinary scientists, including Salmon, McEachran, and McFadyean (in the United States, Canada, and Great Britain, respectively).

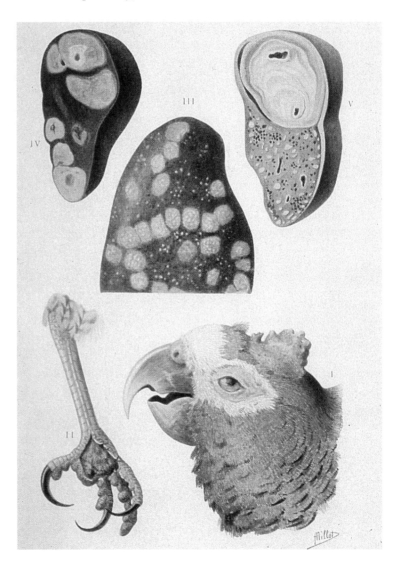

346. Avian tuberculosis. The three upper figures show tuberculosis of the liver in a goose. *Lower left,* Scaly verrucous tubercles on the foot of a goshawk. *Lower right,* a tuberculous lesion on the crest of a parrot. *(From Calmette, 1923.)*

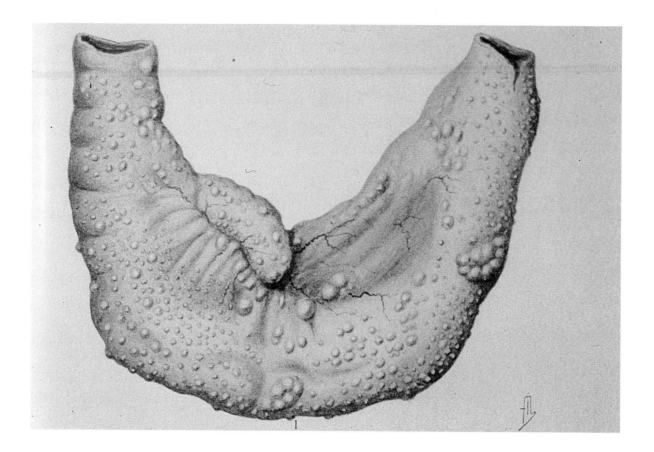

THE INDESTRUCTIBLE SPORE FORMERS

347. Tuberculous infection of the intestine in a child who died some time after drinking milk from a cow infected with the disease. *(From Calmette, 1923.)*

During Pasteur's studies with silkworm diseases he had observed organisms that had sporelike structures. He recognized that these forms in larvae were resistant to situations that destroyed the adults, but he did not clearly state their role and properties. In 1863, as stated earlier, he described a nonpathogenic spore-forming anaerobe, *Bacillus butyricus.*

The British physicist Tyndall, who demonstrated the visualization of particulate matter in air by passing a beam of light through a darkened room, was able to produce sterile air after deposition of particles in a closed container. The particles were the true sources of the life-forms that appeared "spontaneously" in flasks open to the air. He also showed that some bacteria exist in two forms, one heat sensitive, the other heat resistant. The latter could be destroyed by intermittent heating or "tyndallization" (1877). Tyndall provided a practical demonstration both of the role that spores play and of their ability to transform to the vegetative state. His findings helped to clinch the germ theory and put the final nail in the coffin of the theory of spontaneous generation by explaining anomalous results of earlier experiments.

When Koch and Pasteur began to study anthrax, they soon encountered its tendency to form spores (1876). As stated earlier, most of the pathogenic spore-forming bacteria are anaerobic, but the unique anthrax bacillus is aerobic. Ferdinand Cohn described spores in the nonpathogenic *Bacillus subtilis* in 1876, just after Tyndall's work.

During studies of cultures obtained from suspected cases of anthrax Pasteur and Joubert in 1877 isolated a pathogenic anaerobic organism, which Pasteur named "vibrion septique." This microbe, which produced a fatal edematous disease, was later rediscovered and rechristened *Clostridium septicum,* the cause of braxy or malignant edema in sheep. This work set the stage for a special branch of veterinary microbiology involving a number of important animal (and some human) diseases caused by spore-forming anaerobic bacteria of the genus *Clostridium*, including blackleg, black disease, lamb dysentery, gas gangrene, struck, enterotoxemia, botulism, and tetanus.

In 1875 Bollinger discovered the cause of blackleg or blackquarter to be a *Bacillus* organism later identified as *Clostridium chauvoei*. An acute disease that sometimes causes heavy losses in cattle and sheep, blackleg is characterized by fever and crepitating swellings in selected muscles. The death rate is high, especially in cattle. Chabert at Alfort veterinary school in 1783 described the clinical signs and pathology as a type of gangrene with gas formation and crepitation of affected muscles. A heat-attenuated live vaccine was developed in France and Germany. The disease caused heavy losses on the western ranges of North America. Media clippings and postcards from that era reveal scenes of dead and dying cattle. A vaccine was developed by BAI scientists for use as a single dose. O.M. Franklin and T.P. Haslam, graduates of the then new veterinary school at Manhattan, Kansas, made a safer vaccine by filtering cultures of the blackleg organism through a Berkefeld bacterial filter, yielding a nonliving aggressin that induced resistance to the disease. Franklin formed Franklin's Blackleg Serum Company in Wichita in 1916; it evolved later into Franklin Laboratories, marketing a wide range of veterinary products. A new blackleg vaccine based on attenuation of the organism by formaldehyde to form a noninfectious bacteria was developed and became accepted internationally in 1921.

Tetanus, caused by *Clostridium tetani*, was transmitted to rabbits by inoculating them with a suspension of material from a pustule of a tetanus patient in 1884. In the same year Nicolaiev produced tetanus in mice, guinea pigs, and rabbits by injecting them with a suspension of a little garden soil. Pus formed at the site of injection, and Nicolaiev observed a long bacillus that reproduced the disease, although he could not achieve a pure culture. The organism was restricted to the site of the injection and the nerve supplying the area. He assumed that the organism acted via a toxin. Rosenbach in 1886 showed that the organism had a round terminal spore, and in the next year Nocard showed that the horse was susceptible. Shibasaburo Kitasato (1852-1931), a Japanese physician from Ogunigo who had been sent to Berlin to study under Koch, was the first to obtain a pure culture of *Clostridium tetani*, after heating and anaerobic incubation, that retained infectivity. He later returned to his homeland and became Japan's leading medical microbiologist, but not before he had prepared, working with von Behring in 1890, an effective antitoxic antiserum for passive immunization. The feces of animals and humans frequently contain the tetanus organism. The toxin has been attenuated and converted into a toxoid that imparts active immunity and some resistance to subsequent wound infection.

Botulism or "lame sickness" of cattle received intensive study in southern Africa, where Sir Arnold Theiler (1919) showed that it was associated with pica or depraved appetite in cattle that consumed decomposed carcass material and bones on the veld; he attributed the disease to a toxin in the putrefied tissues. This attribution was confirmed in 1927 when Theiler and E.M. Robinson isolated a toxin-forming anaerobe, *Clostridium botulinum*, that proliferates in carcass tissues. The subtlety of the etiological features of botulism is illustrated by the finding that phosphorus-deficient vegetation leads to the depraved appetite and osteophagia. If the organism has multiplied in the carcass tissues, this will lead to signs of botulism in the cattle.

Several strains of the botulinal organism occur. Botulism in humans occurs after consumption of inadequately sterilized canned foods, the spores surviving to allow proliferation and gas formation (in "blown" cans, for example, of tuna fish). Such cases of botulism are usually caused by type A or B of the organism. Type C causes "limberneck" in birds, especially in waterfowl, a type of muscular paralysis often seen during droughts, when various organisms succumb to the disease in or around lakes and pools. Type C also affects farm livestock in Western Australia, especially sheep. The disease in South African cattle was usually caused by type D. Toxicity persists longer in the carcasses of tortoises than in mammalian carrion. Heavy losses can occur in livestock. The toxins are extremely potent and block the neuromuscular junction.

The spore-forming pathogenic organisms present a special problem for eradication programs because the spores of some species can survive at least for several decades and perhaps much longer. Thus after long periods of absence the disease can reappear when a change in environmental conditions or uncovering of the organism makes infection possible.

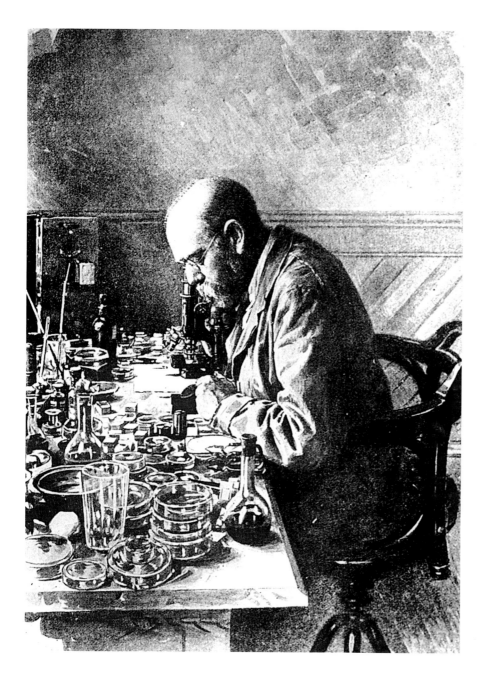

348. Robert Koch using a microscope in his laboratory. He is shown surrounded by flasks of liquid cultures and petri dishes of solid agar. The latter allowed ready separation of individual colonies by subdividing the inoculum with a flamed loop. *(The Wellcome Institute Library, London.)*

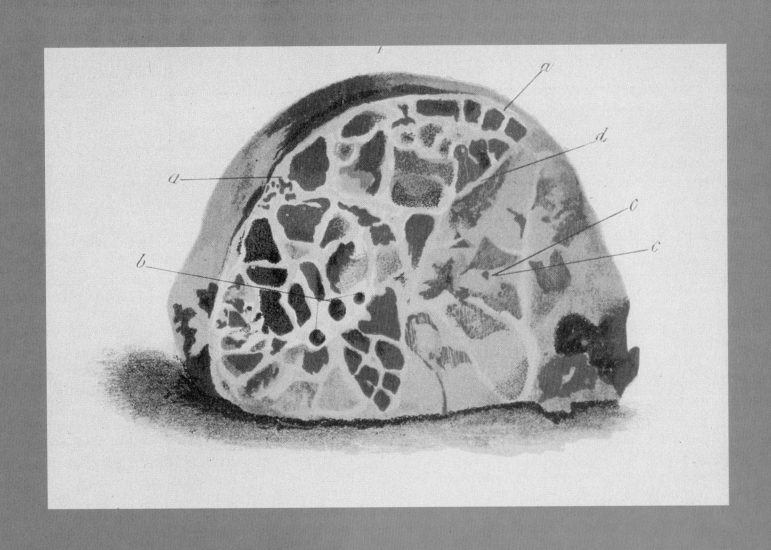

The Heyday of Pathogenic Bacteriology and the Discovery of Viruses

ACCELERATION OF PROGRESS IN BACTERIAL ETIOLOGY OF ANIMAL DISEASES

During the golden age of bacteriology—from the 1860s to the end of the nineteenth century—a myriad of diseases for which a bacterial species is the primary causative agent were characterized by etiology. The case of anthrax in 1876 and 1877 (studied by Pasteur and Koch) provided the template. Pasteur himself demonstrated the agents of malignant edema, pneumococcal infection, staphylococcal infection, and fowl cholera between 1877 and 1880.

Koch and his colleagues paralleled these achievements with the identification of the agents causing typhoid (with Gaffky), streptococcal infection, tuberculosis, and cholera between 1880 and 1884. In 1902 Koch developed a successful strategy for the control of typhoid. Löffler and Schütz finally grasped the elusive agent of glanders, *Pseudomonas mallei,* in 1882. Two years later Löffler also isolated the diphtheria bacillus and showed it to be different from pseudodiphtheritic organisms that affect calves. Kitasato isolated the tetanus bacillus in 1889. In 1892 Welch and Nuttall isolated *Clostridium perfringens (C. welchii),* the cause of gas gangrene, and van Ermengen followed with the identification of the agent of botulism in 1897. The next year Kiyoshi Shiga plucked the bacillus of dysentery (*Shigella* organism). The *Bacillus coli* infectious agent was isolated by Theodor Escherich in 1886; later it acquired his name as the genus *Escherichia*. In addition to the trailblazing approaches and methodologies developed by Pasteur and Koch and their colleagues, other innovations contributed to the rate of progress.

Particularly in the area of optical microscopy, technological advances were important in "seeing" bacteria more clearly. The physicist Ernst Abbe conquered the problem of spherical aberration by developing combination lenses and focusing systems that were manufactured by Carl Zeiss of Jena using Schott's lenses. Much clearer focusing resulted. Abbe also devised a way to deliver oblique angles of light by means of diaphragms, which further improved the visual images. Chromatic aberration, or the distortion of focus resulting from refractions of light of different wavelengths, was overcome by John Dolland in England, who made lenses of two different materials that canceled out the effects of the aberration.

Differential staining was an important technique that enhanced visibility and thus the viewer's ability to identify organisms. Vital staining of living organisms was a prerequisite for visualization of most bacterial species. This technique was developed in the 1870s by Robert Koch, who used aniline dyes such as methyl violet that were introduced by Paul Ehrlich. It was shown

349. *Facing page,* Cross section of the lung of a cow that died in an advanced stage of pleuropneumonia. Coagulated blood and lymph plug the blood vessels and bronchial tubes, and congealed lymph distends the interlobular spaces. The brick-red areas of tissue were called hepatization. Today the disease is known as contagious bovine pleuropneumonia, and is known to be caused by *Mycoplasma mycoides. (From Walley, 1879.)*

350. Foot and mouth disease in a cow. *12* is a posterior view of a lower leg showing dermal inflammation (*a*) and a burst vesicle in the interdigital space (*b, c*). *13* shows part of the tongue several days after bursting of a vesicle and the intense inflammation of the mucous membranes after peeling back. *14* shows the dental pad, which is the most frequent site of vesicles, after rupture of a large one. *(From Walley, 1879.)*

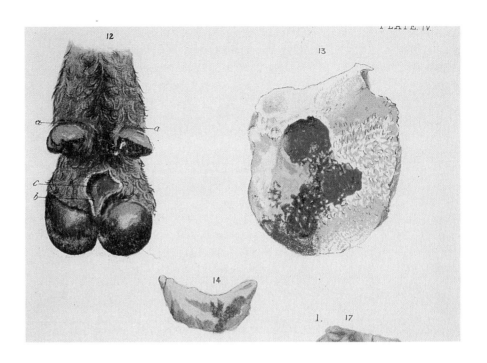

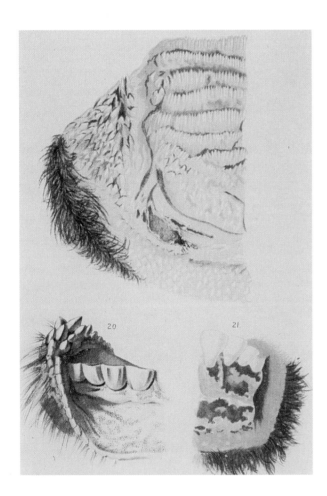

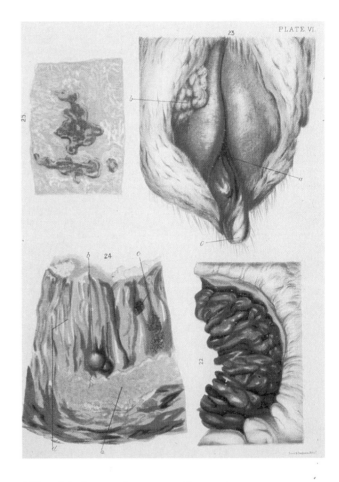

351. Evidence of rinderpest, or cattle plague. *19* shows patchy exfoliation of the epithelium of the hard palate, some denuding cheek papillae, and the dental pad on the sixth day. *20* shows loss of gum epithelium and typical eruption of the mucosa inside the lower lip in an adult. *21* depicts severe loss of the mucous membrane in a four-month-old calf. *(From Walley, 1879.)*

352. Rinderpest in a cow. Severe inflammation causes hemorrhagic rectal folds, *22;* swollen inflamed vulva with a ropy discharge, *23;* inflamed ileum in section, *24;* and sloughing of the ruminal epithelium, *25.* The picture is one of devastating inflammation and erosion of the epithelial surface from os to anus. *(From Walley, 1879.)*

to be helpful in visualizing large bacterial cells but was less helpful in visualizing smaller ones. Löffler introduced other new staining methods.

The Danish doctor Hans Christian Joachim Gram (1853-1938) made the greatest achievement in bacterial staining. His "Gram stain" technique allowed bacteria to be divided into two great groups based on their stains in his system. In his first method, published in 1884, one large class of bacteria was stained purple, including pneumococci, other cocci, anthrax bacilli, and putrefaction bacilli (tubercle bacilli required more than twelve-hour immersion); the other class was decolorized. The former group came to be known as Gram-positive bacteria, and the latter as Gram-negative (these included typhoid bacilli and a few exceptions among the mainly Gram-positive pneumococci). Gram indicated that counterstaining with a red dye was possible: this became a standard part of the method. He became professor of pharmacology in Copenhagen after working with Friedlander in Berlin. The special problem presented by the stain-resistant *Mycobacterium* organisms was solved by Robert Koch, who used a high concentration of dyes with mordanting substances to effect the stain. The tubercle bacilli (and Johne's bacillus), unlike other bacteria, were resistant to subsequent decolorization by acid, which left tuberculosis organisms clearly visible. This resistance was the "acid-fast" property.

DISINFECTION IN THE PREVENTION OF WOUND INFECTION AND THE PROMOTION OF ASEPTIC SURGERY

Separate from the study of bacterial infections as spontaneous diseases was the intractable problem of wound infection. The risk of secondary infection by environmental bacteria—whether it resulted from the ever more horrible maiming of animal and human bodies in combat or from the efforts of the surgeon to intervene in medical problems—was ever present.

The reluctance of the medical profession to admit any defects, as well as its resistance to change, even after evidence became available, was never exemplified more starkly than in its response to childbed fever. Oliver Wendell Holmes (1809-1894) in Boston proposed in 1843 that puerperal fever was a contagious malady, arousing a storm of protest and criticism from the medical profession. A dedicated Hungarian doctor, Ignaz Phillip Semmelweiss (1816-1865), working at the General Hospital in Vienna, then reported in 1847 that mortality rates in obstetrical wards attended by students were much higher than in wards restricted to midwives. He recognized that the disease was a septicemia resulting from introduction of infectious agents by obstetrical workers with contaminated hands. He blamed the high mortality rates on an accepted procedure: the students came to examine the women after performing dissection or postmortem activities. He required that such students scrub their hands with chloride of lime before going into the obstetrical ward. Mortality rates dropped from about 18% to 1%. His colleagues belittled and persecuted him, forcing him to leave Vienna for Budapest, where he became professor of obstetrics and published a classic monograph. Unable to tolerate the continuing persecution, Semmelweiss became insane. Lister later acknowledged Semmelweiss as his forerunner.

An enthusiastic follower of Pasteur's discoveries was the distinguished British surgeon Joseph Lister (1827-1912). Lister was born into a Quaker family in Upton, Essex. He entered the medical profession, then became a surgeon in Edinburgh before holding professorships, first in Glasgow, then in London. Lister concluded that wounds and surgical interventions became septic because of the entry of germs from the air. In 1865 he proposed to overcome this problem in his surgery by spraying carbolic acid (phenol) as an antiseptic agent. Pasteur himself had stated that "if I had been a surgeon I would never introduce an instrument into the human body without having passed it

353. Lister's carbolic acid antiseptic spray from a steam aspirator being utilized in a surgical operation using anesthesia in the nineteenth century. Members of the surgical team are wearing everyday clothes in the disinfectant era that preceded aseptic surgical technique. *(Hulton Deutch Collection Limited, London.)*

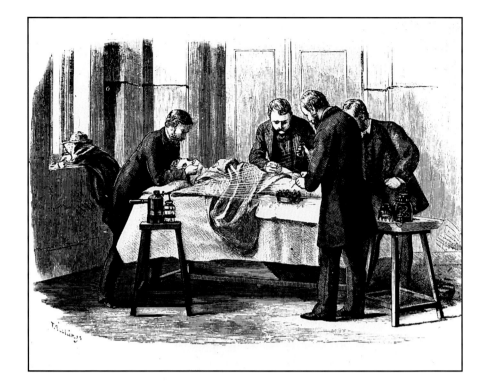

through boiling water." From these seminal thoughts the concept of aseptic surgery was born. Lister had visited Pasteur and witnessed some of his experiments at first hand. He acknowledged a great debt to Pasteur for convincing him of the germ theory with excellent experiments. Lister developed the use of catgut soaked in disinfectant for internal sutures that would digest away without infection after healing had occurred. He worked with James McCall (1834-1915), the founder of the Glasgow Veterinary College, to develop and perfect his methods, using horses and calves in their experiments. The importance of Lister's work for the development of veterinary surgery was enormous. It enabled successful outcomes in many situations for which high risk and frequent failure had been the rule previously.

The most dangerous yet most unpredictable disease of solipeds, chameleon-like in being epidemic, acute, or chronic, which often attained the status of a plague, has been known in its acute form as glanders or malleus and in its chronic form as farcy. A disease primarily of equids, it has plagued the human's long companionship with the horse and can be passed to humans. The name *malleus* is derived from Greek words describing the disease that was called "malignant" by Aristotle (330 BC) and Apsyrtos (fourth century AD), who believed it to be contagious. The words were romanized by Vegetius to the one that was passed down through history, "malleus," that is, "hammer." In 1523 Fitzherbert used the terms *glanders* and *farcy.* During the eighteenth century it gradually became obvious that the disease was infectious, and isolation or slaughter was urged, as well as thorough disinfection of tack and all parts of the stables. The pioneering Danish team of Abildgaard, the first head of the Copenhagen veterinary school, and his colleague Erik Viborg, who succeeded him, established that the acute respiratory syndrome of glanders was one manifestation of the same disease that at other times exhibited itself as the purulent, spreading, eruptive skin disease of farcy.

Erik Viborg in 1797 convincingly established that the acute form was infectious by means of inoculations or intravenous injections of material obtained from diseased horses into healthy ones and by demonstrating the spread of the disease by contact when healthy horses were stabled with diseased ones. This work confirmed Solleysel's observation of 1664. Although researchers at the Alfort and London veterinary schools denied that glanders was infectious, Saint-Cyr and Barthelemy at the Lyon veterinary school in 1849 proved that the chronic form was infectious in horses. Injury and confinement were thought to play a role in initiating infection, and the disease often was exacerbated and spread during military campaigns, when standards of care declined, stress and exhaustion were common, and wounds were frequent. As early as 1812 Lorin showed that humans could become infected with glanders. Pierre-Francois-Olive Rayer (1793-1864) of Calvados wrote a definitive work on clinical glanders and farcy in humans.

Visualization of the organism that caused glanders with the aid of the microscope was at last achieved in 1881 by Victor Babes (1854-1926), a Romanian doctor. The organism, a slender, rod-shaped bacterium, was seen in the pus obtained from human lesions. In the following year Löffler and Schütz obtained the organism in pure culture, then proved that their isolate was infectious (in 1886). The male guinea pig was used as a model for testing because of the predilection of the disease to localize in the testicles and epididymis in that species when infection occurred.

In 1890 and 1891 two Russian veterinarians working independently, Kallning in Dorpat and Hellman in St. Petersburg, used the glanders organism to produce mallein; their work was based on the method Koch used to produce tuberculin. Thus a diagnostic test could be developed that allowed isolation, control, and eventual regional eradication of the disease. Pasteur's colleague, the veterinarian Edmond Nocard (1850-1903), defined and developed the necessary principles and standards for obtaining accurate results with reagents like tuberculin and mallein, which induce hypersensitivity reactions.

McFADYEAN: VISIONARY OF VETERINARY SCIENCE AND MICROBIOLOGY

John McFadyean (1853-1941), the redeemer of the British veterinary profession, was born the son of a tenant farmer at Barrachan, near Wigtown, in Galloway. He left school at sixteen years of age and spent five years as a paid hand on his father's farm. In 1874 he went to the Edinburgh veterinary school, receiving his diploma in 1876. There he accepted a teaching post in anatomy but, enthralled by the discoveries of Pasteur and Koch, he continued to study at Edinburgh University, enrolling concurrently in medicine and science. His lectureship stipend kept him on a maintenance ration and paid his union fees.

McFadyean graduated in medicine in 1882, and in science in 1883. True to his first love, veterinary science, he wanted degrees in medicine and science only to prepare himself for an academic career in pathology and microbiology as a kind of "supervet" grounded in the work of Koch and Pasteur. He wrote a textbook, *The Anatomy of the Horse: A Dissection Guide.* A skillful microscopist, he thrived on laboratory investigations: he wanted to *know.* In 1888 he founded a new scientific medium, The *Journal of Comparative Pathology and Therapeutics,* a quarterly publication of high quality, thereby issuing a veritable challenge to his profession to adopt a rigorous scientific approach to the advancement of veterinary knowledge and avoid distracting, erroneous speculation. His penetrating intellect spanned the compass of the veterinary science of his time, and he communicated all significant advances to his readership, lacing his observations with remarkable editorial commentary.

Not surprisingly, as the best-prepared, most ready disciple of the new microbiology, McFadyean conducted the first test of Koch's tuberculin in Great Britain and published the results under the title "Experiments with Tuberculinum on Cattle" in his *Journal* in 1891, firing the first shot in the veterinarians' war against bovine tuberculosis. Theobald Smith, professor of comparative pathology at Harvard University, differentiated between human and bovine strains of bacteria that cause tuberculosis in 1898.

In 1892 McFadyean was appointed the first professor of pathology and bacteriology and the first dean of the London school. Two years later he be-

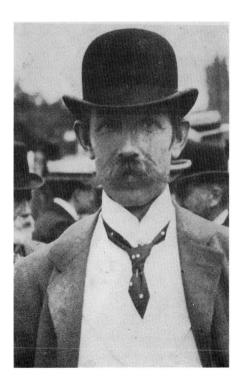

354. John McFadyean (1853-1941), professor of pathology and microbiology at the Royal Veterinary College, London, from 1892 and then its principal from 1894 to 1927. He is regarded as the founder of modern veterinary research and founded the *Journal of Comparative Pathology and Therapeutics.*

came the principal as well. At last the school was in good hands, governed by the most knowledgeable veterinarian in the land. From the day of his appointment the mood and fortunes of the school began to change for the better.

McFadyean did not allow his heavy responsibilities to weaken his zest for science and progress. He grasped the seminal work in Berlin of Löffler and Frosch, who in 1898 were the first to demonstrate that a filterable agent or "virus" was the cause of foot-and-mouth disease. He translated their classic paper and published a summary of it in his *Journal* in 1899. He immediately obtained bacterial filters and was given to examine a blood sample from southern Africa drawn from a horse that had died of the African horse sickness (AHS). He injected a sample of the blood into a horse, which died of the disease in eight days. He took blood and pericardial fluid from the dead animal, combined them, and filtered the concoction through his porcelain filters. He then injected the filtrate into another horse, which also died of AHS in eight days. This study was the second demonstration of a filterable agent that caused an acute disease of animals but was not visible under the microscope.

In recognition of his work on tuberculosis McFadyean was invited to present a paper in the plenary session of the International Tuberculosis Congress that was held in London in 1901. On day one of the congress Robert Koch spoke on combatting tuberculosis; on day two Brouardal, on public health aspects; and on day three McFadyean, on "Danger to Man from Tuberculous Cows." At that time in Great Britain it was estimated that thirty percent of the dairy cows carried infection with tuberculosis and that two percent shed the organism in the milk.

Lister chaired the presentation of Koch's paper. In it Koch expounded his view that far too much importance was placed on the possible hazard to humans of contacts with tuberculous animals. He insisted that the causative agent of human tuberculosis differed from that of bovine tuberculosis and could not infect cattle. He torpedoed the idea that there was a significant risk of the bovine organism spreading to humans via milk or milk products. Therefore he could see no point in taking precautionary measures against such a spread. The audience was startled because these statements were diametrically opposed to current thinking on the subject in Great Britain.

After humbly acknowledging Koch's unsurpassed contributions to understanding of the disease, McFadyean took up the challenge. He "must conclude," he said, that "the almost entire absence of any law dealing with tuberculous udder disease in cows is a scandal and a reproach to civilization." The conflicting views forced attempts to resolve a major medical and veterinary controversy forthwith because the public health was at stake and the Grim Reaper with his scythe was taking an ever expanding toll of human life as a result of the dread disease. In England a royal commission with McFadyean as a member was established within weeks of the fateful Congress to determine whether the human and bovine diseases were the same and whether they were communicable between the two species. Experiments were conducted over ten years, and McFadyean's views prevailed. He was knighted in 1905 for his service to veterinary science and agriculture and for his work on the royal commission on tuberculosis.

John McFadyean was the undisputed leader of the British branch of the veterinary profession for more than thirty years from the date of his appointment to the London school. He quite literally was the founder of effective veterinary research in Great Britain, although he had to accomplish the task on a shoestring budget at the London school. He chaired a committee to investigate contagious abortion in cattle, the first government committee to support veterinary research. A veterinary center was established in Middlesex, and other animal diseases were investigated. Veterinary research attained official recognition belatedly in 1911. A fine research laboratory was not established until 1925, when the Institute of Pathology was opened. McFadyean edited every issue of the *Journal of Comparative Pathology and Therapeutics* from its inauguration until its fiftieth year, 1957, an incredible achievement for such a busy man.

John McFadyean was president of the Royal College of Veterinary Surgeons (RCVS) from 1906 to 1909 and again in 1930, at the age of seventy-seven, because the eleventh International Veterinary Congress was to be held in London that year. Two years later, fifty-seven years after qualifying as a veterinarian, he became the first fellow of the RCVS by election. In his later life, just after retirement, he was angered when the first Agricultural Research Council was established without the inclusion of any veterinary surgeon. He wrote in 1931 to the *London Times* that "the public affront which has thus been put upon the veterinary profession will be deeply resented by all its members." Finally, in 1936, in response to a question in the House of Commons, it was stated that the Council was to be strengthened by the addition of John Smith, the former director of animal health in Northern Rhodesia.

BANG'S DISEASE

Brucellosis of goats was found to cause a serious human disease known as Malta fever. In 1887 David Bruce, a military physician, isolated the causative agent, later named *Brucella melitensis,* from the spleens of infected patients who had died. In 1905 goats obtained on Malta were shipped to the United States. Crew members who drank the raw goat's milk during the voyage developed typical cases of Malta fever. The U.S. Bureau of Animal Industry investigators John R. Mohler and George H. Hart found that the quarantined goats were infected with *B. melitensis.* The goats and their progeny were destroyed. Much later (in 1922) Zammit showed that fifty percent of goats on Malta at that time were infected and that ten percent shed live *Brucella* organisms in their milk. The caprine organism is more infective for humans than is its bovine relative, *Brucella abortus,* although the latter also causes the serious zoonotic disease of undulant fever or brucellosis.

Bernhard Laurits Frederik Bang (1848-1932), of Sjaelland, Denmark, was a veterinarian and microbiologist who made his name in veterinary medicine, microbiology, and public health. At thirty years of age he was appointed to the faculty of the Royal Veterinary and Agricultural College of Copenhagen. He visited the leading veterinary schools in Germany and Austria and became an outstanding clinical teacher who worked relentlessly in his laboratory as well. A special chair in pathological anatomy was created for him in 1887. He focused on two of the greatest zoonotic diseases of cattle, tuberculosis and brucellosis. He showed that calves born of cows infected with tuberculosis could be raised to be healthy if separated from their dams at birth and raised in an environment free of the disease. His work established the effectiveness of tuberculin testing of cattle for early diagnosis, which allowed control of the disease by segregation or slaughter of infected animals. Extraordinary progress was made, first in Scandinavia, where the incidence of tuberculosis in cattle had been high, and then in other developed countries, leading to the virtual eradication of the disease.

Bang is best known for his work on the disease that became known as Bang's disease, contagious bovine abortion, or brucellosis. Bang and Stribolt isolated the causative agent, later called *Brucella abortus,* in 1896 and demonstrated that the disease was contagious. They bought a seven-months-pregnant cow showing prodromal signs of abortion. They characterized the lesions in the placenta, fetus, and uterus in detail, saw the Gram-negative organism in stained smears of these tissues, and established techniques for culturing it. They showed the infectivity of the organism for female bovines, ovines, caprines, and equines but were unaware of its human pathogenicity until Alice Evans of the U.S. Bureau of Animal Industry showed it to have a close serological relationship with Bruce's Malta fever organism.

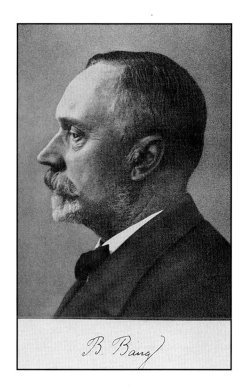

355. Bernhard Bang (1848-1932), who discovered bovine brucellosis or Bang's disease, also known as contagious abortion, enzootic abortion, and slinking of calves. He also played a major role in the eradication of bovine tuberculosis. *(From Adsersen, 1936.)*

Undoubtedly Bang must be remembered as one of the most effective and influential veterinary scientists. By initiating steps to eradicate bovine tuberculosis and making possible the more recent drive to stamp out undulant fever, Bang put the fine veterinary school at Copenhagen at the forefront of veterinary progress and allowed it to realize its potential for contributing in a major way to human safety.

The U.S. Bureau of Animal Industry continued Bang's pioneering work and developed an applied program with the intent of eradication of contagious abortion in cattle. When infection entered a New England herd, the initial abortion storm could affect all pregnant animals within a two-year period, after which it would continue to recur with a lower morbidity rate. In 1911 the veterinary scientists at the U.S. Bureau of Animal Industry isolated the causative organism from bovine milk and from tonsils surgically removed from children with tonsillitis.

When Alice Evans joined the Bureau of Animal Industry in 1915, she started her work on brucellosis by comparing it to Malta fever, which was prevalent on American Indian reservations in the Southwest as a result of consumption of unpasteurized goat's milk that contained Bruce's organism, *B. melitensis.* She established the close correlation between the two *Brucella* organisms, *B. abortus* and *B. melitensis.* In 1914 the Bureau veterinarians had isolated the former organism from aborted fetuses of infected sows. Soon the human disease was found in workers in hog-slaughtering plants. The number of cases detected in humans increased rapidly to more than four thousand in 1938. Undulant fever recurred in infected individuals. Wesley Spink of the University of Minnesota Medical School studied the disease in abattoir workers and showed how precautions could be taken to control its incidence.

John Buck, a veterinary bacteriologist with the Bureau of Animal Industry, developed a live culture of the organism with reduced virulence from a strain isolated from a Jersey cow in 1923, the nineteenth strain studied. In a manner reminiscent of the events leading to the development of Pasteur's vaccine for fowl cholera, "Strain 19" became the approved vaccine strain after it had sat forgotten for two years on Buck's desk at room temperature. On testing in calves it proved to be attenuated enough to protect calves against infection but did not spread between calves. Thus, with a little help from serendipity, Strain 19 was resurrected to become the standard vaccine strain used worldwide. A live culture of the Strain 19 organism was sent to England in 1941, and the strain has never reverted to a more virulent form.

Agglutination tests designed to identify reactors were refined and used to identify infected animals. At the beginning of the cooperative state and federal eradication program in 1934, fourteen percent of the national cattle herd in the United States were reactors. In the next fifty years the reactors were reduced to less than one percent by a policy that included calfhood vaccination, compulsory herd testing and slaughter of reactors, and the incentive of certification. One problem with vaccination with Strain 19 was that it caused protected animals to give a positive reading on the agglutination test. Veterinarians who work with dairy cattle herds have always been a group at high risk for contracting the disease in areas where it is endemic. Many states are entirely free of the disease, but the risk of its reentry persists because of interstate movement and marketing of livestock.

THE FILTERABLE VIRUSES: DEADLY ULTRAMICROSCOPIC PATHOGENS

The ancient term *virus* stems from old Latin usage implying "poison" or "venom." In AD 50 Cornelius Aulus Celsus used it as follows: "Especially if the dog is rabid, the virus should be drawn out with a cupping glass." In thirteenth-century Bologna Soliceto and his pupil Lanfranc in a work on surgery described virus as a poison that comes from the crusts of certain diseases. English usage of the word in the sixteenth and seventeenth centuries referred to the venom of the patient smitten with the plague, the pestilence, or the great plague. By the eighteenth and nineteenth centuries *virus* was used to name any substance that transmitted an infectious disease. Jenner used the terms *cowpox virus* and *variolus virus* for his vaccine and for the fluid that transmitted the disease, respectively.

Despite the success of pathogenic bacteriology, before the end of the nineteenth century it became apparent that some of the great diseases did not fit the model for bacterial origin. In these cases no acceptable causative microbe could be found or implicated, despite convincing evidence of contagion. It was time for a new spirit and new hypotheses. The new direction came with the help of a tool developed in 1884 by Charles Chamberland, one of Pasteur's ablest co-workers—the cylindrical unglazed porcelain filter, which did not allow bacteria to pass through its pores. Chamberland and Emile Roux (1853-1933) developed the filter initially to fit on a water tap in an effort to produce bacteria-free water. Chamberland published a paper called *A Filter Permitting To Obtain Physiologically Pure Water* in 1884. Later the bacterial filter was called a Berkefeld filter.

Dmitri Ivanowski of Russia (1892) used Chamberland's filter to show that sap from plants affected with tobacco mosaic disease was still infective after filtration. He suspected that a toxin was the cause. In 1898 came the seminal discovery, made by two members of the faculty at the Berlin school, Koch's

356. Nineteenth century wood engraving showing Dr. Steven C. Martin taking cowpox virus on ivory points from a heifer at the Vaccine Farm in Brookline, Massachusetts. *(National Library of Medicine, Bethesda, Maryland.)*

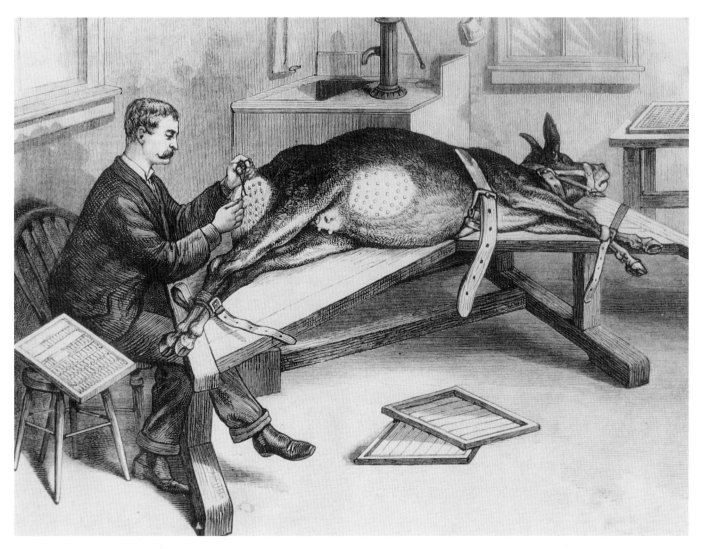

associate Friedrich Löffler and one of his former assistants, Paul Frosch, professor of bacteriology. They subjected the contents of fresh vesicles obtained from the mouths and udders of animals affected with foot-and-mouth disease to filtration through a type of Chamberland's device. The filtrates were shown to be completely free of bacteria, yet they remained infective and produced typical foot-and-mouth disease in cattle three days after injection. The disease in these animals was transmitted to their stallmates by contact, so the possibility that a filterable toxin caused the syndrome was ruled out. These authors' work had been sponsored by a commission set up to investigate the foot-and-mouth disease. The disease can have relatively low mortality rates but high rates of morbidity leading to devastating losses in productivity. Löffler's many contributions to the isolation of causative agents of animal disease are simply phenomenal.

The new concept of submicroscopic "filterable" pathogens triggered a wave of discoveries of agents having similar properties. Sanarelli reported the virus causative of a rabbit plague, myxomatosis, in 1898. As stated earlier, McFadyean demonstrated that a filterable agent caused African horse sickness in 1900. In 1901 Walter Reed's team showed that yellow fever was due to a filterable virus and then demonstrated that the virus was spread by a mosquito vector. In the same year Lode and Gruber found at Innsbruck that fowl plague was caused by a filterable pathogen. The next year Amedee Borrel (1867-1936) at the Pasteur Institute filtered the sheep pox agent. In the same year, Nicolle and his Turkish colleague Adil-Bey showed that the agent of the great cattle plague (rinderpest) was filterable. Thus an avalanche of evidence indicated that specific life-forms, which could not be visualized by the light microscope and passed through filters that retained bacteria, were the pathogens of many of the great epidemic diseases that had for so long defied science. Nonetheless, since these newly identified agents were not culturable by bacteriological methods, their presence was based on circumstantial evidence and their nature remained unknown.

Not all the filterable agents were, in fact, viruses. One of the rampant epidemic diseases was contagious bovine pleuropneumonia (CBPP). The French veterinarians Emile Roux and Edmond Isidor Nocard (1850-1903) showed that the infectious agent was filterable in 1898. They also devised ways to culture it, although it was many years before it could be dependably grown in pure culture. Nevertheless, the organism was the first of a series of pathogens to be discovered, and the genus of these pleuropneumonia-like organisms was named *Mycoplasma*.

New concepts and technologies had to be developed so that the field of virology could advance beyond the knowledge that a whole range of invisible pirates existed and could attack cells; there were no clues to their identity. Martinus Willem Beijerinck (1851-1931) worked in Delft, Holland, as a microbiologist. In 1888 he isolated *Rhizobium leguminarum,* the root nodule bacterium that fixes free nitrogen into a form that can be used by plants. After becoming a professor at the Delft Polytechnical School, he embarked on his great work on tobacco mosaic virus. He was certain that the virus could multiply, but his ideas of a living, reproducing, noncellular material proved difficult for many scientists to accept and were unthinkable to some.

McFadyean suggested that viruses might be obligate parasites of living cells restricted in their reproduction to the body of the host (1908). Steps along the path to understanding included the discovery of inclusion bodies, microscopically visible structures in cells of animals infected with viral diseases. In 1903 Negri reported the presence of Negri bodies in brain cells of animals with rabies. In the same year, Remlinger and Riffat-Bey filtered the rabies virus. In 1909 Benjamin Lipschütz, an Austrian dermatologist, classified the forty-one known filterable viruses by whether they had inclusion bodies (sixteen of them did). The nature of these bodies was not known until 1929, when Woodruff and Goodpasture proved that fowl pox inclusion bodies are bags of elementary bodies, which are the infective filterable virus. This team cultured fowl pox virus in the chicken embryo in 1931, thereby contributing a versatile new technique.

In 1908 in Copenhagen Ellerman and Bang showed that avian leukemia could be spread by cell-free filtrates. In 1911 Peyton Rous at the Rockefeller Institute in New York showed that chicken sarcoma could also be spread by filtrates. These findings sparked a keen interest in the possibility of a viral origin of human cancers and raised new questions about what viruses are and how they act.

At London University's Brown Institution in 1915 Frederick William Twort opened a major new branch of research in virology with his report of a filterable agent that caused lysis of bacteria and was transmissible to future generations, that is, a viral disease of bacteria. This idea was seized upon by a French-Canadian, Felix d'Herelle, who was studying *Shigella* organisms at the Pasteur Institute in Paris in 1917. He found a filterable lytic factor that appeared to be an obligate parasite of the bacillus and christened it a "bacteriophage" ("bacteria eater"), noting that it was a virus.

Edna Steinhardt, Israeli, and Lambert hit upon the idea of growing the virus parasites outside the body in cell cultures. In 1913 they succeeded in growing the vaccinia virus in tissue cultures of guinea pig or rabbit cornea cells. In the same year Levaditi grew polio virus on spinal ganglion cells. There were many pitfalls in the technique, however, particularly bacterial contamination. This problem was not overcome until the arrival of broad-spectrum antibiotics.

Viruses were rendered "visible" (imageable) by the electron microscope. In 1939 Kansche, among others, obtained the first pictures—of the tobacco mosaic virus. In 1930 at Harvard University Max Theiler showed the value of mouse inoculation in the study of virus diseases. New diagnostic tests were developed, and the last fifty years have witnessed an enormous expansion in information about specific viruses and the diseases they cause. The fundamental questions about the nature of the viral diseases, however, have become answerable only since Watson and Crick's revelation of the molecular biology of the gene.

357. Blackleg caused widespread losses of young cattle on the western ranges after 1890. This postcard recorded a typical horrifying scene encountered by farmers or cowboys on their rounds. A Kansas State University veterinary graduate of 1912, O.M. Franklin (died 1973) developed an effective blackleg vaccine after isolating the infectious agent, *Clostridium chauvoei*, in pure culture and making an aggressin by filtering the liquid from infected tissues; he called the product "Germ Free." In 1916, he established his Kansas Blackleg Serum Company in Wichita, and in 1918, another in Amarillo, Texas. He went on to develop a blackleg bacterin in 1923 from the organism killed with formaldehyde to avoid the step of deliberately infecting calves. Later he developed bacterins against other clostridial diseases and renamed his company the Franklin Serum Company, with headquarters in Denver, Colorado. *(Postcard, C. Trenton Boyd Collection.)*

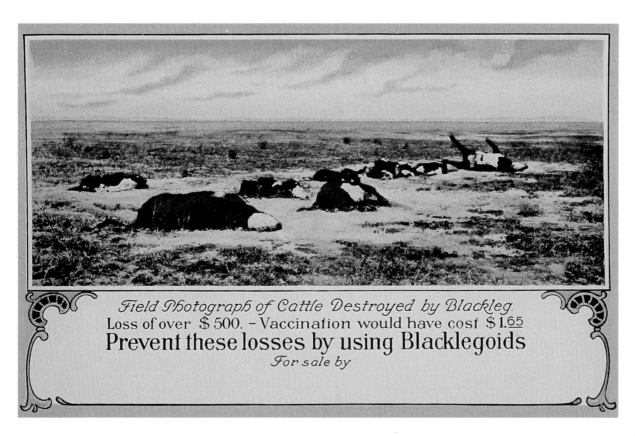

Field Photograph of Cattle Destroyed by Blackleg.
Loss of over $ 500. – Vaccination would have cost $ 1.65
Prevent these losses by using Blacklegoids
For sale by

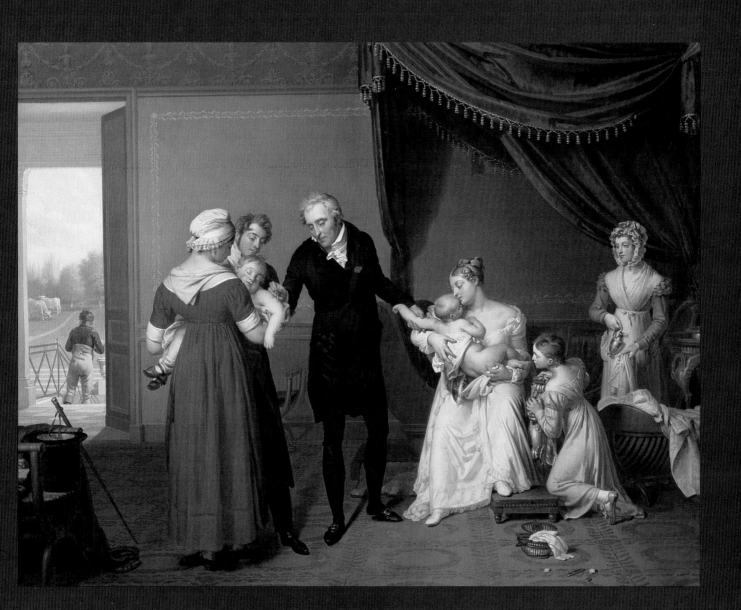

CHAPTER 23

Boosting the Host's Defenses
The Development of Immunological Products

During the eighteenth century five reigning monarchs of Europe died of smallpox. Edward Jenner in 1796 took fluid from a cowpox vesicle on the hand of Sarah Nelmes, a dairymaid, and inoculated it to two sites on eight-year-old James Phipps's arms. The child developed cowpox lesions. Two months later Jenner inoculated him with material obtained from a person with smallpox, with no disease resulting.

Ali Maow Maalin, a cook in Merka, Somalia, contracted the last reported case of smallpox in 1977. Thus in 181 years one of the greatest scourges of humankind was eliminated from the planet, as far as can be determined. This accomplishment has been a vindication of many heroic efforts to achieve safe, durable immunoprophylaxis of epidemic diseases of animals and humans by exposing them to either killed or attenuated live immunogens. Passive immunization using antisera to pathogens prepared in other organisms is still used in prevention or treatment of some infectious diseases of bacterial or viral origin. The special roles of placental and lactational transfer of immunoglobulins in protecting the newborn have become well understood. The veterinary profession and distinguished scientists working at or collaborating with veterinary schools and research institutes have played major roles in many of these achievements. The animals that have been studied in these experiments have saved untold millions of lives.

ASIAN TRAILBLAZING WITH SMALLPOX EXPOSURE

A Chinese medical contribution—surely one of the oldest attempts to protect people against epidemic and contagious diseases—was the deliberate exposure to smallpox. Having recognized that recovered survivors of smallpox infection seemed to be completely resistant to another infection during a subsequent outbreak, the Chinese exploited this idea. They experimented in infants with dermal scratches into which were rubbed materials from the scabs of smallpox patients. Not all survived, but those who did had gained lifelong immunity. The resulting syndrome was said to be less severe if the material for the "variolation" was taken from individuals with mild cases of the disease. Since the mortality rate for the disease was about twenty percent, the rate of variolees—about one percent—appeared to be a very good risk.

Knowledge of the procedure spread gradually westward across Asia and reached Turkey, where the British ambassador's wife, Lady Mary Montagu, was so impressed that she recommended the method to friends in England (1716-1718) and campaigned to have it adopted in her homeland. The Turkish model seems to have involved introduction of the material into veins. The issue was fiercely debated in medical and political circles in England. The Chinese also had an alternative technique of blowing the pox material into the nose through a tube.

358. *Facing page,* Jenner's discovery in 1796 that inoculation with cowpox could impart immunity to the dreaded smallpox led to vaccination clinics for infants like the one depicted in this nineteenth-century painting by Constant Desbordes, which shows Dr. Alibert at work. *(Jean-Loup Charmet/Science Photo Library.)*

407

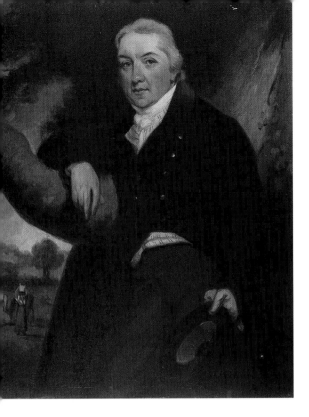

In the mid-eighteenth century, during the rinderpest epidemic that ravaged the cattle of the European continent, a similar technique was tried: a seton soaked in material obtained from an animal with the disease was inserted into the brisket via incisions. The method appears to have been less successful than human variolation.

A SAFE ALTERNATIVE: JENNER'S COWPOX VACCINE

Edward Jenner was one of the pupils of John Hunter, the famous London surgeon and naturalist and forerunner of the experimental approach to medical science. Hunter had a unique impact on the establishment of veterinary medicine as a profession in England, working for the establishment of the London veterinary school, teaching its initial class of students, and training Astley Cooper, who became the leading London surgeon after Hunter's death, as well as the chairman of the veterinary school's first governing body.

Jenner lived with the Hunters for some time and acquired the zealous experimental spirit of his mentor. Overhearing a dairymaid's comment to Hunter that she could not "take the smallpox" because she had had the cowpox, he later asked his mentor what he thought of this gem of rural folklore. Typically, Hunter's response was, "Why think? Why not try the experiment?" The outcome is an early example of an occupational hazard (that is, a mild disease of milkers) being turned to good use by the prepared mind of an investigator.

There is a strange complexity to the story about the milkers' disease that even today is not fully resolved. The pure cowpox vaccines of recent decades appear to have differed from the original strain used in Jenner's vaccine. Jenner conducted his first rigorous test of his cowpox theory in a human subject in 1796. His test involved challenging the human volunteer with virulent smallpox material, not quite as desperate a measure as it sounds because using deliberate infection with the disease was commonly practiced. Jenner published his work in 1798. He included the proposition that a disease of horses known as "grease" may have been the source of the original infection, which was spread by farriers who treated affected horses, then milked cows that later developed cowpox. The dairymaids then caught the disease from the cows. Implicit in Jenner's proposition was the idea that the origin of the disease lay in a form of horsepox that infected the teats of cows and then the hands of milkers. Thus there may have been more than one type of cowpox. In any event, Jenner's method accomplished the goal of protection against the dreaded plague without the risk of acquiring the disease, and "vaccination" replaced "variolation." His name became revered worldwide, except at home, where he came under attack and dire predictions were made about the likely consequences of introducing the "venom of a beastly disease" into children.

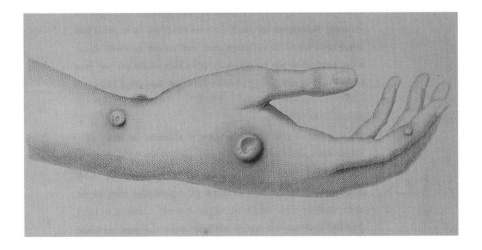

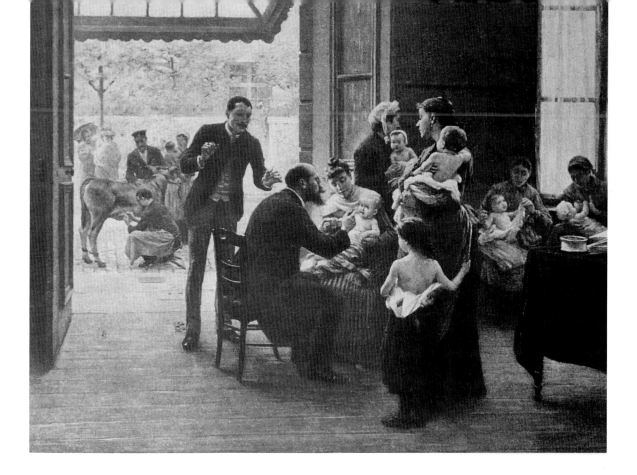

Jean-Baptiste Auguste Chauveau (1827-1917), the son of a farrier, was admitted to Alfort in 1844. He joined the faculty at Lyon after qualifying as a veterinarian. He became one of the greatest scholars and leaders to endow the profession intellectually. His early academic career was in anatomy and physiology; in those fields he was an innovative author. He became interested in microbiology, immunology, and comparative pathology. He demonstrated that tuberculosis was infectious and organized an experiment on relationships between variola and vaccinia. He wrote a thesis for a doctorate of medicine degree on vaccinia and the possible origin of the strain of the Jenner cowpox vaccine. A great experimentalist, Chauveau developed new methods to separate the leukocytes and to culture delicate bacteria and assisted Toussaint in devising ways to attenuate the anthrax organism for safe vaccine production.

361. *Vaccination Gratitude à Paris,* photogravure (1890). After an attendant (visible beyond the doorway) extracted virus from the teats of a cow infected with cowpox, the doctor vaccinated the children brought by their mothers. *(National Library of Medicine, Bethesda, Maryland.)*

PASTEUR'S DISCOVERY OF ATTENUATION AND THE PRODUCTION OF VACCINE STRAINS

There was to be a long wait before Jenner's brilliant (but costly to his personal prestige) idea was exploited effectively in work with other diseases. Jenner in 1798 had published his results and views in a small (seventy-five–page) book with the long title *An Inquiry into the Causes and Effects of the Varolae Vaccinae, a Disease Discovered in Some of the Western Counties of England, Particularly Gloucestershire, and Known by the Name of "The Cow Pox."* The next opportunity seized also had a veterinary flavor: it was Pasteur's development of a vaccine against fowl cholera, a bacterial disease of chickens, in 1879. Pasteur adopted the English term "vaccination," derived from *vacca,* the Latin word for "cow," in recognition of Jenner's pioneering work with cowpox.

Pasteur's primary goal was to study anthrax of sheep and cattle, but rather than go after anthrax directly, Pasteur elected first to study fowl cholera, a contagious disease of chickens that causes them to sicken, become weak, fall asleep, and die. First, he isolated a causative organism. Then he showed that it was lethal for the rabbit but innocuous for the guinea pig. Upon returning to the laboratory from summer vacation in 1879, he found that most of his fowl cholera cultures had died out. The surviving ones failed to induce the

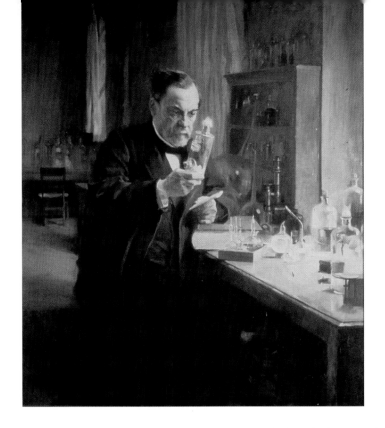

362. Louis Pasteur's work on stereo-chemistry and polarization of light led him to the germ theory of contagious diseases. As a result of his studies of microbes and Jenner's achievements with cowpox, Pasteur developed attenuated live vaccines for anthrax and rabies. *(Institut Pasteur, Paris.)*

disease. Subsequently, perhaps intuitively, he injected the chickens with fresh cultures. Although the fresh cultures were lethal in untreated birds, those previously inoculated with old cultures turned out to be resistant and did not sicken. He then showed that the phenomenon of attenuation required exposure of cultures to air over a long period of incubation at 37° Celcius.

Having established that such attenuation could render a culture effective and safe as a vaccination tool, Pasteur attempted to apply the same principle to anthrax in 1881. The successful outcome is described in Chapter 22. The vaccination of farm livestock was born, and there was a heavy demand for vaccine among farmers and veterinarians. The vaccine, however, was difficult to prepare, and problems were encountered in standardizing the technique. Therefore it could not be readily applied safely in distant regions with different environments.

Pasteur's selection of fowl cholera—the causative organism's genus, *Pasteurella,* was named in his honor—to develop the strategy of attenuation of virulence by repeated subculturing in vitro and by aging the cultures, contained an element of serendipity. He had no clear understanding of the processes of host resistance to infectious disease, which became known as "immunity" (from the Latin word for "exemption"). He had the example, however, of Jenner's intuitive selection of cowpox vaccinia matter to immunize against smallpox about eighty years earlier. Not only did Pasteur show the world a new method for establishing resistance to infection, but also he showed that the syndrome it produced (deep sleep) could be mimicked by injection of an extract passed through a filter that retained bacteria. He interpreted this result as evidence that the organism's detrimental effects were due to the elaboration of a toxin, and in the following year, 1882, he had a vaccine for swine erysipelas.

PASTEUR'S DEVELOPMENT OF SEQUENTIAL VACCINATION AGAINST RABIES

A source of Pasteur's motivation to address the problem of rabies was an emotional childhood experience: he had witnessed a smith sear the wounds of a person who had been bitten by a rabid wolf with an iron spike heated in the forge to the highest attainable temperature. Pasteur decided to seek a vaccine to protect those who had been bitten by a rabid animal. Understanding of the

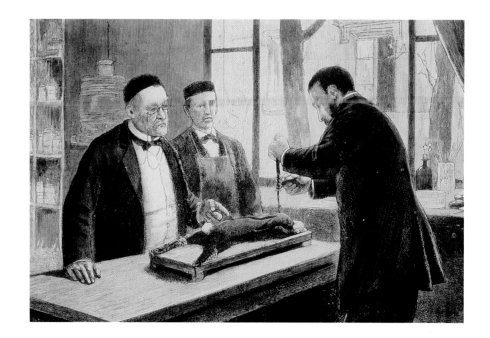

363. After Galtier had shown that the canine rabies virus could be transmitted to rabbits, Pasteur adopted the rabbit as a model to study the disease. He found that virulence of the agent could be attenuated after twenty-five passages through rabbits. Here he is watching as the spinal cord is removed for vaccine preparation. (National Library of Medicine, Bethesda, Maryland/ Science Photo Library.)

disease was increasing. It was known that if a dog devoured the carcass of another that had been rabid, it, too, would succumb. Berndt in 1822 had shown that the saliva was infectious. Victor Galtier (1846-1908), a professor of pathology at the Lyon veterinary school, made the invaluable finding that the disease could be transferred to rabbits by inoculating them with saliva obtained from a rabid dog. Instead of becoming a furious, snapping, infectious menace, as was the case in an infected dog, the rabbit became paralyzed. The rabbit also had the great advantage of having a shorter incubation period for the disease than the dog had.

Although much of Galtier's work was done earlier, he did not publish his results until 1881. Pasteur was quick to recognize the value of the new animal model. His colleague Roux (1853-1933) proposed the idea of intracerebral inoculation with a suspension of infected brain tissue to obtain a more reproducible condition and attempt attenuation by passage. At that time no one had seen the microbe responsible for the disease, nor had it been possible to culture it. It is thought that Pasteur again was able to draw upon folklore for an idea. Shepherds had observed that drying of the matter of sheep pox scabs led to attenuation. Pasteur hit upon the idea that drying the nerve tissue might lead to attenuation of the unseen organism, so his assistants harvested the spinal cords of infected animals and dried them for different periods of time. He showed that some of these preparations were effective as vaccines against rabies in dogs.

Pasteur was under great pressure to transfer his work with animals to humans. In 1885 he began a course of "therapy" on nine-year-old Joseph Meister, who had been mauled by a rabid dog. Pasteur performed a long, unpleasant series of injections using spinal cord tissue that was progressively less attenuated, that is, dried for shorter periods. A second success came a few months later. Jupille, a shepherd lad from the Jura, had been bitten severely by a rabid dog as he was protecting his comrades. Meister and Jupille's survival ensured Pasteur's lasting fame. He became wealthy enough to establish a private laboratory in Paris, the Pasteur Institute, which he directed until his death in 1895. It continues today as a great research center, and a statue of Meister stands on the grounds. Pasteur's home is preserved on the site as a museum. He left a legacy of dedication to the advancement of veterinary and human medicine through his superb generalship in the war against microbes. His skills saved the wine, beer, silk, dairy, and sheep industries of France from disaster, along with many millions of animal and human lives. The impact of his achievements was rapid and global. Many of his colleagues attained distinction in research, and a commercial vaccine industry was born. Perhaps Pasteur's greatest contribution was the recruitment and stimulation of so many great minds to the service of biomedical science.

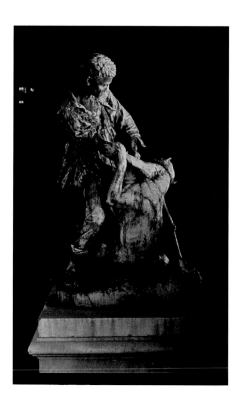

364. The memorial statue outside the Pasteur Institute in Paris is of Joseph Meister, an Alsatian shepherd boy who was savagely mauled by a rabid dog in 1885. He received treatment from Pasteur with the series of injections of attenuated vaccine of increasing strength and survived. (Institut Pasteur, Paris.)

365. As Pasteur watches, a doctor injects the attenuated rabies vaccine into the abdominal muscles of a boy bitten by a rabid dog. *(National Library of Medicine, Bethesda, Maryland.)*

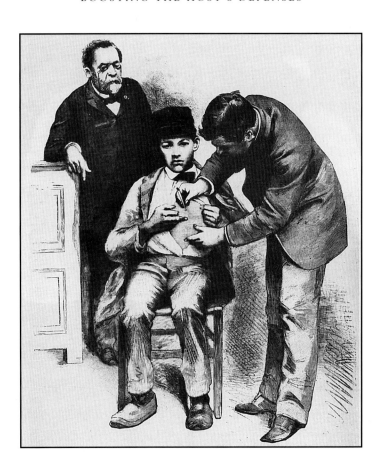

METCHNIKOFF'S DISCOVERY OF THE PHAGOCYTES AND CELLULAR DEFENSE

Elie Metchnikoff (1845-1916), born and raised near Kharkov, Russia, was a child prodigy who started his scientific career in botany and became a great independent thinker. He worked in Germany and switched his interest to comparative embryology of marine organisms and evolutionary biology, becoming a convinced Darwinian. His genius found only frustration in Russia at the universities of Kharkov, Odessa, and St. Petersburg. His devoted first wife died of consumption, and he later remarried. When he moved to Messina in 1882 in the hope of finding the zoological material he needed for his research, his fortunes changed. He demonstrated the phenomenon of motile phagocytic defense cells in the transparent larvae of a starfish after inserting foreign bodies under their skins. He framed the hypothesis that this phenomenon was a general inflammatory defense response of animals against invading organisms. In seeking a more suitable model of infectious disease, he found a fungal disease of the *Daphnia* (water flea) species that fit the bill perfectly and made classic studies of the infecting organisms. He was recalled to Odessa to direct a new bacteriological institute intended to follow the tenets of Pasteur and to prepare vaccines. Ill-suited by temperament to the administrative role of following recipes, he left in 1888. The first product of the Odessa laboratory, an anthrax vaccine, was a disaster, killing thousands of sheep in a field test.

Pasteur invited Metchnikoff to join his laboratory at the Pasteur Institute, and Metchnikoff accepted. There he devoted his energies to studies that led to the elaboration of his theory of cellular immunity as opposed to humoral (antibody) immunity. Although his ideas were long eclipsed by the dramatic progress in humoral immunity made by Paul Ehrlich, Emil von Behring, Shibasaburo Kitasato, and many others, his views were to be vindicated and gained new life in the unraveling of the important roles that cells play in host resistance in the second half of the twentieth century. He shared the Nobel Prize for Medicine with Ehrlich in 1908.

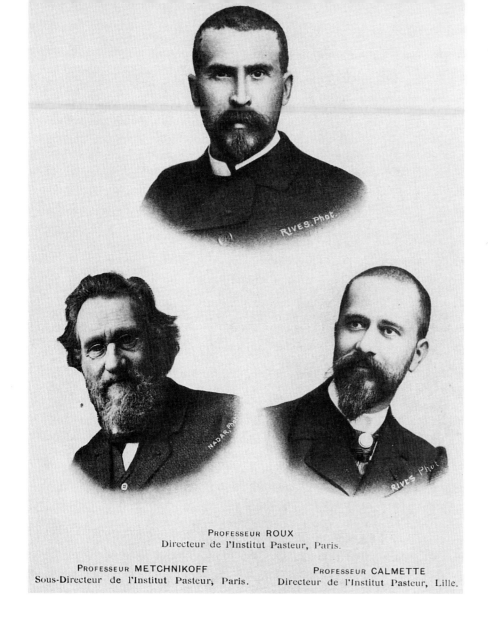

PROFESSEUR ROUX
Directeur de l'Institut Pasteur, Paris.

PROFESSEUR METCHNIKOFF
Sous-Directeur de l'Institut Pasteur, Paris.

PROFESSEUR CALMETTE
Directeur de l'Institut Pasteur, Lille.

366. Elie Metchnikoff (1845-1916), the brilliant Russian invertebrate zoologist, was a disciple of Darwin and the first to grasp the evolutionary significance of cellular immunity. He described the roles of the macrophage and the polymorphonuclear neutrophil as mobile defense forces within the body that combat invading microbes by amoebically engulfing them and imparting resistance to future challenges. Metchnikoff, along with Roux and Calmette, had an enormous influence on the early evolution of immunology. *(National Library of Medicine, Bethesda, Maryland.)*

George Bernard Shaw, in the "Preface on Doctors" to his play "The Doctor's Dilemma," noted the achievement of Almroth Wright: Sir Almroth Wright, following up one of Metchnikoff's most suggestive biological romances, discovered that the white corpuscles or phagocytes, which attack and devour disease germs for us, do their work only when we butter the disease germs appetizingly for them with a natural sauce which Sir Almroth named opsonin.

Almroth Wright (1861-1947) was the great follower of Metchnikoff who showed that there were substances in the body fluids that attached to invading microbes and rendered them more sensitive to phagocytosis by leukocytes. Having an Irish father (a roving clergyman) and a Swedish mother, yet born in Yorkshire, Almroth was much traveled in his youth and attended Trinity College in Dublin, where he studied literature and languages, then medicine. Paralleling the physiologist Claude Bernard, he began his intellectual journey with a trip through "the enchanted streams of literature." This background stood him in good stead because he developed an exceptional ability to express himself. He toured prestigious laboratories in Germany, visiting Cohnheim, Weigert, Ludwig, and von Recklinghausen. Later he spent two years in Australia.

Appointed professor of pathology at the army medical school at Netley, where Bruce had discovered the agent of Malta fever (brucellosis of goats), Wright developed the agglutination test for diagnosis and attempted to develop a vaccine for this unpleasant disease. He foolhardily tested a modified living organism on himself but succeeded only in giving himself the disease. He put the experience to good use, however, by applying rigorous quantitative testing to any subsequent vaccine developments, both of the organism and of the antibody response it induced, and related the latter to the dosage of the organism. He introduced the technique of using capillary tubes in microserology. He applied the new methods and standards in making a typhoid vaccine at about the same time that Pfeiffer and Kolle made theirs, in 1897.

In 1902 Wright moved to St. Mary's Hospital in London with his assistant Stewart Douglas, where they focused on the blood-borne cellular immunity of Metchnikoff's phagocytosis, seeking a bridge between it and the humoral (antibody-based) immunity that had overshadowed it since 1890, when von Behring and Kitasato had shown that immunity to diphtheria and tetanus is due to antibodies against their toxins. Using sodium citrate as an anticoagulant, Wright separated the white blood cells by centrifugation and made stained smears of them. When the serum was inactivated by heating above 60° Celcius for ten minutes before adding the bacteria and the leukocytes, the phagocytosis of the organisms was reduced by almost ninety percent. He concluded that the serum contained substances that modified the bacteria, rendering them much more susceptible as prey to the phagocytes. Wright christened these substances "opsonins" (from the Latin *opsono,* "I prepare victuals for") and showed that vaccination often enhanced opsonic activity. He insisted that the leukocyte is the best antiseptic and that it must not be compromised by pouring potent disinfectants into wounds. He also demonstrated that antiphagocytic substances were a factor in virulence of pathogenic organisms.

THE SEARCH FOR VACCINES AGAINST SWINE PLAGUES

Pasteur's announcement in 1882 of his team's development of a vaccine against *rouget* or *mal rouge* (swine erysipelas) caused a great stir among those in the swine industry and also among veterinarians. A French veterinarian in Bollene, Achille Maucuer, had asked Pasteur to work on the disease in 1877, after the disease had wreaked heavy losses in the swine industry for a decade. It was 1881 before Pasteur could spare Louis Thuillier, one of his assistants, to study the field disease and collect material. The following year the causative germ (a bacterium) was isolated and sent to Pasteur. It was found that the isolate killed rabbits and chickens. Passaging it in pigeons increased the virulence for swine, but when it was passaged in rabbits, the opposite effect was noted: the organism became harmless to swine after a few passages. By first being injected with this harmless strain, then being inoculated at intervals with progressively more virulent cultures, pigs could safely be rendered immune. Thuillier became a casualty of science; he died of cholera while on a mission to Egypt to seek the causative agent of that human plague.

VON BEHRING'S DISCOVERY OF ANTIBODIES

Emil von Behring (1854-1917) was born in West Prussia; like Koch, he was one of thirteen children. He attended the army medical school in Berlin, the high-quality Friedrich Wilhelm Institute, graduating in 1878, two years after Koch's publication on anthrax. In 1889 von Behring was assigned to Koch's laboratory and moved with the master to his new Institute of Infectious Diseases in 1891. Von Behring probed deeply into current views of cellular and humoral facets of immunity. Working with Wernicke, an army colleague, he proposed that an antidiphtheria serum be developed for humans, after experimenting successfully with guinea pigs and rabbits. Then he learned that the toxin was more important for immunity than was the organism. Treating the toxin with iodine trichloride for a few days detoxified it, although it remained immunogenic for sheep. The injected sheep would resist large doses of untreated toxin. Also, their blood had a therapeutic effect. After a great deal of careful experimentation, suitable antitoxic sera were prepared for human use.

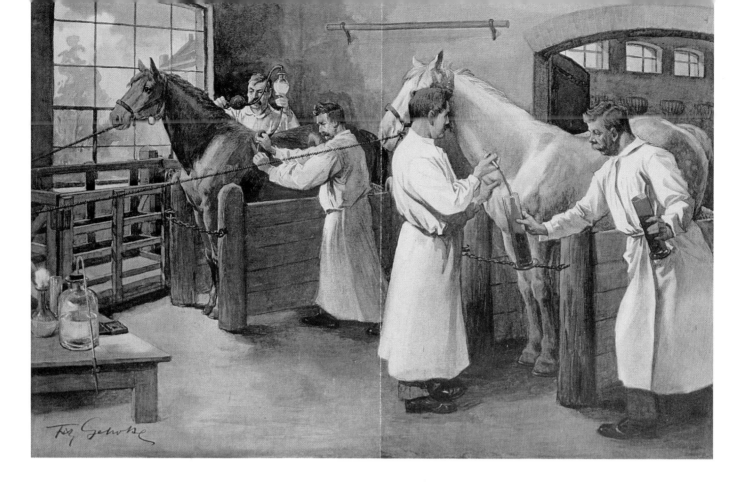

Today it is difficult to appreciate the ancient dread of diphtheria infection and the horror of the disease itself. As long ago as the second century AD, Aretaios of Cappadocia in *On the Causes and Symptoms of Acute Diseases,* under the name "Syrian Ulcer," described the progressive development of a tough diphtheritic membrane over the tonsils and soft palate and into the larynx and trachea. The symptoms included a raging thirst but an inability to drink because of the pain, nausea, and the tendency for the fluid to return via the nose. The unendurable distress made the patient's situation intolerable in any position. The soft palate became paralyzed, and the patient gradually suffocated, often with cardiopulmonary complications. Since the patient was unable to swallow or breathe, only tracheostomy was of any value in therapy.

Edwin Klebs in 1883 visualized the organism in the diphtheritic membrane, *Corynebacterium* ("club-shaped bacterium") *diphtheriae* ("of membrane"). The following year Löffler isolated and characterized the organism. Alexander John Yersin (1863-1943), of plague bacillus fame, and Pierre Paul Roux (1853-1933) made the important discovery that the pathology of the disease was attributable to toxins that the organism produced, which entered the tissues and blood vessels. Building on this finding, Emil von Behring and Kitasato demonstrated an antitoxic effect and prepared antitoxins to both diphtheria and tetanus in 1890. This immune serum could impart passive immunity to the disease when injected into a susceptible individual and also was helpful in therapy. This work was rewarded with a Nobel Prize. The veterinary profession was involved because hyperimmune serum was produced in large volumes, first in sheep, then in horses. Ultimately a toxoid was prepared by treatment with formaldehyde that could be administered safely to infants to impart long-lasting immunity. Behring worked on adjuvants to extend the effective period of sera and by 1913 developed a combined toxin-antitoxin preparation to produce active immunity. About the same time, however, Gustave Ramon developed the principle of using safe formol-toxoids to give active immunity. Lowenstein developed one against tetanus, and Glenny and Sudmersen, one against diphtheria.

Behring became professor of hygiene at the University of Marburg in 1895. He tried in 1895 to produce an antitoxin against the tubercle bacillus but failed, although he did develop a toxin from the organism. Then he attempted to develop attenuated strains that would impart immunity without

367. Emil von Behring (1854-1917) was an army physician who came to work with Koch in 1889, joining Shibasaburo Kitasato (1852-1931) from Japan. Kitasato had joined Koch in 1886 and developed the necessary anaerobic culture methods to isolate the tetanus bacillus. Together Behring and Kitasato showed that the serum of horses made immune by inoculation of tetanus bacteria contained antitoxins that neutralized tetanus toxin. The processes of inoculation and removal of blood containing antitoxins are illustrated. Behring received the first Nobel Prize in 1901 for his work on immunity to diphtheria and tetanus. *(Jean-Loup Charmet/Science Photo Library.)*

disease, proposing in 1903 to use immunized cows to generate sera that would protect humans against tuberculosis. Differing with Koch, Behring believed that cattle were the main source of human tuberculosis via contaminated meat and dairy products; he thought that infants absorbed the bacterium from the intestine, where it lodged in mesenteric lymph nodes, later moving to the lungs. He introduced the concept of "immune milk," the immunized milking cows transferring antibody via the milk. However, he was unable to prove that this method worked. Finally he tried to prepare a vaccine against selected components of the microbe, also without much success. During his career Behring was a consultant with Farbwerke Höchst for many years before branching out on his own in the biologics firm Behringwerke in 1904.

VETERINARY CONTRIBUTIONS TOWARD A VACCINE AGAINST TUBERCULOSIS

A vaccine against tuberculosis was finally achieved, but in France rather than Germany, thanks to the efforts of Albert Calmette (see also Chapter 21). An adventurous naval physician who trained in microbiology at the Pasteur Institute, he was selected by Pasteur to develop an institute to manufacture vaccines in Indochina. He turned his hand to developing a Jennerian vaccine against smallpox by using the water buffalo. He made Pasteur's rabies vaccine, preserving infected attenuated samples of brain tissue in glycerol. By 1891 his was a leading center for making antivenins for snake venoms, which were highly effective if used soon enough. He studied fermentations of rice and opium but became afflicted with a serious case of dysentery and returned to France, where he was asked to establish a new branch of the Pasteur Institute at Lille. He saw a need for a veterinary assistant, and in 1897 Nocard recommended his own assistant, Camille Guerin—sound advice, as it emerged.

Tuberculosis was the major killing disease of humans in northern France when Calmette and Guerin went to work on the problem. In 1924 they published a paper on vaccination of cattle against tuberculosis that described their remarkable study of the attenuation of a virulent bovine strain by repeated biweekly subculture onto potato cooked in bovine bile over a period of thirteen years. They showed that the agent had lost its virulence but retained its immunogenicity. It did not lead to tubercle formation, nor did it regain this capacity. Thus was born the vaccine strain of tuberculosis called, after its developers, Bacillus Calmette Guerin (BCG). The first child was vaccinated in 1921, a baby born of a tuberculous mother. The new vaccine went from strength to strength until 1929, when a culture was sent to Lubeck for preparation of vaccine. Within a few weeks after the product was released for use, 71 of 252 vaccinated children died, and a violent public reaction ensued. BCG's good name was cleared, however, when it was shown that the cultures had become contaminated with a virulent strain in the Lubeck laboratory.

EHRLICH'S MODEL FOR ANTIGEN-ANTIBODY INTERACTION AND SPECIFICITY

Paul Ehrlich (1854-1915) stands out among the many great scholars of immunology. John Hunter in 1823 had noted that blood, compared with most biological materials, was unusually resistant to decomposition. Nuttall in 1888 was the first to show that animal serum has a natural toxicity for many microbes. Hans Buchner attributed this property to substances he called *alexins* ("protective substances"), but Ehrlich renamed them "complement." The discovery of humoral antitoxins ("antibodies") by Behring and Kitasato in the early 1890s was one of the most dramatic developments in the scientific beginnings of immunology.

Ehrlich was a physician with a passionate complementary interest in chemical structure–activity relationships in biology. He worked for some time in that field with Emil Fischer, the noted organic chemist and biochemist. He conceived the idea of unique stereochemical relationships between the active sites of antigen and antibody. Then he proposed the notion that there were both "affinity" and "functional" domains on an antibody molecule. He put forward a new theory of antibody formation involving specific toxin molecules on the surface of certain cells. When binding occurred, the toxin would be assimilated by the cell and the receptor would be released or regenerated. If the challenge was great, these cells might compensate by generating a surplus of side-chain receptors that could be released to circulate as antibody. His famous paper of 1897 described what he perceived as the interaction of diphtheria toxin and antitoxin.

Ehrlich's research career began in hematology and histological staining; he applied new techniques that allowed differentiation of the various types of "white" blood cells in 1879. Then he developed new staining methods for bacteria, including the agent of tuberculosis, contracting the disease himself along the way. He recovered completely after two years in Egypt. He was the first to quantify and standardize antitoxins. His immunological research culminated in his side-chain theory of immune specificity based on stereospecific chemical interactions between antigen and antibody. He was awarded a Nobel Prize in 1908. He switched his focus to the chemotherapy of infectious diseases, undertaking detailed, tenacious research in a quest for "magic bullets." This work led to the development of Salvarsan, the first drug with significant efficacy against syphilis. The latter stage of his career began when he moved to the Institute of Experimental Therapy in Frankfurt in 1899.

Karl Landsteiner of Vienna in 1905 put forward the idea that antibody-forming cells are triggered by exposure to antigen to form completely new substances. He was the first to describe the ABO system of immunological groups of red blood cells (1900) and the rhesus (Rh) antigen system (1926). He was involved in the first experimental models of syphilis and poliomyelitis in monkeys (in 1906 and 1909, respectively). In the field of immunology he favored the idea of cross-reactions between antigens and antibodies, that is, the presence of graded affinities that allow an antibody to react with a variety of related antigens rather than with a single, absolute lock-and-key specificity. Yet his work on blood groups had indicated virtually absolute specificities. The immunogenetics of interspecies hybrids between the horse and the donkey was particularly interesting. Although the serum proteins of the two species showed extensive cross-reactions with the precipitation test, agglutinating reactions clearly distinguished between them. The latter suggested that inherited antigens did, in fact, give rise to specific antibodies. He concluded that there must be two systems of species-specificity and that the one for proteins undergoes gradual change during evolution, whereas the haptens are subject to sudden changes not linked to intermediate stages.

Arrhenius followed Ehrlich's ideas and developed the field of immunochemistry. Tiselius in 1938 demonstrated by using electrophoresis, a technique he developed to separate proteins, that most of the antibody components of plasma and sera are associated with the gamma-globulin fraction.

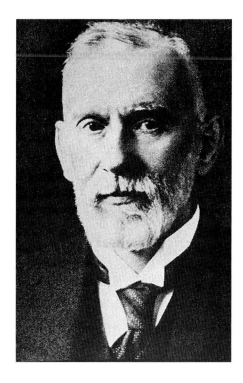

368. Paul Ehrlich (1854-1915). Ehrlich was a genius in vital staining of cells with aniline dyes, using them to classify cells. The founder of immunochemistry, he emphasized that the three-dimensional shape of molecules and active groups was the "lock-and-key" mechanism of specific immunity. He also was the first to propose the concept of selective toxicity as the basis of chemotherapy against infections such as syphilis and trypanosomiasis. *(Science Photo Library.)*

HOG CHOLERA AND THE UNITED STATES BUREAU OF ANIMAL INDUSTRY

When the United States Department of Agriculture (USDA) was founded in 1862, it made no provision for any studies of animal husbandry or veterinary medicine. At that time there was growing concern about importing disease along with livestock brought from Europe. The first USDA head called for legislation requiring quarantine for imported stock. The legislation was passed, but jurisdiction was given to the U.S. Department of the Treasury and no action was taken.

Swine fever or hog cholera, as it became known in the United States, was recognized for the first time in Ohio in 1833. Ten outbreaks had been reported by 1845, and then the virus began to spread rapidly. During the next decade there were 93 outbreaks—nearly a tenfold increase in incidence. In the next five years 173 outbreaks occurred in 23 states. The disease spread throughout the North American continent and around the world. In the U.S. midwest swine belt from 1850 to 1950 hog cholera accounted for an estimated ninety percent of all pig deaths, and more than $30 million of value per year was lost. In the early years hog cholera was not clearly characterized as a disease entity, and diagnosis was difficult.

A physician, George Sutton of Aurora, Indiana, was the first to study the hog cholera epizootic systematically (in Dearborn County). His description of the disease in 1858 was the clearest up to that time, covering both the clinical signs and the postmortem lesions. He conducted transmission experiments, which established that the disease was contagious and that the incubation period was two weeks. He showed that the disease was spread by contact and also induced it by injecting blood taken from a diseased animal. He observed that infected survivors were resistant to a second attack. He found no evidence that the disease was transmissible to humans. One can only applaud the quality and dedication of his investigation.

The disease appeared in England, and John Gamgee sent a specimen to William Budd of Bristol, a noted medical authority on typhoid and cholera. Budd studied the disease and published his findings in 1865, calling the disease pig typhoid because of the clusters of ulcerations he observed in the intestines, especially the colon. He noted that the disease would readily spread via the boots of anyone who entered the pens. Another of John Gamgee's protégés, James Law, became the first professor of veterinary medicine and surgery at Cornell University (1868). He wrote on swine diseases in 1875, differentiating "hog fever," as he liked to call it, from other diseases. He confirmed that a small dose of blood from an infected animal inoculated subcutaneously into a healthy one would induce the disease.

Law attracted brilliant pupils to Cornell's veterinary program. Notable among them were Daniel E. Salmon of North Carolina and Theobald Smith (1859-1934) of Albany, New York, who were responsible for injecting the new scientific philosophy into research on veterinary problems. After consulting Law, Salmon decided to take the agriculture course for the first two years and then pursue the veterinary degree under Law for another two years. However, the clinical facilities at Ithaca were inadequate, so Salmon was allowed to attend the Alfort school in Paris for his last six months of clinical training. In 1872 he gained his bachelor's degree in veterinary science (BVSc) from Cornell. After practicing in Newark, New Jersey, he returned to Cornell to receive the degree of doctor of veterinary medicine (DVM), the first awarded in the United States by a university. In 1878 he was appointed to study hog cholera. He undertook an epidemiological approach and satisfied himself that the disease was contagious.

Commissioner of Agriculture George B. Loring was convinced that a federal bureau of animal industry was necessary so that the serious losses resulting from animal diseases could be curtailed. A veterinary division was established in the USDA, and Salmon became the first chief of the U.S. Bureau of Animal Industry in 1883. He developed a pathology laboratory and a small experimental field station. Because diseases of cattle were to be given the highest priority, early efforts were directed toward the study of bovine lung plague or pleuropneumonia and Texas fever.

Theobald Smith, a physician, was appointed to assist Salmon. He did graduate studies at Cornell under James Law and Simon Gage, who trained

Smith in microscopy. Smith and Salmon applied Koch's new bacterial culture techniques to obtain pure cultures from cases of "swine plague" (hog cholera), then tested them on healthy pigs. A new swine disease appeared in Illinois in 1886, which further confused the researchers. Careful studies of affected pigs revealed cirrhosis of the liver and hepatization of the lungs without the characteristic colonic ulcers of hog cholera.

After testing Pasteur's erysipelas vaccine (1885) by challenging the immunized pigs with blood from hog cholera cases and observing no protection, the researchers at the Bureau of Animal Industry concluded that there were two separate diseases. Daniel Salmon and Theobald Smith intensified their efforts to find a bacterial cause of hog cholera. They isolated a bacterium (1885) in pure culture that they called "Bacillus suipestifer," later named *Salmonella cholerae-suis,* which they claimed was always present in cholera-infected hogs. The workers then attempted to develop a vaccine strain. They experimented with heat-treated killed cultures, administering three injections at eight-day intervals into pigeons. One week later these pigeons and unvaccinated controls were inoculated with an unheated dose of a virulent culture strain. The pigeons that had received the appropriate dose of killed bacteria survived, whereas the control birds, given a single dose of vaccine, died within twenty-four hours. Thus the concept of using a killed "bacterin" as a vaccine was born. Although this principle was to be widely used later in the development of autologous bacterial vaccines in various diseases, its application did not work in pigs against the hog cholera infection. Furthermore, although a small dose of blood from a hog cholera case, given subcutaneously, was invariably lethal, most unvaccinated pigs injected with the unattenuated natural field strain survived. So the herring was red.

While the USDA was experiencing frustrations in its efforts to characterize and devise a means to control hog cholera, the continuing vacuum of understanding led to other initiatives. The University of Nebraska in 1886 appointed Frank S. Billings of Massachusetts as a veterinary pathologist. Billings had trained as a veterinarian in Berlin (1878) and worked under the renowned pathologist Virchow, returning to the United States in 1885 to become a pathologist at the New York Polyclinic Medical School. The following year he took a group of boys from Newark, New Jersey, who had been bitten by rabid dogs, to Paris for vaccine therapy administered by Louis Pasteur. After moving to Nebraska in 1886, Billings began the new Patho-Biological Laboratory; for the first time a state institution had appointed a veterinary researcher to study contagious diseases of farm livestock. Priority was to be given initially to hog cholera. Billings elected to challenge the Bureau of Animal Industry and criticized its work vituperatively through the media. His claims for his own findings, however, failed under scrutiny, and his main contribution was to force the Bureau scientists to become more rigorous and effective. The first full-time American university veterinary researcher turned out to be a bombastic "lemon"; his inappropriate criticisms and provocative role as a stimulus to other laboratories were ill-suited to a university academic appointment.

New reports from Europe (by Selmi of Bologna in 1872 and Briger and Frankel of Berlin in 1890) on the pathogenicity of toxic ptomaines and albuminoids obtained from microbial cultures led the Bureau to establish a biochemistry laboratory headed by Emil Alexander de Schweinitz of North Carolina, who had two doctor of philosophy degrees in chemistry from the universities of North Carolina and Göttingen. Isolation of similar substances in the swine cultures and testing of the substances as candidate vaccines gave inconclusive results.

The field of bacterial toxicology received a great boost from the work of Emil von Behring and Kitasato in 1890 on immunization against diphtheria and tetanus toxins. An entirely new approach to prevention and treatment of

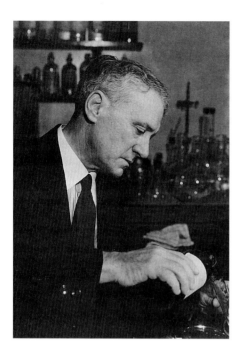

369. Dr. Marion Dorset of the U.S. Department of Agriculture's Bureau of Animal Industry. Dorset pursued the leads developed by Salmon and Theobald Smith in the quest for the causative agent of hog cholera and its control. Dorset's tenacious studies finally revealed that the infectious agent was a filterable virus, and a virus-plus-serum approach to vaccination was developed to protect swine against the disease. *(Courtesy Dr. R. Allen Packer.)*

infectious diseases was unleashed by these exciting discoveries. De Schweinitz seized on the new approach at once and demonstrated in 1892 that the blood serum of guinea pigs immunized against hog cholera provided resistance to the disease. He also showed that the serum would protect guinea pigs when injected two days after they were given an infective dose that would normally have killed them within a week. Although this was an exciting finding, it soon became obvious that the new immune sera could not provide lasting immunity. Losses resulting from swine diseases in 1897 were the greatest in Iowa, so the Bureau conducted a trial there.

DORSET'S MANAGEMENT OF THE SWINE FEVER RESEARCH

De Schweinitz assigned the swine fever research project to his young assistant Marion Dorset, who was born in Columbia, Tennessee, in 1872. Dorset was qualified in chemistry and medicine, and had worked on the serum treatment program. He obtained survival rates of eighty-two percent in serum-treated herds and fifteen percent in control herds. In a larger subsequent trial the rates were seventy percent in serum-treated herds and thirty percent in control herds (1897–98). In some virulent outbreaks, however, the serum was ineffective. As time elapsed and more trials were conducted, the early enthusiasm waned as the overall results became less and less conclusive, until by 1900 and 1901 Salmon had to admit another failure to realize the Bureau's optimistic goals. The sera used in the trials were a mixture of sera that were used against the two organisms representing the two diseases then believed to be the main contagious diseases of American swine (*B. cholerae-suis* and *Pasteurella suisepticus,* representing hog cholera and swine plague, respectively).

With the hindsight of history it seems remarkable that it took so long for such a brilliant team of scientists to accept that their basic tenet was wrong and that their *B. cholerae-suis* was not, in fact, the causative agent of hog cholera, despite the difficulty of inducing disease with the organism and the ease of transmission via contact with an infected animal or inoculation with a small sample of its blood. Not before 1902 was this unfortunate lack of objectivity corrected and the issue of the origin of hog cholera reexamined.

Marion Dorset conducted the reexamination. First, he showed that both blood and serum obtained from infected pigs, even in high dilution, were infective. Then he confirmed the high level of natural infectivity of the disease and that recovered cases were always immune. Subsequently he showed that if an animal survived a low dose (about 0.25 ml) of infective blood, it became permanently immune to subsequent exposure to animals with the disease or to injected blood, even in larger doses. Experiments designed to test the ability of two types of isolated bacteria to cause the disease confirmed the negative results obtained in earlier trials and their inability to provide protective immunity to it. Dorset reasoned that the difference between the infectivities of the blood and of the isolated bacilli must be attributable to the presence of an infective agent in the blood that was lacking in the microbial cultures. At the turn of the century the discovery of filterable animal disease viruses by Löffler and Frosch (1898) provided the necessary clue to progress.

THE DISCOVERY OF VIRUSES AS INFECTIOUS AGENTS

The method devised by Chamberland of passing diluted infective fluid through a filter that held back all bacteria had yielded a filtrate that was still able to transmit foot-and-mouth disease, even at high dilution. Since the agent often induced disease even after several passages, the possibility that it was a filterable toxin was dispelled. Thus the concept of the "filterable virus" of infection was confirmed.

In 1898 Nocard and Roux in Pasteur's laboratory demonstrated that a filterable agent caused contagious bovine pleuropneumonia that could not be cultured by means of the bacteriological methods then available. The filtration technique led to a rush of exciting discoveries of the causative agents of infectious diseases that had formerly defied the best efforts of the bacteriologists. Of veterinary import were the discoveries of the causative agents for the following:

African horse sickness, in 1900, by John McFadyean

Rinderpest, the great cattle plague (at last), in 1902, by Claude Nicolle and Adil-Bey

Sheep pox, in 1902, by Borrel

Fowl pox, in 1902, by Marx and Sticker

Rabies, in 1903, by Remlinger and Riffat-Bey

Except for Walter Reed's pioneering work on yellow fever in Cuba in 1901, such great discoveries as these preceded those of the human infectious disease viruses.

Reed followed the Bureau of Animal Industry's demonstration of vector-borne diseases by implicating a mosquito vector in the transmission of the yellow fever virus from monkeys to humans. When he presented his report in 1901, Reed thanked William H. Welch of Johns Hopkins University for drawing his attention to Löffler and Frosch's work on foot-and-mouth disease in cattle. Having no animal model, Reed conducted the extraordinarily dangerous experiment of inoculating healthy human volunteers with his filtrate, thereby inducing the disease, and he passaged it from them to other individuals to eliminate the possibility of a toxin's being responsible. Reed's team had its martyrs who died for the cause. Discovery of the mosquito vector's role and the demonstration of the presence of a filterable virus that could spread the disease between humans was a great achievement.

Reed's work did not answer the fundamental question of the origin of the virus before it became established in the human species, nor did it provide an experimental animal that could be used as a laboratory model to allow basic investigations of the disease and its resistance in vivo. Reed tried to develop an animal model in macaque monkeys but failed, possibly because he used a Havana specimen that had probably been infected there and become immune. In 1927 Stokes and his colleagues showed that the rhesus monkey was susceptible to the disease. In 1929 South Africa–born Max Theiler (1899-1972), who worked at Harvard University and the Rockefeller Institute, found that mice could be infected by intracerebral inoculation and protected if the virus was given with specific serum. He passaged the virus in both mouse- and chicken-embryo tissue cultures to develop a safe but effective vaccine against yellow fever and received the Nobel Prize in 1951. The answer to the question of an original source was revealed when it was found that the wild monkeys in forested regions of tropical Africa and the Americas carry the virus.

DORSET'S IDENTIFICATION OF THE HOG CHOLERA VIRUS AND A METHOD OF VACCINATION

Dorset conducted filtration experiments on infective blood obtained from animals with hog cholera, with startlingly unequivocal results, and the infective agent was revealed in 1903, after twenty-five frustrating years of effort by the Bureau of Animal Industry scientists. At last it was possible to proceed with a clear sense of direction and a model that really did reproduce the natural disease, although the agent, unlike a good Kochian bacterium, could not be cultured. Unlike the earlier bacterial isolates that were lethal for laboratory animals, the filtered virus was lethal only for hogs. Dorset was at last able to reject the notion that *Bacillus (Salmonella) cholerae-suis* was the primary cause of hog cholera. His dedicated mentor, de Schweinitz, died prematurely of typhoid in his fortieth year, in 1904, just after the breakthrough in the etiology of swine fever. The work was soon confirmed by Paul Uhlenhuth in Berlin and by Ferenc Hutyra and his colleagues in Budapest.

William B. Niles of the Bureau of Animal Industry devised a simple tail-blood method for serial sampling of pig's blood, which made possible the discoveries that the blood became infective on the second day after infection and that *Bacillus cholerae-suis,* clearly in a secondary infective role, did not invade until between the third and the fifth day.

A new wave of research effort began at the Bureau of Animal Industry to exploit the new understanding of the disease with the renewed goal of developing an effective vaccine. Attempts to attenuate the virus directly in the blood were unsuccessful. The next clue came via the 1898 work in South Africa on rinderpest by Wilhelm Kolle and George Turner, who had achieved a state of hyperimmunization in cows by giving a recovered animal repeated, increasingly larger doses of virulent blood over time. The resulting serum was many times more protective than was normal serum. Even more significantly, they showed that a longer-lasting immunity could be achieved when an appropriate dose of hyperimmune serum was given with a small amount of virulent blood.

From 1904 to 1906 the Bureau of Animal Industry team (Dorset, Niles, and William McBryde) developed ways to produce hyperimmunized swine serum against hog cholera. They then tested the serum in combination with virulent blood as an approach to vaccination, with encouraging results. They found that serum alone would protect about two thirds of susceptible pigs for approximately three weeks when the pigs were exposed to infected animals. The principle of combined vaccination with virulent blood and hyperimmune serum was validated: the mortality rate after subsequent challenge was reduced from eighty-two percent to three percent in the laboratory trials.

Dorset was granted a patent on the discovery of anti–hog cholera serum, which gave anyone the right to use the serum without payment of a royalty. An extensive field trial was conducted in 1907 from the Bureau's base near Ames, Iowa, under William B. Niles, a Wisconsin native who was a returning graduate of the Iowa State College. He was engaged in research on infectious diseases of horses, cattle, and swine at the Iowa Agricultural Experiment Station before joining the Bureau in 1898. When serum alone was used in recently infected herds, the mortality rate was about eleven percent, in contrast to the seventy-six percent rate for controls. When the serum was used in herds already badly infected, about seventeen percent died, whereas seventy-one percent of controls died. These encouraging results indicated that serum should be used as early as possible in an outbreak. In herds exposed to diseased animals but not showing any signs of sickness, only four percent of those treated died, whereas eighty-four percent of the controls died. Niles conducted a convincing demonstration for hog farmers at the Union Stockyards Company of South Omaha, Nebraska, and the word spread rapidly. Twenty-one states made hyperimmune sera by 1910, and state agencies made 260,000 inoculations in that year, with satisfactory results.

Congress passed the Virus-Serum-Toxin Act in 1913, which imposed regulations on the use of all viruses, serums, toxins, and analogous products intended for the treatment of domestic animals before interstate shipment or importation into the United States.

When the use of hyperimmune serum alone was compared to the use of a combination of serum and virus in pigs showing no signs of disease when vaccinated but exposed subsequently, the mortality rate in the group receiving the combination of serum and virus was 0.2 percent and in the group receiving serum alone, 0.4 percent. When treatment was given after infection was already present in the herd, the results were 3 percent and 5 percent, respectively. Nationwide between 1913 and 1917 the number of deaths resulting from hog cholera was halved. In 1915 Dorset and Henley developed a pasteurized serum that retained its potency against hog cholera while killing foot-

and-mouth virus. By 1918 more than half a million liters of serum had been produced. The industry now had a technique that allowed it to minimize the losses resulting from hog cholera, although it could not eliminate the virus.

It can be argued that, in fact, the use of unattenuated live virus can only perpetuate the persistence of the virus. Efforts to develop attenuated or inactivated virus vaccines were not made until the 1930s. Dorset used crystal violet dye to inactivate the virus in 1934; results were promising, but Dorset died in that year. McBryde and Cole carried on the work in the hope of developing a safer product. Several inactive vaccines were developed, but with these vaccines immunity of shorter duration took longer to develop and two doses were required. The concept of inactive vaccines was more widely adopted overseas than in the United States. A new approach was required.

MODIFIED LIVE-VIRUS VACCINES AND AN ERADICATION PROGRAM

Two laboratories (those of Baker and Kaprowski) reported independently that the virulence of hog cholera virus could be reduced by passaging in rabbits. By 1951 commercial vaccines were developed from the modified live viruses (MLVs). This approach was timely because "breaks" had occurred in hogs vaccinated by the old, simultaneous method as a result of the emergence of a variant strain that had been used in some commercial virus products. There was a rapid swing to the use of MLV vaccines; they were used ninety percent of the time by 1956. States began to outlaw virulent virus vaccines: twenty-nine states had done so by 1959. These laws were a necessary step toward eradication. President John F. Kennedy signed Public Law 87-209 in 1961 to provide for a national eradication program. Because sound principles of epidemiology were used, hog cholera was eradicated from swine in the United States by 1978. The last case was observed in 1976, one year before the last case of smallpox occurred.

The role of veterinarians whose practices included advising and serving swine farmers deserves mention here. During the phase of serum and serum-virus vaccination of swine against hog cholera, untold millions of doses were administered by veterinarians. This effort allowed them a rare opportunity to profit on a high-volume business, even with a modest markup in prices. More important, the veterinarians felt a sense of accomplishment in participating in a proven program that helped contain the number-one killing disease of swine and kept their clients in business. The federal-state partnership in research of the USDA's Bureau of Animal Industry, in this instance, deserves fulsome praise. This achievement by government laboratories preceded the development of the land grant universities (which had been created in 1862) into major research centers within state colleges and universities, which occurred after passage of the Hatch Act of 1887 and its subsequent implementation. The communication between the farmers and the Bureau of Animal Industry was in the main effective, and both the practicing veterinarians and state governments had opportunities to contribute their ideas and were kept informed of progress. Despite the setbacks and false trails, the story of the eradication of hog cholera stands as one of the great milestones of achievement in American veterinary history.

An even more destructive virus of swine than hog cholera virus is the African swine fever first described by Montgomery in 1921. Hog cholera serum does not protect against African swine fever. The virus appears to enter domestic swine herds because of the presence of reservoirs in the African wild species: the African bush pig, the giant forest hog, and the warthog. African swine fever threatened the Americas when it spread to the Caribbean Islands via the Iberian Peninsula in the late 1970s, and a vigorous eradication campaign was implemented.

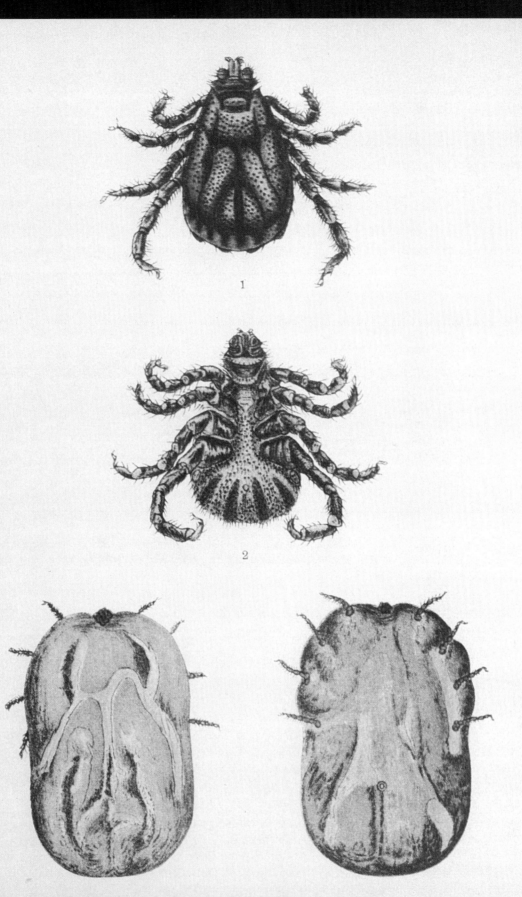

1

2

3   4

C H A P T E R   2 4

Intractable Vector–Borne Hemoprotozoal Parasitic Diseases

VECTOR-TRANSMITTED BLOOD PARASITES

Fulani cavalry from the Sahel region of the Sahara invaded the savanna lands to the south and east in the mid-nineteenth century. The cavalry continued to the bush and forest areas further south until they were met by the tsetse fly, which attacked their horses and gave them trypanoso-miasis. The "centaurs" became foot soldiers, and their advance was checked. When foreign settlers from overseas arrived in African lands south of the Sahara with their livestock, they, too, encountered pests and diseases they had never seen before. As they trekked inland with their imported stock, in river valleys and bush areas the animals were set upon by large, vicious, biting flies known locally by their characteristic buzz, "tse-tse," as verbalized by the Tswana of the Kalahari region. Not only were the animals distressed by the flies' activities, but many also later succumbed to a disease known to the native people as *nagana*. Affected animals, usually cattle, wasted away and died. Humans, too, were affected by the flies; some developed a fatal neurological disorder that came to be known as sleeping sickness. Large regions of the continent were considered unsafe for people and livestock. When Henry M. Stanley, a correspondent for the New York Herald, went to Central Africa in search of British missionary Dr. Livingstone, he started out from Zanzibar with two horses. He was advised that his horses would be attacked by tsetse flies and would become emaciated and die. Stanley caught and studied three species of biting flies. His horses died eight days after they left Zanzibar; he found that they had bots and worms. The cause was probably the viral disease African horse sickness rather than trypanosomiasis. Stanley wrote a book about his experiences: *How I Found Dr. Livingstone: Travels, Adventures, and Discoveries in Central Africa,* in 1872.

EQUINE TRYPANOSOMIASIS: EVANS'S EXPLANATION OF SURRA

To trace the historical development of scientific understanding of these diseases, a diversion is necessary. Griffith Evans (1835-1935) was a remarkable and brilliant veterinarian. After qualifying in London in 1855, he became one of the first veterinary surgeons to be granted entry into the British Army at

370. *Facing page,* Texas fever, or southern cattle fever, was spread by the cattle tick *Boophilus* (formerly *Margaropus) annulatus.* The young ticks on the pasture attach to the skin and ingest a small amount of blood. They molt twice and then mate, and the female greatly increases its intake of blood before dropping to the ground to lay its eggs, which hatch to repeat the cycle. *1* and *2,* Dorsal and ventral views of the male; *3* and *4,* dorsal and ventral views of the female replete with blood. The blood of infected cattle contains the agent that causes the disease in the red blood cells, *Babesia bovis.* It is often paired and can be seen under the microscope. The discovery of this example of a vector-borne hemoprotozoal disease brought scientific acclaim to the Bureau of Animal Industry. *(From a special report of the BAI, Disease of Cattle, revised edition, 1904.)*

425

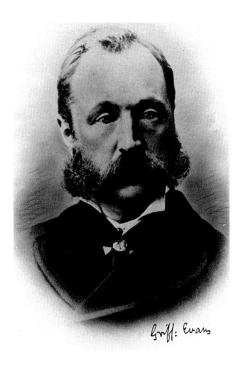

371. Griffith Evans (1835-1935), a veterinary officer in the British Army in Punjab, was studying a febrile disease called *surra* that caused a high mortality in horses, mules, and camels. In 1880 he demonstrated the presence of a flagellated protozoan parasite in the blood of affected animals and established that it was the cause of the disease. The organism had an undulating longitudinal membrane that fit David Gruby's 1843 description of *Trypanosoma* (from the Greek, *trupanon,* a borer, because of its auger-like motion) of a frog. He was transferred before he could clinch his idea, gained from local natives, that a large biting tabanid fly spread the disease. There was no precedent for such vector-borne transmission of a hemoprotozoal parasite at the time. This idea was confirmed by Leonard Rogers in 1899. *(From the Collection of the Osler Library, McGill University, Montreal, Presented by Dr. Erie Evans, daughter of Griffith Evans.)*

officer rank in the Royal Horse Artillery. He was sent to Canada with an army unit and took advantage of the opportunity to train as a physician at McGill University in Montreal. His thesis for the doctor of medicine degree challenged conventional medical views about tuberculosis. Basing his ideas on childhood experiences with consumptives in squalid homes in the mining towns of his native Wales, he insisted that tuberculosis was an infectious disease and that patients with the disease should be segregated, that those who cared for them should take special precautions, and that the patients should be out in fresh air as much as possible. These perceptive views, preceding Koch's discovery of the causative bacterium by eighteen years, were belittled by his examiners, although they passed his thesis after grilling him thoroughly. More than half a century later, McGill University dedicated a section of its Osler Library to the works of Griffith Evans, describing him as "one of McGill's most distinguished sons."

Evans had an extraordinary capacity to get to the center of things and, when addressing a problem, to put his finger on the important questions. Although he traveled as a uniformed British officer, he managed to see President Abraham Lincoln himself, who had granted him permission to visit the federal army's lines and cavalry units during the American Civil War. The two men developed a mutual respect, and Lincoln gave Evans authority to visit all the Union fronts on the condition that Evans return to give Lincoln a firsthand report on his findings.

By a strange twist of fate, Evans's unit was moved to Toronto, where James Bovell, a physician at the University of Toronto, invited Evans to join him in medical research at Trinity College in 1867. The following year Bovell hired a young assistant, William Osler, then a medical student at Trinity. Evans described him as a young man of great charm who had a keen intellect and a remarkable analytical ability. Evans took Osler under his wing. Much later, while Regius Professor at Oxford University, Osler was to recall that he had been inspired in his youth by Griffith Evans, who had with great enthusiasm taught him how to use the microscope. Evans also had an indelible effect on Osler's interest in and outlook on tuberculosis.

In 1877, after spending time back home and informing himself of Pasteur's latest achievements, Evans was sent to India to investigate the outbreak of a lethal disease in army horses at Sialkot. He was soon able to identify the disease as anthrax, the first time it had been diagnosed in India, just one year after Koch had first grown the organism in pure culture. Evans had bought a new microscope before going to the Orient and used it with good effect to study the blood in every case. He ordered deep burial of all affected horses to prevent exhumation and consumption of infected meat.

Looking through his microscope at the blood of animals with anthrax, Evans noted an increase in the number of the large white blood cells. Four years before Metchnikoff described the function of the phagocytes, Evans suggested that the number of white blood cells bore an important relationship to the swarms of bacilli in the blood. His superiors, however, declined his request for support to follow up this lead. Nevertheless, he was soon promoted to inspecting veterinary officer with the rank of major and was assigned responsibility for the entire Ganges River basin in 1878.

Two years later, in 1880, Evans was asked to investigate a severe outbreak of surra, a dreaded wasting disease of horses, in the British Punjab force. Because of heavy losses, with hundreds of horses dead and dying, a transport crisis was looming during the second Afghan War. After reading all available reports on the disease, Evans concluded that evidence pointed to a blood-borne parasite. The term *surra* literally meant "gone rotten," and the syndrome was well known to the native peoples.

The posting was to the dangerous northwestern frontier region on the Indus River and required traveling with an armed escort. Evans had to work outdoors in blistering heat and beset by flies, but again he resolved to deploy his trusted microscope. He observed that the blood of affected horses was teeming with vigorously motile flagellated parasites swimming amidst the red blood cells. With growing confidence in his hypothesis he transferred blood from infected to uninfected animals and was soon rewarded by the appearance of the disease in the latter: just six days later, their blood, too, was teeming with the parasite. He also transferred the parasite from horses to dogs, including a puppy. Thus Griffith Evans, in a remote and hostile outpost of the British Empire, became the first person to associate a serious disease with a trypanosome, a pathogenic protozoal hemoparasite. The organism, *Trypanosoma evansi,* was eventually named after him, and his discovery triggered many studies of other candidates for protozoal blood-borne parasitism.

Evans recognized that a central question remained: How did Surra spread in the field? Again he drew on the experience of natives. The local people attributed the spread to large brown biting flies they called *bhura dhang* (meaning "great needlelike sting"). These aggressive creatures attacked horses until their legs were streaming with blood. Evans assumed that the disease would spread most rapidly when horses were tethered close together and the flies could move from one horse to the next, but the fly season was ending and he could not capture enough specimens to test his theory.

Returning with his infected puppy as a host for the living parasite, Evans was appalled that his ideas and evidence were belittled by the resident expert in Simla, Timothy Lewis, who had been the first person to describe trypanosomes (in particular, *Trypanosoma lewisi*) in rat blood and had concluded that they were nonpathogenic. The Indian medical establishment rejected Evans's views and consigned his manuscript to anonymity by filing it in the government archives, which were later destroyed. The potential disease model for research, the infected puppy, was never studied. Evans, however, had the foresight to send a copy of his report to the *Veterinary Journal* in London, where it did eventually appear in abridged installments. The veterinary profession was angered by the slighting of Evans's work and let its views be known. The importance of his work did not escape the attention of the great scholars of the day, who saw beyond the all-too-often erroneous conventional wisdom. Thus both Pasteur and Koch read Evans's report with great admiration. His work was also publicized by J.H. Steel, another British Army veterinarian in India, who was to launch an Indian veterinary journal and become principal of the Bombay veterinary college. Steel had been sent to Burma to investigate a surra outbreak, but he lacked the special genius that characterized Evans's approach.

After being recalled to England at the age of fifty, Evans planned to revert to his former style and cram research into all his spare time by working with Edgar Crookshank at King's College in London. He particularly wanted to follow up his hunch that trypanosomes might prove to be pathogenic in rats and in monkeys, which served as models for human subjects. In Victorian England antivivisection views were gaining momentum by that time, and Evans had to obtain a license to conduct his proposed research, which he did. He launched the new project with his typical attitude of total immersion. Then suddenly, to the surprise of all, he abandoned it. The explanation for his behavior did not surface until after his death. An emissary from Queen Victoria herself had brought him a directive requiring that he stop the experiments. It is probable that the queen was put up to this action by someone who was jealous of Evans. The most likely candidate was his superior officer and her principal veterinary officer, George Fleming.

Evans, with his new plan thwarted, terminated his brilliant career as a research scientist prematurely at fifty years of age, although he lived to be one hundred. In 1899 Leonard Rogers showed that Evans's hypothesis of nineteen years earlier was correct and that surra was spread via the biting tabanid flies.

TSETSE FLIES AND TRYPANOSOMES IN UNINHABITABLE AFRICA

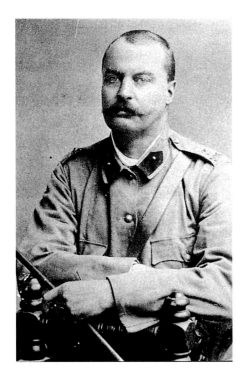

372. Photograph of David Bruce (1855-1931), the British Army doctor who in 1886 discovered the genus of bacteria that was named after him, *Brucella*. The discovery was made in Malta, where the bacterium was present in the goats, the species being called *melitensis*. Zammit extended the study and characterized the risks to the human population of drinking milk from infected goats. Bang in Denmark isolated *B. abortus* from cattle. Both organisms could cause undulant fever in people. Bruce was named a Fellow of the Royal Society. He went to Natal in South Africa in 1894 to study the causes of nagana ("in low spirits") in cattle. He and his wife travelled twenty-eight days by mule-cart and ox-cart from Pietermaritzburg to remote northern Zululand, where he set up a laboratory in a native hut on a hill at Ubombo. He found protozoal parasites he had never seen before in the blood of affected animals (trypanosomes). He established that the disease was spread by a large biting fly known as "tse-tse" (*Glossina* species) and that the flies transmitted the disease only if they had fed on an infected animal. In 1903 Castellani and Bruce found trypanosomes in the cerebrospinal fluid of people afflicted with sleeping sickness in Uganda. *(From Gutsche, 1979.)*

In southern Africa in 1895 David Bruce had established that Evans's ideas about surra held true for the much larger problems of nagana in cattle and sleeping sickness in humans, that is, for diseases caused by pathogenic trypanosomes that were spread by the biting flies, in this case by tsetse flies of the genus *Glossina*. The trypanosomes were discovered by David Gruby (1809-1898) of Hungary, who in 1843 had characterized a flagellate protozoal organism in the blood of a frog and named it the *Trypanosoma* organism.

David Bruce was born in Australia in 1855 but moved to Scotland with his family at five years of age. Despite having left school at fourteen, he went to the University of Edinburgh to study medicine. He graduated and married in 1883, then joined the army medical service. He was first assigned to Malta, where he isolated the agent that caused Malta fever, *Brucella melitensis* (the genus was named after him) and showed that the goat was its reservoir host, spreading the disease to humans via its milk and causing undulant fever. He was recalled to teach in the army medical school at Netley but got the wanderlust again and went to Natal to study nagana, the "depressing disease" of horses and cattle. Traveling with his wife by ox-drawn wagon in 1894, he went to the area of the epidemic in Zululand. By 1895 he had submitted a *Preliminary Report on the Tsetse Fly Disease Nagana in Zululand*. He reported that he had found an infusorial parasite in the blood of affected cattle that closely resembled the one found by Griffith Evans in his studies of surra in India and Burma. He noted that the disease was readily transmitted by a biting fly of the genus *Glossina*. He suspected that wild game species were a reservoir for the parasite. Bruce sent the organism to England, where Plimmer and Bradford named it *Trypanosoma brucei*. Actually, the organism turned out either not to be the one that caused nagana in cattle or to have lost most of its pathogenicity. Subsequent studies revealed that there are at least twenty-two species of *Glossina* flies and many different *Trypanosoma* species with varying host preferences and pathogenicities.

Two *Trypanosoma* species were associated with sleeping sickness in humans. *T. gambiense* was found (by Dutton in 1902) throughout much of the rainforest area in western and central Africa, and *T. rhodesiense* (by Stephens and Fantham in 1910), in drier regions of eastern and southeastern Africa, the latter causing a more acute and more rapidly progressing syndrome. The cattle disease nagana also comprises various diseases caused by different organisms, including *T. brucei, T. congolense,* and *T. vivax*.

Kleine (in 1909) was the first to show that the tsetse fly was the true biological host of the trypanosomes, since the organisms undergo their development in the alimentary tract of the fly and reach the infective stage in about three weeks. The cycle varies with the different species of *Glossina* and *Trypanosoma* organisms.

The traditional strategy for clearing ecological zones of tsetse flies consisted of clearing bush to deprive them of their preferred habitat, killing out all game species that the fly targets for feeding, and saturation spraying by air with potent chlorinated hydrocarbon insecticides. Today this approach seems environmentally threatening, likely to be rendered impotent by insecticide resistance, and unwise because of the persistence of the products in the food chain. More selective destruction of flies can be accomplished with valved fly traps baited with the flavor craved by the flies, and more species-specific sprays are being developed. Implementation of strategic stocking management and movement control can play an important part in zone clearing. After educational programs and incentives designed to gain the cooperation of the cattle ranchers have been implemented, geographical campaign coordination is essential. During the transitional stages development of more productive trypano-tolerant cattle would be helpful, and research directed to this end is under way. Improved chemotherapy for prevention and treatment would also be helpful. Basic research directed at genetic control of the fly and immunological suppression of the hemoprotozoal parasite is advancing knowledge of these challenging diseases. These remarkable parasites have the capacity to modify their antigenic makeup more rapidly than the body's immunologic responses can adapt to them. Although there are drugs that have some efficacy against the parasites, they are far from perfect in terms of selective toxicity.

THE CANADIAN VETERINARY SERVICE AND THE ERADICATION OF EQUINE VENEREAL DISEASE

Dourine ("unclean coitus") is a directly transmitted protozoal infection spread at mating in equids. No insect vector is required. The first signs are swelling of the external genitalia followed by lower abdominothoracic edema. As the disease progresses, neurological signs such as progressive weakness, incoordination, hoof dragging, emaciation, and paralysis frequently follow. An ancient disease, the condition was first described in the West by Ammon and Dickhauser at a Prussian stud at Trakehnen in 1796. It spread through Europe to North America and southern Africa. Rongest in 1896 demonstrated trypanosomes in the blood of an infected stallion. In 1899 Schneider and Buffard in Algeria, using trypanosomes obtained from discharges of infected animals, transmitted the disease experimentally. Doflein in 1901 named the organism *Trypanosoma equiperdum*. In Canada in 1920 Watson achieved, after many attempts, the establishment of a strain of the organism in mice that would reinfect equines and even increased in virulence for the horse, which exhibited much heavier parasitemia than did naturally infected animals. Watson developed an effective diagnostic test based on complement fixation, which allowed the identification of all infected animals, including resistant carriers, and the eradication of the disease in Canada.

A New World Trypanosome-Vector Combination

In South America a different trypanosome-vector combination was discovered. In Brazil in 1910 and 1911 Carlos Chagas found an epimastigote form of a flagellate in the gut of a "cone-nose" or reduviid bug *(Panstrongylus megistus)* that sucked blood aggressively. The organism, which caused trypanosomiasis in animals and humans, was named *Trypanosoma cruzi,* and the disease, Chagas' disease. Medical historians have speculated that Charles Darwin may have contracted this disease when he visited South America during the voyage of the *Beagle*. Although large areas of the continent and adjacent islands are host to the disease, the hypothesis has not been supported by other than circumstantial evidence. The guinea pig, *Cavia porceleus*, a domesticated rodent that is widely kept in the homes of rural native peoples in the Andean mountain chain in South America, is called *cuy* by the Quencha-speaking peoples. These "Indian" peoples cohabit with the guinea pigs—typically eight to fifteen animals per hut are retained by a stone sill. Small holes in the walls of these adobe huts serve as lairs for the reduviid bugs, such as *Triatoma infestans*, that are vectors of Chagas' disease. Guinea pigs and people become infected by entry of infective metacyclic forms of the pathogenic protozoan, *Trypanosoma cruzi*, into the bite wound by contamination with the bug's feces, which are shed as it starts to feed. Infected humans can suffer complete right bundle branch block of the heart. About one hundred and fifty species of mammals have been infected experimentally, including dogs, cats, rats, opossums, and armadillos. At least in the Andes, the main reservoir is probably the guinea pig because people sleep on the floor of their huts and are thus infected. A very high incidence of the disease occurs in rural populations, es-

373. Ernest Edward Tyzzer succeeded Theobald Smith as Professor of Comparative Pathology at Harvard University. He became very famous for his work on fowl protozoal diseases. His beautiful illustrations and detailed descriptions (1929-1932) of each of the important pathogenic species of coccidial protozoa in chickens included diagrams indicating the sites that were affected within the gastrointestinal tract. These classic studies became the standard. He also noted that it was desirable to induce some level of immunity. This illustration showed the site of attack, the small intestine seen here, to be hemorrhagic in the case of *Eimeria necatrix* infection. Tyzzer also showed that the protozoan that affects the liver of turkeys and causes the disease, blackhead, which was discovered by T. Smith, was spread by the helminth *Heterakis gallinae. (From Tyzzer, 1932.)*

pecially in Bolivia and Southern Peru. As a consequence, supplies of blood collected for transfusion tend to be contaminated, and these can lead to further spread of the disease among the people of the region.

Hoare in 1972 reported that at least 125 species of trypanosomes are known from mammals alone and that these species are found in approximately 400 mammalian hosts representing 218 genera and 12 orders.

Epizootic Protozoal Diseases of the Gut and Liver

Although not blood-borne, coccidiosis is a major group of protozoal diseases that affect the gastrointestinal tract or liver. The term *coccidiosis* refers to many diseases of different species of birds and mammals. The bane of the poultry industry, coccidiosis is controlled by a combination of prophylactic chemotherapy and fostered natural immunity. However, the coccidial parasites are ingested from droppings and do not require a vector species for transmission.

Antony van Leeuwenhoek, the Dutch inventor of the microscope, was the first to see a parasitic protozoan, a coccidian oocyst of the later named species *Eimeria stiedai,* in the bile of an old rabbit in 1674. Later, in 1681, he observed *Giardia* organisms in his own stools when he was suffering from diarrhea. *Trichomonas* species were observed in vaginal secretions and in the stool of humans in the mid-nineteenth century. (Much later, *Trichomonas foetus* was found to be a pathogenic venereal parasite of cattle.) There was a long lag between Leeuwenhoek's observations and the recognition that certain protozoa were pathogenic and parasitic. In 1865 Stieda noted that oocysts segmented

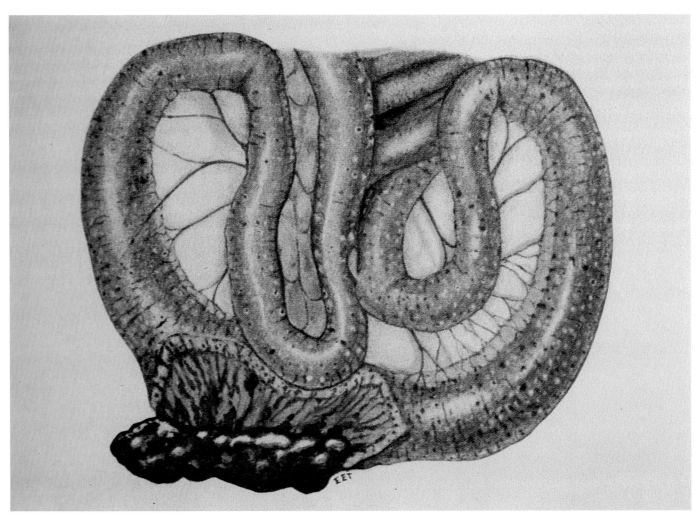

in water and suggested that they were developmental stages of an animal parasite. Then Eimer in 1870 related the oocytes to apparently endogenous structures he observed in the intestinal epithelium of mice. He proposed that these were two forms of the same parasite. Eimer described coccidial infections in several species. In 1869 Rivolta described intestinal parasites in birds that caused an epizootic. He called them "Psorospermes," an early name for such organisms.

Alcide Railliet at the Alfort veterinary school in Paris described *Coccidium* (later, *Eimeria*) *tenellum* obtained from diseased ceca in chickens. He realized that this infection sometimes caused heavy losses in poultry. He also recognized that other, related species caused disease in rabbits. The life cycle was delineated in 1900 by Schaudinn when he was studying an *Eimeria* organism that he found in a centipede. He established clearly the role of the oocyst in transmitting the infection.

Researchers soon realized that organisms similar to those previously mentioned could cause disease in poultry. The complexities were not unraveled, however, until the physician Ernest Edward Tyzzer's classic work at the Department of Comparative Pathology at Harvard University's School of Medicine on *Coccidiosis in Gallinacious Birds* was published in 1929 and 1932. Tyzzer described five pathogenic species in the chicken and one in the turkey. He characterized the pathogenesis of the disease in the digestive tract in each case, showing the life cycle in the gut with brilliant sequential drawings of the microscopic changes in the intestinal epithelium. He was able to demonstrate the specific parts of the gut that were affected and the severity of the changes for each parasite. The resulting diagrams and drawings have been used by avian pathologists ever since. Tyzzer also made the important findings that the host bird developed acquired immunity to the parasite and that this phenomenon could be used as a basis for achieving control of the disease. Earlier, in 1922, he had described another pathogenic protozoan, *Cryptosporidium parvum*.

Theobald Smith in 1895 had discovered the hepatic protozoan parasite that caused the deadly blackhead disease of turkeys, *Histomonas meleagridis*. In the 1920s Tyzzer worked out the details of how it was transmitted via the eggs of cecal worms, *Heterakis gallinarum*.

Tick-Borne Hemoprotozoal Diseases of Cattle

Koch, in his later years (1896-1907), studied several African protozoal diseases, including malaria, trypanosomiasis, East Coast fever (theileriasis), relapsing fever, and piroplasmosis, on site in East and South Africa. The tick-borne group of hemoprotozoal diseases includes piroplasmosis (babesiosis), anaplasmosis, and theileriasis. East Coast fever is a severe bovine disease caused by the protozoan *Theileria parva*. In large areas of eastern and southeastern Africa it is a veritable plague that causes heavy losses of cattle unless intensive tick vector control is practiced. The famous South African veterinary scientist Arnold Theiler characterized the hemoprotozoal disease caused by *Theileria parva*, as well as other protozoal parasites. However, East Coast fever remains a major problem in the eastern part of sub-Sahara Africa.

In understanding the tick-borne diseases it is important to characterize the life cycles in the host mammal and the tick and to define the biology and ecology of the tick species so that control programs can be devised. The U.S. Bureau of Animal Industry, for example, addressed the growing problem of Texas fever (Spanish staggers, or Southern cattle fever) of cattle, and Theobald Smith in 1889 incriminated a microscopic protozoan within the red blood cells of affected cattle as the likely cause of piroplasmosis. (Billings immediately ridiculed this conclusion, providing a stimulus to further research.) Much later it was concluded that Smith must have been working with the blood from animals infected with both piroplasmid *Babesia* and *Anaplasma* or-

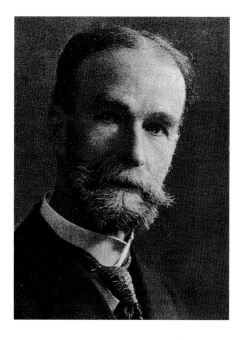

374. Theobald Smith (1859-1934) was one of the most brilliant and focused intellects to interact with the veterinary profession. During a very broad program of study at Cornell University, he acquired enthusiasm for scientific investigation from microscopist Simon Gage and physiologist Burt Wilder that led to his obtaining a doctor of medicine degree at Albany Medical College. He decided on a research career and joined the BAI in Washington, D.C., and Beltsville under Salmon in 1883. His first research there was in bacteriology, isolating *Bacillus* (now *Salmonella*) *cholerae-suis* as the possible cause of hog cholera, which was found later to be due to a filterable virus. His classic work was the orchestration of the BAI team's famous study reported in Bulletin No. 1 of 1893: *Investigations into the Nature, Causation and Prevention of Texas or Southern Cattle Fever.* This was the first model of a vector-borne infection caused by a hemoprotozoal parasite *(Babesia).* Then, in Kingston, Rhode Island, he showed that the devastating blackhead disease of turkeys was due to a protozoan; Tyzzer later discovered that the *Heterakis* worm was the vector. Smith became Fabyan Professor of Comparative Pathology at Harvard University (1895-1915), where he differentiated the human and bovine species of tuberculosis bacteria. He moved to the Rockefeller Institute in Princeton, New Jersey (1915-1934), as Director of the Department of Animal Pathology, where he discovered the immunological protection provided to newborn calves by colostral antibodies (1922-1925), among many other contributions to the understanding of infectious diseases. *(Courtesy Harvard Medical Archives, Francis A. Countway Library of Medicine.)*

375. Arnold Theiler, the founder (1908) of the famous South African Veterinary Research Institute at Onderstepoort, eight miles north of Pretoria. He is shown here in 1935 in front of the Institute with his successor P.J. du Toit (center) and the future director, R. Alexander. Theiler was a Swiss veterinarian who qualified at Berne and completed a doctorate at Zürich, with experience at Munich. He emigrated to South Africa and settled in Johannesburg in 1891. He lost his left arm in an accident involving a maize chopper in his early days there. President Paul Kruger assigned him to control glanders and the rinderpest epidemic of 1896. A brilliant organizer and survivor, he worked first for the Boers and then for the British as chief of veterinary bacteriology for Transvaal, but in reality he worked simply as a dedicated scientist and professional. He was awarded a doctoral degree by Berne. He showed that African horse sickness was due to a filterable virus in 1900, the same year that McFadyean did in London. He worked with Stewart Stockman, a British veterinarian who later established the Weybridge laboratory. Theiler established the causative agent of East Coast fever to be a hemoprotozoal organism that became known as *Theileria parva*. He characterized many other diseases, including botulism, which he showed was acquired by cattle that chewed bones because they needed more phosphorus, and many plant poisonings. He taught at the veterinary faculty that was established at Transvaal University College in 1920 and served as dean from 1923 to 1927. He was truly one of the greatest contributors to veterinary progress, being responsible for more than three hundred publications. *(From Gutsche, 1979).*

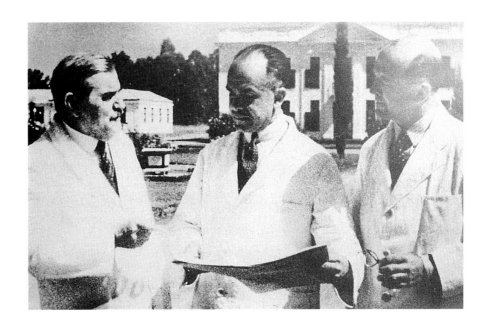

ganisms, since the organisms he described in red blood cells were not of the *Babesia* species. Arnold Theiler differentiated the two diseases in 1910.

Smith and Frederick L. Kilborne, a Cornell-trained veterinarian, published their classic report in 1893, *Investigations into the Nature, Causation, and Prevention of Texas or Southern Cattle Fever.* This work, one of the greatest conceptual achievements of veterinary science, opened up an entirely new category in the etiology of a disease. The authors showed that the organism that caused the disease in the cattle was transmitted by the bite of an infected tick and that a *Boophilus* tick that became exposed by taking blood from an infected bovine then transferred the organism to its progeny via its eggs. Actually Victor Babes had described the protozoan form in Romanian cattle in 1888, and the *Babesia* organism was named after him. The work of the Bureau of Animal Industry scientists included a study of the life cycle of the tick by Cooper Curtice, another Cornellian, whose work clearly showed the principle of transmission of diseases of animals and humans via arthropod vectors and described how these diseases could be contained by vector control.

Cattle tick fever can occur whenever the appropriate *Babesia* species occur and suitable tick vectors for them are present. After infection is transferred from ticks to calves or adult cattle, there is an incubation period of ten days or more before clinical signs appear. These include high fever; enlarged spleen and liver (and gallbladder); hyperpnea; mucous membranes that are red at first and become anemic, then jaundiced; anorexia and depression; and rumen atony. Blood smears are hard to interpret. Morbidity and mortality rates can be high. In some areas seasonal incidence parallels the tick population. In the United States the disease caused enormous losses in the fifteen southern and southwestern states until Bureau of Animal Industry scientists clarified its nature and showed how it could be controlled, thereby eliminating the earlier massive annual losses.

As early as 1889 a federal quarantine order was issued to prevent further spread of the arthropod vector, the tick, via trading in cattle. This order required that cattle from the southern quarantined area in transit to northern markets be yarded separately from the northern stock, and the freight cars had to be disinfested. Control by destruction of the ticks proved to be quite chal-

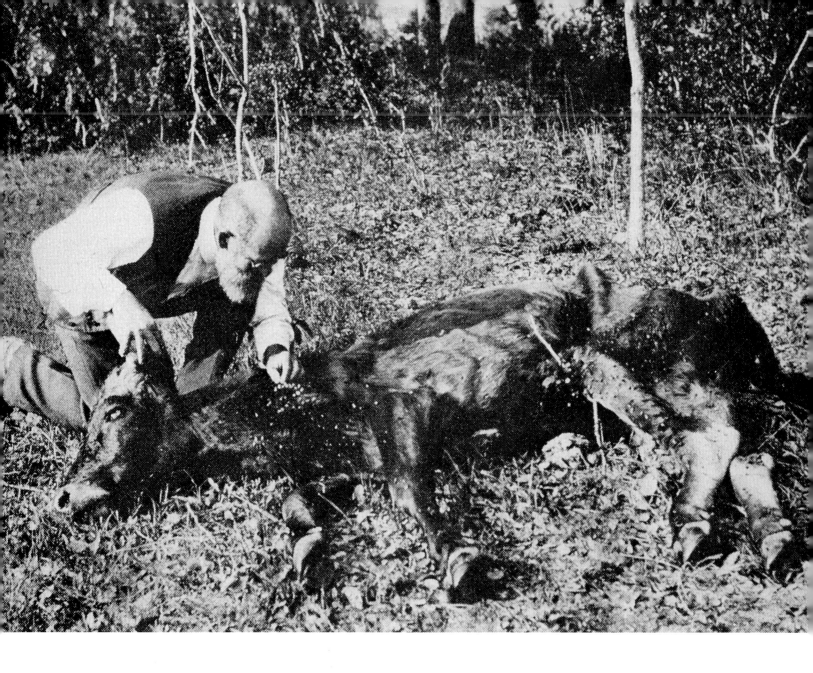

lenging. An English veterinary surgeon, William Cooper, had developed the idea of dipping sheep in a solution designed to kill the parasitic skin mite that caused the devasting ovine dermatitis with loss of wool, known as sheep scab, in 1843. His venture became a commercial success, evolving into the international corporation Cooper, McDougall, and Robertson (purchased by Wellcome in 1959). Experimenting with arsenical compounds as acaricides for cattle in Queensland, Australia, Cooper scientists discovered agents that were effective against the *Boophilus* tick that carried Texas fever. N.S. Mayo, the chief veterinarian for Cuba at the time, used the Australian formulation in 1906, and Joseph W. Parker at the BAI recommended that it be tested in the United States in 1907. A combination of arsenic, soda, and pine tar was developed as a "boiled dip" that was approved for use in 1911. The existing tick eradication campaign that began in 1906 gained momentum with the new dip and was brought to a successful conclusion in the 1920s. Maintaining the efficacy of the dip and detoxifying it before disposal to protect the environment were important developments by the BAI.

376. Dr. Cooper Curtice of the BAI examining ticks on a cow that died of Texas fever. The work of Salmon, Smith, Kilborne, and Curtice (1889-1893) on the causation and mode of transmission of Texas fever is one of the epochal accomplishments in the field of medical history because it was the first to show that arthropods were capable of acting as carriers of agents of diseases affecting mammals. Curtice championed the "tick theory" of the transmission of the disease, and he was responsible in greater degree than any other person for proving that the southern cattle tick *Boophilus annulatus* was the sole carrier of its agent. *(Courtesy* The Nation's Business, *Washington, D.C.)*

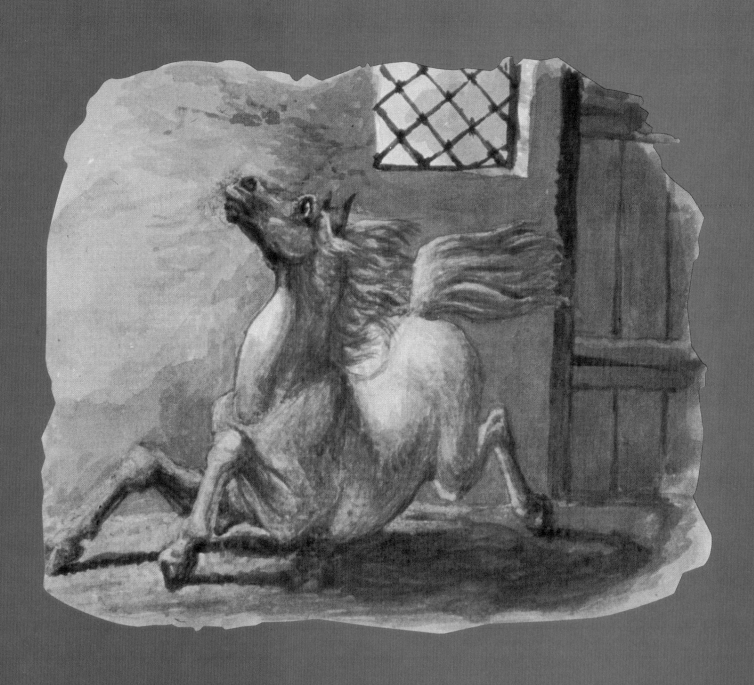

CHAPTER 25

Horse-Doctoring in the Nineteenth Century

The Special Contribution of Edward Mayhew

ARTIST, ACTIVIST, AND VETERINARY SURGEON

Edward Mayhew (c. 1813-1868) came from a prominent artistic family that produced the first editor of the famous humor magazine *Punch*. He was a playwright and an actor before his passionate concern for the welfare of animals drew him to a career in veterinary medicine in middle age. As a student at the Royal Veterinary College in London he was recognized for his outstanding ability and focused application. He was appointed demonstrator in anatomy in his second year and became an excellent teacher and scholar.

Mayhew wrote an excellent paper in 1846, *Distribution and Use of Tendinous Structures As Connected with Muscular Fiber*, which included an explanation of how horses sleep standing up. John Barlow (1815-1856) at the Edinburgh school criticized the paper on the grounds that Dick, a professor of veterinary medicine, had already published on the subject. That paper, however, written fifteen years earlier, had been buried in the *Quarterly Journal of Agriculture*, and Mayhew had not seen it. Barlow, a fine scholar, had brilliantly described the pleuropneumonia epizootic in cattle before he attended Dick's veterinary college. Like Mayhew, he was kept on to teach anatomy and physiology. Barlow was well on his way to a brilliant scholarly career when he died young, at forty-one years of age. Mayhew, on the other hand, was asked to leave the London college because of a dispute with Deputy Professor Charles Spooner, who also taught anatomy. By adjusting the schedule of classes at the London college, Spooner ensured that the students could not attend the private classes in anatomy that Mayhew had planned to offer after his dismissal. The students raised money for a valuable gift and presented Mayhew with a microscope on his departure.

Mayhew opened a veterinary practice with a special focus on dogs and cats but also treated horses. He was an articulate, direct critic of both the London and the Edinburgh schools. He was elected to the Council of the Royal College of Veterinary Surgeons (RCVS) and became a significant voice in the profession. Spooner sued him for libel and lost. Mayhew wrote an accurate article on the state of affairs at the Royal Veterinary College in 1848, exposing Sewell and Spooner's machinations in administering the college and their plots against the RCVS. Sewell had been Principal Coleman's deputy from the start and became a professor after Coleman died, perpetuating the unimaginative drift of the academic institution.

Mayhew condemned all those neglectful or abusive of animals in their charge, whatever their station, and the authorities who turned a blind eye to most of the atrocities perpetrated on dumb animals that they witnessed daily.

377. *Facing page,* Disorders of the neurological system were among the most terrifying to owners and handlers, and Edward Mayhew did much to help people understand the cause of, as well as the behavior associated with and treatment for, these problems. With phrenitis—inflammation of the brain—the horse, in its anguish, may manifest self-destructive violence. *(Courtesy The Royal College of Veterinary Surgeons, Wellcome Library, London.)*

Mayhew was always seeking more effective, humane ways to practice his calling. He was the inventor of the technique of passing a flexible tube through the nostrils of the horse into its stomach without discomfort in 1847. This technique allowed the accurate, safe administration of medicines with minimal restraint, a brilliant advance. Yet the method was not taken up by others because neither of the two veterinary schools would adopt it or teach it, such was their hostility toward Mayhew. Half a century was to elapse before the technique was "rediscovered." In 1849 Mayhew was the first to describe the technique of catheterization in the dog.

Mayhew's zest for humane treatment led him to become one of the first in the profession to use ether vapor as a volatile anesthetic in dogs and cats in 1847. Although he satisfied himself that no pain was evinced by the animal once full anesthesia had been attained, he was troubled because some of the animals vocalized during induction and recovery. He published his results and stated his concern in *The Veterinarian*. To determine the true state of affairs, he, with difficulty, persuaded a dental surgeon to administer ether to him and extract a tooth. Because the tooth he indicated was sound, however, the dentist was unable to extract it, even though Mayhew was anesthetized. After Mayhew recovered, the dentist attempted to extract the tooth without administering anesthetic and failed. The next day Mayhew persuaded the dentist to administer ether and try again, after assuring the operators that he was in no danger from the experiment. As it turned out, they administered ether and failed again to free the tooth but in the process unconscious Mayhew wrecked their operating room and threatened the operators. Remembering none of this happening, he felt satisfied that the cries made by animals entering and emerging from a state of anesthesia were not cries of pain. He was sure that the volatile anesthetic technique would be a great blessing to humanity. He published another paper on the topic, *Observation on the Action of Ether and Chloroform*, in 1848, in which he described administering these agents orally and per rectum as anodynes.

Mayhew's classic monograph, *The Horse's Mouth, Showing the Age by the Teeth*, an accurate, well-illustrated work, appeared in 1849. He revised Blaine's *Outlines of the Veterinary Art* and wrote *Dogs, Their Treatment and Management* in 1854. His interests turned to homeopathy, which he evaluated in 1856. In 1857 his *Dairies of London and Unwholesome Food* exposed the ghastly trade in diseased meat from the debilitated cows of London's dairies. He made a clarion call for the reform of this disgraceful trade and the eviction of dairies from the metropolitan area in the interest of public health.

The veterinary profession, by and large, disliked Mayhew's open, challenging style and the books he wrote for laypersons, such as *The Illustrated Horse Doctor* (1860), which provided information to which only those who could be trusted to use it correctly should be privy, that is, the profession. The hostility he engendered sometimes caused obstructive reactions that had the opposite of his intended effect. Yet in the retrospective view he was a splendid influence on a national profession that was in a sorry state.

NINETEENTH-CENTURY EQUINE DISEASES: MAYHEW'S ILLUSTRATIONS

Edward Mayhew, a rare combination of artist and veterinarian, left the best visual record of the problems facing the horse doctor of his day. *The Illustrated Horse Doctor* contained more than four hundred of his pictures showing features of the diseases of the horse seen with a clinical eye. The illustrations were actually made as wood engravings prepared from the author's own watercolor paintings. Thus they appeared in black and white in the popular book, which went through many editions in the second half of the nineteenth century.

Mayhew wrote his book on the horse doctor to educate the public, who for the most part perceived the horse as an unfeeling working machine. He recognized the true perceivers of the species to be the educated, thoughtful, influential minority, who admired horses and knew that they were capable of a degree of reason and had emotions and sensations, just as humans do. He made a plea for greater concern for the well-being of these fine animals and for improvement in their health care. He observed that during the days of the post chaises the overworked horses survived on the roads for an average of only two years, whereas well-cared-for horses should be capable of work for two decades. The royal stables were full of examples of the latter kind. Mayhew drew attention to the appalling standards of care in the post houses, which he classed as pest houses, characterized by repeated bouts of sickness.

Mayhew argued vigorously for more humane treatment of horses and the use of veterinary assistance for them when required. Not only did he claim that a combination of humane treatment and veterinary assistance was the proper and desirable way to manage the animals, but also he showed that it was sound economically. His book enabled literate persons to acquire a preliminary understanding of diseases so that they could oversee emergency measures and talk intelligently to veterinary surgeons when necessary.

The Illustrated Horse Doctor begins by describing diseases of the nervous system and brain and afflictions of the mouth, nostrils, and throat. It then deals with the thorax, cardiopulmonary problems, and dysfunctions of the stomach, liver, intestines, and urinary organs. Specific diseases receive special attention because they are often not amenable to cure—broken wind, melanosis, water farcy, purpura hemorrhagica, strangles, glanders, and farcy. Diseases of the skin, the limbs, and the feet are covered, and injuries and their treatments, as well as surgical operations, are described.

THE HORROR OF BRAIN DISORDERS IN HORSES

Brain disorders must have been truly frightening to horse owners and grooms. Phrenitis, or inflammation of the brain, often led to violent behavior; the horse's intent was not malicious, but the torment in its head caused the horse

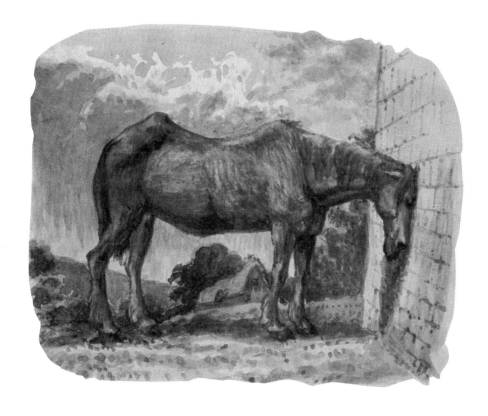

378. Overfeeding often led to a condition called staggers, which featured a "sleepy" stage. *(Courtesy The Royal College of Veterinary Surgeons, Wellcome Library, London.)*

379. Signs of hydrophobia, or rabies, including licking of a skin site, high-pitched neighing, severe mood swings, nervousness, and tremors, culminating in a severely violent phase of biting and kicking. *(Courtesy The Royal College of Veterinary Surgeons, Wellcome Library, London.)*

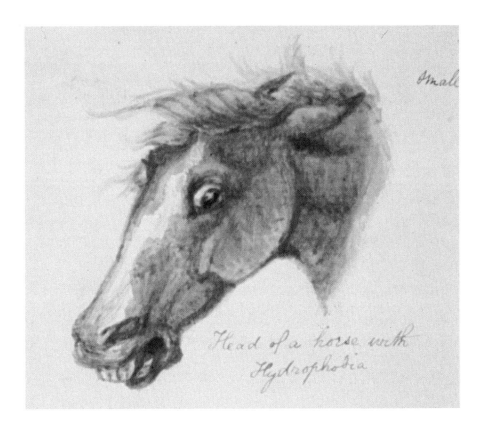

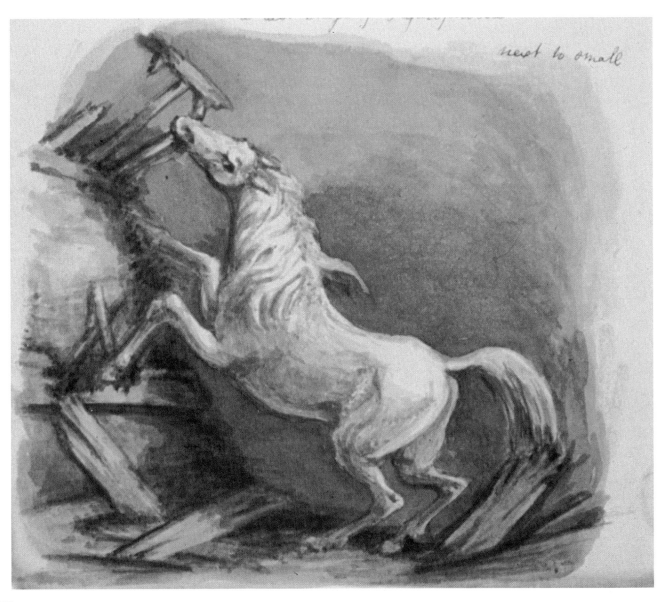

to throw itself around recklessly. Phrenitis was said to be the result of injury caused by the carter flailing the head with the butt of his whip. Brain abscesses resulting from trauma with a skull fracture were considered untreatable. Overfeeding could lead to a condition called staggers, which caused the horse to go through a dumb or sleepy stage and possibly proceed to a stage of mad desperation. Sometimes head-pressing against a wall was an intermediate state. Megrims was considered equine epilepsy and was especially common in draft horses. Various forms were seen, but in its most dramatic form megrims caused the horse to rush up steps into a house or an establishment. Usually there would be convulsions before the fit passed. After several fits a dull, heavy, flaccid, seemingly stupid expression became fixed.

Hydrophobia or rabies was recognized as being attributable to a contagion, usually acquired from a dog or cat. It was known that there was a dormant period after exposure. Early signs might include compulsive, forceful licking at one skin site. Appetite and thirst were deranged, but drinking might induce spasms and fear. The neigh became squeaky, the expression at first one of extreme anxiety but changing to one of cunning. Sudden sweats and phases of grinning ferocity might be manifested. Extreme nervousness and tremors were typical signs. Finally, the furious stage set in and the horse went on a destructive rampage, striking, biting, and kicking at everything in its environment. The only recourse was a bullet.

Other recognized disorders of the nervous system included tetanus, stringhalt, gutta serena, and partial paralysis. It was known that tetanus usually entered via a wound, although in some cases a wound could not be found. The earliest signs were nervousness, excitability, and anorexia. The veterinary surgeon raised the head and saw the haw (third eyelid) projected over the eye, the pathognomonic sign. Muscle spasms set in and became continuous, causing agony and paroxysms. Lockjaw rendered the poor animal unable to eat, and the veterinarian used nasal intubation to pump linseed gruel into horses

380. Tetanus. Reluctance to move because of continuous painful muscle spasms is accompanied by inability to eat. *(Courtesy The Royal College of Veterinary Surgeons, Wellcome Library, London.)*

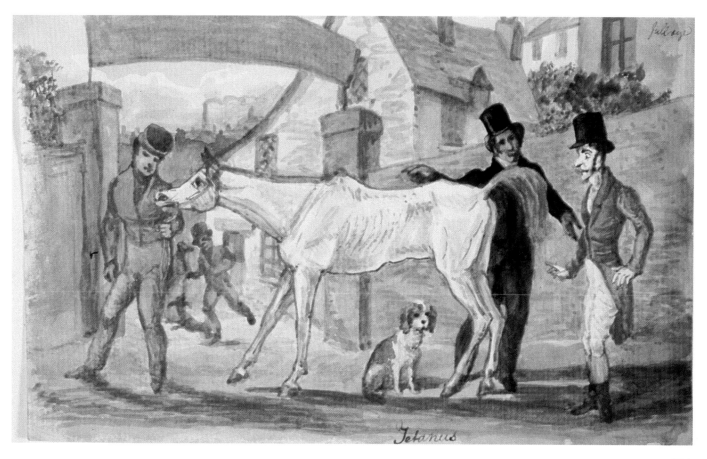

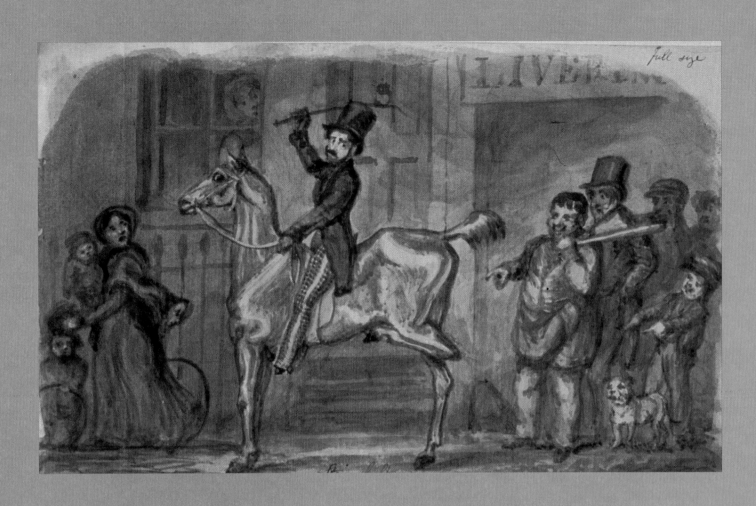

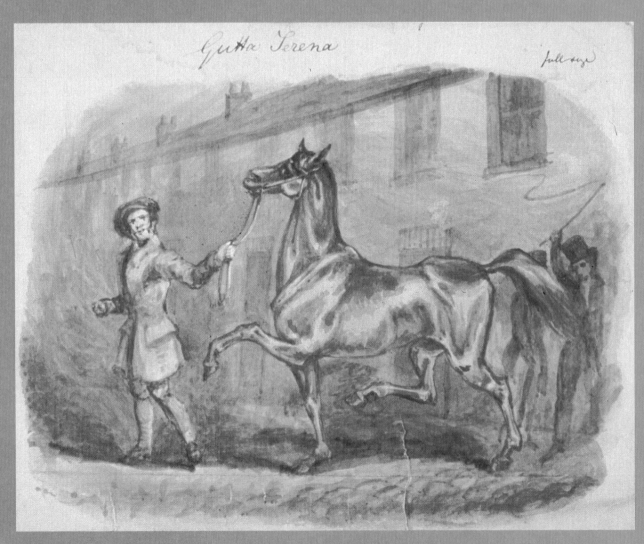

with chronic lockjaw. A strong purgative was thought to be necessary, and no other treatment, but with darkness, quiet, and gentle care by a familiar attendant some horses survived.

Stringhalt was said to be the equine equivalent of chorea in dogs and untreatable. In the horse, however, only the hind limbs manifested the disorder in a rapid, involuntary raising of the hind legs to full flexion a few times in succession. This symptom was usually seen only as the animal started to walk away. The seat of the problem was thought to lie in an injury to the posterior spinal cord that controls the extensor muscles of the rear limbs.

Gutta serena, fixed dilatation of the pupil, was said to be due to paralysis of the optic nerve caused by maltreatment. It involved permanent blindness to one or both eyes. Mayhew depicted the unique gait of a blind horse.

Eye diseases must have been a significant concern because of high incidence and serious consequences for both master and horse. Descriptions included simple and specific ophthalmia or inflammation of the surface membranes (cornea and conjunctiva). The former was considered a result of a foreign body's gaining entrance or trauma with the whip, the latter a result of sealing stables with inadequate space or drainage, thereby allowing irritating ammonia to take its toll. Cataracts, fungoid tumors, blocked lachrymal duct, and lacerations of the lids were also described. Extirpation of the eyeball was necessary for fungoid tumors, which were cancers of the eye.

DISEASES OF THE RESPIRATORY AND CIRCULATORY SYSTEMS

Horses commonly had conditions called colds, with clogged sinuses, then copious defluxions. These were treated by steaming the upper respiratory tract by means of a nose bag containing boiling water. Vascular nasal polyps were frequently seen and were removed surgically. Nasal gleet, a condition caused by filling of the sinuses with pus that became solidified, required surgical opening of the affected sinuses with a trephine and gentle forcing of fluid in, to escape through the nostrils. A seton was then inserted through the hole and out of the nostril and tied. Moving this seton daily assisted in getting the solidified matter to clear.

381. *Facing page, above,* Stringhalt, thought to be caused by injury to the posterior spinal cord, resulted in rapid, involuntary raising of the hind legs to full flexion just when the horse is about to begin walking. *(Courtesy The Royal College of Veterinary Surgeons, Wellcome Library, London.)*

382. *Facing page, below,* The unique gait of the blind horse afflicted by gutta serena, or fixed dilation of the pupils of the eye. The animal steps high and raises its head. *(Courtesy The Royal College of Veterinary Surgeons, Wellcome Library, London.)*

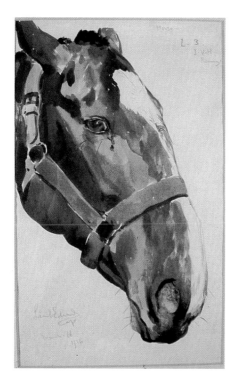

383. Captain Lionel Edwards of the Royal Army Veterinary Corps, painted this picture of a horse at the Romsey Remount Depot in March 1916. The horse had acquired glanders on the Continent during World War I. *(Courtesy The Royal College of Veterinary Surgeons, Wellcome Library, London.)*

384. High choke, a condition of the pharynx and upper esophagus, was caused by the use of concoctions or a whole egg to enhance the horse's appearance. The head is raised, and a nasal discharge is present. In panic, the horse paws and stamps, sweating and heaving in its agony. Unless relief was provided, the horse could suffocate and fall. *(Courtesy The Royal College of Veterinary Surgeons, Wellcome Library, London.)*

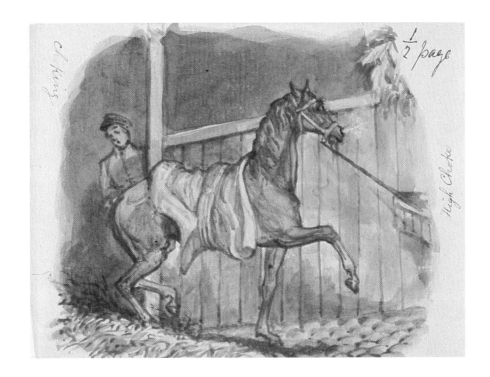

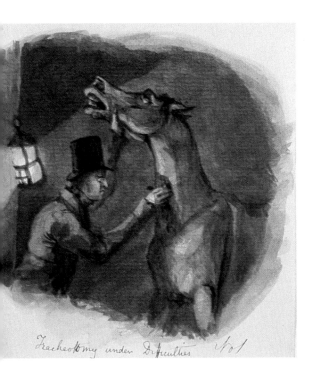

385. Mayhew was ahead of his time in treating respiratory conditions with the use of anesthesia and tracheotomy. Here the operation was being performed on a rapidly failing horse under difficult circumstances at night. The spout of a tea kettle was used to keep the airway open after the incision was made. *(Courtesy The Royal College of Veterinary Surgeons, Wellcome Library, London.)*

442

Sore throat, coughing, and laryngitis were common complaints. Roaring was an especially annoying noisy breathing problem. It was attributed to paralysis of the arytenoideus muscle of the larynx, which allowed the flap of the vocal cords to obstruct the airflow and create the typical sound of roaring. Mayhew attributed many cases of the condition to the fashion of using a bearing rein to pull the head back and up, thereby compressing the larynx for long stretches of time.

Choking was a common, dangerous condition; many cases were due not to disease but to the secret potions in the form of balls used by grooms with a view to enhancing the condition or appearance of the horse. Whole eggs were given for the same purpose and could cause choke. In high choke the object was lodged in the pharynx and upper esophagus. The degree of urgency depended on the severity of the obstruction. If acute, the horse would fidget, stamp, crouch and dance, sweat, and express agony; its neck muscles became tetanic and its flanks heaved. A wire loop could be passed over the object and jerked to dislodge it. If this technique failed, ether anesthesia was resorted to and a temporary tracheotomy tube installed. Mayhew was ahead of his time with such treatments, since few veterinarians would have used ether anesthesia and tracheotomy before the 1890s.

In the case of low choke, when the obstruction had passed as far as the thoracic esophagus, the animal should be given chloroform by inhalation and a probang passed gently to push the obstruction onward into the stomach; Mayhew stressed the importance of patience, saying that it could take twenty minutes to achieve the desired affect. A choking mass that was causing esophageal obstruction was often forced along by a groom with the butt of his whip. The groom's roughness could tear the mucosal lining, which often led to stricture of the tube after it healed. Since the horse was unable to swallow, water, if drunk, returned via the nostrils.

The respiratory tract itself was subject to inflammation in the form of bronchitis, congestion of the lungs, or pneumonia. Mayhew attributed many cases of bronchitis to neglect, for example, letting an animal stand for hours in cold, wet weather after the punishing exertion of riding or drawing a carriage. Exhaustion during overriding could cause a horse to sink and collapse or to pant and droop its head if left standing afterwards. In the former case bleeding was recommended to relieve the evident vascular congestion, fol-

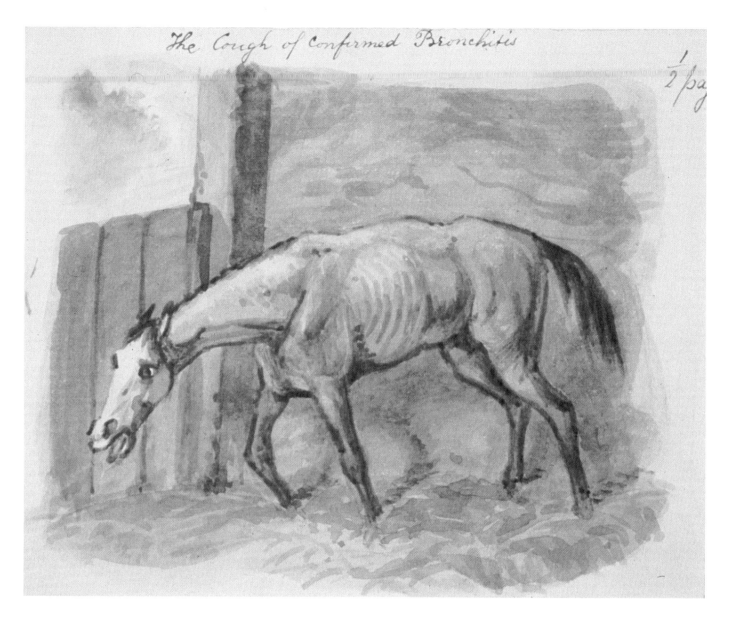

The Cough of Confirmed Bronchitis

lowed by a dose of ether and laudanum. Bronchitis required a more aggressive approach. Continuous steaming was desirable, and a poultice held in place with an eight-tailed bandage around the throat was used for this respiratory problem. A waterproof jacket held in place by holes for the forelegs was applied to the thorax. Flannel kept moist in cold water was wrapped around the chest and kept in place by the jacket. The ether and laudanum medication was used, and only gruel was allowed as food.

Heaves (broken wind) in the horse was seen to be analogous to dry asthma in people. At that time it was thought to originate in the mismanaged digestive tract of working horses, but it soon affected the pulmonary system and other organs. Signs began with a dry hacking cough, ravenous appetite and thirst, indigestion with profuse flatus, and a pendulous abdomen. The diagnostic feature of the condition was the double effort required on expiration, which was due to the emphysema resulting from the loss of elastic recoil by the lungs. Poor-quality feed, overwork, and unsanitary conditions were often partners in the origin of the syndrome. The disease was considered preventable by careful management but never curable. Fatigue could trigger a severe spasm in an affected animal.

Pneumonia was characterized by labored breathing resulting from the loss of elasticity of the inflamed lungs, dejection, and standing with legs spread to help breathing. The treatment was to steam and to dose with a solution of aconite, ether, and belladonna. Lying down was a hoped-for sign of improvement.

386. Mayhew believed most cases of bronchitis were caused by allowing the horse to stand in cold, wet weather after subjecting it to hard labor. Repeated bouts of coughing accompanied by nasal discharge were very bad signs. *(Courtesy The Royal College of Veterinary Surgeons, Wellcome Library, London.)*

443

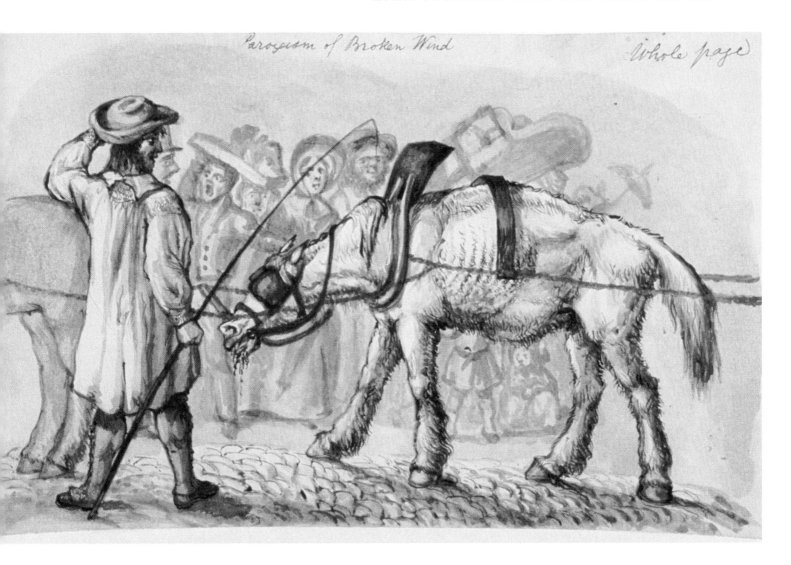

Paroxysm of Broken Wind

Whole page

387. Diagnosis of heaves, or broken wind, was based on the labored second effort on expiration caused by lung emphysema. Fatigue could bring on a convulsive spasm. *(Courtesy The Royal College of Veterinary Surgeons, Wellcome Library, London.)*

Pleurisy was an agonizing affliction, the pain almost on a par with that caused by colic, from which it had to be differentiated. The pain was reflected in the pulse. The rubbing of the inflamed pleural membranes could be heard by listening to the chest. Pressure applied with the fingers to the intercostal spaces caused anguish. Left alone, the animal might lift a foreleg, grimace, and look at its flank as if to locate the cause of its suffering. Oral treatment involved alternating tincture of aconite with ether and tincture of opium. A common sequel was hydrothorax, in which event surgical tapping of the fluid was performed. The outcome was still uncertain, however, and potent drugs were used in the attempt to tilt the odds in the horse's favor. An unusual condition was spasm of the diaphragm in an overexerted horse, which gave rise to a thumping sound. Cardiac disease, seen infrequently, was said at the time to be incurable. Purpura hemorrhagica was a puzzling condition, frequently fatal, involving generalized vascular congestion and swellings that arose on the body. The tongue might protrude, and patches of skin might slough.

Influenza was known to be capable of rapid spread through a stable. It was considered to make its impact felt on every part of the body. Early signs included yellowing of the conjunctiva, the white of the eye, and other mucosa and a sudden onset of weakness. The head was hung down, and respiratory sounds had a grating quality and were accompanied by a copious nasal discharge. Often a leg was held off the floor because of pain. Appetite was lost, the pulse feeble. As the disease progressed, the animal could barely stand or walk. When the discharge from the nostrils flowed more freely and coughing started, the pulse strengthened, becoming less wiry, and the animal usually was turning the corner on the road to recovery.

DISEASES OF THE DIGESTIVE TRACT

Horses were notoriously susceptible to disorders of the digestive tract. Mayhew noted that "abdominal cases are never easy, nor can one be confident of what may occur." Magical powders were commonly marketed by quacks with the claim that they would assuredly improve the condition and performance of the horse, thereby increasing the master's satisfaction. Ignorant carters and grooms added these powders to the oats. The inability of horses to vomit renders them unable to eject a toxic substance once it is swallowed. Affected animals suffered greatly, exhibiting signs of colic, straining, heaving, belching, sometimes squatting, and striking at the abdomen. These signs could progress to convulsions and madness. Treatment included alkalies, opium, and ether; carbonate of ammonia was added if the pulse was weak.

Chronic gastritis might begin with a bout of acute diarrhea followed by constipation and pica, leading to an abnormal, foul-smelling stool. The abdomen became pendulous, the coat rough and dry, and emaciation set in. Bitters, alkalies, sedatives, alkaloids, and minerals were administered in a kind of scattershot treatment. Mayhew attributed the problem to unhealthy, dirty, poorly ventilated stables.

The large larvae of the botfly, called bots, were frequently present in the stomach. The larvae stayed attached to the gastric mucosa for a year. Bracy Clark, a veterinary surgeon in London, described the life cycle of *Oestrus equi,* the botfly, which inhabits pastures and deposits its eggs, usually, on the inside of the knee or the side of the shoulder, whence the larvae were licked after the eggs hatched, swallowed, and attached by hooks to the stomach lining. Clark also described another species, *Oestrus hemorrhoidalis,* that lays its eggs on the hair of the horse's lower lip. The larvae get into the stomach and attach but later are found attached to the rectum or inner verge of the anus, where they cause severe irritation and discomfort. In Mayhew's day no medications were available that would remove the bots, and he recognized that those they tried caused some degree of unthriftiness.

Roundworms and tapeworms were recognized intestinal parasites. Tapeworms in young horses were considered to cause indigestion and abnormal behavior, such as biting the hair off the legs and violently rubbing the nose on a hard object. Quassia in turpentine was said to remove the *Taenia* parasite. The roundworms, such as ascarids, were said to be always in the rectum. Larger ones, called lumbrici, were considered relatively harmless. The strongyli were found to be more harmful, eating through structures and being hard to eradicate, if only because of the large numbers present. The location of some nematodes in the large intestine led to the use of tobacco smoke enemas after other agents failed. The first products to be used were train oil, followed by catechu daily for a week, then a mild physic (aloes and calomel). Should these products not yield the desired outcome, arsenicals and ale were tried. Because of irritation, afflicted horses would disfigure their tail and rump by rubbing violently.

Enteritis and dysentery were known to have many possible causes, but these had not yet been identified. Shallow breathing, along with a hot, dry mouth and a quickened, wiry pulse, was said to be typical of enteritis. The common diagnostic test was to apply manual pressure to the abdomen, but because this was unbearable to the animal with enteritis, it was a dangerous maneuver. The affected horse would attempt to kick and bite. Mayhew considered rectal palpation necessary to confirm diagnosis. Affected animals showed hard, offensive, shrunken fecal balls with streaks of mucus on their surface. The inflammation of the bowels could be sensed as a palpable rise in temperature, the confirming evidence. He recommended a light bleed of up to a quart, following which a pint of water at body temperature was infused into the vein. This treatment induced purgation and perspiration. An aconite drench, followed by repeated doses of an aqueous concoction containing aconite, laudanum, belladonna, and ether, was used. In the event that signs of lingering dull abdominal pain persisted despite these heroic measures, a cloth steeped in liquor of ammonia, diluted one part to six in water, was held against the abdomen for up to half an hour but was removed if blistering occurred.

Dysentery was differentiated from both enteritis and simple diarrhea, being much more violent than the latter. Dysentery was attributed to ingestion or administration of some acrid substance taken into the stomach. Examples given included arsenic, corrosive sublimate, tartar emetic, and blue stone (copper sulfate), all gastrointestinal irritants. Most of these problems arose because of fixed ideas of uneducated grooms or through their consultation with quacks. There was usually a payoff for the groom, which introduced a self-serving aspect. Most masters were ignorant about equine medication and poisons and were easily misled. Mayhew made the point that even the equine purgative in widest use, aloes, had a narrow margin of safety and should not be entrusted to a groom who reveled in violent purgation (sixteen to eighteen defecations) and tenesmus (straining) and hence tended to elevate the dose to a dangerous level. The only treatment for a severe case of dysentery was to give soothing drenches and hope that the poisons could be passed before the damage became irreversible and death ensued. Chronic dysentery was seen in older animals with emaciation, discomfort, and depression. Ascites, or presence of fluid in the abdominal cavity, a hopeless condition that could be detected by palpation, also occurred in old animals as a result of neglectful management.

COLICS AND OTHER MECHANICAL DISORDERS OF THE ABDOMEN

Colic has been forever a hazard for the horse because of a predisposition engendered by the design of its digestive tract. Abdominal surgery was not conducted on horses in the old days because it was believed that the horse was susceptible to lethal peritonitis resulting from operations involving incisions that penetrated the abdominal cavity. Colic is a term for bellyache, but the horse appears to be uniquely susceptible to the severe spasmodic form of colic affecting the small intestine. It started suddenly in most cases. The horse might suddenly stop eating, raise its head, and scrape the floor with a forefoot. If this first pain continued, the back leg might flex to kick the abdomen, the pawing continued, and the horse looked anxiously at its flank.

The bout of pain might pass, but it would recur and worsen; the horse would become more desperate in seeking relief in vain. This stage might culminate in an upward leap followed by a violent fall. The horse then rolled from side to side, kicking and trying to roll onto its back. The horse should be placed in a loose box with straw-truss padding all around the walls and deep bedding on the floor. The first treatment given was ether and laudanum, three doses at ten-minute intervals. If relief was not obtained, the dosages were doubled. A turpentine enema was often used as an adjunct, and the ammoniacal blister cloth applied to the abdominal wall was sometimes deployed. These measures, instituted early, often gave a favorable response. If not, a more serious syndrome than simple colic must have been present. According to Mayhew, "no disease is more quickly dispelled, nor . . . occasions greater agony, is more fearful to witness, or leads to more terrible results than spasmodic colic."

Flatulent colic, a form of painful indigestion, was seen mainly in older horses that gorged on green feed. They appeared sleepy, were reluctant to move, occasionally passed wind (flatus), and had a heavy pulse. After a few days the abdomen became visibly distended and the poor beast became restless, its pupils dilated and vision impaired. Once this desperate stage was reached and early medications had failed to effect a cure, a trocar and cannula

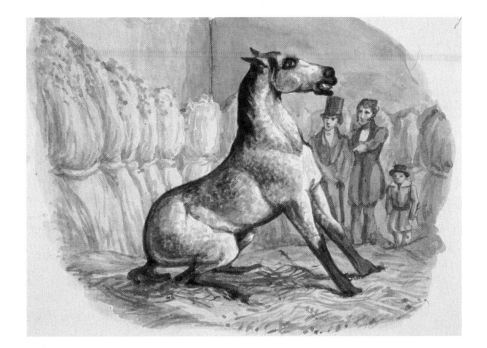

388. Abdominal injuries, often caused by the horses' performing large amounts of work, included damage and rupture of various structures. Unnatural attitudes such as dog sitting or kneeling were commonly assumed. Most injuries were left to correct themselves, with the horse placed in a stall cushioned with straw battens. *(Courtesy The Royal College of Veterinary Surgeons, Wellcome Library, London.)*

were inserted via a small nick in the skin into the cecum and the colon to allow the trapped gas to escape. Although this technique provided relief, it by no means ensured success.

Abdominal injuries were common when vast amounts of work were accomplished by horses. The results were often disastrous; severe damage to or rupture of various structures such as the diaphragm, spleen, stomach, or intestines occurred in some cases. In others, strangulation or intussusception was present. These conditions were agonizing and, except for splenic rupture, were untreatable, although some horses recovered on their own. Large calculi were occasionally seen in the bowel. Hepatitis was an obscure chronic disorder seen particularly in huge, obese brewers' horses fed on the refuse of the tub of fermented mash. Hepatitis also occurred in neglected carriage horses in times of low demand for their services. The severity of the disease might be missed until there was evidence of bleeding from the liver. Typically, repeated attacks were seen until a final, more severe event occurred and a fatal abdominal hemorrhage ensued.

DISEASES OF THE URINARY TRACT

Diseases affecting the urinary tract were thought to have been more frequent in older times but were still a common problem. The medieval practice of grooms was to keep "urine balls" available; these were actually composed of toxic doses of saltpeter and potent diuretics. Mayhew cautioned about the need to educate horsemen to eschew this practice. He made the point that the horse, to the informed observer, will indicate where the problem is. The horse with nephritis or cystitis manifested discomfort by straddling its hind legs, arching the lumbar region of the back, and turning its head repeatedly to look at the quarters with an anxious expression. The test recommended for nephritis was to press down on the loins, causing the affected animal to crouch. The urine production would be scanty, and the fast, hard pulse and rapid, shallow breathing indicated continuous pain. Gentle palpation per rectum allowed the detection of heat radiating from the inflamed kidneys and the pain of any pressure applied around them. An assistant should lift a foreleg to prevent a violent reaction. Unless treatment was initiated soon after onset of signs, the probability of a chronic condition was considered quite high. A

To head Nephritis

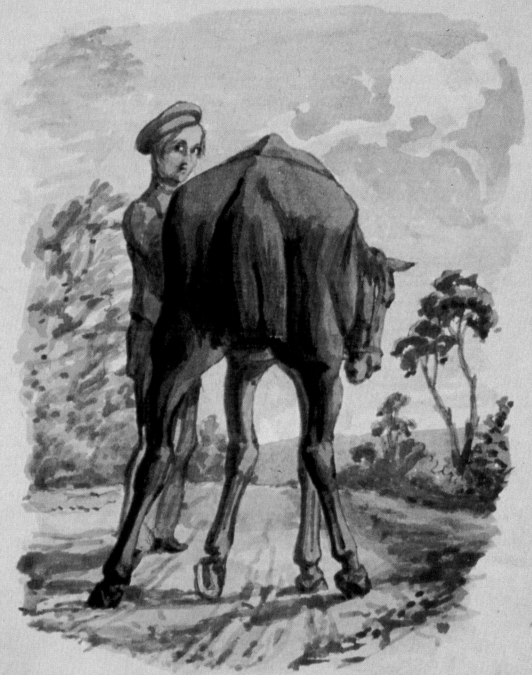

General Symptom of some disease of the Urinary Organs

mustard poultice applied on the loins and overlaid with sheepskins was recommended. This treatment would be supplemented with applications of linseed, croton, belladonna, calomel, and opium. Later, aconite and belladonna were the standbys used to lower the circulation.

Cystitis was a less common, less serious syndrome than was nephritis. Treatment for cystitis was similar to that for nephritis but was supplemented with the ammoniacal cloth, the counterirritant used in cases of severe colic. Calculi might appear in the kidneys, the ureters, the bladder, or the urethra. Extreme pain was observed, and the horse's back was roached. Palpation helped determine the site of the stone. For renal stones the only treatment was to provide water containing hydrochloric acid for the horse to drink, but the prognosis was unfavorable. Stones in the bladder were removed by surgical lithotomy in the male or via Simmonds's instrument for mares. A related condition, spasm of the urethra, was diagnosed by palpation of the greatly enlarged bladder, which could not be emptied, but the cause was not discernable. An extreme remedy used for this desperate situation, which caused extreme anguish, was to bleed the horse rapidly until the spasm relaxed and profuse urination occurred or until the horse fell in a faint and the contents of the bladder could be expressed manually by gentle pressure per rectum. Hematuria was another serious, alarming condition lacking a specific remedy. Lead acetate was used in treatment, along with laudanum or opium. In the event of failure to respond, ergot of rye, considered an experimental agent, was used to arrest bleeding.

Profuse staling, or excessive urination, was already recognized as diabetes insipidus (which resulted in tasteless urine as compared with the sweet urine of diabetes mellitus). It could be induced by a groom's ill-advised use of turpentine or sweet niter. Treatment was potassium iodide, which reduced the extreme desire for fluids and the urine volume while also improving the skin. Albuminuria was an unusual condition rarely seen in the horse, which caused the horse either to adopt a sawhorse position or to bring both hind legs forward but spread. The horse passed a thick urine that produced a precipitate when calomel was added to it.

THE SKIN AND ITS MALADIES

Stable itch or mange, caused by mange mites, was prevalent in neglected and poorly managed horses, especially when horses were taken from a variety of sources. It was recognized to be a highly contagious disease that progressed rapidly when horses were poorly fed and seldom groomed. The lesions commenced as itchiness in the mane, then spread over the whole body, leaving dry, rough bare patches where the hairs dropped out or were rubbed out. Scratching the roots of the affected mane caused the horse to extend its head and neck in ecstasy. Strong liniments or washes were applied several times in a treatment that contained an agent toxic for the parasite such as creosote and turpentine or corrosive sublimate solution with tobacco. A spring itch, known as prurigo, mimicked the signs of mange, but it was not a serious condition and soon cleared up.

In the treatment of ringworm, a cause of hair loss that was not well understood at that time, Mayhew applied a salve composed of glycerine with spermaceti and lead iodide after thoroughly denuding the affected area by washing it with hot, soapy water and drying it carefully.

A variety of lesser evils afflicted the body surface of horses. Surfeit was an eruption of raised heat spots or hives in hot weather that today would be called an allergic reaction. The hives would usually pass in a few weeks. Hidebound was a loss of skin elasticity seen in neglected animals given poor-quality feed and exposed to inclement weather. Lice were a feature of unkempt stock in filthy environments. Larval abscesses in the skin occurred

389. *Facing page,* Horses often exhibited signs of urinary discomfort: straddling of their hind legs, arching of the lumbar region of the back, and turning of the head repeatedly to look at the hind quarters. *(Courtesy The Royal College of Veterinary Surgeons, Wellcome Library, London.)*

when pastured animals were bitten by flies that deposited eggs on the skin or hair. The larval maggots burrowing into the integument caused the abscesses. Multiple warts were an extremely unsightly disfigurement, often appearing first on the head and neck. Two types were discerned, one encased in a cuticle, which tended to be self-bursting, and the other without a surface cap, which tended to keep growing with a rough surface. Treatment was surgical excision or repeated application of caustic substances to destroy the tissue of the growths. A sitfast was a painful, cornlike growth under the saddle that sidelined the animal until a cure could be effected.

Tumors occurred at various sites, many on or under the body surface of the horse. They were to be treated with caution because the outcome was frequently unfavorable after surgery. The worst kind of tumor, known as melanosis in light grey or white horses, was prone to become malignant and incurable. Starting as a small, firm lump, it might remain fairly stable for several years. When it entered the active stage, however, it suddenly enlarged and became soft and fluctuating to the touch. The animal's mood became despondent and slothful. A small pimple at the base of the tail in an old grey horse that was turning white was a giveaway diagnostic sign. The horse became useless and reluctant to move. When it was put down, the internal organs were found to be covered with metastatic tumors.

Stocking, or swelling of the hind limbs below the hock, was a common complaint seen in heavy work horses the morning after Sunday's stagnation in stables and in coach horses after a rest day. It was a circulatory problem that could be avoided by attention to diet and exercise. Water farcy was a related condition seen as dropsy of the hind leg in heavy work horses.

The lower parts of the limbs were frequent sites of dermal disorders, particularly when managerial practices were substandard. Grease, the prime disorder, was an inflammation that started in the sebaceous glands, usually of the rear legs. Unsanitary stalls where the hind feet were always in the urine and fecal wastes predisposed the tissues to the problem. The condition generated a characteristic pungent, foul odor. Swollen fetlocks with exudation and scurf were seen; the uneasy horse stamped noisily because of the irritation and used one hoof to scratch the back of the opposite fetlock. The disease progressed to produce cracks in the affected skin that became ulcerated and purulent. Untreated, the distal limb enlarged and granulation tissue developed in ragged bunches that became hard. The remaining skin became hypersensitive, the hoof enlarged. Early cases were treated with zinc chloride and glycerine after the site was cleaned. More severe cases with cracks were treated with potassium permanganate. If granulations had sprouted, casting and surgical removal of the proud flesh were required, and hot metal was applied to stem the resulting hemorrhage.

Mallenders and sallenders were names applied to the appearance of scurfy patches on the knees and hocks, respectively. Their presence at the points of greatest flexion was suggestive of a period of idleness and neglect. An ointment containing mercurials and camphor was recommended.

Cracked heels were attributed to working in cold, wet conditions and removal of the protective hair behind the fetlock to make grooming easier. The condition bore some similarity to grease and was treated similarly with washes and salves.

DISEASES OF THE LOCOMOTOR SYSTEM

The structure and function of the limbs and hooves were central to the value of the animal that was the key to human transport, traction, sport, and much military activity. Because of the heavy use these parts had to bear, they were vulnerable to many dysfunctions and diseases leading to lameness. One category of problems was the tendency for damaging osseous deposits to form at stress points. Spavins and splints were examples of the transformation of ligaments into bone on the hock and the knee, respectively. The foot of a leg with a bone spavin could not be lifted freely at the trot; instead it scraped the ground as it moved along, leading to excess wear on the toe of the hoof and shoe. The spavin progressively reduced the mobility of the hock joint and might ultimately lead to the joint's becoming locked. The only treatment for the condition was said to be complete rest and good food. Mayhew said that the many devilries of brutal treatments administered or marketed by unscrupulous charlatans for this condition brought great additional suffering to the horse and should be condemned.

Splints occurred in nature, but their incidence was increased by the horseman's desire for a high prancing action. This type of movement placed strain on the fibrocartilaginous tissues of the joints of the forelimbs, such as the union between the splint bones and the cannon bone and between the shin bone and the accessory bones on each side of it. Exostoses formed at these sites and, once initiated, occurred at other related sites. If the bony excrescence was in the vicinity of a tendon, movement caused severe pain.

Spavin and splints were more often diseases of horses bred for speed or a fancy gait than of those used for heavy draft. Ringbone, on the other hand, was a form of exostosis seen particularly in draft horses that had to pull heavy loads up hills. Here the stress came on the joints between the pastern bones and between the small pastern and pedal bones, as well as on the extensor pedis tendon that ran down the front of them. As the osseous deposits developed, pulling hard became progressively more painful and the horse became incapacitated for heavy work. Treatment consisted of rest, powdered opium to allay the pain, and lead iodide applications to the affected leg. Sidebones or ossified cartilages on the wings of the coffin bone were also incurable and caused loss of the elasticity of the rear part of the hoof.

The horse's movements are made possible by mighty muscles drawing on beautifully made strong tendons attached to bones. Even these wonderful tendons, however, are susceptible to strain and tear. The flexor tendons of the forelimbs are particularly subject to strain: bowed tendon occurs frequently, even today. Earlier, tendon strain was also seen in the rear legs of shaft horses that were required to hold back a load while going down a steep decline.

Severe sprains of the tendons in the past were called clap of the back sinews, a confusing term, since it was applied to the forelegs. Foreleg sprains were so severe that the horse could only hobble, resting the injured limb on the toe. Even after prolonged rest and healing, although function had returned, a swelling would persist at the site of the tear in the tendon. Sprain of the back sinews, on the other hand, referred to an injury to the hind limbs of hauling horses caused by the excessive strain imparted when the horses held back loads on the downhill slopes of hilly roads. The damaged horse would hold its heel off the ground to relieve the pain. Such injuries to tendons required many months of rest, and there was always a risk of contraction of the tendon after healing. The ultimate insult to a tendon was seen in racehorses in which the "back sinews" (again, of the forelimb) actually ruptured during the race, causing a complete breakdown. No cure was recognized that would restore the capacity to race, but a degree of healing could occur, although large, unsightly swellings persisted. The only value of the animal would be for breeding or as a pet.

Curb was a result of strain on the tendon of the hock or of its sheath, or both. Undue stresses of the hunting field or stresses resulting from a ridden horse rearing were thought to be factors in the origin of the condition. A swelling was visible on the rear, just below the point of the hock.

The joints of the limbs were subject to a number of lesions resulting from the many stresses and strains imposed on them. In occult spavin there was actual ulceration of the synovial membrane and the underlying cartilage, often within swelling or heat. Clearly this was a serious condition for which there was no specific therapy, but Mayhew tried experimental treatments, including injections into the affected area followed by slinging of the animal. Windgalls was a name given to distentions of synovial membranes, usually on the hind limbs. Although the evidence of their presence was seen as swelling in the groove between the flexor tendons and the suspensory ligaments, dissection revealed that they were, in fact, synovial enlargements of the tendon sheaths, presumably a result of excessive secretion of synovial fluid.

Bog spavin was a distention of the inward and forward part of the upper hock joint caused by an expansion of the synovial fluid thought to result from repeated shocks to the limb such as might occur during rough breaking. Although the horse usually did not manifest signs of pain from the lesion, the animal was blemished.

Thoroughpin was a swelling seen on both sides of a hind leg just ahead of the point of the hock. A synovial swelling, thoroughpin was similar to bog spavin, and sometimes the two occurred concurrently. Blows striking the knees could give rise to synovial swellings. Similarly, blows received by the hocks (as in kicking) and elbows could lead to swellings, but these were of the bursae that protected those sites. Thus capped hock or elbow was a bursitis. Capped elbow might result from the caulkin of the front shoe or the point of the hind foot striking the elbow.

A dramatic, treatable condition was luxation of the patella. The affected animal had one hind leg thrust backward and a lump on the outside of the thigh. The bone was replaced manually as assistants held the horse and pulled the affected limb upward and forward. Relapse could occur.

The advent of rheumatism, said to be a common sequel to influenza, was announced by swelling of the joints accompanied by painful lameness. The sites could shift with time, adding to the suffering and confusing the veterinarian. The swelling of joints and associated pain were protracted. Early treatment consisted of steaming, as for bronchitis, and application of liniment to the affected joints. In severe cases, to relieve the pain of weightbearing, the horse had to be placed in a sling.

390. Lateral luxation of the patella. The horse's entire frame is affected, with the head held erect and the muscles aquiver. Note the marked flexion of the pastern of the affected leg. If forced, the animal can ambulate on only three legs. *(Courtesy The Royal College of Veterinary Surgeons, Wellcome Library, London.)*

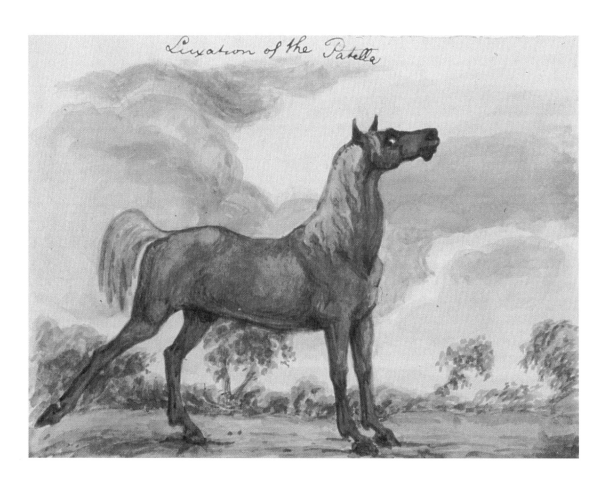

452

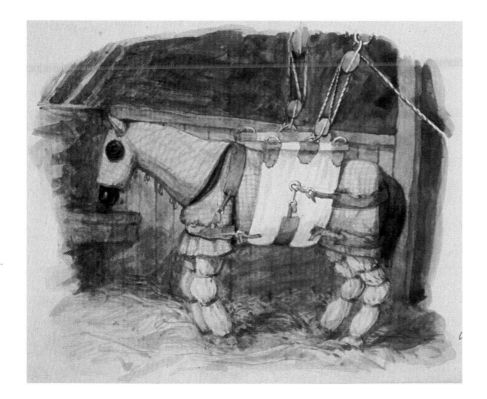

391. Rheumatism was accompanied by severe chronic pain and was thought to be a sequel to influenza. Treatment ranged from steaming and the use of liniment on the limbs, which were then encased in flannel, to covering the body and head along with the use of slings to take the weight off the legs. *(Courtesy The Royal College of Veterinary Surgeons, Wellcome Library, London.)*

DISEASES AND TRAUMATIC INJURIES OF THE FEET

So much wear and tear was imposed on the horse's hooves, its points of contact with the ground against which force-generating movement was applied, that the hoof and adjacent structures were the loci for many problems that led to lameness. Deformities such as "pumice foot" were produced by excessive work on cobbled streets in animals whose hoof structures had become weakened. The pasterns were long and slanting, the crust of the defective hoof chipped and broken by the nails, and the horn showed rings indicative of its irregular formation. The sole bulged and transmitted stress to the coffin bone, which became enlarged, exacerbating the problem. The hoof had to be protected by corrective shoeing to prevent further contact of the sole with the ground and by treating the hoof with glycerine and tar.

Sandcrack was a troublesome condition, the quarter form being seen at the inner quarter of the hoof of light horses and the toe form seen in the horn at the front in cart horses. The trick was to cut off newly forming horn at the coronet, since the stresses of the moving hoof tended to expand the existing crack upward to split the new horn, too. This measure was assisted by special shoe design. False quarter was an incurable state in which a segment of the outer horn failed to form, leaving the hoof vulnerable to injury. Seedy toe involved failure of the union between the outer horn of the hoof and the soft inner layer. The detached portion had to be cut away.

Trauma to the feet of weary cart horses occurred frequently as a result of the hind feet crossing. Failure to lift the hind foot before the forefoot came down on it was seen in light horses, as was overreach, when the inner part of a hind foot struck the outer surface of the coronet of a forefoot.

Corns were a common problem in the forefeet and were considered a consequence of bruises to the sole resulting from movement of the dynamic coffin bone. The corn began as a small hemorrhage or bruise within the sole. Old corns were black and could be trimmed out with a knife. Young ones, however, were infiltrated with fresh scarlet blood and were a more serious problem. Sappy corns were milder, since only the serum and lymph were exuded. The worst corns were those that contained pus and were suppurating; the resulting pressure caused great pain.

Quittor was a devastating condition of the foot in which the pus that formed was contained by the inflexible horn of the hoof, leading to excruciating pain. The infection usually started in the coronet of the hind feet of cart horses and forefeet of light horses, a great swelling developing around the upper rim of the hoof. The pus broke through the laminae and formed internal sinuses that ran down under the sole until the coronet was perforated and the pus could escape to the outside of the hoof. Another form resulted when a prick from a nail during shoeing allowed infection to enter via the sensitive laminae, thence moving upward to the coronet before escaping. Once the pus started to escape, corrosive sublimate was introduced to the sinus via a probe. Mayhew noted that the development of quittor could be avoided in most cases, if wounds and pricks were treated when they first occurred.

Thrush was a foul-smelling decay of the horn underneath the hoof that affected the cleft of the frog. Horses whose hind feet resided in filth were prone to the disease. Thrush also occurred in the forefeet in some cases of systemic disease and was often indicative of navicular disease. The stables had to be cleaned and kept that way, the feet thoroughly cleaned, and all decaying tissue cut away. Canker, a related foul condition, also resulted in fungoid growth that attacked the horn itself. In addition to the decay of the frog, fungoid horn proliferated around the margin at the edge of the sole. This fungoid granulation could be suppressed only with zinc chloride, which was kept dry with flour and compressed with padding that was held in place by pieces of iron under the shoe.

Laminitis, or fever in the feet, was a most injurious condition that could lead to the ruin of a horse. It was attributed to excessive stresses on the feet during long road hauls or long sea voyages. Laminitis might appear the morning after a hard drive, manifested as pure anguish. The horse's head was erect, its eyes glaring, and its back roached; the hind legs were advanced to relieve the afflicted forefeet, which were extended forward and touched the ground only at the heels. The horse was slung to take the weight off the forefeet. The hooves were soaked in hot water to soften them, then the horn was cut around the shoe nails to free them so that the shoe could be removed without force. Belladonna and digitalis were administered orally before this removal. After the horse was bled a quart, a pint of the blood was replaced by slowly injecting a pint of water into the vein. This procedure was invariably followed by copious purgation and perspiration, and the fever rapidly abated. The animal was watched day and night for seventy-two hours, and complete quiet was observed. If the artery by the pastern throbbed, the congestion was relieved by opening the pastern veins and plunging the foot into warm water. The great risk of laminitis was the suppuration, then casting, of a hoof or the descent of the coffin bone from its normal position so that the point pressed down on the sole. Both of these conditions were considered grounds for euthanasia.

Navicular disease was a result of damage to the lower surface of the small sesamoid navicular bone, which is linked to the posterior of the os pedis and rests on the tendon that attaches under the coffin bone. Mayhew attributed an increase in the incidence of navicular disease to the requirement of Principal Coleman of the London veterinary college that there must be pressure on the frog. Coleman's pronouncement caused smiths to shoe horses in a way that brought the frog as close to the ground as possible, and this practice led to the spread of the disease. When the weight of the horse came down on a stone, great pressure was applied through the frog and the tendon to the lower surface of the navicular bone. That bone's surface was susceptible to bruising and ulceration.

Although the initial lameness passed, the lesion often persisted and signs reappeared after a lag period. The horse would point the toe of the affected foot forward and take more weight on the sound one. A peculiar short, groggy gait developed in the effort to protect the painful member, and its

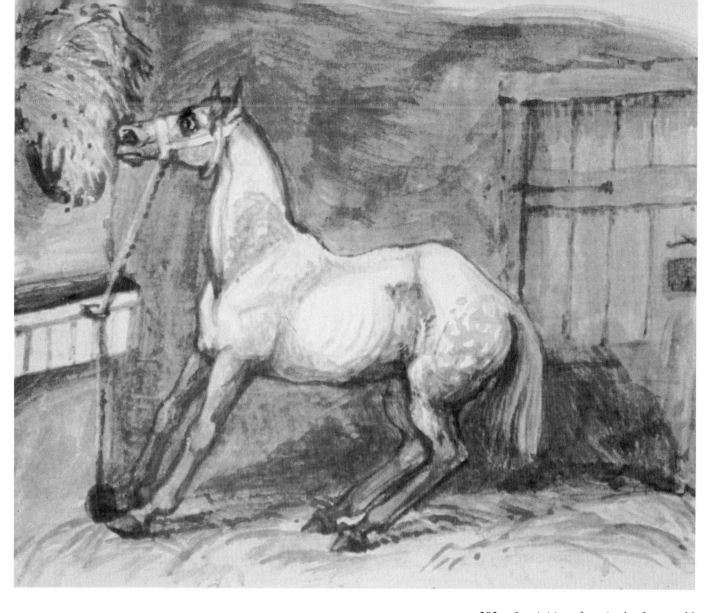

392. Laminitis, a fever in the feet, could have disastrous consequences. It was most often a result of long road hauls, and treatment of the disease was complex. The forefeet are thrust forward to relieve the agonizing pain in the hooves. The horse then settles most of its weight on the hind feet. *(Courtesy The Royal College of Veterinary Surgeons, Wellcome Library, London.)*

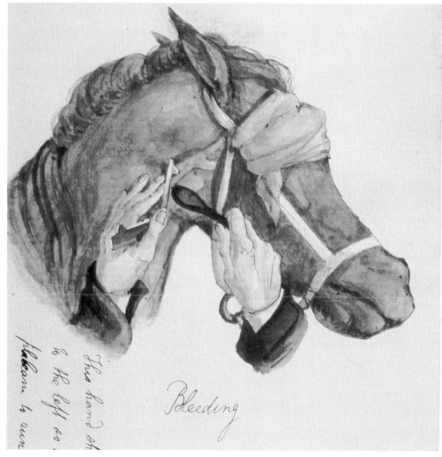

Bleeding

393. Bleeding, or phlebotomy: the art of using a fleam and mallet to bleed a horse from the jugular vein. This common practice was widely used in conditioning and treating horses. *(Courtesy The Royal College of Veterinary Surgeons, Wellcome Library, London.)*

wear was taken entirely on the toe. Avoidance of flexing the leg prevented the tendon from moving across the damaged surface. Mayhew said that the condition must be recognized as chronic and degenerative rather than inflammatory. The only hope for cure was to soak the foot in hot water for an hour on alternating days for two weeks, bandage it, provide a sponge boot, and give the horse a long rest.

TWO GREAT PLAGUES OF HORSES: STRANGLES AND GLANDERS

Strangles developed as an abscess under the jaw mainly in young animals after a vague general indisposition. The animal developed a stiff neck; then a hard, hot, tender enlargement appeared, along with a nasal discharge. The throat became inflamed and sore, breathing difficult. As the animal stood with eyes half closed and a stary coat, the discharge became more copious and anorexia set in. Gradually the swelling softened, and a focal point became discernable. The veterinary surgeon stepped in at this point and lanced the prominence, releasing a pint or more of pus. A prompt recovery ensued in most cases. In extreme cases, however, larger swellings obstructed breathing, and a flow of pus and tears from the eyes, thick drooling saliva, and a copious purulent nasal discharge were evident. Tracheotomy might be required to avoid suffocation. Occasionally the abscess ruptured internally into the guttural pouches, where the material solidified unless flushed out. Yet another form resulted in abscesses elsewhere in the body. Sometimes a horse's condition continued to deteriorate, and the animal had to be destroyed.

Glanders and farcy were widely held to be the most horrible diseases that horses could acquire. At one time the diseases were common in the posting stables and in long-stage teams. Reducing the body's resistance by exhaustion and an excess of stimulating food (oats and beans), coupled with chilling, was enough to allow the diseases to take hold. Glanders was the vigorous, active form of the disease, farcy the slow, progressive form. Not only were the diseases a desperate hazard to horses, but also they were dangerous for humans. It was astonishing to Mayhew that the law allowed the driving or riding of infective glandered animals through the streets. Glanders could kill a horse within a week. On the other hand, if the horse was allowed to rest and was given good food and a dry abode, it could live for years.

The usual pattern was the onset of fever, poor appetite, stary coat, and a rapid pulse. Then a slight nasal discharge started from one nostril, and the lymph node under the jaw on that side enlarged, hardened, and adhered to the mandible. Later the clear discharge became mucoid and started to encrust the parts over which it flowed. The fluid soon turned purulent and increased in volume; it had a characteristic odor. The next stage saw the nasal membranes turn to a dull, leaden color as the nostrils swelled, and the very act of breathing became a challenge. Pieces of decaying tissue and bone appeared in the nasal discharge, indicating the severity of the damage. After death, when the head was split to visualize the nasal septum, small granular tubercles and others that had ulcerated and become confluent could be seen. The pathological process advanced relentlessly back through the fauces to the pharynx and larynx, rendering swallowing impossible and causing the act of respiration to be excruciatingly painful and obstructed, and led to death, probably as a result of suffocation. Mayhew drew attention to a disgraceful trade in glandered horses and pleaded for legislation to prevent it.

Farcy, a version of the glanders contagion that was peculiarly the lot of the poor person's horse, was attributed to utter exhaustion. In cases of farcy, essentially a disease of the skin, "farcy buds" or swellings along the lymphatic channels formed and enlarged slowly, eroded through the surface, releasing matter, and ulcerated. Mayhew cited French work that showed farcy to be not

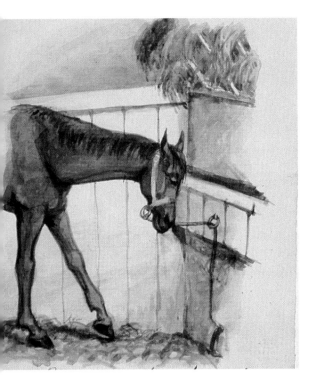

394. Mayhew postulated that changes in shoeing practices, which brought the frog close to the ground, were responsible for an increased incidence of navicular disease. Here the horse was "pointing" with the bad foot; the sound one is bearing most of the weight. *(Courtesy The Royal College of Veterinary Surgeons, Wellcome Library, London.)*

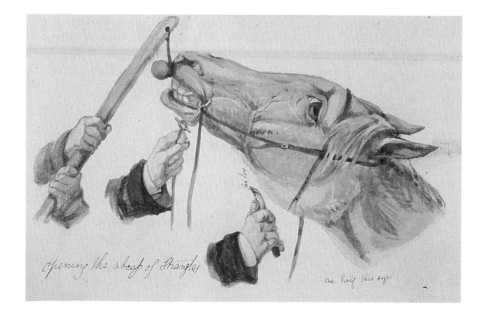

opening the abcess of Strangles

one half this size

395. Horses with strangles exhibited stiff neck, enlargement, nasal discharge, inflamed throat, and anorexia. A large swelling full of pus had to be lanced with an abscess knife. (*Courtesy The Royal College of Veterinary Surgeons, Wellcome Library, London.*)

just a superficial infection but a deep-seated systemic contagion. The disease caused a great thirst that could not be slaked by drinking. Although the superficial lesions of farcy were more accessible and amenable to local treatment than were those of the glanders form, it is unlikely that the infection was ever eliminated. The high-principled Mayhew deplored the treatment of glandered and farcied horses. Both for the humanitarian reason of avoiding further suffering on the part of the horses and to prevent spread of a ghastly disease that required every effort to eradicate, he urged that they be put down.

Horses were susceptible to a number of horrible infectious abscesses resulting from traumatic incidents. Poll evil usually resulted from beating about the head by ill-tempered carters; a great abscess slowly developed in the region of the poll. Fistulous withers began as an injury to one of the bursae that ease the motion of the dorsal projections of the thoracic vertebrae under the skin. The injury was thought to result from saddle pressure. A vile purulent process developed and spread, and surgical drainage and heroic treatment were required.

Despite the censure Mayhew incurred from some members of the veterinary profession for writing and illustrating *The Illustrated Horse Doctor*, it is a unique and priceless legacy that provides a clear and telling image in words and pictures of equine practice in those early times. It certainly enhanced the understanding of disease by horsemen, although it may have revealed the imperfections of veterinary knowledge to an embarrassing extent.

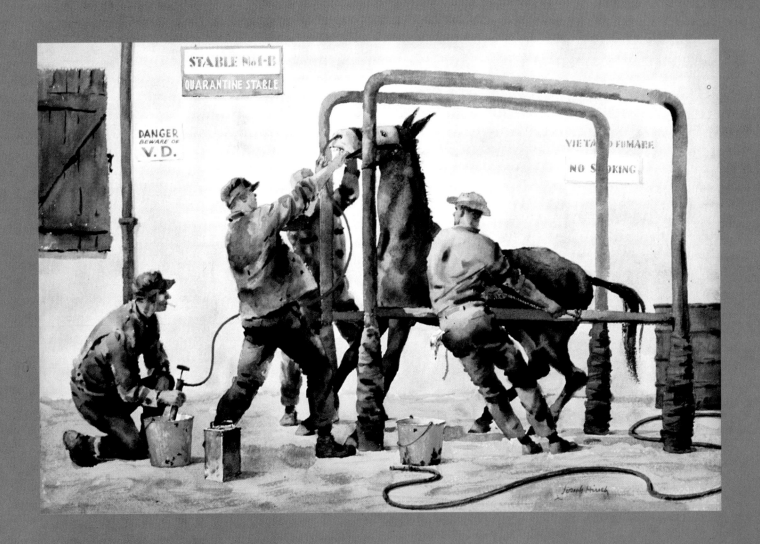

C H A P T E R   2 6

Care of Animals Used in Transport, War, and Sport

THE ORIGINS OF ANIMAL TRACTION IN TRANSPORT

As early tribal cultures evolved into civilizations, the domestication of animals generated clues to the deployment of animal muscle power to assist with the onerous manual tasks of clearing and cultivating areas of land for agriculture. Inventive humans designed and made systems of wooden yokes and leather straps to allow animal muscle energy to be converted into traction power. The idea of using this power to help with transport of goods and people followed the invention of the wheel by the Sumerians of Mesopotamia about 3000 BC. They constructed cumbersome wooden box wagons with four solid wheels, and the motive power was provided by teams of two or four onagers or oxen. Covered wagons and heavy, two-wheeled carts, usually drawn by a team of two, were also made.

The horse was trained to draft work about 2300 BC, and mules became popular for their strength and stamina. The "establishment" or the aristocracy capitalized on the greater speed of the horse by designing lighter carts. Archaeological evidence recently uncovered at sites in Russia, east of the Urals at Sintashta, and in Kazakhstan, two hundred miles east of Petrovka, has shown that light chariots with spoked wheels had been made about 2000 BC. A burial site found at Krivoe Ozero, about one hundred miles north of Sintashta, contained the heads of two horses killed and interred with a chariot and the body of a man. Such war chariots, light, fast, maneuverable vehicles, were used by noble warriors. After learning how to soak wood in water so that it could be bent and molded, the chariot makers fabricated spoked wheels with curved rims. The lightweight chariot soon became an essential weapon of war throughout the Mediterranean region and in West Asia.

It is surprising that a harness suitable for equids was a late achievement. The Chinese introduced shafts by the fourth century BC and led the way in the improvement of harness design, which culminated in the use of collars and traces. Thus the horse was able to advance the art of war and contribute to a popular new sport, chariot racing.

Riding probably began when small equids were first used for backpacking. Donkeys were probably ridden first, then mules. Mounted warriors on horseback did not appear in art until about 1100 BC. The nomads of the Eurasian steppes, probably in the Ukraine, were the first to break and ride horses. By the fifth century BC, mounted cavalry replaced the war chariot. Riders could travel astride from point to point, and progressive cultures developed systems of dispatch riders to hasten communication. Polo and racing on horseback became popular pastimes for warriors. Hunting game animals from the saddle occurred about the same time.

An engineering precursor to the opportunity for efficient travel was the design and construction of roads. The Assyrians developed disciplined armies

396. *Facing page, Treating a Mule,* a dynamic watercolor painting by American artist Joseph Hirsch (1910-1981), shows the U.S. Army Veterinary Corps in action during World War II. Hirsch and eleven other artists commissioned by Abbott Laboratories and accredited by the government produced two hundred and fifty paintings and drawings of the war effort for various uses during the conflict. His travels took him to the South Pacific, North Africa, and Italy. Hirsch's marvelous control of the medium is apparent in this painting, similar to Paulus Potter's *A Farrier's Shop* (Chapter 15), as the viewer is drawn to the action in controlling and treating a reluctant mule. *(U.S. Army Center of Military History.)*

that used chariots and made roads to provide for an expanding empire in Mesopotamia. They even bridged the Euphrates River, a major architectural feat. Earlier, the great rivers had been crossed on rafts made of bundles of reeds or on inflatable rafts made of sewn animal skins, which were more effective in the rapids of the Tigris. The rafts had to be hauled back upstream by towing from the shoreline, except in Egypt, where the prevailing north wind allowed sailing against the current of the Nile. The Assyrians made a partial transition to cavalry in the ninth century BC.

EVOLUTION OF THE DRAFT HORSE IN EUROPE AND AMERICA

The English war-horse was a result of a perceived need in the Middle Ages for bigger horses capable of carrying the great weight of rider, weapons, and armor. A few larger horses probably arrived with the Norman invasion of 1066. King John imported heavy black Flemish horses early in the thirteenth century. Edward I bought *destriers,* trained battle chargers, from France. Many war-horses were caught in concealed pit traps and lost to Robert Bruce's forces at Bannockburn in 1314. Henry VIII was concerned about the declining numbers and size of British war-horses. He passed laws forbidding the sale of horses outside England and requiring landowners to keep at least two mares and breed them to large stallions. During Queen Elizabeth's reign, large horses of the Almaine, Flanders, and Friesian breeds were imported. From all of these imports and efforts emerged the English great horse, usually black, as described by the veterinary surgeon William Youatt in *The Horse* in 1843.

397. The enormous contribution made by animal power to draft work in agriculture is portrayed in this product of photogravure, *A Stiff Pull* (before 1888), by Cuban-born English artist Peter Henry Emerson (1856-1936). Emerson's work frequently portrayed the critical role of the horse in the preindustrial farmer's life as mechanization approached. The two horses plowing the heavy soil of East Anglia are probably of the Suffolk Punch breed. *(National Gallery of Canada, Ottawa, Ontario.)*

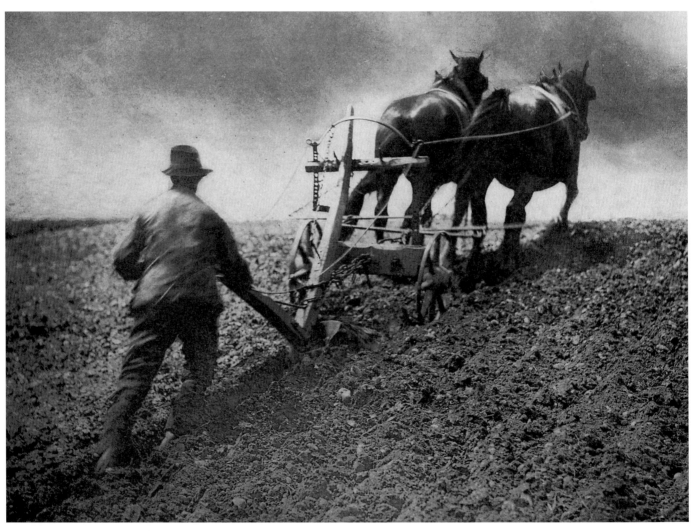

Large horses were used in transport to pull two-wheeled carts and four-wheeled wagons. The wagons were a Dutch development. The English modified them and developed many types of lighter coaches. The coach horse, a mixture of heavy and light horse inheritance, was more attractive and faster for moving people than the cart horse, which had replaced the plodding oxen for road work. Cornelius Vermuyden, a Dutchman who came to England in the seventeenth century to drain the fens, brought large Dutch horses. On the reclaimed land, heavy horses were bred, a nucleus of them in Lincolnshire and Cambridgeshire. In the late eighteenth century Robert Bakewell bred an improved type of cart horse from a base of the Leicestershire black horse, a descendant of the medieval war-horses imported from the Low Countries. Bakewell also imported several Dutch black mares. The great black shire horses drew the heavy, slow coaches and became progenitors of the large horses of English agriculture and the dray horses of London.

Modern breeds emerged. In 1863 the Royal Agricultural Society show identified breeds for the first time: Clydesdales, Suffolks, and a category of diverse breeds that included the old English shire. The English Cart Horse Society and Stud Book, which began in 1878, were precursors of the Shire Horse Society of 1884. The large shire horses had performed well in farm work, which then employed two thirds of England's horses.

The Flemish and Friesian stock contributed to the development of the shire and Clydesdale breeds. The Clydesdale, a leaner, faster animal with less hair on its longer legs, became more popular with overseas buyers. Its use was important in multiple-horse hitches in such regions as the Northwest in the United States and in parts of Australia, where large open areas were broken for wheat farming. Large teams were often used. This breed was also popular for timber harvesting in forested areas.

The old British chestnut-colored Suffolk Punch bloodline has been traced to 1506. The black or grey French Percheron arose in the French district of La Perche. The versatile breed, popular with royalty, was used for military, ceremonial, and draft purposes. Louis XIV sent two stallions and twenty mares to Canada in 1665. After the French Revolution a lighter type, in addition to the larger lines, was developed for coaching. The grey stallions were imported to Ohio in 1851; in time, however, the large black strains were preferred in the United States and many were imported. In France *Le Studbook de la Race Percheronne* was first produced by the Percheron Horse Society in 1883. British breeders imported more Percherons from France, America, and Canada. One goal was to cross the Percheron stallion with the lighter mares to produce the light draft horses needed for artillery and other rapid transport to the front lines in war. This plan was initiated during World War I; the demand declined after the war.

In peacetime the breed proved adaptable as a draft horse on the farm and as a coach and draft horse on the road. During World War II the French breeders exploited the Percheron as a walking, working meat supply in a time of desperate shortage of other meats. The attractive, massive, chestnut-colored Belgian breed, with light mane and tail, became popular in America. It remains popular for show and is often seen drawing brewery wagons.

An interesting analysis of animal draft power was provided by J.O. Williams and S.R. Speelman in the United States Department of Agriculture *Yearbook* for 1934. Their article, *Horses and Mules Meet Need for Cheap Flexible Farm Power, Studies Show,* was a response to the debate concerning the economics of mechanical versus animal traction. The authors acknowledged that one of the major arguments for the use of tractors was speed. The argument for animal draft power was that the speed of the machine could be matched by the use of the multiple-horse hitch, eight or more horses driven with a single pair of lines, which gave speed of operation and the greater flexibility of multiple units. The old walking plows had by 1934 given way to a multiple-bottom gang plow with a seat or sulky.

The authors reported the results of surveys of farmers. Surveys of farmers in the Corn Belt taken in 1929 and 1930 showed that hitches that allowed up to twelve horses in a gang, pulling a four-bottom plow, had been developed to be handled by one person. The most efficient plow was found to be a three-bottom plow drawn by seven horses, which could plow eleven acres a day at minimal cost. Similar results were obtained with other horse-drawn equipment. The average hours worked per head per year was 681. Average feed consumption per head per year was 5166 pounds of roughage plus 3205 pounds of concentrates. The animals were pastured for six months of the year. A similar survey of farmers in the Cotton Belt States of the South indicated that eighty-seven percent of all drawbar work was done by animal power, a combination of horse and mule power. However, there was far less application of large, multiple-hitch gangs in the South; one to four animals per hitch were typical. Although the animals used in the South were smaller, feed consumption per head was comparable, except that the pasture period was short.

Despite the optimistic analysis presented in 1934, the internal combustion engine spelled the doom of horsepower for draft work in developed countries. The passion for power and speed without the potential for perverse animal behavior was addictive. During the 1920s and 1930s the automobile, bus, and truck displaced the horse from the streets, and in the 1930s and 1940s the tractor did the same for the cart horse.

CONTINUING IMPORTANCE OF ANIMAL DRAFT POWER IN ASIA

The developing world still depends on draft animals. Indira Gandhi noted that in India in the early 1980s draft animals provided 30,000 megawatts of power, slightly more power than the total installed electrical capacity at that time, 29,000 megawatts. India's sixteen million ox-carts carried ten times the tonnage of freight carried on India's railways. One old-fashioned wooden cart drawn by two oxen could haul more than a ton for more than fifteen miles in one day in settled areas, interrupted only by extreme conditions such as mud, rocks, or sand. In the last decade the adoption of a new design of a low, cast steel "Animal-Drawn Vehicle" with roller bearings and rubber tires for use on the better roads has increased by two and a half times the weight of the load that can be hauled. Further refinements in yoke and collar design and the addition of a braking mechanism have been under development, since the neck and hump yokes in common use have been another source of inefficiency.

EQUINE COACH AND MAIL SERVICES

The progress in overland transportation made by the Romans depended in part on their planning and construction of major arterial roads, which permitted the movement of people and materials by animal-drawn vehicles or on horseback. After the Roman era the parochial organization of districts led to the development of local networks of roads with less regard for long-distance travel. The common denominator in most forms of road transport was the horse. During the Middle Ages the use of iron horseshoes was widely adopted to protect the hoof and reduce wear. This practice led to a great demand for blacksmiths, and the trade of farriery emerged.

Even by 1700 travel by horse-drawn coach, invented in Europe, was still a slow affair; in Great Britain, for example, the trip from London to Norwich took a week. The widespread implementation of stagecoaches, first introduced in 1640, with the horses changed every ten to fifteen miles, reduced the duration of that trip to less than two days by 1751; the average traveling speed was approximately ten miles per hour. Between 1760 and 1830 the speed of horse-drawn travel by mail coach increased significantly. Travel from

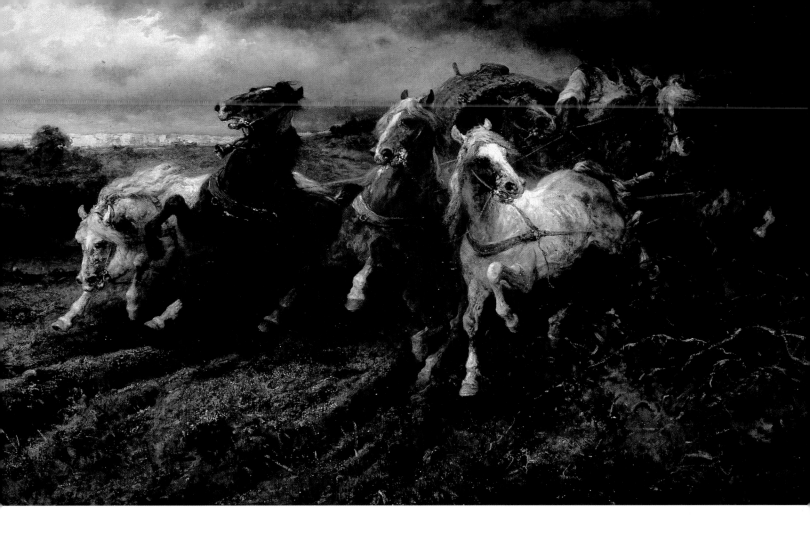

London to Birmingham took only sixteen hours, to Manchester, twenty-eight hours, and to Carlisle, on the Scottish border, forty-one hours. Travel by stagecoach peaked by the 1830s; the system was gradually displaced by railways for long-distance travel. The government mail was handled by a staging system of ten- to twenty-mile intervals run by postmasters who were often innkeepers. Post boys rode the stages until high-speed, four-horse coaches carrying passengers as well as mail started to replace them in the 1780s. Various types of private horse-drawn vehicles were developed, and turnpike trusts were set up to improve roads after 1663, with tolls collected by pikemen at barriers. Turnpikes lasted for more than two centuries, until competition from the railways progressively rendered the turnpikes redundant. The country's freight traveled slowly via the great roads. The introduction of John L. MacAdam's surface material was a great advance. Local travel in many rural areas continued to be horse-dependent until the Second World War.

From 1850 to the 1930s the horse was extremely important. Because its management and health care were primary concerns, the veterinary profession acquired a high profile. At the same time, the number of miles of railroad track in Great Britain increased from 5000 in 1848 to 14,500 by 1875. It had been anticipated that trucks would provide local feeder service to railroads, but trucks also took over most agricultural transport from the horse.

France was able to achieve dramatic changes in the efficiency of horse-drawn transport between 1765 and 1780, when the earliest veterinary schools appeared. In 1765 the trip from Rennes, in Brittany, to Strasbourg took nineteen days by coach, as did a trip from Brussels to Toulouse. By 1780 the former trip took nine days, the latter, eleven. Key factors were the betterment of the roads, the introduction of diligence services and strategic changing points, and improved horse care and veterinary maintenance. The veterinary schools focused attention on the preservation of horse health and the therapy for sick and injured horses at a time when horses were often driven beyond the limits of their endurance in both war and peace.

398. Adolf Schreyer (1828-1899) was a famous German painter of horses in rural and military action. In *The Wallachian Post-Carrier* he depicts the rural post service in a region that today is part of Romania. *(Milwaukee Art Museum, Layton Art Collection, Gift of Washington Becker.)*

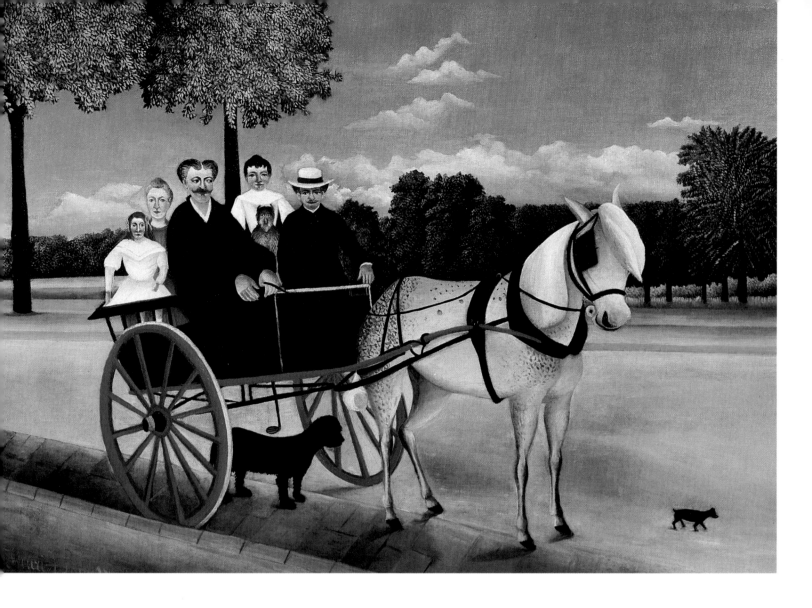

399. *Monsieur Juniet's Carriage* by Henri Rousseau (French, 1844-1910). A grocer's family outing in the Forest of Clamart in the last third of the nineteenth century was painted from a photograph. The attractive dapple-grey pony is led by a tiny dog and followed by a larger one. The privileged position of the family dog in the carriage reflects the family's strong bond with its animal companions. The posed expressions of the people in the cart are in contrast to the bemused charm of the pony. Rousseau is shown seated on the right. *(Lauros-Giraudon, Paris.)*

VETERINARY CARE FOR ANIMALS IN WARTIME

The veterinary profession had its origins in maintaining the animals used in warfare. During peacetime in the late eighteenth and the nineteenth centuries, draft, transport, and sport were priority activities in which animal power was exploited, and military activities involved diversions and training for the next war. When wars broke out, however, the military draft affected animals and their caretakers, the veterinarians.

The numbers of animals sacrificed in fighting the seemingly interminable wars were staggering. The veterinary roles became defined as providing first aid for the wounded, transporting animals to facilities at bases where they received veterinary attention, and assembling army remounts as replacements for the front lines. Although the major species used in wartime was the horse, the dog later played important roles, and in special environments other species were deployed, including the elephant, camel, mule, llama, ox, water buffalo, and homing pigeon. Other species, such as monkeys, bears, goats, and cats, were commonly adopted as mascots. In modern submarine warfare, dolphins and porpoises have been trained for active service.

The most detailed veterinary historical writings in English deal with war. Sir Frederick Smith wrote *A Veterinary History of the War in South Africa 1899-1902,* which was published as a supplement to the *Veterinary Record* on May 25, 1912. He wrote *A History of the Royal Army Veterinary Corps 1796-1919* in 1927. *The History of the Royal Army Veterinary Corps 1919-1961,* written by Brigadier J. Clabby, was published in 1963. *The Veterinary Military History of the United States,* written by Louis A. Merillat and Delwin M. Campbell in 1935, was followed by Everett B. Miller's *United States Army Veterinary Service in World*

War II in 1961. William H.H. Clark wrote *The History of the U.S. Army Veterinary Corps in Vietnam 1962-73* in 1991; he noted the tendency of the United States to demobilize its scout dog program after every war, leaving a disastrous state of unreadiness whenever a new war began. Thus documentation of the detailed history of wars involving British and North American veterinary services is excellent. Only a general perspective need be given here.

British Veterinary Services

The first British veterinary journal, *The Veterinarian,* began publication in 1828 under the editorship of a military veterinarian, William Percivall (1792-1854), who served in the First Life Guards from 1828 to 1854. Since then, a tradition of preserving the record of veterinary military service in war and peace has been upheld. The prolific writer George Fleming (1833-1901), who became Principal Veterinary Surgeon (PVS) of the Army Veterinary Department in 1883, was editor of *The Veterinarian* from 1876 to 1894. Historical records of the profession's role in military activities before 1828 are minimal, in part because James Collins (1830-1895), who was made PVS in 1876 and accomplished many needed reforms, had all previous records of the Army Veterinary Department destroyed.

Early Veterinarians in the British Army. According to Sir Frederick Smith, professional veterinarians first entered the British Army in 1796. Previously cavalry horse maintenance was entrusted to farriers who, in addition to being responsible for all shoeing requirements, were expected to "drench and let blood" when situations required such interventions. Repeated heavy losses of horses during military campaigns in the eighteenth century led to a call for an army veterinary service after the London veterinary school began.

In 1795 the second principal of the Royal Veterinary College, Edward Coleman, was charged by the commander in chief to create an army veterinary service. Coleman was made PVS of the cavalry in 1796 and veterinary surgeon to the Board of Ordnance (Artillery) in a civilian capacity. Coleman's military appointment was lucrative: he received per capita fees and percentages on drugs and supplies. Sir Astley Cooper (1768-1841), a famous surgeon who had studied for two years with John Hunter, dominated the veterinary profession for the four decades of Coleman's leadership. According to Smith, Cooper and Coleman shared a view that the appropriate social status for veterinary surgeons was to be the lowest rung on the medical ladder. Cooper used Coleman as the foil through which to put this view into practice. As principal, Coleman recruited uneducated men considered to be of mediocre or low intelligence. He said sons of farriers, grooms, and stablemen made the best veterinarians—an about-turn from the opinion of his predecessor, Sainbel. Thereby the leaders' alleged view became self-fulfilling.

As PVS, Coleman was required to produce a manual—*Instructions for the Use of Farriers Attached to the British Cavalry and to the Honourable Board of Ordnance*—which he did, in 1796. The savagery of the treatments it recommended is remarkable. These included cautery of the sides for pneumonia, of the belly for enteritis, and of the loins for nephritis, in each case supplemented by the use of rowels in the skin over the affected part. For staggers, four quarts of blood was to be taken, the poll blistered, rowels inserted in the abdominal wall, and *boiling* water poured on the pasterns twice a day. Seven years later these draconian measures were deleted from a second edition. Coleman's one valuable contribution was his insistence on proper hygiene of army stables, including good ventilation, improved feeds and feeding practices, and cleaning and drainage of stalls. Even in this, however, he was merely implementing measures that James Clark of Edinburgh had called for several years earlier. Also, Coleman's design for ventilation of stables was flawed and had to be revised by Karkeek, a practitioner in Truro.

Although the army veterinarians were at first ignorant of glanders, they later instituted measures that brought it under control. The advances came through the efforts of problem-solvers who emerged from the ranks of veterinarians whom Coleman sent to the army. John Percivall (1768-1830) (Willam's father), who qualified at the Royal Veterinary College in 1795, was appointed to assist the PVS and was to reside at Woolwich military base. Percivall started as a civilian and later became a veterinary officer in the Royal Artillery. Although he had to use the officially sanctioned treatments, he was the one who implemented the reforms. Among other effective army veterinarians were James Turner, whom Smith credited with the discovery of navicular disease, and James White and Thomas Peall, who conducted research confirming that glanders was infective. Peall, an Irishman, wrote *Diseases of the Horse* in 1814 and was made professor to the Dublin Society; he later joined the army. He succeeded in infecting a donkey with glanders by placing material from a horse infected with farcy in the ass's nostrils. Clinical signs of glanders appeared after eight days. White proved wrong Coleman's theory that glanders spread by miasma by conducting an experiment in which healthy horses that respired the expired air from a horse with glanders failed to acquire the disease. Ingestion of glandered material, however, readily produced the disease, as did inoculation.

The Royal Horse Artillery Infirmary, constructed at Woolwich in 1804, contained a horse hospital, veterinary stores, and facilities for research. The dedicated John Percivall worked there until 1830, when he died in his quarters. His successor, William Stockley (1776-1860), received his diploma from the Royal Veterinary College in 1794 and entered the army, where he became senior veterinary surgeon of the Ordnance. These two men established the credibility and value of veterinary surgeons in the army by setting high standards. Stockley was elected president of the Royal College of Veterinary Surgeons (RCVS) in 1857.

Coleman came under attack in 1830 both in *The Veterinarian* (William Percivall, editor) and in *The Hippiatrist* (Bracy Clark, editor) for his lucrative contract with the army as its PVS. These comments in the professional media cost Coleman his contract for medicines in 1832. Coleman published one supposedly scientific work on the horse, *Structure and Diseases of the Foot,* in 1798. It appears, however, that he developed strong opinions about how to trim and shoe hooves with no experimental basis, which resulted in the perpetuation of his erroneous ideas and their multiplication through his diplomates from the college and more than one generation of farriers.

The Veterinary Vision of William Percivall. Veterinary surgeons served on active duty with the British Army for the first time with expeditionary forces to Holland in 1799. Five veterinarians went, four with the cavalry and one with the artillery drivers. The first death of a British veterinary officer in war occurred during an expedition to South America: G. Lander of the Ninth Light Dragoons died in the attack on Buenos Aires in 1807. During the biggest campaign early veterinary officers participated in—the Iberian Peninsular War (1808-1814)—the first invasion via Portugal was a disaster. The horses were not conditioned, and the troops were forced to retreat and had to be evacuated from Corunna, in northwestern Spain. The next expedition went to the peninsula in 1809 and stayed five years. A devastating defeat was suffered at Talavera. William Percivall joined the Peninsular forces of Britain and Germany in 1813 and was present at the battles of Orthez and Toulouse. Writing to Lord Liverpool in 1811, the Duke of Wellington (1769-1852) described Spain as "the grave of horses." The Royal Horse Artillery had 1570 horses but received no veterinary support. Percivall also served in Belgium during the prelude to Waterloo in 1815.

William Percivall (John's son) had been appointed a veterinary officer in the Royal Artillery in 1813. After his return to England he trained in medicine at St. Thomas's Hospital under the distinguished surgeon Benjamin Travers, who had apprenticed with Astley Cooper. Travers became president of the Royal College of Surgeons. Percivall also became a licenciate of the Apothecaries Company. Continuing his scholarly pursuits, Percivall published his three-volume *Series of Elementary Lectures on the Veterinary Art* in 1823, five years before he began the first veterinary journal. The first volume was a joint effort by John and William. After these initiatives Coleman cut all further contact with the Percivall family, although John had been careful to preserve a cordial relationship with him. William Percivall also wrote *The Anatomy of the Horse* in 1832; the four-volume *Hippopathology,* published between 1834 and 1852; and *Lectures on the Form and Action of Horses* in 1850.

Percivall's perception was that the Royal Veterinary College in London had been asleep since Coleman's appointment and that the medical profession kept it that way by design, interfering with and governing the veterinary profession. The only hope was that pressure might come from a concerned public. Since only medical men were considered competent to examine the diploma candidates, Percivall took one member of the examining board to see a sick horse in his infirmary and invited him to make a diagnosis, which he was unable to do. Percivall demanded in vain that veterinary examiners be appointed at the London school. He was a visionary and warmly welcomed overtures by the Epidemiological Society in 1851 to seek veterinary cooperation in studying epizootic diseases. He feared for the future of the profession in the time of the advent of the steam engine and the expansion of railroads, which, he foresaw, would reduce demand for horsepower.

Coleman lacked any kind of practical or military experience. During the last decade of Coleman's life he came under repeated public criticism as principal of the Royal Veterinary College and PVS of the army. When William Dick inaugurated his veterinary school in Edinburgh, Coleman blocked Dick's graduates from army service. After 1839, when Coleman died at seventy-three years of age, Dick's much better trained graduates did get appointed to the service and made significant veterinary contributions.

In 1835 a paper written by J.S. Beech appeared in *The Veterinarian*. Beech was with the Anglo-Spanish Legion in Portugal. In *Gunshot, Sabre, Lance and Other Wounds* he included postmortem studies; in one case a horse had died within a few hours after being shot through the abdomen and diaphragm. The four holes in the intestine that resulted were already nearly closed with lymph exudate.

Coleman's stultifying autocracy in veterinary matters in Great Britain ended at his death, which created a long-overdue opportunity for reform that was soon acted upon in the army. Frederick Clifford Cherry (1779-1854) was selected to be the new PVS in 1839. He had considerable military experience and success in private practice before returning to the army. Appalled at the chaotic state of veterinary administration in the cavalry, he admitted graduates of the Dick school in Edinburgh and set much higher standards for veterinary officers than his predecessor had. He published several pamphlets on proper care of the horse's legs and feet. J.W. Gloag, an Irishman of the Tenth Hussars, published an interesting article in *The Veterinarian* in 1839, the year Cherry became PVS, entitled *Hints to Veterinary Surgeons Entering the Army Regarding Their Conduct, Duties, etc.* Despite the prevailing views, Gloag urged the new graduates not to let blood unless the procedure was considered absolutely necessary. He noted that glanders and cataract in horses were common in Ireland and described a special method by which horses should be humanely relieved of suffering by shooting.

Starving Horses in Military Campaigns.   Insufficient feed for horses in war was a major factor in many military campaigns in the eighteenth and nineteenth centuries. British forces in the Peninsular War (1808-1814), the First Afghan War (1838-1842), and the Crimean War (1853-1856) were certainly compromised by the problem, as were Napoleon's forces during his invasion of Russia, where he lost more than 300,000 men and 30,000 French horses. The total losses—of the 150,000 horses in the Grande Armée, which included Prussian and Austrian cavalry—must have been much higher. In 1809 Wellesley, the Duke of Wellington, wrote that losses of horses in the Peninsular War were rising because of a shortage of feed and the low quality of the feed the horses received. They could not work on a handful of barley and a little moldy hay each day. During the campaign of 1812 Murat, one of the French commanders, complained that cavalry charges were not executed with vigor. Nansouty replied, "The horses have no patriotism; the soldiers fight without bread, but the horses insist on oats."

Napoleon Bonaparte defeated Austria, Prussia, and much of Russia but was unable to overcome the British fleet after his invasion of Portugal and Spain. He tried to destroy Britain's economy by enforcing a blockade of all Continental ports. The French troops marched into Portugal in 1807. The next year they captured Madrid in a surprise attack. However, by installing his Brother Joseph on the Spanish throne, Napoleon triggered a massive popular revolt led by a junta. The British sent an expeditionary force to the Iberian Peninsula under Sir Arthur Wellesley, Duke of Wellington. The troops landed in Portugal, initiating the Peninsular War. His force of 13,500 men had only 180 cavalry horses; the three batteries of cannons had no driving horses to pull them. He had several commissaries from which to purchase needed supplies and animals. It took eight days to acquire the five hundred mules and three hundred oxen needed to tow the freight, and some freight had to be left on the beaches, including one gun battery. Only sixty cavalry horses were procured. Nevertheless, Wellington defeated the French attacks led by Marshal Junot. Wellington was recalled to England and relieved of command for allowing Junot to withdraw from Portugal without reprisal. Wellington's replacement, Sir John Moor, was reinforced with more troops and horses. The Spanish revolt, however, was disintegrating, and he was outnumbered ten to one by Napoleon's forces. Moor had to retreat and make a dash for the sea. He succeeded in evacuating his troops but ordered the slaughter of all horses for which no room could be found on board. Only the officers' horses embarked. The butchery of horses was bungled in the confusion, creating a horrifying spectacle.

After Wellington was reinstated, he returned to Portugal with a new, larger force and enlisted a sizable Portuguese army as well. Wellington held off Napoleon's reinforcements and led his troops through a series of victories culminating in the battle of Salamanca in 1812.

Wellington's great victory at Waterloo in 1815 was achieved with the able support of General Blücher, the Prussian commander. Losses of cavalry horses on both sides were heavy before Napoleon's forces were finally beaten. Cannon fire inflicted terrible wounds on horses. Percivall noted that he had never seen so many cases of gastric bloat as when the triumphant army allowed its horses to graze a field of growing wheat on its way back to Paris. Wellington personally rode and lost twelve chargers during the first three years of the Peninsular War. Then he acquired Copenhagen, a fine chestnut Thoroughbred stallion born in 1808, a grandson of Eclipse. Copenhagen survived Waterloo unscathed and was retired to Wellington's estate; the horse died in 1836.

The Afghan campaign of 1838 cost the British the lives of thirty thousand camels. Once again, mismanagement of animals caused huge losses. British forces traversing the Bolan Pass on their way to Kandahar had no animal feed and very little water. The animals wasted away. Half of the horses and virtually all of the camels died of starvation, exhaustion, and exposure. The Russians were faced with a similar catastrophe as their troops moved through central Asia under General Skobeloff, who had mustered a huge

400. *Facing page,* The charge of the Grey Scots. Detail from *Scotland Forever* (1881) by Lady E. Southerden Thompson Butler (English, 1844-1933) captures the courageous style of cavalry charges during the Battle of Waterloo under the Duke of Wellington in 1815. *(City Art Gallery, Leeds/Bridgeman Art Library, London.)*

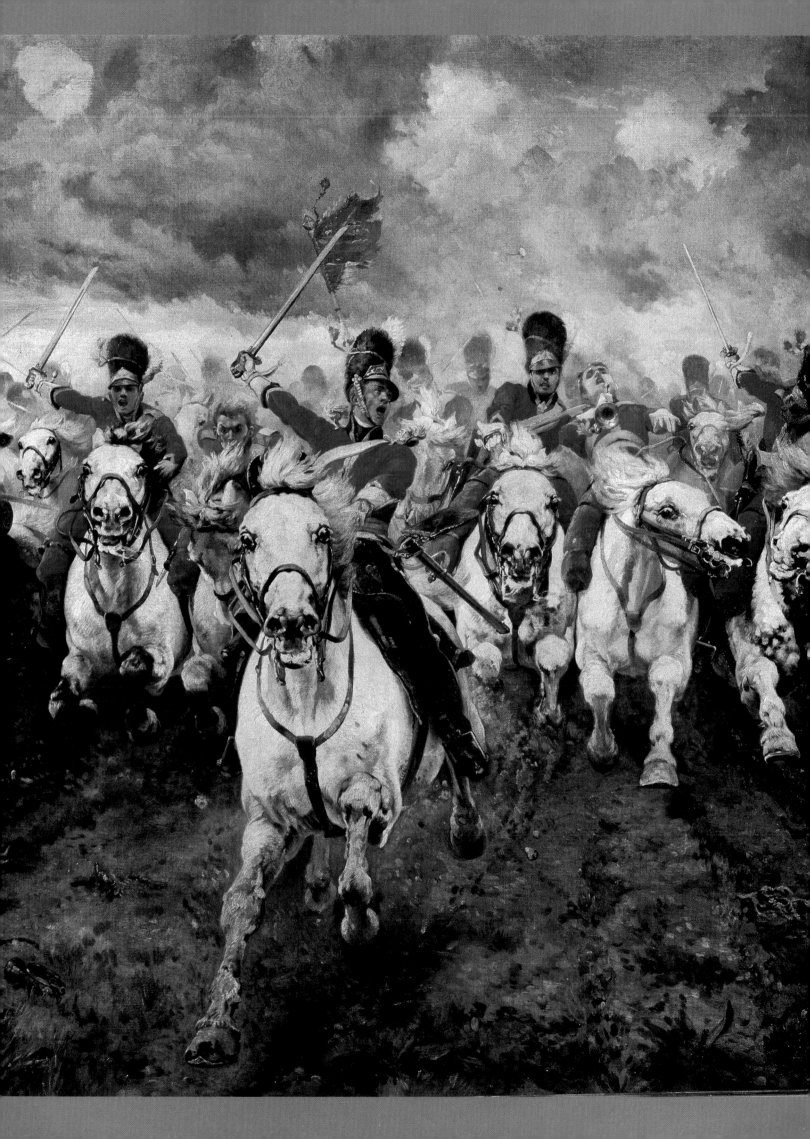

force of twelve thousand transport camels to cope with the arid conditions. Within a few months all but one camel had perished. The British decided to form a camel corps, which was to serve as a "mounted infantry" and take a shortcut across the Bayudu Desert to warn the Sudanese Mahdi's supporters that British troops were prepared to march to Khartoum and relieve the besieged General Gordon. The camels died by the thousands of exhaustion and starvation.

One great success with camels occurred during the First World War, when General Allenby employed the largest, best-organized camel force ever mustered to stop the Turkish advance. T.E. Lawrence (of Arabia), who repeatedly and successfully harassed the Turks with an Arab troop of camel-riding guerillas, participated in that military episode.

The British involvement in the Crimean War against Russia began badly when British forces decided to send their horses on sailing ships. The army had failed to take the advice of its veterinary officers to provide enough medicines and supplies and comfortable quarters with sand floors so that the horses could lie down. They encountered heavy weather on the way and lost many horses. The military target was the great fortress of Sebastopol. In November a storm of hurricane force hit the Sebastopol harbor; thirty Allied ships containing supplies were lost. The horses literally starved to death. So desperate was their hunger that they ate the wooden spokes and floorboards of wheeled vehicles and ate each other's manes and tails. Sebastopol withstood

401. *Entrance to the Bolan Pass From Dadur.* The Bolan Pass, a 60-mile-long pass in mountainous West Pakistan, has been the avenue for invasions of South Asia by various groups over several centuries—all resulting in enormous suffering and death to animals. The first invaders were the Aryan tribes from the steppes of Central Asia, who profited from their advanced use of horses for chariots and transport and caused the decline of the Indus Valley cultures. The British invasion of Afghanistan in 1838 resulted in the deaths of more than 30,000 camels and horses as they traversed the pass on their way to Kandahar. The peril of the pass is dramatically felt in this scene showing the British Army entering the pass during the invasion of Afghanistan. *(Courtesy The Director, The National Army Museum, London.)*

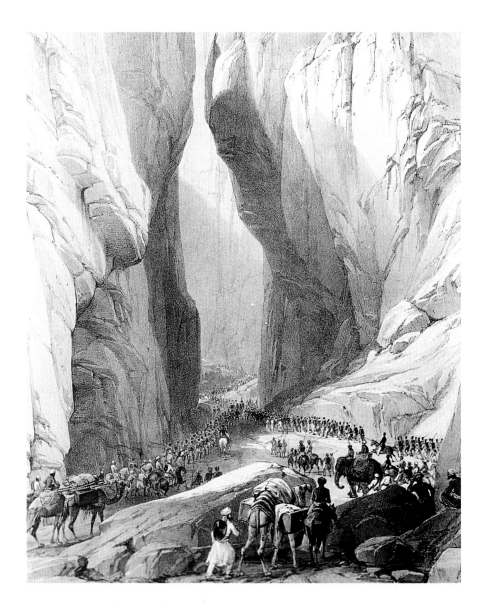

the siege for almost a year, but on September 8, 1855, the French captured the Malakov stronghold and forced the Russians to evacuate the city. The media directed public attention to the terrible suffering of the soldiers and the role of Florence Nightingale rather than to the plight of the horses. More than 400,000 Russian and 300,000 Allied troops died in battle or of disease and malnutrition.

The Crimean campaign is remembered for the futile Charge of the Light Brigade led by Lord Cardigan, which came about because of a miscommunication. Lord Cardigan led his charge to the wrong end of a valley that was well fortified with Russian light artillery. In the space of six minutes the Russian case shots (the hollow iron spheres containing bullets and a timed charge) fired at ranges of 1600, 710, and 300 yards and destroyed the flower of the British cavalry, although the troops rode through and killed all the Russian gun crews. Two hundred and fifty of the 673 men and fifty horses were killed.

The Failure of Moderate Reforms: The Boer War.
The British cavalry and artillery were amalgamated as a single unit under PVS John Wilkinson in 1859. The pattern of appointing a civilian rather than a military PVS persisted until 1890. New grades equivalent to military ranks were introduced for the veterinary service: the grade of veterinary surgeon (VS) was equivalent to the rank of lieutenant, VS first class to captain, and staff VS to major. The grades amounted, at last, to bureaucratic and managerial recognition that adminis-

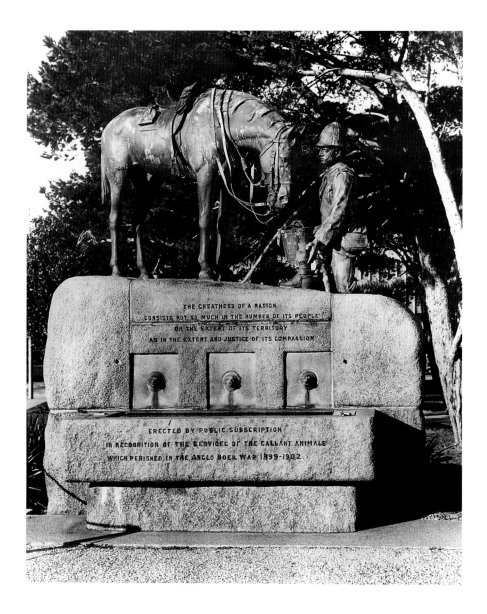

402. This moving commemorative statue in Port Elizabeth, South Africa, honors the memory of the 326,073 horses that died during the Boer War (1899-1902). It was commissioned by Mrs. Gustav Meyer, née Harriet Bunton, of Kings Lynn, United Kingdom. *(Imperial War Museum, London.)*

trative posts within the veterinary services were necessary if the needs of horse maintenance and medical care were to be met. A significant policy change was the authorization of "sick depots" for veterinary care during the Abyssinian (Ethiopian) campaign of 1866. Finally, under James Collins, the PVC from 1876 to 1883, the attachment of veterinary surgeons (VSs) to regiments was ended in two stages, in 1878 and 1881, by a War Office committee led by an informed Edinburgh veterinary surgeon, Major General Sir Frederick Fitzwygram. Fitzwygram was also influential in obtaining authorization for an army veterinary school at Aldershot for the instruction of officers in combat and remount animal selection and in the care, diseases, and treatment of animals used in combat. Special attention was given to exotic, mainly tropical diseases. The school continued to train army veterinary surgeons and farriers to be veterinary hospital assistants until 1938, when it became the Royal Army Veterinary College (RAVC) laboratory. In 1881 the veterinary services were consolidated into the Army Veterinary Department and the PVC became its director general. Thus all VSs were placed on a single list and allowed to wear an identifying uniform.

The Army Veterinary Department was formed to ensure efficient service by qualified veterinary officers. Although sick depots for horses had been introduced during the Peninsular War, not until World War I were sick and wounded horses first evacuated to field and base hospitals where they could receive proper treatment.

Just one year before the Boer War (the second of the South African Wars [1889-1902]), a new edition of "war establishments" incomprehensibly omitted provision for care of sick animals in the field. Thus the war began with no plan for veterinary services, and improvisation on site became the order of the day. Lacking veterinary knowledge, the authorities failed dismally to provide animal care. The director general of the Army Veterinary Department borrowed a few field hospitals from India. Contagious diseases and mismanagement of horses were rampant. The predictable result was a staggering loss of horseflesh: 326,073 horses (sixty-seven percent) and 51,399 mules (thirty-five percent) died. The most revealing statistic was supplied by the veterinary officer (VO) for the Inniskilling Dragoons: of 4170 cases of sickness in horses, only 163 were caused by bullet wounds and only three by shell fire. Despite widespread cases of glanders and epizootic lymphangitis, most of the survivors were sold without veterinary examination, and these diseases were allowed to spread. Horses that were returned to England started an epizootic of lymphangitis that took years to control.

The Twentieth-Century Army Veterinary Corps.

The negative publicity that arose from the sickening wastage of horses and mules in South Africa led to an investigation by a parliamentary committee in 1902. The outcome was a warrant signed by King Edward VII in 1903 creating the Army Veterinary Corps; its leader, formerly a director general and a colonel, was to be ranked as a major general. The man selected to implement this coming of age of the military arm of the veterinary profession, Major General Frederick Smith, was appointed director general in 1907. Condemning previous failures to apply sound principles of animal management and veterinary science, he set about creating a veterinary organization that could provide the necessary support for large, effective mobile field forces. He completed his task and retired in 1910, but he was recalled when the Great War broke out in August 1914.

The veterinary corps performed well during World War I, despite one of the most horrible campaigns in the history of warfare when troops and horses were bogged down in the mud and trenches of Flanders. Mobile veterinary sections had been created in 1913 to get sick and lame animals from the front to the veterinary hospitals. At the beginning of the war, Smith had 164 veterinary officers and 208 veterinary troops of other ranks. By war's end he had

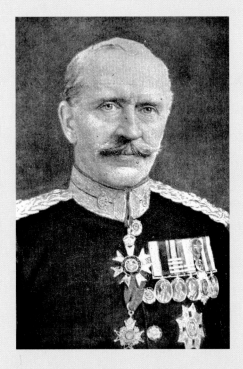

403. Major General Sir Frederick Smith (1857-1929), student at the Royal Veterinary College from 1873 to 1879, head of the Army Veterinary School at Aldershot from 1886 to 1892, and author of textbooks on veterinary physiology (1892, 1895, and 1907 editions) and on veterinary hygiene. Smith devoted his life to the advancement of his profession and the Army Veterinary Corps, of which he became director general in 1907. He wrote a critical veterinary history of the South African War and implemented his ideas for the reform of the corps, which led to effective, humane service in World War I. He wrote the *History of the Royal Army Veterinary Corps: 1796-1919*. His classic, *The Early History of Veterinary Literature*, was published in four volumes (in 1919, 1924, 1930, and 1933). A penetrative, readable treatise, it errs on the side of acerbic judgment of certain individuals. (The Veterinary Record, *1938.*)

1356 officers and 23,146 troops of other ranks. Major Frederick Hobday was consulting veterinary surgeon to the hospitals.

The British Expeditionary Force (BEF) began the war with 53,000 animals and six hospitals. By 1918 there were 450,000 animals and eighteen veterinary hospitals, each with a capacity of 2000. If all fronts were considered, however, Clabby estimated that the army had more than a million animals by 1917; the average daily number of sick animals was 110,000. Between 1914 and 1918, 2,562,549 patients were admitted to veterinary hospitals. Remarkably, seventy-eight percent of these, or two million animals, were returned to duty. Smith certainly accomplished his goals for the veterinary corps and deserved the honor it brought him: he was awarded the title of Knight Commander of the Order of St. Michael and St. George. King George V conferred the title of "Royal" on the Army Veterinary Corps in 1918.

The light draft horses of the artillery that hauled ammunition by night through the watery, mud-filled shell holes sustained the heaviest losses. Because so many of these horses were pushed to exhaustion, the supply of remounts could not replace the numbers of injured and dead animals.

The use of chemical warfare—at first, chlorine gas—led to the effective use of antigas respirators for horses as well as men. Against the later introduction of mustard gas, however, the respirators failed, and troops had to avoid gas-shelled areas by skirting them. During the last two years of the war gunshot wounds killed 77,410 animals; casualties of gas were 211 dead and 2220 injured animals. Bombs began to take a toll in the summer of 1918.

The German campaign used a strategy in Tanzania that was hard to counter. Their commander in chief used his veterinary services to advantage

404. A veterinarian at U.S. Army Veterinary Hospital No. 11 in Gievres, France, in 1919 administering the mallein intraocular test for glanders, the dreaded disease of military horses. After Löffler isolated the infectious agent in Berlin, he developed the test that was crucial for the eradication of the disease. *(National Library of Medicine, Bethesda, Maryland.)*

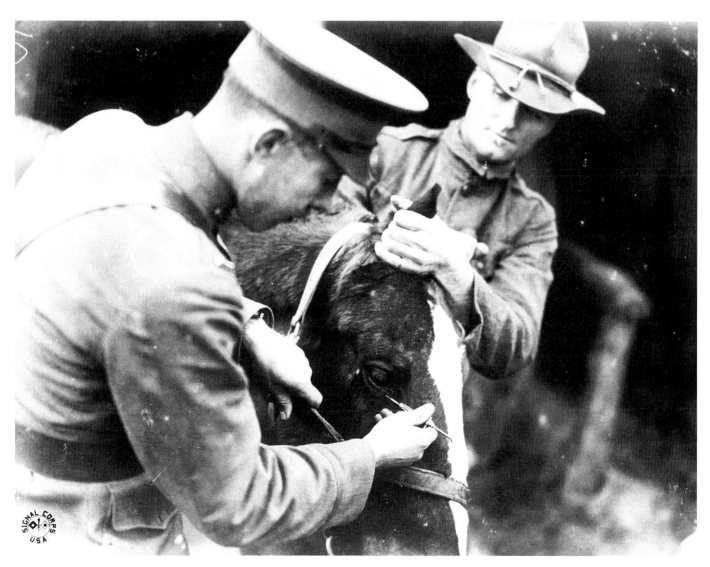

by having them make tsetse fly surveys, and he based his line of retreat on areas containing the worst forms of trypanosomiasis. Despite daily arsenic treatments, these tactics cost the pursuing Imperial forces twelve thousand horses and mules in 1916 and made mounted attacks impossible. Sir Douglas Haig, field marshall and commander in chief, credited the British horses and horsemen and the Army Veterinary Corps that kept them efficient with being far superior to their German counterparts and thereby with being a significant factor in the victory.

During the 1930s, cavalry units were gradually reduced, except in the Union of Soviet Socialist Republics (USSR). The growing firepower of weapons of many kinds, the development of mechanized transport and armored vehicles, and the enormous progress in military aviation made cavalry a high-risk enterprise. The risk was made clear when the gallant Polish Lancers charged the invading German tanks in 1939, suffered heavy losses, and, not surprisingly, failed to slow the advance of enemy troops.

In World War II, mounted troops and equine transport found their niches. The British used pack animals in jungle warfare against the Japanese in Burma in 1943. Brigadier O.C. Wingate and his *Chindits* severed the railroad line between Mandalay and Myitkyina to sabotage the enemy's supplies. They used about a thousand mules, and elephants carried the boats needed for river crossings. In 1942 mules were brought in silently on gliders but were untrained. An operation had to be devised to remove the vocal cords under anesthesia so that the neighing and braying would not disclose their presence to the enemy.

North American Veterinary Services

American Cavalry Before Veterinarians. The American cavalry was formed in 1777. It became the cradle of military veterinary medicine in 1792 when congressional legislation provided each troop of light dragoons (cavalry) with a farrier to shoe and treat horses. Farriers were also assigned to the horse artillery in the War of 1812 (1812-1814) against Canada, then a British colony defended by the redcoats. British support for Native Americans led by Chief Tecumseh was an irritant to the Americans.

The westward migration of settlers from the thirteen former colonies caused battles over territory with the original Native American inhabitants. In 1830 Congress passed the Removal Act, designed to provide all Indians residing east of the Mississippi with a one-way ticket to the west bank of the river. Protection and enforcement were needed, so in 1832 Congress created the U.S. Mounted Ranger Battalion, comprising six companies of one hundred volunteers each. A volunteer had to provide his own horse and equipment and was paid one dollar a day. The companies patrolled the wild country between the great river and the Great Plains. Their main rivals were the Comanche, who had acquired excellent equestrian skills and good horses descended from those of the Spanish invaders. Congress decided a more disciplined army was required and in 1833 approved the establishment of a regular unit, the blue-uniformed regiment of Dragoons, comprising ten companies, A to J, and 750 men. In 1836 a second, light-coated regiment was authorized for Florida because of the uprising led by Osceola, chief of the Seminoles, in 1835. The skirmishes with Indians continued for seven years. Farriers, who had been dropped from the military complement after the War of 1812, were reinstated when the regiments were formed in 1833 and 1836. The term *veterinary surgeon* first appeared in the general regulations of the army in 1834 and 1835; a *Veterinary Department of Cavalry* was mentioned, and the competence of the veterinary surgeon to fulfill the duties of his station was discussed. Since there is no evidence of veterinarians in the army at that time, it is presumed that the new term was being applied to farriers.

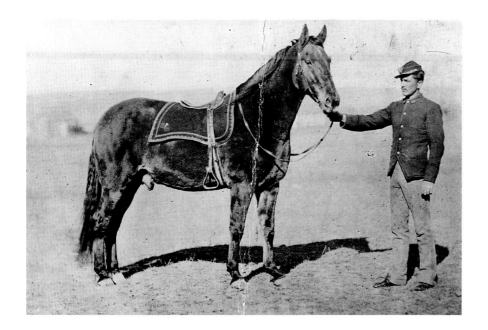

405. Captain Myles W. Keogh's buckskin (light bay) gelding, Comanche, was the only survivor of the U.S. government side in the Battle of Little Big Horn, known as Custer's Last Stand, on June 25, 1876. The horse had received twelve arrow and bullet wounds but made the fifteen-mile trek back to a ship that took him, via Fort Bismarck, to Fort Abraham Lincoln. Nursed in slings for nearly a year, he made a complete recovery, living to age twenty-nine years; he died during a bout of colic. This albumen print from a wet collodion-on-glass negative was prepared in the 1870s by D.F. Barry (American, died 1934). *(Montana Historical Society, Helena.)*

Texas unilaterally declared its independence from Mexican rule in 1836. In 1845 the United States annexed Texas, and Mexico took this action to be a declaration of war. On April 24, 1846, sixteen hundred Mexican horsemen crossed the Rio Grande and attacked two companies of the Second Dragoons. The typical Mexican horseman had a lance, a saber, and a carbine. A combination of Texas Rangers and Second Dragoons armed with six-shot Colt rifles retaliated against the Mexican lancers and routed them. Five Mexicans were killed for each American: the age of firearms had arrived.

Congress authorized the use of more government troops and fifty thousand volunteers. The Dragoons were led by officers trained at the U.S. Military Academy at West Point; the soldiers, also highly qualified, included seasoned European immigrants, English dragoons and hussars, Prussian uhlans, and German cuirassiers. A mighty battle took place at Buena Vista in 1847; the American forces were greatly outnumbered. Nevertheless, they prevailed, but losses were heavy on both sides. Frémont captured California, Kearney took New Mexico, and Scott landed at Veracruz and with his troop of Mounted Rifles marched to Mexico City and captured it. Mexico in 1848 was forced to accept a peace agreement that ceded California, Nevada, Utah, New Mexico, and Texas to the United States. The only horse doctors who participated in the Mexican War were farriers. Limited use of civilian veterinarians in the army began in 1849, the year after the war ended.

Limited Veterinary Services During the Civil War.

The necessity of veterinarians was eventually recognized during the American Civil War (1861-1865). One veterinary sergeant was authorized for each of the three battalions of a cavalry regiment. Use of this initial grade was dropped in March 1862, when an act of Congress authorized a regimental veterinary surgeon with the rank of regimental sergeant major. Abraham Lincoln was elected president in 1860. The eleven states of the South, determined to preserve slavery for their plantation agriculture, seceded from the Union and formed the Confederate States of America, with Richmond, Virginia, as the capital and Jefferson Davis as president. Confederate forces attacked and took Fort Sumter in 1861. The population of the South was about nine million; three and a half million of these Southerners were slaves with African roots. After the Yankees of the North were defeated at Bull Run, Lincoln was empowered by Congress to call up 500,000 volunteers for military service. The Dragoons were renamed the U.S. Cavalry, and twenty-eight new regiments were created. Because more than 100,000 horses were required, six depots for procuring and equipping the cavalry horses were established, each able to stable and train up to ten thousand horses. Within two years the cavalry was increased from five thousand to sixty thousand mounted troopers. This huge increase in the equine base created a compelling need for better-trained veterinarians.

Railroads had expanded dramatically during the mid-nineteenth century to more than ten thousand miles of track. Railroads became the essential supply, troop movement, and communication link that allowed the military to overcome problems that had crippled Napoleon in Russia. The telegraph, too, was a vital new technology. The Southern forces made many raids in an effort to disrupt the rail connections of the Northern forces. The brilliant generalship of Robert E. Lee and J.E.B. Stuart kept the South in a strong position for nearly two years, but the might and sheer numbers of the Union armies gradually took their toll: the cavalry corps of the Army of the Potomac alone, which took the field under General George Stoneman in 1863, had nine thousand men in three divisions.

Lee tried to decide the war in one mighty battle; the chosen site was Gettysburg. The largest cavalry battle had taken place in June 1863 at Brandy Station, where troops on both sides fought to exhaustion. In the preparations for Gettysburg, Stuart's mission of getting behind the Union lines, disrupting supplies, and gathering intelligence about the North's plans and positions was thwarted for the first time by the Union cavalry. Lee was defeated at Gettysburg. On May 11, 1864, Stuart, trying to stop Sheridan's much stronger force, was killed at Yellow Tavern. A man of exceptional energy, Stuart drove his horses and men relentlessly. It was reported that thirty of his fine personal chargers were killed during the war. The war ended a year later. Five-hundred thousand soldiers died, and massive loss of horses to injury and disease occurred. The cost for veterinary civilian staff was about 94,000 dollars. A veterinary hospital was established at Lynchburg in October 1863, but it was said to have been of limited effectiveness because the horses that were sent there were so exhausted that they rarely recovered. By February 1864, 6875 horses had been admitted. Of those, 2844 died, 599 were condemned and cast, and 1483 were classed as unserviceable. Only 1949 remounts remained.

406. *General Robert E. Lee on Traveller,* an albumen print from a wet collodion-on-glass negative prepared in 1868 by Michael Miley (American, 1841-1918). This was the only photograph requested by Lee in Confederate uniform. The iron-grey gelding was a splendid specimen with Thoroughbred and Morgan genes, a potent symbol for Lee's men. It carried the general throughout the four years of the war and followed his hearse in 1870. After Traveller stepped on a rusty nail two years later, the horse had to be destroyed because of tetanus. The original print is uniquely interesting because it shows the faint image of a groom steadying the horse for the long time needed to expose the film. Later, better-known copies of this famous photograph, which were mass-produced in a variety of media, show only the stately Lee astride his famous horse. *(Eleanor S. Brockenbrough Library, The Museum of the Confederacy, Richmond, Virginia.)*

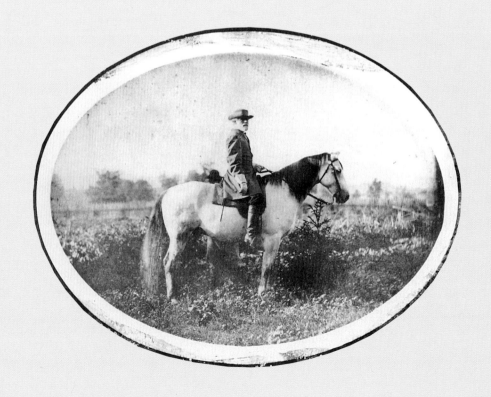

General Robert E. Lee had a magnificent sixteen-hand grey gelding named Traveller as his constant companion throughout the war and in his retirement. Traveller, more than half English Thoroughbred, also had genes from Black Hawk, one of the finest early Morgan horses. Lee bought him as a four-year-old in 1861. After Lee died in 1870, Traveller stepped on a nail and contracted tetanus. He had to be shot, but his skeleton is preserved at Washington and Lee University.

Canine Contributions to Military Actions

The medieval Spaniards were notorious for their use of ferocious mastiff-type dogs in attacking the Native Indian peoples of the Americas after the conquistadors invaded the West Indian Islands and then the mainland.

In Britain during World War I Lieutenant Colonel E.H. Richardson, a noted dog breeder and trainer, persuaded the War Office to establish a military dog training school in 1916. A site was established at Nately Ridge in the

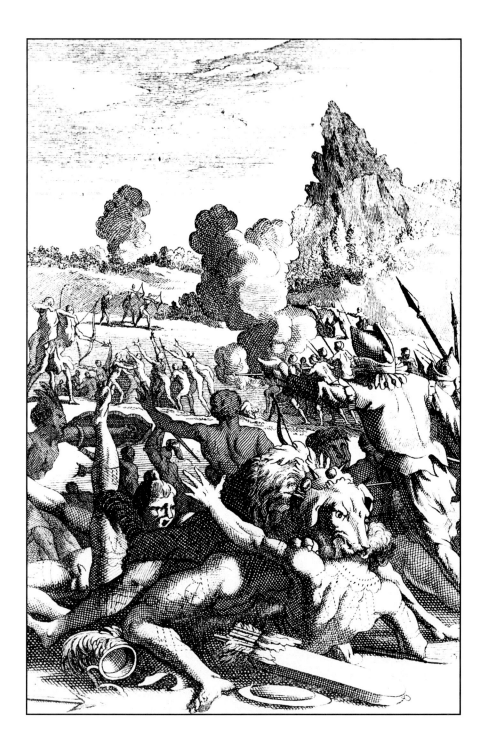

407. A sad commentary on Columbus's discovery of the New World was his decision to unleash dogs on the natives in an attempt to obtain information, which failed miserably. The first "dogging of Indians" took place on the Caribbean island of Jamaica in 1494; "dogging" became a tradition of the conquistadors. This scene is from a 1706 Dutch edition of the original Spanish work (1508-1509) that described this practice. The dogs were fed on cuts from human carcasses. *(Benson Latin American Collection, University of Texas, Austin.)*

New Forest, and training was initiated. The first demand was for a messenger dog service. Private owners were the main source of dogs; the Airedale and the collie were popular breeds. This service was disbanded after the cessation of hostilities.

The modern use of dogs in the military forces grew out of their superior sensory systems (smell, hearing, and sight), which let them detect alien human presence, even in the dark, much more effectively than human guards could. It was estimated that one handler with one trained dog could protect the territory watched by eight sentries. The use of the dog to guard military bases became a common practice. In 1942 the British decided they needed 2500 dogs to enter training for that role immediately.

By 1942 the Allied forces knew that the German forces were using highly trained dogs to locate Allied agents who had parachuted into occupied territory. The first goal of dog training was to use the dogs to help devise ways to baffle these German tracker dogs. Captain D.C.E. Danby was the veterinary surgeon in charge of the operation at Swakley's Farm, near Ruislip, in 1942. Demand for trained dogs expanded rapidly, and the Greyhound Racing Association Kennels at Potters Bar became the headquarters of the War Dog Training School until the war's end. Dogs were trained for guarding premises, for tracking, for messenger duty, and for land-mine detection. Kenneling the dogs outdoors in barrels proved to be effective in minimizing diseases. Barking, always a problem, led to throat infections. Intestinal infections, caused mainly by coccidiosis, were said to account for three fourths of the sick rate. Canine hysteria was related to these intestinal disorders.

Although the training school was run by army veterinary officers, it did not become a unit of the Royal Army Veterinary Corps after the war. The school was operated with the assistance of a strong animal technician service, *Kennel Maids,* whose efforts in nursing care of sick dogs, as well as general kennel management, were outstanding. In the Second World War the predominant breeds used were the Alsatian, for all types of assignments, and the black Labrador, for tracking and casualty detection. Mongrels often made the best mine dogs. Highly intelligent boxers were popular in the Middle East as guard dogs. The use of dogs with patrols to avoid ambushes and surprise attacks by the enemy, especially in difficult terrain, has been an important development. The military role of the dog, unlike that of the horse, whose use in military campaigns is now restricted to special conditions unsuitable for vehicles, shows no sign of declining.

408. During the American Civil War the citizens of Richmond, Virginia, were alarmed by the number of Union prisoners being held in camps in and near their beleaguered city. In an attempt to tighten security after several successful escapes the ferocious guard dog Nero was brought in to hunt down escaped Yankee prisoners. Widely known as "the Castle Thunder Dog," he was named after a prison camp where he helped his Confederate owner, Captain George Alexander, maintain order. Nero, a black Bavarian boar hound, was estimated to weigh 182 pounds. *(Eleanor S. Brockenbrough Library, The Museum of the Confederacy, Richmond, Virginia.)*

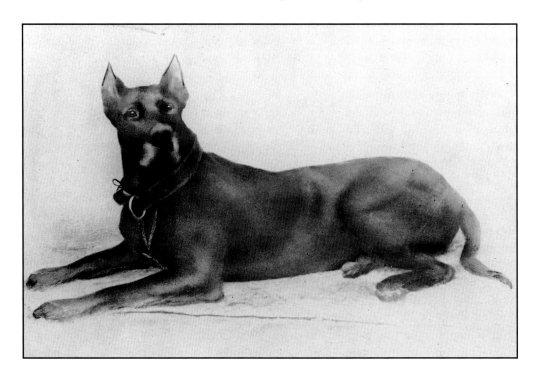

Homing Pigeons As Military Messengers

The American veterinary services in World War II were focused on horses, mules, army dogs, and Signal Corps pigeons. The pigeon service was inaugurated in 1941 under the direction of an officer in the veterinary corps in Fort Monmouth, New Jersey. Signal pigeons were procured, bred, trained, and issued by the Pigeon Service of the army's Signal Corps. About forty thousand pigeons were donated by the American pigeon breeders, fanciers, and owners via an army Pigeon Service agency in Philadelphia, and many were obtained from British and Belgian sources. The Army Veterinary Service endeavored to avoid the entry of contagious diseases and to preserve the general health and efficency of the birds. The most serious diseases were pigeon paratyphoid (a form of salmonellosis), pigeon pox (a viral disease), and canker caused by trichomoniasis. Annual vaccination was carried out to control pigeon pox.

In Europe the pigeon service was a major means of communication. The first news of Wellington's victory at Waterloo in 1815 was sent by homing pigeon. During the siege of Paris in 1870, pigeons became the major conveyors of messages. Nevertheless, by 1908 the British Admiralty saw fit to declare messenger pigeons obsolete because of the invention of wireless transmission. The Germans and the French, however, continued to build up their stocks of trained pigeons. When war broke out, many small boats such as mine sweepers and drifters did not have radios, and field telegraph and wireless systems kept breaking down. The great advantages of the pigeon were its homing instinct and its speed and stamina in flight. Compared to a dog's five-mile range, the pigeon's range of sixty miles or more, regardless of the terrain, was fantastic. Pigeons saved many lives and transmitted much important intelligence information during the war.

THE ENGLISH PASSION FOR NATURE AND ANIMAL SPORTS

The English-speaking world is renowned for its passion for wild nature and its logical sequel, the rural life. Along with these deep-seated interests an attraction developed that grew into an addiction to sports involving animals. A fascinating spectrum of activities evolved, some reprehensible, many admirable. As the opportunities to enjoy wild nature have shrunk with the growth of the human population and the expanding tentacles of technology, the chances of enjoying the appealing features of rural life, too, have become more elusive. The passion for companionship with animals has been part of this history, even for those with few resources. The psychological and physical partnership with a pet has become an important drive that continues to evolve under the changing constraints of society.

The hierarchical structure of British society stemmed from the hereditary divine right of kings, which led to the establishment of a favored aristocracy associated with the royal court. Hunting as a symbol of power over the environment and dangerous beasts is an ancient tradition for royal commanders. Hunting was also considered an important health-promoting activity, although carousing, a frequent offshoot of hunting, probably had a different impact. In Britain the royal quarries, dating to Saxon times, included the stag, the fox, and the hare, but on the Continent the wild boar was preeminent because of its willingness to put up a fight and increase the risk to the hunter. Farther afield, in the time of expanding empires, the focus was on even more dangerous targets such as the lion, tiger, leopard, buffalo, elephant, rhinoceros, and wolf. As technology evolved, hunting became less sporting and more certain, particularly after the development of firearms; their increasing role in the hunt, too, has evolved to meet changing expectations.

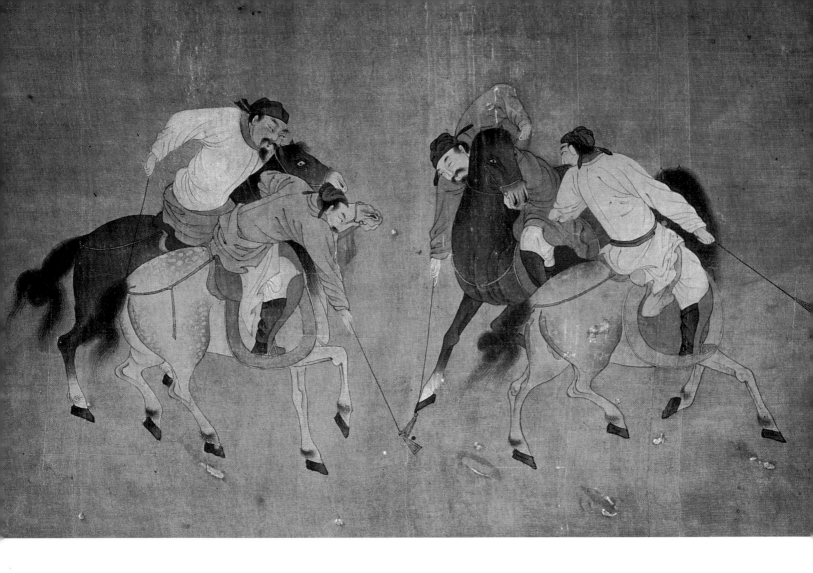

409. The Chinese invention of the stirrup was a necessary precursor to the game of polo, allowing the rider to generate the force and direction needed to effectively use the mallet. This watercolor on silk (c. 1635) by Li-Lin was probably derived from an original from the Yuan dynasty (1280-1368). *(Courtesy The Board of Trustees of The Victoria and Albert Museum, London.)*

Such was the power of emperors and kings that they were able to appropriate lands as special preserves for the royal hunts, which could not be used by ordinary mortals lacking the appropriate genes or favors. Although the aristocrats took precedence, another class—the landed gentry, the country gentlemen who owned property and the successful business owners or nouveau riche—aspired to emulate them by purchasing rural estates. So strong was this motivation that men of standing throughout most parts of Europe adopted the English riding attire between 1700 and 1900, while agriculture was becoming the principal industry, and a characteristic set of sports emerged. The image of the "huntin,' shootin,' and fishin' squire" was a dream aspired to by those in search of the good life and high social status.

Horse Racing: The Sport of Kings

James I (1566-1625), the first king of Great Britain and Scotland (1603-1625) and the only son of Mary, Queen of Scots, gave the country its national flag, the Union Jack, by marrying the cross of St. Andrew of Scotland with that of St. George of England. An enthusiastic supporter of hunting and racing, King James sponsored the breeding of fast horses. He purchased the Markham Arabian, the first pure Arab stallion brought to Great Britain. Other Turk and Barb sires followed, and a trend toward the lighter, fleeter oriental types of horses was initiated. James I, the grandson of Margaret Tudor, claimed succession to the English crown. James proved to be a great internationalist; he planted the colonies in America and harassed the Puritans, many of whom left Great Britain to become an early component of the melting pot of the United States. He is also noted for his strong stance on religious toleration and ordered a revised translation of the English Bible. The result became the authorized version of 1611, the beautifully worded King James Bible.

Charles I (1625-1649), son of James I, inherited his father's hostile relationship with the House of Commons and was overthrown by the Commonwealth that ruled England from 1649 to 1660 and made Oliver Cromwell (1599-1658) Lord Protector in 1653. Cromwell relegated to farm work the large horses that were bred to carry heavy armor. He also issued a decree prohibiting horse racing on the grounds of corruption, an action also motivated to contain wealthy Royalist plotters who had developed stables of swift horses for the evolving sport of horse racing.

King Charles II was made King of Scotland and Ireland after Cromwell and the Commonwealth voted to abolish the kingship in England. King Charles II returned to the throne of Great Britain in 1660. He gave the greatest boost to importation of excellent bloodstock and the promotion of horse racing, even riding in races himself. His studmaster, James Darcy, coordinated the acquisition of Arab, Barb, and Turk strains from North Africa and West Asia.

Three stallions imported in the seventeenth and eighteenth centuries have been identified as profoundly influencing the quality of racing horses in Britain. In 1689, during the reign (1689-1702) of William III (1650-1702), son of William of Orange, the first of the stallions, the Byerly Turk, Colonel Byerly's faithful charger, was imported. In about 1700 the Darley Arabian was brought in from Aleppo, Syria, by Darley of Yorkshire. The third of these founding studs, imported in 1730, was the Godolphin Arabian, a remarkable horse discovered dragging a cart around Paris, having been brought to France from Barbary in North Africa. The horse was presented to the Earl of Godolphin, who had its portrait painted by George Stubbs. These three studs have made genetic contributions to virtually all English Thoroughbred horses. They provided the traits of elegant conformation, coordination, and stamina of the finest horses from the Islamic states.

The preexisting English stock provided great size and length of stride. Eclipse, the most remarkable English-bred horse, was descended from the Godolphin Arabian. He was born during an eclipse of the sun in 1764 and had black spots on his rump. His owner, O'Kelly, started racing him as a five-year-old; he was never beaten in a race, despite never having a whip laid on him. His impact on the national bloodstock was unequalled: he sired 335 winners. Sainbel, the first principal of the Royal Veterinary College, studied Eclipse's conformation as a mathematical model for the desired level of perfection.

Weatherby's *Stud Book* of 1791 became the model of pedigree records. To be qualified to be called a Thoroughbred, a horse's genetic origin must be traceable on both the sire's and the dam's side to animals already accepted in the *Stud Book*.

Commercial Horse Racing in the United States

After the Spanish invaders of North America had reseeded the New World with equine genes, the British brought their improved horses to the colonies. In addition to the horse's contributions to heavy draft work, road transport, and military functions, equestrian sports became important diversions. Before and after the Revolutionary War, racing was mainly a sport for the landed gentry, "men of substance." George Washington and Andrew Jackson were enthusiasts. The main events were individual match races to determine who owned the fastest horse. Bets were wagered in advance. Multiple-entry races held on prepared courses emerged just before the Civil War. These were attended by bookmakers, and all spectators had access to betting.

In retrospect it seems amazing that America's first real racetrack, Saratoga, opened on August 3, 1863, just a few days before the great battle of Gettysburg. The Jockey Club, a central agency similar to the English Jockey Club, was inaugurated in 1894 to manage horse racing. It attracted the most powerful, wealthy, and socially eminent people as patrons. The club allotted racing dates and licensed owners, trainers, and jockeys. It established the rules under which the sport was to be conducted, appointed the stewards, or regulatory officials, and addressed the issue of horse identification. The club, which began in New York and Delaware, came to control breeding and racing of Thoroughbred horses throughout America. From these origins to the end of the Second World War the tradition of horse racing as a social pastime for the wealthy, influential set persisted virtually unchallenged.

The comfortable setting for the sport of kings came to an abrupt halt in 1952 after a New York lawsuit resulted in a ruling that the legislature's delegation of licensing powers to an exclusive social group of sportsmen was unconstitutional. The positive outcome of the decision was a major expansion of the sport: racing became available to the general population. The value of the equine athlete soared, and the number of dollars bet increased dramatically. In 1973 Secretariat's breeding rights were sold to a syndicate for more than six million dollars. The transition of racing from a game of prestige among the elite to just another business competing to make profits was a negative result of the ruling. Thus the status of the great equine athlete changed from that of a beautiful image on a pedestal to that of yet another marketable commodity to be discarded when the dollar flow subsided. The impact on equine veterinary medicine was profound.

Despite the horse having the highest priority among the domestic species served by the veterinary profession, progress in equine medicine, except in

410. This magnificent sculpture of Secretariat was created by John Skeaping (American, born 1901) to honor the chestnut stallion that won the American Triple Crown in 1973. He was rated one of the greatest flat-racing horses of the twentieth century. Sired by the prepotent Bold Ruler, Secretariat's genes went back to the Godolphin Arabian, one of the founders of the Thoroughbred breed. *(Collection of The National Museum of Racing and Hall of Fame.)*

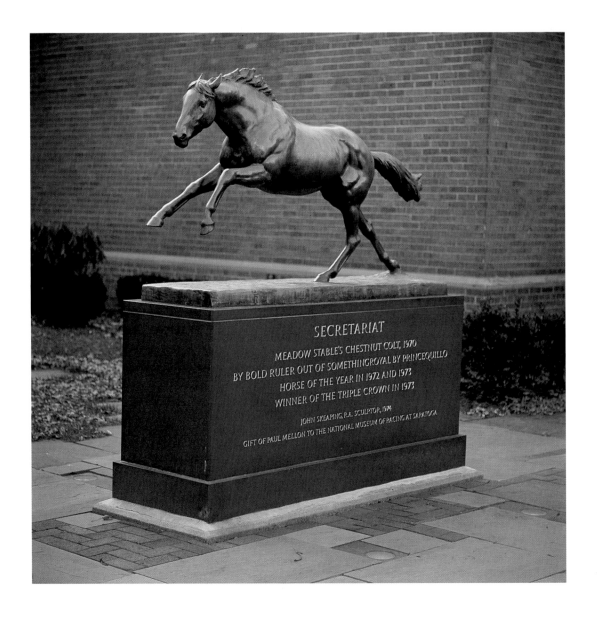

anatomy, was slow. Little progress was made in the internal medicine of the horse until the mid-nineteenth century. Even then, the transition to rigorous scientific analysis, coupled with the growing compendium of knowledge of equine diseases, was accepted with reluctance. The state of therapeutics before the development of general and local anesthetics was disastrous. Much of the pharmacology functioned more to add iatrogenically to the existing burden of disease than to effect cures. Really effective antibiotic and anthelmintic drugs did not arrive until the Second World War; and several major diseases still had no specific treatments.

Veterinary medicine for the racing world was an art form under the old model. It was necessary for an aspiring equine practitioner to apprentice and acquire a reputation by working with established equine specialists who were trusted by the racing elite. The military arm of the profession had a strong presence because of the prior importance of the horse in war. After World War II an enormous economic expansion occurred, and the middle class grew rapidly. The decline in demand for equine energy that followed mechanization in the first half of the twentieth century was reversed by the growing demand for horses in sport and recreation. The growth of veterinary knowledge of food animals and the well-advertised progress in human medicine made the slower progress in equine medicine more obvious, and demands for better veterinary care for the horse increased. The improved economic situation for racing gave the racing community power to push for equine veterinary research. After 1960 research started to yield results, and an exciting period of progress in the understanding of the horse and its diseases began.

Diagnosis and treatment of severe injuries became possible at last. Instead of resorting to the bullet, veterinarians could examine severe injuries in prized animals by means of sophisticated imaging systems; animals could be anesthetized with safer anesthetics after tranquilization and placed on padded hydraulic operating tables that could tilt in any direction. The latest advances in surgical technique were used in the treatment of injuries or fractures. Endoscopic and arthroscopic instruments allowed diagnosis and repair of internal organs and joints. Swimming tanks for horses were devised to promote recovery from fractures and limb injuries by overcoming the problem of weight bearing on injured parts.

Because of the commercialization of racing, however, racehorses became increasingly subject to abuse. More was asked of them by the investors in track operations and all segments of the horse industry. The length of the racing season was extended until racing was offered somewhere in the country throughout the year. Horses were moved from track to track to compete more continuously. The animals were raced too frequently—often before they had recuperated from a previous race—and were started in racing too young. Drugs that had been developed to alleviate suffering during treatment and recovery began to be used to keep animals running when they were already suffering from overuse.

Today few horses run without being given nonsteroidal antiinflammatory drugs to suppress the inflammation of leg tissues that causes pain. Others cannot run effectively without the diuretic furosemide (Lasix), which is thought to reduce the risk of pulmonary bleeding to which many racing horses are susceptible during a race. In many states the use of certain maximum allowable dosages of these agents is legal. Intraarticular steroids such as methylprednisolone have been overused in attempts to return animals to racing prematurely, and joint damage has often resulted. The temptation to use drugs illegally to influence the outcome of races is great. A large industry based on racing chemistry uses sophisticated analytical methods to protect the public. Samples of body fluids are taken from selected animals and submitted for examination after each race. Serious reevaluation of the industry is required. A plan must be developed to preserve horse racing before it self-destructs by pushing its magnificant equine athletes too hard.

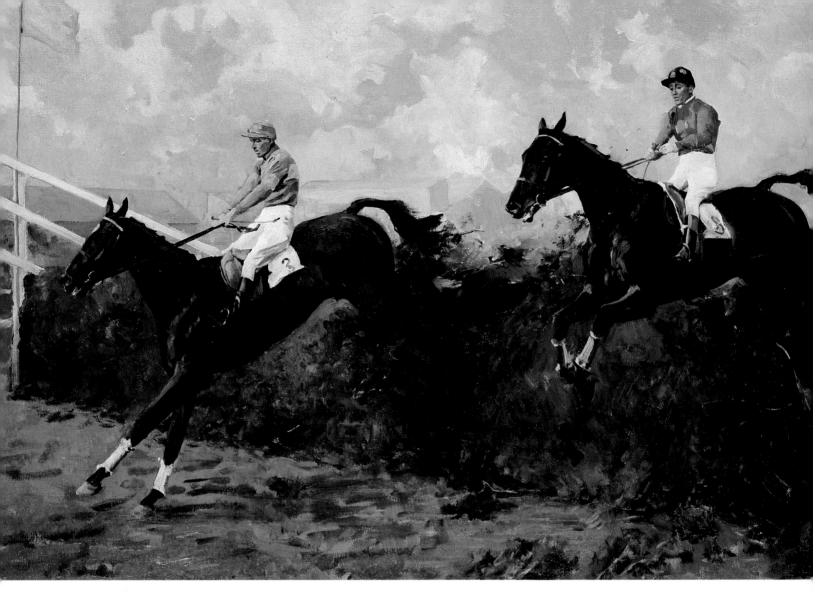

411. Painting by Charles Walter Simpson (English, 1885-1971), *Grand National,* beautifully captures the drama of England's most famous horse-racing event, a grueling test of the fitness and jumping ability of the horse matched with the skill and daring of the rider. *(The Tryon Gallery, London.)*

The Joy of Harness Racing

No story of racing would be complete without mention of the popular sport of harness racing. The key to the development of this exciting sport was the evolution of the Standardbred horse, which became recognized as a breed. The concept of trotting horses derives from the days of road horses, when competition was keen for the best turned out and fastest trotter. Very much an American sport, harness racing traces its roots to the importation in 1788 of Messenger, an English Thoroughbred horse, to stand at stud. He proved to have a remarkable tendency to transfer to his progeny the capacity to trot and pace at high speeds. He is regarded as the patriarch of the Standardbred, the genetic author of speed at the pace. Even the Justin Morgan and Henry Clay lines could not compete with the well-named Messenger's offspring.

Bellfounder, a Norfolk trotting stallion, was imported to Boston from England in 1822. He begat the famous Charles Kent mare, which had genes from Messenger. Undistinguished in racing herself, this mare was bred to Abdallah, another of Messenger's long line, and in 1849 produced a colt, Hambletonian 10, a most fortuitous nick. This magnificent specimen of a trotting horse had the extremely powerful hind legs and the croup higher than his withers that were considered the ideal anatomical arrangement for high-velocity propulsion at the trotting gait. He was not worked to a peak at racing but stood at stud from two to twenty-three years of age. His progency became the pacesetters and studs that set the standards for the industry. Also from Hambletonian 10's line came the magnificent Greyhound, whose burst of acceleration was awesome; Greyhound broke all records with a 1:55.15-minute mile in 1938. This unusual ability to sustain high speeds at the trotting gait was the basis for acceptance of the Standardbred as a separate breed. The mile times required to qualify for the breed have been reduced progressively. The breed became the envy of the world, one of the American breeds that have been sought after in many parts of the world. Standardbred racing is less confined by the weight of the drivers because they have a single-seated, two-wheel vehicle called a sulky. The bicycle or bike sulky with pneumatic tires was introduced in 1892. In 1897 Star Pointer became the first Standardbred to run a mile in less than two minutes. The glamorous Dan Patch in 1905 paced the mile at 1:55.45, and in 1938 Billy Direct pushed the record to 1:55 even. The issue of whether a horse can run faster at the trot or the pace is unresolved. More pacers than trotters are racing today. In the pace the front and rear legs on the same side move forward and backward together, whereas at the trot the opposite hind leg moves in synchrony with the foreleg.

Pacing horses wear leather straps called hopples around their legs, old English devices used to keep trotters in gait, to prevent breaking the gait at high speed. The modern version was invented by an Indiana railroad conductor. Pacers may also wear boots to protect them from hitting themselves with their hooves; the boots are tailored to protect the part vulnerable to the gait of the individual horse.

412. *Greyhound at Goshen,* a fine painting by Richard Stone Reeves (American, born 1919), portrays one of the great trotting horses in action. The trailing horse can be seen breaking stride. After the remarkable speed of this talented grey gelding became known, no one would race against him. *(Trotting Horse Museum, New York.)*

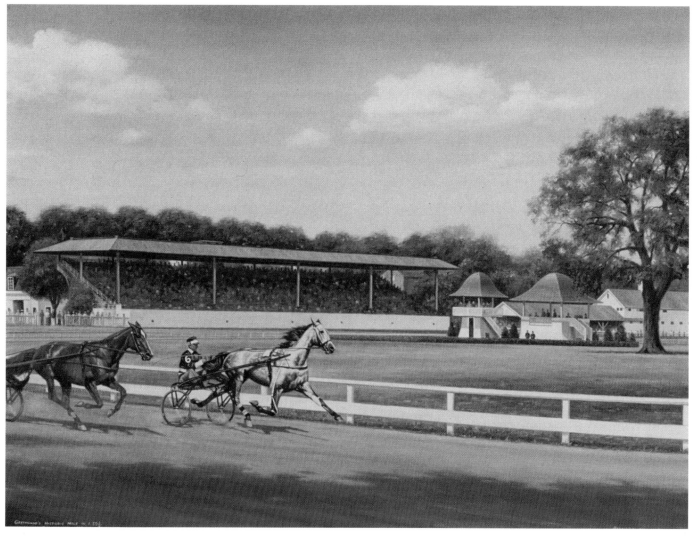

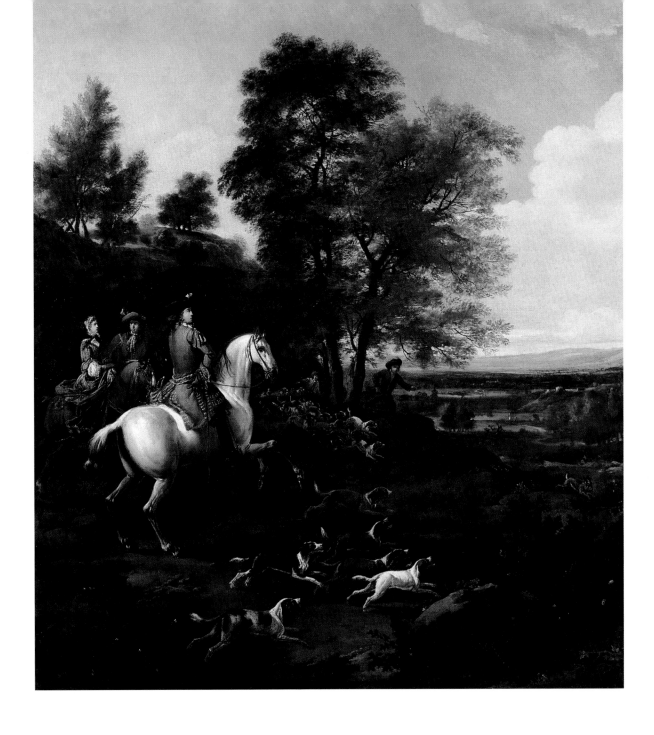

Hunting on Horseback With Hounds

413. Jan Wijck, who was born in Haarlem about 1640, was trained in art by his father, and together they moved to England. There he became known as Jan Wyck or Wycke, and was recognized for his genre paintings of hunting and battle scenes. In this particular oil on canvas, *Hare Hunting* (c. 1690), Wijck has shown the essential elements of the hunt, which has always been a favorite activity of the aristocracy. The hare has been flushed from hiding by the hounds for the chase by the well-dressed hunters and their excited horses. Wijck died at Mortlake in 1702. *(Yale Center for British Art, New Haven.)*

The sport that came to be one of the highlights of the rural scene, foxhunting, may have ancient Saxon roots. Social events in Great Britain were scheduled to mesh with hunting dates, and artists were capitivated by the combination of the social atmosphere, the colors, the fine animals, and the action. Stag hunting and hare hunting had once been popular, but the Enclosure Acts passed after 1709 brought an end to most "green-coated" stag hunting except on moorlands and in forests. The scarlet-coated hunter of foxes became dominant. The early kennels kept for hunting were made up of large, slow, southern-mouthed hounds. Early in the eighteenth century the lighter, faster northern hounds superseded them.

The sport was revolutionized by the Enclosure Acts, which ended the era of open strip cultivation without fencing. Apart from occasional hedges, jumping had not been necessary, but the massive adoption of enclosure confronted the huntsmen with barriers everywhere. Such barriers, depending on local conditions, included planted thorn hedges protected from cattle by stout timber guard rails or "oxers," dry stone walls in the limestone hills, earth banks, and wide drainage ditches and streams; each field had a five-barred gate for access. Jumping over these hazards became a necessity, an added thrill, and the art form of hunting. Jumping also gave rise to the great rural sports of point-to-point racing and steeplechasing, as well as the stylish show-jumping competitions and three-day events. Efficient crop farmers were less than enthusiastic about a great herd of mounted hunters trampling their ripening crops, so hunting was banned in summer until the crops were harvested. Artists captured both the dynamic image of the sport and the exquisite landscape of the countryside.

The nature of the mount had to be upgraded to meet the need for jumping. The motley crew mounted on half-bred cobs, ponies, and equestrian vehicles of all shapes and sizes, often with cropped ears, was replaced with people who could afford the larger bloodstock horses that could and would jump. Unlike the horses bred for racing on flat terrain, the new hunting horses had to be able to carry more weight than a featherweight jockey up hills and down dales for longer periods and to jump with the added weight over formidable obstacles, often in inclement weather. The steeds had to be able to recover quickly from the exhaustion of a hard day's hunting. Hunting created work for veterinary surgeons because of the high-spirited efforts and verve of many riders and the early, inexperienced stages that each horse had to go through. Falls and injuries were frequent in open country and more so on fenced land.

Most of the opposition to foxhunting has been focused on the fate of the fox. During the early days of the sport, when the first huntsman in at the kill was awarded the brush (tail), competition became fierce and tended to corrupt the sport, but reforms were instituted to ensure that only the Master of Fox Hounds was permitted to remove the tail. Considering the array of odds against the fox—scent hounds, huntsmen, huntswomen, and horses— the fox was remarkably adept at keeping the odds even: often the fox escaped completely.

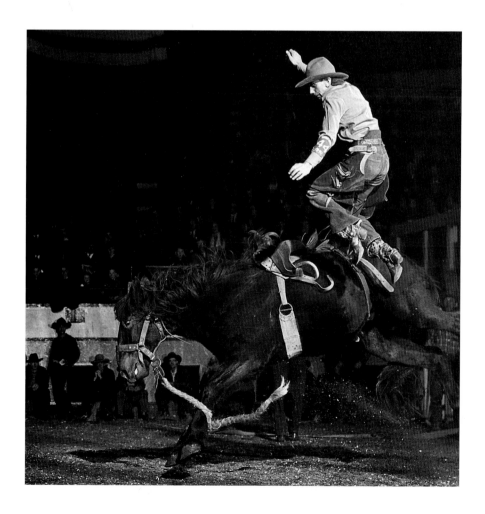

414. The first known rodeo in the United States occurred in 1869. The rodeo had evolved as a sport in Texas during the two decades before the American Civil War. In bronco-busting, a featured event in most rodeos, cowboys attempt to subdue unbroken horses. In *Rodeo,* a 1940 silver print, Dr. Harold E. Edgerton (American, 1903-1990), the inventor of stroboscopic photography, captured the moment when horse and rider are separated. *(The Harold E. Edgerton 1992 Trust. Courtesy of Palm Press, Inc.)*

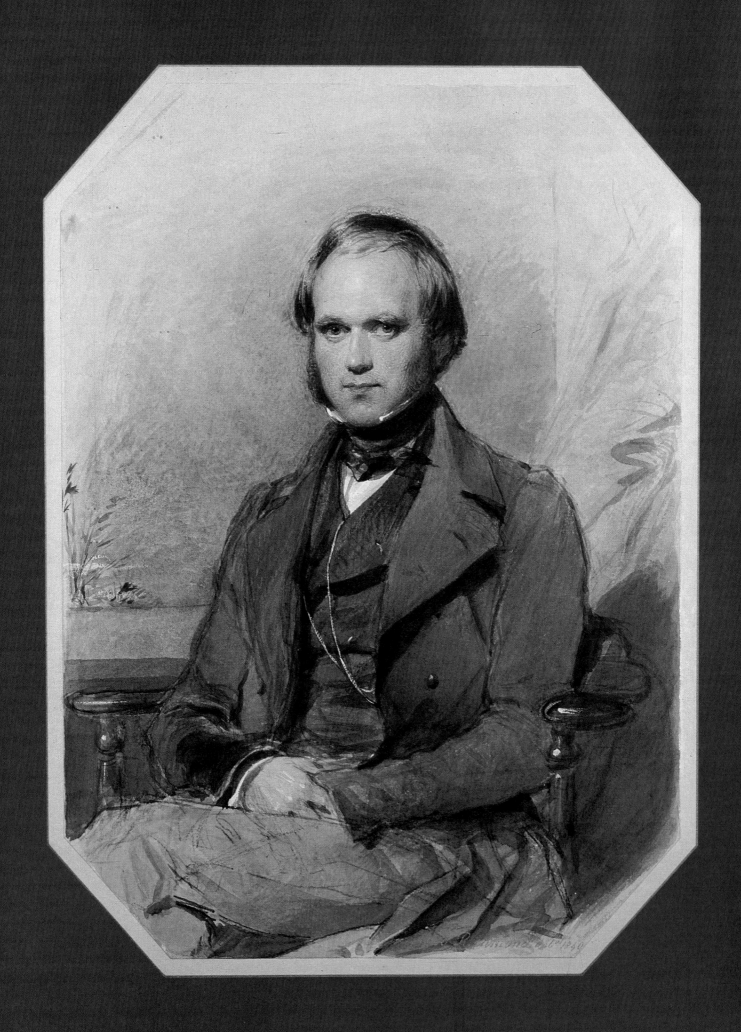

Darwin's Natural Selection and Mendel's Fractional Inheritance

CHARLES DARWIN: REVOLUTIONARY PHILOSOPHER OF NATURE

A mighty book, *On The Origin of Species* by Charles Darwin, appeared in 1859. It developed the concept of biological evolution over a long time scale, which was destined to become the great unifying principle of biology. The extraordinary scope of Darwin's scholarship and of his own investigations made him a significant contributor to geology and environmental science; to microbial, plant, and animal sciences; to animal breeding and biomedical sciences; and to theoretical biology. He stands in historical perspective as the greatest analyst and integrator of biological information, the scholar who made the most significant contribution to the growth in understanding of biology at the macroscopic level.

Darwin proposed a plausible mechanism by which evolution of species could occur—natural selection. This mechanism operated via the intrinsic variability that he realized existed among organisms of the same species. Those best fitted for survival under the environmental conditions of the time would prevail at the expense of those less favorably endowed. Darwin left open the question of the origin of the very first organism (that is, the origin of life itself), except to say that it must have occurred a very long time ago, before the formation of the oldest fossil-bearing rocks or geological strata. Thus he left open the possibility of a "Creator" at the beginning of cellular life. His work and thought have ramifications for medical and veterinary science, and every veterinarian should be aware of at least the essence of his achievements.

THE EXTINCTION AND EMERGENCE OF SPECIES: THE FOSSIL RECORD

Leonardo da Vinci (1452-1519) deduced that fossils were preserved remains of animals that had lived, grown, died, and been deposited on the sea floor long ago and were later uplifted and found in mountains. The Dane Niels Stenscn (1638-1686), known by his Latin name, Nicolaus Steno, was an anatomist who dissected and described the duct of the parotid salivary gland and carried out comparative studies of the teeth. He identified the structures in rocks known as glossopetrae (petrified tongues) to be fossilized sharks' teeth. He proposed that they had been deposited, then uplifted during subsequent conformational changes in the rock strata. The Swiss fossil collector and geologist Jean-Andre Deluc (1727-1817) was the first to correlate the presence of fossils with rock layers. Deluc observed layering of strata where the cliffs of southern England met the sea: chalk over limestone over clay. He no-

415. *Facing page,* Charles Robert Darwin (1809-1882) in his prime; by this time in his career he had found his mission on a voyage of discovery, recorded his impressions, collected his specimens, arranged their evaluation by current authorities, was carrying out research on difficult questions, and was working on a synthesis of his findings in a revolutionary analysis of the nature of biological science in its physical environment. *On the Origin of Species by Means of Natural Selection or the Preservation of Favoured Races in the Struggle for Life* appeared in 1859. Darwin proposed the theory of descent of life-forms and the theory of natural selection from among the spontaneous variations available, and the perceptions of the biosphere were changed forever. His intense, eight-year research study of barnacles resulted in the publication in 1858 of a scientific classic. Darwin's boundless curiosity about nature, his unequalled grasp of the biosphere and its formation, and his intuitive imagination disciplined by meticulous, tenacious attention to detail were used in putting together the pieces of the gigantic puzzle he set out to explain. The pieces filled seventeen books and more than one hundred and fifty articles. Watercolor by George Richmond (1840). *(Robert Harding Picture Library.)*

ticed that the fossils contained in the three classes of layers differed, and he correlated the age of the rock layers with that of the fauna they contained by means of the principle of chronological superimposition. This proposition raised the question of extinction and replacement of species and the need to identify a process or processes by which faunal change occurred and spread around the world.

J.L. Giraud Soulavie (1752-1813) voiced the idea of biological evolution in his seven-volume *Natural History of Southern France,* published between 1780 and 1784, but it was immediately condemned by the Roman Catholic Church. Soulavie used the relative percentages of present-day organisms in rocks as a basis for dating their formation. In 1795 James Hutton (1726-1797), a Scottish physician, wrote *Theory of the Earth,* a fascinating description of the components of the earth's crust moving in a dynamic cycling system. He had switched his interest from medicine to agriculture and concluded that the mountains and highlands were eroded to form the soil necessary for plant growth. However, soil in turn was washed into river systems to reach the sea, where it consolidated to form rocks. The cycle was completed by subsequent uplifting of the rocks, with erosion following again. He also observed that granite intruded into other rocks, an event that would have required that it be in a molten, liquid form.

Georges Cuvier (1769-1832) was born in Montbeliard, near Basel, a French town then in German territory, and studied at Caroline University in Stuttgart. He described the extinction of an entire sequence of mammalian fauna in the Tertiary strata of the Paris Basin in such detail that the concept of extinction became unarguable. Cuvier taught animal anatomy at the Museum of Natural History in Paris. He succeeded Daubenton in teaching natural history at the College de France. When Cuvier was made professor in 1802, his chair was named Comparative Anatomy. His colleague, Alexandre Brongniart (1770-1847), directed the famous Sevres porcelain factory and taught mineralogy at the Faculty of Sciences in Paris. Together they studied the geological layers of the Paris Basin and the fossils they contained, particularly the thick deposits of chalk. In 1812 Cuvier published his *Ossements Fossiles,* or *Fossil Bones,* a four-volume set.

Cuvier believed the faunal changes were a result of "revolutions," that is, catastrophic changes in the environment. Brongniart showed that the deposits alternated between marine and freshwater species. The two professors noted that the oldest layers contained invertebrates and fish, then came the reptiles or oviparous quadrupeds, then marine mammals, and finally, the terrestrial forms. Cuvier created the discipline of paleontology and introduced extinct fossil species into zoological classification. His greatest goal was to establish a general comparative anatomy. Cuvier made a special study of living and extinct species of elephants. He demonstrated that there were major anatomical differences between the African and Asiatic species and that mammoths were closer to the Indian species than the latter was to the African. He knew that the Siberian mammoths were well insulated with hair against the Arctic cold and that a species from America had knobbly, breast-shaped grinding surfaces on its molars, consigning it to a new genus, *Mastodon.*

William "Strata" Smith (1769-1834) was an English surveyor who wrote a succinct book in 1816, *Strata Identified by Organized Fossils,* which listed seventeen strata correlated with their characteristic fauna. These strata ranged from the Jurassic to the Tertiary. He soon added ten more, older strata. He had distributed manuscripts of his work a decade before his book appeared. The period from 1820 to 1855 was a golden age for naming geological stages and estimating their chronology. The use of fossils to assist in this process became known as biostratigraphy, the fascinating field founded by Smith and Brongniart. The Old Red Sandstone, laid down as sedimentary rock in the Devonian period of the upper Paleozooic era, the "Age of Fishes" (306 million to 408 million years ago), was rich in fish fossils and heralded the start of colonization of the land.

William Buckland at Oxford University was a motivating force for budding geologists. He taught Charles Lyell (1797-1875), who became Darwin's mentor, and Roderick Impy Murchison (1792-1871), who named the transition strata on the Welsh border *Silurian* after an ancient Welsh tribe that resisted the Romans. Reverend Adam Sedgwick (1785-1873) was professor of geology at Cambridge University, where he taught Darwin. He named the older strata in southwestern England and Wales beneath the Silurian—the Cambrian strata—after the archaic name for Wales (Cambria). Charles Lyell developed the assumption of "unitarianism"—that the geological processes and natural laws operating to modify the earth's crust act in the same way throughout geological time. This assumption implied that systems were in a "steady state" over long periods. As the pieces of the puzzle were gradually assembled, it became possible to chart the entire geological and biological history of the planet's surface layers.

Eduard Suess (1831-1914) of Vienna, author of *The Formation of the Alps* (1875) and *The Face of the Earth,* published in three volumes from 1883 to 1909, considered the theory of uniformitarianism inadequate to explain all the events that shaped the crust of the earth. He added the concept that the crust was under tension as a result of cooling, which generated lateral thrusts that form rising folds and radial thrusts perpendicular to the surface that cause collapses. His example of the formation of the Alps expressed the idea that a thrust from the south forced an override, while a collapse occurred behind it, forming the Adriatic depression and the western Mediterranean Sea. Marcel Bertrand (1847-1907) extended Suess's ideas and identified the processes that led to the various chains Europe comprises. Bertrand was able to extend his model across the Atlantic Ocean and to include the North American continent. Both Suess and Bertrand recognized that there must be global movements of the earth's crust. Rather than assuming that the land was uplifting because of the collapsing crust, they suggested that all the oceans on the earth must be lowering.

The production of accurate maps of the entire world revealed to the alert observer the congruence of the coastlines of eastern South America and western Africa. Alfred Wegener (1880-1930) was one who made this connection; he then read a report of evidence from rocks and fossils of a former land bridge between Africa and Brazil and uncovered clues from geology and paleontology. He proposed the idea that continents had been connected in the distant past but had "drifted" apart to gradually reach their present positions. In 1915 he published *The Origins of Continents and Oceans.* He joined Danish expeditions to cross the Greenland ice cap between 1908 and 1930 and perished there at fifty years of age while pursuing his interests in meteorology. It took nearly fifty years for his revolutionary theory to be accepted, mainly because of the lack of knowledge of a mechanism that could generate the necessary leverage to shift the vast land masses. Arthur Holmes (1890-1965) of Edinburgh proposed such a mechanism in 1928: powerful convection currents in the fluid substratum underneath the earth's crust. The thermal energy would have been generated by radioactivity in the granites of the continents, causing currents to flow outward toward their peripheries, then downward.

New technologies that permitted studies of the ocean floor allowed revision of Wegener's theory. Harry Hess of Princeton University had made bathymetric studies of the floor of the Pacific Ocean during World War II and conceived the idea of a kind of conveyor belt to account for the behavior of the crust under the ocean. R.S. Dietz suggested that the sliding surfaces be called "sea-floor spreading" and proposed that they were situated far below the lower boundary of the earth's crust at the boundary between the lithosphere and the asthenosphere. Thus the moving bodies were vast plates whose movements could occur because of the fluidity of the asthenosphere. According to the theory of plate tectonics, the ocean crust is consumed into subduction zones of the lithosphere at the same rate as it is generated at mid-oceanic ridges.

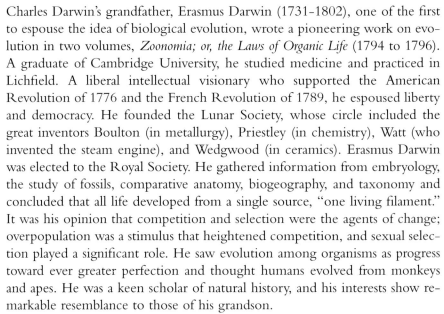

IDEAS AND DEFINITIONS OF EARLY EVOLUTIONISTS

Charles Darwin's grandfather, Erasmus Darwin (1731-1802), one of the first to espouse the idea of biological evolution, wrote a pioneering work on evolution in two volumes, *Zoonomia; or, the Laws of Organic Life* (1794 to 1796). A graduate of Cambridge University, he studied medicine and practiced in Lichfield. A liberal intellectual visionary who supported the American Revolution of 1776 and the French Revolution of 1789, he espoused liberty and democracy. He founded the Lunar Society, whose circle included the great inventors Boulton (in metallurgy), Priestley (in chemistry), Watt (who invented the steam engine), and Wedgwood (in ceramics). Erasmus Darwin was elected to the Royal Society. He gathered information from embryology, the study of fossils, comparative anatomy, biogeography, and taxonomy and concluded that all life developed from a single source, "one living filament." It was his opinion that competition and selection were the agents of change; overpopulation was a stimulus that heightened competition, and sexual selection played a significant role. He saw evolution among organisms as progress toward ever greater perfection and thought humans evolved from monkeys and apes. He was a keen scholar of natural history, and his interests show remarkable resemblance to those of his grandson.

The French natural philosopher Jean-Baptiste de Lamarck (1744-1829), wrote *Zoological Philosophy* in 1809. His idea of evolution was that in every organism there is a force propelling it toward greater complexity and perfection. He also believed in transformism; that is, he thought that the fossil species, rather than becoming extinct, adapted and were transformed into the present species. He claimed that giraffes gained their long necks by stretching—each generation a little longer—toward better forage high in trees and that the change was being inherited. He was not the originator of this concept or of the concept that organs atrophy if unused, yet he is remembered for the idea of the "inheritance of acquired characteristics." The latter became Soviet ideology under Trofim Lysenko, a disaster for Russian genetics.

Sir Charles Lyell discussed and rejected Lamarck's transmutation theory. Rather, Lyell believed that species became extinct one by one, leaving gaps that were filled by new species. Cuvier ridiculed Lamarck, and his ideas did not gain wide acceptance. The Swiss scholar and naturalist Louis Agassiz (1807-1873), founder of the Museum of Comparative Zoology at Harvard University, asserted that a series of fifty catastrophes caused extinctions of organisms that were replaced by new creations of more progressive fauna. He remained a confirmed antievolutionist to his death.

One approach to the idea of evolution came from embryology. Johannes Purkinje (1787-1869), the brilliant Czech physiologist, discovered the germinal vesicle of the chick two years before Karl Ernst von Baer (1792-1876), from Estonia, found the mammalian egg. However, von Baer returned to the hen's egg to study embryological development in detail, then extended his work to look comparatively at many animal forms and develop a general theory of "evolution," although this was a different usage of the word. Nevertheless, the German natural philosopher Ernst Haeckel (1834-1919) of Jena, a committed evolutionist, propounded his "biogenetic law" that "ontogeny recapitulates phylogeny," which asserts that the embryonic development of an individual retraces the evolutionary pathway of its ancestral group. Von Baer's principle was more specific, implying a progression from the homogeneous egg to the heterogeneous embryo, an expanding diversity and complexity of the individual rather than transmutation.

Charles Darwin stated that embryology had provided him with the best evidence for evolution, thereby triggering a surge of comparative studies in the field during and after the 1860s. He saw the embryo as evidence of descent with modification, while recognizing that he had no idea how changes or genetic mutations might come about. Although natural selection can clearly have a negative impact on the losers, how it benefits the winners is not

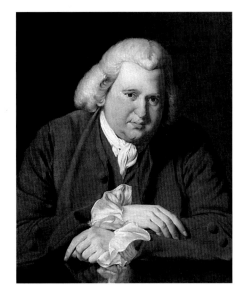

416. Erasmus Darwin (1731-1802) was the father of Robert, the Shrewsbury physician who was Charles Darwin's father. Erasmus, a doctor, trained at Cambridge and Edinburgh and practiced in Lichfield, then Derby. He was also a liberal intellectual thinker, inventor, scientist, and poet. He loved to converse with people who had cutting-edge ideas, and he founded the Lunar Society. Josiah Wedgwood, the famous potter who was destined to become Charles Darwin's maternal grandfather, was a close friend. Erasmus married twice and was grandfather of scientist-statistician and eugenicist Sir Francis Galton (1822-1911), a second cousin to Charles. Erasmus translated Linnaeus's *Genera Plantarum* and wrote *The Botanic Garden*. His most famous work was his two-volume opus on animals, *Zoonomia; or, The Laws of Organic Life* (1794-1796). It included a theory of biological evolution, which noted that change was driven by competition and hunger, lust and sexual selection, and security and survival, one example being adaptation of birds' beaks to handle the available diet. The evidence suggested that all life arose from a single source, "one living filament." *(National Portrait Gallery, London.)*

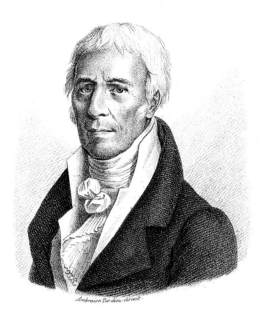

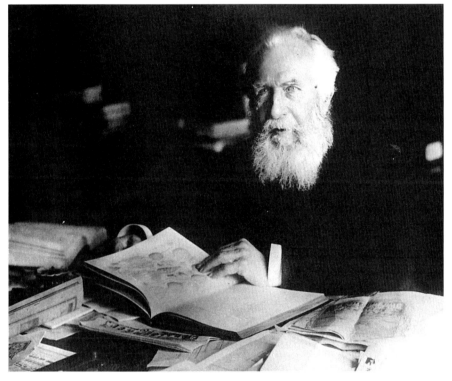

as obvious. Experimental embryology attempted to explain the processes involved. This effort diverted attention away from natural selection to a search for hypothetical chemical "organizers."

The concept of biological evolution addresses the processes of change that lead to the diversity of life systems over time. Today it has been estimated that there are well over ten million genetically differentiable "species" of animals on the planet.

THE SHAPING OF THE MIND OF CHARLES DARWIN

Charles Darwin's father, the eminently successful doctor Robert Darwin, had a fine family home in Shrewsbury. Charles was born in 1809; his mother, a daughter of Josiah Wedgwood, died when he was eight years old. As a boy he developed a strong bent for natural history, riding, and hunting. His father wished him to pursue a career in medicine, and he apprenticed with his father. At sixteen years of age Charles enrolled in Edinburgh, the "Athens of the North" and the mecca for medical education at that time. He was not motivated to study and was appalled by the agony of surgical operations before the days of anesthesia, so he left after two terms, having received a grounding in geology and having fed his interest in natural history with the guidance of Robert E. Grant. Grant was an ardent marine biologist, a committed evolutionist, and an admirer of Lamarck, who wrote *System of Invertebrate Animals* and preached that the higher animals had evolved from worms. Grant went further, tracing both the plant and the animal kingdoms back to simple algae and polyps. He took the chair in zoology at London University. Darwin became deeply involved in invertebrate marine biology at the microscopic level, a field he was to return to later, and presented papers on his findings.

Darwin was sent to Cambridge University to train for the ministry. The idea of becoming a clergyman was appealing. He envisaged serving a quiet country parish and having ample time to pursue his yen for natural history. He led a carefree existence at Cambridge, being active in the sporting set. He showed signs of his later aptitude for scholarship by avidly collecting beetles. Also, he became friends with two professors who recognized a spark of motivation, Sedgwick and John Henslow, in geology and botany, respectively. Darwin walked regularly with Henslow, a naturalist of broad interests, learning the lore of nature. The contact with Henslow, led to the invitation to join the crew of *H.M.S. Beagle* as naturalist and companion to the skipper, Captain Robert Fitzroy.

DARWIN'S UNIQUE OPPORTUNITY: THE VOYAGE OF *H.M.S. BEAGLE*

Emerging awareness of the amazing diversity of the biosphere of planet Earth through marine transport and the exploration of other lands led to a great enlargement of the scope of human thought. In particular, the emerging awareness was a strong stimulus to the development of ideas pertaining to natural philosophy and natural history. Extraordinary achievements resulting from nothing more than the exploitation of natural forces, winds, currents, and directed muscular effort of humans and animals made such development attainable. The ancient Greeks and Phoenicians, too, roaming throughout the Mediterranean and Black Seas, had acquired enlightenment in this way, including the study of the cosmos that was to form the basis of navigation and mapmaking.

419. The voyage of *H.M.S. Beagle* under Robert Fitzroy's command from December 27, 1831, to October 2, 1836, with Charles Darwin as his companion and unpaid naturalist provided a unique opportunity to acquire a near-global perspective of the biosphere in the Southern Hemisphere—its geology, aquatic and terrestrial biology, new glimpses of the fossil record, and even some anthropology. The main focus of the undertaking was charting South America's coasts, including the Galapagos Islands. Darwin, however, poured all his youthful zeal and energy into the study of the natural history of the regions visited; he collected and preserved vast numbers of specimens, recording all his observations daily in large notebooks. After his return he persisted until he got the appropriate experts to review and classify his specimens. Gradually he became convinced of the idea of evolution by natural selection. *(Reprinted by permission from Strickberger:* Evolution, *copyright 1990, Boston: Jones & Bartlett, Publishers, Inc.)*

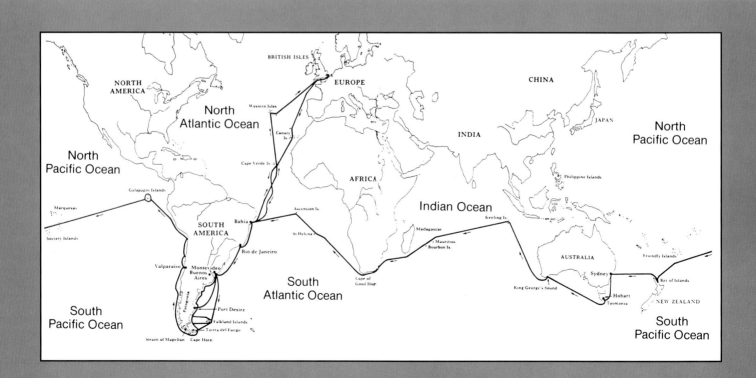

Darwin was extremely fortunate, at the tender age of twenty-two, to have been identified to accompany Fitzroy, already a master mariner, ocean surveyor, and navigator in the Royal Navy, on a voyage around the world. Darwin's father, however, was strongly opposed to his son's departure, and the intervention of his uncle, Josiah Wedgwood, was required before he could be persuaded to allow Charles to accept the offer. Robert Darwin had to come up with the money to make his son's voyage possible, including enough for a microscope and weapons. Charles took with him Humboldt's book, along with the first volume of Lyell's *Principles of Geology,* a parting gift from Henslow, and jars of "preservative spirit." It was December 27, 1831, before the voyagers could depart for the Cape Verde Islands. Darwin suffered terribly and continuously from seasickness during his first three weeks at sea and was virtually incapacitated. The next three weeks, which he spent observing and collecting specimens on the islands, were a heavenly break and a chance to develop his skills. The voyagers then set sail for Brazil and arrived at Bahia within three weeks, after a much smoother voyage.

Darwin's first exposure to a tropical rain forest made an intense impression on him. The first three and a half years of the voyage were spent near the coast of South America, from Bahia to Peru, before the *Beagle* headed toward the Galapagos Islands. Darwin spent much time ashore, studying natural history and assembling a vast collection of unique materials. He kept detailed notebooks but was a poor draftsman. He collected masses of biological specimens and sent them back to Henslow, who sent him the second volume of Lyell's work. The most striking things about Darwin's record are the amazing compass of his knowledge and interests and the tenacity and enthusiasm with which he pursued earth history and biology. It took two decades to identify and classify his specimens after his return to England, but he applied the same persistence to this goal.

The Galapagos, the unforgettable islands named after the giant tortoises that inhabited them, were a great adventure. Darwin's impression was that he was near where new beings appeared on earth. He was amazed to discover that closely related species of tortoises, mockingbirds, and finches differed from island to island and existed nowhere else. At first he failed to grasp the significance of the conformation of the beaks of finches, which were to become a major example of natural selection. It became obvious to young Darwin that, based on his growing awareness of the chronology of geological formations and fossils and the remarkable diversity of species still extant, the animal world could not have been created in a single day.

After leaving the Galapagos, the *Beagle* crossed the Pacific to Tahiti and New Zealand. In Tahiti Darwin started a study of coral reefs that he extended at other Pacific sites; he published his views in a book in 1842. The *Beagle* then traveled to Sydney, Hobart, and Western Australia before crossing the Indian Ocean via the Cocos Islands and Mauritius to the Cape of Good Hope in South Africa. After observing the remarkable differences between Australasian mammals and birds and those he was familiar with in Europe, Darwin was convinced that at least two distinct creators must have been involved. The South Atlantic proved hostile, and the breaks at Saint Helena and the Ascension Islands were welcome as the *Beagle* headed back to Bahia. Then it caught a favorable wind and reached England at last on October 2, 1836; the voyagers were nearly five years older than when they left. Stamped on Darwin's neurons were a vast array of impressions of world natural history such as no person before him had acquired. He worked to put his great talent to use in sorting and evaluating his enormous data base before writing his magnificent opus, consulting experts at every turn to ensure that he achieved the most accurate conclusions attainable at the time.

After returning to his homeland, Charles moved first to London, near his brother, another Erasmus, who lived an exciting intellectual life surrounded by radical reformers. However, Charles had an agenda now; he had been an inveterate recorder and collector on his marathon voyage. He had returned with or sent ahead a diary of 770 pages, notebooks on geology of 1383 pages, and 368 pages on zoology, as well as at least several thousand specimens. He poured all his energy into locating authorities to work on his specimens and writing his *Journal of Researches of the Voyage of the Beagle* while starting a five-volume zoology of the voyage that he edited with the help of the experts.

Lyell introduced Darwin to Charles Babbage, inventor of the hand-cranked computer, and to Richard Owen, hunterian Professor at the Royal College of Surgeons and comparative anatomist at the zoo. Owen agreed to examine some of Darwin's preserved animals and the fossil bones. The latter yielded dramatic discoveries, including giant capybara-like rodents the size of hippopotami, anteaters the size of horses, a giant llama, an armored glyptodon, and a gigantic ground sloth. Unable to tolerate dirty, odious London, the "modern Babylon," Darwin went to Cambridge to reunite with Henslow. He presented papers on his geological findings and interpretations, using fossil specimens to illustrate his points. Back in London, he persuaded George Waterhouse, curator of the zoological museum, to catalog and mount his mammalian specimens. The birds he assigned to John Gould, the great or-nithologist, taxidermist, and animal artist and author of *Birds of Europe* and *Birds of Australia*. He quickly determined that the Galapagos birds included a unique series of thirteen species of finches, and the determination sowed seeds of further feverish thought in Darwin. The four mockingbirds turned out to represent at least three species, each unique to an island, with relatives on the mainland. The Reverend L. Jenyns tackled the examination of the fish and found that all the Galapagos species were new. The plant specimens languished unattended in the British Museum.

DARWIN'S EFFORT TO UNDERSTAND HOW NEW SPECIES ARISE BY NATURAL SELECTION

Charles Darwin's churning thoughts about his exciting discoveries and broadening perspectives had to be recorded and treated systematically. He began a secret new "Notebook B" on the idea of transmutation in July 1837: on the title page, one word—*Zoonomia*. Heresy or not, he was already convinced that transmutation was a fact; how change was brought about was the only question. Usually new traits that appeared in individuals would be merged back into the larger population by crossing, thereby keeping the species more or less uniform: hence the assumption that species were immutable. In isolated stocks, however, such as on the individual islands of the Galapagos, greater inbreeding was possible, and a new characteristic such as a thicker beak could be perpetuated, particularly if it imparted an adaptive advantage, for example, in the efficiency of obtaining nutriments. Darwin made a crude sketch of an irregularly branched, treelike chart; some terminal buds were dying, to become the fossils, and the trunk represented a common organic origin. Intuitively he realized that the idea of life span of individuals did not constrain survival of species and that new forms must be generated continuously to provide candidates for replacing those that failed to survive. A primitive theory was already taking shape in his mind.

Darwin became engrossed in the possibility that the results of artificial selection of domestic livestock might make a valuable contribution to his thinking about evolution. He consulted his friend William Yarrell, a horse and dog specialist who was a veritable fund of knowledge about varieties, crosses, hybrids, foreign escapees, and the like. Darwin came up with the term *descent* for the process of development by transmutation. He filled his notebooks with information gleaned from animal breeders and their publications. He perceived that selection and selective mating were keys to the success of the breeder in producing more useful and productive animals and plants. Would the analogy hold for untended nature as a mechanism for evolution? There must be some inherent variability that would alter the adaptability of an organism to its environment, and isolation would have the effect of fixing new traits.

Darwin noted the opinions of John Sebright, a breeder of poultry who wrote *The Art of Improving the Breeds of Domestic Animals* (1809), and John Wilkinson, who wrote *Remarks on the Improvement of Cattle* (1820). In both pamphlets the power of artificial selection was discussed; Sebright drew the following analogy between artificial selection and its equivalent in nature:

> . . . *There is a strong tendency for like to produce like . . . yet he that is at all conversant with nature must perceive also that there is a certain tendency to change. And this law of nature would soon be assisted by man, who is ever fond of novelty and delights in diversity even for its own sake.*

Sebright also noted that harsh climatic conditions or food shortages destroy the weak and unhealthy first, so they fail to reach maturity and propagate. Darwin extended this thought by writing in the margin as follows:

> *In plants man presents mixtures, varies conditions and destroys the unfavorable kind—could he do this last effectively and keep the same exact conditions for many generations he would make species, which would be infertile with other species.*

At about this point in his thinking about process (1838) Darwin read Thomas Malthus's (1766-1834) *Essay on the Principle of Population* in its sixth edition. Malthus applied the simple, inviolable laws of nature to the understanding of the economy. His thesis was a mathematical principle of human population growth. He noted that population grows at a geometric rate, whereas food resources either fail to increase or grow, at best, at a linear rate. Thus some individuals must die by starvation in the struggle for existence and survival. Both Darwin and Alfred Russel Wallace saw this idea as the basis for a hypothesis concerning the nature of evolution by natural selection. They saw this population pressure as a drive to progress toward perfection.

Ironically the fertile mind that sowed the seed that grew into the concept of the mechanism of evolution rejected evolution as a theory. Malthus cited the experience of breeders to insist that there is a limit to progress. Darwin disagreed, however, insisting with his typical ecological insight that in nature there is continuous pressure from adapting and evolving life-forms to compete and displace others "wedging into any gaps in the economy of nature." Thereby he exposed the weakness of Malthus's argument. Malthus was proposing that people should not have children they could not afford; his message was to contain the burgeoning proletariat, not the rich, to avoid a future revolution of the starving masses. He opposed contraception and had no particular interest in animals. Since the human species had already mastered the ability to expand its food supply through agriculture, it was the one species to which it could be argued that the hypothesis did not apply. Darwin was stimulated by the thought that under the circumstance of overpopulation favorable variations would tend to be preserved and unfavorable ones destroyed. The result would be the gradual formation of new species by natural selection, or the "survival of the fittest," as the theory was to be christened in 1864 by the journalist and philosopher Herbert Spencer.

John Herschel, an astronomer, was the most famous scientist in England from 1830 to 1855. In an appendix to Charles Babbage's *Ninth Bridgewater Treatise* in 1836, Herschel came out in favor of a *natural* rather than a *miraculous* process of species creation. His position settled the question in competent intellectual circles and gave Darwin some assurance that a naturalistic explanation might become admissible. Darwin responded as follows:

> *Hereafter we shall be compelled to acknowledge that the only difference between species and well-marked varieties is that the latter are known, or believed, to be connected at the present day by intermediate gradations, whereas species were formerly thus connected.*

DARWIN'S MARRIAGE, ILL HEALTH, AND WITHDRAWAL TO DOWN HOUSE

While Charles was away on the *Beagle,* his cousin and first love, Fanny Wedgwood, had married. After his return he married her sister Emma in 1839. However, the way he had driven himself since his return to exploit the materials collected had taken its toll. He was stressed severely by overwork. His condition became chronic and deteriorated into a type of nervous crisis with gastrointestinal dysfunction that may have been a cell-mediated multiple allergy exacerbated by stress, mercury intoxication, and foul preservative vapors that affected the immune system and the autonomic nervous system. The condition, waxing and waning, stayed with him. The married couple left London in 1842 and moved to Down House at Downe, in Kent; Darwin settled into a routine to keep productive for the rest of his life.

In 1844 Darwin again met Joseph Dalton Hooker, a botanist and one of his warmest admirers, who had just returned from four years at sea. He revealed to Hooker his dreadful secret: "I am almost convinced that species are not immutable." Hooker agreed to examine the plants collected during the voyage of the *Beagle,* and a regular channel of communication was established between Hooker and Darwin. Charles finished his essay on evolution and showed it to the spiritually devout Emma in September 1844. The very next month an anonymous publication appeared, *Vestiges of the Natural History of Creation.* It was soon traced to Edinburgh publisher Robert Chambers. No doubt stimulated by the fossil evidence of evolving biotas, he espoused the idea that there had been progressive development of life on earth as the planet cooled over time. He proposed that all species arose by descent from common ancestors and that therefore there must be a natural process for the creation of new species. He suggested that the change occurs during reproduction, since this step involved single generative cells. Religious leaders and the spiritually devout denounced the book because it was perceived as a direct challenge to Genesis. Nonetheless, it sold well.

Darwin's versatility showed itself again in 1846, when he had finished processing all but one group of the *Beagle* specimens, an enormous effort that had taken him ten years. He immediately started to work on the remaining group, the unusual Chilean barnacles, which was different in that it required original research. The four-volume work on barnacles, the most focused single piece of research work that Darwin did, was important to his development as a reputable scientist. The research also gave him "breathing space" in which to hatch his evolutionary thoughts while considering the barnacles as a particular example of a group that turned out to be extremely complex. It took Darwin nearly eight years of unremitting toil to work from his initial discovery of a unique parasitic species in Chilean waters to the sorting out of the taxonomy of the entire subclass Cirrepedia. The passage of time allowed the religious furor over *Vestiges* to die down, and his own ideas appeared less revolutionary.

Darwin's health had deteriorated. He gave a copy of his draft essay on evolution, now 231 pages long, to his one confidant, Hooker, to critique. Hooker, who had become his most valued adviser, soon took off on another exploration. They kept in touch, however, and the trip brought more biological food for thought. So desperate did Darwin's health become, and so ineffectual were the doctors, that Charles went to Malvern spa and took the "water cure." Tragedy then struck the Darwin family. His beloved daughter Annie died of a mysterious illness that included severe abdominal pain, causing Darwin to fear that he had passed on a hereditary weakness.

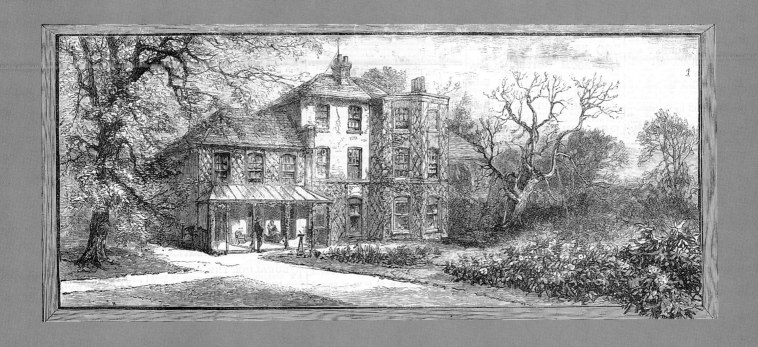

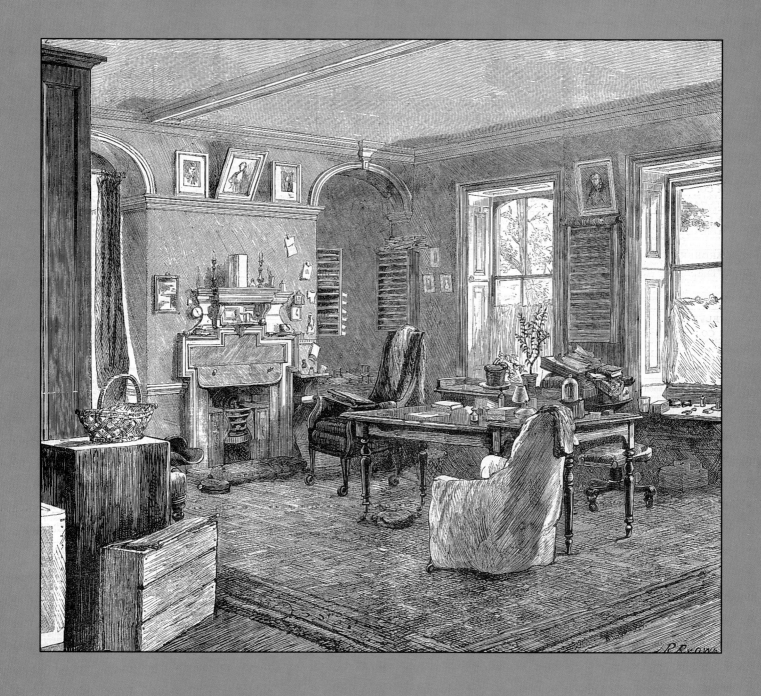

RETURN TO THE SPECIES QUESTION
AND ARTIFICIAL SELECTION

Returning to his great theme of the origin of species, Darwin was awed by the immensity of his accumulating base of data in natural history. Creation as described in the Bible was contradicted by almost every aspect of the natural world, and those who believed in divine creation had no explanations for the fossil record nor for the hierarchy of types of organisms so carefully crafted by Linnaeus. Bishop Ussher's calculation of the date of the creation itself as 4004 BC was clearly absurd. The famous physicist Lord Kelvin (1824-1907), who codiscovered the second law of thermodynamics and developed the Kelvin temperature scale, published a paper in 1866 refuting the doctrine of uniformity in geology. Using elegant calculations, he claimed to have shown that Earth was too young to allow for Darwin's time scale of evolution. His final value for the age of the earth, twenty million years, was based on the rate of cooling of a molten planet. He made an incorrect assumption, however, that there were no renewable sources of heat in the crust. Darwin's own estimate of several thousand million years was incredibly close to the mark accepted today. After Pierre Curie showed in 1903 that radium salts emit heat, Ernest Rutherford shattered Kelvin's long-held theory by proving that the earth generates heat by radioactivity. This new force would later provide the clock to establish the age of the planet and vindicate Charles Darwin.

Darwin was aware of and troubled by the evidence that there had been a rapid expansion of phyla during the early Cambrian period, accompanied by many extinctions. Progress had to await Charles D. Walcott's discovery in 1907 of a marvelous range of fossils in Burgess Shale, which were phyla of soft animals that had been preserved in ancient muds of sudden underwater landslides. The site, dating to about 570 million years ago, was near Burgess Pass in the Canadian Rockies and provided convincing fossil evidence of a "Cambrian explosion" of designs for multicellular organisms.

Darwin's plan was to write a great work on the origin of species. He was working toward that goal by organizing his information about the natural world and expanding his knowledge of livestock breeding. One of his overseas correspondents was Edward Blythe (1810-1873) who worked on zoology in a Calcutta museum. He sent a lot of material on the domestic animals of India that Darwin later used in another book. Blythe's idea of life as a branched tree that subdivides repeatedly was similar to Darwin's; he had envisioned nature as an irregularly branched, treelike formation for a long time. This idea was adopted enthusiastically by Haeckel in 1866. Darwin carried out experiments on the survival of seeds in seawater as a means of spread of life-forms around the world.

As stated earlier, contemplation of the extraordinary diversity of varieties achieved by breeders of domesticated species had long fascinated Darwin as having prospects of yielding clues to the mechanism of natural selection. He had read widely on the subject for many years, and in 1855 he decided to enter into it at first hand by breeding pigeons. He knew already that all domestic breeds of pigeons developed by the fanciers, despite the remarkable diversity of appearance of the varieties, were derived from the wild rock pigeon. His long-standing interest in development led him to focus on the point at which the varietal changes in young birds became detectable. He built a pigeon house and bought fantails, pouters, runts, and tumblers. He mixed with the breeders, picking their brains for every piece of knowledge and lore they would impart. He watched his birds endlessly. Then, after using prussic acid to euthanize them, since it caused the least suffering, he "skeletonized" them and measured them relentlessly.

Darwin recognized that the experienced fanciers had used great skill in detecting almost imperceptible differences to select the traits that became exaggerated to such a remarkable degree in creating the varieties. Applying criteria commonly used by zoologists, Darwin noted that among fifteen varieties that he had bred himself there were the equivalents of three good species and about fifteen good subtypes. Darwin extended his studies to several other domestic species, including ducks, dogs, and horses. He sought out information on varieties of animals of all kinds. Ultimately his message from his intriguing but ghoulish investigation was that the naturalists, who had no difficulty admitting that many domestic races were descended from the same ancestors, should be cautious before deriding the idea that species in nature are lineal descendants of other species.

A professor of botany at Harvard University, Asa Gray (1810-1888), had regularly supplied Darwin with knowledge about plant distribution. Darwin brought him into his confidential inner circle in 1857, providing him with an outline of his theory. Gray championed Darwin's cause in the United States but could not shake his faith enough to omit God from the architectural office of nature. Gray faced a formidable opponent at his own institution in the Swiss naturalist and zoologist Louis Agassiz, a virulent antievolutionist. In 1876, when Gray published a series of essays under the title *Darwiniana,* his genuine support for the theory became clear.

WALLACE'S INSIGHTS ON BIOGEOGRAPHY AND EVOLUTION OF SPECIES

Darwin's meticulous development of the huge canvas of his theory of the origin of species had been shaping slowly but steadily; he had written eleven chapters between 1856 and 1858, about 130,000 words. In June 1858 he received a letter from Ternate in the Molucca Islands, along with a twelve-page memoir on natural selection, written by A.R. Wallace. Independent from Darwin, Wallace had come up with essentially the same concept of a mechanism for evolution. Wallace had been corresponding with Darwin and sending him specimens of fowl tissues. Charles had told Wallace by letter of the great book on species that he was writing and that he had a distinct, tangible idea about how the species came to differ.

The arrival of Wallace's paper caused a crisis for Darwin. He sent it to Lyell, as requested by the author, and turned over to Lyell and Hooker for resolution the question of what, if anything, he should do to preserve his priority. Darwin's personal situation was difficult. Two of his children were deathly ill, and one died. His own health was poor. Hooker and Lyell were able to get the papers of Darwin and Wallace added to the agenda of a meeting of the Linnaean Society on July 18, 1858, and they were read by the secretary. The papers consisted of extracts of Darwin's 1844 essay, part of his 1857 letter to Asa Gray, and Wallace's memoir. Thus after twenty years of labor Darwin was thrust into the open world of communication. The earthshaking revelations of a mechanism for evolution, however, caused barely a tremor in scientific circles. Wallace approved of the way things had been handled; in fact, he said he was gratified if the effect of his memoir had been to galvanize Darwin.

Alfred Russel Wallace (1823-1913) became, as previously described, the codiscoverer of the mechanism of evolution, natural selection. Born in Usk, he had left school at thirteen years of age and acquired an interest in natural history while working as a surveyor's assistant. He met Henry Walter Bates (1825-1892), whose passion was entomology. Both had read Darwin's *Voyage of the Beagle,* Humboldt's *Personal Narrative of Travels to the Equinoctial Regions of the New Continent,* Edwards's *A Voyage up the River Amazon, Including a Residence at Para,* and *Vestiges of Creation* (Anonymous). Bates persuaded Wallace to accompany him on a collecting trip to Amazonia, where Wallace stayed from 1848 to 1852. During that time his brother had joined him, only to die tragically of yellow fever. Wallace himself suffered from repeated fevers and ill health. After Wallace left Bates in his "butterfly heaven," disaster struck

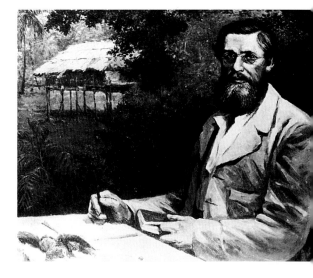

421. Alfred Russel Wallace (1823-1913), a brilliant, heroic, self-taught natural historian, was motivated by Darwin's record of his voyage on the *Beagle.* Wallace explored and collected specimens in the Amazon River basin, including its Rio Negro tributary, from 1848 to 1852 but lost his treasures when his ship burned and sank on the return journey. Rescued, he recorded his unique experiences, then set off in 1854 to roam the Malay Archipelago for eight years, collecting 125,000 specimens and establishing the field of zoogeography. In 1858 he sent Darwin a short essay outlining an intuitive flash he had had that nonhuman species evolve by natural selection, a limited version of the very theory that Darwin had developed two decades earlier but was laboring to substantiate from many angles in his *On the Origin of Species by Means of Natural Selection,* published in 1859. *(British Museum of Natural History, London.)*

501

again. On the journey home, his ship caught fire and most of his precious specimens were lost at sea.

Wallace managed to recollect enough information to write two books. Then he set off for the Malay Archipelago (today Malaysia, Singapore, Indonesia, and New Guinea), where he stayed for eight years. His primary focus became animals and their distribution. He proposed the division of the biosphere's continents and islands into zoogeographical regions and became the leading figure in the emerging field of biogeography. He identified the animal denizens of each of the six regions and acquired respect for his placement of Wallace's line, the imaginary line that runs down the Lombok Strait in Southeast Asia between the island of Bali and the islands of Lombok and Sulawesi (Celebes). Animals in the biogeographical region to the west of the line fell into the Oriental and Southeast Asian group; those to the east were Australasian types.

Wallace had read Malthus's essay, and it may have prompted him, too, to come upon the idea of natural selection. He also wrote *On the Law Which Has Regulated the Introduction of New Species* (1855), *Contributions to the Theory of Natural Selection* (1870), *The Geographical Distribution of Animals* (1876), *Island Life* (1878), and *Darwinism* (1889). He had an original and synthesizing mind but could never quite accept extending the concept of the origin of species to the human race. Instead, he thought that the human mind was injected supernaturally into an evolved ape. Wallace was the first European to study apes in the wild, the orangutans. He received the Royal Medal and was the first recipient of the Darwin Medal.

PUBLICATION OF *ON THE ORIGIN OF SPECIES:* THE FIRES OF CONTROVERSY

Although the book was much shorter than Darwin had originally envisioned, *On the Origin of Species By Means of Natural Selection, or the Preservation of Favoured Races in the Struggle for Life* was a substantial volume of more than five hundred pages when it was first published in 1859. By carefully avoiding use of the term *evolution* in favor of *descent with modification* in the first edition, Darwin tried to minimize the clerical reaction to his theory. Only at the end did he point out that "light will be thrown on the Origin of Man and his History," but there was no direct mention of descent from the apes. Nevertheless, the pundits freely used terms such as *transmutation* and the *ape theory*. The entire first run of 1250 copies was sold on the first day. Several editions later, the book is still in print today. As the ever witty Thomas H. Huxley said, "It was considered a decidedly dangerous book by old ladies of both sexes."

Darwin used his vast knowledge of facts and experimental results to build his case for the idea of evolution (that is, descent with modification) so carefully that his conclusions became inescapable to the reader with an open mind. He then explained the mechanism by which he believed evolution occurred—natural selection. This was the Malthusian concept, that there would be overreproduction of a species, but with Darwin's addition that a variety of traits would affect each individual's ability to adapt to the environment. Individuals with a more favorable combination of qualities would be "fitter," and more of them would survive and reproduce. Despite the delicacy with which Darwin skirted the most controversial issues, Huxley warned Darwin that the work would provoke outrage in some quarters.

In essence Darwin showed that nature, given the appropriate raw materials and environment, was capable of being its own creator, inventing and testing new modifications of designs for life-forms and then selecting from these prototypes the ones that worked best. The much more limited concept that there had to be a divine designer who had created a specific immutable blue-

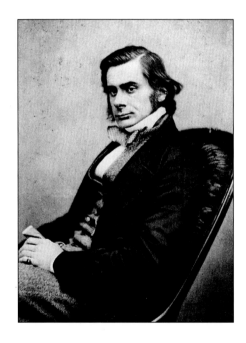

422. When Thomas Henry Huxley (1825-1895) received from Darwin a prepublication copy of *On the Origin of Species,* he was immediately impressed by the quality of the scientific argument and the wide range of coverage. He felt it provided by far the most plausible hypothesis yet developed to explain biological evolution. Knowing Darwin's aversion to controversy and his own penchant for it, Huxley declared himself to be "Darwin's Bulldog." He demonstrated his talent in his debate with Samuel Wilberforce, Bishop of Oxford, whom he overwhelmed at the British Association meeting in 1860. Joseph Hooker, Darwin's confidant with whom he consulted on plant biology, "weighed in" during the debate by showing that the bishop had obviously not read the book and hadn't a clue about the rudiments of botany. *(Hulton Deutsch Collection Limited, London.)*

print for every one of the millions of species was clearly inadequate and at variance with the evidence from the fossil record, from comparative embryology, from species divergence on isolated islands, and from the results of breeder-modified selection and amplification of morphological variation. Darwin left open the question of the origin of life itself, but there is little doubt about his position on the subsequent evolution of the vast diversity of organisms that inhabit the planet. He coined the term *natural selection* for the process of adaptive change within a species that could lead ultimately to a new species. He recognized that because this is such a slow process, it is difficult to demonstrate its occurrence in a scientifically convincing way.

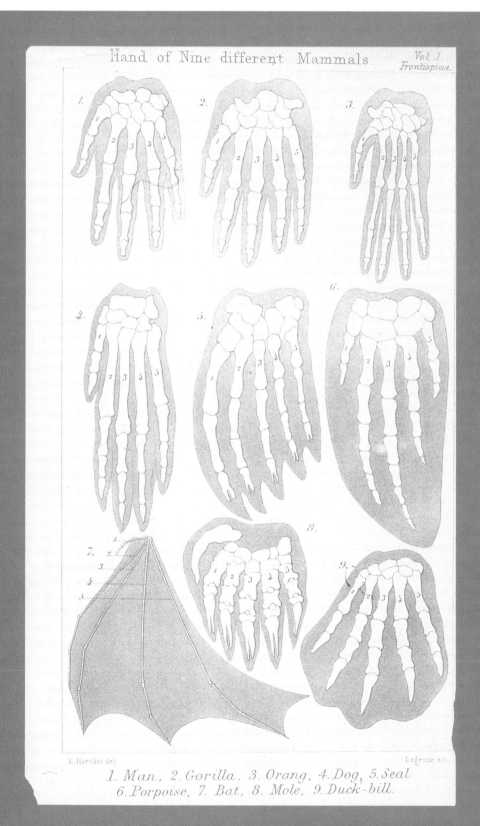

Hand of Nine different Mammals. *Vol I Frontispiece.*

E. Haeckel del.   Lagesse sc.

1. Man, 2. Gorilla, 3. Orang, 4. Dog, 5. Seal 6. Porpoise, 7. Bat, 8. Mole, 9. Duck-bill.

423. Comparative osteology, the study of skeletons of vertebrate animals, gave impressive clues to evolution. This drawing from Haeckel shows the bones of "the hand," or anterior extremity, of nine different mammalian species. It was designed to show their surprisingly uniform skeletal design, despite the remarkable differences in external appearance resulting from functional adaptation. All are shown in the same arrangement with the equivalent of the thumb on the left. Each species has a carpus comprising two transverse rows of short bones, a metacarpus made up of a single bone per digit (*1* to *5*), and five digits, each having two or three phalangeal bones. The magnification varies somewhat in this drawing. (*From Ernst Haeckel, 1911. General Research Division, The New York Public Library, Astor, Lenox, and Tilden Foundations.*)

Surprisingly, perhaps, the initial reviews were respectful, even favorable, but when the second edition arrived one year later, the critics were ready. A famous public clash occurred at the British Association meeting at Oxford in June 1860. Huxley took on Bishop Wilberforce of Oxford and trounced him in a public debate in which the bishop attempted to ridicule Huxley over his descent from the apes. The press had a heyday the following year, when an American of French extraction, Paul Belloni du Chaillu (1835-1903), who had lived as a child in West Africa and returned there to explore as an adult, published a controversial book, *Explorations and Adventures in Equatorial Africa.* He went to London in 1861 and lectured dramatically on the ferocity of gorillas in the wild, and the British public, none of whom had ever seen a gorilla, was fascinated. Du Chaillu brought specimens of stuffed gorillas and gave public demonstrations. Since the existence of the gorilla had only become well known in 1847 from the scholarly reports of two American missionary doctors, Thomas N. Savage and Jeffries Wyman, the chance to see the resemblance of the real thing to the human being created a sensation. Some concluded that Darwin's natural selection justified immorality in humans. Huxley also put Richard Owen, the powerful authority in comparative anatomy and paleontology and the one who coined the term *dinosauria* or *terrible lizards,* in his place in a debate over the structural development of the skull and the similarity of the ape's brain to the human's with respect to the presence of the structure known as the hippocampus minor. Huxley reviewed knowledge of the apes in an important book, *Evidence As To Man's Place in Nature* (1863). Darwin in 1871 published *The Descent of Man,* demonstrating the human's line of descent from apelike ancestors.

VARIATION OF ANIMALS AND PLANTS UNDER DOMESTICATION

Natural selection is affected by the reproductive success of each individual, that is, which genetic endowments achieve fertilization and how many progeny result. The survivability of these genotypes also comes into play, and in this, environment can have a significant effect on natural selection. Darwin was baffled by one implication of his hypothesis: How were characteristics passed from one generation to the next? He devised a provisional hypothesis,

424. Darwin drew on evidence from many sources in developing his ideas about evolution. One of these was comparative embryology, which had revealed the morphological similarity among early embryos of representative species of a great variety of phyla, despite their remarkable disparity later in development. Ernst Haeckel, who was the most enthusiastic promoter of the idea that ontogeny (development of the individual) recapitulates phylogeny (development of the tribe to which it belongs), prepared these drawings to illustrate the concept. He used these eight examples at three comparable stages of development to make the point. The four on the left are representatives of each of the classes of vertebrates below the Mammals; the others are from different divisions of the class Mammalia. (*After Haeckel, from G. Romanes, 1896.*)

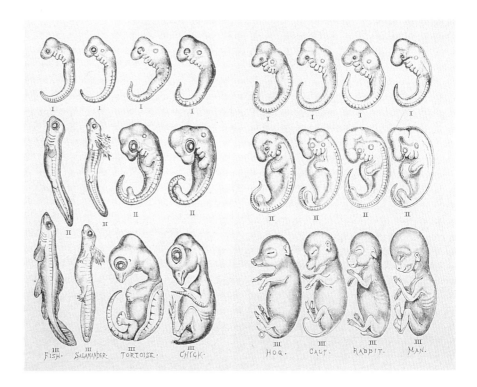

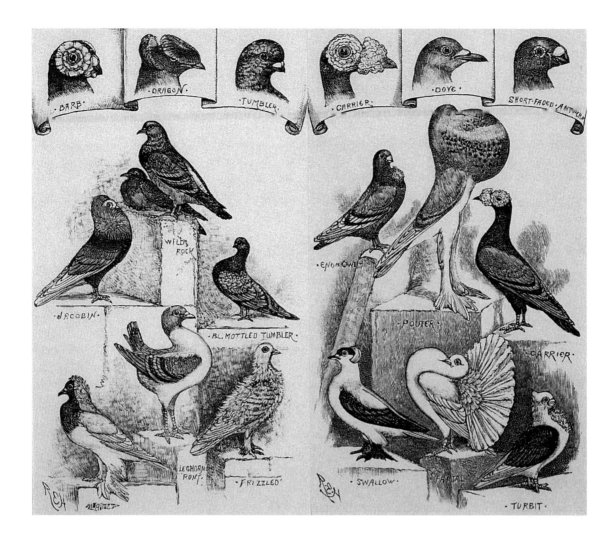

called *pangenesis,* that did not satisfy him, to explain the process. This hypothesis was a derivative of a Lamarckian concept that the more organs were used, the greater their impact on inheritance. At the time, conventional wisdom held that all the cells of the body had particles called *gemmules,* which migrated to the sex cells to be aggregated; only half of these particles were passed on to the offspring at mating. This "tissue democratic model" was shown to be unlikely by Galton, who gave blood transfusions to rabbits from a different strain, with no resulting evidence of genetic adulteration. Darwin was not aware of the nature of Mendel's work of 1866, which probably would have provided the intuitive flash he needed.

Darwin published his theory in *The Variation of Animals and Plants Under Domestication,* which appeared in 1868, thirteen years after he started breeding pigeons; an improved second edition was published in 1875. He was not proud of this work, but its first print run was sold in a week. Although he had performed an invaluable service for anyone interested in breeding domestic species and for veterinarians who need to be informed on such matters, the book did not receive the attention it deserved from the profession. The last chapter of Volume I, which laid out his theory of pangenesis, was controversial.

Although the hypothesis of pangenesis contained a glimmer of the idea of the gene, it missed the mark because Darwin had no mental preparation for the scientific study of hereditary mechanisms. The tragedy for science is that the crucial concept had been developed four years earlier in far-off Brno, in Moravia, Czechoslovakia, then part of the Austro-Hungarian Empire, but the whole world missed its significance. The findings in Moravia did not reach Darwin and in fact failed to reach the attention of the scientific community for thirty-six years.

Darwin's next product was really two books in one, *The Descent of Man and the Expression of the Emotions in Man and Animals* (1871). The first part re-

425. Darwin investigated evolution by artificial selection of domestic pigeons. These drawings from life illustrate the remarkable range of phenotypes that were produced by pigeon fanciers. Darwin learned all the tricks and conducted a massive experiment on breeding them himself, which led him to the conclusion that he had produced the equivalent of three good species and about fifteen subtypes based on morphology, yet all had been created from the wild rock pigeon by the artificial-selection pressure of human whim. Darwin's second edition of the *Variation of Animals and Plants Under Domestication* (in two volumes) in 1875 included information obtained by correspondence with animal breeders around the world. His chapter on *pangenesis* was a speculative attempt to explain genetics by a "democratic" theory that every cell sent "gemmules" via the blood to the reproductive organs. However, Galton showed that transfusing the blood of a black rabbit into a grey one failed to influence the color of the grey rabbit's progeny. *(Romanes, 1896.)*

ceived sustained criticism from St. George Mivart (1827-1900), who wrote critical reviews of the book, then produced a rebuttal, *On the Genesis of Species,* and another view, *Apes and Men.* A devout convert to Catholicism, he embraced the theory of evolution except for its extension to humans; he insisted, much as Wallace did, that God had intervened in human evolution to infuse a soul. St. George Mivart saw himself as a bridge, bringing scientific truth to the theological perspective and a religious perspective back into biology. Although his pandering to both sides earned him some public support, it offended the leaders on both sides of the debate. On one hand, Darwin was extremely disappointed by Mivart's attacks, and on the other, the Catholic authorities excommunicated Mivart. He did, however, write one book of interest to veterinarians, a massive anatomical text, *The Cat.*

Darwin separated his two books, and the new edition of *Emotions* was quite successful. A fascinating examination of the basis of sexual selection and behavior, the book has never attracted the following it should have among the members of the veterinary profession, who have been slow to realize the great importance of the study of behavior to their field. This is strange since veterinarians must use their intuitive grasp of practical aspects of animal behavior every day in their practice. Still stung by the first reception of *Descent of Man,* Darwin published a second edition in 1874. He recognized the extraordinary psychic development of language, thought, and socialization in human evolution and sexual selection. He asserted that "mentally man and animals do not differ in kind although immensely in degree. A difference in degree, however great, does not justify us in placing man in a different kingdom."

George J. Romanes (1848-1894), a Canadian-born graduate of Cambridge University, became a scholar of neuroscience and psychology in 1870. An admirer of Darwin and the *Descent of Man,* Romanes applied evolutionary theory to comparative psychology. He wrote *Animal Intelligence* in 1881, adding humans to the story of evolution in a second edition in 1888. Darwin had been interested in the psychological development of animals and children and had provided Romanes with his forty-year collection of notes and materials on these subjects. He also drafted an essay on instinct that

426. Tree-chart of mental evolution, showing the progress in emotional and intellectual development as a function of organismal evolution and of stages of human development, by George Romanes (1848-1894). Romanes was a Cambridge graduate who worked at the Physiological Laboratory after 1870, studying first the comparative development of reflexes. These studies led to a passionate interest in the evolution of the emotions and the intellect. Darwin was so impressed that he turned over to Romanes the records of his voluminous behavioral studies and notes on this field. Romanes rigorously organized and classified the evidence of animal behavior by zoological categories in a book, *Animal Intelligence,* in 1881, with the main focus on mammals. He extended his analysis in a second book, *Mental Evolution in Animals,* in 1884 in which the original version of this illustration (redrawn) appeared.

EMOTIONAL DEVELOPMENT PRODUCTS	EMOTION WILL INTELLECT	INTELLECTUAL DEVELOPMENT PRODUCTS	PSYCHOGENESIS OF MAN	THE PSYCHOLOGICAL SCALE
Shame, Remorse, Deceitfulness, Ludicrous		Indefinite Morality	15 Months	Anthropoid Apes and Dog
Revenge, Rage		Use of Tools	12 Months	Monkeys and Elephants
Grief, Hate, Cruelty, Benevolence		Understanding of Mechanisms	10 Months	Carnivora, Rodents and Ruminants
Emulation, Pride, Resentment, Aesthetic Love of Ornament, Terror		Recognition of Pictures, Understanding of Words, Dreaming	8 Months	Birds
Sympathy		Communication of Ideas	5 Months	Hymenoptera
		Recognition of Persons	4 Months	Reptiles and Cephalopods
Affection		Reason	14 Weeks	Higher Crustacea
Jealousy, Anger, Play		Association by Similarity	12 Weeks	Fish and Batrachia
Parental Affection		Recognition of Offspring, Secondary Instincts	10 Weeks	Insects and Spiders
Sexual Emotions without Sexual Selection		Association by Contiguity	7 Weeks	Mollusca
Suprise Fear		Primary Instincts	3 Weeks	Larvae of Insects, Annelida
		Memory	1 Week	Echinodermata
		Pleasures and Pains	Birth	

Romanes included in the 1883 book. Romanes regarded the cat as the most intelligent animal after primates and elephants. After learning about Mendel's work, he embraced the new science of genetics.

MENDEL'S MECHANISM OF INHERITANCE AND ITS QUANTIFICATION

Genius emerges in unexpected places, often despite economic disadvantages, as it did in Johann Mendel (1822-1884) born to German-speaking small-holders in the Moravian foothills of Kuhland, then part of Austrian Silesia, now in the Czech Republic. After schooling in Lipnike he went to Olomouc (then Olmutz) University in 1840, where he studied philosophy. A brilliant student but a delicate boy, he was unable to handle stress and was often ill. After the age of sixteen he had to provide for himself by working as a tutor while a student because an injury had left his father disabled. Nevertheless, an inner drive led him to persist in his studies. To gain access to higher education, he entered the Augustinian Monastery of St. Thomas in Brno, Moravia, and changed his given name to Gregor.

Mendel was fortunate that the monastery had a dynamic abbot, Cyril Franz Napp, who had guided St. Thomas to become a leading center of intellectual activity with a special focus on the improvement of agriculture. Napp was interested in gaining an understanding of heredity and breeding. Aware of Bakewell's achievements in improving the Leicester breed of sheep for meat production, he pushed for the British method and its application to quality wool production. His close friend, Rudolf Andre of Saxony, organized sheep research and wrote a book on sheep that was published in Prague in 1815, the first book on genetic improvement of domestic animals.

The abbot sent Mendel to Vienna University for advanced studies in cosmology, which encompassed astronomy, meteorology, and Aristotelian philosophy. Mendel focused on physics and studied under Christian Doppler and the crystallographer Andreas von Ettinghausen.

Christian Doppler was an experimentalist whose elegant studies proved the effect of movement on the pitch of sound, the Doppler effect. A century later the Doppler effect was exploited as a principle in medical research in the development of ultrasonic meters used to measure blood flow, one of the greatest challenges to physiological measurement.

Mendel's grounding in experimental biology began with exposure to Franz Unger, the first professor of plant physiology in the Hapsburg Empire. Unger emphasized microscopy, the new cellular theory, and the importance of studying the nature of fertilization, reproduction, and evolution in plants. He sowed the seeds of physicochemical principles that must govern the inheritance of discernable traits in Mendel's impressionable mind. In 1853, a few years after Mendel's return to the St. Thomas monastery in Brno, Mendel started his experiments on hybridization in peas. Mendel worked from physical concepts and principles in formulating his genetic theory, finding an idea for his model of genetic inheritance in the "sidedness" of crystals. He became convinced that there were structural entities or "factors" (known today as genes) that combined in the process of breeding. Thus the elements would be separated and combined, not merely copied.

In Mendel's period the phenomenon of meiosis, the reduction division that occurs when germinal cells are formed, was not yet known. Yet Mendel intuitively must have grasped that the offspring acquires its full genetic makeup from its parents as two halves, or in other words, that for each trait it received one factor from its male forebear and one from the female. This is the basic mechanism of variation, which sexual reproduction imparts. Mendel used letters in their capital and lowercase representations to indicate this

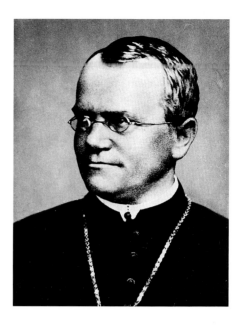

427. Gregor Mendel (1822-1884) was born in Moravia and entered the Augustinian Monastery of St. Thomas in Brno under the direction of Abbott Napp, who was keen on bringing science to benefit agriculture. Mendel was sent to Vienna University, then the jewel of the Hapsburg Empire, and learned experimental biology from Franz Unger, who believed physicochemical principles must govern inheritance in plants. Back in Brno in 1853 Mendel started his experiments with garden peas *(Pisum sativum)*. He conceived of a physical model based on discrete structures or "factors," which are paired so that they can separate and combine during breeding in plants. These factors determined the morphological traits exhibited by the plants. It was his proof of this concept that he presented in two lectures in Brno in 1865 and published in 1866, but his genius passed virtually unnoticed until his work was rediscovered in 1900. *(Mary Evans Picture Library.)*

mechanism. The following diagram shows that this mechanism allows an explanation of the observed ratio of 1A : 2Aa : 1a in second-generation hybrids:

First-generation hybrid pollen cells:	A	A	a	a	
First-generation hybrid germinal (ovule) cells:	A	a	A	a	
Second-generation hybrid off-spring results:	AA	Aa	Aa	aa	$= AA + 2Aa + aa$

Unlike his predecessors who favored a model of blended inheritance, Mendel insisted that there must be a particulate basis to heredity. Therefore there would be no change at the level of the physical elements, but the changes in the combinations of these elements could lead to changes in the nature and form of the organisms that developed from them. Hence there could be a whole spectrum of possibilities. With Napp's support Mendel developed the monastery garden for botanical studies and began his experimental work on garden peas *(Pisum sativum)*. He controlled pollination to produce the hybrids he desired of known parentage. He fostered two types that he knew would breed true, a tall form with smooth, round seeds and a dwarf form that yielded wrinkled peas. Trudy, who became a famous breeder of fuschias in magnificent colors, was his colleague at Brno.

428. Gregor Mendel carried out his classic experiments on genetics using garden peas for hybridization experiments in the garden at Brno monastery, now in the Czech Republic. In this representation of one aspect of his work, the figure on the left shows that crossing a tall plant with a short one yielded offspring that were all tall. He concluded that the factor for tallness was dominant over the one for shortness, which was recessive. These tall hybrids are known as the F1 generation. When they were crossed with other F1 hybrids, the resultant F2-generation hybrids were in a ratio of three tall to one short. He showed that this result was due to one fourth being pure tall, one fourth being pure short, and two fourths being mixed. From these he could obtain true-breeding tall and short strains by selection and further crossing. From this work he concluded that parental factors are transmitted as discrete factors rather than blends. *(Redrawn with permission from* The Human Body: Genetics and Heredity, *1985.)*

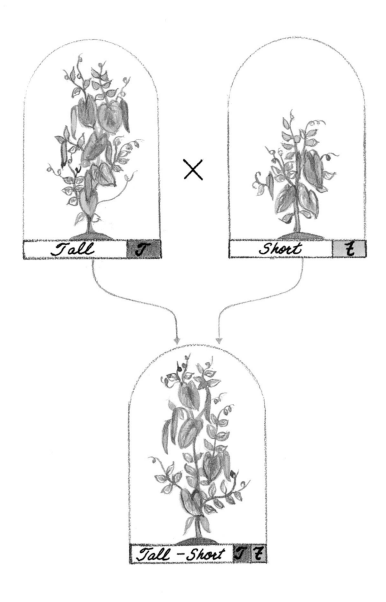

Mendel selected his two pea varieties to differ in eight characteristics such as height (tall or short), pod color (yellow or green), and seed texture (smooth or wrinkled). When a tall plant was crossed artificially with a short one, all the progeny were tall. Thus he said that the trait of tallness was *dominant* and that of shortness was *recessive*. When he crossed the first-generation hybrids, he observed that the recessive traits of parents reappeared in the progeny at a ratio of three tall to one short. This second hybrid generation in turn yielded the ratio of one pure tall to two hybrid tall and one pure short. From these results Mendel concluded that there were paired hereditary factors or *anlagen*—the *genes* in modern thinking—that control the specific expressed characters seen in the offspring.

Mendel put his results and conclusions in writing and sent them to the great authority in Vienna, Nägeli. Nägeli, however, was unimpressed and merely suggested that he conduct studies with the genus *Hieracium,* the hawkweed. Mendel did so and labored on the project for five years, but these hybrids did not follow the pattern established for peas. He had to abandon the project in disappointment. The reason for the disappointment was not discovered until long after Mendel died: the hawkweed is unusual in that its hybrids reproduce parthenogenetically (asexually) and hence remain constant. Mendel presented his work on peas before the Brno Natural Science Society in 1865 in two trailblazing lectures, and it was published in their journal as *Experiments on Plant Hybrids* in 1866, just seven years after Darwin's *On the Origin of Species* appeared in print. In that work Darwin had stated that "the

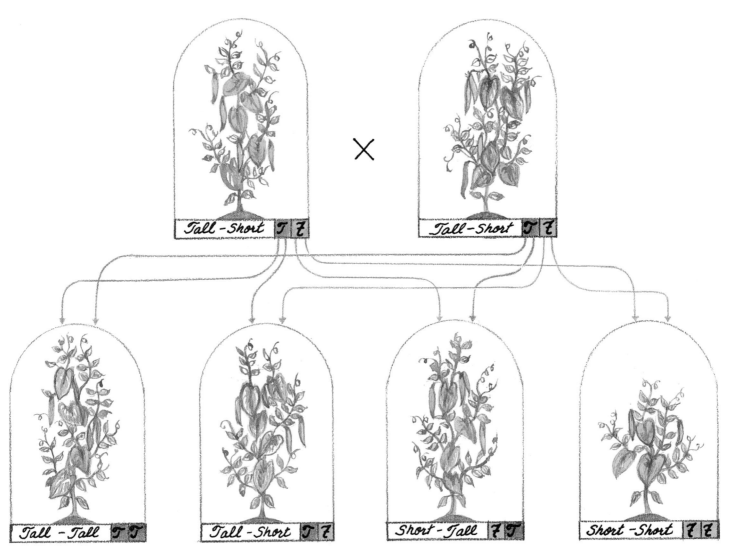

laws governing inheritance are for the most part unknown." The *Origin* had been translated into German in 1862, and an annotated copy was found in Mendel's library, indicating that he had studied it intently. Mendel died in 1884 without receiving scientific acknowledgement of his great achievement. In 1900, when De Vries in Amsterdam, Correns in Germany, and Tschermak in Vienna all rediscovered Mendel's research in the same year, Mendel finally gained the recognition he had always felt would be his due.

Among Mendel's conclusions (not necessarily in the same words) were the following:

1. Each character element is present in two copies (diploid) in the cells of a mature organism. The germinal cells (pollen and ova) have half the number (haploid).
2. The dual genetic character is not always revealed in the phenotype because there are certain alleles (alternative forms) of each element that can be dominant and can mask the expression of other, recessive, alleles (genes).
3. Dominance can be partial, or the combination of alleles can yield a new trait.
4. Complex situations exist in which the action of one allele wholly or partially obscures the effect of a different gene. This action is called *epistasis.*
5. Many traits are determined by the cumulative synergistic actions of many genes.
6. The environment can affect genetic expression.

SEARCH FOR THE CYTOLOGICAL MECHANISMS OF HEREDITY

Mendel said that there had to be physical units governing the genetic process, the working parts of the model of inheritance. Hugo de Vries (1848-1935) of Amsterdam was struggling with the interpretation of his plant hybridization experiments when Professor Martinus Beijerinck, the first to describe a virus (tobacco mosaic), told him about Mendel's paper, which led to the rediscovery of the work. De Vries believed, based on pigmentation changes in members of the genus *Oenothera,* that species changed by mutation, and he wrote a two-volume work on the subject, *Die Mutationstheorie* (1901 and 1903). He also took Darwin's term, *pangenesis,* and used the word *pangens* to define the hypothetical living, self-replicating units; Wilhelm Johannsen at the Royal Veterinary and Agricultural College in Denmark shortened the word to *genes* (Greek for "giving birth to"). He also named the sum of all genes in a zygote its *genotype* and the expressed characteristics of form its phenotype. Over the next two decades de Vries's new species were shown to be freaks caused by abnormal chromosomal combinations rather than new species. As Darwin knew, "nature will deceive you if she can."

Friedrich Schneider in 1873 and Walther Flemming in 1882 made early descriptions of the behavior of chromosomes (colored bodies named by Wilhelm Waldemeyer in 1888) that were seen during cellular mitosis. The crucial discovery of the reduction division of the germinal cells, or meiosis, was made by three microscopists, Edouard van Beneden (1846-1912) of Belgium and Theodor Boveri (1862-1915) and Richard Hertwig (1850-1937) of Munich University, who studied eggs of the genus *Ascaris,* a roundworm of the horse, in the early 1880s. In 1887 August Weisman (1834-1914) of the University of Freiburg proposed that the germ plasm of heredity probably was sited in the chromosomes of the nucleus of the egg and sperm cells, which served as equal partners. T.H. Montgomery in 1901 found that in species of the genus *Hemiptera,* the sequential maturation of sperm along the testis allowed the stages of meiosis to be clearly observed. Walter S. Sutton

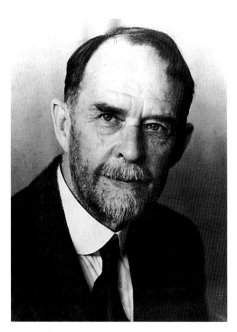

429. Thomas Hunt Morgan (1866-1945) of Lexington, Kentucky, earned a doctorate from Johns Hopkins University in 1890, acquiring a fascination with experimental embryology. He was appointed professor of experimental zoology at Columbia University in New York City, where he joined E.B. Wilson in 1904. Still skeptical about Mendel's concept of heredity, Morgan leaned toward mutation as a basis for understanding evolution. He selected the fruit or vinegar fly, *Drosophila melanogaster,* as his experimental animal model for genetic studies and strove to produce mutations. Studies of massive numbers in his fly-room laboratory proved Mendel right and, with his brilliant team of student colleagues, including Bridges, Müller, and Sturtevant, he characterized the inheritance of morphological features as a function of the fly's four chromosomes. His book, *The Mechanisms of Mendelian Heredity,* which appeared in 1915, paved the way for modern understanding of genes and chromosomes. Morgan was president of the National Academy of Sciences from 1927 to 1931 and worked at the California Institute of Technology from 1928 to 1945. He received the Nobel Prize in physiology and medicine in 1933 for his discoveries concerning the function of the chromosomes in the transmission of heredity. *(The Nobel Foundation, Sweden.)*

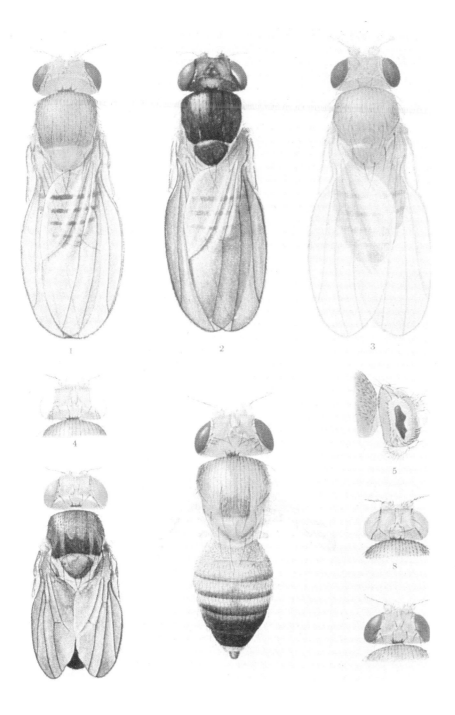

430. Features of the mutant fruit flies that Morgan produced in his fly-room laboratory, which was sixteen feet wide by twenty-three feet long. After a frustrating year of experiments, the appearance of a white-eyed mutant proved crucial to his discoveries. This type was always male, and he used it to establish the concept of sex-linked traits, which led to further evidence that genes were arrayed along chromosomes. Thus Mendel's "discrete factors" were actually the genes. With Sturtevant, Morgan developed the first chromosomal map by analyzing groups of genes that were linked along chromosomes. Morgan's team proved that the chromosomes were responsible for inheritance of morphological characteristics and that these were attributable to combinations of genes. *(From a drawing by E.M. Wallace.)*

(1877-1916) in 1902 and 1903 studied the relative sizes of the individual chromosomes and found in his grasshopper model of the genus *Brachystola* that the twenty-two main chromosomes were composed of eleven pairs, eight long and three short. C.E. McClung in 1901 suggested that there were qualitative differences among the chromosomes and that the accessory or "X" chromosomes of sperm cells might be the determinants of gender.

The great "fly room" experimentalist, Thomas Hunt Morgan (1866-1945), professor of experimental zoology at Columbia University, undertook the massive research challenge to characterize the chromosomal attributes of the fruit or vinegar fly *Drosophila melanogaster*. The fly matures from egg to fertile adult in twelve days, and millions of flies could be produced in bottles at trivial cost. Morgan subjected the flies to various stresses in the hope of inducing mutations and was rewarded with a white-eyed male a year later, in 1909. He believed in discontinuous variation and wrote *A Critique of the Theory of Evolution* in 1916. His research group progressively unraveled the chromosomal rearrangements and the complex relationships between genes and phylogenetic traits. Thus the genome, its paired parental origin, and the traits it gave rise to were defined. Morgan received the Nobel Prize in 1933 for clinching the chromosomal theory of heredity.

BIOMETRIC ANALYSIS AND POPULATION GENETICS

William Bateson (1861-1926) studied variation as a student and then as a professor at Cambridge by means of plant hybridization and rabbit and poultry pigmentation. He worked with his student, R.C. Punnett, on comb morphology in poultry. When he read Mendel's paper of 1866 for the first time in 1900, he immediately recognized its power. He had it translated and published the same year so that its content would be available to the English-speaking world without delay. Because Mendel's ideas had come under attack in *Biometrika,* Bateson wrote *Mendel's Principles of Heredity, A Defense* in 1902. Two years later Bateson said, "Breeding is the greatest industry to which science has never yet been applied."

Archibald E. Garrod (1857-1935), a person of astonishing prescience and insights into the nature of "inborn errors of metabolism," was the first to arrive at the idea of genetic control of biochemical reactions as a result of his interest in the inheritance of metabolic disorders. In 1902 Garrod consulted Bateson about certain congenital malformations and biochemical abnormalities (such as alkaptonuria).

Lucien Cuénot, France's first Mendelian geneticist, at Nancy in a series of publications from 1902 to 1910 showed that inheritance of certain traits of coat color in mice follows Mendel's rules and that some pigment genes are transmitted without expression. Albinism in mice could mask development of coat color—an example of epistasis. Cuénot observed a lethal condition in yellow mice that resulted in dead embryos. He was perhaps the first to propose that gene function is related to production of enzymes and showed that susceptibility to cancer and graft acceptance vary with genotype. In 1924 Guyénot of Geneva wrote a fine book, *Hérédité,* that was published in several editions.

Bateson in 1902 laid the track for a new scientific discipline by introducing the following terms: *allelomorphs* (later alleles), for Mendel's paired hereditary elements that remain distinct; *homozygote,* to denote that each germ cell contributes identical alleles; and *heterozygote,* to denote that the alleles differ. In 1906 he proposed that the name *genetics* be assigned to the new discipline, for which he foresaw a great future of theoretical and applied studies. He became the director of the John Innes Horticultural Institute at Merton in 1910, and Punnett was appointed to the Cambridge chair.

The mathematician G.H. Hardy, responding to a question posed by Punnett, tackled the question of how allele pairs would be distributed in large populations, assuming that no selection occurred. The conclusion of his investigation was that the ratio of dominant to recessive alleles would remain unchanged over generations. A disturbance such as natural selection or mutation would be required to change this equilibrium. Wilhelm Weinberg in Stuttgart arrived at the same conclusion. Hence the resulting equation became known as the Hardy-Weinberg equilibrium of 1908. Even a slight advantage of one form over another would lead to significant change in the proportions of the two alleles over a few generations.

A product of the Columbia University laboratories of Edmund Wilson and T.H. Morgan, Hermann J. Muller of Texas showed in 1927 that ionizing irradiation greatly increases the frequency of mutations and chromosomal aberrations. Muller, a farsighted visionary, once said that "man must eventually take his fate into his own hands . . . and not be content to remain . . . the cats-paw of natural forces." He had generously provided some of his earlier mutant specimens of the genus *Drosophila* and reviews of Morgan's work to colleagues in Russia in 1922. At Koltsov's Institute of Experimental Biology in Moscow Sergei Chetverikov, an authority on the genus *Lepidoptera,* was particularly interested in expansions and contractions of wild populations of *D. melanogaster.* Chetverikov was acclaimed for the classic paper *On Several Aspects of the Evolutionary Process from the Viewpoint of Modern Genetics* (1926),

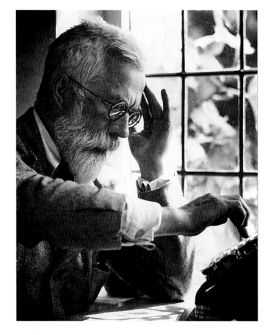

431. Sir Ronald Aylmer Fisher (1890-1962) made massive contributions to science, through his work on biological statistics, and to the development of quantitative genetics. His heroes were Charles Darwin, Gregor Mendel, and W.S. Gosset. Fisher created the concepts of experimental design and the analysis of variance, including the concept of randomization and the development, with Yates, of *Statistical Tables for Biological, Agricultural and Medical Research* (1938) which was produced by hard labor with a hand calculator. His seminal work on population genetics, *The Genetical Theory of Natural Selection* (1930), led to his recognition as a leading genetics scholar, the Galton Professorship at University College, London, in 1933, and the Arthur Balfour Chair of Genetics at Cambridge in 1943. Of particular interest to veterinarians and animal scientists is his *Theory of Inbreeding* (1949). Richard Dawkins anointed him the "greatest of Darwin's successors" in *The Blind Watchmaker* (1946). *(Reproduced by permission of the Fisher Memorial Committee, Gonville and Caius College, Cambridge, U.K.)*

in which he prophetically argued the case for evolution by natural selection that acted on dynamic populations whose genetic variability was generated by mutations. He pointed out that if genes change their nature by mutation, they will be retained by the population, which "absorbs them like a sponge." Lost to science by Soviet political manipulation, Chetverikov was exiled in 1927.

Three brilliant mathematicians developed theoretical models to merge Mendel's genetic concepts with Darwin's natural selection theory: Ronald Aylmer Fisher (1890-1962), John Burdon Sanderson Haldane (1892-1964), and Sewall Wright (1889-1988).

Sir Ronald Fisher (1890-1962) is remembered today for the work on statistics and genetics that he carried out before the computer era. An admirer of Mendel's conceptions and mathematical approach, Fisher published his first paper on genetics in 1918, *The Correlation Between Relatives on the Supposition of Mendelian Inheritance.* He analyzed sixty years of field trial data in plant research while working at Rothamstead Experimental Station and wrote a landmark textbook, *Statistical Methods for Research Workers,* in 1925. He began to focus on genetics and evolution, linking Darwinian and Mendelian concepts in another renowned book, *The Genetical Theory of Natural Selection,* in 1930.

Fisher's growing reputation landed him the Galton Professorship of Eugenics in London in 1933, where he focused on inheritance and classification of human blood groups, with a special emphasis on the theoretical basis of inheritance of the rhesus (Rh) factor. He was appointed to the prestigious Balfour chair in genetics at Cambridge University in 1943. Fisher conducted animal research on inbreeding and recombination in mice and poultry. Fisher said that Mendel's original data were "too good to be true" on statistical grounds. However, Tschermak obtained ratios in his data that were similar to those cited by Mendel. It appears likely that Fisher erred in assuming that Mendel used his experiments with peas to prove a preconceived theory. Mendel himself had published a short paper on his failures with the genus *Hieracium.* The scientific world is indebted to Nägeli's former student, Carl Correns of Tübingen, who obtained permission in 1902 to publish Mendel's letters to Nägeli in which he described his researches in detail. Most of these descriptions are unpublished elsewhere.

Fisher's theory suggested that large populations play a major role in the appearance of new traits that affect survival. He predicted, however, that evolution depends on changes that benefit the individual rather than the population. He revealed his leanings toward eugenics by pointing out that human societies indulge in natural selection against ability and intelligence: the tendency of the ablest individuals to curtail family size set the stage for the ruin of entire civilizations.

J.B.S. Haldane (1892-1964) was a challenging, provocative scholar of physiology and genetics. His father, John Scott Haldane, a distinguished Oxford physician and respiratory physiologist, was an ardent promoter of bridging between theory and practice in science. J.B.S. Haldane took his degree at Oxford in mathematics, was wounded in the First World War, and helped his father develop gas masks for use at the front. He moved to Cambridge to work with Frederick Gowland Hopkins, the leading investigator of enzyme reactions and trace nutrients at the time (1921). Applying mathematical analysis to enzyme reactions, Haldane proved that enzymes adhere to the laws of thermodynamics. His interest in genetics had been awakened when he heard a lecture on Mendel's discoveries in 1901, at nine years of age. By the age of eighteen he was conducting genetic experiments on his sister's three hundred guinea pigs.

Haldane followed Bateson in 1927 at the John Innes Institute. He was appointed to the London chair in genetics in 1933, having calculated for the first time the rate of mutation of human genes and the effect of recurrent harmful mutations. He found the link between hemophilia and color blindness. Haldane worked on air purification systems for submarines in World War II.

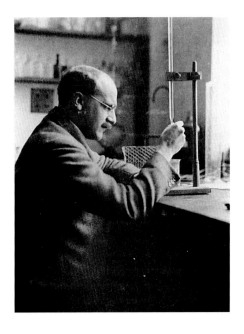

432. John Burdon Sanderson Haldane (1892-1964) was a brilliant mathematician and the son of the distinguished Scottish applied respiratory physiologist John Scott Haldane (1860-1936), who worked at Oxford University for twenty-five years and developed methods to explain the nature of the hazards of carbon monoxide for coal miners, of high pressures for divers, and of low barometric pressures for mountaineers and aviators. John Burden Sanderson Haldane extended his father's work during World War I, improvising gas masks to protect against poison gas, and again in World War II, to make the atmospheric and thermal environment of submarines safe. His training in biochemistry with F.G. Hopkins at Cambridge led to the book *Enzymes* (1930). Even as a child, he became fascinated by genetics after hearing Bateson in 1901 lecture on Mendel's discoveries. By 1910 Haldane was studying inheritance systematically in his sister's three hundred guinea pigs. He extended Bateson's genetic research on plants. In 1922 he described the mathematics of natural selection and in 1932 calculated the rate of mutation of human genes and the effect of harmful mutations on populations. *(Department of Biochemistry, University of Cambridge, England.)*

Ever an activist, he left Great Britain in 1957 to protest the Suez invasion and became an Indian citizen in 1961. Like his father, he espoused bridging basic and applied sciences and was a proponent of unity among scientific fields. Haldane developed a mathematical theory of natural and artificial selection in 1924. He wrote *Enzymes* in 1930 and his famous work, *The Causes of Evolution,* in 1932.

In *The Causes of Evolution* Haldane suggested that one of the principal traits with survival value is immunity to disease. Haldane returned to this idea in the paper *Disease and Evolution* (1949). He noted the existence of a density-dependent selection that limits population growth. He attributed this selection to increasing exposure to a parasite or parasites (bacteria, fungi, viruses, or protozoal and metazoal parasites). He also pointed out that harboring a nonlethal parasite can be beneficial because it is able to suppress the host's competitors. He was particularly interested in the possibility that the host species might attempt to stay ahead of its parasites, which can evolve much faster because of short generation times, by constantly producing new genotypes. Higher animals exhibit surprisingly high levels of diversity, that is, biochemical polymorphism. He noted that this diversity applies to proteins with attached polysaccharide groups that are typically part of cell membranes. The major histocompatibility complex (MHC) is one of these and plays a major role in host resistance to infectious disease. Haldane suggested that natural selection would tend to retain polymorphism to ensure that a diversity of such protective molecules would be available to increase the chance that there would be survivors.

Wright took a more physiological view of genetics, speculating that genes in some way prescribe the chemical reactions of the body, which result in many indirect interactions. His perspective differed from Fisher's in that Wright believed that species comprising many small, nearly isolated populations would be most likely to exhibit adaptive evolution.

William E. Castle at Harvard, working with hooded rats, was one of many who showed that genetics had many more overtones than Mendel's elegant pea experiments had revealed. Sewall Wright (1889-1988), who trained under Castle, worked with guinea pig inheritance. He applied his brilliant mathematical and analytical mind to generate a classic quantitative model for population genetics. Working for more than a decade at the U.S. Department of Agriculture, he had access to a large database of breeding experiments, much as Fisher did at Rothamstead. He considered random mating in large populations of animals to be unlikely, proposing the idea of *demes* or subpopulations within which more rapid changes would be expressed. He applied this reasoning to inheritance in shorthorn cattle. One of his distinguished students, Jay Lush, became the leading scientist in breeding research on domestic livestock. Wright moved to the University of Chicago, and he continued working at the University of Wisconsin long after he retired. His *Evolution in Mendelian Populations* (1931), in which he outlined his shifting balance theory, was a major contribution to genetics.

INTERPRETATION OF LIFE'S BLUEPRINT

J. Friedrich Miescher, a Swiss doctor, studied pus cells and in 1869 isolated a substance he called *nuclein* after he removed the protein. This substance turned out to be nucleic acid. Later it was shown that salmon sperm consists of forty-nine percent nuclein. Edmund Wilson suggested that the substance might be chromatin. Almost sixty years later, in 1928, Frederick Griffith was engaged in research on pneumonia for the British Ministry of Health, studying the causative agent, *Diplococcus pneumoniae,* a type of pneumococcus. He showed that encapsulated strains that had smooth-surfaced colonies were lethal when injected into mice, whereas strains that produced "rough-surfaced" colonies

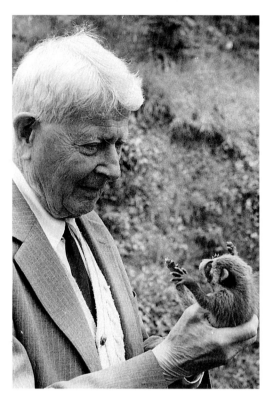

433. Sewall Wright (1889-1988) received a doctorate from Harvard in 1915 after working with William Castle, a pioneer geneticist who used laboratory animals. Wright joined the staff of the U.S. Department of Agriculture, Bureau of Animal Industry, in Washington, D.C., and Beltsville, Maryland, where he matured into a brilliant statistician and mathematical geneticist of growth and pigmentation, working with guinea pigs and Shorthorn cattle. This line of work was applied to animal breeding with great success by his student, Jay L. Lush. Wright also worked on the inheritance of susceptibility to tuberculosis and on histocompatibility. He moved to the University of Chicago in 1926, where he stayed twenty-eight years. He then moved to the University of Wisconsin, where he worked for another twenty-five years. During those periods he developed his creative ideas about evolution and the genetics of populations. He received the Darwin Medal from the Royal Society in 1980. *(Photograph by Doris Marie Provine.)*

were not. When live germs from rough-surfaced colonies were injected into mice, the mice were unharmed. If killed smooth-surfaced organisms were given with the live rough-surfaced ones, however, the mice died and live smooth-surfaced strains could be cultured from their blood, a remarkable transformation.

In 1929 Canadian Oswald Avery (1877-1955) picked up the clue from Griffith's "transformation" and sought the factor that imparted pathogenicity to rough-surfaced pneumococci at the Rockefeller Institute for Medical Research in New York. Avery's team labored for fifteen years on the project, establishing convincingly that deoxyribonucleic acid (DNA) was the genetic messenger molecule that caused the bacterial transformation. Between 1946 and 1950 Erwin Chargaff at Columbia University analyzed the four bases in DNA and showed that the ratios of adenine to thymine and of guanine to cytosine were always one to one, a finding that became a key to the genetic code. E.L. Tatum and Joshua Lederberg showed that biochemical processes in the bread mold *Neurospora crassa* were genetically controlled. Working with George Beadle at Stanford on X-ray–induced mutations, they showed that there is a gene for each enzyme and that collectively the genes are responsible for the network of metabolic pathways. Earlier Beadle had trained with Cornell's brilliant plant geneticist Rollin A. Emerson and with John B. Sumner, the first to crystallize an enzyme (in 1926). Beadle went to California Institute of Technology in 1931 and worked with Morgan, Dobzhansky, Sturtevant, Haldane, and Ephrussi.

Alfred D. Hershey and Martha Chase in 1952 used radioactive isotopes to label proteins in *Escherichia coli* bacteria and a virus *(bacteriophage)* that attacked them. The virus causes the bacteria to make phage rather than bacterial molecules. The phage has a core of DNA and a protein coat, which were labeled differently in the key experiment. The researchers showed that when the phage attacked a bacterium, it injected its nucleic acid component and no protein; hence all the genetic information must have been in the DNA. Therefore the genes were in the DNA.

By the early 1950s it was possible to demonstrate structural features of macromolecules by X-ray crystallography. Maurice Wilkins's department at the University of London applied this technique in the study of the nucleic acids. Rosalind Franklin (1920-1958) made crucial pictures that revealed that DNA had a double-stranded helical structure of uniform diameter. James D. Watson and Francis Crick, working at Cambridge University, put all available information to work and developed a model in 1953 that described the structure of DNA, which comprises bases, sugars, and phosphate. Arthur Kornberg at Washington University synthesized a DNA in 1956.

The field of molecular biology was born, and how the DNA's blueprint was transformed into molecular construction was soon revealed. Francois Jacob and Jacques Monod in Paris proposed that messenger ribonucleic acid (mRNA) was the transient communicator that takes the message from the DNA blueprint to the ribosomes, which receive the building blocks of proteins, the amino acids. In 1965 Robert Holley (1922-1993) at Cornell University completed the decipherment of the structure of a transfer RNA (tRNA) that lines up the amino acids. Crick in 1961 proposed that there must be a specific code composed of a few nucleotides (actually, three) for each amino acid. Marshall Nirenberg at the National Institutes of Health and many others contributed to the final identification of the code. A crescendo of discoveries since then has changed the scope of the veterinary future.

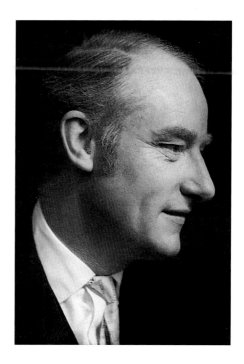

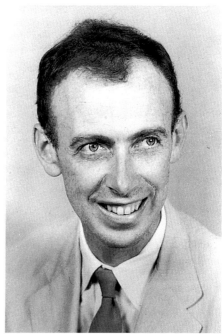

434. One of the greatest landmarks in the development of biological science was the identification and characterization of molecular structures in cells that are responsible for the transfer of the genetic blueprint across generations. After Oswald Avery had identified nucleic acids as the biochemical agents of microbial genetics in pneumococci, it was necessary to determine the specific chemical design of the molecules involved. The key to the solution of this question was provided by Frances Crick *(above)* and James Watson *(below)* in 1953 with their model for the molecular structure of deoxyribonucleic acid (DNA). Their model led to a great explosion of effort in research and its application in genetic bioscience. *(The Nobel Foundation, Sweden.)*

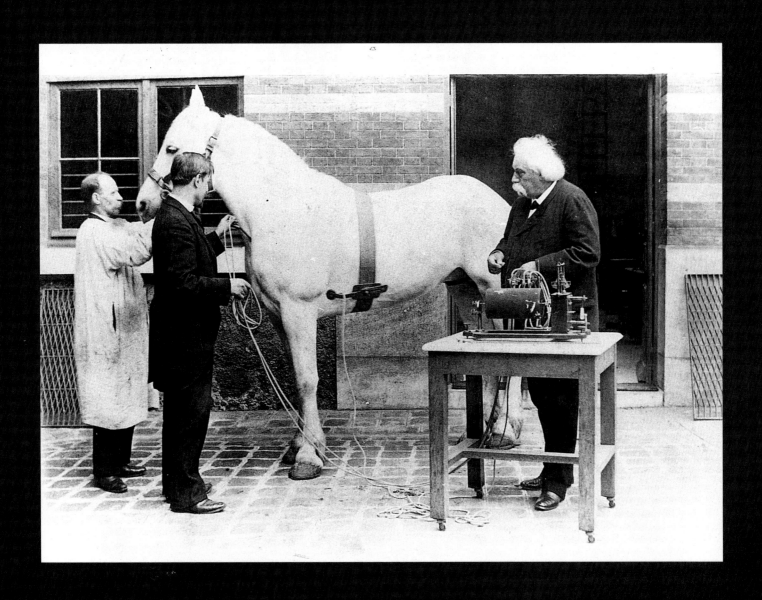

Early Veterinary Contributions to Biomedical Science

∿

A FINE TRADITION IN VETERINARY ANATOMY

Comparative anatomy of vertebrates had emerged as a major field of study before the first twenty-one veterinary schools were established in Europe between 1762 and 1800.

The first comprehensive anatomy of a domesticated animal was Ruini's *Anatomy of the Horse,* published just after his death in 1598. It was written to benefit horses and horsemanship by a passionate admirer of the species. The first complete anatomy of the dog was written by Gerard Blaes or Blasius (1625-1692), a physician at Leyden. Because he prepared his eighty-five-page canine anatomy in 1673 as a model for teaching human anatomy, he focused on the differences between canine and human anatomy to avoid misleading the student. He also described many structural features of other mammals and reptiles. Regnier de Graaf (1641-1673), a Delft doctor, was the first to describe the human ovary. He erred in considering the entire follicle the ovum but correctly anticipated that the ova pass down a fallopian tube. George Stubbs dissected horses in preparation for writing his classic *The Anatomy of the Horse* in 1766, just after the first veterinary school opened, but its scope was limited to the locomotor system. One of the founding pillars of the newly hatched veterinary profession in eighteenth-century France was Philippe-Etienne LaFosse. He published at his own expense the magnificently illustrated *Cours d'Hippiatrique* in 1772.

After Claude Bourgelat launched the veterinary schools, he appointed Honoré Fragonard (1732-1799), whose brother was a distinguished artist, to teach equine anatomy. Fragonard was born in Grasse, a town famous for its role in the development of perfumes. Fragonard was still training to become a surgeon when Bourgelat contacted him in 1762. When Bourgelat moved from Lyon to Alfort, he appointed Fragonard professor of anatomy. Fragonard developed special techniques to preserve equine and human specimens. He injected alcohol laced with spices into the arterial trunks to protect the tissues from putrefaction. Then he removed the skin *(écorché)* and molded the body and limbs into the desired theatrical poses. He dissected muscles, vessels, and nerves, injecting colored wax to create the desired effects. He was discharged on grounds of insanity in 1771 at thirty-nine years of age and disappeared. He resurfaced, however, in 1793 during the French Revolution and worked at the medical school in Paris until his death. Part of his collection of specimens has been preserved at the Musée Fragonard d'Alfort at the veterinary school, including preserved animal monstrosities and intestinal calculi of horses.

As the veterinary schools opened, most developed strong programs in anatomy as the only well-developed veterinary field. Anton Will trained at Alfort and then became professor at Munich. Weber in Dresden wrote on equine osteology; Hernquist at Skara, Sweden, wrote *Anatomia Hippiatrica;*

435. *Facing page,* Jean-Baptiste Auguste Chauveau near the end of his career at the Museum of Paris, repeating the demonstration of the famous experiment of intracardiac cardiography in a standing horse that he had first performed with Marey in 1856, when he was twenty-nine years old. The assistant holds in his left hand the sensors—one going via the jugular vein to the right ventricle and the other via the carotid artery to the left ventricle—that relay the pressures inside the two chambers. An external cardiographic monitor, held in place by a strap around the thorax, allows the precordial impact to be recorded. *(Photograph courtesy of Professor Jack Bost, Ecole Nationale Vétérinaire, Lyon.)*

Neergard and Viborg in Denmark wrote *Anatomie du Cheval;* and Kersting taught anatomy at Hannover. Sainbel (Saint Bel) in London taught anatomy and trained Delabere Blaine, who translated his writings and was a popular teacher. Blaine was not rehired by the professor and left to work in other fields but wrote *The Anatomy of the Horse* in 1799. By the end of the eighteenth century a subdiscipline of veterinary anatomy was taking shape.

A resurgence of comparative zoological anatomy and embryology in the nineteenth century was stimulated by Darwin's collections and fossils. Richard Owen (1804-1892) in London and Georges Cuvier in Paris were dominant figures in those areas of study. Thomas Huxley studied the great apes and became a leading campaigner for Darwin's evolutionary theory. The German anatomists formed a strong society, at first within the Society of German Natural Scientists and Physicians; then they split off on their own to form an international organization, Die Anatomische Gesellschaft, in 1886. Forty percent of its membership was from outside Germany. An important initiative in 1889 was the formation of a committee to standardize nomenclature. A journal that encompassed all the morphological subdisciplines was begun in 1886. Microscopy of tissues had opened exciting new avenues that led to the publication of *Cell Theory* by Schleiden and Schwann in 1838 and 1839, following the peripatetic K.E. von Baer's discovery of the mammalian egg and publication in Königsberg in 1827 of *De Ovi Mammalium Genesi.* The American Association of Anatomists adopted the *Basel Nomina Anatomica* of 1895, recognizing the importance of standardization and the use of Latin as the common anatomical language. Rapid progress was made during the last quarter of the nineteenth century in the development of histotechnique for preserving, staining, and slicing tissue for microscopic study.

As anatomy evolved as a discipline in Europe, it was sometimes, as in Lyon, France, combined with physiology. The greatest of the nineteenth-century French anatomists was Jean-Baptiste Auguste Chauveau (1827-1917), a graduate of Alfort and son of a farrier. He became an assistant at Lyon, chief of work in anatomy and physiology in 1848, then professor in 1864. He wrote *Traité de'Anatomie Comparée des Animaux Domestique* from 1855 to 1857, in which he extended the scope of study from the horse to the other domesticated species by using a comparative approach. He was able to avoid repetition of morphological descriptions, yet to provide understanding of structures and their functional significance. His colleague Saturnin Arloing became a coauthor of subsequent editions. George Fleming translated the work into English in 1873, and it was adopted as the preferred textbook in English-speaking veterinary schools. The *Edinburgh Veterinary Review* noted that

436. Ernst Friedrich Gurlt (1794-1882), an outstanding pioneer of anatomical and descriptive pathological studies at Berlin's Humboldt University Veterinary Medical Faculty published four editions of his *Comparative Anatomy* between 1822 and 1843. This illustration, from a fascinating collection of superb renderings of monstrosities born to domestic animals in *Ueber thierische Missgeburten,* published in collaboration with his brother Ernst Julius Gurlt in 1877, depicts a teratological anomaly described as *Peromelus achirus,* bovine. *(Van Pelt Special Collection of Rare Books, University of Pennsylvania.)*

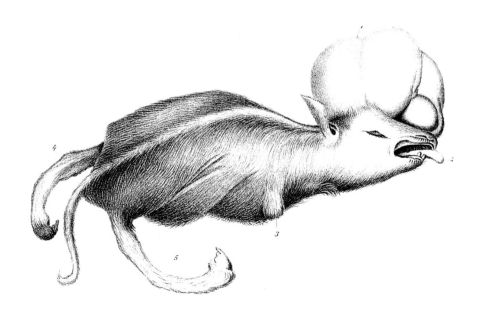

Chauveau had presented a balanced focus among species—horse, ox, sheep, pig, and dog—as well as separate coverage of avian anatomy. Despite the book's length (eight hundred and ten pages), the reviewer found that its information was so well organized and distilled that the work was actually concise. He declared the young anatomist to be in the foremost rank of a new generation of French veterinary scientists. He also observed that Chauveau was already highly distinguished in experimental physiology. Chauveau divided the chairs, giving Arloing the anatomy position after he was appointed director of the veterinary school in 1876. From 1903 to 1905 Lesbre further extended the text by Chauveau and Arloing, and he carried out remarkable investigations of teratology, the study of anomalies and monstrosities.

The establishment of the Royal Veterinary School of the Veterinary Medical Faculty of Humboldt University in Berlin in 1790 had been given a high priority. Germany became the leading nation in anatomical studies, and its veterinary schools produced an outstanding family of veterinary anatomists and anatomical artists. Ernst Friedrich Gurlt (1794-1882) at Berlin published four editions of *Comparative Anatomy* from 1822 to 1843. He and his brother Ernst Julius (1825-1899) published a superbly illustrated book on anatomical monstrosities of domestic animals, *Ueber thierische Missgeburten* (1877). His successor, Leisering, moved to the Dresden school in 1857, where with Müller of Berlin he coedited *Comparative Anatomy* through three more editions.

Wilhelm Ellenberger (1848-1929), a pupil of Gurlt who also studied medicine under Virchow, took over authorship of the microscopic anatomy section of Gurlt's book and moved to Dresden in 1880, where he became professor of physiology and anatomy in 1886. Hermann Baum (1864-1932) was hired to work on canine anatomy for his doctorate under Ellenberger, whom he succeeded to the chair in 1898. By the time of his death in 1932 Baum had prepared for publication the seventeenth edition of the by then magnifi-

437. Wilhelm Ellenberger, Hermann Baum, and Hermann Dittrich produced *Handbuch der Anatomie der Tiere für Künstler (Handbook of Animal Anatomy for Artists)* in Leipzig (1898). Ellenberger had an appointment to teach in the royal academies and train artists in Dresden by presenting the anatomical basis for animal art. Hermann Dittrich, a painter who worked with Ellenberger after 1889, produced the most accurate, exquisite illustrations of animal anatomy, which attracted international acclaim. The great series of anatomical works that flowed from Ellenberger and Baum's laboratory at the veterinary school in Leipzig was derived from this fortunate combination of science and art. Baum completed his doctorate in canine anatomy. *(From Handbook of Animal Anatomy for Artists, 1956.)*

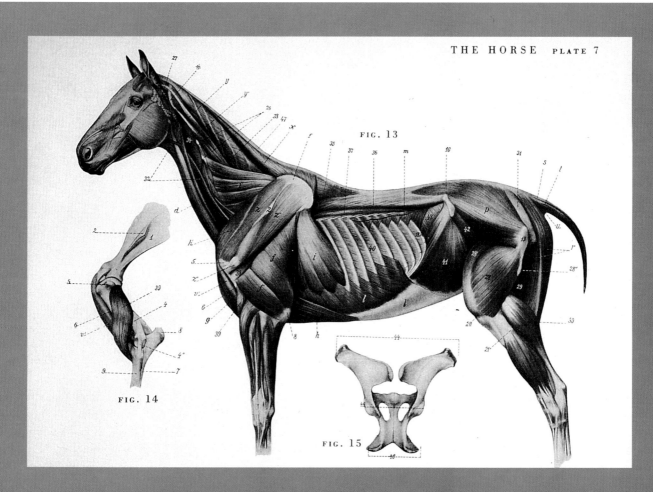

THE HORSE PLATE 7

FIG. 13

FIG. 14

FIG. 15

cent *Handbuch der Vergleichenden Anatomie der Haustiere (Handbook of Comparative Anatomy of Domestic Animals)*. Baum also provided five famous publications on the lymphatic systems of the horse, ox, dog, pig, and chicken. The German anatomists strove for perfection; it is only surprising that so few of the Ellenberger-Baum publications were translated into English in their day.

One wave of excellence in veterinary anatomy stemmed from Paul Martin (1861-1937), who described in depth the ruminant gastrointestinal tract at Zürich in 1891. After becoming professor at Giessen, he produced new editions of his *Lehrbuch der Anatomie der Haustiere* from 1902 to 1923 before teaming with his colleague Wilhelm Schauder to continue this tradition. Another of Martin's protégés, Reinhold Schmaltz, became director of the anatomical institute in Berlin, where he produced a magnificent *Atlas der Anatomie des Pferdes* in five volumes from 1901 to 1929. The Martin tradition at Giessen was extended by August Schümmer, who teamed with Richard Nickel at Hannover and Eugen Seiferle at Zürich to produce a multivolume series from 1954 to 1981. These fine works have been translated into English.

James Law (1838-1921) and John Gamgee (1831-1894) in Edinburgh and London wrote *General and Descriptive Anatomy of the Domestic Animals* in 1862. Law became professor of veterinary medicine and surgery at Cornell University in 1868. John Share-Jones at Liverpool published a four-volume work, *The Surgical Anatomy of the Horse,* from 1906 to 1914. Bradley, a productive anatomist at Edinburgh, wrote books on the anatomy of the horse,

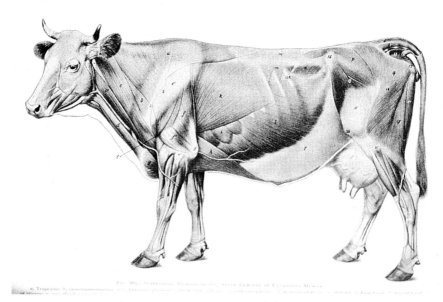

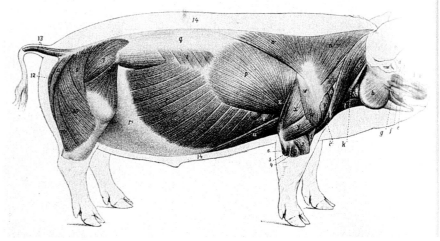

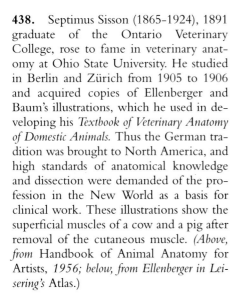

438. Septimus Sisson (1865-1924), 1891 graduate of the Ontario Veterinary College, rose to fame in veterinary anatomy at Ohio State University. He studied in Berlin and Zürich from 1905 to 1906 and acquired copies of Ellenberger and Baum's illustrations, which he used in developing his *Textbook of Veterinary Anatomy of Domestic Animals.* Thus the German tradition was brought to North America, and high standards of anatomical knowledge and dissection were demanded of the profession in the New World as a basis for clinical work. These illustrations show the superficial muscles of a cow and a pig after removal of the cutaneous muscle. *(Above, from* Handbook of Animal Anatomy for Artists, *1956; below, from Ellenberger in Leisering's* Atlas.)

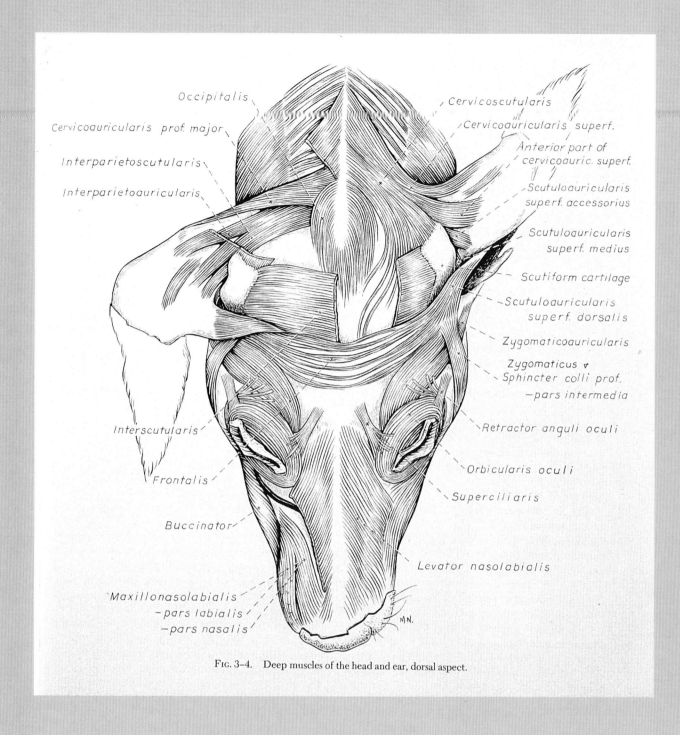

Occipitalis

Cervicoauricularis prof. major

Interparietoscutularis

Interparietoauricularis

Cervicoscutularis

Cervicoauricularis superf.

Anterior part of
cervicoauric. superf.

Scutuloauricularis
superf. accessorius

Scutuloauricularis
superf. medius

Scutiform cartilage

Scutuloauricularis
superf. dorsalis

Zygomaticoauricularis

Zygomaticus v
Sphincter colli prof.
—pars intermedia

Retractor anguli oculi

Orbicularis oculi

Superciliaris

Interscutularis

Frontalis

Buccinator

Levator nasolabialis

Maxillonasolabialis
—pars labialis
—pars nasalis

M.N.

Fɪɢ. 3–4.   Deep muscles of the head and ear, dorsal aspect.

dog, and chicken from 1896 to 1927. In North America Septimus Sisson (1865-1924), an English emigrant to Canada who graduated from the Ontario Veterinary College in 1891, ended up at The Ohio State University. He studied in Berlin and Zürich from 1905 to 1906 and began his great work, *Textbook of Veterinary Anatomy of Domestic Animals.* His successor, James Grossman, produced the third and fourth editions. Sisson, a thorough, demanding teacher, insisted that the veterinary student master the anatomical knowledge that was essential for clinical work. Through his efforts the German tradition of anatomical excellence was transferred to North America. A strong modern tradition emerged at Cornell University under the leadership of Malcolm E. Miller (1909-1960), whose *Guide to the Dissection of the Dog* and *Anatomy of the Dog* were continued by his colleagues Robert Habel and Howard Evans. Habel also produced helpful dissection guides for the large domestic animals. Specialized anatomy texts on the cat were more recent developments.

439. Dorsal aspect of the head of a dog, showing the deep muscles of the head and ear. The strong German tradition in veterinary anatomy was extended to Cornell University, where Malcolm Miller (1909-1960) produced his *Guide to the Dissection of the Dog* and *Anatomy of the Dog.* This picture is from the latter book. Robert E. Habel continued the tradition of excellence in leading the department, and Howard Evans produced later editions of these works. *(Reproduced with permission of W.B. Saunders Company and Dr. Howard Evans.)*

PHYSIOLOGY BASED ON MICROSCOPIC ANATOMY

Johannes Peter Müller (1801-1858), professor of physiology, first at Bonn and then at Berlin, founded a magnificent lineage of talented physiologists. One of his early students was Theodor Schwann, who put forward a general theory of nucleated cells as the basic building blocks of Bichat's "tissues" in 1839. He also demonstrated the presence of a ferment in gastric juice that he named *pepsin*. F.G. Jacob Henle (1809-1885) was another of Müller's students who carried out meticulous work on epithelial tissues, including the intestinal mucosa and the kidney. The *loop of Henle* in the latter organ preserves his name in renal studies, and he coined the term *epithelium*. He described the cellular architecture of the tissues to establish the field of histology or microscopic anatomy based on cytology, which he defined in two editions of *Allgemeine Anatomie (General Anatomy)* in 1837 and 1841. Having settled in Göttingen after being persecuted in Prussia and working in Zürich and Heidelberg, Henle was a prophet of the germ theory before proof was available and set out the essential principles necessary to establish that a pathogenic microbe was the cause of an infectious disease. He also proposed that metastases in cancer arose by seeding from displaced cancer cells. He had a profound influence on several brilliant scholars of the next generation.

Anatomy and physiology overlapped in the areas of histology and embryology. One of the most brilliant comparative physiologists and microscopists, noted for an extraordinary range of interests, was Jan Evangelista Purkinje (1787-1869). A research-oriented physician from Czechoslovakia, he was appointed professor of physiology in Breslau (then in Prussia but today known as Wroclaw, Poland) in 1823 with support from the great German poet, Goethe, who was interested in visual perception. Purkinje's doctoral thesis was titled *Subjective Aspects of Human Vision*. He put to good use the new achromatic lenses on his microscope in describing the axonal cylinder of nerve fibers and the large neurons in the cerebellum that still bear his name. He showed the similarities between animals with experimentally created cerebellar lesions and symptoms seen in human patients. He proposed a hypothesis of a functional hierarchy among nerve cells that set the stage for the neuron theory. Purkinje observed the changes in the position of the eyeballs during the early stage of falling asleep. He described the two phases of sleep far in advance of modern ideas and also classified dreams and their psychological interpretation.

Early in his research career Purkinje was a founder of physiological pharmacology, studying the action of drugs on vision, the action of emetic agents, and vertigo by using himself as the experimental subject. His finding that there is an illusion of continuing turning in space after rotation is stopped, which depends on the position of the head, is known as Purkinje's law of vertigo. The phenomenon of nystagmus that follows rotation was studied in greater depth by Bárány but not until 1914. Müller included Purkinje's observations in his book in 1826. Purkinje then studied binaural hearing and used his findings to develop strategies for the reeducation of deaf children. He was most productive, however, in the study of vision—in his work on the functions of foveal and peripheral vision, the strategies of ocular movements, and the perception of motion. He is also credited with the observation that each person's fingerprints are unique.

Purkinje's histological and embryological studies were remarkable. He coined the term *protoplasm* for the living matter of cells and was the first to make a systematic study of the structure of the tissues. In 1825 he discovered the *germinal vesicle* or cell nucleus when studying the formation of the egg by the hen, concluding that it gave rise to propagation. He proposed in 1837, two years before Schwann's general theory was published, that animal organisms are made up of three primary forms—liquid, granular, and fibrous—and

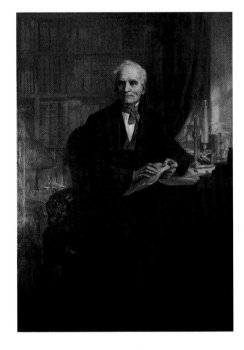

440. Jan Evangelista Purkinje (1787-1869), painted by Czech artist P. Maixner (1831-1884) on commission from his students to honor the fiftieth anniversary of his doctoral degree from Charles University in Prague, where the portrait hangs today. He was eighty-two years old at the time. He had a remarkably creative and productive career; he was appointed to the chair of physiology in Breslau (today Wroclaw, Poland) in 1823, where he stayed until 1850, when he became professor at a new institute in his native Prague. His contributions to comparative microscopic anatomy, pharmacology, and physiology were, truly and without exaggeration, phenomenal. He introduced practical classes into teaching physiology, emphasizing the dynamic nature of the discipline and its role as the foundation of medical understanding. His model of the Physiological Institute in Prague was soon followed in major German university centers, then in other leading European centers, and, in 1871, in the United States. *(Department of Physiology, Charles University, Prague.)*

that the fibrous forms had a nucleus and were analogous to the cells that constituted plants.

Purkinje was acclaimed as a great teacher, and he was the first to develop a laboratory course in which live animals were used to teach the principles of physiology. He supplemented his lecture course with an *experimental collegium* to give students a taste of how research was conducted and how discoveries were made. He finally realized his dream of returning to his homeland in 1850, when he was appointed professor of physiology at Prague with a new research institute. Within five years his educational model had been copied by many German research universities and then was adopted throughout western Europe.

PHYSIOLOGY: THE LEADING BIOMEDICAL SCIENCE

Francois Magendie (1783-1855) made a dramatic but controversial thrust to initiate experimental physiology by using vivisection demonstrations before the discovery of general anesthetics. His successor, Claude Bernard (1813-1878), consolidated the physiological approach to research by using physical and chemical methods. He showed that the exocrine pancreatic secretion (pancreatic juice) was involved in the digestion of lipids and then established that the liver played a central role in carbohydrate and lipid metabolism. He proposed the hypothesis that the organs and tissues of the body functioned to maintain and reset the composition of body cells and fluids. He named this internal environment the *milieu interieur.* Bernard wrote a famous book, *Introduction to the Study of Experimental Medicine,* in 1865 and became influential politically. The outstanding American physiologist Walter B. Cannon (1871-1945), author of *The Wisdom of the Body,* at Harvard expanded the idea of the *milieu interieur,* developing it into his concept of *homeostasis.* Bengt Andersson of Sweden's veterinary school extended these concepts with his brilliant studies of the roles of the hypothalamus in governing the rhythmic ingestive behavior of animals for nutrients and water.

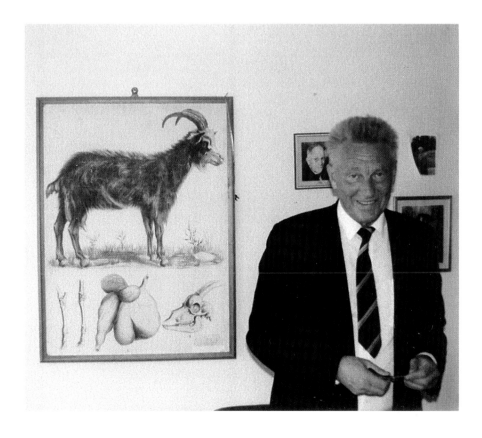

441. Bengt Andersson of Sweden's veterinary school made brilliant studies of the integrating role of the hypothalamus in regulation of intakes of water, electrolytes, and nutrients, using the horned goat as his experimental animal. This trail-blazing research extended Claude Bernard's *milieu interieur* and Walter Cannon's *homeostasis* and sympathetic emotional responses (1915) to show how the brain governs the rhythmic ingestive behavior needed to maintain the body in nutrient balance. In Andersson's work the Horsley-Clarke stereotactic apparatus of 1908 and mapping of the brain nuclei were required, to allow precise lesions in selected nuclei of the brain stem, as developed by Walter Hess (1881-1973) in Zürich to produce rage in cats in the 1920s. Andersson extended this technique to the goat and also developed capillary tube injection to study the humoral factors in hunger and satiety. Hess later showed that stimulation of the grey matter around the third ventricle caused animals to go to sleep. *(Photograph by R.H. Dunlop.)*

Johannes Peter Müller (1801-1858) was the fountainhead of German physiological scholarship. He put forward that each type of sensory receptor responds to the stimulus of a different modality (light, sound, motion, odors [chemicals], touch, temperature, pain, and the like), thereby giving rise to its own specialized sensation (such as seeing, hearing, moving, smelling, feeling, heat or cold, or pain). Müller's durable text, *Elements of Physiology,* appeared in English in 1838. His pupil Emil du Bois-Reymond (1818-1896), who was born in Berlin of French stock, showed that a flow of electricity could be measured in both muscle contraction and nerve conduction in 1843, just as Galvani (1737-1798) had predicted long before. Emil du Bois-Reymond suggested that this flow accounted for the transmission of the excitatory stimulus from nerve to muscle. He succeeded Müller in the chair of physiology, which he held until his death in 1896. Hermann von Helmholtz (1821-1894), who worked at Königsberg, was another from Müller's "stable." He measured the velocity of conduction in nerve fibers and across the neuromuscular junction, showing that conduction in the latter involved a short delay. In 1850 and 1851, he invented the ophthalmoscope, which allowed visualization of the ocular fundus. He attributed color vision to the existence of subsets of the population of retinal light-sensitive, cone-shaped cells in the eye that responded differentially to red, green, and violet wavelengths of light. He proposed that the membranes of the cochlea served as resonators for sound waves and determined the pitch of the sound heard. This thoughtful scholar also established that the law of conservation of energy applied to living tissues and defined the relationship between work and heat.

Carl Wilhelm Ludwig (1816-1895), another Müller protégé, was a remarkable amplifier of physiological research through his generational impact on many students from all over the world. His technological genius transformed the registration of physiological events. For example, he used an indicator arm floating on mercury in a U-tube that was connected to a vascular catheter in a blood vessel to record changes in blood pressure. The indicator point wrote on a smoked-paper surface attached to a drum that was turned by the shaft of a clock-driven kymograph at various rate settings. This was one of his techniques that held sway in laboratories teaching physiology in medical and veterinary schools for almost a century. Another of his notable devices was a stromuhr used to measure the rate of blood flow. His career took him to Marburg, Zürich, and Vienna and finally to Leipzig (from 1865 to 1895), where he developed a famous institute. His own research contribution was to establish that the glomerulus-plus-tubule architecture is the filtration and reabsorption system for renal function. He showed that the urine contained materials that preexisted in the plasma rather than being formed in the kidney. He proposed that the vascular glomerular tufts made an ultrafiltrate of the blood plasma from which the tubules made selective reabsorptions.

The British tradition in physiological teaching and research stemmed from Edinburgh University. William Sharpey (1802-1880), a visionary physician who perceived the need for a biomedical research foundation, visited the dynamic laboratories on the European continent before taking up his professorship of anatomy and general physiology at University College, London, in 1836. One of his legacy of brilliant pupils was Michael Foster (1836-1907), who developed the physiological laboratory at Cambridge from 1870 until he resigned in 1903. John Burdon-Sanderson, another Edinburgh medical graduate, succeeded Sharpey as Jodrell Professor in London in 1874, then moved to Oxford University as Wayneflete Professor in 1884. Edward Schäfer (1850-1935), another Sharpey product, then took the London chair. The Cambridge Scientific Instrument Company, founded by one of Foster's students, A.G. Dew-Smith, in 1881, developed the devices the physiologists needed for research. Foster founded the *Journal of Physiology* in 1878 with one American editor. The *American Journal of Physiology* was initiated in 1898, and the *Journal of Applied Physiology* in 1948.

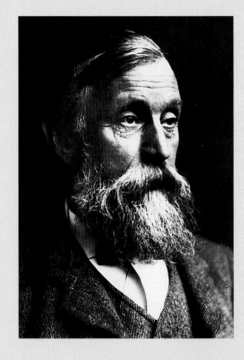

442. The British school of physiologists became preeminent in the second half of the nineteenth century and the early twentieth century. Michael Foster (1836-1907), a brilliant student under William Sharpey (1802-1880) at University College, London, developed the Cambridge physiological laboratory after 1870, founded the *Journal of Physiology* in 1878, wrote a major textbook, and encouraged the founding of the Cambridge Scientific Instrument Company. He gave advice and assistance to aspiring veterinary physiologists, several of whom worked in the laboratory. *(National Library of Medicine, Bethesda, Maryland.)*

The electrochemical properties of the lipoprotein membranes around animal cells proved to be one of the most challenging topics in biological research. Walther Nernst (1865-1933) showed that an electrical potential occurs at the boundary between two different solutions of the same salt. He devised an equation to define this effect. Julius Bernstein (1839-1917), one of Helmholtz's students, used Nernst's concept to propose that the ionic gradients of potassium (high inside and low outside) and sodium (high outside and low inside) across the semipermeable membranes caused a voltage to be present at rest (the resting potential). Because the membrane was selectively permeable to potassium ions, the inside was negative with respect to the outside of the cell. During the action-potential spike that occurred during excitation, the ionic permeability changed sequentially for the different ions.

John Z. Young (born 1907), a famous zoologist and professor of anatomy at London, discovered in 1933 that some nerve fibers of squid were quite large: the giant nerve axons were as large as one millimeter in diameter. Nerve fibers of squid became the experimental tissue of choice in the study of the electrochemical events that explained membrane potentials. Alan L. Hodgkin, Andrew F. Huxley, and Bernhard Katz at Cambridge (from 1947 to 1952) developed formulas and the voltage clamp method to explain the action potential based on changing sodium and potassium ion penetrances through the membrane. H.H. Ussing in Copenhagen developed the chamber that led to the characterization of cyclic carrier systems for electrolytes traversing cell membranes via ion channels in 1951.

Frederick K. Smith, who became a distinguished leader of the Royal Army Veterinary Corps and historian of veterinary medicine, wrote *Manual of Veterinary Physiology* at the turn of the century. He persuaded Charles Sherrington, the Nobel Prize–winning neurophysiologist, to write the section on the nervous system for his third edition. Thus the veterinary profession was introduced to neuron theory as it was evolving. Smith's book was popular and included coverage of the functional histology of the hoof.

Foster's *Textbook of Physiology* entered the field in 1877; Schäfer's, of the same title in two volumes (1898 and 1890), included contributions from John N. Langley (1852-1925), who succeeded Foster as professor, on the autonomic nervous system and from Charles Sherrington (1857-1952) on the central nervous system. Foster insisted on the unity of physiology and pathology, making an apt analogy by ridiculing a science of meteorology that would be divided into two fields of study, one dealing with good weather, the other with bad. Ernest Starling (1866-1927), of "law of the heart" fame, published the first edition of his *Elements of Human Physiology* in 1892 (issued in eight editions) and his more advanced *Principles of Human Physiology*, which included a comparative study of mammals, in 1912. Charles Lovatt Evans (1884-1968) continued the work after Starling's death until 1956. Evans ventured into veterinary matters when asked to investigate sweating sickness in racehorses in Singapore. William Bayliss, who worked with Starling on the first discovery of a hormone (secretin in the intestine), wrote *Principles of General Physiology* in 1915. Samson Wright of the Middlesex Hospital wrote his popular *Applied Physiology* in 1926, which focused on basic explanations of clinical dysfunctions. Sherrington, then at Oxford University, produced an outstanding laboratory manual of surgical skills and physiological methods, *Mammalian Physiology*, in 1919.

Development of a strong base for physiology in Scandinavia began with P.L. Panum in Copenhagen in 1864. Christian Bohr was a theoretician, and his student Karl Hasselbach became a biochemist noted for the Henderson-Hasselbach equation, which defines the relationship between acid dissociation and the hydrogen ion concentration (expressed as pH) once the dissociation constant (pKa) of the acid is known. Holmgren of Uppsala and, later, Robert Tigerstedt of Finland set high standards for the regional research journal *Acta Physiologica Scandinavica*. August Krogh (1874-1949) became the pacesetter in

Danish physiology. He collaborated with Joseph Barcroft, one of Foster's brilliant students at Cambridge, on respiratory physiology. Both had come to the same conclusion—that gases are exchanged between the air in the alveoli of the lung and the blood by diffusion. Krogh's focus on exercise physiology made this field a high point in Scandinavian science. Krogh received the Nobel Prize in 1920 for his discovery that local blood flow is adjustable to the needs of each tissue: in resting muscle few capillaries are open, whereas at work all may be open.

S.C.F. Torup, professor at the University of Lund after 1889, developed environmental and metabolic physiology. He influenced the Arctic and Antarctic polar explorers led by Amundsen and Nansen, who had a doctorate in neuroanatomy and physiology. Environmental and comparative physiology received wonderful leadership from Paul Scholander and Knut Schmidt-Nielsen. Scholander did fundamental research on the remarkable adaptations to diving in seals, among his many stimulating contributions. Schmidt-Nielsen became the quintessential comparative physiologist, studying, among a host of fascinating questions about adaptive and evolutionary physiology, the adaptation of camels to desert environments. Both Scholander and Schmidt-Nielsen moved to the United States.

The North American contribution to physiological research in the twentieth century is too vast to review here. A series of fine books appeared: W.H. Howell's *Textbook of Physiology* in 1905, which was perpetuated brilliantly by Fulton at Western Reserve University; *Physiological Basis of Medical Practice* (1937) by C.H. Best and N.B. Taylor of the University of Toronto; and *Medical Physiology* (1956) by Arthur C. Guyton of the University of Mississippi. The latter two were long popular with medical and veterinary teachers and students because they provided clinical interpretations as well as physiological knowledge. The remarkable challenge undertaken by the American Physiological Society to produce a "comprehensive but critical presentation of the state of knowledge . . . in functional biology" resulted in the massive, many-volumed *Handbook of Physiology* (1959). In 1933 Henry Hugh Dukes, professor of veterinary physiology, first at Iowa State University, then at the New York State College of Veterinary Medicine at Cornell University in Ithaca, produced the text that in later editions became the standard for instruction in veterinary physiology, *The Physiology of Domestic Animals*.

CARDIAC PHYSIOLOGY AT LYON VETERINARY SCHOOL

Following the tradition of Harvey, Hales, Magendie, and Bernard, who made their famous investigations to explain the secrets of the circulatory system, researchers in the French veterinary schools made major contributions to physiological knowledge. Chauveau at Lyon turned his attention from anatomy to the physiology of the circulatory system, choosing the horse as the experimental subject because it had a large heart that would beat slowly, at about forty beats per minute at rest. Initially his procedure was to immobilize the animal and render it free from any pain sensation by severing the spinal cord below the medulla. Respiration was maintained with bellows. The heart was exposed by ablation of a large rib section. At twenty-nine years of age Chauveau published an article in *Gazette Medicale de Paris* (1856), which described all the facts about the beating heart that could be ascertained by observation and by palpation of the actions of its valves by inserting a finger through a small incision in the atrium. He demonstrated these findings at the Alfort veterinary school, where he met E.J. Marey (1830-1904), a physiologist in Paris. These two decided to collaborate in their revolutionary studies of circulatory physiology, and one of the most successful partnerships in the history of physiology resulted.

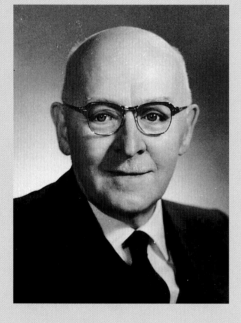

443. Henry Hugh Dukes (1895-1987) was the integrating pioneer of veterinary physiology in America, beginning at Iowa State University. His published notes of 1933 evolved into the textbook used by most veterinary students in North America since then: *The Physiology of Domestic Animals*. Dukes moved to Cornell University in Ithaca, New York, to extend a long, distinguished career in the field. *(Flower Veterinary Library, Cornell University.)*

Marey in 1860 invented a sphygmograph to study the arterial pulse and detect changes of pressure. Chauveau designed a flow meter to measure the velocity of blood flow. Neither of these devices could study phenomena deep inside the heart. Buisson in 1861 devised a new sphygmomanometer, which transmitted pressure by air, that was used to overcome the difficulty. He also invented a simple tambour consisting of a rigid funnel covered by a rubber membrane, which was perfected by Marey and used for recording many types of physiological dynamic changes, including the depth and frequency of respiration.

Chauveau and Marey combined the essential features of these devices with cardiac catheterization to create a cardiographic probe that recorded the sequence of physical events inside the heart during each beat. In 1861 they published graphic proof that the precordial impact occurred simultaneously with ventricular systole. This finding was soon followed by publication of other findings on the details of cardiac hemodynamics. Chauveau also established the chronological relationships between the actions of the cardiac valves and the two principal heart sounds. This accomplishment gave the clinicians a scientific basis for interpretation of the cardiac sounds they heard by auscultation with the stethoscope, which was invented in Paris by René Laënnec (1781-1826) in 1816. These remarkable studies preceded the work of Werner Forssmann, who catheterized his own heart in 1924. For his work Forssmann shared a Nobel Prize in 1956 with André F. Cournand, who had applied the technique in 1944, and D.W. Richards. Forssmann noted that Chauveau and Marey had established the safety of the procedure in the horse long before.

Chauveau studied the pathophysiology of insufficiencies of mitral and aortic valves in the horse by damaging the valve or sectioning its attachments. He then narrowed the aortic and pulmonic valves by incomplete ligation to show the functional consequences of valvular stenosis. He applied a theory of vibration in venous blood that was developed by Savart, a physician, to show that the theory could explain the sounds of breathing engendered by aneurysms (dilations) or localized narrowings of the circulatory system. In 1862 Chauveau used the theory to explain the mechanisms of generation of physiological respiratory sounds and the abnormal sounds of pneumonia. He invented a hemodromograph to record the variations in the speed of blood flow through the coronary arteries (and to estimate changes in volume flow rate) of the horse during the cardiac cycle.

From 1857 to 1862 Chauveau also was engaged in neurophysiological research. He defined the excitability of the equine spinal cord, locating the ascending sensory pathways and establishing the roles of the sensory and motor branches of the vagal nerves in regulating esophageal motility.

Refuting Bernard's idea that utilization of glucose is exclusively pulmonary, in 1956 Chauveau showed that glucose is utilized by muscle; he used the masseter muscle of the horse to measure arteriovenous glucose concentration gradients. This research was a great innovation in concept and technique in the evolution of studies of tissue metabolism. He studied the effects of altitude on exercise physiology, using himself as the subject, during an ascent of Mont Blanc in 1866. Chauveau developed a growing interest in muscular energetics later in life, after he had moved to Paris (1886) and become director of veterinary schools throughout France, and Arloing became director of the Lyon School. Another great achievement of Chauveau's time in Lyon derived from his work on infection and immunity, to be discussed later.

Saturnin Arloing (1846-1911) was a worthy successor to Chauveau. He followed him in the chair of anatomy in 1867 and also in the chair of physiology in 1876, and engaged in physiological research. Arloing studied the sensibility of peripheral nerves and found in 1875 that some forms of neuralgia (pain in an area of distribution of a particular nerve) could be relieved by surgical section of the offending nerve. In 1877 his graphic study of the process of swallowing became classic. He identified the motor points on the cerebral

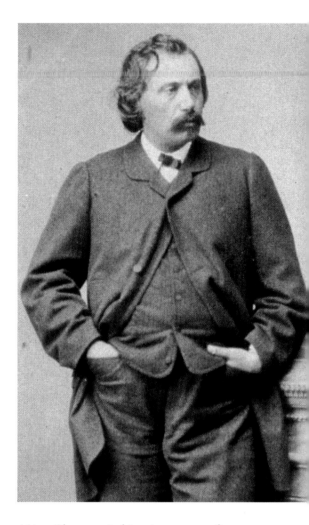

444. Chauveau in his prime, as a professor at the veterinary school in Lyon. He stands tall in history as the most gifted and productive of scholarly veterinarians. He wrote a major textbook on the comparative anatomy of domestic animals that, after translation, became widely used in the English-speaking schools; gave in collaboration with Marey the leading biophysical research thrust to cardiology; and then with his student Rebatek made the first study of the coronary circulation. He applied his remarkable creative skills to many fields of veterinary medicine, notably the physiological sciences, microbiology, and immunology. *(Musée Claude Bernard, Fondation Marcel, Mérieux.)*

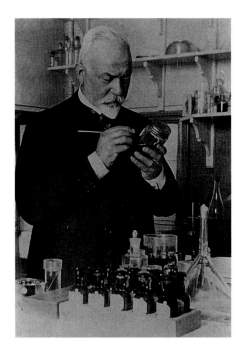

445. Saturnin Arloing was chief of work in anatomy under Chauveau in 1867 and became professor of physiology at the Lyon veterinary school in 1876, when Chauveau became director of the veterinary school. Arloing's studies of sensory nerves led him to therapeutic surgery for neuralgia, and he expanded knowledge of the roles of the cervical sympathetic nerves. He mapped the motor cortex of the brain in the horse and the dog and made classic recordings of the events in swallowing. His doctoral thesis in medicine (1879)—a comparison of the anesthetics chloral hydrate, chloroform, and ether—was a move into pharmacology. He showed the excitatory effects of cocaine in 1885. He later switched his research focus again, this time to the microbiology and immunology of tuberculosis, showing the danger of Koch's tuberculin therapy. He followed Chauveau as director from 1886 to 1911, after Chauveau was named Inspector of Veterinary Schools for France. (*Ecole Nationale Vétérinaire de Lyon.*)

cortex of the horse and the dog. He studied the trophic and secretory functions of the cervical sympathetic nerves. He completed a doctoral thesis in medicine in 1879 that was based on a comparative study of three general anesthetics—ether, chloroform, and chloral hydrate—an early foray into pharmacology. He also studied the excitatory effects of cocaine in 1885. Henri Toussaint, the next in the remarkable dynasty of Chauveau, Arloing, and Toussaint, completed a fine research study on the physiological mechanism of rumination in cattle. The three researchers all progressed from anatomy through physiology to the fields of pathogenic microbiology and immunology.

PHYSIOLOGY OF RUMINANT DIGESTION

The ruminant is the major source of animal products for human foods that are derived from animal feeds that humans cannot digest. Cattle, sheep, goats, the camelids, and farmed game animals such as deer produce edible animal tissues, milk, and tissue extracts, as well as fibrous products such as wool, hair, and hides and residues for animal feeds or supplements. Consequently it was intriguing to discover how the ruminant's digestion worked, in particular, its capacity to degrade plant fibers such as cellulose.

As early as 1685, Peyer studied the structure and function of the ruminant stomach, concluding that fermentation must occur therein. Spallanzani in 1776 carried out experiments to determine the rate of passage of feed. Tiedemann and Gmelin in 1831 made the profound discovery that the two- and four-carbon acetic and butyric fatty acids were formed in the rumen. It was not until 1945, however, that Elsden developed methods that allowed him to demonstrate that the three-carbon fatty acid propionic was formed as well. Haubner in 1837 found that water was absorbed from the third compartment of the ruminant gastric complex, the omasum. In 1855 he showed that cellulose was digested. Wildt in 1874 found that the site of breakdown was the rumen. Reist and Popoff, in 1863 and 1875, respectively, studied the gases in the rumen and found that carbon dioxide and methane were present.

In 1843 David Gruby, a Viennese physician who worked on pathogenic fungi, and O. Delafond observed and made drawings of protozoa in the reticulorumen of cattle and the cecum of the horse. Zuntz in 1879 proposed that anaerobic digestion of fiber took place in the rumen, a significant observation. He noted that such fermentation yielded acids and gases. His student, van Tappeiner, collected saliva from the throat in 1884 and showed that it contained fiber-digesting bacteria. Of course, the organisms from regurgitated boluses of rumen content were the real source of cellulolysis. Dogiel in Russia (in 1927) and Mangold (in 1929 and 1943) reported on the activity of protozoa.

The next major burst of activity developed from the work of Robert Hungate on anaerobic fermentation. Hungate had a long, productive career at the University of California at Davis. In 1939 he demonstrated cellulose fermentation in termites. He cultured rumen protozoa in vitro in 1942 and 1943, and in 1947 he finally succeeded in culturing anaerobic cellulolytic bacteria from the rumen.

In the 1850s Colin and Boulet studied the effects of rumen fermentation on the host ruminant. They showed that the strychnine-containing drug *nux vomica* was absorbed slowly from the abomasum of cattle and more rapidly from the equine cecum. Trautmann in the 1930s found that pilocarpine was absorbed rapidly from the rumen, reticulum, and omasum of the goat. Classic physiological studies then were begun at Babraham Agricultural Research Center near Cambridge under the direction of Sir Joseph Barcroft; Rachel McAnally, who came from South Africa; and veterinary scientist Andrew Phillipson that helped to show that the rumen volatile fatty acids (VFAs) appeared in the blood of sheep after being introduced to the rumen. In 1946 Elsden used partition chromatography to separate the individual lower (shorter chain) VFAs. Andrew Phillipson, along with Innes, had developed the necessary experimental and surgical techniques to carry out these experiments in 1939. McAnally developed the fermentation methods. In 1945 J.F. Danielli worked with Marshall and Phillipson to prove the absorption of VFAs across the rumen wall. Phillipson became the dean of the School of Veterinary Clinical Studies at Cambridge after a productive career in the study of many aspects of digestive physiology in ruminants at the Rowett Institute in Aberdeen. Reginald Moir at the University of Western Australia studied the microbes in the rumen and in the stomach of wallabies.

The study of the physical motility patterns of the ruminant stomach developed separately from the microbial and chemical studies. In Utrecht in 1926 Wester studied the contractions of the rumen and reticulum, using preliminary palpation, then pressure wave recordings. He showed that the reticulum contracts twice at the start of each cycle of mixing contractions. Independently but a little later, in 1928, Schalk and Amadon in North Dakota similarly used a large rumen fistula to show the origin and biphasic contraction of the reticulum, which preceded the wave that spread posteriorly over the cranial pillar and dorsal sac before turning down over the ventral sac. They also found that a second rumen contraction occurred during some cycles. Czepa and Stigler in 1926 used radiology in sheep and goats to study the se-

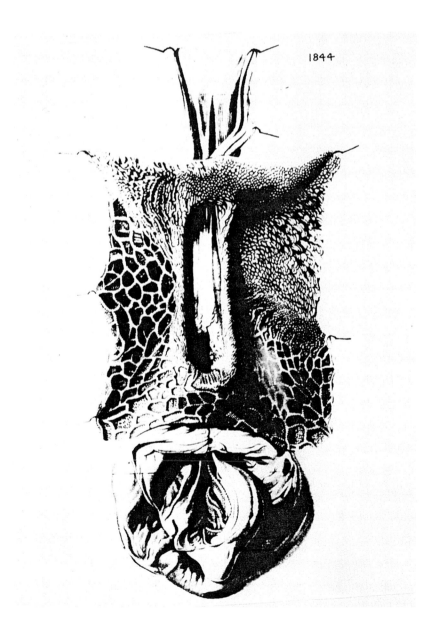

446. The esophageal groove of a sheep, by Flourens (1844). This structure contracts to divert milk sucked by a lamb or a calf directly from the cardia into the omasal canal by creating a tube to the reticulo-omasal orifice, thereby bypassing ruminal fermentation of the milk. Wester in Utrecht, using a cow with a ruminal fistula, showed that this was a dynamic process in the live animal. *(Copy provided by the late Y. Ruckebusch, Ecole Nationale Vétérinaire, Toulouse.)*

quential waves and concluded that some rumen contractions were independent of contractions in the reticulum. The independent contractions were associated with eructation of gas. Robert W. Dougherty at Cornell University and, later, at the National Animal Disease Center in Ames, Iowa, was the outstanding researcher in the field of pathophysiology attributable to the ruminant digestive system. Neural and humoral regulation of the motility of the tract was studied by Robert Comline and Titchen at Cambridge and by Yves Ruckebusch at Toulouse Veterinary School, who also studied sleep patterns.

Leblanc and Trousseau showed the position of the forestomachs in vivo in the sheep in 1823, as well as the site in the flank to be punctured in the event of bloat. Flourens in 1844 claimed wrongly that regurgitation resulted from a contraction of the rumen. In 1874, however, Toussaint recorded pressure waves in the lower esophagus by using an air-filled balloon. He noted that the timing of the rumen contractions did not correspond with that of regurgitation and that the rumen contractions lasted a long time, thereby rejecting the claim of Flourens.

A remarkable feature of the ruminant's design is the esophageal groove. Faber termed the structure the *voie lactée,* and in 1806 Home proposed that its purpose was to divert milk away from the fermentation vat of the reticulorumen. In the newborn calf a reflex triggered by suckling contracts the groove so that it acts like a channel to direct the swallowed milk straight into the abomasum or secretory stomach. Wester showed that the groove closure was blocked by applying a five-percent solution of cocaine to the buccal mucosa. Robert Orskov at the Rowett Institute showed that the reflex closure could be retained much longer if it were kept in training by means of daily suckling stimuli. Other workers in Great Britain showed that the daily flow of saliva in a cow is high—more than one hundred liters—and plays a major role in buffering rumen acids.

GENESIS OF SCIENTIFIC PHARMACOLOGY

The strong focus of early veterinary research on anatomy, microbiology, and cellular pathology led to the setting of the highest priorities on the causes and diagnosis of disease. This emphasis, linked to the need for clinical training, albeit largely empirical at the therapeutic level, contributed to the lower profile of most veterinary aspects of the physiological sciences and pharmacology.

The discipline of pharmacology in medicine began to escape from the traditional "materia medica" approach in Germany. A key figure in this redirection was Rudolf Buchheim (1820-1879), who trained at Dresden and Leipzig but worked initially at Dorpat (later, Tartu), Estonia from 1847 to 1866, with Carl Schmidt. Schmidt demonstrated the presence of free hydrochloric acid in gastric secretions and the unequal distribution of sodium and potassium between the plasma and the interior of the red blood cell. Buchheim dropped the old botanical and chemical classifications and urged a new focus on the mode of action of drugs based on their chemical structures. He called for the development of a new experimental laboratory discipline directed at therapeutic effects. He initiated and edited *Pharmazeutisches Zentralblatt.* In 1845 he wrote on physiological chemistry for Schmidt's *Jahrbücher der Medizin,* and in 1846 he assumed responsibility for revising and editing Pereira's *The Elements of Materia Medica.* Buchheim began by teaching himself the new branch of science he was founding. To achieve his goal, he established a laboratory in his home. He moved to Giessen, Germany, and continued to address his goal of bringing pharmacology into the mainstream of medical science as the logical basis for therapeutics.

The first experimental pharmacologist was Francois Magendie, who studied pharmacological and toxicological mechanisms in the course of his work in physiology. His notable achievement in 1809 was the localization of the site of action for a crude Javan poisonous extract from a plant related to *Strychnos nux-vomica,* from which J.P. Pelletier and J. Caventou isolated the alkaloid strychnine in 1818. Magendie showed that the drug was carried by the bloodstream to its site of action, the spinal cord, where it caused convulsions. Magendie worked with Pelletier, a leader in isolating and characterizing pharmacologically active agents from natural products after F. Sertürner isolated morphine in 1817. They studied emetine from ipecacuanha together, and Magendie carried out experiments on the actions of tartar emetic and prussic acids. Claude Bernard in the 1850s showed that curare acts on the motor nerves to affect voluntary muscle. This finding led to the determination that its site of action was the neuromuscular junction, where it blocked nerve stimulation of the muscle. Bernard also showed that carbon monoxide acted as a toxic agent at the biochemical level, another "first." Francois Tabourin, professor of chemistry and pharmacy at the Lyon veterinary school, initiated comparative pharmacology of domestic animals. Even before Charles G. Pravaz (1797-1853) invented the hypodermic syringe with a hollow needle in 1851, Tabourin advocated the subcutaneous administration of drugs with the aid of a solid needle, which was used to introduce a seton that was supplied with the medication from a small pouch. He indicated that the subcutaneous dose should be four times the intravenous dose, and the oral dose twelve times the intravenous dose.

Oswald Schmiedeberg (1838-1921) was born into a German family in Latvia. He graduated in medicine from Dorpat, where he came under Buchheim's influence and tutelage. He did his doctoral research on the measurement of chloroform in the blood. During the Franco-Prussian War of 1870 and 1871, Strassburg was reincorporated into the new German empire that resulted, and the university was reopened on a wave of enthusiasm. Carl Ludwig at Leipzig recommended Schmiedeberg for the chair in pharmacology in 1872. He joined F. Goltz and F. Hoppe-Seyler, in physiology and physiological chemistry, respectively. Schmiedeberg's institute soon became the leading institution for academic research in pharmacology in the world. Schmiedeberg became a towering figure in biomedical science and was finally able to convert Buchheim's vision to reality. He established the journal *Pathologie und Pharmakologie* in 1873, indicating his interest in the study of drugs in diseased patients as well as in healthy people and animals. His textbook *Grundriss der Arzneimittellehre* of 1883 became a classic that was published in seven editions and was translated into several languages. He drew students to the new discipline from all over the world, training more than one hundred and fifty of them, a marathon performance that led to the adoption of the new discipline in the great universities and centers for medical research.

The bridge for transfer of the new discipline to North America was made by John Jacob Abel of Johns Hopkins University, who studied medicine in Germany from 1884 to 1890. During that period he worked in many of Germany's finest biomedical laboratories, including long stints with Ludwig and Schmiedeberg. He had a flair for biochemistry and with Drechsel isolated calcium carbamate from horse urine. Abel returned to the United States as professor of materia medica at the University of Michigan, although at the time he had acquired a stronger interest in physiological chemistry. Despite the name of his chair, Abel was allowed to transform its role to that of the modern pharmacology of the Schmiedeberg era. He was lured away by Osler and Welch, however, to Johns Hopkins University by the offer of the first chair in pharmacology in 1893. Arthur R. Cushny, a Scot and another Schmiedeberg product, succeeded him at Ann Arbor. After twelve productive years there, Cushny returned to Great Britain in 1905, first to London, then to Edinburgh, where he established a fine tradition in the new discipline of pharmacology. While in Michigan, he produced *A Textbook of Pharmacology and Therapeutics* (1899), the first on the subject in the United States, which lasted through thirteen editions. With Edmunds, his successor, Cushny pre-

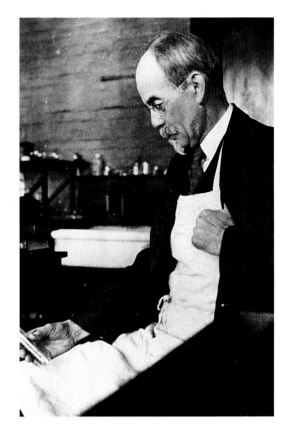

447. John Jacob Abel (1857-1938) was the bridge from German scholarship in pharmacology under Oswald Schmiedeberg (1838-1921) at Strasbourg to North American pharmacology. Abel studied in Germany for six years before becoming professor of materia medica at the University of Michigan. Osler and Welch lured him to Johns Hopkins University, to the first chair in pharmacology in the United States, in 1893. Abel was a brilliant chemist and physiologist. He isolated epinephrine from the adrenal medulla (1897), developed the first vividiffusion device (1913), and was the first to crystallize insulin (1925). He founded the *Journal of Pharmacology and Experimental Therapeutics.* The founder of modern American pharmacology, he guided the discipline to its experimental basis. His model reached veterinary medicine late via L. Meyer Jones, who received his doctorate in pharmacology at the University of Minnesota, taught at Iowa State University's College of Veterinary Medicine, and wrote the first comprehensive textbook in the discipline. *(National Library of Medicine, Bethesda, Maryland.)*

pared *A Laboratory Guide in Experimental Pharmacology* in 1905 based on experiments with drugs in anesthetized rabbits and dogs.

At Johns Hopkins University Abel accepted responsibility for teaching physiological chemistry, which preceded pharmacology in the medical curriculum. He instituted laboratory instruction in pharmacology, as William Howell did for physiology. Abel recruited research-oriented scientists and physicians for further training but did not develop a doctoral program. In fact, the doctoral program in pharmacology at Johns Hopkins was not begun until 1969. Research was Abel's main goal. He is remembered for isolating a derivative of a hormone from the adrenal medulla and naming it *epinephrine* in 1897. Jokichi Takamine claimed to have isolated the pure hormone in 1901 and named it *Adrenaline,* which Parke, Davis and Company perfected as the first hormone to be isolated in pure form. Hence the substance ended up with two names. Much later U.S. von Euler in Sweden showed that norepinephrine was also present in the adrenal medulla.

In 1913 Abel developed an apparatus for vividiffusion that allowed the separation of diffusible substances from the blood of a live animal. He used this technique to prove that free amino acids were present in the blood plasma. He realized that the device had potential for the treatment of kidney failure, but a safe, effective artificial kidney was not applied in renal dialysis until much later. His other great accomplishment was the first crystallization of the pancreatic islet hormone insulin in 1925.

Abel was the founder and original owner of the *Journal of Pharmacology and Experimental Therapeutics,* which was later taken over by the American Society for Pharmacology and Experimental Therapeutics. He created the modern discipline of academic pharmacology in North America and trained several of its early leaders. Two other forces influenced the development of pharmacology: the specialized government laboratories for research on regulation of drugs for efficacy and safety and the burgeoning pharmaceutical industry. Because of the veterinary profession's focus on contagious diseases, the profession during that period was more tightly linked, in view of the lack of effective chemical treatments, to the biologics manufacturers who made preventive vaccines and serums. These became the mainstay of the food animal practitioner during the first half of the twentieth century.

Western Reserve University in Cleveland, Ohio, was the third medical school to take up Schmiedeberg's experimental physiology. Torald Sollman became its spearhead and wrote his classic, the encyclopedic *Manual of Pharmacology and Its Application to Therapeutics and Toxicology* in 1917.

John H. Gaddum, first at Edinburgh, then at the Agricultural Research Council's station at Babraham, Cambridge, wrote a magnificent little book as an introduction to pharmacological research in 1940: his *Pharmacology* remained extremely popular for nearly half a century.

Goodman and Gilman's *Pharmacological Basis of Therapeutics* (1944) became the gold standard for education of physicians and remains at the forefront today.

Henry H. Dale (1875-1968), a student at Cambridge with J.N. Langley and W.H. Gaskell, became fascinated by the concept of neurotransmitters and the autonomic nervous system. Otto Loewi (1873-1961) in Austria in 1921 had shown that, when the vagus nerve of the isolated heart of one frog was stimulated and the fluid perfusing it was allowed to flow over another isolated frog's heart, a *vasgusstoff* was released that caused the beat of the latter to become arrested after that of the stimulated heart. Dale showed that acetylcholine release caused this effect and that it acted at three sites, the autonomic ganglia, the end-organs of the parasympathetic branch of the autonomic nervous system, and the neuromuscular junction. He used a sensitive bioassay system, the ventral muscle of a leech treated with eserine, which extended the life of acetylcholine. Dale also confirmed Elliott's observation of 1905 in the United States that adrenaline given systemically to an anesthetized animal

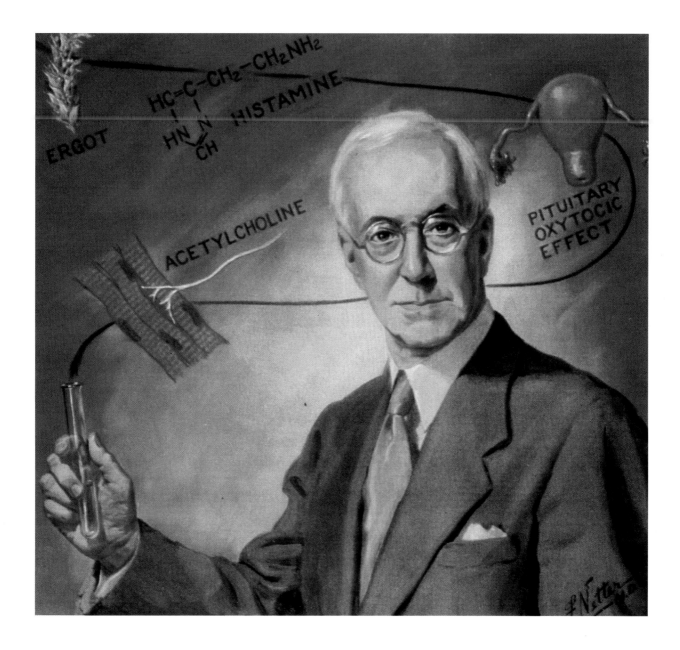

mimicked the effects of electrical stimulation of the sympathetic branch of the autonomic nervous system. With Feldberg in 1933 he categorized synapses as cholinergic or adrenergic. Dale discovered histamine and isolated oxytocin, the hormone that stimulates uterine contraction and milk letdown, in 1928. His work on the brain-modifying effects of ergot alkaloids led to discoveries of neurotransmitters involved in the inhibition of pain, the endorphins. He played a major role in preparing international biological standards.

Veterinary education, with few exceptions, did not follow the human field in adopting pharmacology as an experimental science until after the Second World War. However, veterinary medicine was quick to adopt the use of general and local anesthetics after their discovery in the nineteenth century. The anesthetics were necessary to provide the restraint required during major surgery and to support the humanitarian concerns of the profession. Considerable attention was given to the use of preanesthetic medication in rendering induction of anesthesia easier and safer. The old alkaloids, morphine and atropine, were used, but cats did not tolerate morphine. In large animals chloral hydrate was used, but it was never a completely satisfactory anesthetic when used alone. It was more suitable when used as a hypnotic or sedating agent before inhalation of anesthetic vapor.

The needs of veterinarians were different from those of physicians. Dealing more with acute and infectious diseases for which there were no specific remedies, the profession limped along without a therapeutic armamentarium for most of its first hundred and fifty years. Some pharmaceutical companies developed lines of veterinary products, and some specialty businesses

448. Henry Dale (1875-1968) received the Nobel Prize in physiology and medicine jointly with Otto Loewi in 1936 for isolating acetylcholine (1914) as the active agent involved in the chemical transmission of vagal nerve impulses that inhibit the heart. He graduated in natural sciences at Cambridge in 1898 and in surgery and clinical medicine at St. Bartholomew's Hospital, London (in 1903 and 1907, respectively). As a medical student he engaged in research with Ernest Starling and William Bayliss at University College and with Paul Ehrlich in Frankfurt. He became director of Wellcome Physiological Research Laboratories in 1906, where he worked on ergot and isolated histamine; head of the department of biochemistry and pharmacology of the Medical Research Council in 1914; and director of the National Institute for Medical Research from 1928 to 1942. His many remarkable achievements in the physiological sciences earned him many high honors, including knighthood. Portrait by Frank Netter (1906-1991). *(National Library of Medicine, Bethesda, Maryland.)*

developed and marketed veterinary drugs. The earliest role models for veterinary pharmaceutical research emerged in companies interested in chemotherapy against parasites and bacteria. In the veterinary schools the traditional materia medica and toxicology persisted long after the new approach to pharmacology should have displaced them. The use of external medications was prevalent, especially for the horse: liniments, blisters, ectoparasitic washes, and antiseptic ointments were the order of the day. The use of balls and drenches to purge or soothe the bowel or to break the foam in a bloated rumen was widespread.

In Edinburgh Finlay Dun described, in the ninth edition of his *Veterinary Medicines, Their Actions and Uses* (1895; first edition appeared in 1854), the extremely important differences in responses of the various species of domestic animals to morphine. Dun observed that several species manifested agitation and incoordination, in addition to the desired reduction in sensibility to pain. Overdose could lead to convulsive signs followed by coma and respiratory arrest. Horses became extremely restless, with involuntary movements and staring eyes. Dogs required large doses of morphine and went through a preliminary excitement phase, often with vomiting, before becoming drowsy and unresponsive. Cattle showed excitement and bellowing and had indigestion, sometimes accompanied by bloat. Swine became lively, then dull, with constipation. Cats had the most extreme reactions—agitation progressed to panic behavior and widely dilated pupils.

The Royal Dick College in Edinburgh led the way in bringing the new approach to pharmacology into the veterinary domain. The switch from veterinary materia medica to veterinary pharmacology based on scientific research and experiment got its late start when L. Meyer Jones obtained a doctorate in pharmacology at the University of Minnesota Medical School. He then taught pharmacology at the College of Veterinary Medicine at Iowa State University for twenty-five years. He wrote the first scientifically based work on the subject in the United States in 1954, *Veterinary Pharmacology and Therapeutics.* The work has been continued by his successors and is still in print. Frank Alexander of the Royal Dick School in Edinburgh wrote *An Introduction to Veterinary Pharmacology* in 1960. In the same year G.C. Brander and D.M. Pugh wrote *Veterinary Applied Pharmacology and Therapeutics,* which took a more clinical approach.

THE EMERGENCE OF ANIMAL CHEMISTRY

The establishment of the Society for the Improvement of Animal Chemistry in 1808 as an adjunct of the Royal Society brought together the talents of a group of distinguished scholars in chemistry, physiology, and medicine. Papers were published on blood, urine, poisons, and the role of nerves in animal heat. A kind of clinical chemistry emerged with a goal of using the growing knowledge of chemistry to gain an understanding of physiological and pathological processes. Jöns Jacob Berzelius (1779-1848), the brilliant Swedish atomic chemist and physician, was a trailblazer. British clinical chemists such as William Prout (1785-1850), who proposed the atomic law of whole numbers, analyzed urinary tract stones and considered the role of digestion in their formation. In 1824 he discovered that gastric juice contained hydrochloric acid. Prout also analyzed milk and proposed that because milk was considered the ideal diet for children, foodstuffs should be classified according to their content of the three primary classes of nutrients in milk: fats, carbohydrates, and proteins. Prout proposed a great scheme of chemical transformations in the physiological processes of the body, a speculative precursor to the idea of today's *metabolic pathways.*

The Giessen laboratory group of Justus Liebig (1803-1873) defined the relationships between the inorganic world and the biotic world of plant and animal life. Liebig confirmed the idea that heat was a result of chemical oxidation in the body, the equivalent of combustion. Friedrich Wöhler (1800-1882) discovered that organic acids form salts that are converted to carbonates in the animal body and that urea can be made from ammonium cyanate. Liebig's *Animal Chemistry* was translated into English in 1842, the year it was published in German. A seminal work, it gave impetus to the rapid development of organic chemistry. Liebig thought disease was a result of chemical interactions that led to putrefaction, rejecting Pasteur's idea of pathogenic microbes. In 1897 Edward Buchler (1860-1917) at Bern prepared zymase as an extract of yeast, thereby establishing the specific enzyme catalyst theory of metabolic activity, which led to the formation of the new discipline of biochemistry.

Emil Fischer (1852-1919) in Berlin was the outstanding figure in synthetic organic chemistry. He determined the structure of the purines and showed the role of the peptide bond in linking amino acids in chains to form peptides and proteins. His work was important for pharmacology, since he prepared the first barbiturates, as well as for the foundations of molecular biology. A new class of substances emerged from the work of the microbiologists. Infections gave rise to toxins that damaged the body tissues. Francesco Selmi (1817-1881) showed that microbial decomposition of the tissues of cadavers gave rise to nitrogen-containing organic compounds, which he named *ptomaines*. A search began for the immunogenic and toxicogenic products of pathogenic bacteria. In 1891 the toxin-antitoxin response was discovered by Emil von Behring (1854-1917) and Shibasaburo Kitasato (1856-1931), leading to the concept of using specific antitoxins as therapy against individual bacterial poisons. Emile Roux (1853-1933) in Paris was the first to isolate a bacterial protein toxin.

Tackling the complexities of biological macromolecules and their functions in the animal body and in disease called for new initiatives in physical chemistry. Theodor Svedberg developed the ultracentrifuge that allowed separation of cellular organelles and large molecules. William Thomas Astbury applied X-ray diffraction to the structure of macromolecules. Linus Pauling proposed theories of the chemical bond and valency involving electron sharing. He identified a role for hydrogen bonds in the three-dimensional structure and stability of proteins, as well as the linear coiled structure of some protein molecules in the form of an alpha-helix. Karl Landsteiner (1868-1943) carried out classic work on agglutination and identification of genetic differences in blood groups. This work showed the power of antigen-antibody bonding as a means of stereochemical fitting of chemical groups and receptors, just as Ehrlich had predicted. The new concepts led Pauling into work on nucleic acids and toward the idea that molecular diseases are caused by genetic defects. The older ideas of Archibald E. Garrod (1857-1936) about inborn errors of metabolism were yielding to biochemical progress.

The idea that accessory food substances are necessary for life emerged at the turn of the century and in the early decades of the twentieth century. After demonstrating a dietary need for the amino acid tryptophan in mice, Frederick Gowland Hopkins, the professor of clinical physiology at Cambridge University, noted that a particular class of diseases resulted from a deficiency of one or more of the accessory food substances. At first it was thought that in terms of chemistry they were all amines—a dangerous extrapolation—and Casimir Funk named the accessory food substances *vitamines* as a result. The persistent E.V. McCollum (1879-1967) at the University of Wisconsin uncovered the fat-soluble vitamin A. Later it was shown to be derived from beta-carotene. A British naval surgeon, James Lind, had shown in 1747 that scurvy could be prevented by a daily intake of citrus fruit. The navy prescribed limes, and British sailors were called *Limeys*. Later it was shown that the preventive factor in citrus fruit was ascorbic acid, or vitamin C. Christian Eijkman, a Dutch physician, studied beriberi in the Dutch East

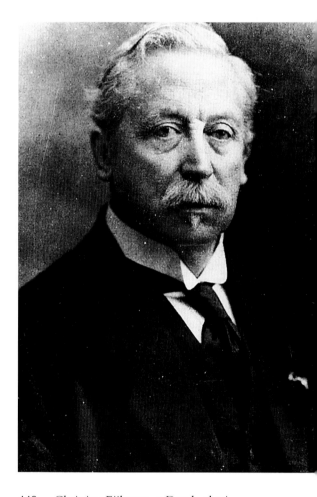

449. Christian Eijkman, a Dutch physician who studied beriberi in the Dutch East Indies. In 1888 he conducted the classic experiment in chickens, which produced disease in groups of chickens that were fed polished rice but not in the groups that were fed unpolished rice. Later, after he joined Utrecht University, it was shown that the missing micronutrient, removed by polishing, was the vitamin B_1 or thiamin. *(National Library of Medicine, Bethesda, Maryland.)*

535

Indies (now part of Indonesia). In 1888 he noticed that in chickens fed on polished rice a similar condition developed, whereas in those fed unpolished rice it did not. The necessary dietary factor, then, was in the polishings, and later, after Eijkman joined the University of Utrecht, the missing factor was shown to be thiamin. Hopkins in 1921 discovered glutathione and its essential role in oxidation-reduction reactions in cells. Hopkins and Eijkman shared a Nobel Prize in 1929. It was known that a dietary factor could prevent rickets. Surprisingly, exposure to sunshine was found to reduce the need for the nutrient, which was called vitamin D. It was found that vitamin D could be formed from precursors in skin exposed to ultraviolet radiation. Several B vitamins were discovered. In 1916 a veterinarian in the United States first proposed that black tongue disease of dogs was analogous to pellagra in humans. The dog was used as the appropriate experimental animal in studying this unpleasant syndrome, and the study led to the discovery of the role of niacin. Carl Arthur Scheunert in the veterinary school at Leipzig conducted important research on micronutrients in Germany between World War I and World War II.

Research revealed the roles of vitamins as cofactors for enzymes. German scholars played a major role in the early stages of unraveling the myriad branches in the vast stem of enzymatic steps and pathways in the mammalian body. Otto Heinrich Warburg developed pressure manometer flasks to aid this search. In 1923 he showed that cancer cells can grow without oxygen when lactic acid is used. While Archibald V. Hill (1886-1977), a Royal Society professor, was studying the biophysics of muscle contraction and the heat it generated, he found that muscle cells require oxygen immediately after but not during contraction. Fritz Albert Lipmann of the Kaiser Wilhelm Institute in Berlin in 1929 isolated adenosine triphosphate from muscle cells; he proposed a role for high-energy organophosphorous compounds in muscle contraction and other energy deployment by cells. He also discovered coenzyme A, which played critical roles in pathways of energy metabolism. David Keith, a Russian working at Cambridge, in 1929 discovered the cytochrome pigments, which play crucial roles in tissue respiration. Hans Krebs received his medical qualification in Berlin in 1925. He then worked in biochemistry there and in Freiburg before leaving Germany for England. He became professor at Oxford University, describing the urea cycle for nitrogen excretion in 1932 and the tricarboxylic acid cycle, or Krebs cycle, in 1937—two of the cornerstones of physiological chemistry. Krebs and Lipmann shared a Nobel Prize in 1953. As knowledge of endocrine regulators advanced, their work gave a great boost to work on mechanisms that underlie metabolic diseases, such as ketosis. Gerty and Carl Cori at Washington University in St. Louis defined the glycogen-glucose-lactic acid cycle, or the *Cori cycle,* which shuttles between liver stores and active muscles; earlier they had identified glucose-1-phosphate and the enzyme phosphorylase, which mobilizes the glycogen. They shared the Nobel Prize in 1947 with Bernardo Houssay of Buenos Aires, Argentina, who discovered the role of the anterior pituitary gland in carbohydrate metabolism. Houssay, a physician, served as a professor of physiology at the school of veterinary science for a decade before moving to the medical school.

EARLY EVIDENCE OF PARASITISM

Parasitism of vertebrate animals and humans is ancient. Pre-Columbian fecal remains from caves in the Americas dated as early as 2500 years ago have revealed evidence of intestinal nematodes and protozoa. Alexander of Tralles (AD 525-605), a physician in Rome in the Byzantine era, left a classic picture in words on the clinical signs of pleurisy. He was also the first to record the differentiation of three types of intestinal parasites: *Ascaris, Taenia,* and

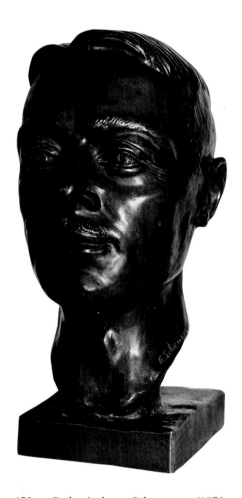

450. Carl Arthur Scheunert (1879-1957), an outstanding physiologist, made major research contributions to the science of vitamins. He made his career at the Dresden and Leipzig faculties of veterinary medicine, separated by three years at the College of Agriculture in Berlin. After 1948 he headed two institutions for nutritional and vitamin research in Potsdam-Rehbrücke, which were merged into the German Democratic Republic's Central Institute of Nutritional Research. His work in vitamin research and testing earned him many honors and a high international reputation. *(Photograph of bust courtesy the Sektion Tierproduktion und Veterinärmedizin der Karl-Marx-Universität Leipzig, Wissenschaftsbereich Tierphysiologie.)*

Oxyuris. He treated them with extracts of male fern and pomegranate. His insightful works were used in Salerno's famous medical school. Avenzoar of Cordova (AD 1072-1162), the greatest of the Moorish Muslim physicians, was the next to write about a parasitic condition. He described the tiny itch-mite, *Acarus scabiei*. The bridge from Spain to France of knowledge of tapeworms was made by a Catalan, Arnaud de Villanova (1240-1311), who taught at Montpellier around 1285. He had gleaned early knowledge of parasitology from Salernitan, Islamic, and Galenic medicine. He introduced the term *solium* (sovereign) for the taenid human tapeworm. The surgical faculty at Montpellier also knew of the scabies mite in the thirteenth and fourteenth centuries.

A French shepherd, Jehan de Brie, provided the first description of the ovine liver fluke. He thought a type of grass found in swampy conditions led to proliferation of a kind of worm in the liver that caused that organ to rot. He presented his thoughts on this disease, the bane of lowland and wetland shepherds, to his king, Charles V, in a written book, *Le Vray Régime et Gouvernement des Bergers et des Bergères par le Rustique Jehan de Brie,* in 1359, although it did not appear in edited form until 1530.

SCIENTIFIC PARASITOLOGY: AN INTERDISCIPLINARY FIELD

Scientific parasitology is unique in that it has evolved since its beginnings as an unfettered interdisciplinary field, a truly comparative branch of both a basic biomedical science and its clinical application in humans and animals. The scholarly Italian court doctor in Florence, Francesco Redi (1626-1697), wrote the first book on parasitology, describing one hundred and eight species. He was interested in ectoparasites and proved that no larvae of flies developed on meat from which adult flies were excluded, a strong disclaimer of the common belief that flies generated spontaneously in meat. Redi described lice and ticks of humans and their domesticated animals. He also gave the first description of liver fluke and the tapeworms of dogs and cats.

Edward Tyson (1651-1708), a London physician and comparative anatomist, made detailed dissections of the round worm *Ascaris lumbricoides* and showed that this species existed in two sexes, another nail in the coffin of spontaneous generation. He was the first to distinguish the apes from other monkeys in *Orang-Outang* in 1699. The French parasitologist Nicolas Andry (1658-1718) wrote an illustrated book on the generation of worms in the human body in 1699. He described the tapeworms of the genus *Taenia* and illustrated the scolex by which they attached to the bowel wall. He believed that the presence of intestinal worms was a consequence of ingestion or inhalation of their seeds. Brera, a medical professor in Pavia, Italy, wrote in 1798 that worms in the gut arose from ingestion of their eggs. He also proposed that they could cross from mother to fetus. He speculated that food could become contaminated by worm eggs from the bowels of animals.

Peter Simon Pallas (1741-1811) was a German natural historian and physician who trained at Leyden, completing his doctoral degree in medicine with a thesis on parasitology. He became entranced with zoology while studying in England in 1761 and shed light on classes of invertebrate animals about which little was known. He was elected a fellow of the Royal Society in 1764. His importance to early parasitology was his contribution to the understanding of bladder worms in his *Miscellanea Zoologica* of 1766. He considered all bladder worms to be a kind of tapeworm and was the first to suggest that the hydatid cysts found in humans were in this category. He considered all bladder worms to be *Taenia hydatigena,* a serious oversimplification, but he was the first to propose that the tapeworms in one animal species might give rise to the cysts in another. His genius was diverted from these intuitive insights in

1767, when Catherine II of Russia picked him for the chair in natural history at St. Petersburg. He dedicated the rest of his life to study of the natural history of the vast Russian empire. He left the empress with a magnificent museum collection.

A German Protestant minister, Johan Göze, wrote the most comprehensive early work on the internal parasites of animals. It was published in 1787 and was dedicated to Pallas. Göze dissected many animal species in his quest for helminths and brought order to their classification for the first time. His many discoveries included *Coenurus cerebellis,* which causes brain cysts in sheep, and the scolex of the genus *Echinococcus* in hydatid cysts. In Berlin M. Bloch extended the classification of the genus *Taenia* and showed that the tapeworm segments contained ovaries.

Swedish-born Karl Asmund Rudolphi (1771-1832) studied medicine at Greifswald, where his talent was recognized and he was made professor of anatomy. He was then called to Berlin, where he founded the Zoological Museum and achieved international fame. A master of histology, he was noted for his comparative studies of the intestinal villi. He wrote *Grundriss der Physiologie,* in which he synthesized the rapid progress in the field, but did not quite complete it before his death. He produced two massive, encyclopedic works on parasitology—the first between 1808 and 1810 (in two volumes) and the second in 1819—that established his reputation as the foremost parasitologist of his time.

Translation into English in 1845 of a revolutionary work written in 1842 by Japetus J.S. Steenstrup, who was appointed professor of zoology at the University of Copenhagen, was a milestone of parasitological thought. His short treatise addressed the issue of alternation of generations. It was known that flukes develop from free-swimming larvae called *cercariae.* In the section on parasites he described for the first time the complete life cycle of parasitic flukes with a multiplication stage in a snail. Steenstrup asked, "Whence come then the free-swimming cercariae?" He showed that they arose in large numbers from saclike structures in the tissues of the snail, which did not resemble their parent flukes. The larval forms were released and eventually penetrated the final host. The cycle was completed by the adult *Trematoda* organisms or flukes, which became oviparous within their host animals such as water birds, their eggs hatching into a form that infected the *intermediate host* (the Ammen or nurse)—the snail—and started a new *generational cycle.* Felix Dujardin (1801-1862), professor of zoology at Rennes, showed between 1847 and 1851 that trematodes and cestodes (tapeworms) pass part of their life cycle in intermediate hosts. He concluded that bladder worms (hydatid cysts) in the tissues were a stage in the life cycle of the segmented tapeworms. He published an excellent work on the natural history of the helminths or intestinal worms in 1845. Steenstrup's model had initiated a new framework of thinking about parasitic infection, which triggered a new wave of investigation that paid enormous dividends for medical and veterinary science.

VETERINARY SCIENCE AND THE ADOPTION OF PARASITOLOGY

Rudolphi said that although Bourgelat founded veterinary schools, it was Philibert Chabert (1737-1814) who founded veterinary *science.* His *Traité des Maladies Vermineuses des Animaux* described the first scientifically developed anthelmintic, *empyreumatic oil,* for the treatment of horse bots and canine tapeworms. He conducted research on fly strike problems and on sheep scab (scabies). He became director of the Alfort school after Bourgelat and initiated the scientific thrust in veterinary medicine.

Casimir Davaine (1812-1882), a French medical practitioner in Paris, carried out important early work on visualizing the organism of anthrax in blood smears. He literally founded medical and veterinary microbiology. In parasitology he was the first to show the value of microscopic examination of feces for the ova of helminths in 1857. In 1860 he wrote a well-illustrated treatise on parasitology of humans and domestic animals. After observing the repeated attacks of biting flies of the genus *Stomoxys,* he suggested that arthropods might be vectors of disease.

Rudolf Leuckart (1822-1898) at the University of Leipzig developed the broader concept of invertebrate parasitology from its roots in helminthology. He established the first major parasite research laboratory in a new zoological institute built for his work. He recognized that the Coccidia were parasitic members of the Protozoa and placed them in the class Sporozoa. He grouped three types of organisms—worms, protozoa, and arthropods—in the category of parasites, thereby creating a new academic discipline, *parasitology.* His great two-volume book of 1876 was translated into English as *The Parasites of Man and the Diseases Which Proceed From Them* in 1886.

Thomas S. Cobbold (1828-1885) was the first important British parasitologist. A physician trained in Edinburgh, he devoted himself to the study of biology. While dissecting a giraffe in 1854, he was struck by the large size of liver flukes in the bile ducts. He named the new species *Fasciola giganta.* He became professor of botany and helminthology at the Royal Veterinary College in 1872, after beginning to dissect all the animals that died in the London Zoo between 1857 and 1860. He wrote a distinguished, lovely book, *Entozoa, an Introduction to the Study of Helminthology,* in 1864.

Timothy Lewis of the British Army Medical Service in India discovered tiny threadlike filarial worms in human blood in 1872. Patrick Manson, a physician working in the customs service in China, showed that the filariae were ingested by bloodsucking female mosquitoes and underwent metamorphosis. He mistakenly thought that humans had to ingest water contaminated by the infected mosquitoes to acquire the disease. Cobbold presented Manson's remarkable report of his discovery of the development of a filarial parasite in the body of a mosquito to the Linnaean Society in 1878. Manson developed a model for his malaria theory of 1894. It was Ronald Ross (1857-1932), however, born in India, who showed in 1898 that the malarial parasite undergoes development within an *Anopheles* mosquito, migrates to its salivary glands, and is inoculated into its human host during a second blood feed. Ross received the Nobel Prize in 1902. He was appointed to a chair in tropical medicine in Liverpool. Cobbold wrote a second book, of much broader scope than his first, in 1879: *Parasites; a Treatise on the Entozoa of Man and Animals Including Some Account of the Ectozoa.* With this work he succeeded in bringing parasitology to the attention of the English-speaking world, which led to its acquiring the status of an academic discipline.

VETERINARY SCIENTISTS: LEADERS IN NINETEENTH-CENTURY PARASITOLOGY

After the fine start provided by Alfort's second director, Chabert, the college became particularly prominent in its achievements in scientific parasitology. Casimir Baillet (1820-1900) described tapeworms and vascular worms in dogs. Jean Pierre Mégnin (1828-1905), a hard-driving, former military veterinarian, published extensively on parasitic mites, providing meticulous illustrations. He wrote more than four hundred articles, including unique studies of the arthropod fauna of corpses and tombs. He compiled his works on mites in a book, *Les Acariens Parasites.*

The greatest figure in veterinary parasitology was Alcide Railliet (1852-1930). He held a chair at Alfort from 1878 to 1920. He influenced many in the field, including the famous Russian parasitologist Konstantine I. Skrjabin, as well as Albert Henry and Gabriel Marotel, who taught at Lyon for more

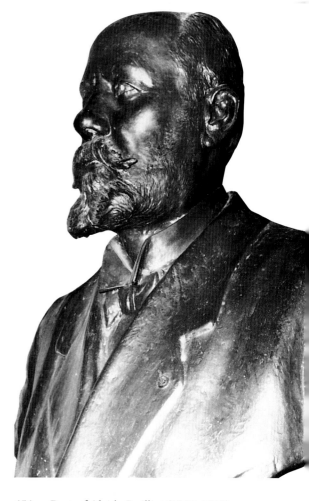

451. Bust of Alcide Railliet (1852-1930) made in his honor. Railliet was professor at the veterinary school of Alfort, Paris, from 1878 to 1920 and a member of the Academy of Medicine. He was perhaps the most significant of the early veterinary parasitologists, setting the stage for all aspects of modern helminthology and making the departmental transition from zoology to parasitology. When microbes were considered the primary cause of disease and death, he established the pathogenic effects of many species of helminths, protozoa, and ectoparasites and introduced extract of male fern as a treatment for liver fluke in sheep. Railliet trained several who became major figures in veterinary parasitology, including Russia's master in the field, Konstantin Ivanovitch Skryjabine (1878-1972); Albert Henry (1878-1943), who followed him in the Alfort chair; and Gabriel Marotel (1873-1951), who became professor at Lyon. Railliet's counterparts at Toulouse were Louis-Georges Neumann (1846-1930), who became the world authority on ticks, and his student André Martin (1876-1954), who discovered the enteropneumotracheal endogenous migration of ascarid larvae. *(Photograph courtesy Service de Parasitology, Ecole Vétérinaire d'Alfort, Paris.)*

than fifty years. Albert Henry (1878-1943) collaborated with Railliet and eventually succeeded him. Henry concentrated on treatment. During the First World War he developed a sulfuration room for the treatment of horses afflicted with mange. Railliet was instrumental in bringing parasitic diseases out of the shadow of the perception then in vogue that pathogenic microbes were the main cause of death. He demonstrated the pathogenic roles of helminths, protozoa, and ectoparasites.

Louis-Georges Neumann (1846-1930), like Henry, was a dominant figure in veterinary parasitology in nineteenth-century France. An orphan, Neumann became an army veterinarian before moving to the veterinary school at Toulouse. He described more members of the family Ixodidae (ticks) than any other scholar and established a type collection in Toulouse. He published a famous textbook on veterinary parasitology, *Traité des Maladies Parasitaires Non Microbienne,* in 1888 and then wrote several volumes on the parasites of domestic animals.

TROPICAL AND SUBTROPICAL PARASITOLOGY

Alphonse Laveran (1845-1922), the most distinguished of French tropical parasitologists, served in the army in Algeria. In 1880 he was the first to describe the hematozoan parasite that causes malaria after inoculation by the infected mosquito. After retiring from the army, he moved to the Institut Pasteur, where he shared a laboratory with Felix Mesnil (1868-1938). Together they wrote *Trypanosomes and Trypanosomiases,* and in 1908 they founded the *Bulletin de la Societé de Pathologie Exotique.* Laveran also confirmed that the genus *Leishmania* was pathogenic. Laveran received a Nobel Prize in 1907 for proving that some protozoans are infectious agents. Mesnil began experiments with organic arsenicals and serum in livestock infected with nagana. Scholars who had worked with him applied his knowledge of malaria and sleeping sickness in devising and implementing effective environmental control programs for the vector insects.

Charles Nicolle (1866-1936) studied under Emile Roux and Elia Metchnikoff. He showed that lice and ticks transmit rickettsial infections such as typhus and relapsing fever. Emil Brumpt studied parasitic diseases in many regions of the world. He studied the mechanisms of transmission of *Trypanosoma cruzi* in South America by reduviid bugs and determined the life cycle of two *Schistosoma* species, *S. haematobium* and *S. bovis.* He also wrote a tome on parasitology; the first edition appeared in 1910. Maurice Neven-Lemaire studied under Grassi in Rome and Ronald Ross in Liverpool before producing his *Traité d'Entomologie Medicale et Vétérinaire* in 1938.

VETERINARY LEADERSHIP IN EARLY TWENTIETH-CENTURY PARASITOLOGY

American parasitology owes its early achievements to a remarkable scholar of German origin at the University of Pennsylvania, Joseph Leidy (1823-1891), the leading professor of anatomy in the land. He was amazing for the breadth of his interests, making his mark in fossil studies and paleontology, mineralogy, botany, and zoology. He wrote on the comparative anatomy of the liver in 1848. James Paget, while a medical student at St. Bartholomew's Hospital in London, had discovered a *Trichinella spiralis* parasite in a human cadaver in 1835. Leidy found a parasite of the same species in a piece of pork he was eating in 1846. After the human disease was characterized, Leidy wrote *The Flora and Fauna Within Living Animals* in 1851. In 1860 Zenker in Dresden traced the source of human infection to raw sausage from a pig.

Two of R. Leuckart's students at Leipzig, Henry Baldwin Ward at the University of Nebraska and Charles W. Stiles of the Public Health Service, were zoologists engaged in parasitological research. Ward became professor of zoology at the University of Illinois in 1909. The Helminthological Society of Washington was formed in 1910 and became the base of the American Society of Parasitologists (ASP), founded in 1925. Eight of Ward's students became presidents of this society. In 1914 Ward founded the *Journal of Parasitology,* which was taken over by the ASP in 1932.

Daniel Elmer Salmon was the first Cornell University graduate in veterinary medicine and in 1876 became the first professional doctor of veterinary medicine who qualified in the United States. He founded the Bureau of Animal Industry (BAI) within the U.S. Department of Agriculture in 1883, which evolved as a research arm of veterinary medicine in the service of agriculture. One driving political motivation for the establishment of the BAI was an embargo that was placed on American swine and pork products by several European nations because of a growing perception of risk from *Trichinella* parasites. The threats of Texas fever to the beef industry and of hog cholera to swine production, both then of unknown origin, were also motivating factors. A microbiological research laboratory, apparently the first in the United States, was set up.

Salmon, an astute judge of talent, was fortunate that three brilliant veterinary scientists were available to join his team at the BAI. The first of these, Theobald Smith, had graduated from Albany Medical College and from veterinary training under James Law and Simon Gage at Cornell University. In 1885 Salmon introduced Smith to the exciting new methods of bacterial culture and strain isolation he had learned in France and Germany. Together they isolated from swine and characterized organisms that came to be known as the genus *Salmonella.* They attempted to create immunity to these bacteria by using multiple injections of suspensions of killed organisms, later called *bacterins.* At first they thought that in *Salmonella cholerae-suis* they had isolated the cause of hog cholera, a devastating new disease of swine that had appeared in Tennessee in 1810 and was spreading rapidly. In time they were shown to have been mistaken, but their early studies placed them at the leading edge of infectious disease research worldwide.

Salmon chose Frederick L. Kilborne, another Cornell University graduate and Smith's classmate in veterinary medicine, to be superintendent of his experimental station in 1885. Kilborne wanted to test the stockmen's idea that ticks might be responsible for Texas fever. Despite advice from scientists who scoffed at the idea, Salmon observed that the northern geographical limits of the incidence of the disease in cattle approximately matched those of the ticks. He gave Kilborne his approval and some of the limited resources available for research. In the first year of study Kilborne established that the cattle tick was essential to the occurrence of Texas fever.

Salmon's third key appointment (in 1886) was Cooper Curtice, yet another member of Law's talent pool at Cornell. Curtice was a man of broad interests who had carried out research in paleontology for the U.S. Geological Survey. Salmon asked him to establish a zoological laboratory for the study of parasitology, including helminth and arthropod parasites of cattle and sheep. Curtice was a highly focused worker. He published reports on fascioliasis, hydatid disease, sheep tapeworm, and myiasis (fly strike) within one year. Curtice was then assigned to work on the biology of the cattle tick. He made the surprising finding that this tick spent its life cycle—from larval stage through nymph to adult—attached to a single bovine host. Later he said that this finding indicated the vulnerability of the disease to control by elimination of the tick vector.

When Curtice resigned in 1891, Salmon hired Charles Stiles to continue the exciting initiative. They collaborated in an important study of sheep scab

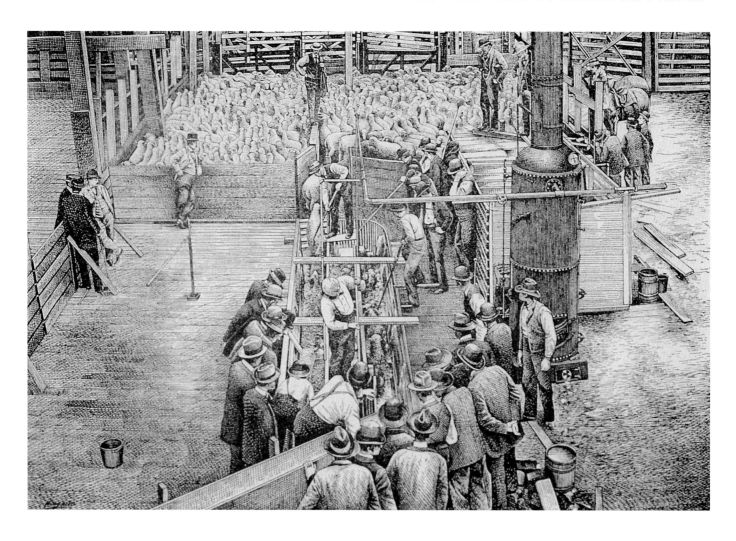

452. View of the sheep-dipping plant at the Union Stockyards in Chicago, Illinois, as illustrated in a report by Salmon and Stiles on the nature and treatment of sheep scab. Dipping was used to prevent the spread of sheep scab. *(Courtesy of the Archives of the National Animal Disease Center, Ames, Iowa.)*

caused by a mite. Albert Hassell (1862-1942) at the U.S. National Museum built a large reference collection of parasites. In collaboration with Stiles he developed an invaluable *Index-Catalogue of Medical and Veterinary Zoology.* The goal of the BAI staff was to understand parasitic diseases so that effective methods could be developed for their prevention or control. The list of diseases under study included bovine piroplasmosis (Texas fever), equine venereal trypanosomasis (dourine), cysticercosis, scabies, swine ascariasis, and the disease caused by the hookworm, *Necator americanus.* The widespread distribution of human hookworm disease in the Southern states gave that disease a high priority in the research. Maurice Hall (1881-1938) developed the use of both carbon tetrachloride and tetrachlorethylene as treatments for hookworm disease after a series of rigorous experimental tests. In 1902 members of the BAI were appointed to the new advisory board of the Hygienic Laboratory, which had been moved from Staten Island, New York, to Washington in 1891. Stiles was appointed to head its zoology division. He isolated a new tick species, *Dermacentor andersoni,* in 1904 when investigating Rocky Mountain spotted fever. Stiles pushed for an eradication program against hookworm disease in the South. When he retired in 1932, Hall was appointed from the BAI to be chief of the zoology division. His special interests were the critical evaluation of anthelmintics in animals and humans and the development of new chemotherapeutic agents against parasites. He was elected president of the American Veterinary Medical Association in 1935. Hall's work initiated a strong tradition of anthelmintic drug testing and development at the BAI, highlighted by Paul D. Harwood's discovery of the broad-spectrum anthelmintic phenothiazine in 1939.

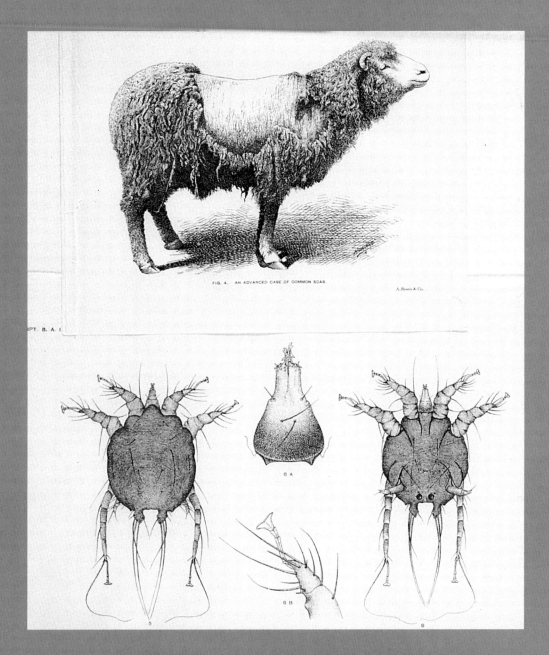

FIG. 4. AN ADVANCED CASE OF COMMON SCAB.

453. Daniel Salmon and C.W. Stiles of the Bureau of Animal Industry published pictures of sheep afflicted with scab and the barely visible mites that cause it in an important report in 1897. After French veterinarian Tessier in 1810 showed that scab could be controlled with an arsenical dip, Gohier isolated the parasite in 1813. Later it was given the genus name *Psoroptes*. With a generation time of only fifteen days, its numbers on a newly infected sheep can reach over a million in three months in winter. Its mouthparts can pierce the epidermis to reach the lymph beneath it, causing intense irritation, scratching, scab formation, and loss of wool. Violations of an 1895 order prohibiting transport led to widespread dispersal of the organism. Nicotine-sulfur and lime-sulfur dips were used to control the disease. *(Fourteenth Annual Report of the Bureau of Animal Industry, 1897, No. 28-17.)*

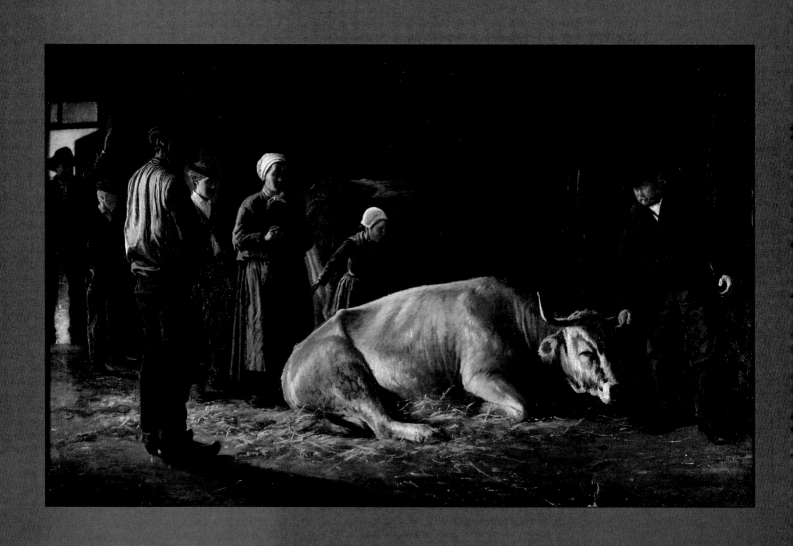

Livestock Production Enhanced by Veterinary Specialists

ENHANCED LIVESTOCK AND THE NEED FOR IMPROVED CARE

Diseases were the most serious causes of economic losses in the breeds of livestock in Great Britain that were improved by intensive husbandry from 1875 to 1925. Sheep on wet pastures were afflicted with foot rot, a bacterial invasion of the softened horn that caused severe lameness. Such environmental conditions also favored infestations with liver fluke, which caused heavy losses in the dense lowland flocks from the midlands westward into Wales during the wet years from 1878 to 1881. An epidemic of contagious bovine pleuropneumonia hit the cattle industry in 1879 and was followed in 1880 and 1881 by outbreaks of foot-and-mouth disease that spread throughout the land. Foot-and-mouth disease was not understood, and because there was no control policy, farmers let it run its course. Although the mortality rate was not high, the costs in lost value of stock and products were enormous. The government tried to reduce the spread by closing markets and fairs, but this action depressed prices even further and did not check the contagion. The national sheep flock was diminished by about twenty percent between 1878 and 1883.

British farmers continued to use the horse as the main provider of energy for farm work, but the expanding network of railways greatly reduced the role of the horse in transport. In the early 1920s steam engines were used in plowing and heavy cultivation on large farms, but the horse continued to be the power source for small farms. When World War II began in 1939, there were still 550,000 horses on farms and fewer than 50,000 tractors. A dramatic increase in mechanization occurred during the war, however, and the number of draft horses declined.

A major development that increased the efficiency of obtaining milk from dairy cows was the *herringbone parlor*. Boyce of Casino, New South Wales, Australia, patented his *echelon stalls* in 1910, the first milking system to apply the principles that became known as herringbone. The idea was ahead of its time; enthusiasm for it waned, and it did not become widely adopted. Hosier in England developed a portable milking bail that he moved around the hill pastures of western England, which allowed a great saving in labor.

Renewed interest in efficient milking began after dairy science professor William E. Peterson of the University of Minnesota, the discoverer of the role of the hormone oxytocin in milk letdown, told the story on an international lecture tour in 1948 of how udder stimulation accelerates milking. Use of a warm washcloth led to relaxation of the udder within a minute, mimicking the action of a suckling calf. A teat cup was used to check the milk manually

454. *Facing page, La Visite du Vétérinaire* (Groteyrolle, 1880). This magnificent painting of an ailing downer cow being evaluated by a veterinarian while a worried family watches is one of the great masterpieces of French art in which the veterinary profession is depicted in action. The veterinarian has felt the ears and horns to determine whether the cow has a fever and has evaluated for other signs of dysfunction. The scene illustrates the tripartite relationship among patient, client, and veterinary surgeon; the case represents a common diagnostic challenge encountered by bovine practitioners. *(Musées de Guéret.)*

545

for mastitis. Ron Sharp, a farmer at Gordonton, New Zealand, developed a modern herringbone milking parlor in 1952. This time the system caught on with dairy farmers, and its use spread rapidly in New Zealand. The design appeared in Great Britain and the United States in 1956. By 1962 parlors were appearing throughout Europe and Australia, and in that year in France the system was adapted for use in milking sheep.

Animal nutrition is too vast a subject to include in this text, except to note the enormous importance of pastures and forages (hay, silage, and by-products of cash crops). Frank B. Morrison of Cornell University and the University of Wisconsin left a legacy of knowledge of animal nutrition. The idea of feeding standards for all classes of livestock developed.

TECHNOLOGY: ENHANCEMENT OF THE SENSES IN CLINICAL EXAMINATION

The techniques of physical diagnostic examination in medicine and veterinary medicine are an exercise in pathophysiology crudely tested through the subjective senses of doctor or veterinarian. These techniques include palpating, listening, observing, and testing reflex responses. Percussion was developed as a technique by Leopold Auenbrugger (1722-1809) in 1761. Texture of hair and elasticity of the skin were examined to assess health. Indelicate application of the doctor's ear to the body wall over the thoracic and abdominal organs was replaced by auscultation after Laënnec began using a stethoscope in 1816. Visual observation for evidence of differences from normal appearance, function, and behavior was a core component of the development of medical reasoning. Observation of the rate of vascular refilling after compression was used as an indicator of circulatory function.

Physical measuring devices were gradually developed to increase the precision of physiological measurement. An important step was the application of thermometry, described by German physician Carl Wunderlich (1815-1877) in 1868 in his work *On the Temperature in Diseases: a Manual of Medical Thermometry.* This manual was an early venture into objective, numerical precision of measurement to aid diagnosis. Despite the great start Hales gave to the measurement of blood pressure in the horse, a practical instrument for the measurement of blood pressure in humans, the sphygmomanometer, was not invented until 1876 by Ritter von Basch. In 1896 Scipione Riva-Rocci introduced the prototype of the instruments used today to measure systolic arterial pressures. N.S. Korotkoff showed that the diastolic pressure could also be determined by combining use of the instrument with the use of a stethoscope. He used as an endpoint the point at which sounds associated with arterial constriction by the cuff ceased, a less precise endpoint than that of systolic pressure. However, more than a century was to pass before reliable techniques were developed for clinical use in animals. Before real sense could be made of the dysfunctions detected by physical examination, a deeper understanding of disease processes was necessary.

The progressive study of clinical signs of disease obtainable by physical examination now includes about one hundred and fifty observable manifestations. The art of the diagnostician lies in interpreting these signs in the context of a much more vast body of knowledge about diseases and animal dysfunctions so that a differential diagnosis can be made.

The book in English that is most valuable as an aid to the clinical diagnosis of bovine diseases, *Clinical Examination of Cattle,* was compiled by Gustav Rosenberger at the Hannover Veterinary School in 1979. This book was the second edition (1977) of a German text that appeared first in 1964. The coauthors were Gerrit Dirsken at Munich, Hans-Dieter Gründer at Giessen, and Eberhard Grunert, Dietrich Krause, and Matthaeus Stöber at Hannover. Rosenberger also published a compendium of diseases in cattle in 1970.

It is impractical to attempt to review the evolution of the field of internal medicine in veterinary medicine. The awesome scale and scope of this burgeoning field indicate that about eleven hundred diseases have been described for cattle, a similar number for horses, about seven hundred and fifty for sheep, and six hundred each for pigs and goats. Douglas C. Blood of Australia and James A. Henderson of Canada published a compendium of the diseases in these species, *Veterinary Medicine,* at Guelph in 1960. Otto Radostits from Saskatoon has assumed responsibility for the production and editorship of this valuable book. In 1990 Bradford P. Smith of the University of California produced a massive work with one hundred and thirty authors, *Large Animal Internal Medicine,* which is restricted to diseases of horses, cattle, sheep, and goats. The first major textbook on swine diseases, written by H.W. Dunne in 1958, was expanded under Allen D. Leman's orchestration and editorship to a comprehensive volume, *Diseases of Swine,* with ninety-nine authors from nine countries by its sixth edition in 1986. All three of these books provide comprehensive bibliographies of the relevant literature in English but not in other languages.

VIRCHOW'S REFORM IN CELLULAR PATHOLOGY

Johannes Müller (1801-1858), the famous physiologist at the University of Berlin, was instrumental in the evolution of the discipline of pathology in Germany from 1830 to 1858. He used the improved achromatic microscopes of 1830 as tools that allowed pathologists to visualize beyond the evidence gathered by their eyes in dissection and gross pathology to the new level of magnification—×300—needed for histopathology. Müller personally showed the power of the microscope by using it to study the fine structure of tumors.

Müller's brilliant protégé Rudolf Virchow (1821-1902), a farmer's son from Pomerania who trained in medicine in Berlin and was appointed to the Charité Hospital there, gave pathology a dynamic perspective by declaring, as expressed in his famous saying, *omnis cellula e cellula,* that all cells arise from cells. He emphasized that the cell is really the *ultimate morphological element* in which there is any manifestation of life. Thus he was able to make the transition from tissue pathology to write *Die Cellularpathologie,* his famous text of 1858.

Virchow saw clearly the need for a new approach to pathology. Even as a young man he challenged the medical profession in Germany to drop its habit of deductive speculation about disease. He urged a focus on thorough gross postmortem examinations at autopsy, with sampling of affected organs for subsequent microscopic examination, to reach a factual evaluation of the changes that are present. Since not all questions could be answered, he urged that a physiological approach to experiments on animals be made so that the factors leading to observed pathological lesions could be determined. Because his methods provided knowledge and assurance not achieved by others, he soon became recognized as a credible authority.

The greatest descriptive pathologist in Europe in 1846 was Carl Rokitansky, a Czech who worked in Vienna. In that year he completed his famous *Manual of Pathological Anatomy,* which was translated into English in 1854. The manual was the distillate of his experience of thirty thousand meticulously conducted autopsies. Nonetheless, he was still caught up in the old model of speculative deduction. This limitation was anathema to Virchow, who, while applauding the master for his brilliant anatomical pathology, declared the book to be dangerous for medicine because it espoused a false pathology of humors and wrong thinking about disease. Conservative pressure forced Virchow to leave Berlin for Würzburg in independent Bavaria. Journal editors were unwilling to publish Virchow's views

455. Rudolf Virchow (1821-1902), born in Pomerania (now part of Poland), transformed medical thought with his revolutionary book, *Die Cellularpathologie* (1858). He slew the resilient old dragon of humoral pathology with his dictum, *omnis cellula e cellula* (all cells arise from cells). His compass was vast: in addition to his medical scholarship he founded physical anthropology in Germany (he is shown in this picture studying craniology), participated in archeological explorations, was a distinguished advocate of liberal political and social reform, and led the charge to improve life and prevent disease through his activism on measures to enhance nutrition and public health, including the recognition of a major role for veterinary medicine. As early as 1850 he showed that living larvae encysted in the human muscles of cadavers developed into the ephemeral adult worms in the intestine if fed to dogs. Zenker at Dresden in 1859 completed the story by discovering how the worm in humans arose from the consumption of infected pork or sausage. Virchow coined the term *zoonosis* and won compulsory examination of pig meat for trichina in Berlin in 1865. He was appointed to the Imperial Animal Health Deputation of the Ministry of Agriculture.

His curiosity seemed infinite, as did his capacity to work systematically for defined goals and to record his findings. He insisted on rigor in scrutinizing questions, methodical pursuit of solutions, and never going beyond experience, settling for defensible, limited conclusions. He saw medicine as a dynamic evolution from cookbook techniques to a science-based application of supportable theory driven by the theoretical biomedical sciences that should be coordinated as experiment-derived pathological physiology. Consequently medicine needed awareness of its historical roots more than any other field of science. His famous journal, *Virchow's Archives,* is still published. *(Francis A. Countway Library of Medicine, Boston.)*

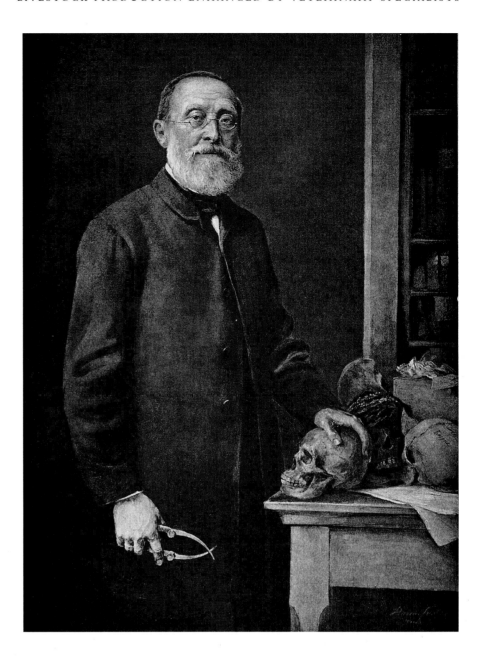

after his devastating review of Rokitansky's book. His response was to found his own journal in 1847, *Archives for Pathological Anatomy and Physiology and Clinical Medicine,* which became known as *Virchow's Archives.*

Another of Müller's scholars, Robert Remak, challenged in 1842 the widespread idea that cells formed from some primitive exudative fluid or *blastema.* Ten years later he declared forcefully that this concept of the extracellular creation of animal cells was not credible, and it was Remak who convinced Virchow on this point. Virchow seized on the vital point that traditional pathologists had missed: pathological changes did not need to be morphological in the sense of being anatomically visible. From the anatomical approach was born the physician's simplistic perspective of two categories of illness, "organic" versus "functional" problems. Virchow's point, however, was much more visionary. He noted the error of the strict morphologists' approach and stressed that molecular changes and degenerations that might not be detectable could occur. Subsequent reductionist techniques of biomedical science have vindicated Virchow's prescient view. It can be argued, however, that the molecular changes are still structural to some extent, although they are invisible with technologies currently available.

Virchow was recalled to Berlin as professor and given a splendid Pathological Institute in 1856. He joined the Prussian Lower House in 1862 and served in the Reichstag from 1880 to 1893. He made enormous administrative contributions to public health in war and peace. The area of bio-medical science that gave Virchow the greatest difficulty was the explosive development of pathogenic microbiology that followed the seminal work of Pasteur and Koch. Pasteur had little time for cellular pathology because techniques were not yet available for experimental study. Some pathologists confronted Virchow on the issue of his concept of intrinsic dysfunction of cells versus the microbiologists' view of attack by alien pathogenic organisms. Edwin Klebs, one of Virchow's pupils, was a leader in this criticism. Klebs had worked with Koch and with Löffler and had discovered the bacterial agent that causes diphtheria. A remarkably insightful person, Klebs forged a strong bridge between the microbiological and pathological approaches. Virchow fought back, arguing that Klebs confused the initiating cause, a microbe, with the disease process itself. He claimed that parasitic agents are never more than inciting causes and that the behavior of the tissues determines the nature of disease. Although there was truth on both sides, both scientists carried their arguments too far and thus lost credibility.

Virchow developed a strong interest in comparative medicine and zoonotic diseases after observing epidemics of trichinosis in Germany. He showed that consumption of infected pig meat led to direct infection of humans if the parasitic agent was living. He pressed for and won compulsory examination of pig meat for the presence of *Trichina* organisms in Berlin in 1865. Ten years later he was appointed to the Imperial Animal Health Deputation of the Ministry of Agriculture and became engaged in the development of animal health legislation.

As a medical student in London, Paget found the *Trichina* organism in human muscle. Leydy in the United States was the first to identify it in pig meat in 1847. Zenker showed that *Trichina* organisms were responsible for a serious epidemic of human disease near Dresden in 1861. The organism could cause death.

Virchow studied hydatid disease and showed that the multilocular form arose from infection by *Echinococcus* organisms. Kuchenmeister and Siedel revealed the life cycle of the parasite in 1853. They found that the incidence of hydatidosis in humans was directly correlated with the incidence of the adult worms in dogs. Control measures were implemented to break the cycle by preventing infection in the dog.

William Osler (1849-1919), the creative Canadian genius of internal medicine, studied in Berlin in 1873, when Virchow was fifty-two years old. Osler found Virchow to be a great inspiration for his ideas of correlating signs evident on clinical examination of patients with terminal illnesses with the gross and microscopic findings on autopsy to advance understanding. Osler declared that the scientific medicine of Germany in that period was in the forefront worldwide. He particularly admired Virchow for the breadth of his interest and knowledge, as well as for his reforming zeal and remarkable commitment to the improvement of human life.

Julius Cohnheim (1839-1884), who had worked at Kiel, Breslau, and Leipzig, discovered the vascular role in inflammation. He showed that circulating white blood cells gave rise to pus cells by diapedesis (transmigration) across the walls of microscopic blood vessels into an injured tissue.

William H. Welch (1850-1934) was one of the great visionary leaders of the health sciences in the United States. He had studied zoology under Leuckart in Leipzig, pathology with Cohnheim at Breslau (just before the latter went to Leipzig), and microbiology and pathology with Theodor Kitt at Munich's veterinary school. After his return to the United States he studied salmonellosis in swine and reported his findings to the International Veterinary Congress in 1894. Welch is known for his identification of *Clostridium welchii (C. perfringens),* the organism that causes gas gangrene. He was the mentor of Walter Reed of yellow fever fame. So intense was Welch's admiration that he regarded Virchow's establishment of the principle of cel-

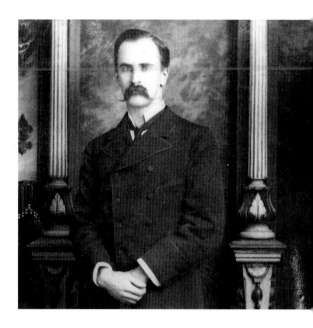

456. Sir William Osler (1849-1919) was one of the leading architects of the evolution of the medical professions. His development into one of the most distinguished physicians, teachers, and scholars of his time was influenced by several people connected with the fledgling veterinary profession in Canada. Under James Bovell in Toronto he studied the parasite *Trichinella spiralis.* Griffith Evans, discoverer of pathogenic trypanosomes, was working in Bovell's laboratory at the time and showed Osler how to use the microscope. Osler fed encysted larvae to animals to determine whether he could transmit the disease. Bovell joined the faculty of OVC in 1864. Osler went to McGill medical school in 1870. Another friend of Bovell's, Duncan McEachran, founded the Montreal Veterinary School in 1866 and built a new place to house it in 1875. He appointed Osler to teach veterinary students in 1876. Osler gave the inaugural lecture that fall, *The Relations of Animals to Man,* addressing comparative anatomy, embryology, and Darwin's studies on evolution. McEachran welcomed enthusiastically Osler's proposal that the veterinary faculty be named the *Faculty of Comparative Medicine and Veterinary Science.*

Osler discovered a pulmonary parasite, *Filaroides osleri,* in dogs during a lethal disease epidemic from 1876 to 1877. Although the cause of death was probably canine distemper, animal viruses had not yet been discovered. He learned much about tuberculosis from McEachran and Evans. Osler went to Europe again in 1884 and consulted several outstanding veterinary scholars and physicians in Germany. He left McGill for Philadelphia that year, having left an indelible stamp of quality, a new thrust in pathology, and a commitment to comparative medicine and research on the Canadian veterinary profession. *(McCord Museum of Canadian History, Notman Photographic Archives.)*

lular pathology as the greatest advance in the history of scientific medicine. In the United States Welch became a professor of pathology and, with William Osler, one of the architects of the Johns Hopkins Medical School.

Theobald Smith (1859-1934) had left the Bureau of Animal Industry (BAI) in 1895 to be head of the Massachusetts State Board of Health Laboratories and Harvard's first professor of comparative pathology. He and Welch were appointed to the board of directors of the Rockefeller Institute for Medical Research that Welch had conceived. Welch's goal was to create an institute for human disease research like the BAI veterinary research operation for animal diseases. Welch spoke at the American Medical Association in 1904. His presentation was entitled *The Bureau of Animal Industry: Its Service to Medical Science*. Welch had sought to hire Smith as director of the new institute, but Smith declined consideration. He joined the Institute later, however, in 1914. Ernest E. Tyzzer took Smith's former position at Harvard and did classic work on coccidial diseases of chickens. Smith recruited H.W. Graybill, a veterinary parasitologist from the BAI.

NORTH AMERICAN VETERINARY FOCUS ON PATHOGENESIS

Joseph Woodward, a physician at the Army Medical Museum in Washington, published the first scientific report in veterinary pathology in North America in 1870, which described the histopathologic features of contagious bovine pleuropneumonia, but this was an isolated event. A more fruitful initiative occurred in Montreal, Canada, however, when William Osler began teaching in Duncan McEachran's Montreal Veterinary College in 1876. This remarkable school became the Faculty of Comparative Medicine at McGill University. Osler applied his special magic to teaching physiology and pathology and put the course of study at McGill on the high road to academic motivation and excellence before departing to the University of Pennsylvania in 1884, where he had a similar impact.

In 1862 McEachran and Andrew Smith, both from Edinburgh, were partners in founding the Ontario Veterinary School, then at Toronto. Today, based sixty miles further west at Guelph, where it moved in 1910, it is the oldest surviving educational institution for veterinary medicine in North America. McEachran was a great scholar and visionary in his chosen profession and could not accept the pragmatic Smith's expedient political maneuvers. Smith opted for a shorter course and lower standards to ensure large numbers of students. McEachran left in disgust and began the Montreal college as a private initiative to seek to attain his higher aspirations for the profession. This remarkable man had a great capacity for work. He accepted an appointment as Chief Inspector of Livestock by the Dominion government in 1876, a post he held until 1902, while continuing as principal of the Montreal college.

No doubt McEachran was influential in persuading the Ministry of Agriculture for Canada to open the first quarantine station in North America at Point Levis, Quebec, in 1902. Because he inspected imported livestock there, Canada was kept almost free of the epidemic diseases that recurred in Europe and the United States. Not satisfied with the finest veterinary curriculum and the beginnings of an outstanding government service, McEachran also saw the need for research. Osler, too, was a spearhead in research, investigating hog cholera in 1878 and Pictou cattle disease of Nova Scotia in 1883. J. George Adami studied tuberculosis, and one of his trainees became the first Dominion animal pathologist. The only comparable quality of pathology instruction was at Harvard Veterinary School, which opened in 1882 with L. Frothingham, who had trained with Albert Johne (discoverer of Johne's disease) at Dresden. The Harvard School closed in 1902. Pathology

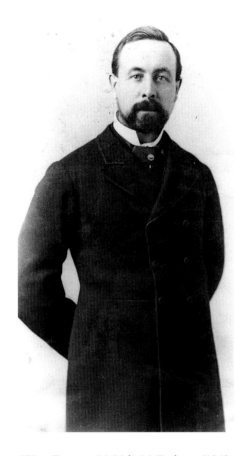

457. Duncan McNab McEachran (1842-1924) graduated from Dick's Edinburgh college in 1862, then emigrated to Canada, where he assisted Andrew Smith in founding the Ontario Veterinary College but despaired over the low standards Smith set to attract students. Moving his practice to Montreal in 1865, he set up a new college with a three-year curriculum and built a new building for it ten years later. He persuaded the government to establish a quarantine station at Levis in 1875 to prevent the entry of European animal plagues. He recruited McGill physician William Osler to join the faculty in 1876 to teach and to initiate research in comparative pathology. He appointed one of his French-born graduates, Victor Daubigny, to lead the French section in 1879; Daubigny established a French school with Orphyr Bruneau in 1885 that merged with the one at Laval University in Quebec in 1895. McEachran was appointed Chief Veterinary Inspector for Canada in 1884. He introduced the tuberculin test as an early foray into population-based diagnosis for a plan to eradicate tuberculosis, emphasizing the need for compensation. His ideas and ideals were carried forward by John Gunion Rutherford, who was the first veterinary director general for Canada and became president of the AVMA in the 1908-1909 session. *(McCord Museum of Canadian History, Notman Photographic Archives.)*

was not taught at Cornell University until 1896, one year after it became a veterinary college. Thus Osler was a conceptual parent of veterinary pathology in North America.

VETERINARY CLINICAL PATHOLOGY AND DIAGNOSIS IN THE LIVING

After the strong focus on rigorous necropsy followed by microscopic tissue examination that flowed from Virchow's leadership in pathology to the German veterinary schools after 1850, the next challenge was to advance knowledge of pathogenesis, which required the development of a research thrust with laboratory methods and experimental animal models. The parallel development of pathogenic microbiology and parasitology greatly enhanced the specificity of diagnosis in cases of infectious disease. For study of the noninfectious diseases such as nutritional, metabolic, and endocrine disorders, as well as most cancers, physiological, biochemical, and cytological approaches were needed. Even with the infections, hematological, immunological, and chemical analyses of body fluids could be used in elucidating the pathogenesis and course of the host response to disease. The result was the birth of a field of veterinary clinical pathology or clinical laboratory medicine.

Hematology of domestic animals may have stemmed from observations made on blood drawn as a standard therapeutic practice, that is, bleeding. W. Nasse in 1842 noted that equine red blood cells (RBCs or erythrocytes) tended to settle rapidly in a tube, leaving a layer of yellowish plasma above the sedimented RBCs. The blood of other species did not behave in the same way. Theobald Smith and F.L. Kilborne saw the agent that caused Texas fever in RBCs in blood smears on microscopic study in 1893. The researchers noted the pathognomonic sign of port wine–colored urine, which resulted from renal damage. Kilborne found that the infectious agent was transmitted by bloodsucking ticks. Arnold Theiler in South Africa studied the immense problem of blood-borne parasitic diseases on the African continent and discovered *Theileria parva* in the blood cells in East Coast fever.

In the United States S.H. Burnett studied the blood cells of the main domestic species in the first decade of the twentieth century. At Kansas State College W.E. King and R.H. Wilson reported the observation of leukopenia in hog cholera in 1910. Habersand in 1921 showed that the red blood cells were hemolyzed in equine infectious anemia. J.P. McGowan and A. Crighton in Great Britain in 1923 made the important discovery that a form of anemia in intensively housed piglets was due to iron deficiency and responded to treatment with iron preparations. The field of hematology became popular as an important adjunct to diagnosis in the living animal, and D. Wirth in 1931 wrote *Essentials of Clinical Hematology of Domestic Animals.* In the United States D.L. Coffin published his *Manual of Clinical Pathology* in 1944, and in Great Britain G.F. Boddie presented a broader scope in his *Diagnostic Methods in Veterinary Medicine* in the same year. In 1961 O.W. Schalm's *Veterinary Hematology,* published by the University of California, was more comprehensive with respect to hematology of domestic animals.

Leukemia was diagnosed in a horse in 1891, in a dog in 1904, and in a cow in 1906. In 1916 lymphoma in cattle was seen as a herd problem by Du Toit, who made diagnoses on the basis of changes in leukocytes. This was the foundation on which subsequent efforts to eradicate viral enzootic leukosis in Europe were made. Unlike leukemia, in which the blood may be swamped with excessive numbers of proliferating leukocytes, a virulent condition in cats with the opposite effect was described by J.S. Lawrence and J.J. Syverton in 1938. This condition was panleukopenia, in which a specific virus caused aplasia of the bone marrow. Another devastating viral disease of cats was explained by the studies of W.F.H. Jarrett and his team at the University of

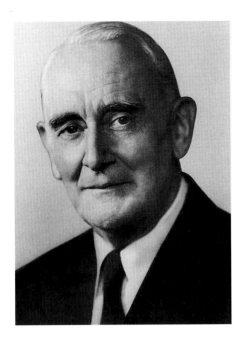

458. Francis William Schofield (1889-1970) was born in Rugby, England, and emigrated to Canada at sixteen years of age. He graduated from the Ontario Veterinary College with the bachelor's degree in veterinary science at the University of Toronto in 1910. He caught poliomyelitis, which weakened him physically but did not cripple him. He joined the faculty of OVC and completed a doctorate in veterinary science in 1911. As a Presbyterian missionary he taught in Seoul, Korea, from 1916 to 1919, and returned there on his retirement.

Schofield was renowned as an inspiring teacher and an intuitive researcher. He showed that "bleeding disease" of cattle was attributable to ingestion of moldy sweet clover, which contained a substance that inhibited coagulation of the blood and caused hemorrhages. This clue led to the discovery of dicoumarol at the University of Wisconsin, and then warfarin. He proposed that lethal mink enteritis was caused by a virus akin to the one causing feline panleukopenia and that a toxin from certain strains of *Escherichia coli* caused edema disease of swine. *(Ontario Veterinary College.)*

Glasgow veterinary school. That disease proved in 1964 to be another cancer induced by a retrovirus called feline leukemia virus.

E. Kaiser in Frankfurt in 1909 reported on the study of the animal cells in transudates and exudates as a diagnostic aid. B.S. Parkin in South Africa in 1931 described the application of lymph node aspirates in the diagnosis of trypanosomiasis in livestock. Special instruments were devised that could sample a small piece of living tissue; that is, a biopsy could be performed. This procedure allowed speedy examination, in some cases while the surgeon waited, using quick-frozen, stained specimens, needle aspirates, or imprints. Decisions could then be made based on factual cytopathological information; for example, characteristics of lesions in proliferative diseases such as cancers and bone marrow or lymphatic responses could be assessed. In the veterinary field this technique of cytology has become particularly important in companion animal practice.

F.R. Page, a Canadian veterinary practitioner, reported in 1922 an unusual occurrence in which cattle fed on sweet clover bled to death after a standard dehorning procedure. Frank Schofield, pathologist at the Ontario Veterinary College, followed up on Page's report by conducting feeding trials with sweet clover. In 1924 he reported that moldy sweet clover was the cause of the problem and investigated the blood changes. He proposed that a compound called coumarin was formed in the moldy material. A brilliant research study at the University of Wisconsin led to the discovery that the mold converted the coumarin in the plant to a toxic dimer, which the researchers named dicumarol, a potent anticoagulant. Studies of its molecular structure led to the synthesis and study of related compounds. One result was *warfarin,* which was found to be an effective rat poison and an invaluable aid to patients at risk for intravascular coagulation, as in coronary thrombosis. The discovery proved to be lucrative and generated the resource base that made the Wisconsin Agricultural Research Foundation a major player in funding research at Madison, Wisconsin.

Immunology has always fascinated veterinarians because they were in on it from its early days and recognized its importance and application in host resistance to infections. As far back as the mid–nineteenth century Chauveau was proposing the mechanism of immunity. C. Todd and R.G. White, while producing immune sera against rinderpest, observed adsorption of immune sera onto red blood cells and their capacity to induce agglutination. Prophetically they noted that the specificity of the method had potential for use in differential diagnosis and that the difference in red blood cell antigens might have potential as a way to study heredity. Australian scientist R.R.A. Coombs moved to Cambridge University and described the antiglobulin test for isoagglutinins. The *Coombs test* became a vital tool in detecting immune-mediated anemias.

CLINICAL PATHOLOGY OF METABOLIC DISEASES

During the early years of the twentieth century great strides were made in quantitative clinical chemistry, and progress in the understanding of metabolic diseases of animals resulted. Until crucial discoveries were made, milk fever, grass staggers, acetonemia, and aphosphorosis lacked specific treatment.

Milk fever was a strange choice of title for the syndrome of parturient paresis in dairy cattle, in which cows became weak and unable to rise around the time of calving. J. Schmidt in 1898 reported successful treatment of the condition by means of the simple physical act of pumping air into the udder via the teats. C.E. Hayden and L.B. Sholl at Cornell University in 1924 found that affected cows had hyperglycemia with glycosuria. The next year W.L. Little and N.C. Wright in Great Britain made the crucial discovery that a profound hypocalcemia was present. The logical step of administering calcium salts as therapy was attempted soon afterward, attended by dramatic recovery in many instances. P.A. Fish at Cornell University showed that elevating the hydrostatic pressure in the lumen of the mammary gland increased the concentrations of calcium and phosphorus.

A related disorder known as grass tetany, grass staggers, or lactation tetany was described that manifested tetanic signs rather than the paralysis seen in milk fever. B. Sjollemo in Holland in 1930 showed that a major decline in serum magnesium concentration was usually present in affected animals. H. Dryerre measured fourteen plasma constituents in blood samples solicited from practitioners in forty-two cases and reported in 1932 that the only consistent change detected was hypomagnesemia. Dryerre's study is the earliest example of a concept that became known as a *metabolic profile* based on blood chemistry. Payne at Compton, England, coined this term as an approach to the study of production-related diseases. Treatment of the disorder involved administration of magnesium salts intravenously to control the tetanic twitching and muscle spasms.

Acetonemia or ketone body accumulation (ketosis) in the blood accompanied by hypoglycemia was found to be present in another condition of lactating dairy cows as they came into high production after calving. O. Stinson in Great Britain treated this *postparturient dyspepsia* with intravenous infusions of glucose in 1929. J. Sampson and others at Cornell University in 1933 described a similar condition in late-pregnant ewes. Sir Hans Krebs at Oxford University, discoverer of the Krebs cycle, became intrigued by the metabolic disorders that led to acetonemia in ruminants after E.J.H. Ford and J.W. Boyd at Liverpool revealed the sequence of events in bovine ketosis in 1960. Krebs explained the genesis of the disorder as resulting from inadequate supply of glucogenic substrates at times of high demand for energy in ruminants.

Arnold Theiler in South Africa in 1918 provided an ingenious explanation of the factors that led to two syndromes commonly seen in cattle, lamsiekte and stiffsiekte. Low content of phosphorus in forages grown on phosphorus-deficient soils led to metabolic disorders and a craving to eat bones, a type of pica. One consequence was the ingestion by cattle of anaerobic *Clostridium botulinum* bacteria that caused the syndrome of botulism in lamsiekte. Other studies in South Africa showed that a disease of sheep on range that was characterized by jaundice and photosensitization with skin lesions was a result of ingestion of poisonous plants. C. Rimington and J. Quin described the toxic extract in 1937, a finding that led to explanations of other diseases of humans and animals involving toxic cholestasis and photosensitization. H.W. Bennetts in western Australia characterized several diseases associated with mineral imbalances in the diet that were investigated in the laboratory by Underwood. Bennetts also characterized many poisonous plants.

As early as 1889 M. Heip found glucose in the urine of a horse that he suspected of having diabetes. An anonymous French report in 1900 of a dog excreting large volumes of urine free of sugar suggested that the dog might have had diabetes insipidus. M. Dorras in Great Britain in 1907 reported a case of canine diabetes mellitus that featured glycosuria. Eighty years later, basic veterinary research on a similar condition in cats revealed the presence of a specific protein, the mysterious *amyloid* seen on histological study in a number of diseases, in the pancreas of such cats.

P.E. Howe in 1922 used early protein fractionation techniques to study the plasma proteins of cattle and showed that the concentration of fibrinogen was increased in inflammatory conditions. Orcutt and Howe in the same year reported evidence that colostrum ingestion in newborn calves led to the transfer of maternal immunoglobulins to the blood plasma of the calf and might thereby impart resistance to infectious disease. This finding proved to be of enormous importance in the management of newborn animals, particularly calves. Today every effort is made to ensure that the calf receives sufficient colostrum or a replacement antibody cocktail in the first day of life.

The preceding few examples provide a flavor of the exciting discoveries in the field of clinical investigation, from which the application of the clinical laboratory has extended from the university to the teaching hospital and to the level of the practice laboratory. Clinical pathology has become a mainstay of internal medicine.

THE INTEGRATION OF VETERINARY SCIENCE AND CLINICAL MEDICINE: HUTYRA AND MAREK

The veterinary college of Budapest, Hungary, had a golden era during the first third of the twentieth century. The architect of its rise to excellence was Ferenc (Franz) Hutyra (1860-1934), who was born in Szepeshely. While a medical student at the University of Budapest, Hutyra became an award-winning demonstrator in physiology, then a research student in the Institute of Pathological Anatomy and an assistant in that institute upon receiving a doctoral degree in medicine in 1878. He was an associate professor in the veterinary school in 1886 and acquired a veterinary diploma. He received professorships in pathology, internal medicine, and epidemiology. The school was elevated to college status, and Hutyra became its rector. He oversaw the transition of the veterinary profession from an empirical art to a challenging scientific career of enormous opportunity. His primary focus was on infectious diseases—their pathology, microbiology, and immunology. Tuberculosis, brucellosis, glanders, and swine fever were accorded high priorities. His work with Köves led to wide implementation in Hungary of the serum-virus vaccination against swine fever developed by the BAI scientists in the United States.

Hutyra worked most closely with another brilliant veterinary scholar, Jo'zsef (Josef) Marek (1868-1952), who was born in Vagszerdahely. A graduate of the veterinary school, Marek entered practice and participated in controlling the epidemic of swine fever then raging in Hungary. Hutyra noticed his remarkable talent and hired him as his assistant. Marek obtained a doctoral degree from the University of Berne in Switzerland. He then was appointed associate professor under Hutyra and director of the clinic of medicine. Together, Hutyra and Marek wrote a two-volume text, *Special Pathology and Therapeutics of the Diseases of Domestic Animals,* that had an enormous impact in enhancing the progress of the veterinary profession. Hutyra focused on the infectious diseases, Marek on the organic, noninfectious ones. The book, a major advance from the traditional, single-discipline books that preceded it, integrated knowledge from all basic and applied disciplines based on the latest scientific works. It also took into account public health and sanitary regulations. It was exceptionally well illustrated with pertinent examples from clinical cases and laboratory findings. Originally published in Hungarian and German, it was translated into Italian, Spanish, Russian, and English, which indicates its global demand and impact. The early English editions were translated in the United States by John R. Mohler, when he was assistant chief of the BAI, and Adolph Eichorn, who was chief of its pathological division. Later editions incorporated into the authorship Rezso Manninger, another brilliant protégé of Hutyra.

Hutyra was an active founder of the Office Internationale des Epizooties (OIE), which was based in Paris. He was elected president of the Permanent Committee of International Veterinary Congresses. Marek wrote another major work, *Klinische Diagnostik der Inneren Krankheiter der Haustiere,* that went through several editions. In that work he focused on pathogenesis, using a physiological approach to physical diagnosis. He introduced electrical stimulation of muscles and nerves as an aid to diagnosis. Also, he was a pioneer in therapeutics of colic in horses, using gastric lavage in selected cases. He demonstrated the genesis of the form of colic that arises from thromboem-

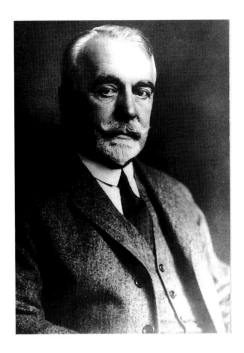

459. Ferenc Hutyra (1860-1934) graduated as a physician in 1878 and later was appointed rector of the veterinary school in Budapest, Hungary. He had been engaged in research in the medical faculty and was a man of broad intellectual perspective. He obtained a veterinary diploma. In 1890 he published *Reforms of Our Veterinary Education,* identifying the then-current weaknesses and charting a new reorganization plan. Reforms were implemented, the school was accorded university status, and a golden age of scientific and clinical productivity resulted under his leadership. His disciples included Marek, Manninger, Köves, and Jármai, and in 1905 Hutyra was appointed "rector for life." Aujesky showed in 1902 that pseudorabies was infectious.

Hog cholera (swine fever in Europe) was introduced to Hungary in 1895, and Josef Marek described its pathology. Hutyra had followed Dorset's work at the Bureau of Animal Industry and was the first in Europe to prove that the primary cause was a filterable virus, with *Salmonella* and *Pasteurella* as secondary invaders. He developed the standardized hyperimmunized serum to protect swine by 1907. The Phylaxia Serum Institute was founded in 1912 to mass-produce veterinary sera and vaccines. He combined inoculation of virus and serum, which led to a mild infection and the end of virus excretion within a month. The famous book by Hutyra and Marek was awarded the book prize of the World Veterinary Congress for the best veterinary publication of the previous twenty-five years. Hutyra was one of the founders of the Office Internationale des Epizooties in 1921 and was elected president of the permanent committee of veterinary congresses. *(Royal Veterinary College, Budapest.)*

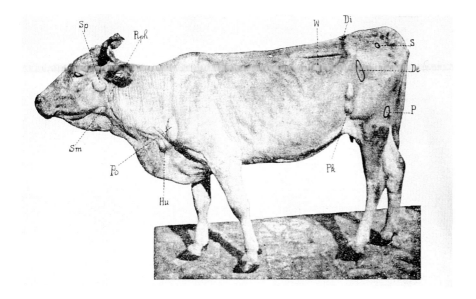

460. Generalized enlargement of the lymph glands in a cow with pseudoleukemia (today, bovine leukosis). The letters refer to the anatomical names of the individual superficial lymph nodes that can be identified. From the first volume of *Special Pathology and Therapeutics of the Diseases of Domestic Animals,* fourth German edition, by Franz Hutyra and Josef Marek of the Royal Veterinary College at Budapest. The work was translated by John R. Mohler, who became director of the Bureau of Animal Industry (1917-1943), and others as the second American edition in 1920. Marek graduated from the Budapest school, received a doctorate from the University of Berne, Switzerland, and is renowned for his pioneering work describing the lesions of the syndrome known as fowl paralysis or neurolymphomatosis. The condition was found to be infectious and became known as Marek's disease of poultry. Modern research led to development by Biggs and others of a vaccine against the herpes-type virus discovered in 1962. Marek made major contributions to bring science to bear on clinical veterinary medicine, including gavage to prevent gastric rupture in horses, demonstration of verminous mesenteric arteritis as a cause of colic, and surgery for strangulated colon. *(From Hutyra et al, 1920.)*

bolic mesenteric arteritis caused by strongyle larval invasion and leads to necrosis of parts of the bowel wall. He operated successfully on horses with strangulated colon. He elaborated the pathogenesis of dourine. After careful research Marek developed treatments and preventatives for liver fluke of sheep and for rickets in all species. He introduced radiological examination as an important aid to diagnosis and was avant garde in developing clinical specialty fields such as dermatology, neurology, clinical pathology, and clinical pharmacology. Marek's disease, an important disease of poultry, is named after him. This disease, caused by a virus, leads to a form of neoplasia.

RECOGNITION OF THE NEED FOR RESEARCH: THE CENTRAL VETERINARY LABORATORY AT WEYBRIDGE

Great Britain established a state veterinary service in 1865 as the veterinary department of the Privy Council during the rinderpest crisis. After 1850 it became progressively more obvious in countries with well-developed livestock industries that scientific investigations would be needed to reduce the risk of contagious animal diseases. Advances in pathology and pathogenic microbiology led to the recognition that disease control would be greatly enhanced by more accurate diagnosis. Great Britain established a diagnostic laboratory in a single basement room in 1893 to address concerns arising from an epizootic of swine fever (hog cholera). The laboratory was able to address other scheduled reportable diseases of animals.

After Stewart Stockman (1869-1926) was appointed Chief Veterinary Officer (CVO) in 1905, he emphasized the need for postgraduate training and research into pathology and epidemiology in controlling infective diseases. He was awarded funds in 1913 to erect the Central Veterinary Laboratory where it stands today, at Addlestone, New Haw, near Weybridge, now in the Southwest London metropolitan region. Stockman, a visionary, was a graduate of the Dick veterinary college in Edinburgh in 1890. He then studied under Nocard at Alfort in France before returning to the Dick to teach pathology, attaining the rank of professor. He resigned to join the Boer War in 1900, then worked on rinderpest control in India before returning to South Africa as Principal Veterinary Office for the Transvaal. He collaborated with Arnold Theiler, who was Veterinary Research Officer for the Transvaal, in eliminating rinderpest, glanders, and epizootic lymphangitis. This experience was to stand him in good stead after his appointment as CVO for Great Britain in 1905. In addition, he took on the role of director of research. Stockman's mentor at Edinburgh had been John McFadyean, whose daughter he mar-

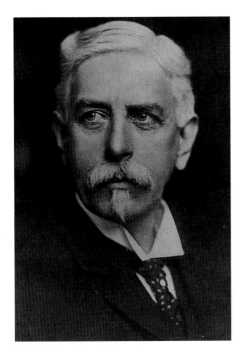

461. Daniel Elmer Salmon (1850-1914), the founder of the United States Federal Veterinary Services, became chief after Congress established the Bureau of Animal Industry in 1884. He had been a member in 1868 of the first group of students taught by James Law at Cornell University, receiving his bachelor's degree in veterinary science in 1872 after being allowed to attend the Alfort school in Paris for six months to acquire clinical experience then unavailable in Ithaca, New York. He also used that opportunity to become familiar with Pasteur's new methods of microbiology. Cornell awarded him the first degree of doctor of veterinary medicine in the United States in 1876.

Salmon set high goals for the new agency, including the suppression and extirpation of contagious diseases of domestic animals, the protection of the nation's livestock industries, the production of high-quality foods of animal origin, to guard the public against zoonoses and contamination, and to promote research. Salmon introduced population medicine and orchestrated the eradication of contagious bovine pleuropneumonia by 1892. He launched attempts to eradicate trichinosis and hog cholera from swine and Texas fever from cattle. He came under attack from the powerful meat-packing industry and resigned in 1905, before the Meat Inspection Act was passed in 1906. He went to Uruguay to establish scientific veterinary medicine there. William Welch was a great admirer of Salmon's Bureau of Animal Industry and drew on his ideas in planning the Rockefeller Institute for Medical Research in Princeton, New Jersey. *(Archives of the National Animal Disease Center, Ames, Iowa.)*

ried in 1908. Together McFadyean and Stockman created a strong scientific program in veterinary research, virtually from scratch. They transformed the profession.

One building at the Central Veterinary Laboratory was set aside for production of swine fever antiserum. Early research projects addressed aspects of tuberculosis, brucellosis, and redwater disease of cattle, as well as the foot-and-mouth disease that affected several species and two diseases of sheep, scrapie and louping-ill. Rabies, which had been eradicated by 1902, returned in 1918, and a new campaign eliminated it in four years. The special problem of containment of foot-and-mouth disease had the result that all further work on the disease was conducted at a new laboratory at Pirbright in 1925. Stockman died the following year.

The Agricultural Act of 1937 allowed expansion and the establishment of research departments in bacteriology, biochemistry, parasitology, pathology, and diseases of poultry, as well as a satellite laboratory for Scotland at Lasswade. The Second World War forced a switch of priorities to preparation of agents to protect against anthrax in the event of biological warfare. The Strain 19 *Brucella abortus* vaccine for cattle was introduced from the United States in 1942 to prepare for a campaign to reduce the incidence of undulant fever in humans and to work toward its eradication, along with that of tuberculosis, from cattle.

As new diseases were characterized, virology and genital diseases became areas for research, and biochemistry tackled metabolic and toxic diseases. A major effort to explain *Turkey X disease* in the early 1960s led to the finding that imported groundnut (peanut) meal contaminated with specific mycotoxins was responsible. Safety and efficacy standards for biological and chemotherapeutic products were developed. The viral plagues that affect poultry, such as Newcastle disease and avian influenza, were mastered. The epidemiology department tackled enzootic bovine leukosis, maedi-visna, and bovine spongiform encephalopathy, a disease that was traced to the recycling of rendered sheep tissues containing the scrapie agent as a protein source for dairy cattle. Swine fever and pseudorabies were eradicated.

PLAGUE CONTROL: THE BUREAU OF ANIMAL INDUSTRY'S PRIORITY TO SAFEGUARD LIVESTOCK

The Bureau of Animal Industry came into being after a vote in Congress on May 29, 1884. The legislation did not have an easy passage because of the issue of states' rights versus federal jurisdiction. The infant veterinary profession was still struggling for acceptance in the United States, and detractors ridiculed the idea of having a horse doctor at the head of a federal bureau. However, the forward-looking chairman of the Committee on Agriculture in the House of Representatives, the Honorable William H. Hatch of Missouri, gave strong support and arguments for the bill.

Hatch pointed out to those who would belittle the horse doctors that Henri Bouley, a veterinarian who had been a professor at the Alfort school, was then the leading scientific figure in France. He noted that Bouley had been the first, the most able, and the most persistent advocate and exponent of Pasteur's investigations and discoveries and thereby had produced a revolutionary change in medical views about contagious diseases. Hatch also noted that a brilliant veterinary scholar, Professor Chauveau at the Lyon veterinary school, had demonstrated that contagious diseases were caused by living germs several years before either Pasteur or Koch did so. Hatch reported that Chauveau's protégé, Saturnin Arloing, and his colleagues had succeeded in isolating the causative agent of black-leg disease, then a major concern of American cattle producers. Hatch went on to cite achievements by many other European veterinarians; he had certainly studied the historical record.

He also defended the fledgling American veterinary profession, noting the contributions of men such as Law, Liautard, and Salmon. Hatch cited specifically Daniel Salmon's report, as veterinarian of the Department of Agriculture, on bovine pleuropneumonia. The House voted to uphold Hatch's views by 155 to 127. The bill was then passed by the Senate and signed by the President.

The remarkable success of the BAI's investigations of Texas fever and its hard-won battle with hog cholera were described earlier. The European struggles with rinderpest, too, have been identified. One of the most daunting of the plagues has been foot-and-mouth disease, caused by the smallest yet perhaps the most contagious of viruses. The disease has visited the United States nine times in the last one hundred and twenty-five years, and Canada once. The three outbreaks in the nineteenth century were all traced to importation of infected stock in 1870, 1880, and 1884 and were arrested within a few months. The 1902 invasion, however, affected two hundred and forty-four herds and took a year to erase by the slaughter policy. The invasion was believed to have arisen from a shipment of cowpox virus imported from Japan to be prepared for smallpox vaccine. A similar scenario played out in an episode in 1908. Its origin was traced to the same batch of contaminated cowpox virus.

The outbreak of foot-and-mouth disease in 1914 and 1915 was by far the biggest and most devastating outbreak. It hit more than 3500 herds in 22 states and the District of Columbia. Its origin remains unknown, but a suspected source was tanning material imported to Niles, Michigan. The final toll was about 77,000 cattle, 85,000 swine, 10,000 sheep, 100 goats, and 9 deer. A 1924 eruption in California was on a similar scale, affecting more than 900 herds and involving more than 100,000 domestic animals and 22,000 deer. Its entry was attributed to raw garbage from ships. A smaller outbreak in Texas in the same year was associated with sailors from foreign ships in Galveston. California was hit with foot-and-mouth disease again in 1929. Quarantine was enforced and kept it contained within the state. Garbage from ships returned from reservoir countries was the source. A law was passed by Congress in 1930 that included strict regulation to strengthen the measures used to exclude the disease. There has been no subsequent outbreak.

462. Early scene at a Bureau of Animal Industry laboratory. Although modest by today's standards, creation of such a laboratory was a revolutionary development before the turn of the century. The science of pathogenic microbiology had been created in France and Germany and promoted by the genius of Pasteur and Koch and their colleagues. Daniel Salmon brought insights on the French methods of the bureau and launched Theobald Smith on their application to animal diseases. Smith moved ahead by adding Koch's sophisticated methodologies and became one of the leading bacteriologists and protozoologists in the world. *(National Agricultural Library, Boltsville, Maryland.)*

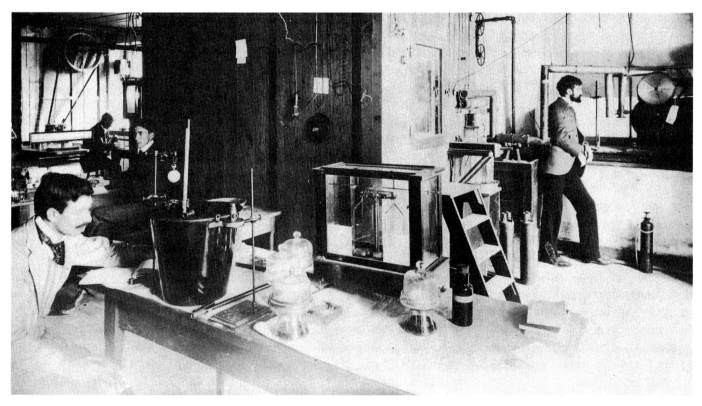

The United States adopted an aggressive policy to protect its southern border with Mexico from virus invasion during an outbreak in Mexico in 1926. Mexico kept American surveillance for foot-and-mouth disease in a state of high alert for nearly three decades after 1925. Teams of Mexican and American veterinarians investigated the first of the series of outbreaks in 1926. Perhaps entering the state of Tabasco in cattle brought there on a banana boat, the disease soon spread to adjoining states. The most disastrous outbreak occurred in 1946 in the state of Veracruz after zebu cattle had been imported from Brazil. Misdiagnosed at first as *yerba* or vesicular stomatitis, the disease was diagnosed as type A foot-and-mouth disease at Pirbright in December. Because of the failure to implement controls, however, it had already spread rapidly. A Mexico–United States Commission to Eradicate Foot-and-Mouth Disease was established, but a vast territory of 260,000 square miles across the full width of Mexico became infected. A huge campaign had to be mounted to eradicate it.

The slaughter policy for infected and exposed animals was devastating for the small farmers, despite the payment of indemnities. Their livelihood was gone after they lost cows for milk, oxen for plowing, pigs for meat, and goats for milk and meat. Nearly 900,000 head of stock were slaughtered. To reduce the impact, a vaccination scheme for quarantined areas was added in June 1948 because the affected area contained seventeen million head of susceptible livestock. Acquiring sufficient type A virus vaccine from international stocks was a challenging assignment. Adding to the difficulty, revaccination every four months was recommended. Sixty million doses of vaccine were administered by August 1950. Nevertheless, another outbreak of a different virus, type O, occurred in 1949 in one herd, but it was eradicated promptly. Yet another such event occurred in 1951, exacting more losses. By September 1952, however, Mexico was finally declared free of the disease, after more

463. Slaughtering and burying cattle to eradicate foot-and-mouth disease in the United States. *(USDA Plum Island Animal Disease Center.)*

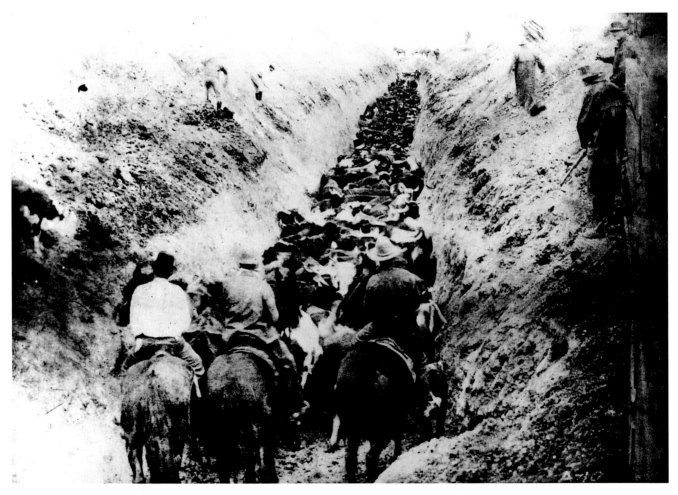

than one million head of stock had been slaughtered and nearly a hundred times this number vaccinated. Massive amounts of time, money, and vaccine had been invested, and many farmers were left destitute. Although implementation of the slaughter policy was a painful experience for some of the American veterinarians who participated, the goal of keeping at bay this devastating disease was accomplished. Foot-and-mouth disease broke out in Western Canada, in 1952, but effective measures soon brought it under control.

The total program of the BAI from its inception in 1884 through its closure in 1954 is an impressive story of achievement. The box below provides a

DISEASE CONTROL BY THE BUREAU OF ANIMAL INDUSTRY (1884 TO 1954)

1885	First *Salmonella* bacteria are isolated by the Bureau of Animal Industry (BAI).
1886	Bacterins, or killed bacterial cultures, are shown to act as vaccines.
1888	BAI shows that Texas fever is spread by ticks transmitting a protozoan. First proof of arthropod-borne infection.
1889	The concept of protozoa-tick vectors is confirmed and refined.
1891	First tuberculin test of cattle in the United States is administered in Pennsylvania.
1892	BAI announces eradication of contagious bovine pleuropneumonia.
1895	Difference between bacteria causing human and bovine tuberculosis is demonstrated.
1902	C.W. Stiles defines hookworm disease in the South.
1903	Dorset and de Schweinitz discover hog cholera virus.
1905	*Brucella melitensis* (Malta fever) is found in imported goats.
1907	Hyperimmune serum is developed to prevent hog cholera.
1909	BAI begins traceback of tuberculous cattle and swine to farms.
1914	BAI discovers that *Trichina* organisms of pork are killed by controlled refrigeration.
1914	*Brucella suis* of swine is discovered.
1918	*Brucella* organisms of cattle, goats, and swine are defined.
1925	Sewall Wright completes twenty-year study of guinea pig genetics that lays the foundation for population genetics.
1929	BAI eradicates foot-and-mouth disease.
1929	Fowl plague is eradicated, and field test for pullorum is developed.
1930	Strain 19 vaccine is developed to protect cattle from brucellosis.
1930s	Anthelmintic properties of phenothiazine and hydrocarbons are described.
1931	Stained-antigen blood test for pullorum in poultry is developed.
1934	Equine glanders is eradicated.
1935	Crystal-violet killed vaccine is used against hog cholera.
1939	BAI supplies standardized *Brucella* antigen to state diagnostic laboratories.
1942	Dourine is eradicated.
1943	Cattle tick fever is eradicated.
1947	BAI awards first license for vaccines for the fur industry.
1949	Variant strain of hog cholera virus is discovered.
1951	New tests differentiate foot-and-mouth disease, vesicular stomatitis, and vesicular exanthema.
1952	Cause of bovine hyperkeratosis is discovered.
1953	Vibriosis is identified as a cause of bovine infertility.
1954	Research on foreign animal diseases begins on Plum Island.

464. *Facing page, above,* Inspecting a herd of sheep for foot-and-mouth disease. Herders drove the sheep slowly between automobile and fence while the inspector watched for lameness, drooling, and other visible signs of the disease. *(USDA Plum Island Animal Disease Center.)*

465. *Facing page, below,* A young cow is released from a holding chute. This scene illustrates the equipment that was developed to meet the needs of large-animal veterinarians, particularly bovine practitioners. They must handle, make pregnancy or health examinations on, and treat or inoculate large numbers of powerful beasts in a hard day's work. Before the development of devices for restraint such as chutes and tilting operating tables, the physical strength of several men was required to make such routine examinations and surgeries possible. *(United States Department of Agriculture.)*

skeletal list of the tactics and the accomplishments in one aspect, control of contagious diseases. By bringing the great plagues under control, the BAI allowed the livestock industries to advance to their full potential without fear of catastrophe. Recently, for example, African swine fever, which is spread by *Ornithodorus* ticks, spread westward from the Iberian Peninsula to Cuba, the Dominican Republic, and Haiti, where it had to be eradicated by another traumatic slaughter policy.

Since the disbanding of the BAI and the continuance of its functions under the aegis of the Agricultural Research Service, repeated changes in administration of veterinary matters at the federal level have created many problems for those responsible for setting and responding to changing priorities for animal disease control. The established tradition of surmounting infectious disease, however, has been maintained (see the box below).

CONTINUING PROGRESS IN CONTROL OF CONTAGIOUS DISEASES (1954 TO 1984)

1955	New fowl cholera organism is isolated and identified.
1957	Vaccines are developed to prevent fowl cholera.
1958	Virus that causes bovine rhinotracheitis is discovered.
1959	A virus involved in the bovine shipping fever complex is isolated.
1959	Screwworm flies are eradicated from the American Southeast.
1959	Vesicular exanthema is eradicated.
1960	Twenty-year program proves the role of *Mycoplasma gallisepticum* in chronic respiratory disease in chickens and infectious sinusitis in turkeys.
1961	Domestic animal health research and diagnostics are consolidated at the National Animal Disease Laboratory (now the National Animal Disease Control Center) in Ames, Iowa.
1965	Rapid test for hog cholera is developed.
1966	In vitro culture is developed for protozoan and helminth parasites.
1968	Complement fixation test for anaplasmosis is developed.
1970	Pooled-sample technique is used to identify *Trichina* organisms in hog carcasses.
1971	Venezuelan equine encephalitis is eradicated.
1971	A vaccine for Marek's disease in chickens is developed and licensed.
1972	Parasites are identified in tissue cross-sections.
1972	Work begins on *Sarcocystis fusiformis* parasite of livestock.
1973	Sheep scabies is eradicated.
1974	Exotic Newcastle disease of poultry is eradicated.
1978	First killed virus vaccine against pseudorabies in swine is licensed.
1978	Hog cholera is finally eradicated.
1981	A parvovirus is identified as a cause of swine infertility.
1982	A subunit vaccine against foot-and-mouth disease is developed by gene splicing.
1982	Joint foot-and-mouth disease vaccine bands are established for the United States, Canada, and Mexico by tripartite agreement.
1982	Eradication of African swine fever from Caribbean Islands is begun.
1983	Recombinant vaccine against coccidial infections of poultry is developed.
1984	High-mortality strain of avian influenza is eradicated in poultry in Pennsylvania and Virginia.

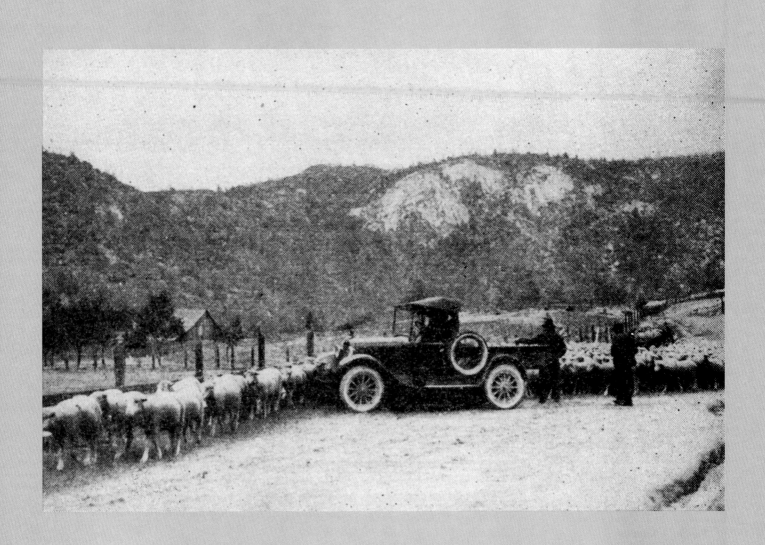

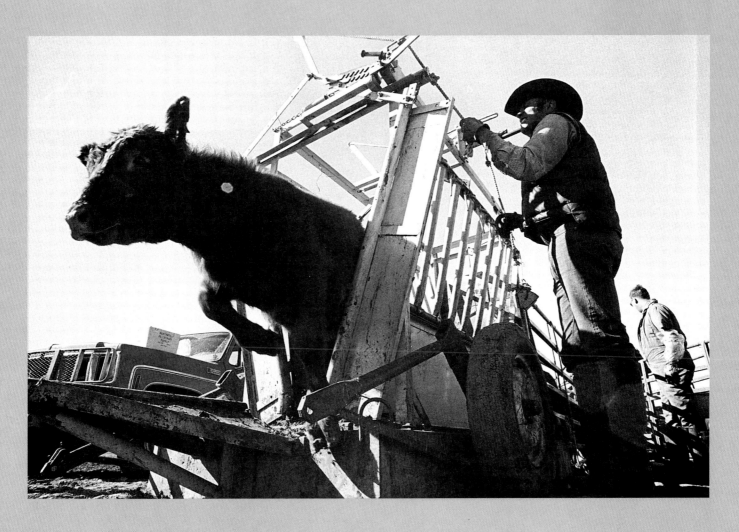

466. A research veterinarian vaccinating a steer with a strain of foot-and-mouth disease vaccine. The potential for devastation of the entire livestock industry that resides in the several strains of foot-and-mouth viruses led to the enforcement of a successful eradication policy in the United States and Canada and to cooperation with Mexico to protect the southern border from reinvasion. However, the disease is prevalent in many parts of the world where it is endemic, and losses are controlled by vaccination with appropriate strains of killed virus. At the Plum Island isolation facility, the U.S. Department of Agriculture continues in the search for more effective and safer vaccines. Today genetic engineering is being used to expedite this approach. *(United States Department of Agriculture.)*

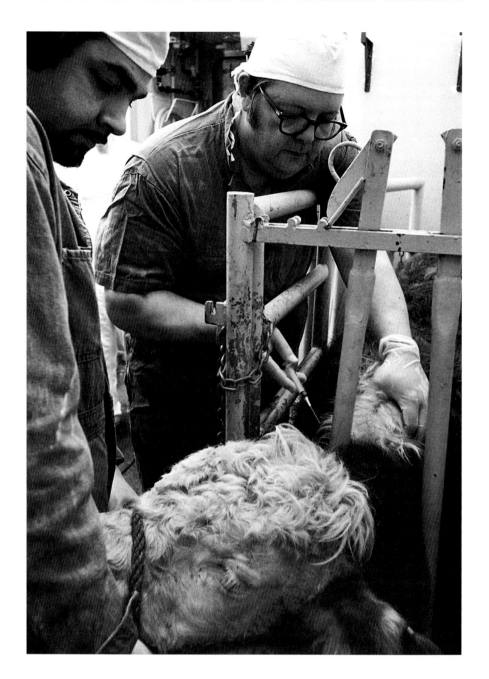

VETERINARY ACHIEVEMENTS IN OBSTETRICS AND DISORDERS OF REPRODUCTION

The earliest role of the veterinarian in disorders of animal reproduction was in obstetrics of domestic animals. Several early texts in this field were written by European authors, often as part of broader coverage of surgery and clinical veterinary medicine. W.L. Williams of Cornell University was the leading American figure in the field of reproductive disorders of animals. He authored a highly regarded text, *The Diseases of the Genital Organs of the Domestic Animals,* that was in use for a long period, with several editions. Dystocia of the mare and cow and ways to effect delivery of the fetus (or fetuses) that was malpresented or deformed were major focuses. Franz Benesch of Vienna developed his universal fetotome, which was imported to North America and widely used by veterinary practitioners during the first half of the twentieth century. This device allowed the veterinarian to dismember the fetus for delivery in pieces when delivery of the intact, living fetus had proved impossible. Benesch also introduced the technique of epidural anesthesia in 1926 to relieve pain at parturition and prevent straining when that interfered with manual assistance to delivery. He wrote *Veterinary Obstetrics* in English in 1938, which was revised by J.G. Wright of Liverpool University in 1951 and then by G.H. Arthur in Bristol in 1964. Many instruments were developed to assist delivery, particularly of the lodged fetus: various fetotomes, including an ingenious one by Thygesen in Denmark, as well as finger knives, Colin's scalpel, and cutting hooks. Internal dissections have been displaced to a large extent in the modern era by the development of cesarean section in 1940 by E.R. Frank of Kansas State University and Stephen J. Roberts of Cornell University. Veterinary students have been taught manual obstetrics of cattle by means of rubber phantoms, which are used to represent the uterus in which a dead fetus or calf could be arranged in various abnormal presentations that the student rectifies for delivery.

ARTIFICIAL INSEMINATION: AMPLIFICATION OF GENETIC POTENTIAL

Arabs may have used artificial insemination (AI) in the horse as early as the fourteenth century. After successful AI experiments in amphibia, Spallanzani in 1780 in Italy used freshly collected canine semen to inseminate a bitch in heat directly into the uterus: three puppies were born sixty-two days later. He also showed by filtration that fertilization was attributable only to the spermatozoa in the semen. In addition, in 1803 he found that stallion semen could be frozen and later thawed and that the sperm regained their motility. John Hunter succeeded in fertilizing a woman by means of AI in 1799. An English dog breeder, Everett Millais, used Spallanzani's method between 1884 and 1896 to inseminate nineteen bitches, and fifteen of them produced puppies. Heape noted that AI simplified crossbreeding in animals of different sizes and recommended that it be used to study genetic and telegenic factors. Professor Pearson of the University of Pennsylvania's veterinary school wrote to Heape, advising him of his team's success with AI in the mare. Repiquet, a French veterinarian, in 1890 applied AI in horses to enhance fertility, which was at low levels in some studs. Hoffman at Stuttgart recommended that semen be collected from a mare's vagina by syringe after mating and injected into the uterus as a form of supplementary AI, often with a milk diluent added. Danish veterinarians in 1902 used AI to breed several mares from a single ejaculate, thereby extending the genetic influence of famous stallions.

After E.I. Ivanov in Russia in 1899 was asked by the chief of the Royal Russian stud to explore the potential of AI, he practiced AI on horse-breeding farms and showed the importance of rigorous technique. He extended the practice to cattle and sheep, and successful work was conducted at a station at Askaniya-Nova. He was also successful with AI in birds. A research facility was established to study the physiology of reproduction in domestic animals and to train veterinarians and technicians in the use of AI. Steady progress resulted, and by 1938 more than a million cows, fifteen million sheep, and forty thousand mares in the Union of Soviet Socialist Republics were inseminated by AI in a single year.

In 1914 Milovanov and others collected semen from rams, bulls, and stallions by means of an artificial vagina based on a design used for dogs that was developed by G. Amantea, a professor of physiology at the University of Rome. A Cambridge model was developed in England by Arthur Walton between 1934 and 1935. He shipped a Suffolk ram's semen to Prawochenski at Pulawy Institute in Poland in 1936, using a vacuum flask and cracked ice to hold the temperature below 10° C. Although fifty-one hours elapsed from the time of collection to the time of AI of the ewes, two of the five ewes conceived and one gave birth to a ram lamb of distinctive Suffolk appearance. Eduard Sorensen of the Royal Agricultural and Veterinary College in

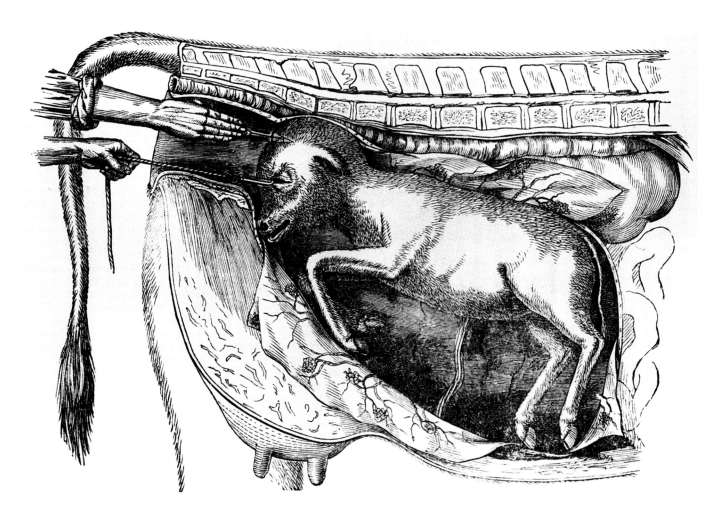

467. James Beart Simonds was the first professor of cattle pathology at the veterinary college in London, appointed in 1842 on the urging of the Royal Agricultural Society, which provided financial assistance. While he was principal (1872-1881), the RVC received its royal charter (1875). He had studied rinderpest in Europe before it arrived in England in 1865 and was placed in charge of control when it did arrive, becoming the first chief officer in the Veterinary Department (precursor of the State Veterinary Service) of the Privy Council. He was also involved in the campaign to free the islands of sheep pox and bovine pleuropneumonia. The RVC has a large file of documents relating to his many services to the profession. He was belittled acrimoniously and unfairly by Sir Frederick Smith in his *Early History of Veterinary Literature*, fourth volume, which was published posthumously. Simonds had experience in agricultural practice before joining the college and had an exemplary career. This illustration, method of delivery of a stillborn calf with water on the brain, as well as the one on the facing page, is from one of his works on bovine obstetrics. *(National Library of Medicine, Bethesda, Maryland.)*

Denmark followed the Russian developments with great interest and developed an artificial breeding cooperative association with Jens Gyllingholm in 1936. It was so successful that by 1960 almost all cows were bred by AI in Denmark. After World War II AI was widely used to restore depleted herds in Europe.

In the United States, after early work at the Pennsylvania Veterinary School, L.L. Lewis at the Oklahoma Agricultural Experimental Station published a bulletin on AI in horses in 1906. He used a device called an impregnator. A similar technique was used in cows: semen was collected from the vagina after mating, and it was put into a capsule that was inserted into the uterus of another cow in estrus. Using a similar technique, Hughey in 1910 bred many mares to a single stallion.

Thomas C. Webster used AI in cattle at Fort Steilacoom, Washington, and at Winnebago State Hospital in Wisconsin in 1930. Howard Clapp of Pabst Farms in Oconomowoc, Wisconsin, used AI between 1934 and 1938. In 1937 it was used in the dairy herd at the University of Missouri, Columbia, and the practice was rapidly adopted for use in the station herds at land grant colleges. C.L. Cole at the North Central Experiment Station at Grand Rapids, Minnesota, was the first to show that large numbers of cows could be bred successfully by AI in 1937 and 1938. G.W. Salisbury at Cornell University developed AI as a practical technique between 1938 and 1944. Successful AI units were soon developed in New York State. Salisbury and N.L. Van Denmark wrote the first important text, *Physiology of Reproduction and AI in Cattle,* in 1961.

The first cattle-breeding organization to use AI in the United States, the Cooperative Artificial Breeding Association No. 1, was set up by Enos Perry of Rutgers University, New Brunswick, New Jersey, who had visited Sorensen's operation in Denmark. The first technical adviser was James A. Henderson of Canada; he was assisted by A.F. Larsen of Denmark for the first

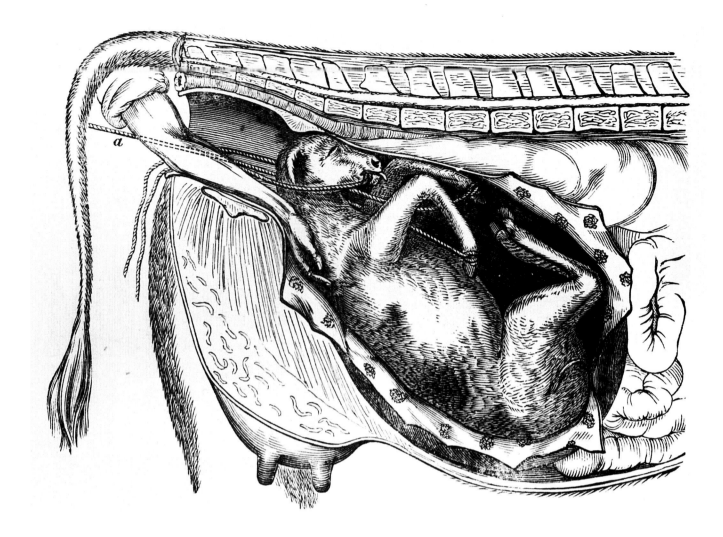

two months. Henderson became the professor of clinical veterinary medicine at the Ontario Veterinary College at Guelph and, later, dean of the College of Veterinary Medicine at Washington State University at Pullman. In December 1954, the Waterloo Cattle Breeding Association of Ontario became the first in the world to operate a program based entirely on the use of frozen semen and developed much of the equipment that was required. The American Breeders Service began as the American Dairy Guerney Associates of Northern Illinois, founded by J. Rockefeller Prentice in 1941, adding Holstein bulls in 1945 and Jerseys in 1948, followed by many beef breeds. It moved via Madison, Wisconsin, in 1946 to its present magnificent site at De Forest, Wisconsin, in 1965. The first live calf sired by AI with frozen semen was born in 1953. Through the progeny test program since 1952 and genetic trait analysis since 1975, ABS has had phenomenal impact improving the quality and performance of dairy and beef cattle. It continues to be a spearhead for the application of advances in reproductive and genetic technology.

The first successful embryo transfer in a mammal was achieved by W. Heape in a rabbit in 1890. The first viable transfer in a bovine was reported by E.L. Willett and others in 1951. The technique attained practical application with the prevention of infection and the work of a group at Cambridge University led by L.E.A. Rowson in the late 1960s and early 1970s. R.P. Elsden of Australia developed a nonsurgical approach via the cervix at Colorado State University. The technique is now well established commercially and allows multiplication of a desired bovine genome by superovulation of a high-quality dam, fertilization of her ova by semen from a high-quality bull, and transfer of the embryos to synchronized surrogate cows of lesser quality to carry the embryos to term. Elsden and G.E. Seidel developed a technique of freezing bovine embryos for prolonged storage with an attainable survival rate of more than fifty percent.

THE VETERINARY EQUIVALENT OF GYNECOLOGY

The pathogenesis of reproductive disorders and the optimization of reproductive performance in herds are major concerns of veterinary medicine. A century of studies of the estrous cycle of female mammals has provided a picture of the endocrine regulation of reproductive performance. F. Lataste at Bordeaux, France, reported early studies of reproductive cycles in rodents in 1887. W. Heape showed in 1900 that ovulation in the rabbit is induced by coitus. In 1903, F.H.A. Marshall at Cambridge University differentiated the functions of the Graafian follicle and the corpus luteum and described the estrous cycle of the ewe. He established the effect of changing light gradients in mammals that reproduce seasonally. In 1910 he wrote *The Physiology of Reproduction*. F.F. McKenzie at Missouri characterized the estrous cycle of the sow in 1926. John Hammond, also at Cambridge, wrote *The Physiology of Reproduction in the Cow* in 1927. Sydney A. Asdell, who had been Marshall's first doctoral student at Cambridge, also worked with F.G. Hopkins. Asdell did postdoctoral work with Marshall and Hammond before going to Massey University in New Zealand; he then returned to join the Cornell University Department of Animal Husbandry in 1930. He unraveled the roles of the ovarian hormones and pituitary gonadotropins in reproduction and the role of prolactin in lactation, starting with rabbits and goats, then studying the cow. Since these early studies, particularly since 1945, there has been a remarkable expansion in studies of reproduction and infertility. Highlights include the development of the radioimmunoassay of protein hormones by Solomon Berson and Rosalyn Yalow at the Downstate Medical Center of the State University of New York, which led to many advances in endocrinology. A.V. Nalbandov at the University of Illinois established the concept of releasing hormones that control the hormones of the anterior pituitary. Roger Short studied reproduction and lactation in a wide range of species with a special focus on the regulation of seasonal behavior. Hugh Tyndale-Biscoe of CSIRO, Canberra, carried out pioneering investigations of reproductive physiology and seasonal mating behavior in marsupial mammals of Australia. Colleges of veterinary medicine, agriculture, medicine, and biological sciences in many countries have collaborated in discovering the complex endocrinology involved in the reproduction of all types of livestock.

The College of Veterinary Medicine at Colorado State University has long been a leader in animal reproductive biology and disease. Heavy losses encountered in the severe blizzards of the winter of 1949 and 1950 were accompanied by frostbite of the scrotum in most range bulls. As a result, Harold J. Hill and Lloyd C. Faulkner and the clinical faculty developed techniques of estimating breeding soundness of bulls, including those of a politically influential client of an innovative black veterinarian, G.W. Cooper of Roggin, Colorado, who later joined the faculty at Tuskegee University's veterinary college in Alabama. Funding for equipment followed, and a mobile laboratory was obtained; this allowed for the initiation of the Colorado bull testing program. Hill was the prime mover in establishing the Rocky Mountain Society for the Study of Breeding Soundness in Bulls in 1954, which evolved into the Society for Theriogenology in the 1970s; the sacred bull "Nandi" was its logo. Literally translated, *theriogenology* means the scientific study of reproduction; this ambitious title was probably a bit broader in scope than the combined range of practice of the society's members.

The Colorado group developed the W.G.R. Marden electroejaculator in collaboration with a Denver electronics company. This device greatly enhanced the process and speed of performing soundness examinations on bulls. The Colorado group became a powerhouse of research on reproduction in horses as well as cattle; a strong laboratory support arm focused on basic physiology and pathobiology.

A disciple of Nils Lagerlöf in Sweden was Raimunds Zemjanis, a Latvian who worked in Russia before migrating to Sweden and then to the United States, where he became a master of herd reproductive examinations at the University of Minnesota. He attracted outstanding graduate students and wrote a superbly practical clinical text, *Diagnostic and Therapeutic Techniques in Animal Reproduction.* Graduates of his clinical training could make a living by performing pregnancy and gynecological examinations in cattle. The story of the evolving competence of the bovine practitioner in reproductive work was told well and regularly by Elmer Woelffer of Oconomowoc, Wisconsin, who edited the veterinary page of *Hoard's Dairyman,* a popular monthly magazine for dairy farmers. Kenneth McEntee at Cornell University's Veterinary College held a unique chair of reproductive pathology and gave research in theriogenology a major boost.

A HARD ROAD TO THE USE OF CHEMOTHERAPY AGAINST MICROBES

A major problem faced by the veterinary and medical professions was the lack of effective weapons against infection. The idea of chemical warfare against infectious diseases belongs more to Paul Ehrlich than to anyone else. Ehrlich (1854-1915) had been present at the meeting of the physiological society in Berlin in 1882 when Robert Koch presented his earthshaking findings on the bacteria that cause tuberculosis. Koch described how he overcame the difficulties in staining the causative agent, which had a waxy protective coat. Ehrlich had developed expertise in vital staining of organisms and tissues with the new dyes that had been developed in Germany. He improved Koch's stain for the organisms that cause tuberculosis.

Ehrlich elaborated on Chauveau's idea that microbial poisons are produced by the host, proposing that the animal body produced "magic bullets" or antibodies that are tailored to bind to the proteins of the invading parasite and destroy it. He shared a Nobel Prize with Elie Metchnikoff in 1908 for their contributions to the understanding of immunity. Erhlich, a great medical scholar, himself a survivor of tuberculosis, became obsessed with the idea that synthetic chemistry could provide the answer to infectious diseases and systematically searched for selectively toxic agents that would kill invading bacteria without harm to the host. Ehrlich and Kiyoshi Shiga of Japan, discoverer of the *Shigella* organism that causes dysentery, found that trypan red cured one mouse (but not a human) of sleeping sickness caused by trypanosomiasis. Ehrlich focused on the great scourge shown by Schaudinn and Hoffmann in 1905 to be caused by the spiral organism *Treponema pallidum.* After considering the historical development of high-risk mercury in syphilis therapy, Ehrlich, in pursuit of his goal, conceived that organometallic compounds containing arsenic might be more tame for the host, yet more permeable to the bacterium. After a marathon series of modified compounds were tested, Ehrlich and Hata reported in 1910 that *No. 606 salvarsan* had proved effective against the venereal agent. The drug was not without risk, however, and in 1914 he developed a modified version, *neosalvarsan,* that was more soluble and safer to administer. A related product, *arsphenamine,* was developed and used in the United States in 1917, but none of these agents had the desired selectivity, although cures were achieved.

The German dye industry was destined to make the next significant advance in this frustrating battle with the microbes. Gerhard Domagk (1895-1964) of the Bayer Company, himself a survivor of the trench warfare of Flanders in the First World War, was a medical student when he enlisted in military service and witnessed many horrifying *gas gangrene* infections in soldiers who suffered open wounds. He made a personal vow to help overcome such problems if he survived to complete his medical education.

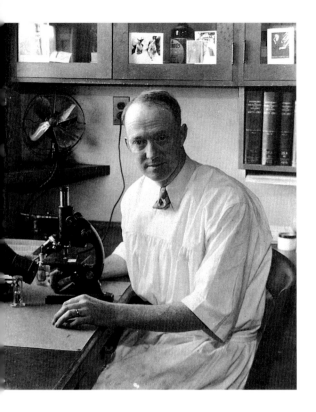

469. William H. Feldman (1893-1974) received his doctoral degree in veterinary medicine from Colorado State University at Fort Collins in 1917. He joined the faculty there and taught materia medica, pathology, and microbiology while engaging in research on tuberculosis and oncology. He selected Mark Morris, then an outstanding second-year student, to assist him part-time. The high quality of Feldman's work led to his recruitment by the Mayo Foundation in Rochester, Minnesota, in 1927 to work on tuberculosis in the Division of Experimental Medicine. He developed an experimental-model tuberculosis infection in guinea pigs. With H. Corwin Hinshaw, a specialist in pulmonary medicine, he embarked on a massive program of screening all sulfonamide drugs for efficacy, without real success. Alfred G. Karlson was another distinguished veterinarian who joined Feldman's team.

Studying the new sulfones, they achieved some efficacy for the first time in human patients, but hemolysis was a problem. In 1944 they were the first to test Selman Waksman's newly discovered streptomycin and found it effective, even against highly pathogenic strains. Feldman contracted tuberculosis himself in 1948. Jorgen Lehmann in Sweden showed that para-aminosalicylic acid had antitubercular activity, and the Rochester group found that the combination of streptomycin and para-aminosalicylic acid was more effective but that resistance could still be a problem. *(By permission of Mayo Foundation.)*

Domagk worked with Hoppe-Seyler, a famous professor of applied chemistry at Kiel University at the City Hospital, where he became acutely aware of the powerlessness of the medical profession against pulmonary tuberculosis. Moving to Greifswald University's Pathological Institute and working under Gross, Domagk studied phagocytosis by Kupffer's cells in the liver. He showed that injected *Staphylococcus* bacteria were taken up by cells of the reticuloendothelial system more effectively if the organisms were damaged by prior immunization or by some external treatment.

Carl Duisberg, president of Bayer, created a great new initiative to develop a laboratory for research and organic chemical syntheses in the search for new drugs that would be effective against infectious diseases. He hired Wilhelm Roehl, who had worked with Ehrlich on trypanosomiasis, and a team of chemists working under Heinrich Horlein. By 1916, they had developed *germanin* to treat sleeping sickness and by 1924, *Plasmoquine* to treat malaria, but Roehl died in 1929 of acute streptococcal infection in the midst of this exciting vindication of Ehrlich's ideas.

Bayer hired Domagk in 1927 to develop a pathological program to guide the next phase of research. Domagk selected the ubiquitous hemolytic streptococcus, cause of the devastations of childbed fever and scarlet fever and the very germ that had killed his colleague, Roehl. He established a lethal experimental model in mice, using a "hot" strain of pathogenic streptococci. A brilliant chemist, Joseph Klarer led the synthetic chemistry research team and produced an array of new agents to be tested, culminating in 1932 in a red dye, Kl-730. In this substance a sulfonamide was attached as a side chain. Although the substance was ineffective against the streptococci in in vitro cultures, when Domagk injected it into his mouse model in which all untreated mice died, it provided one hundred percent protection. The agent's red crystals were christened *Prontosil rubrum*. A water-soluble form that was tested in humans proved to be remarkably effective in 1935, but only against streptococcal infections. French scientists showed that the true efficacy of the agent was due to the sulfonamide side-group. This finding triggered a new wave of research, and a long series of related *sulfa drugs* were developed. Domagk was awarded the Nobel Prize for medicine in 1939, but Hitler's Nazis did not allow him to travel to Stockholm or to accept it. His work had begun the new era of chemotherapy against bacterial diseases.

ANTIBIOTICS: WEAPONS OF WAR AMONG BACTERIA EFFECTIVE IN THERAPY

Alexander Fleming (1881-1955), a physician and microbiologist, was a protégé of Almroth Wright at St. Mary's Hospital in London. Fleming discovered lysozyme, an antibiotic formed by animals and humans, then released into their body secretions as a general antibacterial agent. Lysozyme was ineffective against most pathogens. Working with cultures of pathogenic bacteria in 1928, he observed that an airborne contaminant organism had entered one culture plate and caused a zone of lysis of the bacteria growing on the plate around its opportunistic colony. Serendipity was at work again. The contaminant strain and the lysis it caused on the plate became visibly detectable only because research on molds was going on in the same building and Fleming had left the inoculated Petri dish unattended in an unheated lab while away on a three-week holiday. The prevailing thermal conditions had allowed both the contaminant and the bacterial strain to grow. Fleming's genius was to recognize the importance of the evidence before his eyes upon his return.

Fleming studied the contaminant and found that it was a strain of *Penicillium* mold. He speculated that this particular strain had produced a chemical that diffused out from its colony and suppressed or killed the surrounding bacteria, which had been inoculated onto the plate and formed colonies. He subcultured the mold and extracted a substance that he found would prevent the growth of many species of pathogenic bacteria in vitro. He named the new agent penicillin and inadvertently launched the antibiotic era. He showed that his discovery did not appear to harm white blood cells in vitro. Also, when it was injected into healthy laboratory animals, there was no evidence of toxic effects. He published his findings in 1929. No one followed up on this exciting lead by treating infected animals until Howard Florey at Oxford initiated a program to search for antibacterial substances in the late 1930s.

Florey and the brilliant biochemist Ernst Chain screened the literature and found evidence of two agents that were made by microbes and attacked other microbes, penicillin and pyocyanin (made by a strain of *Pseudomonas* bacteria). Florey selected penicillin for the first series of experiments. After succeeding in isolating the active agent, the researchers conducted the first crucial experiment in 1940, using mice inoculated with a lethal strain of streptococcus. Half of the mice were treated with penicillin; the others were untreated, infected controls. All the untreated mice died, whereas one hundred percent of those treated with penicillin survived. The drug was soon used successfully in humans.

Mass production of penicillin required American assistance via the United States Department of Agriculture regional research laboratory in Peoria, Illinois, where Andrew Moyer was briefed by Norman Heatley of the British team. The drug was given priority in the treatment of those seriously wounded in the war. The drug was remarkably effective and safe for such conditions and for the treatment of gonorrhea. At last an effective weapon against many lethal bacterial infections was available to the health professions. Many other antibiotics with varying spectra of antibacterial activity and efficacy in vivo have since been discovered.

The applications of antibiotics and chemotherapeutic substances against bacteria, helminths, fungi, and ectoparasites provided veterinarians with weapons against many of the diseases they were called upon to diagnose, treat, and prevent. Reversal of the diseases caused by viruses by means of therapy has proved to be much more challenging. A similar situation exists in cancer therapy. Progress has been made, but an enormous research effort will be needed to find treatments for these diseases. Vaccines are extremely important in the interim. It is important to remember the historical feeling of impotence in the face of bacterial and helminthic diseases before the discovery of sulfonamides and antibiotics. It must also be noted, however, that some of these trusted weapons are losing their edge because of genetic transfer of resistance among microbes and because of an increasing incidence of immunosuppression that lowers natural host resistance to pathogens.

SYSTEM MODELING AND HEALTH MANAGEMENT IN ANIMAL PRODUCTION

As systems of livestock farming became more intensive and business oriented, the monitoring and recording of events became necessary. With the advent of the modern computer it became possible to manage vast amounts of data and generate models to define production systems. Progressive refinement of these models led to software development in the form of programs that could be used to test the system and identify weak links in the production process. An early conceptualizer of the potential of this approach was Peter Ellis of the Department of Veterinary Epidemiology and Economics at Reading University in England. One of his graduate students, Roger Morris of Australia, returned to Melbourne and, working with Douglas Blood, developed a graduate program in veterinary epidemiology based on Ellis's concept.

Calvin W. Schwabe at the University of California, Davis, developed a master of science degree program in veterinary preventive medicine and focused on the veterinarian's role in public health. He produced a classic text, *Veterinary Medicine and Human Health* (1964, 1969, and 1984).

Morris has taught brilliant graduate students who have carried the concepts through to the practical level of application to dairy cattle and swine. Morris has applied the same principles to the control and eradication of contagious diseases, working with OIE to improve their computer systems for monitoring such diseases globally and regionally. Ellis and others have applied these approaches to defining terrestrial and aquatic animal production systems. This new approach to information management and analysis, as predicted by its pioneers, has had an earlier impact on productivity and profitability of domestic animals than has genetic engineering and its application through biotechnology.

The previously described conceptual approach to animal production systems will become increasingly crucial to the goal of maintaining an adequate supply and a diversity of food to feed the burgeoning human population while trying to protect the environment. Inevitably these advances will place more pressure on the veterinarian to master evolving complex technologies as well as the evolving veterinary knowledge.

Douglas Blood, Roger Morris, Norman Williamson, and others had developed health programs for dairy herds in Victoria, Australia, by 1978. Tremendous progress has since been made in developing "production medi-

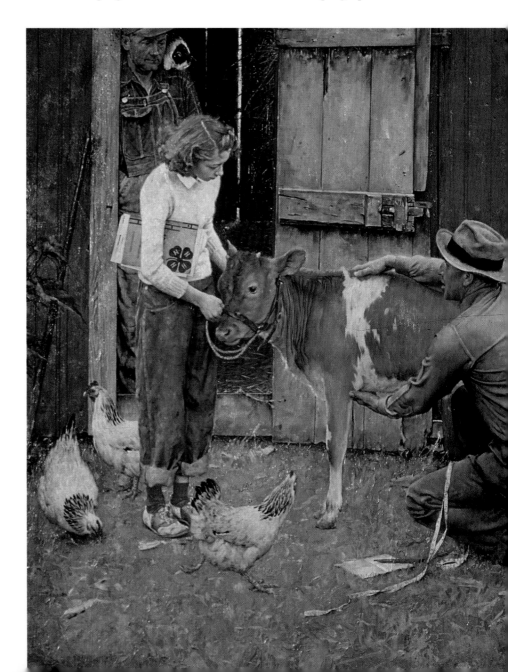

470. After Vermont Congressman Justin Morrill's second try at a Land Grant College Act in 1861 was passed by Congress and signed by President Abraham Lincoln in 1862, this uniquely American initiative established higher education at the state level that emphasized the study of agriculture and the industrial arts without excluding scientific and classical studies and included military tactics. Advocate William Hatch of Missouri convinced Congress to pass the Hatch Act in 1887, which funded the agricultural experiment stations to engage in research that included the study of livestock diseases. In 1914 the Smith-Lever Act created the cooperative state-federal extension service, institutionalizing the outreach agricultural technology transfer programs of the land grant universities and colleges to be conducted by off-campus instructors, typically the county agricultural extension agents aided by campus specialists. This wonderful scene, *County Agriculture Agent,* painted by Norman Rockwell (1894-1978) in 1948 captured the flavor of the outreach process and the hunger of farm families to learn and acquire new ideas. This process led to the concept of continuing education for adults. Children of rural families were encouraged to participate in livestock improvement through the U.S. Department of Agriculture's program of instruction in useful skills for young people, the 4-H program, named for the fourfold aim of improving the head, heart, hands, and health. *(UNL–Gift of Mr. Nathan Gold, Sheldon Memorial Art Gallery, University of Nebraska–Lincoln. 1969. U-563.)*

cine programs" to guide decision making in dairy and swine production enterprises. The concept has been widely adopted in Australia, the United States, the United Kingdom, New Zealand, Canada, and elsewhere. The University of Guelph's Ontario Veterinary College has developed a Department of Population Medicine, and postgraduate and continuing education courses in this field have been developed at several colleges of veterinary medicine. Great effort has been invested in development of computer software systems that define the animal production and health process.

As the business of livestock production has intensified, the goal at the working end of livestock production has been reminiscent of Descartes—to convert the animal into a machine that converts feed into food. That the humanitarian aspect of this goal is questionable was identified by Peter Singer and Jim Mason in *Animal Factories* in 1980. A continuous effort is required to ensure that ethical issues of animal well-being are kept in the forefront in planning modifications of complex animal handling and slaughtering systems. Ronald Kilgour, who worked at the Ruakura Agricultural Research Center in New Zealand, was one of the most committed scientists to apply rigorous studies of behavior to the husbandry and welfare of farm livestock. With his colleague, Clive Dalton, he published an excellent book in 1984, *Livestock Behavior: A Practical Guide*. D.G.M. Wood–Gush (1922-1992) in Great Britain took an innovative approach in developing proposals for systems designed to meet the behavioral needs of poultry and swine in the 1970s and 1980s.

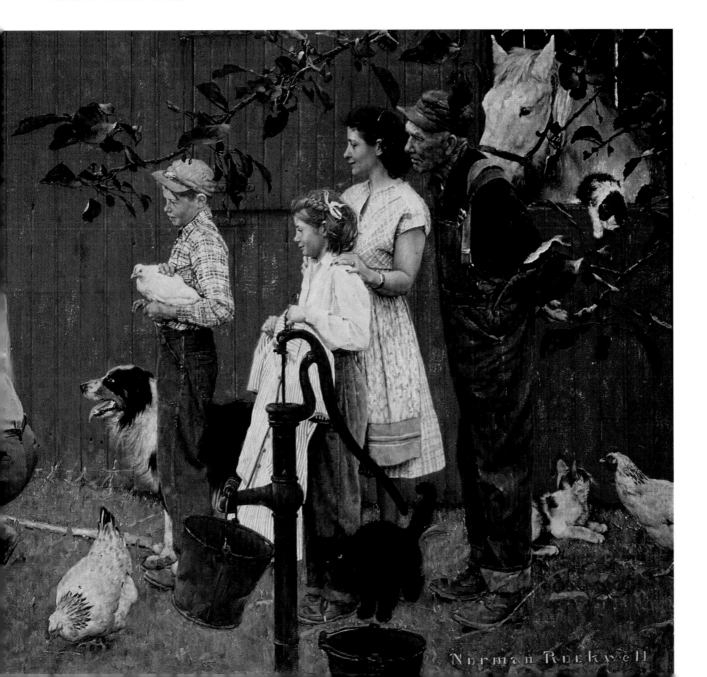

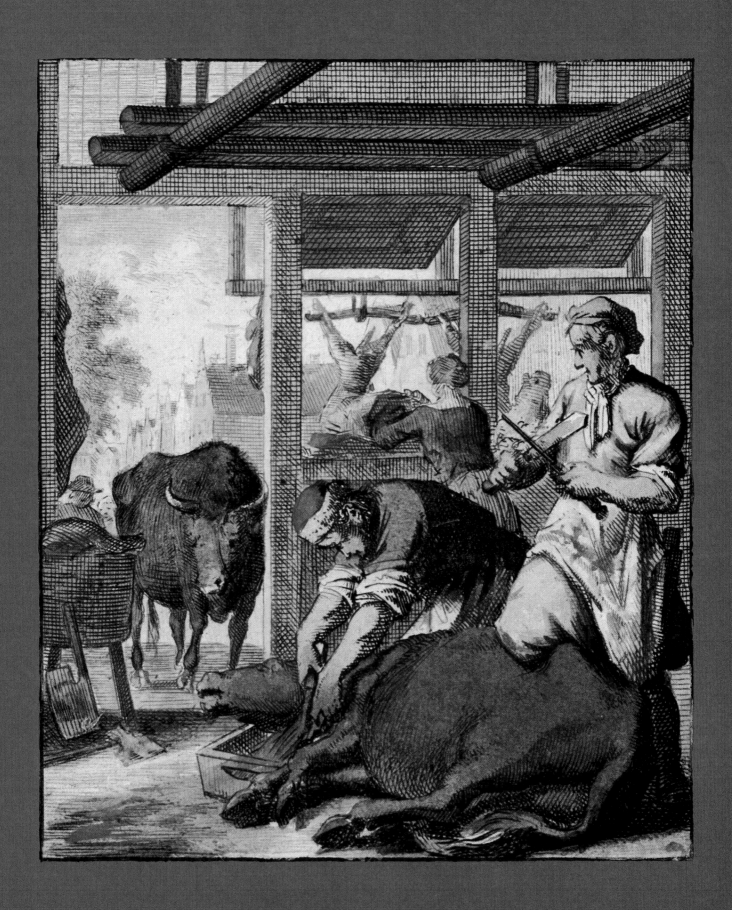

C H A P T E R 3 0

Veterinary Roles in Human and Ecosystem Health

THE BEGINNINGS OF EPIDEMIOLOGY AND VETERINARY PUBLIC HEALTH

Gaining understanding of the nature of diseases required the correlation of events that had been carefully observed and recorded so that a conceptual model could be developed, analyzed, tested, and revised. A London haberdasher, John Graunt, first perceived the importance of this epidemiological approach. He analyzed the weekly reports of births and deaths in the city, a seemingly small but crucial step in quantifying the patterns of disease in populations. His book, *The Nature and Political Observations Made Upon the Bills of Mortality,* which appeared in 1662, was the first such use of routinely collected statistical data on disease incidence. His analysis revealed that birth rates were higher for males than for females but that infant mortality rates were also higher for males. He also showed that seasonal variations in mortality were considerable, which suggested the presence of environmental factors, and he was able to demonstrate the effect of an epidemic of plague, a zoonotic disease.

In America rabies was the first zoonosis to be recorded—in the *Archives of Virginia* in 1753. It became an epizootic, and the people knew it could occur from dog bites. The next major zoonotic disease was yellow fever, which entered repeatedly via ports. An epidemic of yellow fever occurred in Philadelphia, then the national capital, in 1793 after an influx of Haitian refugees. John Adams and Thomas Jefferson appealed for a national quarantine system, which became law in 1799. The act was published in the first American medical journal, the *Medical Repository,* which had been inaugurated two years earlier by three visionary young physicians, Samuel Mitchell, Edward Miller, and Elihue Smith. They were the first to express the importance of veterinary medicine in the public health, albeit before the profession existed in America. For their journal they requested information about "histories of such diseases as appear among Domestic Animals" and "accounts of insects—whether any uncommon death or numbers of them; whether troublesome or noxious to man, beasts or vegetables," as well as data on "the state of the atmosphere." Their goal was to assemble the history of health in the United States on an annual basis. The 1799 issue of the journal contained a report entitled *Jenner on the Cowpox,* which cited the findings presented in a paper that was published in England in 1798. Cowpox, another zoonotic disease, was used to provide the first vaccine against smallpox.

The Philadelphia Society for Promoting Agriculture was founded in 1785 in a period of great intellectual ferment. One of the founders, the lexicographer Noah Webster, had a passionate interest in public health and called for sanitation to prevent pollution and for examination of animals to be used for food. Judge Richard Peters, who became president of the society in 1805,

471. *Facing page,* Portrayal of the career of butchering or slaughtering animals for meat. The animal has been stunned with a traditional poleax. This piece comes from a collection of engraved copperplates of a hundred different arts, trades, and professions collected and published in Amsterdam in 1694. The translation of the title is *The Human Industry: Shown in 100 Illustrations of Handycrafts, Arts, Actions, and Industries, With Verses,* done by Johannes & Caspares Lukin, a father and son team. Johannes Lukin (1649-1712) was a famous engraver. For each field, the name of the trade, a Biblical text, the illustration, and a semi-religious moralizing verse are provided. The verse for this piece reads

The meat market is open by turns,
So that you can buy the meat you need;
If you desire a leg of mutton,
You can eat it safely, on my word.

(Atlas Van Stolk, Rotterdam.)

called for the establishment of a veterinary profession. In 1807 the physician Benjamin Rush urged that veterinary education be initiated and that attention be paid to the safety of foods derived from animals. Another member and physician, James Mease, presented a course on the "Comparative Anatomy and Diseases of Domestic Animals" from 1812 to 1813. He had insisted in 1792 that the only way humans could acquire rabies was from the bite of an infected animal.

Virchow selected the term *zoonosis* to describe infections of animals that are in turn contagious to humans. Such diseases, when they occurred in domestic animals, represented an occupational hazard to rural livestock workers and those in the butchering trades. Because these infections may not be apparent in the host animal, their hazard to humans may be masked. It was imperative that a system be devised to report the occurrence of infectious diseases of animals and human communicable diseases so that correlations could be detected. In 1920 an epizootic of rinderpest, an animal disease that was not considered a zoonosis, led to the establishment of l'Office Internationale des Epizooties, based in Paris, to start data collection on infectious diseases of animals and to notify government veterinary services whenever a reportable disease was detected.

In the United States the Massachusetts legislature was the first to pass laws to ensure the quality and safety of milk, prohibiting its adulteration in 1856 and, in 1864, forbidding the use of milk obtained from diseased cows. Montclair, New Jersey, began the regular bacteriological examination of milk in 1900. In 1908 Chicago was the first city to require pasteurization of all milk except that obtained from tuberculin-attested herds. The American Public Health Association was begun in 1872 with the stated goals of advancing sanitary science and promoting public hygiene. Daniel E. Salmon in 1881 presided over its ninth meeting, for which the theme was veterinary medicine in public health. The U.S. Congress in 1879 established a National Board of Health. The board retained James Law of Cornell University as a consultant to report on animal diseases of importance to public health. He proposed that the board should establish a veterinary committee to address the control of animal contagia and parasites that also affect humans, and he prepared the first list of ten major zoonotic diseases. The National Board of Health, however, did not survive.

DISTURBING PERCEPTIONS OF MEAT INSPECTION IN AMERICA

The horrors of the Chicago stockyards—for both humans and animals—were portrayed by Upton Sinclair in *The Jungle,* a misleading and provocative book that was published in 1904. The book was grossly unfair to the federal meat inspection service of the Bureau of Animal Industry (BAI), and Salmon was dismissed. Cattle streamed into Chicago on trains from the railheads all over the Great Plains west and south of the city. The cattle had been driven overland to railheads in great herds by the drovers on horseback. As the population of beef cattle on the prairies increased, the markets in the eastern states expanded and export demand grew. The slaughtering and packing plants became saturated and adopted assembly-line systems; steam power was used to hoist the shackled carcasses to the overhead rails after the cattle had been stunned and bled. Sanitation and the health of the animals received scant attention until the Pure Food and Drug and the Meat Inspection Acts were passed in 1906. The acts provided the necessary federal funds to empower the U.S. Department of Agriculture to launch a system of meat inspection that could work. The Public Health Service Milk Code of the 1920s required that veterinarians be employed to ensure that milk was safe. Brucellosis became a major occupational hazard of workers in the meat trade until Wesley Spink at the University of Minnesota developed guidelines for infection prevention.

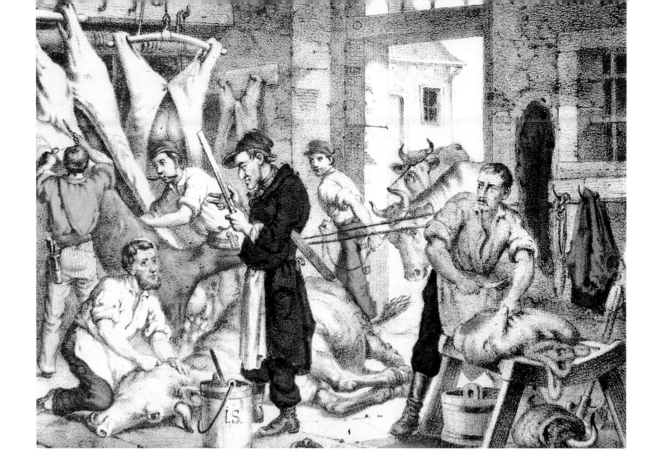

THE CASE FOR A VETERINARY ROLE IN PUBLIC HEALTH

The new approach of disease prevention, as well as the meat and milk inspections, required a much more analytical and impersonal epidemiological methodology than that required for clinical practice. Biostatistics became more important. In the established veterinary profession few role models were applying these population-based methods. Because the actual inspection of animal products tended to be a boring task compared with the challenge of handling a clinical case, it was difficult to recruit promising students and graduates to work in the field. The need was compelling, but leadership was necessary to articulate it and to generate the case studies in a way that would catch the imagination of the dedicated scholar. In addition, acquiring curricular "turf" by means of concessions from traditional established disciplines to make room for the new fields was, as always, difficult.

Although the methodological requirements were similar for control of animal diseases in herds or populations and for control of zoonotic diseases and food safety, the latter had a more compelling protective and regulatory basis. Since this was also less directly appealing to the animal owners, they were less willing to pay for it. Consequently, as with central policies implemented to eradicate or control epizootics, a state-funded authority was required for it to be effective. The "free market" would not provide the desired level of protection for the public health. Unscrupulous traders have always existed around the edges of towns and cities to foster a market in uninspected, unsound, or diseased meats, often after processing into pies, sausages, and salted products. These products, cheaper than unprocessed meats, were particular hazards for the urban poor, just as the unsanitary disposal of wastes from the meat trade was hazardous for the environment.

As the urban centers began to develop controls over food safety in the last third of the nineteenth century, traders became more evasive. In Great Britain John Gamgee was commissioned in 1862 to report on the meat and livestock trade. He estimated that about twenty percent of the meat consumed in the 1850s and early 1860s came from diseased animals. He recommended that a national system of specially trained veterinary inspectors be established. First,

472. Ritual slaughter scene in an eighteenth century Friesian town. The long knife is typical of those used for the ritual method, and the animal on the floor is in the position used for cutting the throat without prior stunning with a poleax in accordance with religious regulations. Two skinners are at work on the left, aided by ropes to pull the hide; one has a knife between his teeth. A small animal, probably a sheep, is slaughtered on the table on the right. *(Nederlands Openluchtmuseum, Arnhem, The Netherlands.)*

however, it was necessary to overcome a widespread political tenet in Great Britain that the consumers themselves were the best judges of their self-interest and that a system involving inspection and regulation was both undesirable and unnecessary. The psychological milieu was more favorable in Europe, where France, Austria, and Prussia had accepted systems for state intervention in both agriculture and public health.

In Europe the initial thrust toward state intervention came from physicians such as the German pioneer of social medicine, Johann Peter Frank, whose six-volume *System of a Complete Medical Policy* was published between 1779 and 1819. He believed that controls were necessary to protect the health of both the individual and the human "herd" and emphasized the importance of meat inspection. He regretted the lack of a scientific basis for inspection of animal products and called for a system of centralization of slaughter in public abattoirs, where the meat inspection was carried out by trained members of the veterinary profession.

On the other hand, research in French veterinary schools indicated that meat from animals with rinderpest could be consumed safely, and there was a tendency to extrapolate from this finding without proof to conclusions about the safety of meat from animals with other diseases. Few veterinarians were prepared to campaign for the establishment of a meat inspection program to protect the population. Although the Paris Council for Public Hygiene created an opportunity for veterinary participation in developing a program of veterinary public health, progress was slow.

SCIENTIFIC MEAT INSPECTION

The application of a scientific approach to inspection of meat began in 1855 when Friedrich Küchenmeister in Dresden showed that a relationship existed between the agent that caused pig pimples, *Cysticercus cellulosae,* and the human tapeworm, *Taenia solium.* In Leipzig in 1861 Rudolf Leuckart found a similar connection between cattle pimples and a human tapeworm attributable to them. Ernst F. Herbst in Göttingen followed Joseph Leidy's observation of *Trichinella spiralis* in pig meat in Philadelphia by showing that the organism could penetrate the intestinal wall after ingestion. In the 1850s, Virchow showed that the tiny larvae in muscle develop into adult worms in the canine intestine. In 1860 Friedrich A. Zenker, a Dresden pathologist, traced the path traveled by the *Trichinella* organism that is encapsulated in pig muscle. He noted that after consumption, the organism enters via the human intestinal wall, then migrates to human muscle, based on studies of a fatal case in a woman who made sausages. At last a scientific basis was established for the transmission of disease from animals to humans via infected meat. This work aroused forward-looking veterinarians to call for their profession to assume responsibility for meat inspection.

The discoveries of pathogenic bacteria led to findings that bacteria could multiply in meat and other foods and cause "food poisoning." Public recognition of this risk was a decisive factor in the acceptance of a need for meat inspection. The early acceptance of the germ theory of disease by the veterinary profession gave it a strategic position in meat hygiene. Previously unexplained episodes of serious illness could be understood and, perhaps, prevented by "sanitary police." By the early 1880s bacteriology laboratories were started in some public slaughterhouses, and scientific meat inspection evolved rapidly. The role of veterinarians in public health was gradually accepted by the medical profession, demanded by society, and implemented into law by politicians. Because veterinary education prepared a person to recognize and diagnose diseased animals, veterinarians could engage effectively in premortem inspection. Similarly, their growing expertise in animal pathology made them the logical authorities on immediate postmortem meat inspection

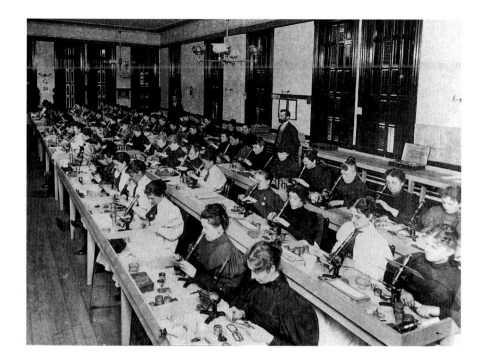

473. Two Bureau of Animal Industry veterinarians overseeing sixty persons engaged in microscopic examination of tissues for trichinella parasites from hog carcasses destined for export. This disease was the first zoonosis identified as a reason to curtail export of U.S. pork to European destinations. The Meat Inspection Act of 1890 provided for the inspection and certification of salted pork and bacon for export and was followed by a more stringent law the next year that applied to both export and interstate shipment. The enormous task of inspecting one to two million hog carcasses per year required many such inspection centers. Meat from other species, involving even larger numbers, was inspected. *(Courtesy of the Archives of the National Animal Disease Center, Ames, Iowa.)*

at the abattoir. The local authorities began to consult veterinarians who were prepared to develop expertise in food hygiene. Such specialists participated in drafting legislation for the state control of food quality. By about 1900 veterinarians were employed in policing the legislation as inspectors and even as directors of public slaughterhouses.

Achieving uniform standards of meat safety was a problem in a system that was made up of many small businesses with private slaughterhouses and butchers' shops, which were the main avenue for the meat trade. Regular inspection of such establishments was impractical, and naturally the owners of small businesses resisted efforts to replace them with central municipal abattoirs where all meat could be inspected. Thus a long period of transition was required in some countries. Although in Great Britain the Public Health Act of 1875 gave urban sanitation authorities the power to establish a public slaughterhouse and many did so, the town corporations were reluctant to disrupt the traditional system of small, private abattoirs. In Europe, particularly in French- and German-speaking regions, the town councils did acquire the authority to prohibit all slaughtering except in the central public abattoir, where inspection could be carried out and humane methods could be enforced. As a result their public abattoirs became self-supporting, whereas the British and Dutch abattoirs tended to lose money and in their towns a large proportion of uninspected meat was marketed.

A leading figure in the development of a rigorous scientific approach to meat inspection was Robert von Ostertag (1864-1940) in Berlin. Ostertag wrote books on meat hygiene in the 1890s. He was appointed to the Hygiene Institute in Berlin in 1903 and taught animal hygiene at Humboldt University. He investigated tuberculosis in cattle in 1905. Writing about the role of the veterinarian in human health, Ostertag stated that "the times in which the job of veterinarians is only curing diseased animals are over. Now they must do the important tasks of food hygiene for public health." Not only was he the scientific founder of the field, but also he had a great effect on public policy. In 1908 he became the first director of the Department of Veterinary Medicine in the Kaiser's Health Office. He became extremely influential and was known in Germany as the "Father of Meat Hygiene." An institute was erected in his name and contains an exhibit honoring his life and achievements.

AVOIDANCE OF SUFFERING DURING SLAUGHTER

Those who were concerned about the treatment of animals wanted oversight of standards of animal care during shipment. Also of central importance was the actual procedure of animal slaughter. In England John Galsworthy wrote *The Slaughter of Animals for Food* for the *Daily Mail* in 1912, which was copied and distributed by the Royal Society for the Prevention of Cruelty to Animals (RSPCA). The piece was a plea for the use of more humane methods in the abattoirs. He noted that more than eight million sheep were killed each year in England and Wales without prior stunning by having a knife thrust into the neck, then the tip inserted between two vertebrae to sever the spinal cord. Starling, the famous physiologist (discoverer of Starling's law of the heart and of the first hormone, secretin), estimated that the time for loss of consciousness as a result of this procedure varied from five to thirty seconds and was even longer if the butcher was not skilled. Galsworthy recommended stunning the animal by carefully aiming a blow from a club with a heavy head to land on the top of the head between the ears.

Procedures that were used for killing food animals had become controversial in the nineteenth century. The focus of concern stemmed from the perception that slaughtering was performed in a manner that was cruel to the animal. At the time only cattle were stunned by a blow from a hammer; other species simply had their throats cut or were "stuck." The fledgling veterinary profession did not take an active position on this issue. Individual veterinarians, however, did voice concerns and propose reforms. A special hammer with a projection on it was developed to stun swine. This device was followed by an explosive spring-pistol stunner with a bell-shaped end that stabilized its position on the head. The most dependable sudden effect was achieved by the captive-bolt pistol, which could be adapted for use in most species. Electrical stunners were invented but required precise application. The method of choice for the slaughter of hogs became carbon dioxide anesthesia; the pigs were moved on a conveyor through a chamber filled with the gas and were bled before consciousness returned.

Veterinary research on electroanesthesia appeared promising, but dependable loss of consciousness was difficult to achieve. Humanitarian concerns still exist about methods of ritual slaughter in orthodox Jewish and Muslim religious practices, in which slitting of the great vessels of the neck and complete bleeding without prior stunning are required. One of the earliest laws of Hitler's National Socialist regime in Germany disallowed ritual slaughter, apparently with anti-Semitic intent. The methods have not been banned in other cultures, although witnessing their performance is quite disturbing to most people.

Many animals continue to be killed in inappropriate ways. Continuing efforts and research are required in this field. It is also imperative that the handling of animals before slaughter be conducted in ways that prevent apprehension, fear, and abuse.

ENHANCEMENT OF MEAT SAFETY IN MODERN TIMES

Concentration of slaughtering into a few large operations was mandated in Great Britain during the Second World War, and effective meat inspection was attained. However, the private butchers who made this concession won government assurance that they would be allowed to reopen their businesses after the war. This did not happen until 1954, when 3500 businesses opened, and more opened the next year. Veterinary inspection was again rendered impractical for part of the meat supply. Full inspection was not achieved until 1968, when it became illegal for meat to leave a slaughterhouse without post-mortem inspection.

The European Community heightened standards further with a set of Fresh Meat Regulations. This development caused a trend toward large private slaughterhouses because they could adapt to new technologies more rapidly than could the centralized public abattoirs. Laboratories were required to provide specific analyses for the veterinary inspectorate, who had to make greater use of lay inspectors to contain costs. As the old plagues were eliminated, public confidence in the meat trade was increased but new challenges emerged. *Salmonella* organisms and other enterotoxic enterobacteria, including some strains of *Escherichia coli,* proved particularly troublesome as contaminants that could cause food poisoning. The emergence of infectious antibiotic resistance that could be transferred among these organisms became a major public health concern.

BRUCELLOSIS OF ANIMALS AND HUMANS IN THE NEW WORLD

Although brucellosis is believed to have been absent from the New World before the conquest that followed the arrival of Columbus, it could have entered at any time since his arrival with livestock brought from Europe. The bovine form of the disease is suspected to have been the cause of an abortion "storm" in cattle in Louisiana and Mississippi in 1864. Franck showed that the disease was infectious by placing pieces of placenta from a cow that had aborted into the vaginas of healthy, late-pregnant cows, which soon aborted.

Brucellosis in humans is thought to have occurred in Cuba at least as early as 1885. The goat strain was proved to be present in Jamaica in 1912. Strong concerns existed about the probable presence of the bovine brucellosis organism in Canada by 1914, and the presence of positive reactors was demonstrated by 1922. By 1945 brucellosis was considered the most common disease in Canada that was transmitted to humans by animals. However, a strong government campaign succeeded in eradicating it by 1985.

Argentina, with its huge populations of cattle (57 million in 1983) and sheep (30 million), has suffered from epizootic bovine abortion at least since the late nineteenth century. It was described in Buenos Aires in 1892, and a high percentage of dairy cattle became infected with brucellosis. Unpasteurized milk was sold in Buenos Aires province until 1966. Large numbers of cases of brucellosis in humans have been recorded.

Gutierrez Oropeza reported a diagnosis of the disease in humans in Venezuela in 1898. Alberto Barton in 1909 indicated that a human epidemic occurred in Peru from 1907 to 1908; the condition was associated with long-term, irregular bouts of fever but low mortality. He attributed the disease to consumption of fresh goat cheese. A little earlier, in 1906, a New Jersey quarantine station isolated *Brucella melitensis* from the milk of goats that had arrived from Malta. The same goats had infected most of the passengers and crew of the ship *Joshua Nicholson,* which had arrived the previous year.

THREE ARCHITECTS OF VETERINARY PUBLIC HEALTH IN THE UNITED STATES

Although many have contributed substantially and tenaciously to veterinary public health in the United States, three towering figures have dominated the profession. All three have had long, productive careers. Karl F. Meyer, a Swiss graduate of the fine veterinary school at Zürich in 1909, worked with the Swiss veterinary pathologist Arnold Theiler in South Africa. Meyer emigrated to the United States and became professor of pathology and bacteriology at the University of Pennsylvania's School of Veterinary Medicine. In 1914 he went to the University of California, where he built the Hooper

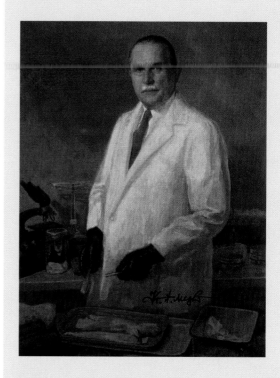

474. Karl Friedrich Meyer (1884-1974), a Swiss who trained in veterinary medicine at Berne, worked there with Kolle in microbiology, then completed a doctorate at Zürich and worked with Theodor Kitt in Munich's veterinary school. He moved to Pretoria, South Africa, to work with Arnold Theiler from 1908 to 1910 on hemoprotozoal diseases, particularly East Coast fever (on which they did not see eye to eye), and other tropical and zoonotic diseases. Meyer then moved to the School of Veterinary Medicine at the University of Pennsylvania for three years before going west to join the small Hooper Foundation of Medical Research at the University of California as associate professor of tropical medicine. He stayed there for more than fifty years, becoming the director in 1924. The Hooper Foundation began in a building that had housed the veterinary school before it closed. Meyer's focus was the epidemiology of infectious diseases of animals and humans. Under his leadership the Hooper became one of the world's leading research institutes of comparative medicine and zoonotic diseases.

Meyer established the viral origin of equine encephalitis. His work in establishing the risk of botulism in humans from *Clostridium botulinum* was derived from his experience in South Africa, where the organism was cultured from animal feces. This work saved the American food-canning industry from disaster. Meyer became the national authority on many infectious diseases, particularly pneumonic plague and psittacosis, and the world's leader in progress in understanding zoonoses. He developed the curriculum for California's School of Public Health. *(Special Collections, University Archives, University of California at San Francisco.)*

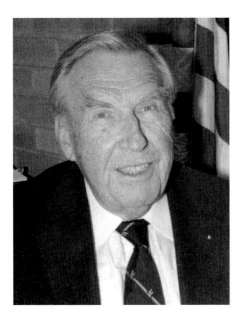

475. James H. Steele emerged as a leading figure in shaping a veterinary role in public health from within the U.S. government. A visionary, he had an unusual grasp of the historical role of the profession in epidemiology, focusing on the burgeoning field of zoonoses from rabies onward. He developed a remarkable competence in organizing the available knowledge in the field and using it to influence planning and decision making. As a veterinary sanitarian in the Public Health Service he was assigned to zoonoses epidemiology and control in the Communicable Disease Center in Atlanta. He was appointed the first chief of the new, specifically veterinary officer corps in 1947. He created a veterinary public health unit in the epidemiology branch of the Communicable Disease Center and helped establish graduate education in public health as a new veterinary specialty, opening new avenues for participation. By secondment of new federal public health veterinary officers to state health departments, he had a major impact on participation at the state level. He worked with W.Z. Zimmerman of Iowa State University, who had shown a high incidence of trichinosis in garbage-fed hogs, and Irving Kagan of the Communicable Disease Center to promote evaluation of human diaphragms for trichinosis. Opposition from the meat-packing industry made eradication unattainable. Steele urged that the socioeconomic consequences of zoonoses be more actively assessed, and he obtained support for this position from the World Health Organization, which formed a veterinary public health unit. He retired as assistant surgeon general in 1971 but was still bubbling over with progressive ideas and became professor of environmental health at the School of Public Health of the University of Texas, Houston. *(Courtesy J.H. Steele.)*

Foundation into one of the world's leading centers for infectious disease research. He earned a doctorate in zoology in 1924 for a thesis on botulism and was awarded an honorary medical degree in 1940 for his many contributions to public health. He is the only veterinarian known to have been nominated for a Nobel Prize, but the outbreak of World War II caused a hiatus in the presentation of the Nobel awards.

James H. Steele served as a sanitarian in the military until the end of World War II. He was then charged with drafting a program encompassing the control of animal diseases that were transmissible to humans and otherwise significant for public health. He developed a bibliography of titles relevant to public health in 1945. The Bureau of States' Relations in Washington, D.C., established a Veterinary Public Health section in 1946. Steele was asked to prepare an overview of animal diseases and zoonoses of public health interest. He produced the Zoonosis Chart, which initially listed fewer than forty diseases, but little was known of the epidemiology and control measures except for a few high-profile diseases. The status of veterinarians in the U.S. Public Health Service was changed from that of scientists or sanitarians to that of a new class of veterinary medical officers. Steele's great contribution was made through the Communicable Disease Center.

The third of the small group of scholars and visionaries who took a global view of veterinary public health is Calvin W. Schwabe of the School of Veterinary Medicine at the University of California at Davis, and the School of Medicine in San Francisco. He has worked in many parts of the world tracking the epidemiology and pathogenesis of zoonotic diseases. He developed an outstanding masters' program in Veterinary Preventive Medicine at Davis, which opened new vistas of opportunity for the profession. He is renowned worldwide for his magnificent book, *Veterinary Medicine and Human Health,* which was first published in 1964; every aspiring veterinary student should read the latest edition. Schwabe's perspective is both scholarly and historical as he outlines the contributions of leading veterinarians to the progress of knowledge and action in the pursuit of human health and well-being. He is the leading philosopher of the veterinary profession.

EMERGING ZOONOSES AND THE INSECURE SPECIES BARRIER

A strange disease of humans that involved neurological disorders, organ damage, and arthritis was described at Lyme, Connecticut, in 1975. Lyme disease was caused by infection with a spirochete organism, *Borrelia burgdorferi,* which was first isolated by W. Burgdorfer in 1982, and was spread by the bite of a tiny tick, *Ixodes dammini,* which overwintered in the fur of white-tailed deer. This creature, *Ixodes dammini,* is now considered to be responsible for more human illness than any other arthropod vector of disease in the United States: there are four thousand cases of Lyme disease per year in New York State alone. The tick is also a vector for babesiosis. A Harvard entomologist, Andrew Spielman, proposed that the disease may have originated on Naushon Island, Massachusetts, which became a privately owned haven for mainland deer after the forests were cut and the deer were harvested by Native Americans and immigrants. Only in the 1960s, after regrowth of dense shrub and tree cover in areas reforested earlier, did the deer return to the mainland states of Massachusetts, Connecticut, and New York and multiply. Lyme disease occurs in about twenty states, and people now live closer to deer than ever before. The white-footed mouse was found to be a key reservoir species. The tick bite introduced the *Ixodes* organism into other hosts such as dogs and humans, an initial erythematous lesion followed by migrating erythematous lesions signaling the site. Penicillin therapy was found to be successful if treatment was started early. Eradication of the mice and deer was effective in preventing further cases of the disease on Great Island. Vaccines against the spirochete are becoming available.

Arboviruses are arthropod-borne RNA viruses that are spread by infected blood-sucking insects such as mosquitoes, ticks, and sandflies. Original sylvatic (forest or jungle) life cycles of arboviruses such as yellow fever and dengue did not require a human host, but once the virus gains entry into a human population where suitable vectors such as mosquitoes and breeding sites such as old tires are present, a human cycle can become self-sustaining. The viruses that cause equine encephalitis can establish multiple vertebrate reservoirs and recur seasonally. Other viruses can be arthropod sustained, spreading transovarially from a female tick to her progeny, as in tick-borne encephalitis.

Scrapie, an unusual disease of sheep, has been known since the eighteenth century. French scientists J. Cuillé and P.L. Chelle showed that it was a transmissible disease in 1939. A brilliant Icelandic physician, Bjorn Sigurdurson (1915-1959) showed that the disease was a spongiform encephalopathy and christened it a *slow virus disease.* Sigurdurson established Keldur, the Comparative Research Center, about ten kilometers from Reykjavik, with help from the Rockefeller Foundation in 1948. While he was director, from 1948 to 1959, he traced the epidemiology of scrapie (*Rida* or ataxia with trembling) and another ovine disease, *Maedi-visna,* in Iceland. Scrapie arrived in 1878 via an infected English Oxford Down ram that was imported by way of Denmark. It spread in a local area, causing losses of sheep on a few farms, then stabilized until 1953, when it spread widely and the itching sign of the disease became more evident. Sigurdurson was followed as director of Keldur in 1959 by veterinarian Páll A. Pálsson, who was chief of the Veterinary Health Service for Iceland. He implemented a control program in 1978 to eradicate the disease from all the newly infected areas, slaughtering all flocks with confirmed cases after 1982. The disease was eradicated by 1990.

Other transmissible spongiform encephalopathies—the human diseases kuru and Creutzfeldt-Jakob disease and the animal diseases transmissible mink encephalopathy and bovine spongiform encephalopathy—have also been described. Bovine spongiform encephalopathy became an epizootic in the United Kingdom in the 1980s, and the Central Veterinary Laboratory traced its likely source to recycled offal from sheep that was used in cattle feed after rendering. The infectious agent of scrapie is not a typical virus, and some researchers have labeled it a *prion,* indicating that it is proteinaceous. This agent, whatever its true nature, is remarkably resistant to thermal sterilization and solvent treatment. Elimination of the source of infection is leading to a progressive decline in the number of cases. This condition is an object lesson in the need to monitor changes in husbandry practices so that no new opportunities for infectious agents to cross the species barrier are permitted. Bovine spongiform encephalopathy has not been shown to be a zoonosis, and elaborate precautions have been taken to deny it any opportunity to become one.

Influenza of humans and animals is caused by a group of RNA viruses that can be characterized by means of immunological and molecular study. The "A" strains are perpetuated in aquatic birds, particularly in migratory waterfowl. When the ducks congregate on bodies of water before their seasonal departure to warmer areas, there is a rapid buildup of infection via ingestion. As the organism infects the gut epithelium in these species, it multiplies rapidly and multiple subtypes of two series of antigens can form. If one of these subtypes happens to be a highly pathogenic strain for other species, devastating epizootics can occur. It is possible that the decimation of chicken stocks in Pennsylvania in the early 1980s originated in that way. The enteric agent in one species can become a cause of severe respiratory disease in others. Influenza is a zoonosis, and in the twentieth century many epidemics have spread around the world from East Asia. Intensive integrated systems of waterfowl, swine, and farmed fish coupled with a dense human population may

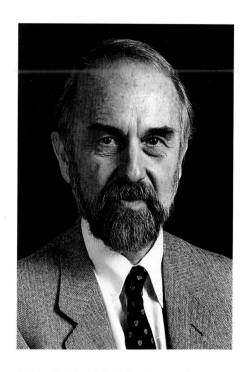

476. Calvin W. Schwabe is the most philosophical of veterinarians and has the broadest appreciation of the profession's potential contribution to human and animal well-being, derived from a profound historical and ecological perspective. In addition to the degree of doctor of veterinary medicine, he holds graduate degrees in zoology, tropical public health, and parasitology. He made great contributions to international public health during a decade at the American University in Beirut. He became an authority on hydatid disease and many other zoonoses and chaired the World Health Organization's Expert Committee on Veterinary Public Health, as well as being a member of its Division of Communicable Diseases. Based at Davis, he has been professor of epidemiology in the Schools of Veterinary Medicine and Medicine at the University of California since 1966. He founded the successful Masters of Veterinary Preventive Medicine program. At the twentieth World Veterinary Congress in 1975 in Thessaloniki, Greece, he was selected to be the inaugural lecturer for the first observance of World Veterinarian's Day. He was the fourth Wesley W. Spink lecturer on comparative medicine at the University of Minnesota. His topic was *Cattle, Priests and Progress in Medicine* (1978). He is renowned for his magnificent treatise, *Veterinary Medicine and Human Health,* which has evolved through several editions. *(Courtesy School of Veterinary Medicine, University of California at Davis.)*

477. Accredited veterinarian attaching an identifying tag to the ear of a steer certified to be clear of a reportable zoonotic disease based on immunological tests. The eradication of tuberculosis and brucellosis from most of the United States and Canada required that dependable diagnostic tests be carried out methodically at intervals. Certificates were required for interstate shipment. The accredited veterinarians were the delivery system responsible for testing, tagging, and certification, including vaccination with Strain 19 *Brucella abortus* vaccine in the case of brucellosis. This photograph illustrates one of these campaigns in progress. *(United States Department of Agriculture.)*

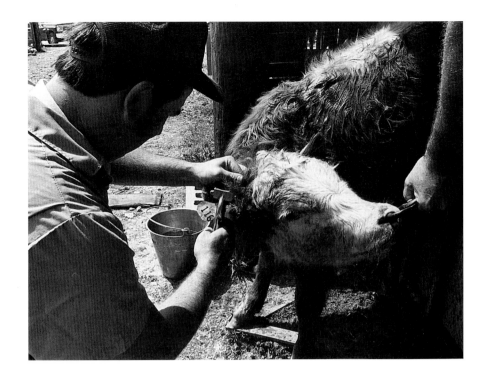

promote the appearance of new strains. It is alleged by some scientists that all major human epidemics since 1957 began in China or nearby territories, where similar practices are employed. Even the equine influenza virus can undergo reassortment with the swine virus.

Immunodeficiency-inducing retroviruses have emerged as the most formidable of the new human plagues. Several human immunodeficiency viruses (HIVs) have been isolated as causes of acquired immunodeficiency syndrome (AIDS), the delayed outcome of HIV infection. Simian immunodeficiency-inducing viruses have been isolated that may be innocuous to one primate species, yet lethal to another. It has not been established, however, that AIDS is a zoonosis derived from monkeys. Other retroviral diseases affect domestic animals and have been controlled with vaccines. A massive effort is under way to seek a vaccine for the human disease. The serious protozoal or fungal infection that often affects immunocompromised patients with AIDS was discovered long before by a Brazilian veterinarian, Antonio Carini, in rat lungs in 1909 and 1910. The organism, *Pneumocystis carinii,* was named after him.

THE CONQUEST OF SCREWWORM MYIASIS

In myiasis flies lay their eggs on the skin or in wounds and their larvae invade and consume the tissues. The penal colony of Devil's Island in French Guiana, South America, was the site of the discovery by French naval surgeon Charles Coquerel in 1858 of a myiasis-causing parasitic fly, *Cochliomyia hominivorax,* the New World screwworm fly. After the fly deposits its eggs in the nostrils or on an open wound, the resulting larvae emerge in about twelve hours and quite literally devour the living flesh for about a week before they drop out. The spiral ridge with spines running the length of the larva gave it the appearance of a screw, hence its common name. On Devil's Island the fly found an attractive human medium for deposition of its eggs, or "fly strike," which led to myiasis or consumption of the tissue by the insatiable growing larvae. Once recognized, the screwworm fly was soon found in domestic livestock and in humans elsewhere. From the southern third of the United States through Mexico into South America it became a dreaded pest. One county in North Carolina suffered ten thousand cases in a single outbreak. The human sites of screwworm entry were mainly the nose, eyes, and skin, and multiple larvae were involved. The larvae (up to three hundred) in the nasal passages may defy detection for some time and can be difficult to eradicate.

The screwworm fly is considered one of the most important pests of farm livestock. In the southern United States and Mexico strenuous efforts were made to avoid infestation. The seasonal behavior of the fly in North America was exploited by breeding to avoid calving, branding, and castrating during periods when the fly was active. Labor cost of surveillance, prevention, and treatment of individual animals was high. In fact, it was a major role of cowboys in susceptible areas. The screwworm may also have been a limiting factor for deer populations in the southern United States.

The great idea of eradicating the fly by mass production and release of male flies sterilized by irradiation was proposed by E.F. Knipling and H.T. Rainwater in 1937. The monogamous female flies, after mating with a sterile male, would fail to produce fertile eggs, and gradually, after repeated releases of the males, the population of flies would decline. Knipling tested the technique on a small island off the Florida coast and followed the successful outcome with a large test on the Caribbean island of Curaçao. A major program was then applied in 1957 to the enzootic area of southern Florida from which annual spread through the southeastern United States occurred. In just two years the fly was eradicated from the region. The producers in the southwestern United States campaigned for a similar program. It began in 1962, and an attempt was made to establish a fly-free barrier along the nearly two-thousand-mile length of the Mexican border. The barrier was penetrated by flies migrating northward from the enzootic areas of Mexico. A joint Mexico–United States screwworm eradication commission was needed to launch a program in the enzootic area. A plant was developed in southern Mexico that produced half a billion sterile male flies per week by 1982. It used about a hundred tons a week of dried blood, milk, and eggs. The sterile pupae were distributed to strategic sites for hatching and release by as many

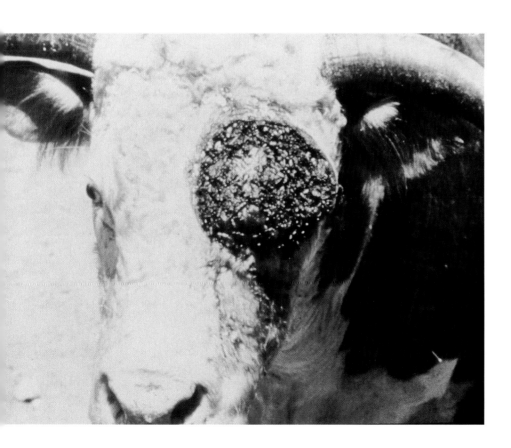

478. The New World screwworm fly, *Cochliomyia hominivorax,* laid its eggs in the eye of this cow. After hatching, the voracious larvae devoured the eye and surrounding tissues, an example of myiasis. The name *screwworm* is derived from the narrow row of backward-facing spines that spiral around the body of each larva. After four to eight days the larvae drop and burrow into the ground, then pupate. The pupae turn into adults after one to eight weeks, depending on ambient temperature. The flies live a few weeks and mate monogamously; then the female lays its eggs in wounds or body orifices to repeat the cycle. Dr. Coquerel, a naval surgeon in a penal colony in Cayenne, French Guiana, discovered the larvae in the sinuses of five patients (four were transportees) in 1858. Three of them died, although he had flushed up to three hundred larvae from their sinuses. A true zoonosis, the fly may have regulated the deer populations of the southern United States by depositing eggs on the navel stump of the fawn, resulting in a lethal infestation. Eradication by Knipling and Rainwater's idea of controlled breeding, irradiation, and release of sterile males in massive numbers stands as perhaps the greatest achievement of applied entomology. *(Food and Agriculture Organization of the United Nations, Rome.)*

as sixty aircraft. Livestock movements were controlled by inspection and quarantine stations. The barrier was then extended further south, and by 1988 releases were made in Guatemala and Belize, with the ultimate goals of creating a sterile-fly barrier at the narrow isthmus of Panama and allowing no flies north of it. The cost seems enormous, but it has been estimated that if the pest were reestablished in the United States and Mexico the annual cost would be of the order of 600 million dollars. The cost of the campaign was about 750 million dollars. This campaign has been the most impressive demonstration of exploiting entomological knowledge to achieve global control of an insect pest that caused losses of animal and human lives.

Spread is always a possibility with a highly mobile pest. One American soldier who was wounded in the Panama campaign in 1990 acquired screwworm infestation, which was discovered on his return. A dog arriving in France from South America was found to be infected. A really startling development was the appearances of the "New World" pest in Libya in 1988. Apparently it arrived with cattle from South America. Fears were aroused that it might spread through Africa, the Middle East, and the European side of the Mediterranean Sea. The United Nations began an eradication program in collaboration with several governments. The Food and Agriculture Organization's Screwworm Emergency Center for North Africa coordinated the campaign, with headquarters in Rome and field operations managed from Tripoli. Fourteen countries provided assistance. Training courses were provided, and the Libyan veterinary service mounted ninety field teams to inspect all animals in the area at risk. The number of cases increased to ten thousand in the second half of 1990. Sterile pupae were shipped from the Mexican plant in December 1990, and the flies that emerged were dispersed. Within a few months vast numbers were being dispersed, and by October 1991 eradication was officially declared.

THE ACCLIMATIZATION MOVEMENT

In eighteenth-century Great Britain the aristocracy competed to establish private menageries and aviaries with specimens imported from the expanding Empire. Isidore Saint-Hilaire founded the Société Zoologique d'Acclimatation in Paris in 1854 to exploit exotic animal species for agriculture and commerce. An early initiative was the importation of Chinese silkworm eggs. Later the idea was expanded to help the French colonies by introducing mongooses from Asia to Martinique in the Caribbean to control the fer-de-lance, the venomous viper.

The idea of "acclimatization" societies soon caught on internationally. Frank (Francis) Buckland (1826-1880) was the leading force in founding the Acclimatization Society of the United Kingdom in 1860. His enthusiasm had been aroused after he was invited to attend an "Eland Dinner" at the Aldersgate Tavern, with Professor Owen carving, which was designed to promote eland farming in Great Britain. Buckland proposed an amazing list of candidate species for acclimatization in Britain. The society, mainly composed of the aristocracy, foundered in 1867.

The concept of acclimatization societies was taken up more vigorously in Australia and New Zealand. Ecological disasters sometimes resulted from importations to these dominions. The brush-tailed possum that was taken from Tasmania to New Zealand, for example, became a major pest there and a reservoir of disease. From the deer importations, however, a new cervid industry was to arise, and trout and salmon imports brought these regions a great reputation for fishing. Australia, with scant concern for the native fauna, set out to stock the "new country" with important, useful, ornamental animals. The secretary bird was brought from South Africa to combat the venomous snakes. The European rabbit importation failed when the rabbit became a major pest.

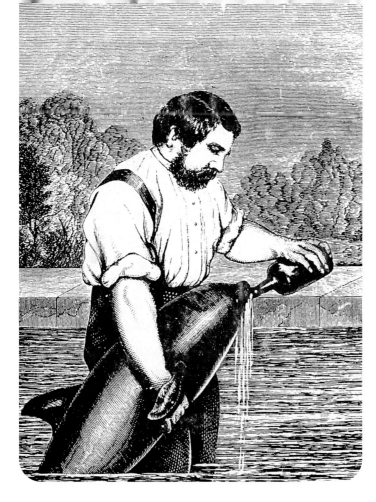

479. Frank Buckland physicking an ailing porpoise. "There was only one way; so I braved the cold water and jumped into the tank with the porpoise," he said. "I then held him up in my arms (he was very heavy) and, when I had got him in a favorable position, I poured a good dose of sal-volatile and water down his throat with a bottle." *(From* The Curious World of Frank Buckland *by G.H.O. Burgess, 1867.)*

The translocation of zoological species has had enormous educational value but has tended to lead to international homogenization of ecosystems, with serious consequences. The acclimatization movement and other importations of organisms achieved few lasting benefits. They brought in their wake disastrous consequences for native fauna through competition and introduction of exotic diseases. The steady growth in popularity of zoos that were open to the public and the general lack of support from the Zoological Society and the British Association for the Advancement of Science weakened the case for the Acclimatization Society. The movement, except in Australasia, was over before the end of the nineteenth century.

A GROWING VETERINARY ROLE IN THE CARE AND MANAGEMENT OF UNDOMESTICATED SPECIES

The study of diseases and ecology of undomesticated or "wild" animals is a field of almost infinite scope. Only a few of the possible avenues of inquiry can be addressed here.

The popularity of zoological gardens led to a demand for safer methods in the initial capture of animals from their ecological habitats. Once selected species had been caught, their health care could be studied. Hence a specialized field of veterinary care of captive wild species emerged. In addition to protecting the investment in establishing and maintaining zoos, the gradual expansion of veterinary clinical care, animal husbandry, and physiopharmacological and pathobiological knowledge of wild animal management and diseases led to significant research programs, which had application to many facets of comparative medicine that offered new research models. This progress was recorded annually in the *International Zoo Year Book*.

The zoological gardens became important in education and in the conservation of animal species. Despite recent criticism, zoos play a special role in arousing curiosity, particularly of children, in natural history. This role cannot be replaced by films and television documentaries. Zoos must continue to improve the attractiveness of their exhibits and the conditions for the animals so that the animals' innate behavioral drives can be satisfied. Murray E. Fowler has edited a book bringing together much of what is known about diseases in nondomestic species: *Zoo and Wild Animal Medicine,* first published in 1978.

The study of diseases of wild animals that threaten human health because the animals are reservoirs or vectors of infectious diseases that can spread to humans—the study of zoonoses—is a field of veterinary public health of major importance. Well over two hundred such diseases have been identified. The reverse situation, or zooanthroponosis, such as the infection of animals with human tuberculosis, is also common. In some situations a disease exists in both animal and human populations but can be transferred between species. Additional zoonoses are identified regularly. Biological diversity is so great that discoveries of new diseases and opportunities for diseases to be transferred to the human species from the "natural" environment can be predicted to continue.

There are major arguments for expanding research in zoological medicine and animal ecology to enlarge understanding of the interaction of infectious diseases among species. The intensive studies of diseases will grow gradually in response to specific situations that affect such interactions via changes in population dynamics of species that increase the hazards to human health. This intensification of study will lead to further attempts to manipulate ecological situations to enhance safety. Similarly, where feral species become a hazard to human or native faunal species, control programs will be required. Gary Wobeser at the University of Saskatchewan has made a valuable contribution through his work in this field and points the way for others in *Investigation and Management of Diseases in Wild Animals* (1994).

Discoveries of the spread of infectious agents from wild species to humans provided the initial stimulus for studies of wildlife diseases. The discoveries of many bacterial diseases in the late nineteenth and early twentieth centuries, for example, along with the demonstrations of vector-borne protozoal and viral diseases and the life cycles of helminthic parasites, occurred after the spread of infectious agents. Wildlife disease studies received a boost from the finding that arbovirus diseases often have reservoirs in wild species of birds and mammals.

480. William Hornaday was chief taxidermist at the Smithsonian's U.S. National Museum. A leading advocate of protection and display of native animals, he played a major role in lobbying Congress to support the establishment of the National Zoological Park in Washington, D.C. He was successful in 1889, two years after he had developed a small menagerie at the museum. The zoo was created on 175 acres of Rock Creek Valley and opened in 1891. The goals were to exhibit and study animals. The New York Zoological Society (now the Wildlife Conservation Society) was formed in 1895 and made preservation of native animals a high priority. The Bronx Zoo opened in 1899 with William T. Hornaday, who had left the Smithsonian, as director. This early photograph shows him participating in an operation on a Mexican grizzly bear in 1904, outside a makeshift hospital. The veterinarian in the white coat performing the surgery is Dr. W. Reid Blair, the first full-time zoo veterinarian in the United States. An enclosed veterinary hospital was not constructed at the zoo until 1916. Blair graduated from McEachran's college in Montreal in 1902 and joined the New York zoological park that year, serving until 1940. He wrote *In the Zoo* in 1929, in which he described zoo practice from the point of view of the clinician, surgeon, and pathologist. *(The Wildlife Conservation Society, Bronx, New York.)*

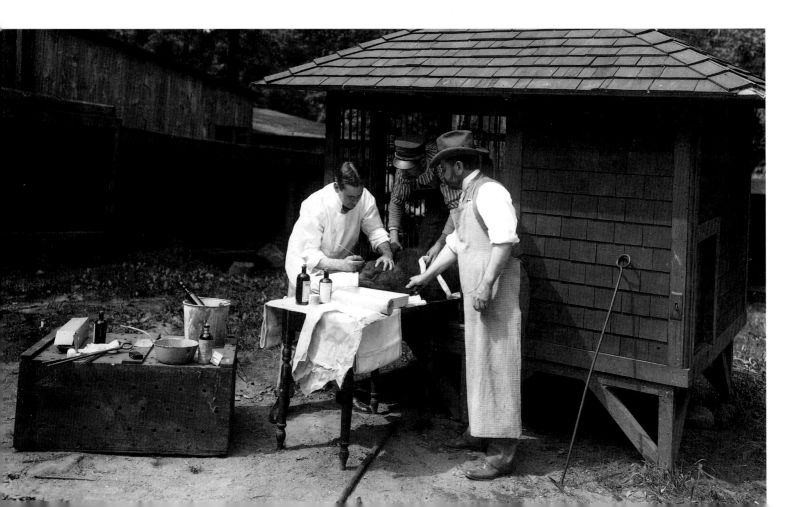

FOOD, FIBER, AND TOURISM: MANAGEMENT OF WILD SPECIES

Since World War II, efforts have been made to increase protein intake by expanding the use of harvested meat from wild species in Africa. Game meats are exported to supply demands for the luxury of exotic dishes, but care must be taken to manage these species to avoid population declines.

David Hopcraft of Kenya attended London University and Berea College, Kentucky, graduating with degrees in animal sciences and agriculture. He then studied wildlife sciences, ecology, population dynamics, and rangeland agronomy and received a doctoral degree at Cornell University, for which he compared the productivity of cattle and Thomson's gazelles in Kenyan savanna ecosystems in 1975. This study was supported by the National Science Foundation. The gazelles were many times more productive than the cattle in lean meat production per acre, did not cause degradation of the pasturelands, and did not require inoculations, dips, or watering points. Costs were much lower with the gazelles, and net income per acre was eight times higher. Subsequently Hopcraft developed a game ranch at Athi River in Kenya and worked with twenty species of animals. He studied the effect of interaction of multiple species in an attempt to encourage use of the entire spectrum of rangeland vegetation.

The game meat of gazelles is lean and has a low lipid content. The hides are also a valuable product. Hopcraft's proposition is that the natural ecosystem is richer and more stable than the human-cattle system that has largely displaced it, and he urges a return to that long-adapted system. One advantage of such an approach is that the landscape for tourism would be improved by the conservation of wild species. The culture of many African tribes, however, is oriented to placing value on cattle and small ruminant species. Some tribes have taboos against eating the flesh of wild animals such as the wildebeest.

The veterinarian has special skills that are valuable in animal capture and handling, wildlife population management, and disease diagnosis and control. The call for these skills is increasing, as it must, in the policymaking arena to protect and conserve the species by avoiding excessive cropping or losses. Most of the field studies of wild animals have been conducted by zoologists who have been interested in mammals, birds, or lower life-forms or in ecology. These people are an invaluable resource in understanding the behavior, nutrition, and reproduction of the animals they have studied in nature.

WILDLIFE STUDIES CONDUCTED BY THE UNITED STATES FISH AND WILDLIFE SERVICE

Two agencies of American government, the Office of Public Lands and the Commissioner of Indian Affairs, were merged to form the Department of the Interior. Under Lincoln the United States Department of Agriculture was formed from the Interior Department. The American Organization of Ornithologists was formed in 1883. In 1885 the Division of Entomology and Economic Ornithology, which became the Division of Economic Ornithology and Mammalogy the following year, was formed in the U.S. Department of Agriculture. The Division of Biological Survey was developed in 1896 and became a bureau in 1905. The bureau proposed three areas of study: the effects of birds on agricultural production, the distribution of birds in the western states, and the migration of birds and associated problems.

The first topic to be addressed was the effect of the house sparrow on agriculture. This bird, introduced in 1873, spread throughout the United States. When the ornithological division was first formed, the first ornithologist was C. Art Miriam, a physician. A distinguished scholar, he was known for Miriam's "life zones," which categorized the effect of temperature on the distribution of living organisms based on latitude and altitude, and for the biological survey from Alaska to Baja California, Mexico.

The Lacey Act of 1900 prohibited interstate movement of illegally taken game and regulated avian and mammalian importation. It also established the concept of avian reserves and the difference between game and nongame species.

In 1910 a massive die-off of hundreds of thousands of ducks in Utah and California was attributed to "western duck disease." The problem recurred in 1912. Zoologist Alexander Wetmore in 1914 and 1915 thought that at least two entities were involved in the disease. One entity was identified as *"alkali disease"* because of the alkali salts around western lakes. Wetmore, who focused on mineral toxicology, also proved experimentally that birds died of lead poisoning after eating lead shot. A pioneering avian pathologist, he observed the resulting tissue lesions as streaks on the heart muscle, which were not identified to be infarcts until 1970. He described the characteristic signs of lead poisoning in animals as a function of time and the duration of survival of birds. If placed on a regimen of clean water that was free of lead, the animals recovered. Wetmore became the secretary of the Smithsonian Museum and a great authority on birds, publishing *Birds of Panama* (four volumes) and birds of New Guinea. Cases of lead poisoning in waterfowl in Utah were confirmed in 1919. In 1927 a breakthrough occurred in the study of western duck disease when a gull was poisoned by food. By 1931 Kalmbach had confirmed that the disease was attributable to type C botulism.

Prairie dogs were poisoned in 1905, and a terrifying outbreak of rabies in coyotes occurred in the Great Basin of Nevada, Idaho, Oregon, and California in 1915 and 1916. The National Parks Service did not hire a veterinarian until after 1990.

The illegal capture, export, and import of wild specimens, especially ornamental and song birds, for the pet trade is particularly destructive. It is estimated that more than twenty million specimens a year are sold, and many more die in the trapping, holding, and shipping stages. Cage bird medicine has become a significant specialty within veterinary medicine. Although such birds are susceptible to a range of diseases similar to those of domestic birds, special knowledge and appropriate equipment and techniques are necessary to examine, diagnose, and treat them.

Wild birds can be important reservoirs of viral diseases that can infect poultry, such as the viruses of Newcastle disease, avian influenza, and duck plague. *Chlamydia* is the new name for the tiny intracellular bacteria that cause psittacosis and ornithosis. These agents are infective to humans as well as poultry; hence the conditions they cause constitute serious zoonotic diseases. Aspergillosis is a serious fungal disease that affects the respiratory tract and liver of birds. One of the most successful veterinary roles in wild bird conservation involves the management of species of raptor birds, including the American symbol, the bald eagle.

EXPLOITATION OF MARINE MAMMALS AND FISH

Marine mammals of the order Pinnipedia—the seals, sea lions, walruses, and sea elephants—have been put in jeopardy by intense hunting. Massive harvests of fur seals were taken by the Russians in the Pribilof Islands between 1786 and 1834. The decline in numbers resulted in restrictions that allowed rebuilding of the stocks to several million by 1867. The American hunting period began in 1870 with the leasing of sealing rights for twenty years. By 1890 two million seals had been harvested on the islands. The seals were also hunted recklessly at sea, and restrictions had to be implemented again. Hunting for seal pelts was big business but it always seemed to become excessive. The Orca or killer whales also take a large number of fur seals.

The Guadalupe fur seal, once abundant off the California coast, received similar treatment of overharvesting. The Newfoundland harp seal was hunted initially for its blubber, but the pelts, especially those of the newborn pups, then became more valuable. In the modern era a public outcry was orchestrated against the harvesting of the baby seals on the ice floes of the estuary of the St. Lawrence River. Some European countries placed trading sanctions on seal pelts and fish sales from Canada. Harry Rowsell, a veterinarian from the Canadian Council on Animal Care, was asked to report on the industry and to conduct an on-site inspection during the seasonal kill.

There has been a tremendous boom in the keeping of ornamental fish in aquaria. This requires mastery of the aquatic environment and knowledge of breeding myriad species. When diseases occur, veterinary knowledge is needed; thus a new area of specialization has opened up for the profession.

EMERGING DISEASES AND THE ENDANGERMENT OF WILDLIFE

A lethal disease appeared in seals in Siberia in 1987 and in northwestern Europe in 1988. The cause of the deaths was traced by scientists in the Netherlands to morbilliviruses that were shown to affect pinnipeds and cetaceans. This category of viruses includes those that cause measles in humans, rinderpest in cattle, peste de petits ruminants in sheep and goats, and canine distemper in dogs. The deaths of Baikal seals in Lake Baikal were thought to result from phocid distemper, since the virus resembled that of canine distemper. The devastating European outbreak, caused by a different strain of virus, killed an estimated seventeen thousand harbor seals. Other seal species were infected, but their mortality rate was low. Harbor porpoises stranded on the Irish coast in 1988 were suspected of having had a morbillivirus infection. More than a thousand Mediterranean striped dolphins died of morbillivirus in 1990 and 1991.

Among land animals, recent deaths in wild lions have been attributed to newly appearing strains of morbillivirus. Previously the Felidae had not been known to be susceptible to viruses in this group. Since vaccines can be prepared against morbillivirus infections, a new vista, the vaccination of wildlife, has emerged in response to the new virus strains.

IMMOBILIZATION OF GAME FOR STUDIES AND TRANSLOCATION

Antonie M. Harthoorn was born in England and graduated from the Royal Veterinary College after his education had been interrupted by several years of service in the army in World War II. He became interested in the effects of stress, trauma, shock, and surgery on the circulatory system and traveled to Utrecht and Hannover to pursue this interest. He worked in physiology and pharmacology, later completing a doctoral program in these fields in London. He joined the veterinary faculty at the University of East Africa, first in Kampala, Uganda, and then in Nairobi, Kenya. After developing courses for veterinary students, he turned to his real avocation—studying the ecology of large African mammals—with a goal of learning enough to protect them. He became a vegetarian.

Harthoorn decided to conduct field studies of large African game mammals and was interested in developing a pharmacological method to immobilize them so that samples could be taken and antidotes administered and the animal would then be able to get up and walk away with no ill effects. Studies were initiated in the Semliki area of Uganda. Harthoorn was joined in this undertaking by his counterpart in the medical faculty, Cecil Luck, and a Fulbright Fellow in wildlife management from Washington State University

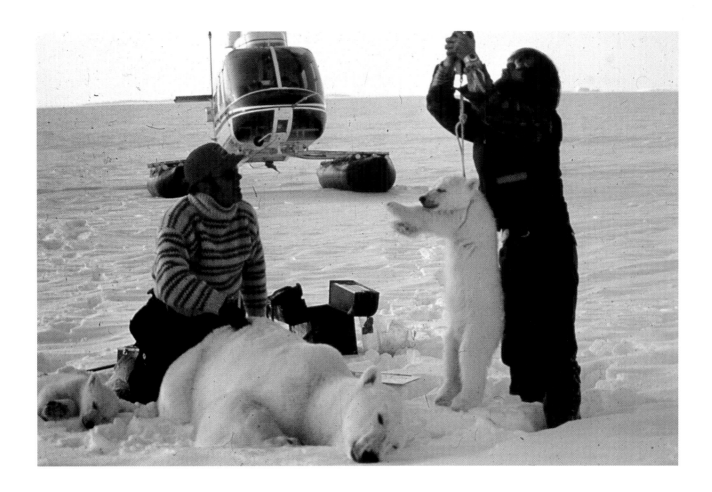

481. Veterinarian Antonie Marinus Harthoorn pioneered the development of potent pharmacological agents and combinations delivered by "flying syringes" to facilitate the safe capture of large wild animals. As head of physiology and biochemistry at the University of Nairobi, he was motivated by the goal of relocating endangered African species. He moved to the Transvaal Nature Conservation Division in Pretoria, South Africa. His techniques have been adopted in zoological population studies world wide. Here two veterinarians are participating in ecological field research on Baffin Island's polar bears, sponsored by the Canadian Wildlife Service and the Northwest Territorial Government. These studies address the efficacy and safety of anesthesia immobilization during drug capture and reversal, growth and development measurements, and seasonal migration patterns. Well-being and survival of both mother and cub are always a high priority; the cub is placed beside the mother's nose to minimize anxiety and to expedite resumption of normal behavior upon arousal. *(Courtesy Dr. Jerry Haigh, Saskatoon, Saskatchewan.)*

at Pullman, Helmut K. Buechner. Buechner brought a prototype of a pneumatic-powered gun that would project a syringe at animals to allow the injection of drugs into unrestrained animals from a distance. Harthoorn had been considering the possibility of incapacitating large mammals with a dart gun like that used with curare by native South American peoples, but the prospect did not seem feasible. He also had been conducting experiments with drugs in captive and domesticated mammals to determine whether the pharmacological goal of reversible paralysis was attainable. Buechner's "flying syringe" seemed the conceptual answer to delivery of a measured dose of the agent to the tissues of the animal. However, modifications were needed for use with large mammals over longer distances.

Harthoorn and his colleagues carried out experiments with bows and syringe-type arrows, including powerful steel hunting bows and Archer crossbows. The crossbows were more effective because they were more powerful and arrows were unnecessary. Another advantage of the bow was that it did not make a loud noise. Eventually the Capchur gun, powered by released carbon dioxide gas, was developed in the United States by the Palmer Chemical Company. The original projectile syringe was developed by J.A. Crockford in Georgia and was adapted for veterinary use by Frank Hayes. Harthoorn made further modifications so that it could be effective for use in large animals with thick hides.

Buechner's initial experiments with the use of nicotine sulfate in Uganda Kob antelope were not successful. The team developed a bow and syringe-arrow technique for use with the short-term muscle-paralyzing agent succinylcholine. After the drug was absorbed, the animal would lie down and be unable to rise. Helmut could mark his animal, and it would recover and be up grazing within about thirty minutes. He tagged fifty animals without a fatality.

Harthoorn faced a much greater challenge because of the size of his targets and his goal of relocating them to areas where they might be able to survive. He was able to hit hippopotami in the early dawn as they returned from grazing areas to their wallows. He also targeted some of the animals in shallow water, but he had to time a drive to get them back on land before they lost the ability to walk. Interestingly, the hippopotami that received succinylcholine did not lose the ability to swing their heads and necks or to chomp with their dangerous jaws.

Succinylcholine was less successful in the giraffe and African buffalo because the dosage had to be estimated and delivered accurately. Other drugs for which antidotes were available were tried, such as tubocurarine and gallamine triethiodide. Gallamine was used in the large elephant. Although onset of paralysis was slow, the paralysis was reversible with the use of prostigmine in a quarter of an hour. Its performance in the wild rhinoceros was unsatisfactory, and a new "cocktail" of drugs comprising a narcotic (morphine), a tranquilizer (phencyclidine), and a hypnotic (hyoscine) was developed. The breakthrough came in 1963 with the discovery of a new opiate derivative, M99, later called etorphine, with ten thousand times the effect of morphine. New tranquilizers were tried, and an effective combination requiring very low doses was selected. More than three hundred rhinoceros were captured by means of the tranquilizer, and Harthoorn's goal of being able to ensure the survival of species by relocating them to safer parks became attainable. Etorphine, xylazine, and hyaluronidase and more effective antidotes have been used recently to hasten induction of paralysis and help ensure survival. Harthoorn summarized the result of his chemical immobilization studies in *The Chemical Capture of Animals* in 1976.

PROGRESS IN WILDLIFE PREDATION AND RABIES CONTROL

Predator-prey dynamics have fascinated ecologists for a long time, but where wild predators and livestock interact, the threat of stock losses becomes a dominant chord. In North America the coyote has a bad reputation with sheep farmers. Today some farmers use llamas to protect their flocks. In Eurasia wolves and brown bears take adult sheep and goats; frequently wolves take the young of equids and of cattle, too, although cows exhibit vigorous antipredator behavior.

Feral dogs and cats can become a menace to native species and have caused extinctions of native species when introduced to islands. Feralization is a process in which individual animals become desocialized and learn to fend for themselves. When these animals breed, the young do not become bonded to humans and are essentially wild, although they may learn how to use foods or wastes derived from human habitation. In Australia feral cats seem to grow larger and are a real threat to native mammals, birds, and other fauna. Feral dogs form packs and hunt species of food animals. Feral pigs are extremely destructive to the environment and multiply rapidly. A strong capsule containing cyanide that only pigs' jaws are strong enough to crush has been developed in Australia. Veterinary specialists have become involved in the problem of feral animal control.

Although in Western Europe and North America most dogs are well-kept and vaccinated against rabies, there is still a surplus puppy problem. The situation in other parts of the world is often quite different. In large regions of Asia dogs receive little supervision and tend to multiply. In some regions there is a vague community responsibility for them rather than direct ownership. Staggering population densities can occur: one estimate for southwestern Sri Lanka yielded a result of three thousand dogs per square kilometer. Venereal infection with *Brucella canis* appears to help contain further population expansion. In such areas the dog may become the reservoir species for the rabies virus. Several hundred people die of rabies annually after dog bites. Some people still resort to traditional medicine instead of the Pasteur vaccine for treatment.

Despite the preponderant Muslim religion in North Africa, especially in the Maghreb region, most rural families tend to keep dogs, and ownerless dogs, too, are common. Rabies has been a real concern, and mass vaccination campaigns have been conducted. In Nepal, where ninety-five percent of the people live in rural areas, the French charitable organization Vétérinaires sans Frontières sponsored a remarkably successful vaccination campaign in the city of Lalitpur, reaching about seventy-five percent of the urban dogs. It is much more difficult to achieve control in rural areas.

It has been estimated that there are more than half a billion dogs in the world. About three and a half million people a year are given postexposure treatment to prevent rabies, mostly after dog bites. Nonetheless, about 35,000 people die of dog-transmitted rabies each year, most of them in developing countries.

Vampire bats in South and Central America and Trinidad can carry the rabies virus. Although insectivorous bats elsewhere occasionally carry the virus and have been known to infect people, the hematophagous vampire bat is a much more dangerous beast. It has a preference for cattle blood. Epidemics of rabies in cattle in Mexico were reported by Piso in 1658, although the nature of the disease was not confirmed until between 1908 and 1911. It is estimated that more than a million cattle die of paralytic rabies in Central and South America each year. Human blood was found in the stomachs of vampire bats in Mexico, which indicates that a serious hazard exists.

An epidemic of paralytic human rabies in Trinidad was mistakenly diagnosed as poliomyelitis in 1927 because the patients had no history of bites. J.L. Pawan in Trinidad in 1936 first showed that in humans who were bitten by vampire bats paresthesias developed at the site of the bite and that excitability, paralysis, and death followed. The bats were shown to be infected with the rabies virus, and although most of them died, some survived. Thus it was established that the vampire bat was unique because some of the bats could be carriers. The epidemic took nearly a hundred human lives and did not recur, so unanswered questions remain.

In Western Europe the reservoir species for the rabies virus is the red fox. In Switzerland a rabies vaccine for foxes has been developed for oral intake in bait. This vaccine has been quite effective, and the method is being used in several European countries and has been initiated in Eastern Europe. In North America the reservoir species group in the Midwest is the skunk, and in the Southeast, the raccoon. The raccoon, however, has migrated north and has brought the virus with it to New England. In 1994 in a trial conducted at the Tufts University School of Veterinary Medicine a genetically engineered rabies vaccine composed of oral vaccinia-rabies glycoprotein and designed for wild raccoons was distributed in fishmeal baits along the Cape Cod Canal to create a vaccine barrier. Almost all the baits were taken within a week, three quarters of them by raccoons. Although rabies in raccoons is widespread in Massachusetts and is causing concern among cat owners, it has not been reported south of the canal. An initial trial was conducted earlier in an unpopulated part of New Jersey.

VETERINARY ZOOTOXICOLOGY COMES OF AGE

Poisonous, sometimes lethal, bites and stings of venomous animals have always been a source of human fascination and fear. For example, the story of Cleopatra's suicide, in which she used an asp, *Cerastes vipera*, to bite her arm, has captured the imagination. The veterinary practitioner is in a particularly difficult diagnostic situation when the recipient of the venom is a vertebrate animal that cannot recount the event of the strike. Making matters even worse, there has been no comprehensive coverage of poisonous bites and stings in books in English. Roger Caras wrote a valuable introduction to the general subject, *Venomous Animals of the World,* in 1974 from the viewpoints of scientific knowledge and public interest. Recently Murray E. Fowler has provided the veterinary perspective in his *Veterinary Zootoxicology* (1993), which emphasizes clinical management of animal victims of envenomation. Fowler provides an invaluable global perspective of both the terrestrial and marine organisms, vertebrate and invertebrate, that are equipped to deliver toxic substances to other animals, and he addresses the difficulties of diagnosis and treatment.

The books previously mentioned draw from a large body of knowledge about the dangerous species and their biology, and the authors review important advances of the last few decades in the study of the specific ingredients of the venoms and their detrimental effects on animals and humans. Only a small number of biologists have participated deeply in field studies of venomous animals. Some of them have carried out the in-depth studies that are needed to collect venom and make it available to research laboratories and for antivenin production. One of the most famous laboratories for antivenin production is the Butantan Institute, which was initiated and organized under the brilliant, tenacious leadership of Vital Brazil in 1899 at the veterinary school at the University of São Paulo, Brazil. The institute collected and solicited collections of venomous snakes from all over Latin America and prepared antivenins that were distributed to the farms and plantations where workers were at risk. Similar approaches have been developed on other continents where the risk of snakebite envenomation is high.

482. Painter Jose S. Perez (born 1929) has special affection for animals of every kind. This fondness and fascination led him to create this unique piece of art honoring the veterinarian. His idealized veterinarian is shown completely integrated in the animal world, attracting the empathy, curiosity, and trust of all the many species represented, except his immediate patient. The veterinarian is seated at the base of a tree, surrounded by a great variety of mammals and birds, wild and tame, including even an invertebrate snail. His patient is a young orangutan who is very unhappy, bawling as he clutches onto the veterinarian's pants during the procedure to remove a splinter. Perez has created a vivid scene that catches the mood and the focusing of each animal's attention. The veterinarian, a regular "Dr. Doolittle," looks as concerned, knowledgeable, and wise as a doctor in *All Creatures Great and Small*. (From Perez on Medicine, *W.R.S. Publishing, Waco, Texas.*)

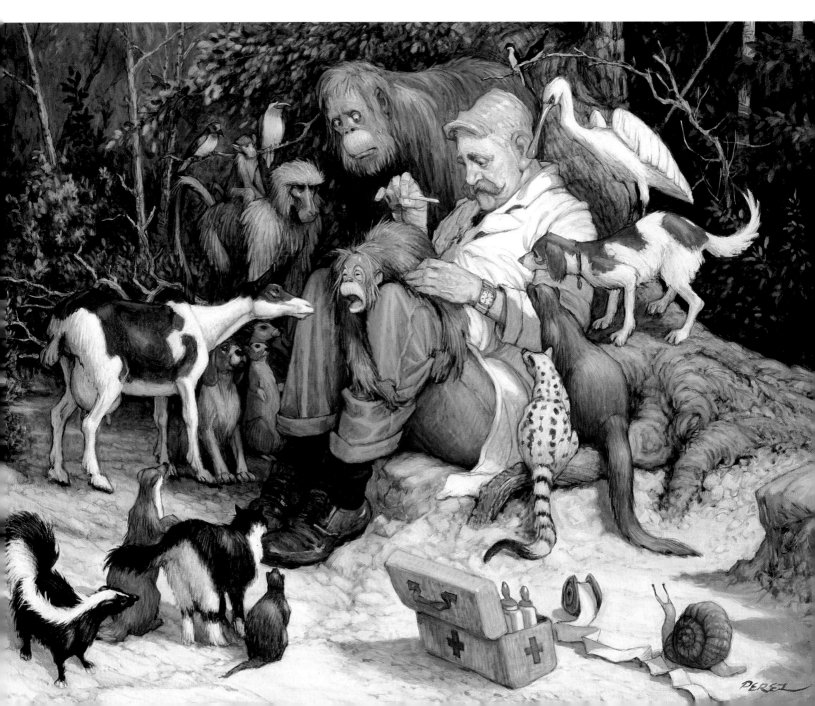

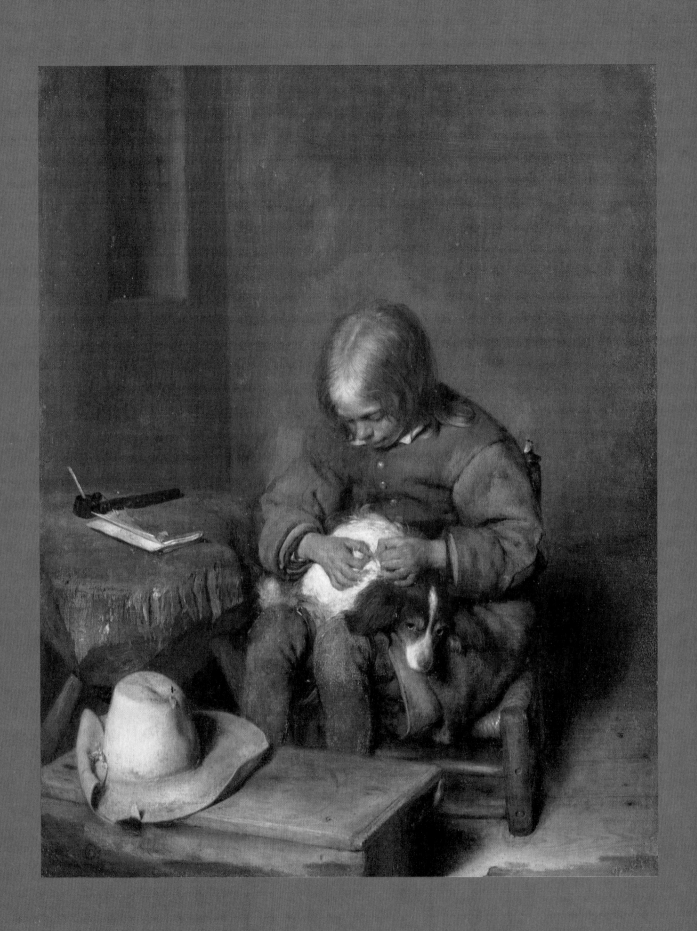

Companion Animal Medicine

ROOTS OF THE BOND WITH COMPANION ANIMALS

The two species of animals that evolved into the first familial pets or companions were both carnivores, which can be attributed to their larger, more complex brains relative to body size. Successful predation of other animal species required considerable intellectual capability, as well as its application in the hunt itself. The earliest domesticate was almost certainly the dog. Human adoption of captured wild cubs (wolf pups) may have been the first step in taming, or attraction to the odors of meat, raw or cooking, or food refuse may have been the magnet that drew the wild carnivores to the campsites. At some point a relationship was established in which each side had something of value to offer the other. The dog became a servant in the hunt and a guard; dogs were useful for traction, for herding, even for warmth in northern climes, and progressively, for recreation and companionship.

The earliest groups to be exploited must have been tamed from wild populations of wolves, of which several species exist. By the time of the earliest urban civilizations several specific roles had been established, with conformations and behaviors to match the roles. Thus the early fleet-footed sight hounds such as the Afghan and various types of greyhound were developed in West Asia and Egypt. At about the same time the mastiff types—the dogs of war—hunting dangerous game and guarding, appeared in Mesopotamian works of art. Evidence from Egyptian tomb art shows that spaniel and hound types were available to assist in the hunt of smaller mammals and birds. Cats, too, were used in Egypt for this purpose, especially for hunting wild fowl and other birds; they also helped control the rodent population. Small toy-breed types also emerged early; clearly the human craving for companionship has existed for a long time. When the dog was first used for traction of sleighs and travois is not known. Herding-dog types emerged after the hunting instincts were converted to shepherding and rounding-up behaviors. A wide spectrum of specialized pet breeds emerged much more recently, in the past two hundred years.

THE LEGACY OF DELABERE BLAINE

London-born Delabere Blaine (1770-1845) was apprenticed to a Buckinghamshire surgeon for seven years, then attended the medical school at the Borough Hospital under Dr. Haighton, a physician who was working on neurophysiology in the dog. Blaine became a fine anatomical artist and depicted the results of Haighton's experiments on transection of nerves to relieve pain. During the same period the London veterinary school opened. When the principal, Sainbel, needed an assistant and an anatomical demonstrator, he appointed Blaine, who taught anatomy, physiology, and pathology and translated

483. *Facing page,* Undoubtedly, the dog was the first domesticated animal. Dogs, used for hunting, guarding, herding, recreation, and especially companionship, have been "man's best friend" since earliest times. The Dutch painter Geraert Terborch, or Gerard ter Borch (1617-1681), specialized in portraits and genre scenes like this oil painting, *Ein Knabe Floht Seinem Hund.* A boy is carefully examining his dog for fleas while the dog sits impassively on his lap. Such scenes by Terborch demonstrate his elegant, subtle use of color and texture in his personal style of depicting familial tranquility. In this particular painting the boy's implied affection for his dog only heightens this warm feeling, and we are reminded of the power of the human-animal bond. *(Artothek.)*

484. Delabere Blaine (1770-1845) is a classic study in contrasting personalities. Never a qualified veterinarian throughout his remarkable career, he was, however, the first to concentrate on canine diseases, leading directly to the development of this specialty. Originally an anatomical artist, Blaine studied briefly with Sainbel, the first principal of the newly opened London veterinary school. After a brief stint as a surgeon with the horse artillery, Blaine built a highly successful veterinary practice, specializing in the treatment of dogs. Blaine wrote and illustrated several books, including *A Concise Description of the Distemper in Dogs: With an Account of the Discovery of an Efficacious Remedy for It,* first published in London in 1800. The book was popular with the public and went through several editions, with Blaine making additions to each. However, his alleged quackery guaranteed his shunning by the veterinary profession, including the Royal Veterinary College, which denied him the diploma he felt he deserved. Despite his success, Blaine's place in the history of his profession is flawed by his mercenary nature, perhaps best displayed in his hawking of remedies he knew to be worthless. *(The Science Museum/Science & Society Picture Library, London.)*

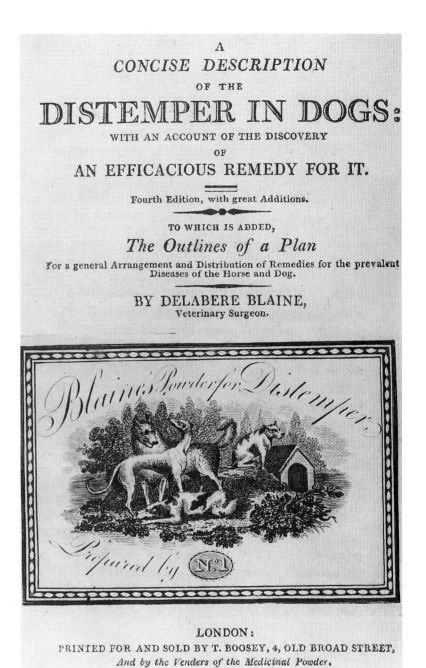

A
CONCISE DESCRIPTION
OF THE
DISTEMPER IN DOGS:
WITH AN ACCOUNT OF THE DISCOVERY
OF
AN EFFICACIOUS REMEDY FOR IT.

Fourth Edition, with great Additions.

TO WHICH IS ADDED,
The Outlines of a Plan
For a general Arrangement and Distribution of Remedies for the prevalent Diseases of the Horse and Dog.

BY DELABERE BLAINE,
Veterinary Surgeon.

LONDON:
PRINTED FOR AND SOLD BY T. BOOSEY, 4, OLD BROAD STREET,
And by the Venders of the Medicinal Powder.
1806.

Sainbel's lectures into English in his spare time. A promising beginning ended when Sainbel terminated Blaine's appointment, perhaps because Blaine appeared the more competent and knowledgeable to the students.

Blaine moved to Lewes, Sussex, where he established a veterinary practice that attracted those whose animals, in particular, dogs, were not attended to by farriers. He conducted experiments and claimed to have found an effective remedy for canine distemper. Because he failed to make ends meet, he had to close his practice. He reverted to the practice of surgery and was appointed assistant surgeon with the horse artillery. He gained not only human surgical experience but also, since he was responsible for all sick horses, further veterinary experience.

Blaine did not adapt well to military life and resigned to take up the practice of surgery in London. He spent his considerable spare time writing a book on *The Anatomy of the Horse* (1799) and making drawings for it that were poorly colored in the printed book. His experience as a dissector was evident: even the clitoral sinuses were described. His acquaintance with the scholarly literature of comparative anatomy and physiology enriched the text. Blaine's fortunes changed for the better when he inherited an estate in Essex and for a short period became a sporting aristocrat with horses and dogs. He then rejoined the army and served during combat in Ireland and Holland; at the end of 1799 he resigned again, retiring to Northumberland to enjoy the sporting life and to write.

In 1800 Blaine published *A Concise Description of the Distemper in Dogs, With an Account of the Discovery of an Efficacious Remedy for It*. Because the disease was dreaded, the book quickly went through several editions, but it was an unworthy promotion of his treatment. The public was fooled to such an extent that he was consulted widely, and he decided to reenter practice, specializing in the care of dogs and horses. He returned to London and published more books, including *A Domestic Treatise on the Diseases of Horses and Dogs* and *The Outlines of the Veterinary Art* (1802), which addressed the diseases of the horse and dog. He advertised himself as "Professor of Animal Medicine," an invalid title because he was neither a qualified veterinarian nor a professor at the time. Nevertheless, his practice was a success and outgrew its original premises. His alleged quackery and unwarranted self-assurance alienated him from the veterinary profession, including the Royal Veterinary College (RVC) and Coleman, its principal, and prevented him from receiving the diploma from the college that he felt he deserved, having been a founding teacher there. Although Blaine was the leading canine veterinarian, Coleman shunned him, and it is unlikely that he would have signed a graduation diploma for Blaine.

The successful Blaine practice took on a partner about 1812, the remarkable William Youatt. Probably the two best veterinary intellects in London at the time, they made a formidable team. The practice, veterinary historian F. Smith estimated, saw two to three thousand canine cases per year and quite a few horses. At the age of forty-six, Blaine retired from practice. He was offered but declined the directorship of the St. Petersburg veterinary school in Russia. In 1817 he published *Canine Pathology,* which Smith rated to be outstanding. Blaine employed the experimental method, even in his practice cases, and advised others to do the same but not to talk about it. He considered it essential to conduct postmortem examinations and was an authority on rabies. According to Blaine, "No dog has rabies but such as have been bitten; nothing short of the actual bite can produce it." Yet Principal Coleman continued to preach his faith in the spontaneous generation of the disease.

Blaine's knowledge of the drugs then available for clinical use was based on his scholarship and experience. His works on equine medicine were considered inferior to his trailblazing works on the dog. In both cases their strongest point was his awareness of gross pathology gleaned from postmortem examinations. This awareness was particularly valuable in the diagnosis of colic, which led to a growing competence in gastroenterology in the veterinary profession. He became convinced that glanders was contagious. He claimed a special competence in foot diseases, which Smith doubted, and in the treatment of laminitis or founder.

In 1832, long after Blaine retired from practice, he wrote a fourth edition of his *Outline of the Veterinary Art*. Reflecting the progress that had been made in veterinary clinical medicine in thirty years, it was a vast improvement over the earlier, disappointing efforts. Blaine's appetite for knowledge was enormous. He read every veterinary work in English and continental languages and had an aptitude for history and illustration. After retirement he wrote *An Encyclopedia of Rural Sports,* a huge work. Engraved on his burial vault at Newport on the Isle of Wight is the following: "Distinguished by the improvements he effected in the Veterinary Art." His weak point was his mercenary nature; in the brazen manner of a patent medicine salesman he advertised some remedies as efficacious that he must have known to be, in the main, worthless. His legacy to his profession stems from his being virtually the first to focus on diseases of the dog and to develop on a large scale the market in canine medicine, an area in which the demand for veterinary skills was destined to become the greatest in the second half of the twentieth century.

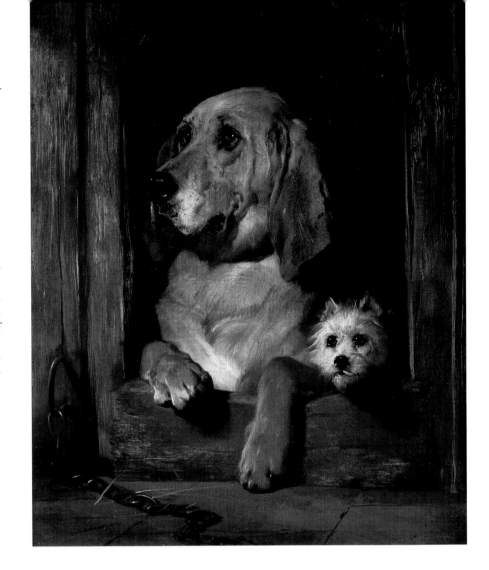

485. Sir Edwin Henry Landseer (1802-1873) is recognized as a gifted painter of animals. Many consider this painting, *Dignity and Impudence* (1839), his best work. Jacob Bell owned the dogs and commissioned the painting. What makes this particular Landseer painting so compelling, in addition to the great skill in putting brush and paint to canvas, lies in the contrasts Landseer has built into its composition. Grafton, the noble bloodhound, has been captured in perfect repose, his massive paws lending to this dignified stature. Scratch, the Scottish terrier whose eyes betray the dog's anxiety, is in perfect contrast to the pose of the bloodhound. Also, the disparity in size of the two breeds is apparent by the nestling of Scratch's head on Grafton's left forelimb. Landseer was criticized by some for imparting human characteristics to his animals. *(Tate Gallery, London; Art Resource, New York.)*

THE AMAZING YOUATT: REINVENTION OF THE PROFESSION

William Youatt (1776-1847) left the Nonconformist ministry and a school headship to become a veterinary surgeon at the mature age of thirty-seven. He began as an apprentice in Delabere Blaine's practice in London in 1813. Blaine urged him to avoid Blaine's own error and enroll in the RVC to obtain a qualification. The unscrupulous Principal Coleman, however, persecuted Youatt mercilessly after he enrolled and eventually succeeded in driving him out without a diploma. Youatt went into partnership with Blaine until the latter's retirement and waited until after Coleman's death in 1839 before finally arranging to take his diploma from the London college. He finally received it in 1844, three years before he died.

Youatt was extremely enthusiastic and strove to build the credibility and image of the profession. He shared Blaine's love of dogs; they became his strongest area of interest. He also wanted to become a "vet for all species," however, and he developed his knowledge in all areas. He hoped to convince the RVC to accept that it should teach the diseases of all domestic animals, not just those of the horse.

Like his predecessor and later partner Blaine, Youatt took a special interest in rabies. Both men were far ahead of Coleman and most of the medical profession in their conception of the disease. Before them, Bardsley in 1793 had been ahead of his time in insisting that rabies was a contagious disease. Youatt built his knowledge through reading, working at the British Museum, and writing on veterinary matters. He had a strong interest in livestock agriculture. He joined the Royal Agricultural Society of England in 1838, the year it was founded, and was appointed to the council. He is believed to have been responsible for the insertion of a clause in the society's charter giving it power to improve the veterinary art in its application to cattle, sheep, and pigs.

Working through the council, Youatt formed a subcommittee "For the Improvement of the Veterinary Art" with himself as chairman and several leading faculty members of the London school as members. Coleman, however, manipulated the outcome, first supporting recommendations in the subcommittee to expand the curriculum to encompass the food-animal species, then opposing them in the college, where he knew he could count on the support of his board of governors. Nonetheless, the society persisted in its goal of adding cattle pathology to the curriculum of the veterinary college for four years. Finally the governors gave in but would not hire a specialist, so the deputy principal had to teach the course. After Coleman died, Sewell, too, tried to prevent change, but eventually a specialist in the field was appointed, with funding from the Agricultural Society.

Youatt is distinguished by his many contributions to the logical development of the veterinary profession in Great Britain. He also published a series of books, one on each of the major domestic species, blazing the trail for broadening the profession's role in society, particularly in agriculture. He edited the important periodical *The Veterinarian,* which became a major force in the evolution of the profession. It was founded in 1828 by William Percivall, another great reformer of the profession, who served as veterinary surgeon to the Life Guards.

It is extraordinary that neither Blaine nor Youatt, two of the most influential men in the early stages of the evolution of the veterinary profession in England, was considered a graduate or a licensed veterinary surgeon throughout most of the productive years of his association with the profession.

EARLY FOCUS ON EXTERNALLY ACCESSIBLE CONDITIONS

After the work of pioneers Blaine and Youatt, the great innovator and humanitarian Edward Mayhew (died 1868) left his mark with his early experiments on the use of ether anesthesia in dogs and cats. His many contributions to companion animal medicine included the use of the urinary catheter in both male dogs and bitches, which contradicted the current dogma that the os penis prevented its passage in the male. He also advanced techniques for canine obstetrics. He revised Blaine's book, *The Outlines of the Veterinary Art,* and wrote others on the management and treatment of dogs.

John W. Hill, Fellow of the Royal College of Veterinary Surgeons (FRCVS), of Wolverhampton wrote an illustrated text, *The Management and Diseases of the Dog,* in 1878. He observed that in those days the medical care of dogs was frequently entrusted to the care of the individuals who professed knowledge of subjects of which they were on all scientific points totally ignorant. His illustrations included drawings of a severe case of rickets and of the front teeth of dogs in various stages of growth and decay. Henry Gray (1865-1939) graduated from the RVC in 1885 and specialized in small animal practice. A prolific author and reviewer of texts, he performed an invaluable service by translating Eugene Nicholas's French text of 1914, *Ophtalmologie Vétérinaire et Comparée,* into English. This translation was the first specialized publication on veterinary ophthalmology in English.

Exciting veterinary developments on the Continent began in Vienna when the physician and veterinarian Hugo Schindelka took charge of the canine clinic from 1893 to 1911. He had studied under the renowned professors of the second Viennese medical school. He introduced "grand" clinical lectures accompanied by demonstration of clinical cases. An outstanding diagnostician, he was the founder of veterinary dermatology. His work established a Viennese tradition of excellence in that field, which led, via David

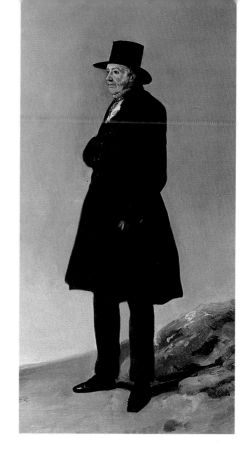

486. William Youatt (1776-1847), like Delabere Blaine, was not considered a graduate or a licensed veterinary surgeon throughout most of his highly productive career. After briefly apprenticing in Blaine's London practice, and approaching forty years of age, Youatt enrolled in the Royal Veterinary College only to be driven out without a diploma. Although he developed his knowledge in all areas of veterinary medicine, he shared Blaine's strong interest in dogs and was well in front of the medical profession of his time in his understanding of rabies. He was a prolific writer, publishing books on each of the major domestic species. Youatt also edited *The Veterinarian,* a journal that became a major force in the evolution of the veterinary profession. He was finally awarded his diploma in 1844, three years before his death. *(By the Kind Permission of The Royal Agricultural Society of England.)*

Wirth, who built the Vienna Small Animal Clinic in 1932, to Kral, who brought this speciality field to America via the University of Pennsylvania. Also in Vienna, a great tradition in veterinary ophthalmology began with Joseph Bayer, author of *Augenheilkunde (Ophthalmology).* A medal in his honor recognizes veterinary ophthalmologists of unusual proficiency. Similarly Rudolf Berlin began a tradition in this comparative field at the Stuttgart Veterinary College in 1875, although the college closed in 1893. Excellence in ophthalmology in the Utrecht veterinary school in the Netherlands derived from the work of Heinrich Jacob, a Munich graduate appointed to head the Small Animal Clinic in 1911. He wrote a major text in the field in 1920.

Canine dentistry had a surprisingly slow start in the second half of the nineteenth century. George Fleming, writing on *Rabies and Hydrophobia* in 1872, illustrated a technique of cutting off the tips of the canines and incisors, then filing them, which he claimed would prevent the spread of rabies. False teeth were fitted in an old collie in 1897. Real progress, however, was not made in oral medicine on the dog until Hobday.

EUROPEAN LEADERSHIP IN CANINE INTERNAL MEDICINE

As a precursor to canine and feline internal medicine, vast knowledge of physiology and of the genesis of the dysfunctions that result in pathology was required. Since dogs and cats were only late accorded a priority in investigation for their own sakes, progress in understanding their diseases was acquired indirectly via research directed toward human needs.

Physiological investigation of digestion and metabolism was conducted in the dog by the Dutch physician Regnier de Graaf (1641-1673). He, along with Swammerdam, was an ardent supporter of the comparative philosophy of medical research. In 1664 de Graaf reported on studies involving continuous collection of canine salivary and pancreatic juices via fistulas leading outward from their ducts. More than two centuries elapsed, however, before J.

487. Scientific progress in companion animal medicine in the nineteenth century awaited the development of veterinary pathology, microbiology, and immunology, but the battle against parasites was being waged in the trenches, as this advertisement demonstrates. *Buchan's Carbolic Disinfecting Soap No. 11, The Best Dog Soap in the World* was reputed to "kill all parasitic life on man or beast." In this color chromolithograph it is difficult to determine who is enjoying this large dog's bath the most: the two children administering the scrubbing or the dog. *(National Library of Medicine, Bethesda, Maryland.)*

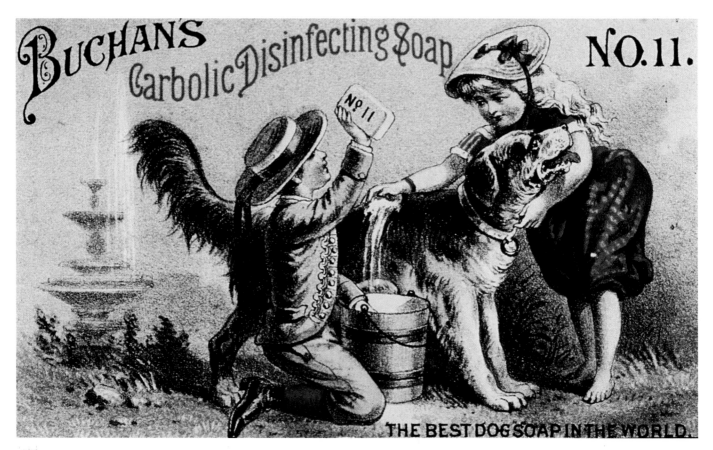

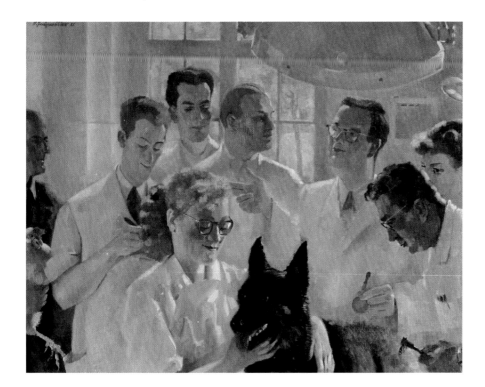

488. The portraits of professors of veterinary medicine, particularly from the school in Leipzig, and paintings of veterinarians working with farm animals are well known to the countrymen of German painter Conrad Felixmüller (1897-1977). *Clinic Lesson in Leipzig* is a striking example of his expressionism. Clinicians are examining a dog while students and the dog's owners look on, listening to an observation resulting from percussion and palpation. Careful history taking and physical examination were stressed in early European works on canine medicine. *(Courtesy Prof. Dr. Dr. h. c. mult. Schulze, Tierärztliche Hochschule Hannover.)*

von Mering and O. Minkowsky in Strassburg in 1889 showed that dogs could not live after complete surgical removal of the pancreas. It was noticed that their urine contained sugar, their stools became pale and greasy, and their livers showed fatty degeneration. They became excessively thirsty, drank copious amounts, and urinated frequently (diabetes). Since the urine was sweet the condition was named diabetes *mellitus (honeylike)*. It was concluded that the pancreas put out a factor that was necessary for the utilization of sugar by the tissues. The factor was shown to be absent from the duct secretion, yet to be produced by the gland even when the duct was tied off. Thus was endocrine secretion revealed and the stage set for a range of discoveries about digestion and intermediary metabolism, culminating in the famous experiment in dogs by Banting and Best in Toronto. That experiment led to the isolation of insulin from the beta cells of the islets of Langerhans, for which a Nobel Prize was awarded in 1923. There was a long interval before such physiological discoveries were applied effectively in cats and dogs.

Scientific progress in companion animal medicine had to await the development of veterinary pathology and in the case of infectious diseases, the emergence of veterinary microbiology, immunology, and parasitology. Surprisingly the promising field of immunology was slow in focusing on the opportunities it presented in protecting pet animals, especially against viral diseases. The late appearance of the use of chemotherapy and antibiotics against bacteria, as well as truly effective, safe vaccines and anthelmintics as developed by the pharmaceutical and biologics industries, left the small animal clinician with few effective weapons against microbial annd parasitic infections until after World War II.

Early works on canine medicine stress careful history taking and physical examination. The dramatic progress in comparative pathology after Virchow and in microbiology in the second half of the nineteenth century led to remarkable advances in understanding the origins and causes of febrile conditions. After René Laënnec's great work on auscultation the stethoscope was developed and soon became the visible symbol of a practitioner of medicine or veterinary medicine. Improved mercury thermometers used to measure the intensity of fever provided the "other arm" to the clinician's repertoire of physical aids in the art of diagnosis. Percussion and palpation allowed manual and aural skills to be expanded. The adequacy of reflex activity was tested by pinching or pricking appropriate sites and by using rubberized mallets to check reflex tendon responses. When added to the spectrum of visual impressions, these techniques expanded the ability of veterinarians to define the physiological status of their patients.

Study of the development of detailed descriptive pathology and symptomatology allowed the clinician to acquire the art of differential diagnosis. Much effort was put into the idea of pathognomonic changes as a key to diagnosis of internal disorders. Thus each disease was considered to have its particular trademark of clinical signs that facilitated its recognition. Georg Müller, professor and director of the clinic for small animals at the veterinary school in Dresden, Germany, assembled his vast experience in a textbook, *Diseases of the Dog and Their Treatment,* just before the start of the twentieth century. Alexander Glass at the University of Pennsylvania acquired rights of translation and developed five English editions that were published in the United States in 1896, 1908, 1911, 1916, and 1926. The First World War virtually arrested progress in Europe, and the pendulum of progress in small animal medicine swung progressively toward Great Britain and North America after the war. Müller's work, arranged on a body-systems basis, was a remarkable achievement that demonstrated great progress in diagnosis and classification of diseases but also revealed the deplorable status of canine and feline therapeutics during the early decades of the twentieth century.

The most disheartening of canine diseases, because of its high mortality rate and lack of effective remedies or preventatives, was distemper. Distemper was recognized early to be a highly contagious disease that spread readily from

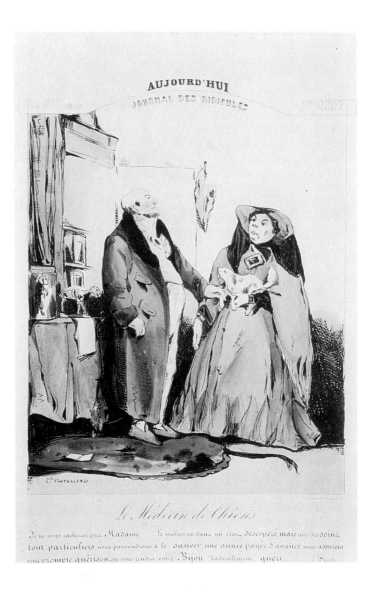

489. In this hand-colored lithograph by Camille Fontallard, *Le Médecin de Chiens,* published in *Aujourd' Hui, Journal des Ridicules* in 1839, a veterinarian is taking the pulse of a little dog in the arms of its owner. The veterinarian remarks, "I will not hide from you, Madam, this sick dog is in a hopeless state. But, with very particular care we will save him. A year's fee in advance would assure a quick cure and we will give back your 'Bijou' totally recovered." Veterinarians, like other professionals of their time, were not immune to being ridiculed by the public. *(National Library of Medicine, Bethesda, Maryland.)*

an infected animal to an animal in normal condition. For example, three spectacular outbreaks of distemper swept through the canine population of Greenland in 1888, 1889, and 1904 and caused extreme hardship by disrupting the sled transport on which the people depended. The disease also caused economic devastation when infection entered fur farms.

In areas densely populated by dogs, few young animals escaped the infection; the signs usually started to appear within a week of exposure. The first detectable change was a fever. The animal soon became anorexic, shivery, restless, depressed, and lacking in energy. The nose was hot and dry, the skin lost its elasticity, and the hair coat became dry and harsh. The manifestations included mucopurulent nasal and ocular discharges accompanied by a persistent cough; vomiting and mucopurulent diarrhea; pustules on the abdomen and inner thighs; and severe neurological disorders progressing to chorea and convulsions.

Despite many claims to have isolated and cultured specific causative bacterial agents, understanding of the nature of the disease did not become possible until Carré reported in 1905 that there was an ultrafilterable agent in nasal secretions of infected dogs that could reproduce the disease in experiments in dogs. The attempts to develop an effective vaccine against the virus at the Pasteur Institute were unsuccessful. The only hope was that the patient would recover by virtue of its own constitutional resistance aided by nursing care. Real progress was not made in development of an effective vaccine against canine distemper until the classic work of Patrick Laidlaw and G.W. Dunkin. Once this was accomplished, the owners' worries about loss of valued puppies were greatly reduced and veterinarians were able to focus on the wide range of other diseases that afflicted the canine species. The special case of rabies is addressed in Chapter 30.

Hoffer in 1850 described a disease in dogs that he labeled *dog typhus.* In 1898, almost fifty years later, Klett demonstrated that this canine plague of Stuttgart was caused by a microscopic bacterium. *Stuttgart disease* of dogs spread rapidly in Europe, and the mortality rate was high. Clinical signs included oral bleeding and ulceration. A spirochete organism was observed in the kidneys. Several species were isolated; in 1925 in England, Thomas Dalling and L.P. Pugh showed that *Leptospira icterohaemorrhagiae* caused jaundice and bleeding. Antiserum against the organism was prepared in horses and used in the treatment. McIntyre and Stuart in 1947 showed that another agent, *L. canicola,* caused the common, insidious canine disease, chronic nephritis.

AT LAST: THE BOON OF ANESTHESIA

The early days of veterinary surgical interventions, before the discovery of the anesthetic properties of certain substances, called for forceful restraint and considerable anguish for both humans and beasts. The goal of attaining a state of insensibility and relaxation in the patient before surgery had been sought throughout history. Application of the depressant and hypnotic properties of materials containing ethanol, opium, hemlock, mandrake, or hyoscyamine had been tried with varying degrees of partial efficacy and risk of serious side effects. As the chemical ingredients of natural or fermented products were purified, a wide range of almost pure chemicals became available for pharmacological study.

Eventually the following classes of substances were identified that had pain-preventing effects: inhalation anesthetics, agents that had a general effect after intravenous injections, and substances that paralyzed nerve trunks and local branches after being injected adjacent to them (local anesthetics). The three goals of anesthesia were insensibility, muscular relaxation, and safety. Achieving muscle relaxation was tricky because it was necessary to maintain respiration while the other muscles were being relaxed.

COMPANION ANIMAL MEDICINE

The new veterinary profession in London was ahead of the medical profession in trying the South American muscle-relaxing arrow poison, which contained curare, for possible therapeutic value. At the London veterinary college in 1835 William Sewell used it to treat a horse with tetanus, and alleviation of the locked jaw and other clinical signs was remarkable. However, its use required several hours of artificial respiration. The horse ate ravenously after its breathing was restored, but it died the next day of distention colic without recurrence of the tetanic signs. The enterprising William Youatt in 1838 tried curare in a rabid dog. The excited animal became still but continued to breathe, dying during the night. Youatt persisted with pharmacological experiments and used curare in demonstrations to the profession. Although he considered the drug promising, he had to resort to prolonged artificial respiration on occasion.

The great French physiologist Claude Bernard cautioned on humanitarian grounds against using curare as a substitute for anesthesia. He observed that the animal could become completely paralyzed but that feeling and consciousness, with a full capacity for suffering, persisted.

Opium was one of the few agents in the physician's bag that had a readily discernable effect against pain. Consequently it tended to be overused, with disastrous consequences of addiction and side effects. Elsholz induced hypnosis and analgesia in humans with intravenous transfer of a crude solution of opium in 1665. However, a series of deaths resulting from blood transfusions rendered use of the intravenous route unacceptable. Boerhaave administered opium to minimize the pain of surgery. Serturner isolated the active ingredient, morphine, in 1806. He demonstrated its painkilling action in the dog and on himself. Tragically he became an addict and died. Experiments with morphine continued after the development of the hypodermic syringe. Tabourin, a veterinarian in France, made an improved syringe in 1851, adding significantly to the tools available to the veterinary surgeon. Morphine in the dog induced vomiting and a soporific effect with some analgesia, but not true anesthesia. Morphine was found to be unsuitable in the cat, causing extreme pupillary dilation, apprehension, and excitement or terror.

Early experiments with ether were conducted by Paracelsus in the sixteenth century. He found that chickens would drink ether and become unconscious or fall asleep. Taken orally, ether acted as an anodyne in humans,

490. Early surgery. The use of anesthesia at Angell Memorial Hospital between 1935 and 1940 is shown. The medical profession benefited from veterinarians' early use of various substances for anesthetic properties. In 1835 William Sewell used curare to treat a horse with tetanus at the London veterinary college. The clinical manifestations of the condition were relieved, but the horse died of colic. Three years later William Youatt used curare on a rabid dog with mixed results. Opium, morphine, ether, and chloroform were all used on various species, the results ultimately contributing to the understanding and correct usage of these products. Pierre-Cyprien Oré advanced intravenous anesthesia by testing the action of chloral hydrate in animals in 1872, and its use was adopted by equine veterinarians throughout Europe at the end of the nineteenth century. Eventually barbital, sodium hexobarbital, pentobarbital, and sodium thiopental were developed and used during the first half of the twentieth century. *(Archives of the Massachusetts Society for the Prevention of Cruelty to Animals.)*

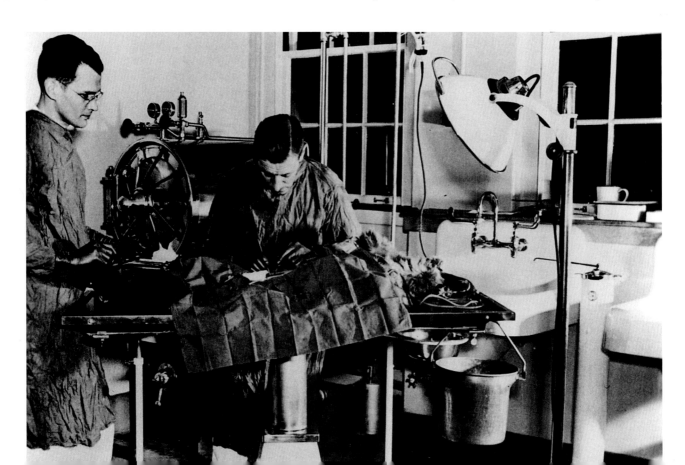

relieving pain and suffering. Much later, in 1847, Crawford in India was reported to have introduced ether vapor into the rectums of three dogs, which induced vomiting and incoordination with diminution of sensitivity.

Inhalation anesthesia was launched by Humphrey Davy, who showed that breathing Priestley's newly discovered gas, nitrous oxide, induced a state of euphoria and mirth and also relieved pain. In 1779 Davy reported placing a cat in a large jar containing nitrous oxide. The animal soon exhibited violent movements that ceased within two minutes, after which the cat lay quietly. After the cat was removed from the jar, there was a bounding pulse and the animal revived in a few minutes. Davy showed that the agent could be used safely as an anesthetic in animals and recommended its use during surgery. His proposal, however, was essentially ignored until 1844, when a dentist in Connecticut, Horace Wells, used it for painless extraction of one of his own teeth. After battling with the discoverers of the anesthetic effect of ether vapor for priority, Wells committed suicide. "Laughing gas" lapsed as an anesthetic until after the 1860s, when it again found application in dentistry; in 1868 it was tried in surgery. After a mixture of oxygen and nitrous oxide was introduced to reduce the risk of asphyxia during long operations, the mixture became popular in human obstetrics.

Henry Hickman, an English doctor with an experimental bent, found that carbon dioxide gas inhalation had an anesthetic affect on dogs in 1824. Carbon dioxide was considered unacceptable for human use by his peers because of disturbing side effects. Klemm in 1864 resurrected the idea and reported using it for anesthesia in cats, but his veterinary peers also found it unsuitable. It did not come into significant practical use as an anesthetic until its utilization in rendering swine insensible as they passed through a chamber before slaughter.

After the gases carbon dioxide and nitrous oxide failed to achieve acceptance as human or veterinary anesthetics in the first half of the nineteenth century, the field was open to a new class of agents: the volatile liquids whose vapors were sufficiently potent to induce anesthesia after inhalation. Michael Faraday showed that ether vapor had effects like those of nitrous oxide, which triggered a trend of "ether parties." During such a diversion an American doctor, Crawford Long of Jefferson, Georgia, observed that the participants felt no pain. He decided to test this effect in a patient in 1842 and successfully excised cysts from a boy's neck while the boy was under ether vapor–induced insensibility. Long did not publish this finding until 1849.

A former partner of Wells, William Thomas Morton opportunistically picked up where Wells had left off. He, too, was a dentist but also owned a plant that manufactured false teeth and was studying medicine. He consulted his chemistry professor, Charles Jackson, about an alternative to nitrous oxide. Jackson recommended diethyl ether as having a longer-lasting analgesic effect. Morton tested ether vapor on his pet spaniel, on himself, and then on one of his dental patients. He persuaded a surgeon to let him use ether on a patient during surgery for removal of a cervical tumor before an audience in 1846. Unlike his predecessor's attempt with nitrous oxide, the procedure with ether was successful. The business-minded Morton applied for a patent and added a dye to the colorless ether to give it color and a different odor, announcing the resulting product as a new anesthestic gas, *Letheon*. The surgeons, however, saw through his scheme and discredited him. It was even alleged by some of them that he might have been the cause of Wells's suicide.

Jackson disputed Morton's patent claim and had an article published attributing the discovery to himself. Jackson in 1853 published fabricated accounts of experiments on animals purported to have been performed as early as 1841 (to achieve precedence over Long's belated entry into the race) to substantiate his claim to be the discoverer of surgical anesthesia. A bitter fight ensued, but shortly thereafter the infuriated Morton died of a stroke. The title of inventor of surgical anesthesia was not to be won easily or yet rewarded: Jackson became an alcoholic and was committed to an insane asylum. Of particular interest, however, was his claim that a mixture of four or five parts of ether to one part of chloroform gave the best results in animals. Similar mixtures became popular in Europe, and it is not clear who deserves the credit. Jackson made the point that use of a mix of ether and chloroform was safer in animals that perspire than in those that do not, such as the cat. Dogs, which depend on panting for cooling, were considered more vulnerable than ruminants or horses. Jackson also stressed the importance of preventing anoxia by allowing air to mix with the vapor.

The discovery of chloroform in 1831 was followed by James Simpson's demonstration of its effectiveness as an anesthetic in 1847. He collaborated with a professor at the Glasgow veterinary school in testing it on domestic animals. Simpson was dissatisfied with the dependability and ease of induction with ether anesthesia and also was concerned because it was explosive. Chloroform gave faster, more effective induction than ether anesthesia but carried a greater risk of respiratory or cardiac arrest. Combinations of chloroform, ether, and ethanol became popular in Europe, whereas in North America use of preanesthetic medication with morphine before the administration of ether was preferred in the dog.

The veterinary profession moved quickly to adopt inhalation anesthesia as an aid to surgery. However, reaction soon set in against the technique after a series of fatal anesthetic accidents and negative publicity, including cautionary remarks in professional journals in Great Britain. As described earlier in this text, Mayhew tested ether and had it administered to himself during dental extraction to reassure himself that animals were not suffering during the excitement stage and were genuinely insensible during deep anesthesia for minor surgery. He showed that inhalation of pure ether rendered a cat unconscious in about ten seconds, a dog in fifteen to forty-five seconds. In cows a long period, more than fifteen minutes, was required to attain anesthesia by means of ether inhalation, but the anesthesia was effective, for example, in a case of amputation of a hind leg. In horses two or three minutes was required, and it was soon recognized that an admixture of oxygen or air with the vapor was necessary. Inhalers had to be developed.

The idea of local anesthesia developed through the recognition that cold (rubbing a part in snow or ice) led to numbness and loss of local pain sensation. This process was mimicked much later, when spraying ethyl chloride was found to have a rapid cooling effect. Carl Keller in 1884 discovered the anesthetic properties of cocaine for topical use in the eye. William Halstead, surgeon at the Johns Hopkins Medical School, realized at once the opportunity to inject it around nerves to achieve selective local or regional anesthesia. The goal was achieved, but because of experiments conducted on himself, Halstead became addicted to cocaine. In New York, Liautard injected ether, chloroform, and, later, cocaine in horses as aids to diagnosing the seat of lameness in horses.

The discovery of the nonaddictive synthetic agent procaine in 1904 was followed by its rapid adoption in clinical practice. Spinal anesthesia was tried but was considered too risky until veterinarians Retzgen in Berlin and Benesch in Vienna developed epidural anesthesia in 1925. Farquharson developed the paravertebral nerve block technique for standing surgery of the abdomen in cattle in 1940.

The goal of safe, effective intravenous anesthesia was approached by one small step with the synthesis of chloral hydrate. Pierre-Cyprien Oré discovered its anesthetic action in animals and then tested it in humans in 1872, but it was considered unsuitable because of its extended recovery period and questionable safety. The use of chloral hydrate was adopted by equine veterinarians, however, to depress and even partially anesthetize the horse when given orally, rectally, or intraperitoneally in facilitating brief surgical procedures like castration. In Belgium chloral hydrate was used intravenously in horses after 1908 as a general anesthetic, but the procedure was risky; nonetheless, such use was adopted elsewhere.

In 1903 the German genius of organic chemistry, Emil Fischer (1852-1919), among his myriad discoveries and syntheses (purines, amino acids and proteins, enzymes, and carbohydrates), synthesized diethylmalonyl urea, or *Veronal,* a stepping-stone hypnotic and sedative agent that led to the barbiturate series of intravenous anesthetics. He trained with Kekulé in Bonn and von Baeyer in Strassburg and Munich before taking professorships in Erlangen, Würzburg, and finally, Berlin, where he reached the full flowering of his creativity. After barbital the next step was sodium hexobarbital, an intravenous barbiturate anesthetic, in 1932, widely used for a time in human surgery. Auchterlonie used it in Britain for anesthesia in the dog. Pentobarbital and the shorter-acting sodium thiopental displaced barbital, and other derivatives were developed.

HOBDAY TRANSFORMS VETERINARY SURGERY AND PRACTICE

Frederick G.T. Hobday (1870-1932) of Burton-on-Trent graduated from the RVC in 1892. In recognition of his promising talents he was appointed by Principal McFadyean to be house surgeon. He worked as a *locum tenens* in several practices to gain experience and became a lecturer in materia medica and therapeutics, as well as in animal hygiene and dietetics. Ever zestful for experience, he worked in the free outpatient clinic for the poor. He studied the deployment of local and general anesthesia in animals and developed the "Hobdaying" operation for roarer horses, those suffering from a condition in which the vocal cords relax and partially occlude the airway, causing a roaring sound. Hobday used topical cocaine for eye surgery. He was awarded fellowship in the Royal College of Veterinary Surgeons in 1897. He recorded events in a series of 1200 canine anesthesias. He developed a humane method for securing animals before induction and a bellows mechanism for controlling delivery of chloroform vapor to the dog. His approach led to a dramatic reduction in deaths during anesthesia. Hobday left the college to join a large equine practice with Frank Ridler in Kensington in 1899. Hobday gave outstanding service during the First World War, when he was responsible for treatment and care of many military horses.

After the war Hobday developed a small animal consultative service and infirmary in the Kensington practice. He had a remarkable flair for developing techniques of surgery and apparatuses to facilitate the process. His many notable contributions included lendectomy for cataract, intestinal anastomosis for intussusception, limb amputations, and correction of hernias.

A strong proponent of comparative medicine, Hobday played a large part in persuading the Royal Society of Medicine to establish a section on comparative medicine. He became its second (and first veterinary) president in 1924. With the support of the association of the Masters of Foxhounds, Hobday and the editor of *Field* magazine made a public appeal in 1925 for funds for research into the great dog plague, canine distemper. The successful campaign led to the breeding of the disease-free dogs needed for the experiments by James B. Buxton at the Medical Research Council. Buxton became professor of comparative pathology at Cambridge University. Sir Patrick Laidlaw and Major G.W. Dunkin developed an effective distemper vaccine by 1928. A canine antiserum was also developed that protected exposed dogs if given promptly. In those early days vaccination was accomplished either by a dose of killed vaccine followed by a dose of live virus a week later or by simultaneous administration of live virus and serum at different sites. These developments were essential to breeders and to exhibition of dogs at shows.

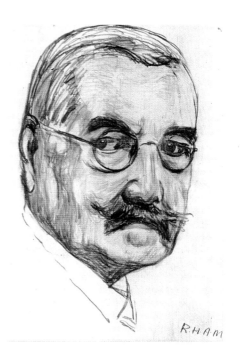

491. Sketch (from a photograph) of Sir Frederick G.T. Hobday (1870-1932), by R.H.A. Merter, MRCVS, 1930s. Hobday, an 1892 graduate of the Royal Veterinary College in London, made enormous contributions in the evolution of anesthesia and radiology and advances in surgical technique during his highly productive career. Today's small animal hospital is a direct outcome of his idea of an infirmary for small animal medicine and surgery. Hobday was principal of the Royal Veterinary College from 1927 to 1937. *(Historical Collections, The Royal Veterinary College Library, London.)*

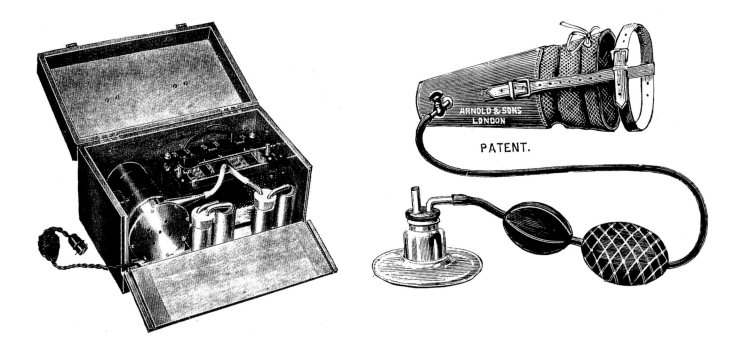

492. Two of the many items of anesthetic equipment designed and developed by Sir Frederick Hobday. *Left,* An electrical motor pump used for administering anesthetic vapor. *Right,* His design of an anesthetic inhaler. The mask was preferably made of aluminum or another metal for facility in sterilization. Hobday's interest in and involvement with anesthesia contributed to its development and safe use with lower mortality rates. *(Historical Collections, The Royal Veterinary College Library, London.)*

Hobday had introduced the X-ray machine to the College while still a houseman. His excellent text, *Canine and Feline Surgery,* was first published in 1900. Through several editions it showed the evolution of anesthesia and radiology, as well as the advances he made in surgical technique. His idea of an "infirmary" for the small animal branch of a practice was the precursor of the small animal hospital of modern practices. More than any other single individual, he showed the way to the development of effective small animal medicine and surgery.

On McFadyean's retirement in 1927, Hobday was appointed principal of the RVC, a position he held for ten years. He was extremely popular with students, who recognized his genius and commitment to the advancement of the profession. He also conducted a major renovation of the college's buildings at the site in Camden Town.

SMALL ANIMAL PRACTICE IN NORTH AMERICA

During the profession's early years in North America, few veterinary schools offered classes in small animal medicine and surgery or had suitable hospital facilities for pet animals. Cecil French, a doctor of veterinary science from McGill University in Montreal, published *Surgical Diseases and Surgery of the Dog* in 1906, which contained chapters on body regions, components of the locomotor system, and neoplasms. In this remarkable book, each section had a bibliography of relevant published veterinary literature. These included the contributions of the early French authors, such as those of Cadiot in 1893.

The book provided a comprehensive listing of all surgical conditions known at that time. It also described international developments in anesthesia, including the popular Billroth mixture from Germany containing chloroform (ten parts), ether (three parts), and ethanol (three parts). It could be administered by compressor devices such as those devised by Hoare, Junker, and Hobday. The mixture was considered to induce a short excitement phase and to be safer than pure chloroform. If the dog was given atropine as a preanesthetic, the use of a simple mask sufficed for delivery of the vapors.

Louis A. Merillat wrote a multiple-volume *Veterinary Surgery;* the first volume (1905) dealt with animal dentistry and diseases of the mouth. A significant contribution to the veterinary literature was the monthly *Journal of*

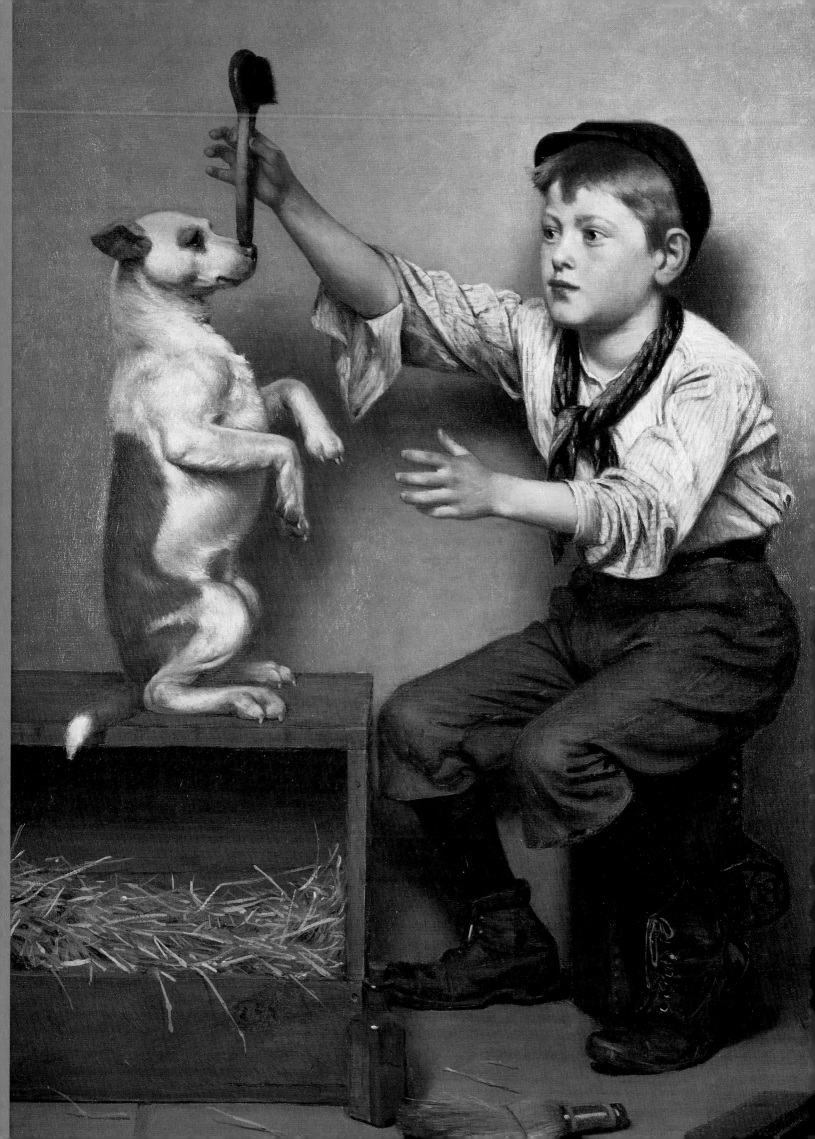

493. *Previous page, The New Trick,* oil on canvas, was painted in 1903 by John George Brown (1831-1913). Born into a poor family in Durham, England, he emigrated to the United States when he was twenty-two years old, settling in Brooklyn. He painted sentimental scenes of children and developed the street urchin figure, which remained popular throughout his career. His Horatio Alger–like depiction of the youthful American spirit of self-help proved highly inspirational and reveals much about the American culture of the late nineteenth and early twentieth centuries. His paintings of what appeared to be an uncomplicated urban environment romanticized the poverty of street life, something he would have been familiar with. In this scene during a moment of frivolity the bootblack is attempting to balance his brush on the nose of his dog, which is doing its best to cooperate in the venture. The companionship of the dog provides the youth a respite from his work. Brown's paintings remain popular today. *(Courtesy Galleries Maurice Sternberg, Chicago.)*

Comparative Medicine and Veterinary Archives, which was begun in the late nineteenth century in Philadelphia with the goal of providing leadership to veterinary journalism. It was edited by an Alfort graduate, Rush Shippen Huidekoper, who was assisted by Horace Hoskins and H.D. Gill. The journal was remarkable for its many advertisements, which indicated the keen competition for students among private and public colleges, as well as the growing range of products available to the veterinarian. It abstracted new information from both Europe and North America.

Although painful to relate, the crude methods that were employed in earlier times must be recalled so that the enormity of the progress that has been made can be grasped. Male cats were castrated without anesthetic after being thrust head first into a long rubber boot for restraint. After Lister introduced surgical antisepsis, it was adopted by the veterinary profession on the recommendations of J.A.W. Dollar in Britain in 1908 and G. Muller in Chicago the following year. German veterinary surgeons introduced absorbable catgut sutures and insisted on anesthesia and analgesia with chloroform and morphine by 1914. The standard technique of restraint for abdominal surgery in the dog, however, was still to suspend it by the hind legs from a hook on the wall or on a steeply tilted table. Pressure from the viscera on the vital organs in the thorax compromised cardiopulmonary functions. A turning point in North American practice came when Charles G. Saunders provided a model description for ovariohysterectomy in 1915, but infection continued to be a major sequel to surgical intervention.

THE AMERICAN ANIMAL HOSPITAL ASSOCIATION

The idea of small animal practices based on high-quality purpose-designed hospitals was a development of the top echelon of American practitioners. Early in the twentieth century, J.C. Flynn in Kansas City pioneered small animal hospital design and spread the word around the country. Frank Miller in New York City was another enthusiast for sophisticated small animal practice, which caught the attention of the pet-loving public. After the First World War, J.V. Lacroix developed an outstanding practice at the North Shore Animal Hospital in Evanston, Illinois, and published the influential *North American Veterinarian.*

The culmination of the impressive drive of the leading small animal practitioners of the early twentieth century and their insistence on high standards was the founding of the American Animal Hospital Association in Chicago in 1933. Mark L. Morris, Senior, of Shelton, New Jersey, was installed as the first president. The other distinguished charter members were Donald A. Eastman of Moline, Illinois; Stanwood W. Haigler of St. Louis, Missouri; John V. Lacroix of Evanston, Illinois; Louis H. LaFond of Detroit, Michigan; John F. McKenna of Hollywood, California; and Arthur R. Theobald of Cincinnati, Ohio.

The first annual meeting of the American Animal Hospital Association was held in Cincinnati in 1934. It included a seminar on distemper immunization and presentations on fracture repair. The purpose of the association was to promote the best possible veterinary service, hospital facilities, personnel, and methods of practice for the care and treatment of small animals. Because most of the members were self-employed practitioners, the initial thrust was toward setting out the described standards for hospitals, each represented by a director, and depending on the principle of self-help in seeking improvements. A system of inspection of hospitals was established, which gradually evolved into a comprehensive evaluation of the practice. A system of evaluation of pet foods was offered to manufacturers. Thus the goals of achieving credibility of standards for hospital premises, equipment, and veterinary services on one hand and for pet foods on the other were imple-

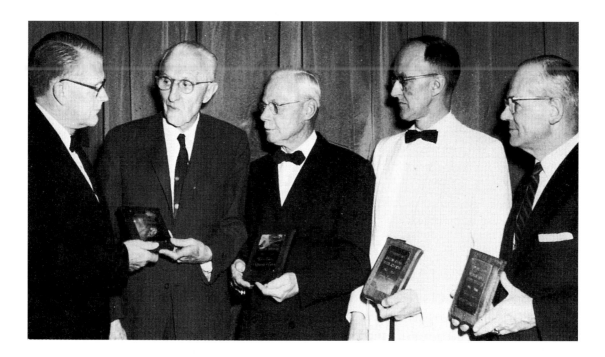

mented to provide confidence to the pet-owning clientele. The American Animal Hospital Association provided leadership in urging the veterinary profession to become involved in recognition of the importance of the bond between humans and companion animals. Membership now exceeds 14,000, and the association has acquired an enormous influence on issues affecting small animal medicine and surgery.

THE ANGELL MEMORIAL HOSPITAL

George Thorndike Angell was the founder of the Massachusetts Society for the Prevention of Cruelty to Animals (SPCA). The president of the society, Francis H. Rowley, conceived the idea of creating a fitting memorial hospital for animals in Boston to honor Angell. It would illustrate the humane principle in action by providing a facility where animals would receive proper veterinary medical and surgical treatment. Construction began in 1913.

The timing was right to attempt the introduction of the important principle of aseptic surgery and healing of incisions by first intention. A major advance in the pharmacology of anesthesia arrived in 1931 with intravenous pentobarbital sodium, which gave greater control of anesthesia and relaxation of the patient. These results allowed the surgeon to concentrate on perfection of surgical technique. The goal of aseptic surgery was met at the Angell long before it was adopted generally in private practices or even in the veterinary colleges. Major advances in radiology aided accuracy of diagnosis. Gerry B. Schnelle gave outstanding leadership in this field and wrote *Radiology in Canine Practice* in 1945. Erwin F. Schroeder developed the Schroeder version of the Thomas splint for use in pet animals. He became a leading authority on fracture repair.

A special contagious disease ward, mainly for distemper cases, was developed in 1940. In the same year an outstanding initiative of accepting high-quality veterinary graduates into a fifteen-month internship program was launched. Many distinguished small animal clinical scholars and practitioners have benefited from this splendid, challenging opportunity. After World War II a department of pathology was established under David L. Coffin, who focused on clinical applications. A fellowship in pathology was created that attracted several stars from Europe. T.C. Jones later became pathologist and director of research. C. Lawrence Blakely was noted for diaphragmatic and perineal herniorrhaphy.

494. American pioneers in small animal practice, such as J.C. Flynn in Kansas City, Frank Miller in New York City, and J.V. Lacroix in Evanston, Illinois, helped establish the need for an organization to set the high standards necessary for the practice of small animal medicine. The American Animal Hospital Association was founded in Chicago in 1933. The founding members of the American Animal Hospital Association were honored at the organization's thirty-fifth annual meeting in 1958. In this photograph from that meeting are, *left to right,* Dr. Joseph A.S. Millar, in 1958 president; Dr. J.V. Lacroix, who conceived the idea for the organization; Dr. Stanwood W. Haigler, one of the original members; Dr. Mark Morris, the first president; and Dr. Arthur Theobald, the first treasurer. *(Courtesy the Morris Animal Foundation, Englewood, Colorado, and the American Animal Hospital Association.)*

611

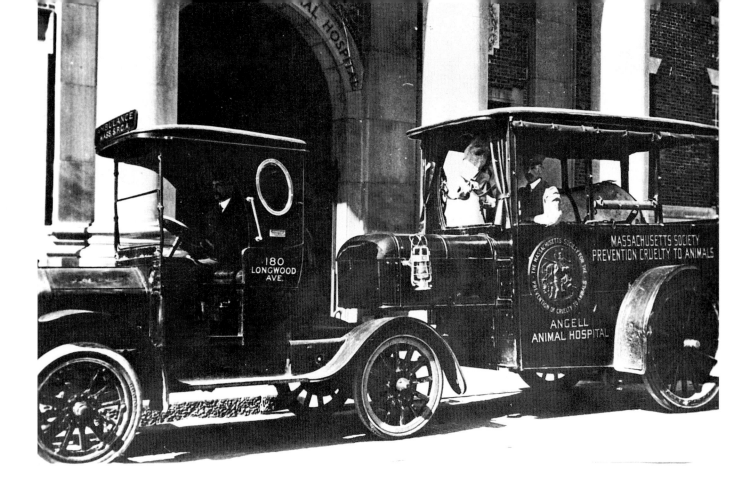

495. The Angell Memorial Animal Hospital in Boston was created to honor George Thorndike Angell, who had founded the Massachusetts Society for the Prevention of Cruelty to Animals (SPCA). The hospital has been associated with many advancements in veterinary medical care, including anesthesia, aseptic surgery, radiology, and fracture repair. The hospital has never used experimental animals in research, a reflection of the influence of the SPCA, but is committed to any other research that will contribute to the quality of small animal medicine. In this early scene in front of the hospital a horse is being delivered for care. *(Archives of the Massachusetts Society for the Prevention of Cruelty to Animals, Boston.)*

Because of the Angell's derivation from the SPCA, the hospital developed a policy of never using experimental animals in research. However, the hospital is strongly committed to any other facet of research that may contribute to the advancement of knowledge in small animal medicine. Feline cases and the quality of feline medicine have increased progressively. In 1931 a smaller version of the Angell was established in Springfield, Massachusetts—the Rowley Memorial Animal Hospital.

SMALL ANIMAL SURGERY ATTRACTS TALENTED VETERINARIANS

After the way ahead was initiated by Hobday and Wright in England, North America produced excellent surgeons who brought small animal surgery up to the standard of its human counterpart. Anesthesia, asepsis, radiology, pathophysiology, and surgical technique made possible sophisticated surgical interventions that would not have been countenanced in the first three decades of the twentieth century. Visionary pioneers appreciated the vast amount that could be learned from their colleagues in medical education and research. Carl F. Schlotthauer, staff veterinarian for the Institute of Experimental Medicine at the Mayo Clinic and Foundation, was a leading figure in this effort. He was able to persuade leading medical scholars from Mayo to speak and demonstrate state-of-the-art approaches at the American Animal Hospital Association meetings, which promoted interest in establishing clinical specialties in the veterinary profession.

A major boost to the largely neglected area of small animal clinical sciences and services in the veterinary schools was realized when the national accrediting body for the colleges, the American Veterinary Medical Association Committee on Education, was initiated. The activity resulted from the appointment of the relentless perfectionist James Farquharson of Colorado State University. He awakened the committee to its responsibility to be rigorous in its inspections and evaluations and to call for the changes that would have to be made if small animal medicine and surgery were to meet attainable, expected standards.

The medical figure who had the most continuous, direct impact on small animal surgery was Jacob Markowitz. He had received postgraduate training in the human and surgical research laboratory at the Mayo Foundation, where he had worked with Carl Schlotthauer and surgeons who performed human surgery. After returning to the University of Toronto, Markowitz took James Archibald of the Ontario Veterinary College (OVC) at Guelph as a graduate student. The collaboration between Markowitz and Archibald in small animal surgery, and Harry Downie in physiology led to dramatic developments in clinical and experimental surgery at OVC. This team updated Markowitz's fine text *Experimental Surgery,* and Archibald edited the 1965 edition of *Canine Surgery.*

The University of Pennsylvania made major commitments to specialties in small animal and comparative medicine. Clinical pathology, cardiology, orthopedics, oncology, ophthalmology, and anesthesiology were developed to high levels of expertise. Ellis P. Leonard at Cornell University promoted the highest standards in aseptic surgery as a necessary commitment to successful outcomes. Addition of clinical internships and residencies in the colleges had a major impact on small animal veterinary practice. The construction of the new Animal Medical Center (an old one had existed since 1914) on New York's East River in 1962, near the Rockefeller and Sloan-Kettering Institutes and Cornell's New York Hospital, gave a boost to the aims of collaborative medical research and provided ultramodern facilities for pet medicine. The center has a teaching affiliation with the University of Pennsylvania.

A SPECIAL FLAIR FOR COMPARATIVE ORTHOPEDICS

Veterinarians have been responsible for many inventions and advances in technique in orthopedic surgery and therapeutics. The high incidence of automobile accidents involving animals with serious trauma to the locomotor system, which regularly challenge the veterinarian, has contributed to this development. The X-ray machine and fluoroscopy were major contributors to accurate diagnosis of such conditions. The profession and its technological support staff, however, paid an awful price in radiation burns to the hands before this hazard was recognized and appropriate precautions were taken. Just one year after Wilhelm Roentgen discovered X-rays, five papers were published on their application in veterinary medicine. In Vienna the Physiology Institute installed an early apparatus and collaborated with the clinic to publish results. Richard Eberlein in Germany was one of the first to use and develop the techniques of radiology. Under Wirth in Vienna, A. Pommer was appointed to lead the first veterinary radiological institute in the world in 1927, which he did until his death in 1958. He was selected for the first independent chair in veterinary radiology. Pommer's contributions spanned a broad front, and many foreign visitors went to Vienna to train under his tutelage. Much later, Sten-Erik Olson in Sweden developed an outstanding reputation and superb facilities for veterinary radiology.

Since the first half of the twentieth century phenomenal progress has been made in radiology and radiotherapy, and computed tomography scans, ultrasonography, and magnetic resonance imaging have been developed. Improved imaging of both soft and hard tissues has resulted—at a price, of course, since these were expensive technologies. Schnelle at Angell and William Carlson at Colorado State University in Fort Collins, Colorado, led the way, and outstanding successors have followed them.

Erwin F. Schroeder in 1933 adapted the old Thomas traction splint of 1875 by tailoring it to fit any size animal of the canine species. It applied the extending force to both the proximal and distal ends of the fractured bone to prevent overriding. Remarkably, his design allowed the animal to remain ambulatory while healing was progressing. During the 1930s adoption of sterile techniques in the pursuit of truly aseptic surgery was promoted by leading canine surgeons. Otto Stader studied the technique of a Swiss surgeon, Gadvilli, who brought the Steinmann pin to America. Stader adapted pairs of such pins in supporting blocks to bring the ends of fractured bones into proper alignment and hold them there by fixation. His technique was extremely effective and was adopted in human as well as veterinary orthopedic work.

Studies of implantable support materials to fix fractures began in the nineteenth century. In 1936 the quest for an inert material that was strong enough for the task led to vitallium, an alloy of cobalt, chromium, and molybdenum. In another, "stainless steel," nickel replaces the cobalt. New developments involve plastic-coated metals and sintered (porous) metals that permit bone cells to invade them. H. Hansmann was testing nickel plates screwed into the bone as early as 1886, and Svend Larsen of Copenhagen plated fractures with high-carbon steel plates between 1920 and 1927 with encouraging results. By 1951 G.C. Knight in England and C.I. Chappel and Archibald in Canada used vitallium plates successfully in dogs.

Cerclage or bone wiring techniques developed early. Emerson A. Ehmer (1895-1954) used such a technique in canine fractures, and J. McCunn in London was a notable user of the technique. Ehmer of Seattle developed the Kirschner-Ehmer half-pin splint, which became extremely popular with small animal veterinary practitioners.

Molded splints and casts were used to fix fractures from early times and underwent considerable refinement in the first half of the twentieth century. Jacques Jenny (1917-1991), a Swiss, developed the technique of making removable plaster casts in two half-shells to fit perfectly the contours of the limb and was among the first to venture into modern bone plating.

Pioneers of the application of intramedullary pinning of fractured limb bones included Ellis P. Leonard of Cornell in 1935, author of *Orthopedic Surgery in the Dog and Cat* (1960), and Wade O. Brinker of Michigan State University, who wrote *Canine Surgery*. A new, self-retaining, spring-loaded extension splint, available in a variety of diameters and lengths, was invented by Salo Jonas in 1949 and improved a few years later. The splint became popular until tissue reaction set in after healing, and it was extremely difficult to remove after it was inserted.

DEGENERATIVE BONE DISEASE AND HIP DYSPLASIA

Besides traumatic injury, the problem of degenerative lesions affecting bones and joints received little attention until the Second World War. The redoubtable Gerry Schnelle (1904-1976) discovered from pelvic radiographs that many large-breed dogs had deformed coxofemoral joints, although they showed no gait defects. Little attention was paid to these lesions until the war, when Schnelle was asked to procure German shepherd dogs for sentry duty. Dogs with hips showing the lesions on X-ray broke down quickly during training. The condition became known as hip dysplasia and was a cause of great concern to breeders. Sophisticated approaches were developed to correct the condition by means of plastic or stainless steel femoral head prostheses. Moltzen-Neilson in Denmark showed that a similar condition also affected small dogs.

PROGRESS IN CANINE DISEASES OF NUTRITIONAL ORIGIN

Fits in dogs were reported in the United States in 1916 and in Great Britain in 1924. This condition became known as canine hysteria. After Carl Schlotthauer in Rochester, Minnesota, showed that it occurred in dogs fed nothing but bread and skim milk, E. Mellanby in England reported in 1946

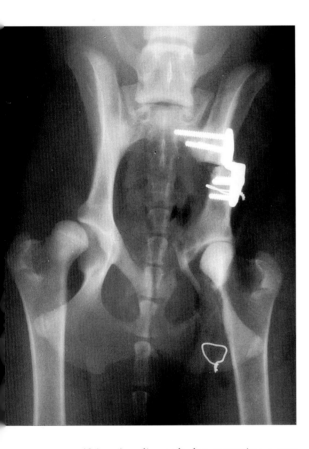

496. A radiograph demonstrating a case of canine hip dysplasia in which the right side has been treated surgically with a triple pelvic osteotomy using a Slocum plate. Although Gerry Schnelle (1904-1976) had shown from pelvic radiographs that large-breed dogs were susceptible to this condition, it was not until the Second World War that attention was finally brought to these lesions. Because German Shepherd dogs with hip dysplasia were unable to complete their training for sentry duty, the veterinary profession developed means to correct the condition. This condition was later shown to be present in smaller dogs by the Dane, Moltzen-Neilson. *(Courtesy Diagnostic Imaging, Purdue University School of Veterinary Medicine, West Lafayette, Indiana.)*

that the condition was produced regularly in about two weeks if animals were fed on cooked white flour bleached with nitrogen trichloride but not if the flour was unbleached. The problem was found to be attributable to the gluten modified by the *agene* process, which was attractive to the baker because it eliminated the need to store flour for at least two weeks to achieve the degree of "rise" desired by most consumers.

THE CAT BOOM: DEMAND FOR FELINE SPECIALISTS

Early attention to diseases of cats tended to focus on feline infections that carried a zoonotic risk for humans. C.O. Jensen reported on tuberculosis in dogs and cats as early as 1891. Hamilton Kirk, who wrote *The Diseases of the Cat* in London in 1925, described tuberculosis. Ear mange caused by a tiny mite was a significant problem. A.S. Griffith provided a detailed description of tuberculosis in *Tuberculosis of the Cat* in 1926. Similar emphasis was given by Oscar V. Brumley in his *Textbook of Small Animals,* published in Philadelphia in 1931. Peter Olafson and W.S. Monlux at Cornell were the first, in the article *Toxoplasma Infection in Animals,* to describe feline toxoplasmosis, which came to be recognized as an important protozoal zoonosis. Only gradually did studies come to address the cat's disease problems. Significant progress in feline health was slow in coming to a developed world recovering from two devastating world wars.

No other branch of small animal medicine has accelerated as rapidly as feline medicine has in the last few decades. The popularity of cats as pets has surged in a time of changes in life-styles such as both spouses working and crowded housing units, for example, apartment blocks and condominiums, being developed. Cohabitation with the cat is much easier than with the dog under such circumstances. The number of cats in the United States surpassed that of dogs for the first time in the early 1990s.

Feline specialists had emerged slowly during the previous decades, with the Angell's Jean Holzworth leading the way. A class of veterinarians who were prepared to train specifically in cat care and diseases emerged. The cause of the feared cat plague, panleukopenia, or infectious gastroenteritis, as it was known earlier, did not start to yield to science until 1928. In that year J. Verge

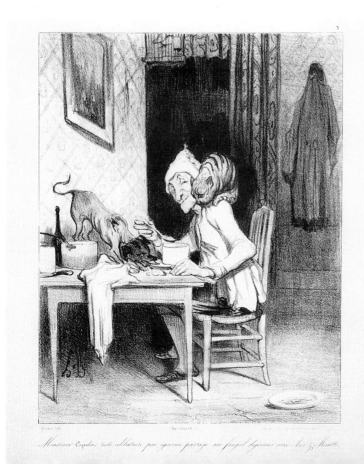

497. *Monsieur Coquelen Partage son Frugal Déjeuner avec Azor et Minelle,* by Honoré Daumier (French, 1809-1879). In this lithograph by the great satirist and cartoonist, Monsieur Coquelen is seen sharing his frugal breakfast with his two small animal companions. Azor, the dog, has the audacity to actually find a place on top of Coquelen's table for his scraps, with Minelle, the cat, perching herself on Coquelen's shoulder, eyes a spoonful of his meal. From the expressions on their faces it is difficult to determine who is the master of the house, a not-uncommon occurrence for many small animal owners. *(New York Public Library.)*

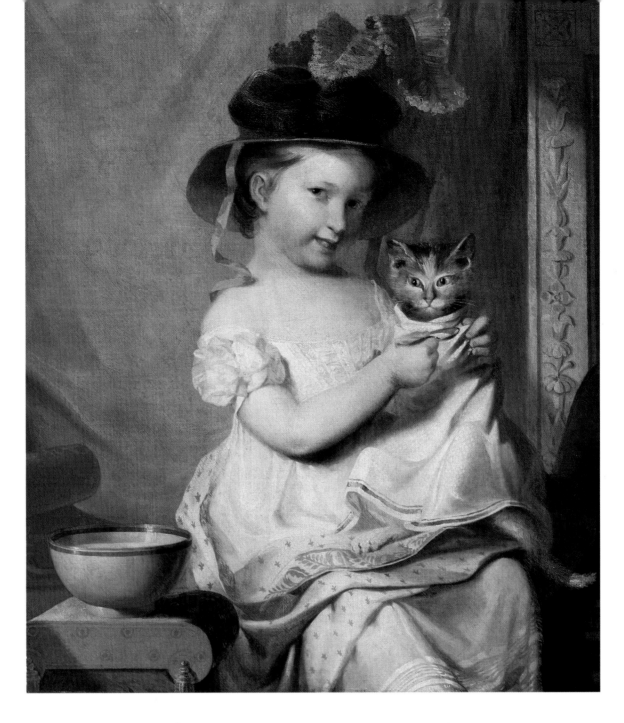

498. Samuel Breese Morse (1791-1872) is widely known for inventing the telegraph and the Morse code. Before his scientific endeavors, however, Morse had a successful career as a painter of forceful, realistic portraits between 1815 and 1837. He was also instrumental in organizing the National Academy of Design in New York City. Morse painted *Little Miss Hone* in 1824. The elegance of this composition and its subjects is in sharp contrast to the behavior of the participants in the preceding figure by Daumier. The well-dressed young girl is about to give a spoonful of milk to her well-mannered cat. The look of concern in the cat's eyes expresses its uncertainty about the forced generosity of Miss Hone. Morse has beautifully captured in this scene the unpredictable nature of cats. *(Gift of Martha Karolik for the M. and M. Karolik Collection of American Paintings, 1815-1865; Courtesy Museum of Fine Arts, Boston.)*

and N. Cristoforoni demonstrated the presence of a filterable infectious agent or virus in clinical cases in France. E.E. Leasure and colleagues in the United States prepared an effective vaccine from a formolized suspension of tissues obtained from infected cats in 1934. A few years later, J.S. Lawrence and J.T. Syverton at the University of Rochester isolated a virus from infected cats in a research colony. They found that the virus caused enteritis and agranulocytosis. The virus appeared to be the same as the original virus isolated from field cases of infectious enteritis. From the finding that the white blood cells virtually disappeared from the blood for about a week after the onset of clinical signs, the name *panleukopenia* was coined. The virus was shown to be related to the one that causes canine parvovirus infection, which appeared as an international epidemic that started in 1977.

Cats are susceptible to rabies, pseudorabies, feline infectious peritonitis, feline viral rhinotracheitis, and several other acute or chronic viral infections. The viral disease of cats that has drawn the most scientific interest, however, is the oncogenic (cancer-causing) virus. This virus is of great interest in medical and veterinary research because, like the virus of AIDS, it is a retrovirus (that is, it contains reverse transcriptase enzyme) that copies the virus RNA into a matching single strand of DNA. It is thought that the feline leukemia virus originated in rats and infected ancient members of the cat family. A re-

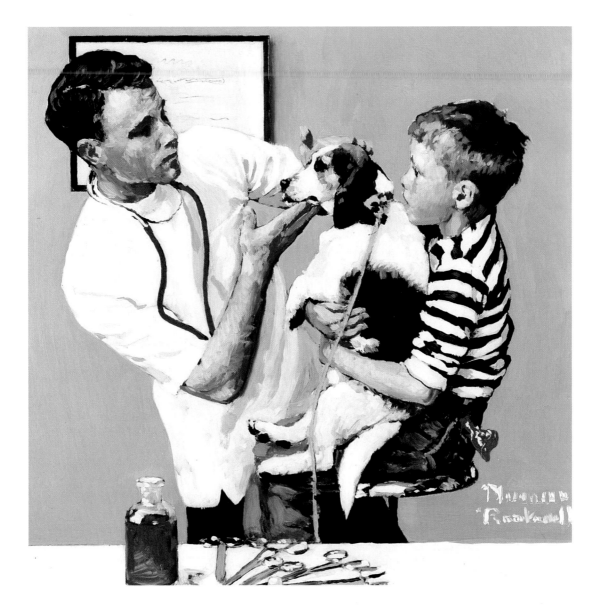

search group at the Glasgow Veterinary School led by W.F.H. Jarrett in 1964 first implicated the virus in a cat with lymphosarcoma. The virus replicates in rapidly dividing cells of lymphoid tissues and bone marrow. The possibility of a public health risk from feline leukemia virus has not been resolved but there is concern because some strains of the virus grow in human cells in tissue culture. The disease is spread mainly via saliva. A hantavirus is thought to be a cause of urolithiasis. Cases of spongiform encephalopathy (such as bovine spongiform encephalopathy) have appeared in cats in the United Kingdom.

Cats are susceptible to many bacterial, fungal, and parasitic diseases. Nutritional problems such as deficiency in the amino acid taurine are starting to yield to high-quality scientific research, but a much greater research effort must be invested in studies of the nature, pathogenesis, and management of feline diseases.

Because of the popularity of the cat and the intimate nature of the relationship between cat-owning families and their pets, growth in demand for advice on cat care, feeding, and management has been rapid. An even greater challenge, however, exists in the field of feline behavioral consultation. The veterinary schools, with a few exceptions such as the school at Tufts in Boston, have been slow to give this aspect of feline care a high priority. The resulting vacuum is being filled by other groups, and specialized programs are emerging, such as the program at the Anthrozoology Institute at the University of Southampton in England. Individual veterinary practitioners, on the other hand, have developed a strong interest in this field and a few have written books on the topic.

499. Perhaps the best-known and most often reproduced artwork in American veterinary medicine is *The Veterinarian* by Norman Rockwell (1894-1978). Rockwell created nearly four thousand paintings and illustrations during a career that lasted seven decades. His work is a record of contemporary American life—so much so that his name alone has come to suggest a certain atmosphere of the acceptable sentiments of his time. The practice of companion animal medicine, especially the veterinarian's relationship with the patient and client, is captured in this work, originally commissioned by the Upjohn Company in the early 1960s and reproduced on the cover of the 1963 program booklet for the American Veterinary Medical Association's centennial convention. One need not be a dog lover to feel the compassion of the veterinarian as he gently begins his physical examination or the concern of the young boy for his dog. Rockwell has captured perfectly the human-animal bond. *(Courtesy Dr. and Mrs. William V. Ridgeway, Jr.)*

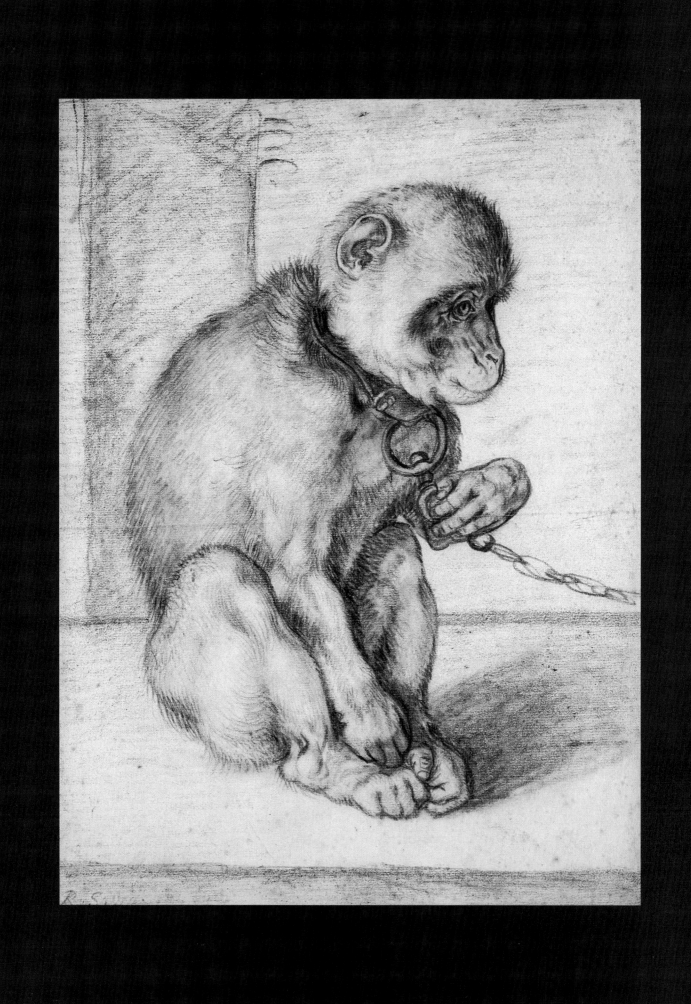

Bioethics, Animal Experimentation, and Sentience

EARLY ANIMAL EXPERIMENTATION

Before effective medical care of sick or injured animals and humans could be achieved, methods had to be developed for the investigation of the nature of disease processes in the body and their reversal by therapy. This development required the application of scientific experimentation.

Dissection allowed description of the appearance and relationships of the many parts of the body. The ethical challenge here was the existence of religious taboos against dissection, even of cadavers, in many societies. After this challenge was overcome during the Italian Renaissance, progress in anatomy was rapid. Physiology was a much more challenging ethical issue because it involved intervention and, often, surgery on live animals. In the days before anesthetics this procedure became known as vivisection. Suffering was entailed, and the investigators' desire to solve clinical problems or their level of scientific curiosity had to be strong to undertake such studies in animals that were forcibly restrained and expressing their anguish.

Early efforts to gain an understanding of functional and disease processes by applying the scientific approach expounded by Francis Bacon met with ridicule in the media. Bacon (1561-1626) proposed methods of observation and careful compiling of case histories to develop a consistent perspective of individual diseases. He also emphasized the need for experimentation and reasoning from the results in working toward a conceptual basis for the practice of medicine. These ideas were an extension of the Hippocratic tradition toward understanding the natural world and discerning its general laws via induction.

René Descartes (1596-1650) was a French natural philosopher who claimed that the bodies of humans and animals obeyed the laws of mechanics and hence that they could be compared justifiably with machines. He noted that the animal body had to operate without rational, noncorporeal guidance, whereas for the human being, endowed with the faculty of language and an imperishable rational soul, there might be such guidance as well as immortality. This concession may have protected him from charges of heresy while leaving him open to charges of having created the concept of a *beast-machine*.

The new science received a major boost in Great Britain when King Charles II chartered the Royal Society of London for the Improving of Natural Knowledge in 1662. The fellows (each a Fellow of the Royal Society, or FRS) became known as the *virtuosi* and were subjected to scorn and satirical attacks. They also were accused of propagating atheism and undermining university education. They were defended by Bishop Thomas Sprat in 1667.

500. *Facing page, A Young Monkey,* chalk drawing by Roelandt Savery (Flemish, 1576-1639). Savery trained in Amsterdam and, along with several of his Dutch contemporaries, made numerous drawings of a wide range of animals early in the seventeenth century. This chained monkey with no tail is probably a specimen of the *Macaca silvana,* which live on the Rock of Gibraltar. Where Savery actually saw this monkey remains a mystery, but the artist's career took him throughout Europe, including the courts of Emperor Rudolph II in Prague (1604) and Emperor Matthew in Vienna (1614). Savery was one of many artists heavily influenced by Albrecht Dürer's realistic portrayal of animals in nature, as can be seen in the warm manner in which he has captured the resignation of this chained animal. Like the work of Dürer, Savery's drawings of animals, both small and large, influenced Dutch animal artists for centuries after his death. *(Rijksmuseum, Amsterdam.)*

Early experiments on the properties of air and its role in the physiology of respiration in animals by Robert Boyle became a favorite target of the mockers. He placed animals in a glass vessel and pumped out the air, with results that would be predictable today but were not then. Samuel Butler in 1664 poked fun at Robert Hooke's biological experiments with the microscope. Butler mocked the doctors' newfound methods of examining the pulse and considered all animal studies a waste of time. He expressed no concern, however, for the well-being or suffering of the animals subjected to experiments. Hooke and Lower showed that a dog could be kept alive with its respiratory muscles cut by pumping air into the lungs via regular, gentle use of bellows of which the tip was inserted into a cut in the trachea. Thomas Shadwell wrote a popular comedy, *The Virtuoso,* in 1676 in which the main character, the virtuoso Sir Nicholas Gimcrack, described Hooke's experiment with the bellows, only to have it ridiculed by one of the other characters.

After initial successes with blood transfusions from animal to animal, another target emerged. Among others, Jean Denis (1635–1704), a French physician, tried the technique from animal to human with lethal results. In Shadwell's play the virtuoso's uncle says:

> . . . *I believe if the blood of an ass were transfused into a virtuoso, you would not know the emittent ass from the recipient philosopher.*

A damaging image of physicians as incapable, unscrupulous, and avaricious was frequently created by the witty entertainers. Strangely, it was not the critics but the scientists themselves who were the only ones to express concern about the suffering of the animal subjects of their experiments and remorse after the infliction of pain to gain knowledge.

The sensitive Haller in Göttingen in 1752 wrote that his studies of animal function involved:

> . . . *a species of cruelty for which I felt such a reluctance as could only be overcome by the desire of contributing to the benefit of mankind.*

Joseph Addison in 1711 reported having witnessed an experiment on a late pregnant bitch in which the abdomen and uterus were incised and a puppy was removed and held under its mother's nose. She immediately began to lick it and only vocalized a cry when the puppy was removed. He called it a barbarous experiment but appreciated that it was an impressive demonstration of the power of the mother's maternal instinct to overcome pain to protect her young.

It is necessary to be aware of the public attitudes and perceptions of a given historical period when evaluating responses. Before the eighteenth century, animals were considered a low form of life, and their suffering was seldom perceived to be a cause of concern. Cruel treatment of animals in everyday life was common.

CONCERN FOR EXPERIMENTAL ANIMALS

The pendulum started to swing away from satire and toward concern about the validity of hurting and killing animals for scientific studies with Susanna Centilivre (1669–1723). In Centilivre's comedy *The Basset-Table* in 1705 Valeria, the enthusiastic experimenter, and Lady Reveller, her critic, examined the issues. Suffering and death of animals had to be weighed against any advancement of knowledge obtained. Lady Reveller foresaw the horrifying prospect of human vivisection as a likely sequel to experimentation on living animals.

Richard Steele attacked the blood sports that were in vogue in 1709: cockfighting, cockthrowing, dogfighting, bullbaiting, and bearbaiting. He

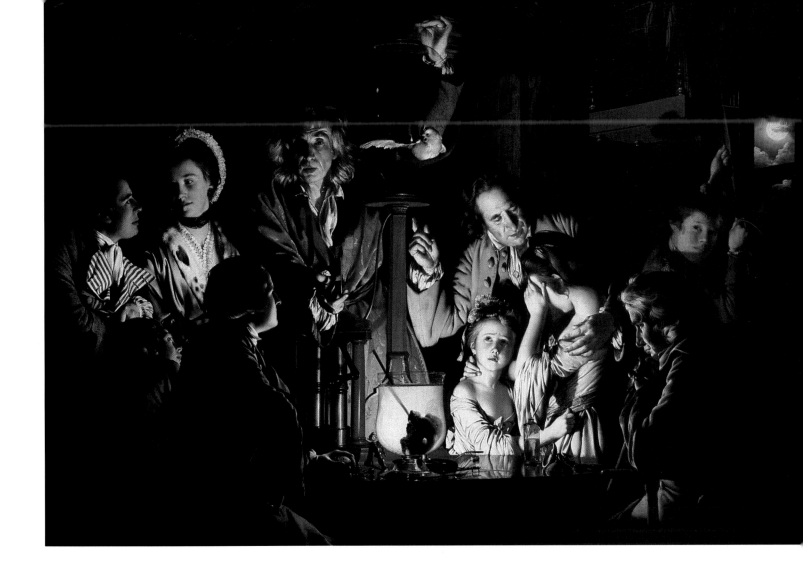

urged their replacement by tenderness, compassion, and humanity. Killing innocent animals was allowable only for the purposes of human safety, convenience, and nourishment. The distinguished poet Alexander Pope, an animal lover, wrote an essay, *Against Barbarity to Animals*, in 1713 in which he quoted Plutarch (AD 46-120), the Greek philosopher who lived in Rome: "Humanity may be extended through the whole order of creatures, even to the meanest." Pope castigated abuse of animals for entertainment and in the process of slaughtering. Pope attributed a rational soul to some higher animals, such as dogs. A contemporary of Stephen Hales, the brilliant curate who established the scientific basis of hemodynamics, Pope opposed vivisection and felt it unjustified, either to improve physiological knowledge or to obtain medical benefits. In his *Essay on Man* he supported a higher status for animals.

John Gay in *Trivia*, a poem written in 1716, imagined a vicious coachman's soul being reincarnated in a hackney horse in atonement for his brutalities. Through the remainder of the eighteenth century a major transition evolved in societal attitudes. The most impressive depiction of human insensitivity and brutality toward animals as a step in the progression to similar callousness with respect to fellow humans was William Hogarth's series of engravings, *The Four Stages of Cruelty*, published in 1751. The leading figure, Tom Nero, begins as a juvenile tormentor of animals and progresses through the practice of brutality as an adult to become a murderer who is hanged, then dissected in the anatomy theater. Oliver Goldsmith deplored the willful massacre of harmless dogs in 1760 by a mob rampaging under the guise of stamping out rabies. He also contrasted the growing compassionate attitude toward animals with the widespread desire for a meat diet. Sara Trimmer (1741-1810) wrote *Fabulous Histories Designed for the Instruction of Children Respecting Their Treatment of Animals* in 1786. It was realized that compassion should be instilled at a young age.

501. *Experiment on a Bird in the Air-pump* (1786), an oil painting by Joseph Wright ("Wright of Derby") (1734-1797). Wright was one of the first English painters to take his subject matter from the Industrial Revolution. In this instance he shows by dramatic lighting a cockatoo being suffocated in a vacuum chamber. Wright has captured the reaction to the cruelty of these popular eighteenth-century "experiments" in the facial expressions of the participants. The indifference of the "scientist" in the center of the painting is contrasted by the children's expressions of shock. *(Reproduced by courtesy of the Trustees, The National Gallery, London.)*

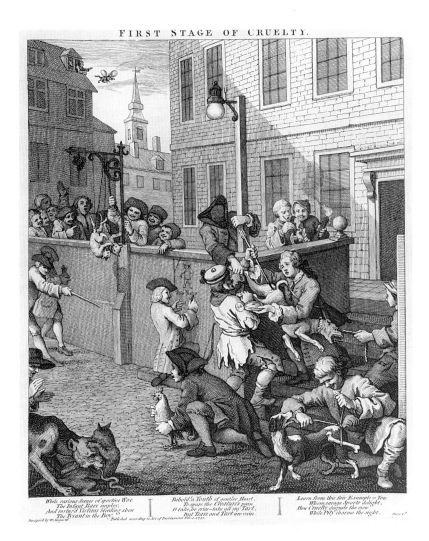

FIRST STAGE OF CRUELTY.

While various Scenes of sportive Woe
The Infant Race employ.
And tortur'd Victims bleeding shew
The Tyrant in the Boy.
Design'd by W. Hogarth.

Behold! a Youth of gentler Heart,
To spare the Creature's pain,
O take, he cries—take all my Tart,
But Tears and Tart are vain.
Published according to Act of Parliament Feb.y 1.1751.

Learn from this fair Example—You
Whom savage Sports delight,
How Cruelty disgusts the view
While Pity charms the sight.
Price 1.s

502. William Hogarth (English, (1697-1764) was the first eighteenth-century artist to develop a kind of picture dramatizing the corrupt moral values of the period, which he described as "modern moral subjects." First done as a series of paintings, Hogarth's "progresses," which dealt with a variety of topics, were later made into engravings for popular sale. In one of his later progresses, *The Four Stages of Cruelty,* Hogarth follows the life of one main character, Tom Nero, an orphan. Each scene in the series is full of visual clues showing cruelty to animals, which demands our attention. The verses following the engravings are by the Reverend James Townley. Hogarth wrote as follows of this "progress":

The four stages of cruelty, were done in hopes of preventing in some degree that cruel treatment of poor Animals which makes the streets of London more disagreeable to the human mind, than any thing what ever, the very describing of which gives pain.

In *First Stage of Cruelty* (1751), several species of domestic animals are being cruelly treated by young boys, especially Tom Nero, who, with two other boys, is inserting an arrow up the anus of a dog in the center of the print. *(Yale Center for British Art, Paul Mellon Collection, New Haven, Connecticut.)*

503. In *Second Stage of Cruelty* (1751) Tom Nero has become a coachman and can be seen beating his horse after it has broken its leg as a result of being overburdened with too many passengers to pull. He has also savagely gouged the crippled animal's eye. The posters in the background advertise legal forms of human cruelty. *(Yale Center for British Art, Paul Mellon Collection, New Haven, Connecticut.)*

SECOND STAGE OF CRUELTY.

The generous Steed in hoary Age
Subdu'd by Labour lies;
And mourns a cruel Master's rage,
While Nature Strength denies.
Designed by W. Hogarth.

The tender Lamb o'er drove and faint,
Amidst expiring Throes;
Bleats forth its innocent complaint
And dies beneath the Blows.
Published according to Act of Parliament Feb.y 1751.

Inhuman Wretch! say whence proceeds
This coward Cruelty?
What Intrest springs from barbrous deeds?
What Joy from Misery?
Price 1.s

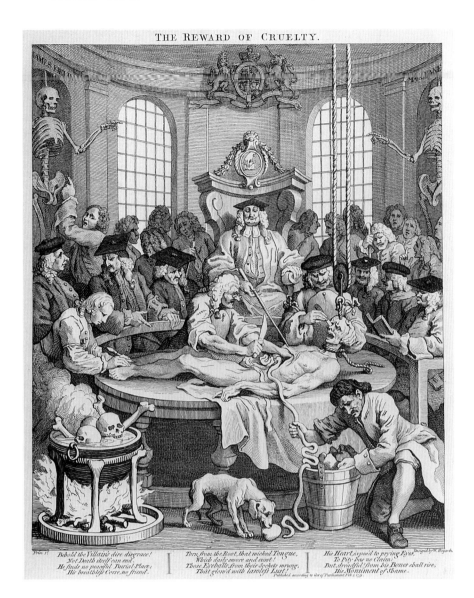

THE REWARD OF CRUELTY.

Behold the Villain's dire disgrace!
Not Death itself can end.
He finds no peaceful Burial-Place;
His breathless Corse, no friend.

Torn from the Root, that wicked Tongue,
Which daily swore and curst!
Those Eyeballs from their Sockets wrung,
That glow'd with lawless Lust!

His Heart, expos'd to prying Eyes,
To Pity has no Claim:
But, dreadful! from his Bones shall rise,
His Monument of Shame.

504. *The Reward of Cruelty* (1751) is the final scene in Hogarth's *Four Stages of Cruelty*. After a lifetime of cruelty to animals, Tom Nero has died and is being autopsied by a group of sadistic surgeons. Although dead, Tom appears to be in pain. As a final symbolic act of revenge, Tom's heart is being eaten by a dog. *(Yale Center for British Art, Paul Mellon Collection, New Haven, Connecticut.)*

Francis Coventry (1725-1754), a vicar, wrote *The History of Pompey or the Life and Adventures of a Lap-dog* in 1751 (it was rewritten in 1752), a caustic reflection and dog's-eye view of a contemporary dog's fate in being passed from master to master and eventually being obtained by an ambitious medical student, who seeks to impress his peers by vivisecting it to demonstrate the motion of the bowels. Pompey escapes, but Coventry does not spare the ladies who pamper their lap-dogs, the hypocrisy of society, those who perform vivisection for medical education and research, the philosophers who speculate on animal souls, or the lawyers who weigh the legal status of pets.

Samuel Johnson (1709-1784) admired fine doctors but was appalled by vivisection experiments and doubted that they would lead to therapeutic benefit. His denunciation of such experiments in 1754, echoing Shakespeare's, was mainly anthropocentric, angrily fearing the possibility of detrimental effects on the moral standard of humans rather than being concerned about the suffering of the animals. Johnson acknowledged the scientific value of experimentation in natural history. He also insisted that good could come from pain because it quickened the mind.

The French philosopher and writer Jean-Jacques Rousseau (1712-1778) deplored the idea that animals were sentient but could not reason. In *Emile* (1762) he claimed that animals could form ideas. He also asserted that great eaters of meat are generally more cruel and ferocious than other humans. He argued romantically for a return to a simpler life closer to nature, a theme that has persisted in human thought.

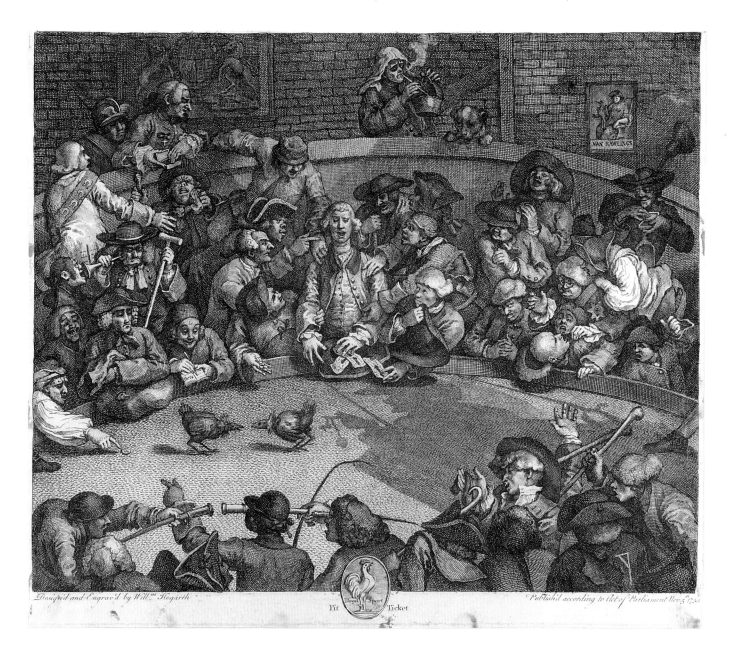

505. Much of what Hogarth intended to portray in his "progresses" can also be found in many of his other engravings. Full of artistic detail, they provide a wordless narrative of the cause and effect of corrupt behavior. *Pit Ticket: The Cockpit* (1759) portrays the eighteenth-century British attraction to animal blood sports. Here Hogarth has intermingled men from all classes to illustrate the consequences of drunkenness and gambling. *(Yale Center for British Art, Paul Mellon Collection, New Haven, Connecticut.)*

Thomas Percival (1740-1804) expressed eloquently the concern about becoming callous after repeated exposure to horrific spectacles of animal experimentation in *A Father's Instructions* (1789):

Beware my son . . . of observing spectacles of pain and misery with delight! Cruelty, by insensible degrees, will steal into your heart; and every generous principle of your nature will be subverted . . . .

He also wrote *Medical Ethics* in 1803. The thoughtful Percival praised the value of experimentation for the progress of medicine but insisted that its goals must be beneficial and that animal suffering must be minimized.

ANTHROPOCENTRIC AND UTILITARIAN PHILOSOPHIES

Immanuel Kant (1724-1804), the renowned German philosopher from Königsberg, in 1785 espoused the anthropocentric Christian view of animal exploitation. He stated that a legal relationship could exist only between rational beings, namely, humans. Animals were mere objects, but humans should abstain from violence and cruelty toward them, lest they demean themselves. He is said to have illustrated this point in his talks by showing

Hogarth's engravings. He considered slaughtering permissible but asserted that it must be accomplished quickly and without torture. Painful experiments were allowable in pursuit of medical benefits but not to satisfy mere speculation.

The classical Greek philosopher Epicurus had claimed that all creatures seek pleasure and strive to avoid pain. The British philosopher Jeremy Bentham (1742-1832), himself a great cat lover, resurrected this idea and proposed a calculus of utility or utilitarianism. Utility was defined as any property in an object that tends to produce an advantage or to prevent the happening of a mischief. He postulated a teleological end, which should be sought by everyone, of universal happiness. This proposition invoked a theory of moral sensibility and subjugation of self-interest. Bentham broadened the compass of compassionate concern to include nonhuman animals. Thus he urged an end to wanton cruelty toward animals because he perceived them to be just as vulnerable to suffering as their human counterparts. According to Bentham, *"The question is not, Can they reason? Nor, Can they talk? But, Can they suffer?"* The Christian and Kantian religious criterion that humans could exploit animals because they lacked a rational soul was replaced by an awareness of their capacity to suffer. Bentham accepted the practice of slaughtering on the grounds that animals could anticipate neither their future nor their impending death. It was also considered legitimate to kill animals that are dangerous or cause damage.

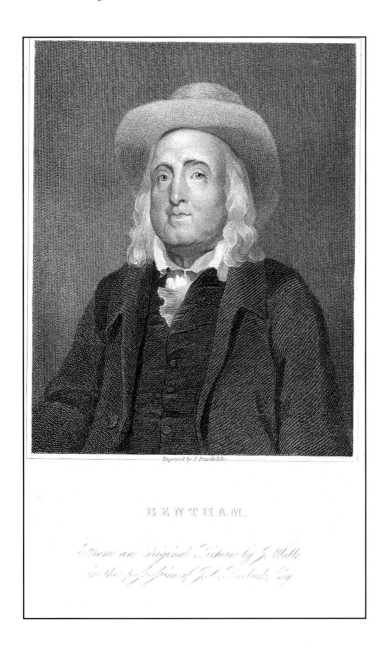

BENTHAM.

506. Jeremy Bentham (1748-1832) applied his theory of utilitarianism to animals. As one of the most influential British jurists and philosophers of his day, he preached abhorrence of cruelty to animals, likening their vulnerability to suffering to that of humans. *(The Mansell Collection, London.)*

Bentham urged that the 1826 legislation about procurement of human bodies be reformed to allow a supply of cadavers for medical dissection from the destitute classes, as had been allowed in post-Revolutionary France. The goal was to end the practice of grave robbing by "resurrection men," which evolved to meet demand because the only legal source was the gallows. The resulting Anatomy Act of 1832 replaced those thus released from their graves with the unclaimed bodies of paupers who died.

The German philosopher Arthur Schopenhauer (1788-1860) urged the restriction of animal experimentation and condemned its abuses. He deplored the assumptions that animals are without rights and that human treatment of them had no moral significance. Schopenhauer was an advocate of universal compassion as the only guarantee of morality.

EARLY ACTIVISTS PROTEST ABUSES OF ANIMALS IN SOCIETY

Bullrunning and baiting were abominable "sports" practiced in Great Britain. Bulls were aroused to anger by various preliminary atrocities, then turned loose and chased by courageous dogs and crazed men who beat them unmercifully before the final baiting.

The barbarity of abuses perpetrated on animals in society in the eighteenth century makes gruesome reading. Gradually, education started to make children aware of the horrors of cruelty they witnessed virtually every day. A few observers became convinced of the need for action to protect animals from maltreatment. John Lawrence (1753-1839) was a gentleman-farmer who argued that natural justice entitled beasts to the right of protection under the law. They had life, intelligence, and feeling, which implied that they had rights. His focus was on animals used in agriculture, transport, and sport. Humane treatment was a duty, and he called for legislation.

507. *The Knacker's Yard,* or *The Horse's Last Home,* wood engraving from an etching by George Cruikshank (English, 1792-1878). From *The Voice of Humanity* (London, 1831). The inhumane manner in which animals were treated during the eighteenth century is captured in this gruesome scene, supposedly sketched by Cruikshank on the site. A knacker's yard would be analogous to an automobile junkyard, where worn-out domestic animals (or their bodies) were purchased to be sold for fertilizer or animal feed, much like a worn-out automobile would be "parted out" today. Cruikshank's piece shows an end, however profitable, unbefitting a lifetime of servitude by the horse. *(Mary Evans Picture Library.)*

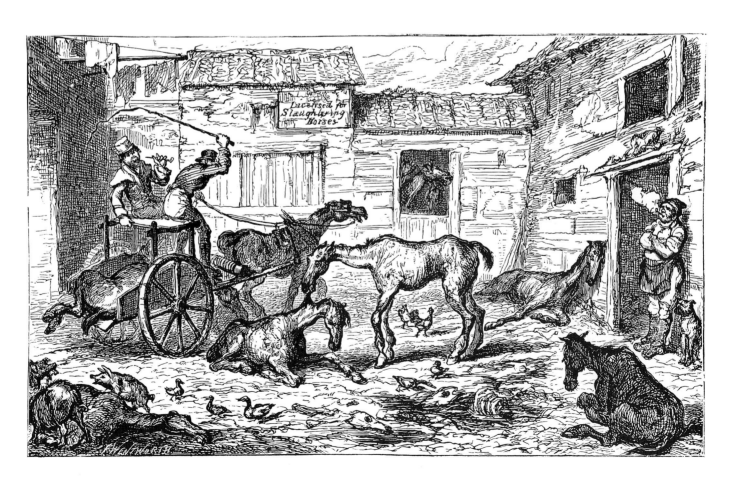

Edinburgh-born Thomas Erskine (1750-1823) was a contemporary of Lawrence's who held similar views. A wealthy lawyer, Erskine became Lord Erskine of Restormel and introduced a bill to prevent wanton cruelty to animals in the Upper House in 1809; it was passed in the Lords but failed in the Commons. Later, Erskine joined forces with Richard Martin (1754-1834), an ebullient Irishman who owned great estates in Galway and was elected to the British House of Commons. Martin, Erskine, and Lawrence planned a new legislative initiative on behalf of animals in 1821. It proposed that if any person who had charge of any horses, cattle, or sheep wantonly beat, abused, or mistreated any of them, that person should be brought to justice. Since the bill's authors left intact a widely held traditional opinion, the right of owners of animals to do as they liked with their own animals, the bill was passed on the second attempt in 1822, *An Act to Prevent the Cruel and Improper Treatment of Cattle.* Martin himself brought the first prosecution under the act, that of a costermonger charged with cruelty to a donkey. Martin insisted that the abused ass be brought into the court so that its wounds could be visible to all, a fine publicity stunt. His goal was to be an agent of change toward a more compassionate society and a more acceptable human behavior toward animals in society's care.

Martin introduced other bills aimed at protecting animals from such forms of cruelty as bullbaiting and dogfighting, the general protection of cats and dogs, and the avoidance of maltreatment of animals in slaughterhouses. All of these efforts were narrowly defeated, however, which is remarkable by today's standard but evidence of a deep-seated tradition. In 1835 Joseph Pease's act was passed, which outlawed any cruel treatment of domestic animals and the keeping or using of any site for running, baiting, or fighting any animal.

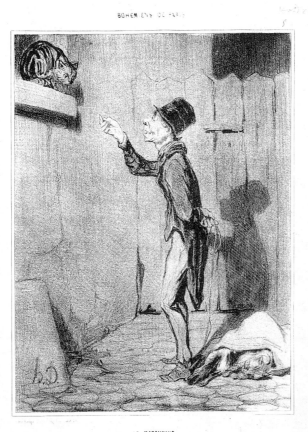

LE MARAUDEUR

M. Minet entrepreneur general des gibelottes de Paris (Diners à 52 sous)...

508. The skill of the great French cartoonist, satirist, and caricaturist Honoré Daumier (1808-1879) is evident in this lithograph, *L'Entrepreneur des Gibelottes (The Stewed-Rabbit Contractor).* The cat is being enticed from the safety of its perch on the window sill to be added to the "catch of the day." *(New York Public Library.)*

The Society for Prevention of Cruelty to Animals (SPCA) had been formed in London in 1824 by a group of twenty-one individuals, who elected the Reverend Arthur Broome (1780-1837) as secretary. Two committees were established initially, one to develop ways to influence public opinion, the other, on which Richard Martin served, to be responsible for inspection of animal-related activities in the metropolis. Within four years the SPCA was in dire straits financially. Lewis Gompertz replaced Broome and established sound fiscal policies. During its first few years the SPCA had brought about a hundred and fifty prosecutions, mainly of drovers and others connected with Smithfield market. Gompertz, an inventor and a vegetarian, was strongly opposed to any exploitation of animals whatsoever, even declining to ride. He authored *Moral Inquiries Into the Situation of Man and Brutes* in 1824 and *Fragments in Defense of Animals* in 1852, in which he attacked cruelty to horses and cattle, hunting, whaling, and vivisection. He developed a system of inspectors. After Princess Victoria came to the throne in 1837, she awarded to the SPCA the prefix "Royal" (in 1840), which increased the profile of animal welfare and enhanced the society's standing with the aristocracy. The royal support continued through the First World War. During that period a decline in the anthropocentric view of animals and a growing sense of a unity of nature and feeling a part of it were noticeable. The aristocratic pastimes of hunting, shooting, and fishing, however, were sacrosanct, and meat eating and horse racing were also off limits to the reformers.

Early in the nineteenth century, books began to appear on abstinence from animals as food for humans. The word *vegetarian* was coined in 1842, and William Metcalfe's followers established the Vegetarian Society of England in 1847. Their role model emigrated to America and was a founder of the movement there. Another vegetarian, Howard Williams, wrote an influential book, *The Ethics of Diet,* in 1883.

The main thrust of actions taken by the RSPCA in its first few decades was limited to suppression of bullbaiting and cockfighting, cruelties participated in mainly by the working class. This tactic alienated the famous political philosopher, John Stuart Mill.

Progress was slow; in 1854 an act prohibited the use of carts drawn by dogs, and in 1869 wild birds were granted protection. The big issue of vivisection was finally addressed in 1876.

509. A beautiful watercolor painting, *Fighting Horses* (c. 1820), by the renowned French painter Théodore Géricault (1791-1824). The unruly horses are being beaten by the keeper in an attempt to bring them to order. This particular work is interesting in that it is obviously related to Géricault's famous lithograph of 1818, *Horses Fighting in a Stable. (Copyright The Cleveland Museum of Art, The Charles W. Harkness Endowment Fund, 29.13.)*

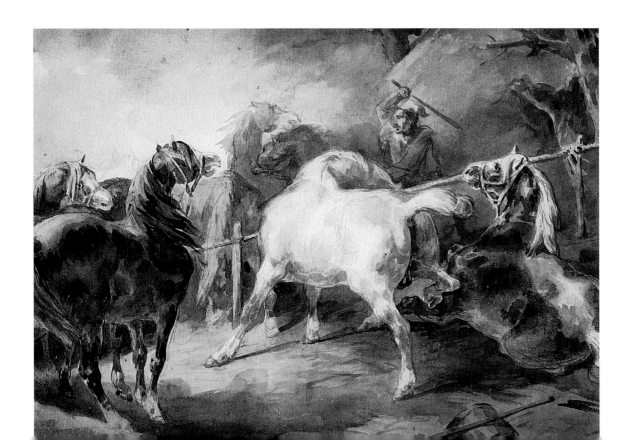

Charles Darwin was torn in his view of the complex issues arising as a result of the campaigns for and against vivisection. Darwin denied having participated in the British Association's initiative in favor of vivisection (1871) and the development of the Scientists' Bill. He did state to a royal commission, however, that he approved of its language *"in the main,"* although it did not exactly express the physiologists' conclusions. He confirmed that he had never performed an experiment on a living animal. However, he believed that such experiments were necessary to physiology and that physiological research in the future *"would confer the highest benefits on mankind."* Nonetheless, it was his belief that most experiments could and should be performed while the animal was rendered insensitive to pain. When asked about his view on inflicting any pain that was not absolutely necessary on any animal, he was quoted as saying, *"It deserves detestation and abhorrence."* His responses have been quoted out of context by manipulators of both sides of the argument. Undoubtedly, however, he admired the achievements of many medical and scientific researchers.

John Colam became Secretary of the RSPCA from 1860 to 1906, and the primary focus of the society became education of the public about the avoidance of cruelty. By 1878 the number of inspectors had grown to forty-eight. Colam had a truly remarkable touch with problem solving. The RSPCA inspectors were based in London and were uniformed after 1856; the police were pleased to leave the enforcement of anticruelty laws to them. They traveled the country investigating complaints and following up on information. Colam required them to be respectable and disciplined. He improved the society's favorable public image while maintaining the reforming thrust of its effector arm. He held true to the fundamental principles of animal welfare while being prudent both in keeping government support and in avoiding negative repercussions. When a Spanish bullfight was to be staged in London in 1870, he terminated it by jumping into the ring to demonstrate the strength of his convictions. He edited *Animal World,* the society's publication, and frequently conducted prosecutions. Colam may have been too preoccupied with respectability, however, to keep the more progressive and radical elements satisfied. This traditionalism cost the RSPCA the glue that had held the Utilitarian and Evangelical arms together and led to splintering of more activist groups.

THE PAINFUL FRENCH FOCUS ON EXPERIMENTAL PHYSIOLOGY

Xavier Bichet (1771–1802) was a prodigy who held a clinical professorship in Paris but brought a new perspective to bear on the function of tissues and organs. He wrote a book in 1802 reviewing his physiological researches on life and death. He classified the tissues based on direct observation and primitive biochemical tests. He injured specific organs in experiments and studied their resulting decline in function and death. This work was an early venture into pathophysiology and the study of the nature of death.

The man who launched the French thrust in physiology was François Magendie (1783–1855). He qualified as a physician in 1811 and started teaching anatomy, physiology, and surgery in Paris but left the university after two years. He established a medical practice but privately offered courses in experimental physiology laced with vivisection demonstrations. A prolific author and researcher in physiology and pharmacology, he trained several excellent researchers. Within fifteen years, his growing reputation led to his election to the French Academy of Sciences. However, physiology had not yet attained the status of a discipline in its own right. Magendie was appointed to the chair of medicine of the Collège de France in 1830. Two years later he assumed the chair of human anatomy at the Museum of Natural History;

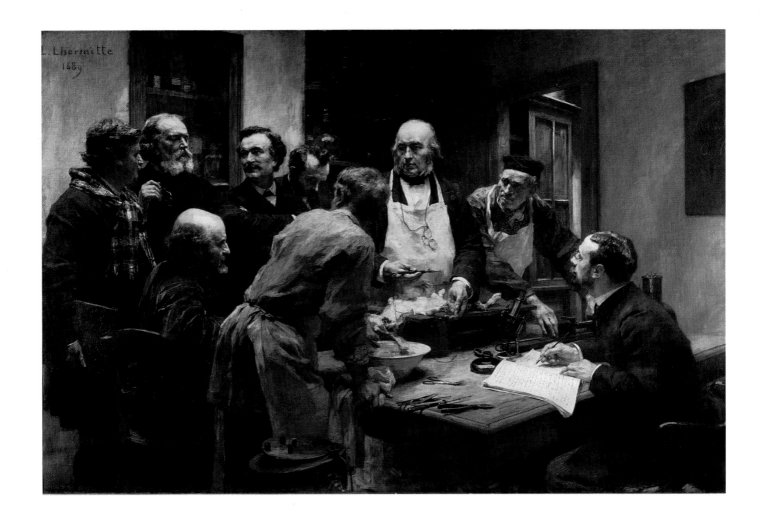

510. Claude Bernard (1813-1878), who studied under the great French physiologist François Magendie at the Collége de France, is vivisecting a rabbit in his laboratory in this painting, *Claude Bernard dans son Laboratoire* (1889) by Léon Augustin L'Hermitté. Bernard's integration of studies in histology, pathobiology, physiology, biochemistry, and pathophysiology resulted in his famous text *An Introduction to the Study of Experimental Medicine* (1865), which proposed that conclusions could be drawn only from experiments, leading to further questions and experiments. Although his experiments frequently involved vivisection (he and his antivivisectionist wife separated over this issue in 1870), his studies, especially in the role nerves play in regulating the diameter of blood vessels and his concept of the unchanging internal environment (which eventually came to be known as *homeostasis*) contributed greatly to modern medicine and saved many lives. *(Jean-Loup Charmet.)*

then, after Cuvier's death, he exchanged it for his coveted chair of comparative physiology. Magendie's physiology was based on vivisection experiments aimed at answering questions about the mechanisms of animal function. In the days preceding the discovery of general anesthetics, he set a standard for callousness in surgical intervention that horrified most observers. Since he performed public demonstrations, he acquired a notoriety for cruelty. His visit to London in 1824 triggered strong protests about his demonstrations, in which frogs, rabbits, cats, and dogs were used. He made significant contributions to physiological understanding. His last, most distinguished pupil was Claude Bernard (1813-1878).

Bernard investigated beyond the mainly physical aspects of physiology studied by his mentor, studying biochemistry under Jules Pelouze and medical reasoning with Pierre Rayer. Several times Bernard won the Montyon prize established in physiology by Laplace; he was appointed to the Academy of Sciences in 1854. This appointment led to the creation of a new chair for him in general physiology in the faculty of sciences at the Sorbonne. Magendie died the next year, in 1855, and Bernard assumed his chair, which had become the chair of experimental medicine at the College of France. Bernard combined Bichat's histology and pathobiology, Magendie's mechanistic scientific physiology, and his own initiatives in biochemistry and pathophysiology into an integrated approach to experimental medicine. This work led to his famous text, *An Introduction to the Study of Experimental Medicine,* and his insistence that physiology should be accorded the status of an independent discipline in academic research.

Bernard acquired a passion for the deployment of vivisection in testing his scientific ideas similar to that of his mentor, Magendie. His fame led to the adoption of research on animals in Europe and North America. The triumvirate of Magendie, Bernard, and Louis Pasteur led the public to a widespread expectation that animal experimentation would lead to important progress in understanding the function of the body and the treatment and prevention of diseases.

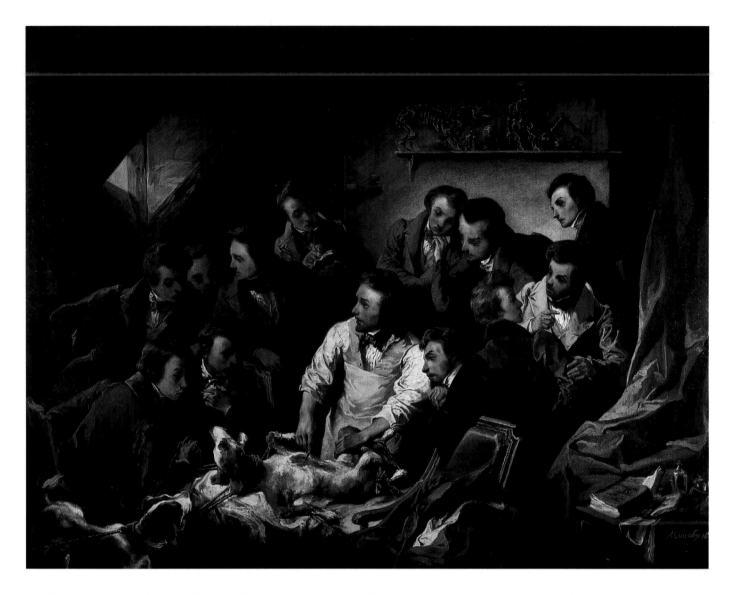

Research in physiology, pharmacology, pathology, and microbiology progressed remarkably in the second half of the nineteenth century. The French pioneers resorted to barbarous methods in achieving their goals before anesthesia made possible further progress with reduced suffering.

511. Painting by Emile-Edouard Mouchy (c. 1802-1870) of the dissection of a living dog (1832). *(The Wellcome Institute Library, London.)*

A RESEARCH DIMENSION: NEW FRENCH VETERINARY SCHOOLS

A new academic field of veterinary science began at Lyon and Alfort (1762 and 1764, respectively) for the training of equine veterinarians. After the Revolution, horse medicine was caught in the general zeal for reform that swept through French institutions. One result at Alfort was the appointment of three distinguished, influential professors: comparative anatomist Louis Daubenton in ovine genetics and wool production, Felix Vicq d'Azyr, and Antoine Fourcroy.

Lower faculty salaries, in addition to lower academic standards for acceptance of veterinary students compared with those in other academic fields, were negative factors. Nevertheless, brilliant scholars were nurtured in these colleges. The most significant development was the appointment of an Alfort professor to one of the chairs of the Section of Rural Economy of the Academy of Sciences, in which Lyon representatives became corresponding members. Alfort also dominated the six seats granted to veterinary medicine in the Academy of Medicine.

The importance of the horse in war had been a major factor in obtaining royal support for creating the veterinary schools. Support for research to enhance the health and effectiveness of horses continued through the period of revolution and reform. The two veterinary schools received from the army stables the horses cast off because of disease, crippling, or old age. The result was a new approach to animal experimentation distinct from that of Parisian physiologists, surgeons, and microbiologists.

When Pierre Flandrin (1752-1796) became director of the Alfort school, he conducted physiological research on equine gastrointestinal physiology. In 1790 he sought to establish whether absorption from the gut contents occurred via the lymphatic vessels or the bloodstream. The Parisian scientific establishment was impressed. When Flandrin died prematurely, his pupil Alexis-Casimir Dupuy (1775-1849) continued the experimental thrust. He also invited Guillaume Dupuytren and Magendie to join him in a series of experiments on equine physiology. In 1828 Dupuy went to Toulouse to direct the new, third veterinary school. His two best pupils and colleagues at Alfort, Jean Bouley and Urbain Leblanc, also left the Alfort school and went into practice. They continued to engage in equine research, including neurophysiology and studies on the origin and causes of glanders. Both had sons, Henri Bouley and Camille Leblanc, who followed in their fathers' academic and professional tradition and became founding members of the Society of Biology, along with Armand-Charles Goubaux, who became professor.

A graduate of the Lyon school, Gabriel Colin (1825-1896) moved to Alfort to dedicate his prodigious energy to the study of animal physiology. He collaborated with the human physiologist Pierre Bérard, who edited the tenth edition of Richerand's important manual of medical physiology, *New Elements of Physiology,* which first appeared in 1801.

The greatest of the early veterinary physiologists in France was Auguste Chauveau (1827-1917), who trained at the Alfort veterinary school, then joined the Lyon faculty. The breadth of his academic genius was remarkable. A brilliant anatomist, he wrote the finest veterinary anatomy text in French. In physiology, too, he was a genius of technique and research ideas. He designed equipment that allowed certain sophisticated physiological studies to be carried out without major surgical intervention, including a special instrument he devised for the first cardiac catheterization conducted in the horse. A towering figure in physiology, Chauveau also became a great authority in microbiology and immunology.

THE EFFORTS OF MARSHALL HALL AND BURDON-SANDERSON

Marshall Hall (1790-1857) was a research-oriented Nottingham physician. A graduate of the Edinburgh school, he toured continental centers, where he acquired knowledge of current medical research before moving to London. He accumulated animals of various kinds in his home, where he set up a laboratory. He developed devices for his physiological studies, which included chronic temperature monitoring of bats during hibernation. He was a medical reformer who challenged his profession to justify its practices and attempted to gain understanding of function so that more effective therapies could be evolved.

One of Hall's targets was the widespread practice of patient bloodletting (bleeding). He was interested in the effects of hemorrhage during obstetrics, publishing papers such as *On the Effects of Loss of Blood* in 1826 and ". . . *the Morbid and Curative Effects of Loss of Blood,*" in 1832. The latter was based on experiments with dogs and on observations he made while patients were bled for medical reasons. He set forth guidelines for safe bleeding to avoid risks, which helped wean the medical profession from its pernicious tradition of using bloodletting as a cure-all.

Hall early recognized the public concerns about animal experimentation and urged that a society of physiological research be formed to oversee the conditions under which such investigations were conducted. *"Unhappily for the physiologist,"* he wrote, *"the subjects of animal physiology are sentient beings and every experiment is attended by pain or suffering."* Therefore he felt that such investigations should be legally regulated or their perpetrator would be accused of cruelty. Consequently he laid out five principles for discussion as a template for decision making before a proposed experiment could be authorized. These included lack of an alternative way to address the question that would not require intervention; requirement of a clearly stated objective; avoidance of unnecessary repetition; minimization of suffering, which included selection of less sentient subjects; and careful observation and recording of results with publication so that the public and other scholars could be made aware of them and so that duplication would be avoided.

Hall worked in the period before general anesthetics were discovered and was committed to minimizing suffering. Wherever the experimental goal permitted, he used prompt decapitation or transection of the spinal cord to ensure that sensation and volition ceased. He commended this practice to those who skinned eels alive, then a common practice. He studied the capillary circulation in vivo with a microscope, then studied neurophysiology by means of a truly comparative approach encompassing specimens from many vertebrate phyla. He made many significant contributions to the study of the nervous system. He also insisted that a code of medical ethics be required. Nonetheless, Hall became a main target, after Magendie, for attack from antivivisectionists. Moreover, his case was unusual in that he was criticized by members of his own profession who opposed vivisection and he never obtained an academic post; hence he left no legacy of scholars.

The central problem of the ethics of physiological research relates to the *means* by which its innately desirable *ends* have been reached. The difficulty arises because the subjects of the experiments are sentient creatures that feel pain and have learning capacities that evolved to promote survival. The latter include emotional reactions and awareness of danger that heighten apprehension and fear or aggression. Thus, in addition to the more immediate sensation of pain and discomfort, there is the psychological reaction of suffering resulting from perception of signals that cause fear. It is paradoxical that in the very mid-nineteenth-century period when the means to avoid suffering through the use of analgesic and anesthetic drugs had arrived, the antivivisection movement in Great Britain gained momentum and became a *cause célèbre*.

A remarkable figure who entered the scene in the second half of the nineteenth century was John Scott Burdon-Sanderson (1828-1905), an Edinburgh medical graduate who served on the Privy Council and the Cattle Plague Commission in England from 1865 to 1866. Burdon-Sanderson was appointed the first professor superintendent of the new Brown Animal Sanatory Institution established by the philanthropic bequest of Thomas Brown to the University of London. Burdon-Sanderson appointed William Duguid to be his resident veterinary surgeon, having used his services earlier while working on the cattle plague epidemic for the Privy Council. The Institution's stated goal was *to investigate and endeavor to cure maladies, distempers, and injuries of quadrupeds or birds useful to man.*

Burdon-Sanderson had prepared himself well for a career in pathophysiological research and animal experimentation. After gaining his medical qualification in Edinburgh, he studied organic chemistry and embryology in Paris and physiology with Claude Bernard. Burdon-Sanderson had a strong interest in pathology and microbiology and said that he was really a pupil of Chauveau, from whom he learned many of his great ideas about comparative pathology, infectious agents, and immunology. He put all his experience of continental ideas and methods to good use at the Brown Institution.

Accepting the ethos of the bequest, Burdon-Sanderson tackled one of the major cattle scourges, contagious bovine pleuropneumonia, and did some preliminary studies of foot-and-mouth disease and anthrax. Burdon-Sanderson addressed the issue of the infectious agents and attempted to develop vaccines, whereas Duguid characterized their epidemiology. However, the work was plagued by the growing criticism of antivivisectionists. Since the work was aimed at developing ways to protect livestock from devastating contagious diseases, the hostility of the protestors seems to have been misdirected.

Burdon-Sanderson left the Brown Institute in 1878 to become professor of physiology at University College, London, for seventeen years and then was appointed Wayneflete Professor at Oxford. He had a major influence on animal experimentation in British universities. He followed Michael Foster, who went to Cambridge University and founded the Laboratory of Physiology there, which became the focal point of Great Britain's reputation in physiological research in comparative physiology. This reputation was amplified for the veterinary profession through the Agricultural Research Council's Centre on Animal Physiology at Babraham and, later, by the establishment of a veterinary school at Cambridge.

Burdon-Sanderson had a profound impact on the development of professional animal physiology and its application to pathophysiology of diseases in Great Britain. His *Handbook for the Physiological Laboratory* of 1873 gleaned the best approaches to the subject from the several fine laboratories in Europe. This work made available to the budding British scholarly elite the most current technology (such as Ludwig's kymograph of 1846) and experimentation applied to the field. He was appointed to the first independent chair of physiology, the new Jodrell Professorship, in London. The seminal influence of Professor William Sharpey was recognized in the dedication of the text, and the Viennese Emanuel Klein and Lauder Bruxton (on histology and on digestion and secretion, respectively) were major contributors to the book. Bruxton became the leading British pharmacologist. The major criticism of the book by competent reviewers was that it failed to give an adequate coverage of and insistence on the need for anesthesia. However, Burdon-Sanderson did insist that the field of physiological research should be restricted to experienced investigators and the trainees under their expert supervision working in suitably equipped laboratories. He also stated that living animals should never be used in veterinary education in the mere pursuit of manual dexterity.

After Burdon-Sanderson moved to Oxford University as Wayneflete Professor of Physiology, he modernized the teaching of physiology, pharmacology, and pathology. He also served at the Infectious Diseases Hospital and on a royal commission on the consumption of tuberculous meat and milk. He helped orchestrate a judicial compromise between the experimenters and the antivivisectionists that facilitated the inauguration of Oxford's faculty of medicine in 1885. His successor was Sir William Osler, who also was interested in animal diseases and was an active participant in comparative medicine.

BRITISH ANTIVIVISECTIONISTS DEMAND LEGISLATION

The deplorable image of vivisection created by François Magendie and later, by his pupil Claude Bernard triggered the antivivisection activist movement in Great Britain. The apparent complete insensitivity toward animal suffering under the surgeon's scalpel became a traditional view of French biomedical science. Since Magendie had conducted similar experiments on cast-off cavalry and haulage horses, the veterinary school at Alfort was watched by British humanitarians. As early as 1846 individuals petitioned the French government to suppress vivisection at Alfort, without effect. By 1857 the tales of brutal practices there provoked the RSPCA to seek an audience with the king. He met with its representatives in 1861 but did not take the necessary action. The tensions heightened when the *Times* of London reported in 1863 that a culled horse would be turned over to students for experimentation and that it could be tortured for hours, having as many as sixty surgical interventions performed on it before it died. The British veterinary profession signed a mass protest; even French newspapers joined the clamor for reform. The *British Medical Journal* chimed in, noting that *". . . now that we possess the means of removing sensation during experiments, the man who puts an animal to torture ought to be prosecuted."* (Inhalation of ether had been shown to produce general anesthesia in Boston in the late 1840s.)

Exposure of the French practices aroused British public opinion and the traditional anti-French animus of the British. The Anglo-Irish aristocrat and writer Frances Power Cobbe (1822-1904), who had been scoffed at for advocating university places for women in 1862, joined the fray with an essay on *The Rights of Man and the Claims of Brutes.* While vacationing in Florence, she learned that Moritz Schiff was conducting a wide range of vivisection experiments on dogs and other species. She was disturbed to hear firsthand from Dr. Appleton, a visiting scholar from Harvard, that frightful things were being perpetrated on these animals. She went to work with remarkable zeal and put together a memorial petition signed by 783 people urging Schiff to spare his animals as much pain as possible. This first initiative of organized opposition to vivisection had little immediate result but had the effect of arousing local aristocrats to continue the pressure. Schiff departed for less hostile environs in 1877.

Another impact of the news of Alfort was the offering of prizes by the RSPCA for the best essays on vivisection. An army veterinary surgeon to the Third Hussars, George Fleming, and a physician won prizes for essays calling for the use of anesthetics in experiments on animals. Fleming's essay was entitled *Vivisection—Is It Necessary or Excusable?* and was used by the antivivisectionists in Europe. After the publication of these essays in 1866 the British Association for the Advancement of Science published four guiding rules for vivisection: it was not to be used for acquiring operative skills; it was always to be performed by qualified experts suitably equipped; the patient was to be under anesthesia wherever possible; and it was never to be demonstrated when suffering was involved. The controversy resurfaced in 1874 when a French surgeon, Eugène Magnan, performed operations on dogs to demonstrate the effects of injected alcohols at the British Medical Association Congress. Magnan fled to France to escape the resulting prosecution by the RSPCA.

Cobbe was again aroused to action and wrote another of her famous *"memorials,"* announcing her concern about the growing number of experiments conducted in Great Britain and alluding to the disgraceful Magnan affair. A distinguished group signed the document, including Browning, Carlyle, Lecky, Ruskin, Tennyson, Lord Shaftesbury, and seventy-eight physicians. The queen expressed her support for the RSPCA and her concern over the treatment of animals in science. The RSPCA set about documenting evidence of painful experiments based on published research. A letter from George Hoggan, who had been a student of Claude Bernard for four years, was published in the *Morning Post* in 1875. He claimed that none of the experiments was justifiable and that their primary goal was to get ahead of one's contemporaries in science, even at the price of an incalculable amount of torture.

Cobbe, Hoggan, and others drafted a bill for regulation of the practice of vivisection later that year. However, the scientists developed a contradictory bill, promoted by Burdon-Sanderson and Thomas Huxley, designed to maintain freedom of research. The government appointed a royal commission of enquiry with representation from both sides of the issue. After taking testimony from a long slate of distinguished witnesses, the commission reported that a total ban would be unreasonable, since the research sometimes mitigates human suffering and a ban would cause a "brain drain" of the best scientists to other countries. However, it also called for state licensing of original research and teaching demonstrations. The result was redrafting of new bills by both sides in the dispute.

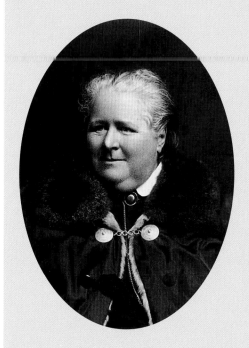

512. Frances Power Cobbe (1822-1904), outstanding antivivisectionist and leading feminist of the period, was responsible for the first organized opposition to vivisection. Her initial efforts, which included an essay, *The Rights of Man and the Claims of Brutes,* did not lead to an immediate result, but the Anglo-Irish aristocrat did arouse other aristocrats to continue pressuring for humane guidelines for vivisection. *(Hulton Deutsch Collection, Limited, London.)*

Cobbe had been disappointed with the position taken by the RSPCA, which she considered overly cautious, and assembled a new group, the Victoria Street Society. The president was Anthony Ashley Cooper (1801-1885), seventh Earl of Shaftesbury, who led a delegation to see the home secretary early in 1876. The delegates were invited to submit suggestions for legislation. The Victoria Street Society drafted a new bill that disallowed experiments on dogs, cats, and the equid species. Other animals could be subject to experiment only under conditions of complete anesthesia. The Earl of Carnarvon presented the bill, but its passage had to be delayed because of a serious illness in his family. Meanwhile, the General Medical Council obtained three thousand signatures from medical practitioners urgently petitioning the home secretary to modify the bill. The result was passage of the Cruelty to Animals Act of 1876. Although the act made important restrictions on animal experimentation, these could be annulled by special certificates issued by the home office.

BIOMEDICAL SCIENTISTS SEEK PUBLIC SUPPORT FOR RESEARCH

It seems odd that the extreme antivivisectionists deemed it morally wrong to follow up *"mere"* or *"morbid"* scientific curiosity with experimentation. Unless the overarching argument that any exploitation of animals is evil can be sustained, it seems irrational to selectively suppress bioscience in an age when most of its scientific hypotheses can be tested without causing suffering. Also, as biomedical research has evolved, the process has become more complex and sophisticated. There is little doubt today that the role of a biomedical scientist has become more exacting and that clinically relevant outcomes have become more dependent on the efforts of professional scientists. One has only to recall the catastrophic loss of life to epidemics of contagious diseases of people and domestic animals throughout history or, today, the existence of the acquired immunodeficiency syndrome (AIDS) in humans and epizootic virus diseases of domestic vertebrates, to realize that all available motivation and skill must be harnessed if deaths are to be minimized.

The Physiological Society of Great Britain was established in 1876, the very year in which the Cruelty to Animals Act was passed. It was paradoxical that the remarkable scientific successes of a small group of distinguished scholars in this field should have been accompanied by a major action of public policy designed in part to limit their freedom to continue to perform the experimental methods on which their achievements had been based. A royal commission had been appointed in 1875 to conduct an inquiry into the allegations that the British physiologists inflicted cruelty upon the animal subjects of their experiments. The commission reported, after thorough investigation, that it had been unable to find evidence in support of the charges. Nevertheless, the antivivisectionists used the media and any other means available to generate public outrage at the physiologists who, they believed, were deliberate torturers of animals.

The tactics of antivivisectionists finally provoked the scientists to retaliate with a publicity campaign in an effort to set the record straight in the eyes of the public and their political representatives. The scientific and medical journals carried a large number of articles on animal experimentation between 1875 and 1890. A high point in the debate occurred in 1881 at the International Medical Congress in London. The participants included many authorities who were heralding the powers of the new wave of research in biomedical science to develop solutions to the medical problems that caused so much misery to humankind. The list of scholars was formidable and included Owen, Huxley, Koch, Pasteur, and Virchow. The congress made a major focus of the vivisection issue and concluded with a resolution to the effect that experiments on living animals are indispensable to medical progress and that, in the interests of both man and animal, it would be undesirable to restrict competent persons from performing them. The British Medical Association promptly echoed the congress's position by stating that prohibition of experimentation on animals would *"prevent investigations which were calculated to promote the better knowledge and treatment of disease in animals as well as man."*

It was anomalous that the debate over vivisection was mainly a cause sustained by middle-class and upper-class women. They were the activists for protection against perceived licentiousness in animal cruelty, whether it be in brutal working-class sports or in the scientists' laboratories. The scientists pointed out the inconsistency of these traditional aristocrats attacking well-intentioned scientific research while their families were actively engaged in the blood sports of stag hunting, fox hunting, and game-bird shooting. The effect of the debate was a proliferation of provivisection and antivivisection views rather than an attempt by the groups to work constructively to develop a sound policy that would let society have the best of both worlds—a kind of *progressus sine noxa* (progress without harm)—rather than Hippocrates' more inhibitory *primum non nocere* (above all, do no harm).

AMERICAN INITIATIVES TO STOP CRUELTY TO ANIMALS

During the mid-eighteenth century in Germany, legal actions were taken against people who had committed acts of vicious cruelty toward animals. Several German states and Swiss and German cities developed societies and laws condemning cruelty to animals. The Scandinavian countries soon followed suit. The Latin Roman Catholic countries were less sensitive to animal suffering. Influential figures in Europe's humane movement included Frederick the Great (1712-1786), who had great affection for his animals, and Pastor Albert Knapp in Stuttgart, who founded the first German animal welfare society in 1837. Emperor Joseph II had put an end to animal baiting in 1789.

Adolf Nordvall in Sweden presented a strong philosophical argument against vivisection. Victor Hugo was the first president of the French Anti-Vivisection Society in 1883. An international network of leading figures in the movement to prevent cruelty to animals developed.

The United States developed codes of animal protection that closely followed their precedents in Great Britain. Cruelty to horses, cattle, and sheep was made a misdemeanor in New York by 1828. Other centers soon adopted similar laws, but it was reported that enforcement was rare. Reverend Charles Lowell in Boston preached against cruelty to animals in 1837. After the Civil War a New Yorker, Henry Bergh (1813-1888), who had just returned from being U.S. ambassador to Russia during the Civil War, attended the RSPCA meeting in Great Britain and set out to emulate the English example in the United States. He succeeded in mobilizing influential citizens to join him in a campaign to create an American Society for the Prevention of Cruelty to Animals. The state of New York approved the proposal in 1866. The very next year Philadelphians led by Caroline Earl White formed an SPCA in that city. Bergh enlisted Emily Appleton in Boston, who joined forces with George Angell, a wealthy lawyer and a slavery abolitionist who shared her concern about cruelty to racehorses. In 1868 they formed the Massachusetts SPCA, which published a journal, *Our Dumb Animals,* and drafted state anticruelty legislation. The remarkable spread of the influence of the Anglophile reformers Bergh and Angell was indicative of a more receptive substrate, at least among the influential urban middle and upper classes in the United States than in Britain.

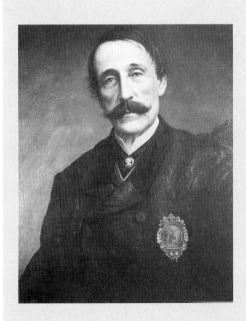

513. Emulating efforts in Britain, Henry Bergh (1813-1888) founded the American Society for the Prevention of Cruelty to Animals (ASPCA) in New York in 1866. Thereafter, many state associations were soon established for the protection of animals. *(Reproduced by Kind Permission of The American Society for the Prevention of Cruelty to Animals, New York.)*

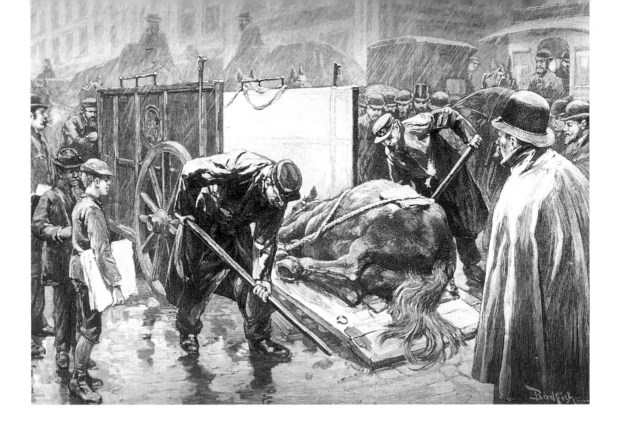

514. In this engraving by Standenbaur from a drawing by W.P. Bodfish a sick horse is being placed in an ambulance in the streets of New York in 1888. Humane care of horses became a top priority, and legislation against abuse, overuse, transportation, and other practices was passed. *(National Library of Medicine, Bethesda, Maryland.)*

Prevention of abuse of horses was a top priority in legislation prohibiting the beating of horses, the use of the bearing rein, and the suffering imposed on food animals neglected in long-distance rail transport. Thousands of animals, often unfed and unwatered, died in trains on the way to the slaughterhouses. The American SPCAs federated as the American Humane Association (AHA) in 1877 in a campaign to stop this inhumane treatment. Early in the twentieth century, the AHA under William Stillman founded the Red Star to aid army animals in much the same way that the Red Cross aided people. The AHA also placed equal concern on preventing cruelty to children and animals. In 1884 Bergh had helped found the New York Society for the Prevention of Cruelty to Children (SPCC), an idea that soon echoed around the world, as well as in Great Britain, where the RSPCA was directly influential in creating a national SPCC. It is a reflection of the societal attitudes of the period that it took the more visible atrocities suffered by animals to arouse concern about and action to prevent the less apparent abuses of children.

The previously mentioned pioneers were less successful in campaigns for legislation against vivisection than those for protection of children from abuse. Bergh later received articulate support in this effort from the physiologist Alfred Leffingwell, who had witnessed some of Claude Bernard's experiments and quoted Harvard professor of medicine Henry Bigelow as follows: "It is the blood and suffering, not the science, that rivets [the students'] breathless attention . . . vivisection deadens their humanity and begets indifference to it."

While the preceding events were unfolding, the 1862 Land Grant Act was passed. It encouraged the formation of universities in each state to offer instruction in "agriculture and the mechanic arts." Animal use in research increased progressively thereafter and gained another boost with the passage of the Hatch Act in 1887, which funded research at the Agricultural Experiment Stations.

A NEW VETERINARY FIELD: LABORATORY ANIMAL SCIENCE

The American Public Health Association was founded in 1872, and in 1879 a National Board of Health was established by the United States Congress. Quarantine stations were erected near major international seaports to block the entry of contagious diseases of humans and animals. John Shaw Billings was the army's Inspector of Hospitals. He later organized the Library of the Surgeon General of the Army, which evolved into the mighty National Library of Medicine; created the marvelous bibliographic service of the *Index Medicus;* and designed two famous hospitals, The Johns Hopkins Hospital in Baltimore and the Peter Bent Brigham Hospital in Boston.

The Ransdell Act of 1930 created the National Institutes of Health (NIH) to replace the former Hygienic Laboratory. The NIH, as the designated research body of the Public Health Service, was to grow into the world's largest funding system for medical research and the training of medical researchers. Its focus became progressively directed toward advanced laboratory-based studies of basic biomedical processes and chronic diseases. This focus left a void in the area of infectious diseases. A Communicable Disease Center was established in 1946; its name was changed to the Centers for Disease Control (CDC) in 1980. It was the CDC's routine surveillance systems that in 1981 noted the emergence of a new syndrome of *Pneumocystis carinii* pneumonia, which led to the identification of the acquired immunodeficiency syndrome (AIDS). The CDC needed veterinarians with advanced training in contagious diseases, and they played a significant part in its development under the guidance of James H. Steele. William T.S. Thorp became chief of the Laboratory Aids Branch of NIH and played an important role in the design of animal facilities to meet the needs of animal welfare in the rapidly expanding medical and biological research.

The far-sighted planners at the Mayo Clinic in Rochester, Minnesota, perceived a need to strengthen their research capability. They established a Division of Experimental Surgery and Pathology in 1914. The following year they hired Simon D. Brimhall (1863-1941), a veterinarian who graduated from the University of Pennsylvania, to manage their research animal operations. He was responsible for development of the animal facilities and breeding colonies, for the investigation of diseases of laboratory animals, and for assisting in research involving experimental animals and ensuring that only healthy animals were used and that they received excellent postsurgical care. This animal research center proved to be a momentous step for the veterinary profession and evolved into a major supporting arm for biological and medical research.

Carl F. Schlotthauer (1893-1959) followed Simon Brimhall and John Hardenbergh in the role of animal research manager. Schlotthauer was also appointed professor in the University of Minnesota graduate school in 1945, the first professorship in the field of laboratory animal medicine in the United States.

Charles A. Griffin (1889-1955) was a veterinarian and microbiologist at the New York State Board of Health Laboratories in Albany from 1919 to 1954. He masterminded the development of pathogen-free animal colonies, the raising of rabbits free of the dreaded *Pasteurella* infection, and the development of diets free of contaminating *Salmonella* organisms. The American Association for Laboratory Animal Science established a memorial award honoring his name and achievements. The first president of this association was Nathan R. Brewer, the veterinarian in charge of animal facilities of the University of Chicago in 1950.

Karl F. Meyer (1884-1974), the famous Swiss veterinary comparative epidemiologist whose global reach extended to the George Williams Hooper Foundation at the University of California at San Francisco, developed a model institutional facility for experimental animals; he was assisted by Bernice Eddy. As early as 1928, he had written a review of *Communicable Diseases of Laboratory Animals.*

Later developments included the design of systems that allowed the production of entirely germ-free, or *gnotobiotic,* animals by veterinary teams. In 1963 the NIH developed a *Guide for Laboratory Animal Facilities and Care,* which set high standards for the management of the animal units. The National Academy of Sciences developed an Institute of Laboratory Animal Resources in 1953. The institute developed guidelines for training in laboratory animal medicine, a field that was recognized as a specialty board by the American Veterinary Medical Association in 1957. A number of distinguished medical schools began to offer NIH-sponsored residency programs in laboratory animal medicine for veterinarians. These included the medical schools at The Johns Hopkins University, Yale University, Bowman Gray, Michigan, Washington, and Texas. In addition, in 1966, Congress passed the Laboratory Animal Welfare Act (now known as the Animal Welfare Act), the first law to offer protection to laboratory animals in the United States. An important development in Canada was the establishment of the Canadian Council on Animal Care under veterinary pathologist Harry C. Rowsell in 1968.

CHARTING THE MORAL COURSE: LESSONS FROM HISTORY

The fundamental question about animal experimentation is whether it is morally justifiable. What criteria would make it justifiable or unjustifiable? To attack this issue, the question of its purposes must be aired, along with the interpretation of their degrees of necessity. Overcoming ignorance of how the human body works has been a central value and goal in the conduct of experiments on animals. These gave rise to the widely perceived necessity to address this question so that progress can be made in overcoming the myriad diseases to which human flesh is heir. Since most societies and cultures have deemed it unthinkable to carry out such experiments directly on the beneficiary human species, animals with comparable functions and dysfunctions have been used. Has the goal withstood the test of time? The majority of individuals would agree that it has and that humans have much greater understanding of their processes and diseases as a result of this comparative research. Often a long time lag and many intermediate steps and experiments have been required in finding answers to complex questions and coming up with effective therapies and preventive measures for diseases.

An important question is whether these gains at the expense of animal lives and well-being were justified and can continue to be so. Philosophers, scientists, and thinking persons have debated loud and long on the issue of the moral value attached to animals and whether this value can be prioritized by species, depending, for example, on their degree of neural capacity or sentience. At each end of the spectrum of debate there are persons with extreme, "black or white" views for whom the issue is clear-cut. There is no doubt that there was a shameful era in history when animals were vivisected without concern for suffering. In the societies of that time various atrocities were inflicted on animals. The Roman authorities even promoted such activities as entertainment to distract the masses, thereby defusing political activism. This promotion was an appeal to the baser side of human nature, a degrading maneuver in an age when human slavery and exploitation were rampant.

Neglected by many commentators is the possibility that without the horrible efforts of the early vivisectors little progress might have been made toward the sparing of suffering in subsequent generations of animals. The most critical period for the practice was the first half of the nineteenth century, when French scholars, whose hearts were undoubtedly hardened by post-Revolutionary excesses, took the initiative of using animals in trying to answer biomedical questions. The discovery of anesthesia and better analgesics made possible the removal of suffering from many experiments, and euthanasia could be performed without recovery from anesthesia. The mounting tide of concern about the early experimenters' insensitivity peaked after this technical problem was well on its way to resolution in the second half of the nineteenth century.

Many of the protagonists in the debate have argued in terms of absolutes. A more sensible approach might be to examine the issues in the light of historical change. At one time, just to survive, poor, hairless humans living at high latitudes had to make themselves clothing of pelts or hides at the expense of the original animal owners. Few humans are in that situation today, although the use of leather, especially for footwear, is widespread. What could be rightly asked is whether the evolving cultures considered such issues with sensitivity and made appropriate adjustments. There is real concern that animal experimentation has become a major industry involving vast numbers of animals that would not even exist but for well-funded biomedical research. Ultimately the right of the researcher to conduct a given experiment depends on laws enacted to govern the process and the regulations created to implement them. To allow for change as new challenges and opportunities for research arise, an adaptive attitude is required. The question of moral concern must be expanded to encompass issues like overpopulation, environmental degradation, and the creation of new life-forms. Catastrophic situations, whether the result of epidemic diseases or other planet-threatening events, require heroic actions and sacrifices. Animals may be expected to be made to contribute to the resolution of such catastrophes, with insistence on humane treatment.

Important initiatives have been made in developing alternatives to replace the use of animals in testing, such as computer models, synthetic fibers and even synthetic skin, although they do not always serve as well and can lead to unforeseen problems. Significant progress in the methodology and statistical evaluation of techniques such as the LD50 is leading to major reductions in the numbers of animals used in testing of pharmaceuticals and products used in the home.

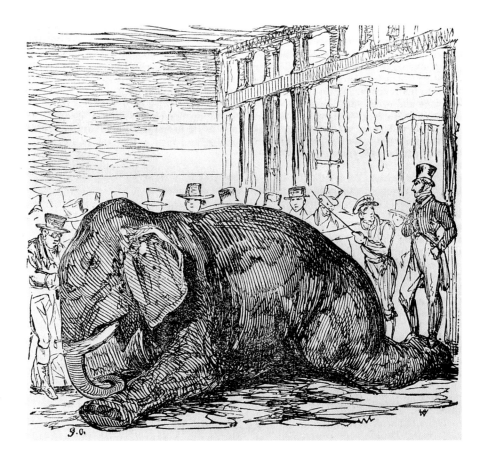

515. *Dead Elephant at Cross's Menagerie, Exeter Change,* engraving from an etching by George Cruikshank (English, 1792-1878), published in the second volume of William Hone's *The Every-Day Book: Or the Guide of the Year* (London, 1826). Cruikshank, known for his satirical drawings attacking the savage ethical code of his time, captured the plight of this captive elephant's death with great dignity and grace. According to the entry in Hone's *Book* for May 9, this Indian elephant had been kept stationary in a den at the Royal Menagerie at Exeter Change on the Strand in west central London by its owner, Mr. Cross, from 1814 to 1826. The animal had annual paroxysms, becoming infuriated, which were undoubtedly musth. In India the elephant would have been allowed to rampage in the forests until the condition ran its natural course, but in this poor creature's case he was kept confined in his den and drugged with "24 pounds of salts, 24 pounds of treacle, 6 ounces of calomel, an ounce and a half of tartar emetic, and 6 drams of powder of gamboge. To this was added a bottle of croton oil."

In 1826, the last year of the elephant's life, the medicine produced no effect on the annual rage. After the elephant attempted to escape his den, which was precariously located on the second floor of the building, his handlers, fearing he would crash through the wooden floor and get into the Strand below, attempted to poison him with arsenic. This attempt failed, and he was subsequently shot at least one hundred and twenty times before a sword, affixed to a pole, was thrust in him to the hilt, finally ending his life. The illustration was accompanied by the following poem:

THE ELEPHANT
As he laid dead at Exeter Change

In the position he liked best
He seemed to drop, to sudden rest;
Nor bowed his neck, but still a sense
Retain'd of his magnificence;
For, as he fell, he raised his head
And held it, as in life, when dead.

(Courtesy the Charles Major Collection, Purdue University Libraries, West Lafayette, Indiana.)

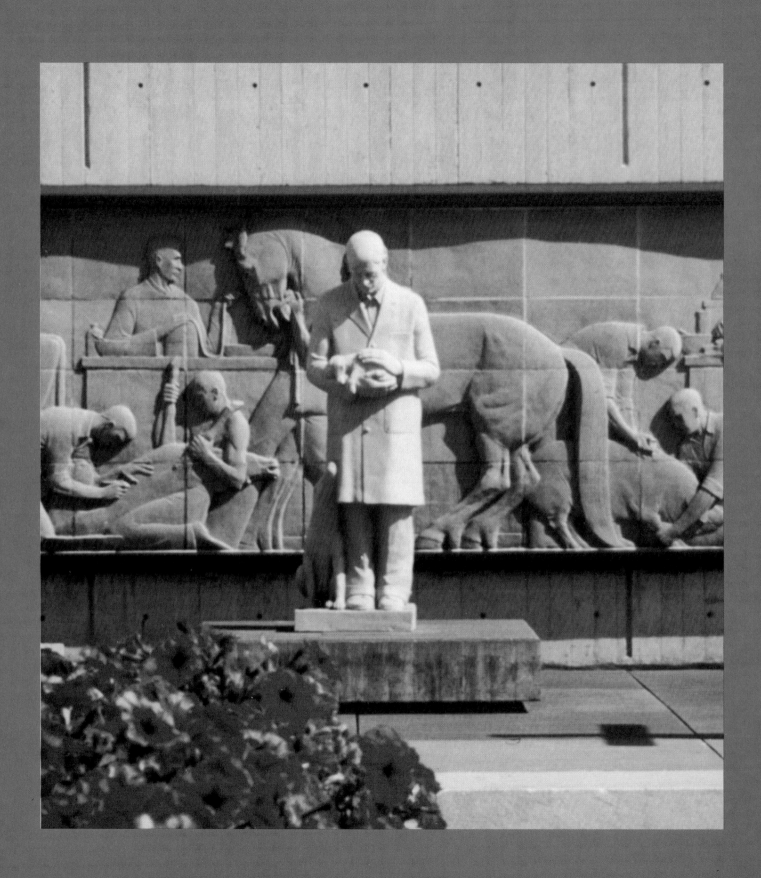

Evolving Veterinary Careers

A Spectrum of Opportunity

THE NEW PROFESSION FROM 1762 TO THE EARLY NINETEENTH CENTURY

It can be argued that the modern veterinary profession was born of the aggressive nature of humans: the need to fight and dominate. People in good standing with their royal courts in the second half of the eighteenth century were the prime movers, horsemen who knew about breeding, training, and maintaining horses and educated young aristocrats to whom the art of riding was second nature. The focus on the horse was both practical and symbolic. The horse was important in war, both when ridden by the cavalry and for transporting necessary weapons, personnel, and supplies. In fact, the perceived need to exploit the motive power of the horse was a vital factor in creating a demand for horse doctors. A trade for horse foot-maintenance mechanics, the farriers or blacksmiths, was already in existence. These usually burly men were used to handling large horses and working red-hot iron into functional horseshoes and other equine equipment. Although Bertin focused on the need to find ways to control the epidemic diseases of agricultural animals that were threatening the peasant economy, his ideas were not translated into action at the veterinary schools.

The earliest veterinary graduates had to make the transition from farrier to veterinarian. The former trade required familiarity with the ways of horses and the ability to restrain, handle, shoe, and dose them. The new professionals added knowledge of anatomy and a cursory awareness of equine diseases and treatments, a sketchy empirical tradition. The occupational hazards included risk of physical injury from frightened or vicious animals that had to be restrained or cast and trussed to allow surgical intervention in the days before anesthesia. The horrible affliction of glanders led to terrible sores with little hope of recovery. A number of veterinary students at Alfort became infected and died of the disease.

It was a challenging period for veterinary faculty. Creating a base of knowledge about animal function and disease virtually from nothing but a base of equine anatomy was a formidable task. The art of performing examinations and surgical interventions, however, required special heavy-duty equipment, which brought out ingenuity in instrument design and manufacture. Manual dexterity and physical coordination were also essential skills for the veterinary surgeon.

Two of Bourgelat's important contributions were to seek educated, intelligent students and to plan a rigorous course of study. His successor, Chabert, turned these features to good advantage by articulating the need for research and setting a fine example by conducting a strong program of research in veterinary science. This emphasis on research earned the graduates respect for having a scientific attitude and being competent (for the times) as horse doctors.

516. *Facing page,* This larger-than-life sculpture is one of the best known works of Danish-born artist Christian Petersen. Petersen became the first artist-in-residence at Iowa State University in 1937. *The Gentle Doctor,* depicting a veterinarian caring for a female dog and her pup, resulted from many years of interaction between Petersen and the faculty and students of the College of Veterinary Medicine at this institution. The original work now stands in the Scheman Continuing Education Building on the main university campus, while a full-scale replica welcomes visitors at the entrance to the College of Veterinary Medicine. *(Courtesy of the College of Veterinary Medicine, Iowa State University.)*

517. This horrifying picture depicts an actual case of glanders in a veterinary student in Alfort, France, who died of the disease in 1836. Sainbel, the principal of the London school had died of the disease in 1793, but it was not diagnosed at the time. It gradually became realized that glanders was a zoonosis and a serious occupational hazard for people who dissected or worked with horses. A French military surgeon, Lorin, diagnosed two cases of human farcy in 1812 after Jean Hameau had observed in 1810 that the disease could affect people. In 1817 a London veterinary student was infected via a cut while dissecting. Pus from his lesions was inoculated into a donkey, which contracted the disease and died. John Elliotson in London in 1830, unaware of the nature of the disease, described the signs in gory detail—abscesses, pustules, purulent nasal discharge with gangrene of the nose, prostration, and death. Rayer in Paris wrote the most complete monograph on the zoonosis in 1837 and was appointed to France's first chair in comparative medicine in 1862. The cause of the disease was proposed by Chauveau and the bacterium *Pseudomonas mallei* was isolated by Löffler and Schütz in 1886. Strauss's preparation of an extract called mallein allowed the development of a test to be used in eradication of the disease from equidae. William Hunting, editor of the *Veterinary Record,* wrote a clinical treatise on glanders in 1908 that included an appendix on glanders in humans that described a number of cases and published reports. He noted that *Carnivora* had become infected by eating the flesh of glandered horses. *(Reproduced from Théoridès:* Des miasmes aux virus histoire des maladies in fectieuses, *Editions Louis Pariente, Paris, 1991.)*

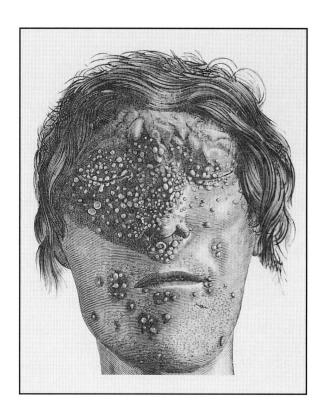

In modern parlance, Bourgelat made the paradigm shift that, although far from perfect, was necessary to allow the intellectual seeds of a new profession to germinate and progress to fruition. LaFosse, on the other hand, tried to build on a foundation (farriery) that was inadequate to support the necessary intellectual development for veterinary medicine. Despite a valiant effort based on his own contribution to a scientific thrust, his approach was doomed to fail because the farrier trade was composed of people ill-prepared for the challenge. Nevertheless, by exploiting the state of the farrier art attained by LaFosse and others, the new veterinary profession was able to acquire skills it needed to command a degree of respect. This gave the profession a launching pad, albeit a seriously flawed one because of the lack of a scientific base. Before the end of the eighteenth century, France became distracted from orderly events by the French Revolution of 1792, which was followed by carnage and strife that set back progress. The Lyon veterinary school survived only because of the tenacity of director Louis Bredin, who evacuated it to his estate.

A remarkable story developed when the doge (duke) of Venice corresponded with Bourgelat about the possibility of starting a veterinary school at Padua in the state of Venezia. Bourgelat at first proposed that two students be sent to Alfort to study the new field of veterinary medicine there but later wrote to the duke that it would not be necessary to send students because he had a very good Italian student, Guiseppe Orus, whom he would send to Padua. Orus started the Padua school on September 9, 1773, the second veterinary college in Italy, after Turin. The Turin school, a military school, was established to produce horse veterinary surgeons for the army, but it had a difficult initiation after it was named. Consequently, people wishing to be veterinarians came to Padua from other Italian states, so the Padua school considered itself to be in contention with Turin for the site of the first effective school. There was an important difference in the motivations for the two schools. Venice had been a great center for international trade by ship, but trade with the East stopped because of the plague (black death). The adaptable Venetians observed the successful development of livestock agriculture and bought cattle from Hungary and Russia at high prices. Thus the agricultural animals were given a higher priority at the Padua school, as Venice became the first Italian state to acquire a bovine focus and study diseases of cattle.

The most striking feature of the Padua school was its name: Orus christened it *Collegium Zoojatricum Patavinum* and enshrined the name on the school's seal. Evidently he was a visionary who foresaw that veterinary medicine applied to all animals, perhaps, at first, to all domestic animals. Tragedy struck the school after Napoleon invaded Italy. First he took Lombardy and Emilia, and later Venezia. His army entered Padua in 1797, and the war moved in a seesaw fashion between France and the Austro-Hungarian Empire. Padua changed hands several times, and the veterinary school was closed between 1794 and 1796. The founder, Guiseppe Orus, died prematurely in 1792 at forty-two years of age. He wrote two books, *Osservazioni fisico-pratiche sopra alcuni animalia domestici villerecci* (1779) and *Trattato medico pratico di alcune malattie delgi animali domestice,* which his wife published one year after his death. Only about forty students had graduated from the school, but they were a different breed from the army horse doctors, being trained in the scientific and medical ideas of Padua and in the clinical veterinary medicine of all domestic species. The medical faculty of Padua survived and kept a part of the spirit of the veterinary school, saying that the physicians should study something of veterinary medicine to be competent in public health.*

Progress in veterinary service for the equine community was held back by its traditions and established ideas. Lacking the farriery tradition, the intellectual innocence of the approach to the medical needs of food- and fiber-providing species allowed a more direct scientific thrust to develop. Each country had its own priorities, attitudes, and policies, but the emerging scientific approach transcended national borders. An important societal development of the late eighteenth and the nineteenth centuries was the advancement of private and public transport and communication. The stagecoaches reached their peak in the 1830s, then the railroads began to displace them. The various armies that fought across Europe in the early decades of the nineteenth century required army veterinarians. Most of the diplomates of veterinary schools ended up in the army until greater stability was achieved in rural areas. The military actions and invasions increased the spread of infectious diseases in horses and other livestock.

The British Profession's Efforts to Gain Official Recognition

The young profession in Great Britain was frustrated by its lowly status and lack of parity with human medicine. Veterinarians perceived the control of the London school by governing and examining bodies composed solely of representatives of the medical profession to be a major factor in suppressing their aspirations. In 1823, when William Dick opened his school in Edinburgh, at least there was an alternative. The founding of the first veterinary journal in English, *The Veterinarian,* allowed concerns to be aired and ideas to be shared among the one thousand (approximately) who were in the profession by Coleman's death.

The father and son veterinary team of Thomas Mayer (1791-1848) and Thomas Walton Mayer (1814-1887) organized a committee to campaign for a change in the official status of the profession. Led by Thomas Turner, the committee petitioned the Privy Council in 1841 to confer upon the veterinary profession the title *Royal College of Veterinary Surgeons* (RCVS). The case was based on the need for a new system for regulating the educational examination of those who would become practitioners. A Charter of Incorporation was submitted and, after imposing certain regulations, Queen Victoria granted a Royal Charter of Incorporation in 1844. All the existing graduates of the London and Edinburgh schools thus became members of the RCVS, although colleges fought this transfer of their authority.

---

*The full story will be told in a book by Professor Alba Veggetti of the Bologna Faculty, to be published by the Institute of the History of the University of Padua.

No sooner was the charter approved than the heads of the colleges and the governors of the Royal Veterinary College (RVC) realized that the monopolistic authority of their fiefdoms had been lost to the new royal college. They protested and petitioned the new RCVS, but to no avail. William Sewell, the principal of the RVC who had followed Coleman, was in a particularly tight corner as a pawn of the RVC's governors, who were surgeons or physicians. Professor Dick in Edinburgh declared independence from the charter, but Sewell could not obtain support of the Royal Agricultural Society of England for such a bold move. The breach was not repaired in London until 1852, when Professor Sewell was appointed president of the RCVS. He died the following year.

During the 1840s, turbulent years for Britain's veterinary establishment, the profession started to expand its scope. John Gamgee traveled to the Continent and reported that only nine percent of the horses he saw in Paris were lame, as compared with a tragic forty-two percent in Great Britain. *The Veterinarian* published its first article on diseases of cats in 1841. By 1850 it reported that "many practitioners" were restricting their practice to dogs—the beginning of urban companion animal medicine.

The effect of the royal charter for the veterinary profession was profound. As stated earlier, it made the existing graduates of the London and Edinburgh schools members of the RCVS, although they failed in their bid to gain an exclusive right to the title of veterinary surgeon. All new graduates received the diploma of membership. The most important change, however, was the breaking of the stranglehold the medical profession had on the London college. All six members of the board of governors resigned. Five of the doctors on the board agreed to serve temporarily as part of a transition team on a mixed board that included veterinary examiners for the first time. At last the veterinary profession was achieving command of its own destiny. The RCVS set about creating a register of qualified veterinarians, but the Edinburgh data were not provided. Professor Dick chose to work with the Highland and Agricultural Society of Scotland instead, having seceded from the RCVS.

There was much to do to break out of the previous defective traditions of student selection and curriculum. In London in the 1850s veterinary education was still in a dismal state. Facilities and laboratories were cramped and entirely inadequate. Although a good supply of horses was brought to the RVC for soundness examinations, professors gave students little insight into the process of evaluation. The students were not even entrusted to perform duties such as casting for surgery or administration of medicines, let alone being allowed to participate in the operations themselves. No books were provided, no instruction in shoeing was given; only in dissection were the students given reasonable opportunities to learn.

William J.T. Morton (1800-1868) was appointed professor of chemistry and materia medica at the RVC in 1839 and was the first to take the RCVS diploma examination in 1844. He was considered a fine teacher. He wrote *Veterinary Pharmacopoeia,* and after Youatt died, he became a coeditor of *The Veterinarian.* He seems to have been a positive force in the school. He retired in 1860. A long-standing concern about the weak educational background of students entering the college was finally addressed by the institution of a matriculation examination in 1864 that required evidence of ability to read, write, and do some elementary arithmetic. When the RCVS became responsible for the curriculum and examination in 1844, they immediately decreased the duration of study to two years. Sainbel's original duration of three years was not restored until 1876; in 1885, it was increased to four years. It was common practice in England, as in many parts of Europe at the beginning of the nineteenth century, for students to choose when they were ready for examination.

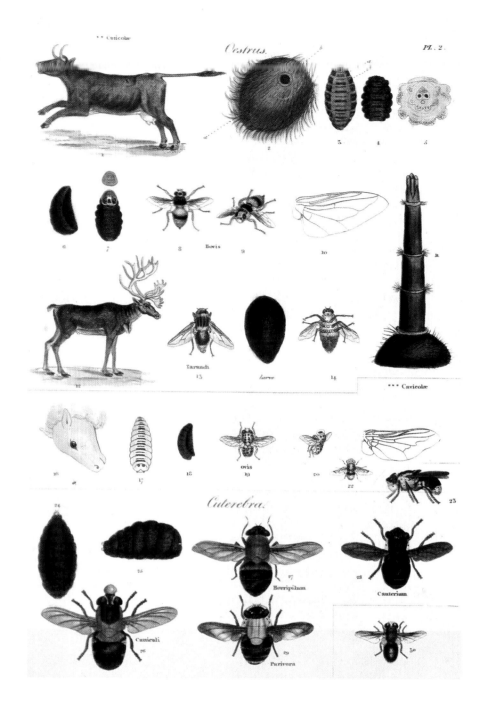

518. Bracy Clark (1771-1862) from west-central England was a brilliant young man with a classical education who apprenticed in medicine and surgery before opting for the new Royal Veterinary College in 1792. A good linguist, he helped his mentor Sainbel, the founding principal, who set high standards and shared his enthusiasm for equine studies. Clark also led in the first equine patient when the RVC's infirmary opened in 1793. He graduated in 1794, just after the new principal was appointed. He deplored Coleman's policy of lowering standards for the profession and criticized him harshly in *The Farrier and Naturalist.* He toured veterinary facilities on the continent, then established a very successful London practice specializing in draft horses. A prolific author, he wrote on the veterinary art, equine anatomy, and bits and shoes, including *Hippodonomia,* which dealt with the natural movements of the hoof when bearing weight. He designed hinged shoes to allow for expansion. He condemned the "blacksmith physicians" for their ignorance and use of vile medications. He acquired the skeleton of the famous racehorse *Eclipse,* which Sainbel had studied. As this illustration shows, he became very interested in stomach bots of horses, and this led to studies of the life cycles of the bee-sized parasitic flies that worry livestock and can cause gadding when they deposit their eggs or larvae. Today they are known as *Gasterophilus* in horses, *Hypoderma*-type in cattle and reindeer *(Oedemagena),* and *Oestrus* in sheep, their larvae becoming gastric bots, subcutaneous warbles, or nasal bots, respectively. The genus term *Cuterebra* is now used for those that affect rodents and lagomorphs. *(From Clark, 1824.)*

Perhaps the most revealing evidence of the attitudinal problem of the RVC's board of governors was given in their response to a request in 1840 from veterinary practitioners who sought to become subscribing members of the college (as any other person was allowed to do): the governors adamantly rejected the request "because they might learn some of the secrets of the College thus becoming more skillful and successful and might interfere with the interests and profits of the College."

Veterinary Attention to Food Animals

James Beart Simonds, a rural practitioner at Twickenham, was appointed in 1840 by the RVC to meet a growing demand, backed by a grant from the Royal Agricultural Society of England, that lectures be instituted on anatomy and treatment of diseases of cattle, sheep, and other domestic animals.

Curiously, the principal and the governors of the college had resisted this demand for a long time. As a result, the chair of cattle pathology was named. The initial focus was to be on the infectious diseases. Although frequently the subject of criticism by veterinary commentators such as Smith and Gamgee, Simonds played a crucial role in expanding the scope of the profession to encompass the food animal industries. He demonstrated by simple experiments that foot-and-mouth disease was contagious for both cattle and pigs, then showed how strict isolation could prevent its spread. He diagnosed sheep pox in 1847, showed that it was contagious, and pressed for an act to control the disease by destruction of affected stock and regulation of imports. The authority was granted in 1848. His experiments established that cowpox vaccine failed to give protection against sheep pox but that "lymph" fluid from infected sheep ("ovination") provided protection. The disease was eradicated, recurred in 1862, and was eradicated again in 1866. Simonds diagnosed swine fever in Berkshire in 1862. His role in the 1865 rinderpest outbreak in Great Britain is discussed in Chapter 29. Simonds was principal of the RVC from 1872 to 1881. He conducted a detailed review of the educational system and also completed the incorporation of the college in 1875 by Royal Charter.

GROWTH OF THE PROFESSION IN THE MID-NINETEENTH CENTURY

It should be realized that most of the schools on the Continent received state support, whereas in Great Britain they were dependent on tuition, fees, and sponsors and therefore tended to be impoverished. The middle decades of the nineteenth century were an exciting period on the European continent during which veterinary scientists moved into the mainstream of biomedical research. The horse and the ruminant species received special attention. The centralized government system in France allowed veterinary research to be funded and effective control measures for epizootics to be implemented. In England, under its private funding system, this did not happen.

Into clinical practice came improvements in methods and devices to facilitate the handling of horses, such as Abildgaard's casting harness, which facilitated the safe casting of horses. Then came the discovery and application of the anesthetic effect of certain volatile organic chemicals: diethyl ether and chloroform. Other developments led to great improvement in surgical technique: improved needles and suturing materials, instruments that could ensure hemostasis, and sterile absorbent sponges. Lister's disinfectant spray with phenol followed, and the sterilization of surgical instruments by boiling in water or holding in a flame was introduced. Charles Pravaz's invention of the hypodermic syringe and needles to permit injections into subcutaneous tissues or muscles or directly into the venous blood was a major advance. Much more precise control of the dosage of medications became possible. Many of these advances were superbly captured in a major work by an artist at the royal veterinary school in Copenhagen in 1898.

John Gamgee, at his Albert veterinary school in London in 1865, introduced the use of a thermometer during clinical examination to show that fever was a feature of the cattle plague. The enterprising George Armatage at Glasgow demonstrated the value of the instrument by reporting considerable data that had been obtained with the thermometers made by L. Cassella in a pamphlet, *The Thermometer As an Aid to Diagnosis in Veterinary Medicine,* in 1869, and the thermometer was soon adopted by practitioners.

William Hunting (1846-1913), a Londoner who graduated from Gamgee's New Veterinary School in Edinburgh, became a brilliant clinician with a flair for writing. He decided to establish a new scientific veterinary journal to represent the views of the regional veterinary associations. He founded his weekly *Veterinary Record* on borrowed funds in 1888. It focused on news and comment with an emphasis on clinical material. The journal was an immediate success, and it continues today as one of the most influential veterinary journals. In 1908 Hunting wrote *Glanders: A Clinical Treatise,* a brilliant description of the history and clinical features of the disease, including the use of mallein in diagnosis. The book has excellent color illustrations of the lesions and an appendix on the disease in humans. The histories of numerous human cases are cited.

Development of Surgical Instruments: The Ingenuity of Brogniez

A prominent contributor at the level of intervention in the surgical treatment of the horse was a Belgian who had trained at Alfort but did not complete the course or receive his diploma because of illness: André-Joseph Brogniez (1802-1851). He had experience as an instrument maker and became a great leader in veterinary surgical technique and instrument design. Brogniez was awarded a veterinary diploma by a commission in Brussels in 1832. He joined the veterinary faculty at Cureghem in Brussels at its beginning. He wrote a three-volume book in 1839, *Traitée de Chirurgie Vétérinaire,* in which he reviewed most of the published works on veterinary surgery, mainly by French authors, of the first eight decades of the profession. The book outlines the initial curriculum used at Cureghem. A marvelous feature of the book was the set of illustrations of the finely made surgical instruments he designed and of operations he devised while working at the Cureghem site in Brussels. A detailed picture is provided of the technique for *désabotter un pied,* evulsion of the sole and the vasculature of the corium, which was popular at the time but later discredited. His interest in equine locomotion extended to human mobility; he was an early developer of articulated prostheses for humans. He founded the *Journal Vétérinaire et Agricole de Belgique* and, with his colleague Delwart, the first Belgian veterinary society. He became a member of Belgium's Royal Academy of Medicine in 1841 and in 1847 was awarded the rare honor of Chevalier de l'Ordre de Léopold. Recently the magnificent Brussels buildings were closed and the faculty was moved to Liège.

519. Plate XXXII from the three-volume text, *Traité de Chirurgie Vétérinaire* (1839-1845), by Professor André-Joseph Brogniez (1802-1851) of the Belgian veterinary school when it was sited in Cureghem, Brussels. After training and teaching at Alfort, Brogniez was a leading figure in the establishment of the Brussels school. An extremely skillful instrument-maker, he was a leading developer of new methods to address the formidable problems facing veterinary surgeons, especially with large animals such as horses. This plate diagrams some of the ingenious devices he designed to cope with major obstetrical delivery problems in the mare, including hydrocephalus and monstrosities affecting the fetus. *(Faculté de Médicine Vétérinaire, Université de Liège.)*

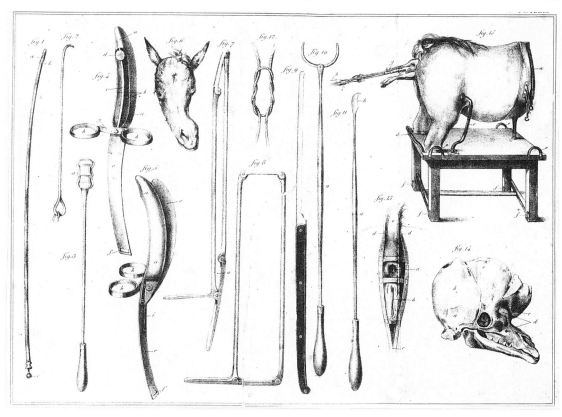

Renewed Campaign for Recognition of the Profession in Great Britain

The medical profession in Great Britain gained the privilege of a monopoly over medical practice under the Medical Act of 1858. The Veterinary Surgeons Bill, designed to obtain similar privileges for veterinary surgeons, was brought forward in 1866 but was abandoned because of government opposition after H.A. Bruce, the spokesperson for the Privy Council, found that the state of veterinary science was not sufficiently advanced to merit this privilege. The knowledge of many diplomates of the RCVS was considered inadequate. Armatage successfully lobbied the profession for support for an entrance examination in 1867. It came into practice in 1870, and the requirement of a practical examination for graduating students was added in 1872.

The quality of veterinary journalism became more scientific when George Fleming founded *The Veterinary Journal* in 1875. Sir Frederick Fitzwygram became president of the RCVS in the same year. These two military veterinarians pushed through a number of educational reforms and were able to expand a number of powers of the RCVS under a supplemental charter in 1876. However, the goal of control of unlicensed veterinary practice was denied. Fitzwygram was also successful in ending the rift between the Edinburgh school and the RCVS and bringing Dick's school into the fold of the Royal College, at last unifying the profession.

The final chapter in the struggle for professional recognition through public policy was written in 1881 when George Fleming became president of the RCVS with a mandate to pursue an act of Parliament. He first gained the support of the Royal Society for the Prevention of Cruelty to Animals (RSPCA), which supported the protection of the title *veterinary surgeon* to help the public avoid the evils of quackery. The RSPCA's president agreed to introduce the proposed act to the House of Lords, and Fleming persuaded Earl Spencer, Lord President of the Privy Council, to take charge of the bill. In the face of vocal opposition from unqualified persons who styled themselves as veterinary surgeons, the proposed bill was amended to allow unqualified practitioners who had continuously practiced veterinary medicine and surgery for five years to claim registration and to petition the RCVS for entry as "Existing Practitioner" under a separate register, although they could not claim to be members of the RCVS. The Veterinary Surgical Act received the Queen's assent on August 27, 1881, and the full legal protection of the professional privileges of veterinary surgeons was attained ninety years after the opening of the London college.

The Era of Private Veterinary Colleges in the United States

Veterinary medical education within the United States began in private veterinary schools with the Veterinary College of Philadelphia in 1852. The era in which they operated has been reviewed by Everett B. Miller in the article "Private Veterinary Colleges in the United States 1852-1927" in the *Journal of the American Veterinary Medical Association* in 1981. Some of the twenty-six colleges played an important role in the development of the veterinary profession in North America, training 9388 veterinarians. Five of the twenty-five schools trained 7171 veterinarians, or seventy-six percent of them, according to the combined figures for the New York College of Veterinary Surgeons (NYCVS) and its virtual successor, the American Veterinary College (AVC) in New York. These five schools were the NYCVS and AVC, the Chicago Veterinary College, the Kansas City Veterinary College, the Indiana Veterinary College (Indianapolis), and the McKillip Veterinary College (Chicago). Clearly they had economic difficulty because their average life span was only fourteen years.

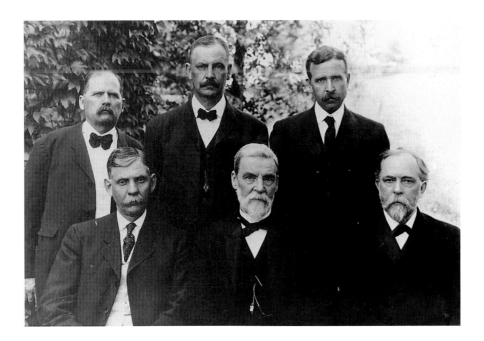

520. James Law (1838-1921), the foundation professor of veterinary medicine at Cornell University in Ithaca, New York, is shown with the original veterinary faculty he recruited to start a college as seen in 1896. *Back row, left to right,* Walter Long Williams, a graduate of Montreal Veterinary College in 1879, chair in surgery including zootechnics, obstetrics, and jurisprudence; Pierre Augustine Fish, who had a doctor of science degree from Cornell and veterinary doctorates from the National Veterinary College, Washington, DC (1896) and Cornell (1899), physiology and pharmacology; and Grant Sherman Hopkins, anatomy, who received his DVM from Cornell in 1900. *Front row, left to right,* Veranus Alva Moore, a doctor of medicine dedicated to veterinary medicine and bacteriology; James Law, who graduated from Edinburgh Veterinary College in 1857 at age nineteen and became professor of anatomy, physiology, and materia medica in John Gamgee's Edinburgh Veterinary College in 1860; and Simon Henry Gage, who received a bachelor of science degree from Cornell (1877) and became one of the finest microscopists of his day and a devoted enthusiast of science, anatomical methods, histology, and embryology. This formidable team and its great achievements are testimony to James Law's wisdom and judgment of people. *(Courtesy of The Flower/ Sprecher Library, Cornell University.)*

Eleven private veterinary schools, the greatest number of such schools to be open at the same time in the United States, were in operation from 1913 to 1916. Failure to attract pupils was the primary reason for the demise of schools. An interesting distortion occurred when Robert McClure developed a diploma mill in Philadelphia, issuing for one hundred dollars apiece forged diploma certificates that purported to certify graduation from the Philadelphia College of Veterinary Surgeons (PCVS). An authentic PCVS had come into existence after Robert Jennings's school, the Veterinary College of Philadelphia (VCP) of 1852, had closed in around 1866 and a PCVS had been chartered in an attempt to replace it. The PCVS appears to have operated only as an apprentice system and had no connection with McClure.

Two years after Jennings began his school, the Boston Veterinary Institute opened its doors when the Massachusetts legislature granted a charter to a Boston physician, D.D. Slade. The prime mover for the school, however, was an English immigrant (in 1845) who had trained as a surgeon in England and stated that he was also a veterinary surgeon, signing himself George H. Dadd M.D., V.S. After he had written *The Modern Horse Doctor* (1855), his school closed, in 1860. Previously he had written *The Reformed Cattle Doctor* and another book on the anatomy and physiology of the horse.

Of the first three private veterinary schools, only the NYCVS of 1857, led by Alexandre Liautard, who arrived from France in 1860, and the AVC, to which Liautard led a faculty exodus from the NYCVS in 1875, could be considered viable. Chicago Veterinary College produced the most graduates, including A.D. Melvin, the Chief of the Bureau of Animal Industry (BAI) from 1906 to 1918. The reputation for providing the highest-quality education was earned by the Kansas City Veterinary College. By 1905, forty percent of the veterinarians working at the prestigious BAI were alumni of the Kansas City school. The other Chicago faculty, the McKillip Veterinary College, had the largest clinical service.

Because of the growing concerns about standards, storm clouds were brewing for the private veterinary schools. Even Harvard's veterinary program had lower standards for admission than other programs at the university had. This was an unhealthy tradition and a bad omen for the profession, despite a period of growing prosperity for veterinary practitioners and the increasing diversity of veterinary roles, from the care of horses and agricultural and companion animals to new opportunities for careers in teaching, research, and

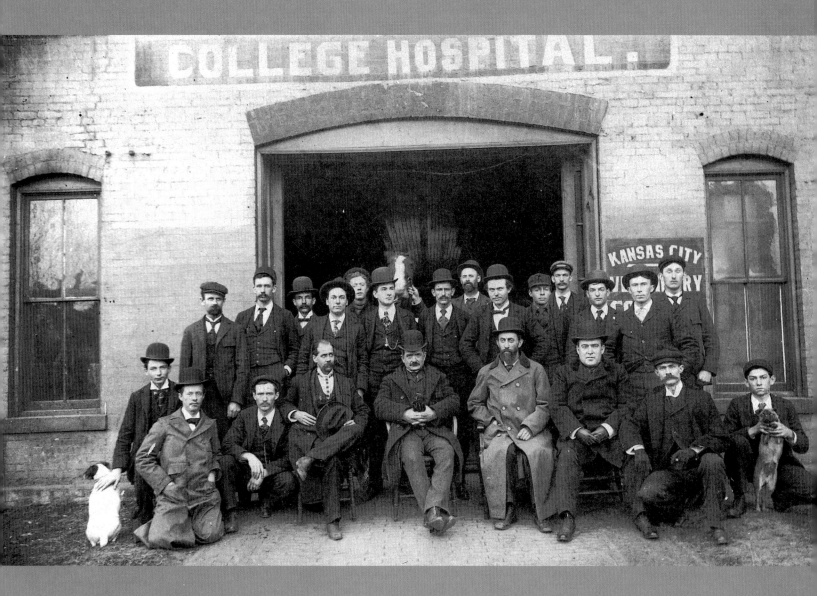

521. Kansas City Veterinary College faculty and students, along with two dogs and a horse, photographed at some time between 1896 and 1902. The college began in 1891 but made slow progress at first and moved several times, until, during R.C. Moore's presidency of the College Corporation, a site was purchased and fine buildings were constructed in 1902, with well-equipped laboratories. Enrollment of students improved rapidly because of the adoption of a three-year course, the excellent facilities and the twenty competent faculty. The college met USDA standards for a curriculum that rendered its graduates eligible for appointment to the BAI. A strong mentoring program for students included social and athletic activities. The statesmanship and competence of Sesco Stewart, MD, DVM, is credited with guiding the college to its position of eminence. He served as dean from 1896 to 1918 when the school closed and all its records were transferred to Kansas State University at Manhattan where college status was conferred on the veterinary department in 1919. Many leaders emerged from the ranks of the 1789 graduates of the Kansas City College, including William L. Boyd (class of 1909) who became the founding dean of the college of veterinary medicine at the University of Minnesota, fifteen state veterinarians, numerous BAI staff members, and three AVMA presidents. *(Photograph, C. Trenton Boyd Collection.)*

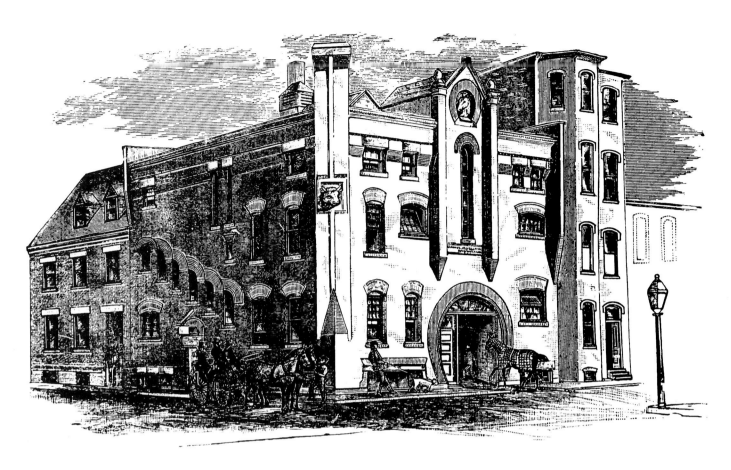

government service. The American Veterinary Medical Association (AVMA) sought ways to induce higher standards in the schools. It established a Committee on Intelligence and Education. Surveys were conducted, and it was determined that the school catalogues claimed more then they could possibly deliver. The association sought to ensure that the schools lived up to the announcements in their literature. A voluntary on-site inspection system was created, and six private and several public schools were inspected. The committee report of 1906 endorsed five of the six schools that were eligible for the AVMA membership: the Chicago, Kansas City, Indiana, McKillip, and Cincinnati veterinary colleges. This was a timely act when consumer concerns were rising.

The U.S. Department of Agriculture (USDA) was facing severe criticism of the nation's meat inspection program after the publication of Upton Sinclair's *The Jungle* in 1906. The federal response included examination of the adequacy of training that BAI veterinarians received for meat inspection. Training was considered satisfactory, and the Meat Inspection Act of 1906 became law. However, the USDA decided to continue the system for inspection of establishments providing veterinary education that the AVMA had initiated. The USDA visited eighteen American sites and one school in Canada. The report of 1908 found only four private schools to merit a class A rating: the Chicago, Kansas City, Indiana, and San Francisco veterinary colleges. Graduates of these schools were eligible to take the civil service examinations for the BAI. Three other colleges were awarded class B status: the McKillip and Cincinnati colleges and the U.S. College of Veterinary Surgeons in Washington, D.C. The ranking did not mean the schools had to close, but it affected the employability of graduates in government service. As a result of the rating system, the BAI produced *Circular 150,* which specified nineteen regulations for entrance to the veterinary inspector examination. The rating system was adopted by the AVMA when it resumed the inspections in 1912.

522. The attractive setting of Harvard University's short-lived (1886-1901) school of veterinary medicine. Charles Parker Lyman, FRCVS (c. 1848-1918), graduated from Edinburgh Veterinary College on 1874, emigrated to America, and served as professor of veterinary medicine of the Agricultural College of Massachusetts. He was president of the USVMA from 1877 to 1879. From 1879 to 1881 he investigated bovine pleuropneumonia epidemics in Britain and the United States for the USDA. In 1882 he was appointed professor of veterinary medicine at Harvard University's Veterinary Department and dean in 1886 when it became a School. He was dean for the entire life of the School, which closed in 1901. He was an advocate of compulsory tuberculin testing of cattle to protect the health of the public. During its short existence, the Harvard School of Veterinary Medicine had a significant impact on the veterinary profession by insisting on a more rigorous education along with a greater focus on professional goals and responsibilities. Harvard maintained a research thrust in diseases of domestic animals by maintaining a department of comparative pathology, where very important studies of infectious diseases were carried out by Theobald Smith and Tyzzer. Lyman's son, Richard P. Lyman, became the first dean of Michigan State University's College of Veterinary Medicine at East Lansing in 1910. *(Francis A. Countway Library of Medicine, Harvard University.)*

Justin Morrill's Educational Paradigm

The Farmer's High School (which evolved into Pennsylvania State University), the first agricultural school in the United States, was chartered in 1854. Michigan State University began an agricultural college the next year, and the University of Maryland followed in 1856. These institutions became land grant colleges under the Morrill Act of 1862.

The Morrill Land Grant Act, passed by the U.S. Congress and signed by President Abraham Lincoln in 1862 (after his predecessor, Buchanan, had vetoed it in the previous administration), was landmark legislation. It established a unique system of education, research, and service in agriculture and the mechanical arts. Most states took up the option of accepting a grant of federal land in return for creation of an institution of higher education.

The land grant initiative led to the establishment of veterinary schools in many states with the intent of serving the needs of animal agriculture. At that time the focus was to be on the horse for its draft and transport value and on the species that produce food and fiber. This bias has changed with the mechanical replacement of equine energy and the reduced focus on animal fiber, but state legislatures have held firm to the goal of food and hide production. As a result, discrimination occurred against funding for the techniques and research that were needed for the care of the companion and nondomestic species.

In the growing enlightenment of the last few decades of the twentieth century the value of animals, along with the importance of conservation of the natural environment, has finally been recognized. Animals are prized, not only for their own worth, but also as members of families, in which they have intrinsic educational value and provide a priceless bonding in partnership and fun with human fellow-spirits of any age, race, or gender. However, this advance does not yet include a societal and political commitment to public funding of research for their well-being.

Eastern Canada was ahead of the United States in developing veterinary academic programs. Andrew Smith's Ontario Veterinary College, after it opened in Toronto in 1862, was extremely popular with American students. For many years it was the major training center for veterinarians in North America. McEachran's college, which was started in Montreal in 1866 and had William Osler on its faculty, set the highest standard in veterinary training.

James Law at Cornell took his first student, Salmon, in 1868, but Salmon took part of his studies in France. The full veterinary program was not opened until it was established as the New York State Veterinary College at Cornell University in 1894, but in the intervening twenty-six years Law taught the entire program. The first land grant college to open a state-supported veterinary program was Iowa State University in Ames, Iowa, in 1879. Private veterinary colleges opened at Harvard in 1882 and Pennsylvania in 1883. Then the land grant system added Ohio State University in 1885 and Washington State University in 1899. The private colleges could not provide the same quality for the same price as the subsidized land grant colleges. In most cases the private colleges could not withstand inspection or continue to attract sufficient students to stay solvent. Gradually the pendulum swung away from a phase when nearly all veterinary education establishments were private to a period when all but the University of Pennsylvania and Tufts University were public, that is, state universities and land grant colleges. Special provision had to be made to meet the needs of black students in the United States, and the Colleges Act of the 1890s was passed to ensure their competitive access to education, eventually including the veterinary medicine program established in 1945 at Tuskegee University in Alabama. This institution played a unique role in recruiting and educating black students from North America to become veterinarians.*

---

*The Legacy, by Dr. Eugene Adams, documents the history of Tuskegee University.

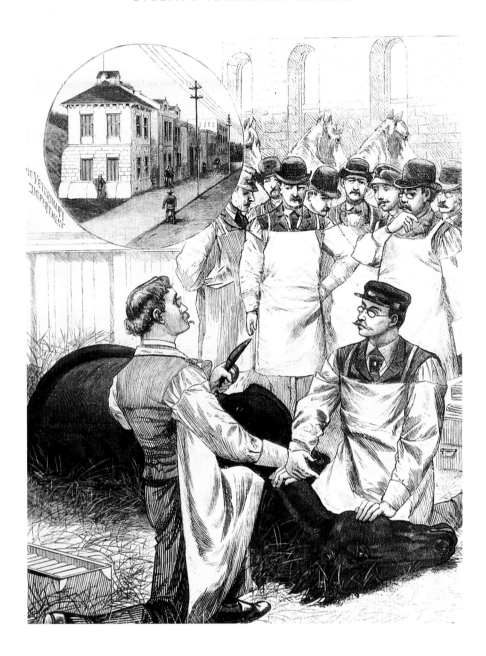

523. A clinical session at the School of Veterinary Medicine at the University of Pennsylvania as sketched by J. Shaw. A visionary physician and a signer of the Declaration of Independence, Benjamin Rush addressed the medical students at the University of Pennsylvania in 1807 on *The Duty and Advantages of Studying the Diseases of Domestic Animals and the Remedies Proper to Remove Them* at the request of the Philadelphia Society. He called for establishment of a veterinary chair that could grow into a faculty of veterinary science. It was seventy-seven years later that the school of veterinary medicine was established in that city under Rush Shipper Huidekoper, a leading physician, although James Mease had taught a course in veterinary studies as early as 1813. This particular school was unique because of its close link to a medical faculty at a major private university. It was able to establish strong academic opportunities at the graduate level in basic medical sciences, clinical specialties, and comparative research in a spirit of "one medicine." The scene shows faculty discussing a critical case in a recumbent horse before a very concerned group of students. Part of the school's buildings are shown in the inset. *(National Library of Medicine, Bethesda, Maryland.)*

The French Connection to New York

A Parisian veterinarian, Alexandre Francois Liautard (1835-1918), emigrated to the United States in 1860, as mentioned earlier. Having lost his mother when he was five years old, Liautard had been forced to develop an independent nature. He became a highly motivated student in high school. Influenced by an uncle who was a veterinarian in the artillery, he was admitted to the veterinary school at Alfort in 1851 at sixteen years of age. It was a good time to attend Alfort, which had a favorable international reputation, a strong curriculum, and outstanding research faculty, including Delafond, Nocard, Colin, and Bouley, as well as collaboration with Pasteur. It had a new building for anatomy and busy clinics: more than eleven hundred animals (mostly horses and dogs) received care at the hospital, and more than seven thousand were seen as outpatients from 1850 to 1851. The excellent training prepared Liautard well, at least for urban veterinary practice.

The Alfort school imposed draconian discipline on virtually a military model. This did not sit well with the intellectually motivated Liautard. Yvart was inspector-general of veterinary schools, and the director of the school itself was Renault. The curriculum was heavily weighted toward anatomy, farriery, and surgery. Liautard was consistently ranked between tenth and twentieth in a class of about fifty students. A few days after his father died in 1855,

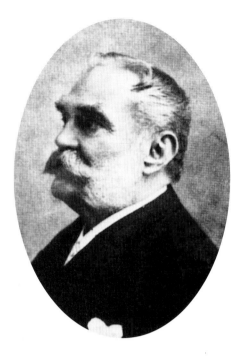

524. Alexandre Francois Liautard (1835-1918) was a French veterinarian (Toulouse, 1856) who emigrated to the United States in 1860. He helped salvage the failing New York City Veterinary School in the 1860s and then founded the American Veterinary College and Hospital in 1875. He headed it for twenty-five years, then retired and returned to his native France. Rigorous but popular, his program was a beacon for advancing urban veterinary medicine. In 1877 he became editor of the *American Veterinary Review,* which bridged the Atlantic for information on professional developments worldwide. Even after returning to France, he provided a monthly feature until 1918. He was a tremendous force in uniting professional standards internationally and for building cohesion and high standards in the American profession. He was a strong proponent for the establishment of the USVMA in 1863, a time when there were no American graduates, and for its maturation into a national body; it was christened the American Veterinary Medical Association in 1898. (*From* American Veterinary Review.)

however, he was dismissed for "a very serious disciplinary infraction." The specific infraction was not recorded. He became ill, could not take the semester examinations, and was expelled from the school. He was later admitted to the veterinary school in Toulouse and was allowed to finish his fourth year, receiving his diploma in 1856. His activities after graduation, from 1856 to 1860, have remained mysterious. Although he was thought to have been in the army, there appears to be no record of military service.

Liautard, a doctor of veterinary medicine and a medical doctor, lived in the United States from 1860 to 1900, then returned to spend his old age in his native France. He gave his most productive years to American veterinary medicine but never became a citizen. His contribution was enormous. He salvaged Busteed's failing NYCVS in the 1860s, but when it deteriorated again he left, taking most of the students with him to form the AVC in 1875, also in New York. He headed the AVC for twenty-five years, when it was a beacon for advancing veterinary education. Although demanding and strict, he was articulate and was admired by his many students. In 1877 he became editor of the *American Veterinary Review,* which provided an overview of developments in veterinary science worldwide. He became its proprietor and publisher from 1881 to 1900 and continued to provide a monthly feature from France until he died in 1918.

The Establishment of the U.S. Veterinary Medical Association

During the tumultuous times of the Civil War, just before the Battle of Gettysburg, a coterie of loyal members of the veterinary profession assembled on June 9, 1863, in the Astor House in New York to found the U.S. Veterinary Medical Association (USVMA). Josiah H. Stickney, who had graduated from medical school in Boston and qualified in London as a veterinary surgeon, was elected president of the association, and Alexandre Liautard, secretary. Only seven states were represented: New York, Massachusetts, Pennsylvania, New Jersey, Delaware, Maine, and Ohio. Those present were all practitioners, mostly self-educated—few were veterinary graduates. There were no American graduates in 1863, so the few who had qualified had received degrees overseas. Representatives of medical and agricultural professions were present. Thirty-nine persons attended. A seal with a picture of a centaur and a motto *Non Nobis Solum* (not for us alone), was adopted. The clear intent was to extend the association to the entire country. To promote the attainment of this goal, it was later decided to vary the site of the annual meeting, alternating between New York and other cities. In 1889 the association formally agreed to become a national body.

The USVMA met in Chicago in 1890 and began to plan for a national association of veterinarians of America. The First International Congress of American Veterinarians was held during the Columbia Exhibition of 1893. The rechristening of the USVMA as the American Veterinary Medical Association (AVMA) took place in Omaha, Nebraska, in 1898. The AVMA became the largest veterinary organization in the world. In 1900 there were approximately 8163 veterinarians in the United States. Only about forty percent were North American veterinary graduates, and less than five percent of them (only 385) were active members of the AVMA.

THE ETHICAL DIMENSION OF VETERINARY WORK

The practice of veterinary medicine is not a right but a privilege, a monopolistic professional authorization granted by law to treat sick animals belonging to another person. In the United States the individual states, not the federal government, decide who merits this privilege within a given state under the conditions of a practice act. One weakness of this model is the need to

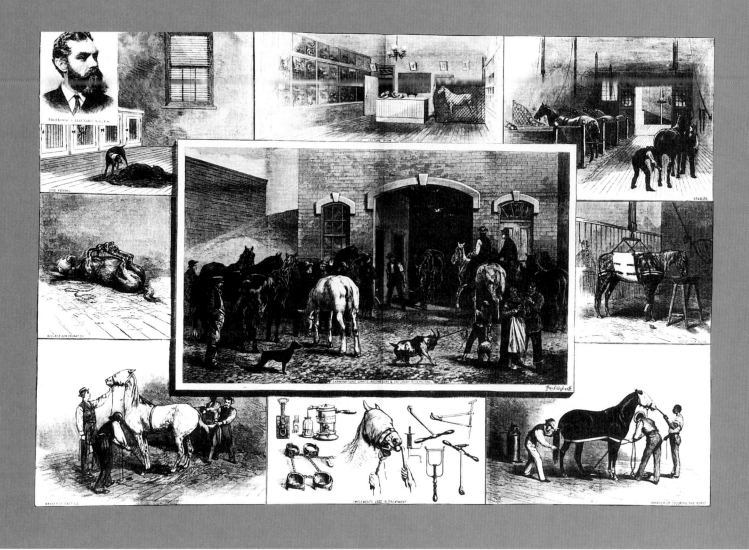

pass licensure examinations for every state in which practice privileges are sought. The privilege can be revoked as a disciplinary measure by a state's board of examiners. To be worthy of the trust implied under the monopoly, a licensee must be of "good moral character." Because there are many examples of "unprofessional conduct," a code of appropriate conduct, derived from the oath of Hippocrates, has been held up as a standard for aspirants to professional licensure. In the United States, guidance on ethics is given by the national professional body, the AVMA. Some ethical standards come under federal jurisdiction and must be complied with. A system has evolved in which there are national and state board examinations and clinical competency tests.

A primary concern of the early profession was the problem of competition with quacks. The magnitude of this problem was evident in data obtained for Great Britain in 1851. The national census of that year recorded that 5979 persons supplied some sort of veterinary services, whereas the survey of the RCVS revealed that only 1018 veterinary surgeons were in practice. In the United States the practicing veterinarians became activists to protect their own interests and the public from competing, unqualified lay persons. The USVMA wrote its first code of ethics in 1867, when the veterinarians were not required to be licensed, mainly with the view to the suppression of quackery. The code evolved gradually as the knowledge gap between quacks and veterinarians widened. Maintaining harmony and cooperation among competing practitioners brought rules governing professional etiquette. Some of these were more in the vein of proper business practices rather than in the ethical domain.

525. Scenes from the veterinary hospital of the private American Veterinary College in New York around 1880, in the time of Alexandre Liautard. The college began in 1875 when Liautard withdrew from the New York City Veterinary School with most of the students, and he led the American Veterinary College to prominence for twenty-five years. It is apparent from this illustration that the horse was the dominant species studied. This was a time when equine power was essential for urban transport. The facilities were spacious, and the scenes depict the various activities engaged in by faculty, staff, and students to care for their equine patients. Despite the fact that it was a private institution dependent on fees for its income, free clinics were held one afternoon each week. *(National Library of Medicine, Bethesda, Maryland.)*

The AVMA has developed the *Principles of Veterinary Medical Ethics,* reviewing and revising it at regular intervals, as a general behavioral guide for the profession. In 1989 Jerrold Tannenbaum wrote *Veterinary Ethics,* a valuable contribution to the evolution of professional insights into an important area that touches on everything veterinarians do in the course of their professional activities.

One ramification of ethics that is a cause of deep concern for scholars trained in pathogenic microbiology or toxicology concerns biological and chemical warfare. Mass production of pathogenic organisms or toxic chemicals with a view to their potential distribution in warfare represents an ethical challenge. For example, during the Japanese invasion of China in the 1930s, the Japanese developed a top secret research unit (Unit 731) for biological warfare at PingFan, near Harbin, Manchuria, around 1938. The toxic agents were tested on human prisoners, and the work continued until the end of World War II, when all survivors were executed. Toxicology is affected by the international ethical constraints on warfare. The use of radioactivity in weapons and potent toxins or poisonous gases raises similar concerns.

DRAMATIC PROGRESS IN INFECTIOUS DISEASE RESEARCH AFTER THE 1880s

As the 1890s drew to a close, veterinary medicine adapted to the remarkable progress in microbiology, pathology, and immunology of the previous decade. In practice the horse continued to be the main focus of veterinary work in peace and war, but the horse was becoming a serious problem in large cities. As numbers of horses increased, so did the volume of manure dropped on the street, and the problem of its disposal reached nightmare proportions. There was a massive swing by the public away from the horse transport to the bicycle fitted with Dunlop's pneumatic tires, which in Boston led to a substantial decline in the number of horses.

Swine were a source of meat and other products, but they were also the first agent of recycling in the modern era. Swine were fed on kitchen and table wastes, thereby becoming a garbage disposal service. In Great Britain this waste, called swill, was collected and in many swine units was a major component of the diet. The problem with swine in the eastern United States was their prolificacy. They had large litters and multiplied rapidly, becoming a major pest that had to be controlled. The garbage-feeding system was considered unsanitary and was thought to increase the risk of diseases that could spread to the human population. Such fears were amplified with the advent of knowledge about pathogenic microbiology.

The late nineteenth and the early twentieth century was a time of rapid expansion of the dairy industry, particularly in and around large cities, where the demand for milk grew rapidly. The improved safety of pasteurization was an important factor, along with the development of refrigeration. Tuberculosis became the greatest concern. The veterinarians developed a major employment niche by providing health care and treatment for dairy cattle.

Veterinary trends in North America included the opening of the West and the westward expansion of cattle and sheep on the pastures of the prairies and plains and through the intermountain plateaus to the coast. The productivity of the rich midwestern soils led to cultivation of heavy crops that provided a basis of feed for fattening swine and cattle, which in turn led to strong family farms that needed veterinary services for their livestock. However, the development of effective products against infectious diseases, particularly vaccines, was a prerequisite. The development of the BAI brought recognition of the scientific potential of veterinary medicine for agriculture and growing career opportunities in the public sector as well as in rural practice.

Veterinary services for companion animals were growing slowly. A few veterinarians began to specialize in urban pet practice, but it was very much a private operation to meet the needs of those willing to pay. Neutering was becoming important. Although there was an urgent need for a vaccine to protect against distemper, the main concern about the dog was the growing incidence of rabies and fear of its zoonotic potential.

PROGRESS IN THE EARLY 1900s: INTERRUPTED BY WAR

The horse had lost ground to the bicycle in the cities and to the railroads for distance travel, and then came the internal combustion engine, which generated "horsepower" for vehicles. Horses held their own on the farm and for local transport, as well as for riding and sport for those who could afford them. The creation of powerful, totally controllable vehicles that could reach exciting speeds, however, was to set the stage for the progressive demise of the equine species in developed countries, except for sport. Enormous numbers of horses were used during World War I in Europe, so the veterinary corps of the participating nations were in demand, although the Great War disrupted many veterinary developments. The decline in the numbers of horses started gently but became precipitous after World War I, and doomsayers were forecasting the end of the veterinary profession, which had overspecialized its talents to meet the horsemen's needs.

The BAI did make a commitment to attend to diseases of the horse because of its importance in agriculture and published a state-of-the-art book on the subject. The label *horse doctor,* however, did not go away. It became a pejorative term in the rivalry between the "vets" and the "aggies" (or "plow jockeys") on the land grant college campuses and in Canada after the Canadian veterinary college moved from Toronto to Guelph, the site of the Ontario Agricultural College. Earlier chapters have recorded the enormous effort that was expended in applying microbiology and immunology to the epidemic diseases of food animal species.

The veterinarians had been involved in the work of rabies control, which no one else wanted. A great new issue was the relationship between bovine tuberculosis and the safety of milk and meat. The veterinary researchers led by McFadyean at the RVC in London and Theobald Smith at Harvard won the day by establishing the high risk of tuberculosis, especially to infants. As a result, programs were initiated to eradicate the disease, respect for the profession increased, and career opportunities became available in public service. Meat inspection came under veterinary supervision. Towns and cities were expanding and, with them, the number of dogs and, to a lesser extent, cats. The humanitarian movement grew in political significance, and veterinarians began to set up urban pet hospitals.

VETERINARY CAREERS BETWEEN THE WORLD WARS

The most challenging adjustment after 1918 was to the precipitous decline in the role of the working horse as it was replaced by engine-driven vehicles. The last of the narrow-spectrum private veterinary schools closed their doors. One benefit, however, was that rural practitioners could travel the rounds of their practices more quickly and comfortably by car. The veterinary schools at land grant colleges were quick to modify their curricula to decrease the equine focus and greatly raise the commitment to food animals. Universities promoted agricultural research in animal breeding, nutrition, housing, and animal product processing. There was a huge expansion in the marketing and consumption of animal products. World trade in meat, wool, and animal feeds expanded explosively. The private sector of industries that developed products for use in farm livestock became profitable. Vaccines, serums, bacterins, and toxoids were produced by biologic companies in response to the extraordinary progress in microbiology. One example was pullorum disease of chicks. L.F. Rettger had isolated the cause, *Salmonella pullorum*, in 1900. Later, it was shown that the infection localizes in the ovaries, infecting the eggs. The chicks then died of bacillary white diarrhea (BWD). The BAI developed a blood agglutination test in 1927 that was used in a national plan in 1935 to establish pullorum-free flocks. Joseph Edward Salsbury (1887-1967) from England, attended the Kansas City Veterinary College, graduating in 1914. After building a fine horse practice in Nebraska, he settled in Charles City, Iowa, and became a poultry-disease specialist. He then established Dr. Salsbury's Laboratories, selling specialty pharmaceuticals and biologics to the poultry industry. He was aided in this latter venture by Oliver Peterson. John G. Salsbury took over his father's company in 1961. Benjamin S. Pomeroy, of the University of Minnesota, was one consultant to the firm who helped keep it at the forefront of poultry disease product development.

Pharmaceutical corporations developed a wide range of veterinary products that were of variable efficacy because rigorous testing was not yet required. The first effective tick-killing products were marketed and the development of effective safe anthelmintics was initiated. The range of products available for the treatment of metabolic diseases grew steadily, and some proved very successful. Anesthetics were in big demand; new, injectable products replaced, in part, the old inhalational chemicals. A range of pharmacodynamic agents that affected pathophysiological changes was offered to combat, if only temporarily, the symptoms and discomfort of the animals. The spectrum of surgical instruments and other interventional equipment expanded to include restraining devices, operating tables, lights, and X-ray machines. A few kits and techniques to aid diagnosis in practice or at wardside started to appear.

Referral by practitioners of difficult cases to hospitals at the colleges, or of specimens to veterinary diagnostic laboratories or veterinary science research departments, became standard. Modifications in the armed services created roles for veterinarians in war-related research, canine medicine for guard and messenger dogs, pigeon health, and food safety as the role of veterinarians in equine care declined. A growing need for regulatory veterinary services emerged as international sea and air travel and trade posed heightened threats of epidemics to domestic stocks of animals. Veterinarians were also needed full-time and part-time (after federal accreditation) to participate in brucellosis and tuberculosis eradication campaigns and to serve as emergency response professionals if penetration of an exotic disease caused an epizootic or if an environmental catastrophe occurred.

Small animal practices advanced and expanded rapidly, and high standards were proposed for hospital operation. Limited use was made of technicians, and women veterinarians were almost unknown. Until the sulfonamides arrived in the late 1930s, coping with cases of bacterial disease tended to be disheartening.

WORLD WAR II AND RURAL PRACTICE ACCORDING TO HERRIOT

The First World War had been fought mainly on foot and horseback. Transport horses were used to move supplies, troops, and guns. The Second World War, a much more technological war, was fought by means of guns, armored machines, naval ships and submarines, air forces, and bombs. Horses, mules, camels, and elephants had specialized roles in difficult terrain.

Veterinary "devoicing" was needed in the Burmese jungle. Fear of chemical and microbiological warfare led to veterinary research in military laboratories. Guard dogs and other useful animals such as message-carrying homing pigeons required veterinary attention and supervision. Ensuring safe food and water supplies for the troops was a major military role for veterinarians in World War II.

Good news for practicing veterinarians was the arrival of a range of antibiotics, anthelmintics, and new vaccines. Practice efficacy was transformed, and practice became much more enjoyable with more effective general and local anesthetics and analgesics to minimize suffering in the animal patients; better vaccines against viral diseases and spore-forming, toxin-producing bacteria; antibiotics that were effective against bacterial infections, including septicemia and mastitis; and a wide range of pharmaceutical products and instruments for the treatment of noninfectious diseases or for operations.

These were the golden days of the James Herriot stories written by Yorkshire veterinarian James Alfred Wight (1916-1995), which still fascinate audiences today, on screen or in story. No more wonderful advocate of the veterinary career has ever appeared. Wight's stories reveal why the career is rewarding, frustrating, satisfying, and challenging in the face of the three-way interaction between animal, client, and veterinarian. The tales are woven with a wonderful instinct for and memory of how this balancing act is conducted in veterinary practices with a clientele ranging from the individual pet owner or child to the small-farming family and the efficient operator of a large enterprise, and cooperation with bureaucratic government agents while identifying the misdeeds of nefarious characters who must be brought to justice. The quirks of the individual veterinarians are included in the mixture. Always present is Wight's infatuation with the beautiful but harsh environment of his Yorkshire Dales.

OVERCOMING THE EXCLUSION OF WOMEN

Veterinary medicine, like human medicine, was perceived to be an exclusive professional preserve for men of the genus *Homo*. If any policy ever justified the exclusion of the species-defining term *sapiens,* this was surely the one. Mothers are by tradition the doctors of ninety percent of children's health problems during their early years. Women frequently become the main caretakers of elderly parents or grandparents. Not until about one hundred and twenty-five years from the origin of the veterinary profession did two women gain access to veterinary education in the modern era; two years later, those two women graduated. One graduated from Alfort, the other from the school in Zürich—both in 1889.

The case most revealing of the attitudes of men was that of Aleen Cust (born 1868), who was admitted to the liberal New Veterinary College of Edinburgh, from which she passed all examinations and graduated in 1900. The legal advisor to the Royal College of Veterinary Surgeons (RCVS) found that the RCVS could license only "persons"—and a woman did not fit into that category! Aleen went to the far western part of Ireland and practiced veterinary medicine. Although the RCVS at that time technically had jurisdiction over veterinary practice in Ireland, it evidently chose not to chance its powers in that fierce environment. She worked in a mixed practice, and her clientele and her employer thought well of her. During World War I she worked in a military veterinary hospital in France. She then returned to Ireland and worked as an inspector in the Department of Agriculture.

Enlightenment came to the British Parliament in 1919, when it passed the Sex Disqualification (Removal) Act. As a result, the professions had to allow women to register forthwith, but the pill was so bitter that it took the

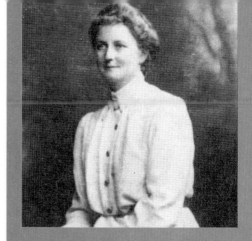

526. Aleen Cust (1868-1937) wanted to be a veterinarian and succeeded in becoming Britain's first female veterinary surgeon after overcoming the enormous odds because of male chauvinism. It took a principled principal, William Williams, FRCVS, who created the New Veterinary College in Edinburgh in 1873, to admit her (under the alias surname I.A. Custance to shield her mother; this was actually the surname of a famous jockey) in 1894. She was considered one of the best students in her class, but the all-male Council of the RCVS refused to allow her to sit the first professional examination for licensure ("They did not have the power to do so!"). As a consequence, she graduated with only a testimonial that she was fully competent in all subjects. Nevertheless she obtained an assistantship with William Byrne in Roscommon, Ireland, and proved to be a very capable and popular practitioner; only the Catholic Church found her role improper. Hobday from London met her at the Budapest World Congress in 1905 and was favorably impressed. The Galway Council appointed her veterinary inspector in 1907; the RCVS tried to block the appointment, but she prevailed under the compromise term "inspector." When Byrne died in 1910 she ran the "four-horse" practice over an eight-mile radius on her own until 1915, procuring horses for the British Army in the last year. She then went to France with the YMCA. Again she had to bypass many hurdles to be allowed to use her professional expertise. After the war, the Parliament passed the Sex Disqualification (Removal) Act in 1919, and in 1920 the solicitor for the RCVS said "Women are now entitled to enter the veterinary profession," and Edith Knight (thirty years junior to Cust) succeeded in being admitted to the veterinary school at Liverpool that year. Aleen Cust was permitted to take the RCVS examination in 1922 and passed to become the first female MRCVS. Knight passed the next year. Remarkably, Cust wrote in an article in the *Veterinary Record* regarding women in the profession in 1934, when the number of registered women veterinarians had soared to thirty-one, that "You have chosen the Best Profession in the World." *(Courtesy J. Moran, Roscommon, Ireland.)*

RCVS three years to swallow it and allow Aleen Cust to take the final examination for membership, that is, for licensure to practice. With this heroic act the veterinary profession became the last of the major professions to admit the previously adjudged nonsapient women to its ranks. Extraordinarily clever, productive men like Sir John McFadyean, principal of the RVC from 1894 to 1927, consistently opposed the entry of women into the profession. Full women's suffrage was not obtained in Great Britain until 1928. None of the dire consequences prophesied by the naysayers were fulfilled in the first decade after women acquired the right to vote or after they were allowed to practice veterinary medicine.

Edith Knight, who graduated from the Liverpool school in 1923, became the second woman to be a member of the RCVS. When Hobday followed McFadyean in 1927 as principal of the RVC, women were admitted for the first time to the London veterinary school. Hobday had a major influence in changing attitudes about women entering the profession, and their numbers climbed steadily. Many practitioners, however, resisted letting women who were students "see practice" with them and even, as reported in 1934, made women pay a premium to do so. When hired as assistants after graduation, women were usually offered lower salaries, a trend that has continued to the present day.

Many women made great achievements in the profession. For example, Conne M. Ford (London, 1933), a specialist in bovine infertility, wrote a biography, *Aleen Cust, Veterinary Surgeon,* in 1990. Olga Uvarov, who graduated in 1934 and worked in the pharmaceutical industry, became president of the RCVS in 1976. Mary Brancker (RVC, 1937) became the first woman to preside over the British Veterinary Association. The proportion of women entering the British veterinary profession grew annually from less than six percent in 1960 to fifty-six percent by 1992. The tables are turned, well and truly, because most veterinary colleges in democratic countries report a majority of women in their annual entry. In the United States the majority has reached more than seventy-five percent in many colleges of veterinary medicine. The only concern is that of greater health risk to the woman veterinarian during pregnancy. Women have entered the profession from which they were excluded for so long; now employers must become more vigilant in policing any discrimination against further advancement on the basis of gender.

The first American woman to receive a veterinary diploma and succeed in a practice career was Massachusetts native was Elinor McGrath, who graduated from the Chicago Veterinary College in 1910. Florence Kimball graduated from Cornell in the same year, but she became a nurse. The first Canadian woman to receive the degree of doctor of veterinary medicine was Jean Rumney, who received her degree in 1939. In Quebec, however, the first woman graduated in 1965 from St. Hyacinthe. A dramatic increase in the admissions of women to North American veterinary colleges began in the mid-1970s and has continued. Roy Thompson in *The Good Doctors* (1986) tells the following American success story. Sandra O. Karn of Gaithersburg, Maryland, graduated as a doctor of veterinary medicine from Michigan State University in 1965, after a five-year leave during which she had three children. She became president of the District of Columbia Academy of Veterinary Medicine, which served the Middle Atlantic states with veterinary continuing education. She became the first woman to serve on the Maryland Veterinary Medical Associations's board of directors (in 1973) and the first women to serve on the state's Board of Veterinary Medical Examiners: she was appointed by the governor in 1984. She also became the first woman in the forty-eight contiguous states to serve as president of her state's Veterinary Medical Association (from 1980 to 1981). A brilliant spokesperson for her profession, Karn made herself available for call-in radio programs on veterinary concerns and conducted a press conference in 1980 at the peak of public concern about the canine parvovirus epidemic. Helen Fairnie of Curtin University in Perth, Western Australia, became the first woman to preside over the Australian Veterinary Association (from 1982 to 1983).

THE CHANGING SCENARIO DURING THE SECOND HALF OF THE TWENTIETH CENTURY

During the 1950s major funding opportunities for research and postgraduate training in the health professions and related sciences allowed more academically competitive veterinary schools to expand research and advanced training, which was overdue. Although the National Institutes of Health at first allowed funds to be used for research to benefit animals, this opportunity was constricted as attention was focused on areas of clinical benefit to humans or important discoveries in relevant basic sciences.

The USDA closed the BAI in 1954 and transferred veterinary research operations and veterinary regulatory functions to the Agricultural Research Service and the Animal and Plant Health Inspection Service, respectively. The Food and Drug Administration managed the federal regulation of veterinary pharmaceuticals through its Bureau (later, the Center) for Veterinary Medicine. Regulatory roles became more tightly defined and more specialized.

The number of veterinarians in the military services was reduced, but retention of veterinarians was considered necessary. The horse made a strong comeback as a recreation and companion animal, but competition from other sports and gambling opportunities is eroding the economic viability of horse racing.

Colonel William H.H. Clark has written *The History of the United States Army Veterinary Corps in Viet Nam 1962-1973* (1991). The U.S. veterinary corps was asked to help the Army of the Republic of Vietnam (ARVN) develop a veterinary care system for its military dogs. The ARVN did not have any veterinarians on staff, and the American planners had no experience with military dogs or their health care. Although the U.S. military had found it needed dogs in previous wars, it always disbanded the expert canine scout units that were developed during each war after it ended. To a limited extent the French had used dogs based at a training center in Go Vap in its military activities in Indochina. The British had developed a jungle warfare school in Johore Bahru to counteract the Communist insurgents in the jungles of Malaya. Dogs were trained and used with considerable success. The American veterinary corps had used dogs for military purposes in the South Pacific Islands in World War II and again in the Korean War. They were used as scouts to detect hidden enemies, as sentries to guard missile sites and other strategic facilities, and as tracker scent-dogs to seek out the enemy or lost persons.

Because the U.S. Department of Defense did not have enough dogs to meet the estimated numbers that were needed in Vietnam, it had to purchase dogs in Europe and begin to train people and animals. Facilities had to be built, dog food obtained, staff trained, dog training initiated, veterinary care made operational, laboratory support provided, and vaccines and drugs supplied. Health problems included heat exhaustion and malnutrition, rabies, distemper, leptospirosis, an unfamiliar rickettsial disease, tropical canine pancytopenia, and parasites. Several thousand dogs were lost during the war. Zoonoses included rabies and leptospirosis.

The veterinary corps played a major role in human food procurement and safety inspection and also worked with the care of other species. There were signal pigeon units, pack mules, and elephants. The corps collaborated with USAID to assist the Vietnamese through a Participating Agency Support Agreement. The experience was unique because several major exotic diseases were present, including rinderpest, foot-and-mouth disease, hog cholera, and

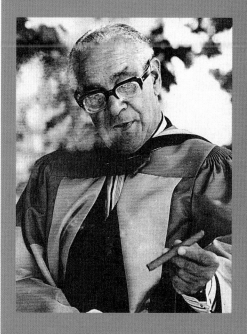

527. Emmanuel Cyprian Amoroso (1901-1982), universally known as *Amo*, was born in Port of Spain, Trinidad. He became a brilliant student of science and medicine at the National University of Ireland before earning a doctorate at University College London in 1934. He was appointed to teach histology and embryology at the Royal Veterinary College, where he became professor of physiology in 1947, a post he held until retirement in 1968. His research activities in many aspects of reproductive morphology and function were legion, and his classic work on placentation earned him the title of Fellow of the Royal Society (FRS). An inspiring lecturer, he brought the cutting edge of relevant scientific research into the college, thereby having a major impact on the development of the British veterinary profession. Amo's insatiable curiosity led to his appointment as visiting scientist at the Institute of Animal Physiology, Babraham, where his stimulus continued for many years. *(Historical Collections, The Royal Veterinary College Library, London.)*

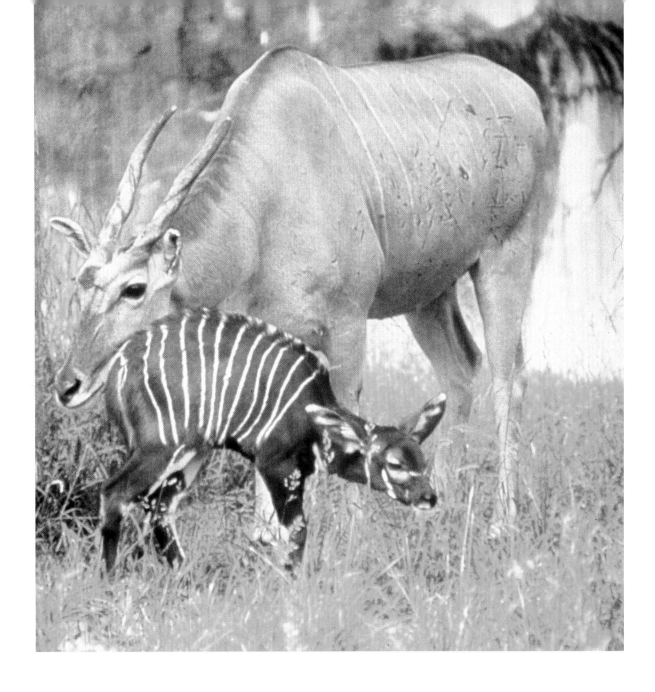

528. Veterinary researchers in theriogenology made many breakthroughs in reproductive biotechnology of domestic animals that are now being applied in humans and nondomestic species. Their achievements include the collection, dilution, and freezing of semen for later use in artificial insemination (AI); and multiple ovulation, fertilization, and embryo transfer (ET) to synchronized surrogate mothers to multiply the most desirable genomes. A spin-off has been application of AI and ET to preserve the genomes of endangered species. This photograph shows a successful outcome from the collection of a rare bongo embryo in Los Angeles and its subsequent implantation into an eland by a research team led by Betsy Dresser at the Center for Reproduction of Endangered Wildlife at the Cincinnati Zoo. The next phase is a plan to produce multiple bongo embryos and implant them into an entire herd of elands in Kenya. Each species at risk will be a major challenge. *(Center for Reproduction of Endangered Wildlife, Cincinnati Zoo.)*

Newcastle disease. Vaccines against Newcastle disease, hog cholera, and rinderpest were made. Many bacterial infections were prevalent. One lasting achievement was sending Vietnamese students to Thailand for veterinary training so that a nucleus of well-qualified people could return to help their country.

The poultry industry became the leader among animal industries in intensification. Extraordinary progress has been made in breeding, nutrition, management, processing, and standardization. Vaccines were developed for the major virus infections, including Marek's disease. The demand continues for veterinary research on poultry diseases and human food safety issues, as well as the health management of production farms. The vulnerability of the industry to infectious disease epidemics becomes detectable from time to time. The swine industry is following the lead of the chicken, egg, and turkey industries. Veterinary swine specialists and researchers are actively involved in protecting swine health and productivity.

The adoption of artificial insemination has led to a fantastic increase in milk productivity of dairy cattle. The best Holstein genes have been selected to this end. The approval of Bovine Somatotropin (BST) for use in dairy herds allows its deployment to reduce the rate of decline in milk production after peak lactation is reached. There have been international movements of the gene pool for beef cattle as beef producers compete with those of the other species. Specialized veterinary surgeons have used embryo transfer extensively. Health and productivity computer modeling systems have been developed by veterinary faculty with great success in achieving mastery of animal production systems. Similar techniques are being applied in an effort to gain control of animal waste recycling, a major problem for large production units. Genetic engineering and molecular manipulation of cells are creating an infinite spectrum of possibilities for further progress. One cost has been the progressive retrenchment of small farms and farmers as animal production has become more and more business oriented.

The first vaccines against cancers were veterinary achievements in the control of such devastating viruses as Marek's disease and feline leukemia virus. Veterinarians are participating in the research on acquired immunodeficiency syndrome and other emerging diseases. As the farms and processing plants become larger and more mechanical, problems have increased with zoonotic diseases and food safety. Toxic conditions continue to appear, and newly recognized biological toxins such as mycotoxins and algal toxins continue to present challenges to humans and animals. Feral animal populations must be controlled, or natural wildlife will be displaced. Wildlife veterinary medicine is needed to conserve species. Animal capture and behavioral studies are expanding. Because aquaculture is growing dramatically, increasingly specialized veterinary knowledge of fish, mollusk, and shellfish health and safety for human consumption is needed. The need for care of captive animals in zoos and aquaria and those used in circuses and other exhibitions is increasing.

Companion animal veterinarians have become the largest group within the veterinary profession. Companion animal medicine has been a great success story: the standard of care for pets has increased steadily. Also, the expansion of care for exotic pets, cagebirds, aquarium fish, and miniature pigs has been remarkable. A range of specialists patterned after those in human medicine is developing, but promotion of fields such as neurology and behavior is needed. Veterinarians today must be very good at what they do. The diversity of opportunity is still there, and the magic of working with animals and those who enjoy them remains a perennial attraction.

Veterinary Neurology Lags Behind the Human Field

Early studies in neuroscience were conducted in animals but mainly by medical researchers. Rolando (1773-1831) at Sassario in Sardinia in 1809 ablated the cerebellum in several species, noting that unsteadiness resulted. Flourens (1794-1867) in Paris used fine neurosurgery to show in 1820-1823 that the semicircular canals maintained equilibrium. Charles Bell (1774-1842) showed in 1811 that only the ventral roots of spinal nerves led to muscle contraction on galvanic stimulation and conceived of the concept of a proprioceptive neural system to maintain posture. François Magendie (1783-1855) exposed the spinal canal and the lumbosacral nerve roots in six-week-old puppies in 1822 to show that the dorsal roots were sensory and the ventral ones were motor; this led to the *Bell-Magendie Law*. He also discovered that strychnine acted on the cord.

Marshall Hall (1790-1857) was an observant, scholarly physician who recalled that Gilbert Blane in 1788 had shown that some neural functions persisted after loss of consciousness in a kitten. He reported that a pole-axed horse had temporary convulsions then relaxed and began to breathe again despite a lack of reflex response of the limbs to pricks or cuts. Eye-protection reflexes persisted unless the rostral medulla was destroyed. The sphincters of bladder and anus depended upon intact spinal reflexes. Jan Purkinje (1787-1869) gave the first microscopic description of the brain with its neurons, axons, and dendrites. He conducted classic research on vision and on centrifugal effects on eye movements and equilibrium. M.H. Romberg (1795-1873) in Berlin was the first clinical neurologist and described many functional impairments and their progression. Robert Bentley Todd (1805-1859), an Irish physician at Westminster Hospital Medical School, wrote a description of the neurological effects of lead poisoning, one case showing the convulsions, coma, and death observed later in cattle.

Guillaume Duchenne (1806-1870) used a Faraday induction coil to stimulate the muscles of facial expression, recording the outcomes photographically. Charles Darwin used some of Duchenne's pictures in *The Expression of the Emotions in Man and Animals* in 1872, adding his own photographs of children's emotions and drawings of those of animals. John Hughlings Jackson (1835-1911) in Britain built on this framework and applied his ideas to the study of drunkenness, epilepsy, and insanity as loss of higher control of neural function. Sigmund Freud (1856-1939) in Vienna drew on Jackson's ideas in evolving his early psychoanalytic theory: the *id* as the part of self characterized by animal instincts and drives, the *ego* as the controller of these lower passions that prevents them from taking over conscious behaviors and aspires to the higher ideals of sensitivity and reason.

Turning to veterinary matters, the distinguished neurologist William Richard Gowers (1845-1915) with Sankey described two cases of distemper myelitis in *The Pathological Anatomy of Canine Chorea* in 1877. Sir David Ferrier experimented on the brains of monkeys and lower animals. He exhibited a monkey with a large lesion of the left motor cortex that manifested hemiplegia at the Seventh International Medical Congress in London in 1881. When the Congress ended he was charged with operating on the animal without a license and in a way caused pain under the Cruelty to Animals act. He was tried and acquitted because his colleague Gerald Yeo had performed the surgery under anesthesia for him and held a government license to do it.

Richard Caton (1842-1926) at Liverpool was the first to record the spontaneous electrical activity of the brains of rabbits and monkeys in 1875. However it was Hans Berger (1873-1941) in Jena who published his treatise on electroencephalography in 1929, after which the technique became popular. Camillo Golgi (1843-1926), an Italian physician, developed the silver nitrate staining method to stain nerve cells, after which he moved to the University of Pavia. Santiago Ramón y Cajal (1852-1934) of Spain improved on Golgi's methods and showed the cellular and fiber architecture in more detail, firmly establishing that neurons were independent elements rather than parts of connected networks. Sir Charles Sherrington (1857-1952) recognized the gaps between neurons, as well as between neurons and muscle cells. In consultation with Michael Foster of Cambridge and a European scholar there, Verrall, they agreed on the term *synapse,* from the Greek for "clasp." Golgi, Cajal, and Sherrington each received a Nobel Prize.

Ivan Pavlov (1849-1936) was a Russian physiologist who won a Nobel Prize in 1904 for his work on digestive secretions in dogs. He became most famous for his work on conditioned reflexes. By pairing an unconditioned stimulus, food, with a conditioning stimulus, the sound of a bell, he was able to get dogs to salivate at the sound of the bell alone. Subsequent studies have revealed that the brain's responses are much more complex than this simple demonstration implied.

Herman Dexler (1866-1931) was the outstanding pioneer of veterinary clinical neurology. He graduated as a veterinarian in Vienna in 1888 with a keen interest in neurology. He worked under Heinrich Obersteiner (1847-1922) at the Viennese Institute for Brain Research and acquired the state of the art in human neurology. Also he worked on the neuroanatomy and neurophysiology of domestic animals he used as a basis to study their neurology. He authored *Die Nervenkrankheiten des Pferdes, (Neurologic Diseases of Horses)* in 1899 and was the first to describe disc protrusion with compression of the spinal cord in a dog. He moved in 1898 to become chair at the German University of Prague and developed a unique laboratory of comparative neurology. He published many papers on animal neurology and behavioral problems. He became dean of the Medical Faculty the year he died.

E. Frauchiger (1903-1975) was a human neurologist in Berne who worked with Professor of Buiatrics W. Hofmann on clinical and pathological aspects of neural diseases in domestic animals. Frauchiger completed a veterinary Ph.D. at Zurich and then worked part time at the veterinary faculty in Berne. He wrote *The Nervous Diseases of Cattle* in 1941 and began an institute that evolved into the Institute of Berne. J.R.M. Innes from Scotland, who moved to America, and Leon Z. Saunders wrote their classic text, *Comparative Neuropathology,* in 1962. Contributions to the work were made by Ludo van Bogaert of Antwerp; R. Fankhauser from Berne; William J. Hadlow from Hamilton, Montana; and Kenneth V.F. Jubb from Guelph, Ontario and then Melbourne, Australia. B.F. Hoerlein (1922-1987) from Auburn, Alabama, brought radiology and surgery to bear on the diagnosis and treatment of spinal disease of dogs.

The study of the autonomic nervous structures of the ruminant gastrointestinal tract and of the higher centers in the nervous system that govern their activity has been a major field for veterinary and physiological research. M. Dussardier in Marseilles studied vagal effects on forestomach motility and the medullary centers in the brain that control it via the vagus nerves. He also developed an ingenious technique to allow fibers growing from a cut vagus nerve to reinervate a cut phrenic nerve, supplying striated diaphragmatic muscle. This allowed recordings to be made in conscious sheep; J.P. Rousseau applied the technique to study afferent and efferent autonomic fibers. Ainsley Iggo, a New Zealander at the Dick veterinary college in Edinburgh, studied the firing patterns of individual nerve fibers of the vagus. With Barry Leek, now in Dublin, he characterized mechanoreceptors and chemoreceptors in the stomach wall as well as efferent fibers supplying its smooth muscle. Donald A. Titchen in Sydney and Robert Comline in Cambridge used decerebrate preparations to differentiate central and peripheral mechanisms. Alvin F. Sellers, Charles E. Stevens, and Alan Dobson at Cornell investigated gastric blood flow as a function of motility and food intake. Ruckebusch and colleagues studied the neural and humoral regulation of abomasal and intestinal motility, including the migrating myoelectric complex. Ralph Kitchell at Davis studied taste in ruminants among his many neuroanatomical investigations. Fred Bell at the RVC and his student, Basil Baldwin, who is now at Babraham, explored the relationships between neural function and behavior. Bengt Andersson in Uppsala, Sweden, characterized the roles of the hypothalamic nuclei in the intake of food and water.

Chabert at Alfort first described sleep with rapid eye movement (REM) in cattle in 1796. There is also evidence that cows dream. Eugene A. Serincky and Nathaniel Kleitman first recorded REM sleep in 1953, in which eye movements were associated with electroencephalogram patterns. Using electroencephalography to record brain electrical activity and obtaining physical recordings of muscle activity, French neurosurgeon Michel Jouvet showed that cats lose their muscle tone during REM sleep periods. He found that the brain stem effectively paralyzed the body at the onset of a REM episode. Because this type of sleep is associated with dreaming, it may have been necessary to avoid acting out the dreams that could render an animal vulnerable to predators. Thus while the rapid eye movements that gave rise to the acronym REM occur, the other muscles only twitch, although some minor vocalizations may be heard, especially in dogs. Blood pressure and heart rate increase, and the frequency of the brain waves rises to close to that of the awake brain. Jouvet called the state "paradoxical sleep" because the brain appeared to be very active yet the body was immobilized. REM sleep has been observed in the fetus in utero and by the time of birth composes up to half an infant's sleeping time. When Bill Dement in New York awakened subjects repeatedly just when they entered REM sleep, the REM periods increased in frequency. When the subjects were allowed undisturbed sleep later, the time of lost REM sleep was made up, indicating that it has a significant role in body function. REM-deprived cats manifest behavior changes, some ceasing grooming themselves, others becoming restless. During non-REM or slow-wave sleep, various growth hormones are secreted to restore the somatic systems. This stops during the REM sleep stages. Ian Oswald in Edinburgh put forward the hypothesis that the dreams are a consequence of the repair and restoration process of the brain itself. The most active researcher of sleep in ruminants was Yves Ruckebusch (1931-1989) at Toulouse veterinary school. Animals exhibit a wide range in the proportion of each twenty-four hours given to sleep. Some bats sleep twenty hours a day, while some antelopes are lucky to sleep one hour. Hibernation is probably dreamless; it has to be energy-conserving since there is no food and water intake. It is also presumed that there is less need for restoration of tissues, including those of the central nervous system.

In the 1930s Konrad Z. Lorenz and Nikolaas Tinbergen began to study animal behavior objectively in natural habitats. They followed their field observations with laboratory research and animal modelling. Tinbergen moved to Oxford to establish a Department of Animal Behavior, where his group investigated the stimuli that influence behavior. Veterinarian Michael W. Fox wrote *Integrated Development of Brain and Behavior in the Dog* in 1971. Oskar Heinroth summed up the field of animal behavior when he remarked that "animals are very emotional people with little ability to reason."

The Trend to Specialization (1950 to 1993)

Specialty groups with advanced professional training in clinical or paraclinical specialty fields began to appear after the Second World War in several countries, mostly in North America, where there were 5061 diplomates by the end of 1993. These specialists are in the applied veterinary fields in which a diploma of specialization by examination carries judicial weight. The usual route to specialty board qualification is through a residency at a veterinary college where training in the applied field is offered at an advanced level. After several years of specialized study and experience, usually including a research paper or a thesis, the examinations are taken. The specialty fields recognized by the AVMA and their numbers of diplomates are listed in the table on p. 669.

There are nine veterinary academies that do not grant diplomas but represent discipline or specialty groups. These groups are feline medicine, veterinary allergy, cardiology, consultants, dentistry, comparative toxicology, dermatology, nutrition, and pharmacology and therapeutics. The scholars in more basic disciplines tend to belong to national academic societies and may have a more loosely knit veterinary society or association as well. Many other associations and societies exist, including groups of species or discipline specialists in areas relevant to the veterinary profession, veterinary education, or veterinary technicians. Some of these groups are large and meet regularly (for example, bovine practitioners and parasitologists). Government agencies and international organizations such as the World Health Organization, FAO, OIE, ILRAD, ILCA, and the Heifer Project are important in veterinary relations with the developing world.

The growth of specialization has been a major factor in improving the standards of veterinary medical services. Specialization has worked against the small town model of the mixed practice, however, in which the practitioner is expected to be a generalist and capable on all fronts. Some consider this expectation unrealistic, and in rural areas large practices with several veterinarians and some specialization within the group by species and technologies have been emerging. The work of companion animal practitioners has evolved and

Specialty Board and Colleges Recognized by the American Veterinary Medical Association (1993)					
Name of Specialty	Date of Recognition (Year)	Number of Diplomates	Name of Specialty	Date of Recognition (Year)	Number of Diplomates
Veterinary pathology	1951	1056	Veterinary anesthesiology	1975	104
Veterinary preventive medicine (1951, Public Health)	1978	513	Veterinary practitioners	1978	332
Laboratory animal medicine	1957	523	Subspecialties		
Veterinary radiology	1962	152	Canine and feline	—	258
Veterinary microbiology	1966	239	Equine	—	36
Veterinary toxicology	1967	83	Dairy	—	8
Veterinary surgery	1967	538	Swine health	—	3
Theriogenology	1971	259	Veterinary dermatology	1982	83
Veterinary ophthalmology	1971	162	Zoological medicine	1983	33
Veterinary internal medicine	1972	726	Veterinary dental college	1988	27
Subspecialties			Veterinary nutrition	1988	35
Cardiology	—	66	Veterinary emergency and critical care	1989	30
Internal medicine	—	545	Veterinary clinical pharmacology	1990	16
Neurology	—	56	Poultry veterinarians	1991	142
Veterinary medical oncology	—	59	Veterinary behaviorists	1993	8
			TOTAL		5061

continues to evolve along the lines of that of their counterparts in human medicine. Equine practice was late in becoming scientific but has progressed rapidly to meet the demands of the racing, eventing, and companion horse industries. Because of the rapidity of intensification in production units, food animal practice is difficult. Adaptation to emerging needs is a major challenge; the priorities are changing as food preferences and food safety tend to overshadow productivity through consumer-driven market forces. Also, considerations of animal welfare and waste disposal are limiting the concentrations of animals that will be tolerated. Thus the food animal species specialist must not only be a genius at analyzing every facet of the production system and a state-of-the-art clinician, but must also be knowledgeable enough about the industrial developments, societal changes, legal constraints, and market forces to provide philosophical guidance to the entire enterprise.

Students are always interested in the emergence of new fields and challenges. Conserving wildlife and helping the developing nations surmount their veterinary problems are two areas in which there is considerable enthusiasm. The expansion of the profession into the arena of the health management of farmed aquatic animals is surely one of great potential. Veterinary medicine's potential to contribute to safeguarding the public health has not nearly been fully exploited. Protection of food is becoming more challenging and scientific, and new zoonoses continue to emerge. Protection of the environment from hazardous pollution is a high priority, as is the protection of endangered species. The veterinary profession is well suited to the protection of animal welfare, and behavior studies must be given a much higher priority.

Strengthening Training in Veterinary Research

The American profession in 1992 was reported to be dominated by its clinical arm of private practitioners, who make up eighty-one percent of the profession (sixty-nine percent of these in small animal practice exclusively or predominantly), whereas nineteen percent were in public or corporate practice. The proportion of veterinarians who are women rose steadily to reach nearly twenty-nine percent by 1992. Among those who are veterinarians, the men are nine years older (median age) than the women. A serious concern is that the proportion of veterinarians engaged in research is too low. This situation is partly attributable to a shortage of opportunities and funding for research training.

The pace of growth in national biomedical research has expanded dramatically during the second half of the twentieth century, but the veterinary component has not shared proportionately in the growth because veterinary-motivated research made possible by funding through the National Institutes of Health became progressively more excluded by the growing restriction of funding to research related to problems in human health. The U.S. Department of Agriculture has failed to give an adequate priority to veterinary research. Consequently, the pool of funds for research training and research on veterinary concerns that scientists can compete for is far too small. Specific funds for veterinary research were approved once by Congress in the 1970s but were vetoed by President Ford on the advice of the secretary of agriculture, a devastating political setback. It is imperative that the research arm of the profession be strengthened by the colleges and by major increases in funding for veterinary research priorities.

The veterinary colleges are in a difficult situation because most of them have given their highest priority to professional education and specialty board certification. They deserve great credit for their accomplishments in these aspects. The modern North American doctor of veterinary medicine is well trained to commence a career in private practice. Standards are high because the colleges must be accredited by the AVMA after periodic inspection and program evaluation. Growing opportunities to take elective courses before graduation and to gain an introduction to a chosen field through externships have strengthened the applicability of the training. The residency and board certification model with a modest introduction to research has produced an array of elite specialists in many fields. The collective veterinary research effort in the colleges and veterinary science departments, in the national institutes, and in industry is simply not yet at an adequate level to sustain the progress that is needed.

Postgraduate academic training to the doctoral level must be strengthened at most colleges. Faculties must recruit strong research scholars who can build teams, including predoctoral and postdoctoral research scientists. For trainees to be successful, stipends and research funds are needed. Trainees need mentoring to begin to prepare themselves to venture into and participate in the mainstream of biomedical research. If progress in the area of veterinary research is to catch up with the rate of progress in laboratory and clinical veterinary service, funding opportunities must improve.

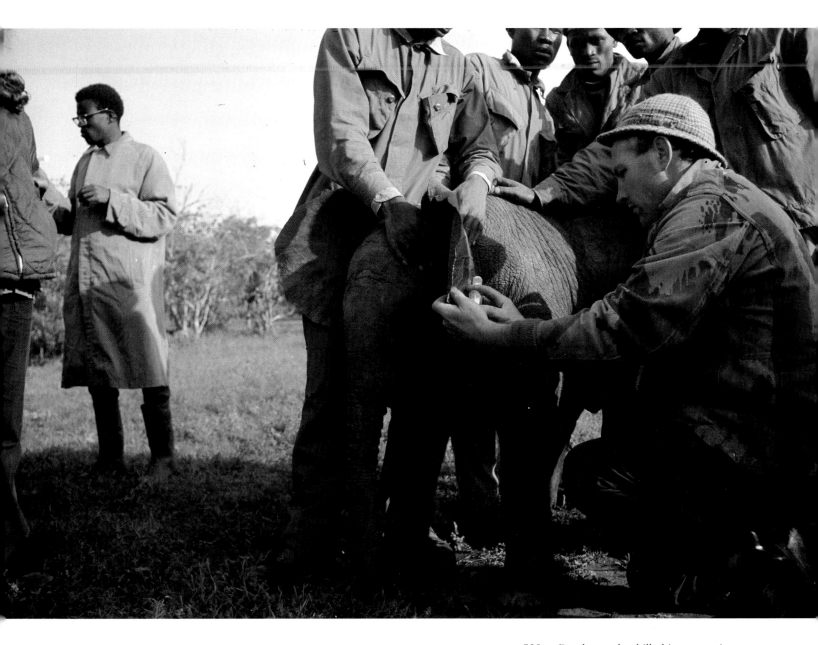

529. Poachers who kill rhinoceros simply to collect the valuable horn have caused a precipitous decline in rhinoceros populations in the last twenty-five years. During a rhinoceros translocation effort in Kenya, a veterinary team discovered this young elephant that had fallen into a pit. A prompt emergency effort to remove it from the pit, treat its injuries, and provide nursing care led to a complete recovery. *(Courtesy Dr. Jerry Haigh, Saskatoon, Saskatchewan.)*

200 Jahre Tierärzliche Hochschule in Wien. Vienna: Tierärtzliche Hochschule, 1968.

200 Jahre Tierärzliche Lehre und Forschung in München. New York: Schattauer, 1990.

Aaris-Sørenson, Kim. *Danmarks Forhistoriske Dyreverden*. Copenhagen: Gyldendal, 1988.

Abou Bekr Ibn Bedr. Le Nãcéri: Traité Complet D'Hippologie et D'Hippiatrie Arabes. Traduit de l'Arabe par Perron, M. Paris: Mme. V. Bouchard Huzard, 1852.

Ackerknecht, Erwin H. *Das Reich des Asklepios*. Bern, Switzerland: Huber, 1963.

Adahl, Karin. *A Khamsa of Nizami of 1439*. Acta Universitatis Upsaliensis: Figura Nova Series 30, 1981.

Adsersen, Vald., ed. *Selected Works*. Copenhagen: Levin & Munksgaard, 1936.

Ainsworth, G.C. *Introduction to the History of Medical and Veterinary Mycology*. Cambridge: Cambridge University Press, 1986.

Akurgal, Ekrem. *The Art of Greece*. New York: Crown, 1966.

Alder, Gary. *Beyond Bokhara: The Life of William Moorcroft 1767-1825*. London: Century, 1985.

Allen, G.E. *Thomas Hunt Morgan: The Man and His Science*. Princeton, NJ: Princeton University Press, 1978.

Anderson, John K. *Ancient Greek Horsemanship*. Berkeley: University of California Press, 1961.

Anderson, John K. *Hunting in the Ancient World*. Berkeley: University of California Press, 1985.

Anderson, Sigurd, ed. *P.C. Abildgaard*. Copenhagen: Kandrup, 1985.

Anderson, E.N. *The Food of China*. New Haven: Yale University Press, 1988.

Andrews, Michael A. *The Birth of Europe*. London: BBC, 1991.

Anthony, David, Telegin, Dmitri Y., and Brown, Dorcas. "The Origin of Horseback Riding." *Sci. Am.* 265 (1991): 94-100.

Aristotle. *Selected Works*. Trans. Hippocrates, G. Apostle and Gerson, Lloyd P. Grinnell, Ia: Peripatetic, 1982.

Armatage, G. *The Thermometer as an Aid to Diagnosis in Veterinary Medicine*. Leighton Buzzard: Muddiman, 1869.

Arnold, Thomas and Guillaume, Alfred. *The Legacy of Islam*. London: Oxford University Press, 1931.

Athar, Shahid, ed. *Islamic Medicine*. Karachi, Pakistan: Pan-Islamic, 1989.

Attenborough, David. *The First Eden*. Boston: Little, Brown, 1987.

Attfield, Robin. *The Ethics of Enivronmental Concern*. 2nd ed. Athens: University of Georgia Press, 1991.

Ayala, Francisco J. *Population and Evolutionary Genetics*. Menlo Park, Calif: Benjamin/Cummings, 1982.

Babcock, Ernest B. and Clausen, Roy E. *Genetics in Relation to Agriculture*. New York: McGraw-Hill, 1918.

Baldry, Peter. *The Battle Against Bacteria: A Fresh Look*. 2nd. ed. Cambridge: Cambridge University Press, 1976.

Bang, Bernard. *Selected Works*. Adsersen, Vald. ed. Copenhagen: Levin & Munksgaard, 1926.

Barclay, Harold B. "Another look at the origins of horse riding." *Anthropos* 77 (1982): 244-249.

Barfield, Thomas. *The Perilous Frontier*. Cambridge Mass: Blackwell, 1989.

Barker, C.A.V. "John G. Rutherford and the controversial standards of education at the Ontario Veterinary College from 1864 to 1920." *Can. Vet. J.* 18 (1977): 327-340.

Barker, C.A.V. and Crowley, T.A. *One Voice: A History of the Canadian Veterinary Medical Association*. Ottawa: Canadian Veterinary Medical Association, 1989.

Barlow, John S. *The Electroencephalogram*. Cambridge: Massachusetts Institute of Technology Press, 1993.

Barnabe, Gilbert, ed. *Aquaculture*. Trans. Lindsay Laird. 2 vols. New York: Horwood, 1990.

Bartley, Mary M. "Darwin and domestication: Studies on inheritance." *J. Hist. Biol.* 25 (1992): 307-333.

Basham, Arthur L. *The Origins of Development of Classical Hinduism*. Zysk. G. ed. Boston: Beacon, 1989.

Basham, Arthur L. *The Wonder That Was India*. 3rd ed. London: Sidgwick, 1967.

Bataille, Georges. *Lascaux*. Trans. Austryn Wainhouse. Lausanne: Skira, 1955.

Beaver, Paul C. and Jung, Rodney C. *Animal Agents and Vectors of Human Disease*. 5th ed. Philadelphia: Lea & Febiger, 1985.

Beckett, J.V. *The Agricultural Revolution*. Cambridge: Blackwell, 1990.

Beddall, Barbara G. "Wallace's annotated copy of Darwin's *Origin of Species*." *J. Hist. Biol.* 21 (1988): 265-289.

Bellamy, David and Pfister, Andrea. *World Medicine*. Oxford: Blakewell, 1992.

Beltran, Antonio. *Rock Art of the Spanish Levant*. Trans. Margaret Brown. Cambridge: Cambridge University Press, 1982.

Benedict, Francis G. *The Physiology of the Elephant*. Washington: Carnegie Institute, 1936.

Berenger, Richard. *The History and Art of Horsemanship. Including a Translation of Xenophon's The Art of Horsemanship*. 2 vols. London: Davies, 1771.

Bergler, Reinbold. *Man and Dog: The Psychology of a Relationship*. Oxford: Blackwell, 1988.

Bernstein, Ralph E. "Darwin's alter ego: Co-originator Alfred Wallace." *Pers. in Biol. and Med.* 27 (1984): 234-238.

Berry, Wendell. *The Unsettling of America: Culture and Agriculture*. San Francisco: Sierra Club, 1977.

Bibby, Cyril. *T.H. Huxley*. New York: Horizon, 1960.

Bibel, Debra J. *Milestones in Immunology*. Madison: Science Tech, 1988.

Bierer, Bert W. *American Veterinary History*. Typed manuscript, 1940.

Binford, Lewis B. *In Pursuit of the Past*. London: Thames, 1983.

Bishop, Jerry E. and Waldhol, Michael. *Genome*. New York: Simon & Schuster, 1991.

Bisseru, Balideo. *Diseases of Man Acquired From His Pets*. London: Heinemann, 1967.

Bitel, Lisa M. *Isle of the Saints: Monastic Settlement and Christian Community in Early Ireland*. Ithaca, New York: Cornell University Press, 1990.

Blaisdell, John. "Andrew Snape (1644-1708) and the beginning of veterinary anatomical instruction in England. *Vet. Hist.* (NS) 6 (4) (1990/91): 134-153.

Bliss, Michael. *The Discovery of Insulin*. Chicago: Chicago University Press, 1982.

Blum, Deborah. *The Monkey Wars*. New York: Oxford University Press,1994.

Blum, Jerome, ed. *Our Forgotten Past*. London: Thames, 1982.

Boakes, Robert. *From Darwin to Behaviorism: Psychology and the Minds of Animals*. Cambridge: Cambridge University Press, 1984.

Boardman, John. *Greek Art*. Rev. ed. New York: Praeger, 1973.

Boardman, John. Griffin, Jasper, and Murray, Oswyn, eds. *The Oxford History of the Classical World*. Oxford: Oxford University Press, 1986.

Boitani, Francesca, Cataldi, Maria, and Pasquinucci, Marinella. *Etruscan Cities*. Trans. Catherine Atthill. New York: Putnam Publishing Group, 1975.

Bokonyi, Sandor. "Development of early stock rearing in the Near East." *Nature 264* (1976): 19-23.

Bonnard, Andre. *Greek Civilization*. Trans. Lytton Sells. Vols. 2 and 3. New York: Macmillan, 1961.

Borek, Ernest. *The Code of Life*. New York: Columbia University Press, 1965.

Bost, Jacques. "Les écoles vétérinaires françaises (Lyon et Alfort) face aux épizooties du XVIIIéme siècle." Institut d'Histoire de la Médecine, *Cycle de conférences* 1979-1980, 133-162. Collection Fondation Mérieux.

Bost, Jacques et Gerbaud, O. "L'enseignement vétérinaire à la fin du XVIIIe siècle: de la tentation médicale au réalisme agricole." Institut d'Histoire de la Médecine, *Cycle de conférences* 1984-1985, 37-68. Collection Fondation Marcel Mérieux.

Bost, Jacques. *Lyon, Berceau des Sciences Vétérinaires*. Lyon: Editions lyonnaises d'art et d'histoire, 1992.

Bostock, Stephen St.C. *Zoos and Animal Rights*. London: Routledge, 1993.

Bouchet, Alain, ed. *La Médecine a Lyon*. Lyon: Hervas, 1987.

Bowlby, John. *Charles Darwin*. London: Pimlico, 1991.

Bowler, Peter J. Evolution, *The History of an Idea*. Rev. ed. Berkeley: University of California Press, 1989.

Boyd, Lee and Houpt, Katherine A. ed., *Przewalski's Horse*. Albany: SUNY Press, 1994.

Boyle, Robert. "New pneumatical experiments about respirations." *Philosophical Transactions of the Royal Society*, vol. 5, nos. 62-3 (1670) 2011-2031, 2035-2056.

Bradshaw, John. *The Behavior of the Domestic Cat*. Wallingford, Oxon: CAB International, 1992.

Brainard, Daniel. *On the Nature and Cure of the Bite of Serpents and the Wounds of Poisoned Arrows*. Washington: s.n., 1855.

Brentjes, Burchard. *African Rock Art*. Trans. Anthony Dent. New York: Potter, 1969.

Brereton, John M. *The Horse in War*. New York: Arco, 1976.

Bridge, Antony. *The Crusades*. New York: Franklin Watts, 1982.

Briggs, John C. "A cretaceous tertiary mass extinction: Were most of Earth's species killed off?" *Bioscience* 41 (1991): 619-624.

Brock, Thomas, ed. *Milestones in Microbiology*. Englewood Cliffs, NJ: Prentice Hall, 1961.

Brodrick, A. Houghton, ed. *Animals in Archaeology*. New York: Praeger, 1972.

Brogniez, A.J. *Traité de Chirurgie Vétérinaire*. Brussels, Belgium: Société Encyclographique des Sciences Médicales, 1839.

Bronowski, J. *The Ascent of Man*. London: Futura, 1981

Brooks, Lester. *Great Civilizations of Ancient Africa*. New York: Four Winds, 1971.

Brown, Evan. *World Fish Farming: Cultivation and Economics*. Westport, Conn: AVI, 1983.

Brown, Jonathan. *Agriculture in England*. Manchester: Manchester University Press, 1987.

Brumme, Martin F. "Tierärzt und Tierschutz in Deutschland in der ersten Hälfte des 20. Jahrhunderts. Eine Skizze zur Historisierung einer aktuellen Diskussion." *Argos Speciale uitgave* (1991): S29-S39.

Bucherl, Wolfgang. *"Das Hans der Gifte: die Geschichte von Butantan Institut Sao Paulo"*. Stuttgart: Kosmos Gesellschaft der Naturfreunde, 1963.

Budiansky, Stephen. *The Covenant of the Wild: Why Animals Chose Domestication*. New York: William. Morrow, 1992.

Bulliet, Richard W. *The Camel and the Wheel*. New York: Columbia University Press, 1975 and 1990.

Bunker, Emma C., Chatwin, C. Bruce, and Farkas, Ann R. *Animal Style Art from East to West*. New York: Asia Society, 1970.

Busvine, James R. *Disease Transmission by Insects*. Berlin: Springer, 1993.

Butler, Stella V.F. "Centers and peripheries: The development of British physiology, 1870-1914." *J. Hist. Biol.* 21 (1988): 473-500.

Bynum, William F. and Porter, Roy, eds. *Companion Encyclopedia of the History of Medicine*. 2 vols. London: Routledge, 1993.

Cadiot, P.J., translated and expanded by Dollar, J.A.W. *Studies in Clinical Veterinary Medicine and Surgery*. New York: William R. Jenkins, 1901.

Calaby, J.H. and Tyndale-Biscoe, C.H., eds. *Reproduction and Evolution*. Canberra: Australian Academy of Science, 1977.

Calef, George. *Caribou and the Barren-lands*. Ottawa: Canadian Arctic Resources Commission, 1981.

Calmette, Albert. *Tubercle Bacillus Infection and Tuberculosis in Man and Animals*. Trans. Williard B. Soper and George H. Smith. Baltimore: Williams & Wilkins, 1923.

Campbell, Bernard. *Human Ecology*. London: Heinemann, 1983.

Campbell, Joseph. *The Mythic Image*. Princeton: Princeton University Press, 1974.

Caras, Roger. *Venomous Animals of the World*. Englewood Cliffs, NJ: Prentice-Hall, 1974.

Carcia-Carrillo, Casimiro. *Animal and Human Brucellosis in the Americas*. Paris: OIE, 1990.

Carroll, Harry J., Jr., et al. *The Development of Civilization*. Chicago: Scott Foresman, 1961.

Carruthers, Peter. *The Animals Issue*. Cambridge: Cambridge University Press, 1992.

Castle, W.E. "Piebald rats and the theory of genes." *Proc. Nat. Acad. Sci.* 5 (1919): 126.

Carter, H.E. "Vivisection and the British veterinary profession in the 19th century." *Friskies Veterinary International*. 1 (1) (1989) 59-64.

Chadwick, John. *The Mycenean World*. Cambridge: Cambridge University Press, 1976.

Chard, Chester S. *Man in Prehistory*. 2nd ed. New York: McGraw-Hill, 1975.

Chauveau, A. *The Comparative Anatomy of the Domesticated Animals*. Revised and enlarged with Arloing, S. 2nd. Engl. ed. translated by Fleming, George. New York: D. Appleton Co., 1905.

Chauvois, Louis. *William Harvey*. London: Hutchinson, 1957.

Chetverikov, S.S. "On certain aspects of the evolutionary process from the standpoint of modern genetics." *Proc. Am. Philosophical Soc.* 105 (1961): 167-195.

Childs, B. "Sir Archibald Garrod's conception of chemical individuality: A modern appreciation." *N. Eng. J. Med.* 282 (1974): 71-77.

Chiodi, Valentino. *Storia Della Veterinaria*. Milan: Farmitalia, 1957.

Chukaszian, Babken L. *Le Traité d'Hippiatrie du XIII siècle*. From: *Armenian Studies in Memoriam to Haig Berberian*. Dickran Kouymian, editor. Lisbon: Calouste Gulbenkian Foundation, 1986.

Clabby, J. *The History of the Royal Army Veterinary Corps*. London: J.A. Allen, 1963.

Clark, Bracy. *A Short History of the Horse and Progress of Horse Knowledge*. London: Adlard, 1824.

Clark, J. *A Treatise on the Prevention of Diseases Incidental to Horses*. Edinburgh: W. Smellie, 1788

Clark, Kenneth. *Animals and Men*. New York: William Morrow, 1977.

Clark, Ronald. *The Life and Work of J.B.S. Haldane*. Oxford: Oxford University Press, 1984.

Clark, William H.H. *The History of the United States Army Veterinary Corps in Vietnam 1962-1973*. Roswell, GA: W.H. Wolfe, 1991.

Clarke, Cyril, "Mules must come to science." *New Scientist,* February 3rd. (1983).

Claster, Jill N. *The Medieval Experience 300-1400*. New York: New York University Press, 1982.

Clendening, Logan. *Source Book of Medical History*. New York: Dover, 1942.

Close, Angela E., ed. *Prehistory of Arid North Africa*. Dallas: Southern Methodist University Press, 1987.

Clutton-Brock, Juliet. *Domesticated Animals From Early Times*. London: British Museum (Natural History), 1981.

Clutton-Brock, Juliet. *Horse Power*. Cambridge: Harvard University Press, 1992.

Cochrane, Willard W. *The Development of American Agriculture*. 2nd ed. Minneapolis: University of Minnesota Press, 1993.

Cockrill, W. Ross. "The water buffalo." *Sci. Am.* 217 (1967): 118-125.

Cole, F.J. *A History of Comparative Anatomy*. New York: Dover, 1975.

Coleman, J., ed. *The Sheep and Pigs of Great Britain*. London: "The Field" Office, 1877.

Colenbrander-Dijkman, Anne-Marieke. *Dieren in Wetenschap en Samenleving: een bibliografie voor veterinairen*. Utrecht: 1983.

Collard, Andrée and Contrucci, Joyce. *Rape of the Wild: Man's Violence against Animals and the Earth*. Bloomington: Indiana University Press, 1989.

Collins, Desmond. *The Human Revolution*. New York: Dutton, 1976.

Combe, Iris. *Herding Dogs*. London: Faber & Faber, 1987.

Comben, Norman. *Agriculture Husbandry Farriery and the Veterinary Art*. Berkhamsted, UK: n.p., 1991.

Connah, Graham. *African Civilizations*. Cambridge: Cambridge University Press, 1987.

Consortium for International Development. *Range Livestock Production in the Peoples Republic of China*. Proc. Int. Symposium, New Mexico State University, 1983.

Convegno Sulla Storia della Medicina Veterinaria. Reggio Emilia: 1994.

Craven, Roy C. *A Concise History of Indian Art.* New York: Oxford University Press, 1976.

Cooper, Jilly. *Animals in War.* London: Heinemann, 1983.

Cope, Zachary. *Almroth Wright.* London: Nelson, 1966.

Corcos, Alain F. and Monaghan, Floyd V. *Gregor Mendel's Experiments on Plant Hybrids.* New Brunswick, NJ: Rutgers University Press, 1993.

Cornell, Tim and Matthews, John. *Atlas of the Roman World.* New York: Facts on File, 1982.

Cornford, Francis M. *Before and After Socrates.* Cambridge: Cambridge University Press, 1932.

Cotchin, Ernest. *The Royal Veterinary College London.* Buckingham: Barracuda, 1990.

Cotterell, Arthur. *China: A Cultural History.* New York: New American Library, 1988.

Cox, J. Charles. *The Royal Forests of England.* London: Methuen, 1905.

Crawford, Michael and Marsh, David, *The Driving Force.* New York: Harper & Row, 1989.

Creel, Herrlee G. *The Birth of China.* New York: Ungar, 1937.

Crosby, Alfred W., Jr. *The Columbian Exchange.* Westport, Conn: Greenwood, 1972.

Cummins, John. *The Hound and the Hawk.* New York: St. Martin's Press, 1988.

Cushing, Harvey. *The Life of Sir William Osler.* Oxford: Oxford University Press, 1940.

Dadd, George H. *The Modern Horse Doctor.* Boston: John P. Jewett, 1855.

Dahanukar, Sharadini A. and Thatte, Urmila M. *Ayurveda Revisted.* Bombay: Popular Prakashan, 1989.

Dahmus, Joseph H. *A History of Medieval Civilization.* Indianapolis: Odyssey-Bobbs, 1964.

Dale-Green, Patricia. *Dog.* Chatham: W. and J. Mackay, 1966.

Dampier, William C. *A History of Science.* 3rd ed. Cambridge: Cambridge University Press, 1942.

Darby, William J., Ghalioungui, Paul, and Grivetti, Louis. *Food, the Gift of Osiris.* 2 vols. London: Academic, 1977.

Darwin, Charles. *The Collected Papers of Charles Darwin.* Ed. Paul H. Barrett. 2 vols. Chicago: University of Chicago Press, 1977.

Darwin, Charles. *The Red Notebook of Charles Darwin.* Ed. Sandra Herbert. London: British Museum (Natural History), 1980.

Darwin, Charles. *On the Origin of Species by Means of Natural Selection, or the Preservation of Favored Races in the Struggle for Life.* London: John Murray, 1859.

Darwin, Charles. *The Variation of Animals and Plants Under Domestication.* 2nd ed. 2 vols. London: John Murray, 1875. (1st edition 1868)

Darwin, Charles. *The Expression of the Emotions in Man and Animals.* London: Murray, 1872.

Daumas, Eugene. *The Horses of the Sahara.* Trans. Sheila M. Ohlendorf. 9th ed. Austin: University of Texas Press, 1968.

Davidson, B.R. *European Farming in Australia.* Amsterdam: Elsevier, 1981.

Davidson, T.D. "A survey of some British veterinary folklore." *Bull. Hist. Med.* 34 (1960): 199-232.

Davis, R.H.C. *The Medieval Warhorse.* London: Thames, 1989.

Davis, Simon J.M. *The Archaeology of Animals.* New Haven: Yale University Press, 1987.

De Beer, Gavin R. *Vertebrate Zoology: An Introduction to the Comparative Anatomy, Embryology, and Evolution of Chordate Animals.* London: Sidwick and Jackson, 1959.

Dembeck, Hermann. *Animals and Men.* Trans. Richard and Clara Winston. New York: Natural History, 1965.

Department of Antiquities, Ashmolean Museum. *Animals in Early Art.* Oxford: Ashmolean Museum, 1978.

Desmond, Adrian. *The Politics of Evolution.* Chicago: University of Chicago Press, 1989.

Desmond, Adrian and Moore, James. *Darwin.* London: Joseph, 1991.

Diesner, Hans-Joachim. *The Great Migration.* Trans. C.S.V. Salt. Leipzig: Leipzig, 1978.

Dincer, Ferruh. Editor: *Proceedings of the 25th International Congress on the History of Veterinary Medicine.* Ankara-Cappadocia-Istanbul, Turkey, 1992.

Dingley, Pauline. *Historic Books on Veterinary Science and Animal Husbandry.* London: HMSO, 1992.

Dobzhansky, Theodosius G. *Genetics and the Origin of Species.* New York: Columbia University Press, 1937.

Dodge, Theodore A. *Riders of Many Lands.* New York: Harper & Row, 1894.

Dodgshon, R.A. and Butlin, R.A., eds. *A Historical Geography of England and Wales.* London: Academic, 1978.

Dogra, S.C. "Microbial agents used in ancient India." *Indian J. Hist. Sci.* 22 (1987): 164-169.

Douglas, Norman. *Birds and Beasts of the Greek Anthology.* London: Chapman, 1928.

Dowling, Harry F. *Fighting Infection.* London: Harvard University Press, 1977.

Dozier, Rush W., Jr. *Codes of Evolution.* New York: Crown, 1992.

Drew, Isabella M., Perkins, Dexter Jr., and Daly, Patricia. "Prehistoric domestication of animals: Effects on bone structure." *Science* 171 (1971): 280-282.

Driesch, Angela von den. *Geschichte der Tiermedizin: 5000 Jahre Tierheilkunde.* München, 1989.

Driesch, Angela von den. Kulturgeschichter der Hauskatze, in Schmidt, Vera. und Horzinek, Marian, C. editors, *Krankheiten der Katze.* Stuttgart: Gustav Fischer Verlag Jena, 1992. pp 17-40.

Drum, Sue and Whitely, H. Ellen. *Women in Veterinary Medicine.* Ames: Iowa State University Press, 1991.

Duffey, John. *The Sanitarians: A History of American Public Health.* Urbana: University of Illinois Press, 1992.

Dunn, Leslie C. *A Short History of Genetics.* Ames: Iowa State University Press, 1991.

Duvernay, Bernard. "The progressive history of the farrier profession." *Hoofcare and Lameness* 93-1 (1993): 20-24.

Dykstra, Ralph R. *Animal Sanitation and Disease Control.* 6th ed. Danville, Il: Interstate, 1961.

Edwards, Elwyn H. *Horses: Their Role in the History of Man.* London: Willow, 1987.

Egana, C. Sanz. *Veterinaria Española.* Madrid: Espasa-Calpe, 1941.

Eibl-Eibesfeldt, Irenäus. *Ethologie die Biologie des Verhaltens.* Frankfurt: Athenaion, n.d.

Eisler, Riane. *The Chalice and the Blade.* San Francisco: Harper & Row, 1987.

Eldredge, Niles, ed. *The Natural History Reader in Evolution.* New York: Columbia University Press, 1987.

Eliot, Elizabeth. *Portrait of a Sport: A History of Steeplechasing.* London: Longmans, 1957.

Eliot, Simon and Stern, Beverley. *The Age of Enlightenment: An Anthology of Eighteenth Century Texts.* Volume 2. Open University Press with Ward Lock Educational, 1979.

Ellenberger, Wilhelm. *Leisering's Atlas of the Anatomy of the Horse and of the Other Domestic Animals.* Transl. from 3rd German ed. By Peters, A.T. and Sturdevant, L.B. 2nd. ed. Chicago: Alexander Eger, 1908.

Ellenberger, Wilhelm and Scheunert, A. *Lehrbuch der Vergleichenden Physiologie der Haussäugetiere.* Berlin: Paul Parey, 1910.

Ellenberger, Willhelm, Baum, Hermann, Dittrich, Hermann, and Münch. *Handbuch der Anatomie der Tiere für Künstler.* Leipzig: Theordor Weicher, 1911.

Ellenberger, Wilhelm and Baum, Hermann. *Lehrbuch der Topographischen Anatomie des Pferdes.* Berlin: Paul Parey, 1914.

Ellenberger, Wilhelm and Baum, Hermann. *Handbuch der Vergleichenden Anatomie der Haustiere.* 14th ed. Berlin: August Hirschwald, 1915.

Eluere, Christiane. *The Celts.* Trans. Daphne Briggs. New York: Abrams, 1993.

Enggass, Robert and Brown, Jonathan. *Italy and Spain 1600-1750.* Englewood Cliffs, NJ: Prentice Hall, 1970.

English, P.B. and Cao, G.R. "Veterinary education in China." *Australian Vet. J.* 64 (1987): 180-183.

Epstein, Hellmut. *Domestic Animals of China.* New York: Africana Publishing Corp. 1971. (Published in United Kingdom by CAB, 1969).

Epstein, Hellmut. *Domestic Animals of Nepal.* New York: Holmes & Meier, 1977.

Ercolani, Giovanni Batista. *Carlo Ruini: Curiosita Storiche e Bibliografiche Intorno Alla Scoperta Della Circulazione del Sangue.* Bologna: Zanichelli, 1873.

Ereshefsky, Marc, ed. *The Units of Evolution.* Cambridge: Massachusetts Institute of Technology Press, 1992.

Espersen, Gert. *Danske Dyrlaegeinstrumenter Gennen 200 ar 1773-1973.* Frederiksberg: 1981.

Evans, A. Margaret and Barker, C.A.V. *Century One: A History of the Ontario Veterinary Association 1874-1974.* Guelph, Ont: A.M. Evans, 1976.

Evans, G.H. *Elephants and Their Diseases.* Rangoon, Burma: Govt. Print., 1910.

Evans, Herbert M. and Cole, Harold H. *An Introduction to the Oestrous Cycle of the Dog.* Berkeley: University of California Press, 1931.

Evans, Hilary and Evans, Mary. *The Life and Art of George Cruikshank.* London: Frederick Muller Ltd., 1978.

Ewald, Paul W. *Evolution of Infectious Disease.* Oxford: Oxford University Press, 1994.

Fagan, Brian M. *The Great Journey.* London: Thames, 1987.

Fahimuddin, M. *Domestic Water Buffalo.* 2nd ed. New Delhi: Oxford, 1989.

Fairbank, John K. *China: A New History.* Cambridge, Mass: Belknap-Harvard, 1992.

Fairley, John. *Racing in Art.* New York: Rizzoli, 1990.

Fankhauser, R. and Vandevelde, M. "Veterinary neurology—Past, present and future." *J. Comp. Path.* 98 (1988) 275-286.

Fanti, Mario and Chiossi, Rosa. *Ricerche su Carlo Ruini 1530-1598.* Bologna: Li Causi, 1984.

FAO. *The New World Screwworm Eradication Programme.* Rome: FAO, 1992.

Farb, Peter. *Man's Rise to Civilization.* New York: Dutton, 1968.

Feldman, William H. *Avian Tuberculosis Infections.* Baltimore: Williams & Wilkins, 1938.

Feldman, William H. *Proceedings of the Staff Meetings of the Mayo Clinic.* Vol. 19: 1951

Fenner, Frank and Gibbs, A., eds. *Portraits of Viruses.* Basel: Karger, 1988.

Ferrill, Arthur. *The Origins of War.* London: Thames, 1985.

Fiedel, Stuart J. *Prehistory of the Americas.* Cambridge: Cambridge University Press, 1987.

Finley, M.I. *The Ancient Greeks.* York: Viking, 1964.

Fischer, Klaus-Dietrich. "Two notes on the *Hippiatrica*." *Greek, Roman and Byzantine Studies* 20 (1979): 371-379.

Fisher, John R. "British physicians, medical science, and the cattle plague, 1865-66." *Bull. Hist. Med.* 67. (1993): 651-669.

Fisher, John R. "Professor Gamgee and the farmers." *Vet. Hist. 1.* (1979-80): 53-55.

Fisher, John R. "Animal health and ecological disaster in nineteenth century Australia." *Veterinary History,* Vol. 3 No. 4 (winter 1984/85).

Fisher, John R. "Not quite a profession—The aspirations of veterinary surgeons in England in mid-nineteenth century." *Hist. Res.* 66. (1993): 284-302.

Fisher, Ronald A. *The Genetical Theory of Natural Selection.* Oxford: Clarendon Press, 1930. (rev ed. 1958, New York: Dover).

Fisher, Ronald A. *Statistical Methods of Research Workers.* Edinburgh: Oliver and Boyd, 1925.

Fisher, Ronald A. "Dominance in poultry." *Phil. Trans Royal Soc. Bull.* 225(1935): 195-226.

Fleming, George. *Animal Plagues: Their History, Nature and Prevention.* London: Chapman, 1871.

Fleming, George. *A Text-Book of Veterinary Obstetrics.* 2nd ed. London: Baillière Tindall & Cox, 1896. (1st ed. 1878).

Flew, Antony. *Darwinian Evolution.* London: Paladin, 1984.

Flexner, Simon and Flexner, James T. *William Henry Welch and the Heroic Age of American Medicine.* New York: Viking, 1941.

Fogle, Bruce. *Pets and Their People.* London: Collins Horvill, 1983.

Fong, Wen. *Beyond Representation: Chinese Painting and Calligraphy, 8th-14th Century.* The Metropolitan Museum and Yale University Press, 1992.

Forbis, Judith. *The Classic Arabian Horse.* New York: Liveright, 1976.

Ford, Connie M. *Aleen Cust Veterinary Surgeon, Britain's First Woman Vet.* Bristol: Biopress, 1990.

Foster, William Derek. *A History of Parasitology.* Edinburgh: E & S. Livingstone, 1965.

Foster, William Derek. *A History of Medical Bacteriology and Immunology.* London: Heinemann, 1970.

Foucart-Walter, Elisabeth and Rosenberg, Pierre. *The Painted Cat.* New York: Rizzoli, 1987.

Fountain, Robert and Gates, Alfred. *Stubbs' Dogs.* London: Ackermann, 1984.

Fowler, Murray E. *Veterinary Zootoxicology.* Boca Raton, Fla: CRC Press, 1993.

Francis, John. *Bovine Tuberculosis.* London: Staples, 1947.

Freeman, Leslie G. *Altamira Revisited and Other Essays on Early Art.* Chicago: Institute for Prehistoric Investigations, 1987.

Friedberger, Franz and Fröhner, Eugen. *Veterinary Pathology.* Trans. M.H. Hayes. 6th ed. 2 vols. Chicago: Chicago Medical, 1909.

Friedlander, Walter. *The Golden Wand of Medicine.* New York: Greenwood, 1992.

Froehner, Reinhard. *Kulturgeschichte der Tierheilkunde.* Kontstanz: Terra-Verlag. Vol.1 1952. Vol.2 1954. Vol.3 1968.

Fruton, Joseph S. *A Skeptical Biochemist.* Cambridge: Harvard University Press, 1992.

Futuyma, Douglas J. *Evolutionary Biology,* 2nd Ed. Sunderland, Mass: Sinauer Association, 1986.

Gaffney, B. and Cunningham, E.P. "Estimation of genetic trend in racing performance of thoroughbred horses." *Nature* 333 (1988): 722-724.

Galsworthy, John. *The Slaughter of Animals for Food.* London: RSPCA, 1913.

Gamble, Clive. *The Paleolithic Settlement of Europe.* Cambridge: Cambridge University Press, 1986.

Gamgee, John. *The Cattle Plague.* London: Robert Hardwicke, 1866.

Gardener, Helen. *Art Through the Ages.* 8th ed. San Diego: Harcourt Brace Jovanovich, 1986.

Gardner, Eldon J. *Principles of Genetics.* 5th ed. New York: John Wiley & Sons, 1975.

Garner, Robert. *Animals, Politics and Morality.* Manchester: Manchester University Press, 1993.

Garrett, Laurie. *The Coming Plague: Newly Emerging Diseases in a World Out of Balance.* New York: Farrar, Straus and Giroux, 1994.

Garrison, Fielding H. *An Introduction to the History of Medicine.* 4th ed. Philadelphia: WB Saunders, 1929.

Gauthier-Pilters, Hilde and Dagg, Anne I. *The Camel.* Chicago: University of Chicago Press, 1981.

Ghiselin, Michael T. *The Triumph of the Darwinian Method.* Chicago: University of Chicago Press, 1984.

Gilbert, Martin. *The Dent Atlas of British History.* 2nd ed. London: Dent, 1993.

Gillispie, Charles G., ed. *Dictionary of Scientific Biology.* Vols. 3, 9 and 13. New York: Scribner, 1970-1990.

Ginsberg, H.S. Editor. *Ecology and Environmental Management of Lyme Disease.* New Brunswick, NJ: Rutgers University Press, 1993.

Gittleman, John L., ed. *Carnivore Behavior in Ecology and Evolution.* Ithaca: Cornell University Press, 1989.

Glahn, E., "Signs and meanings." In Toynbee, Arnold. ed. *Half the World.* New York: Holt, Rinehart and Winston, 1973.

Glubb, John. *A Short History of the Arab Peoples.* New York: Stein & Day, 1970.

Gohau, Gabriel. *A History of Geology.* Trans. Albert V. Carozzi and Marguerite Carozzi. New Brunswick, NJ: Rutgers University Press, 1990.

Goodall, Vanne M., ed. *The Quest for Man.* New York: Praeger, 1975.

Goodfield, G. June. *The Growth of Scientific Physiology.* New York: Arno, 1975.

Gotthelf, Allan, ed. *Aristotle on Nature and Living Things.* Pittsburgh: Mathesis, 1985.

Gould, Stephen Jay. *Ontogeny and Phylogeny.* Cambridge, Mass: Belknap Press of Harvard University Press, 1977.

Gowlett, John A.J. *Ascent to Civilization.* New York: Alfred A. Knopf, 1984.

Grafe, Alfred. *A History of Experimental Virology.* Trans. Elvira Reckendorf. Berlin: Springer, 1991.

Grande, Paul M. *Prehistoric Art, Paleolithic Painting and Sculpture.* Greenwich, Conn: New York Graphic Society, 1967.

Grant, Michael. *The History of Ancient Israel.* New York: Scribner, 1984.

Grant, Michael. ed. *The Birth of Western Civilization.* New York: McGraw-Hill, 1964.

Grbasic, Z. and Vuksic, V. *The History of Cavalry.* New York: Facts on File, 1989.

Greer, Thomas H. *A Brief History of Western Man.* 3rd ed. New York: Harcourt Brace Jovanovich, 1977.

Griffin, Donald C. *Animal Thinking.* Cambridge: Harvard University Press, 1984.

Grmek, Mirko D. *Diseases in the Ancient Greek World.* Trans. Mireille and Leonard Muellner. Baltimore: Johns Hopkins University Press, 1989.

Gros, Francois. *The Gene Civilization.* Trans. Lee F. Scanlon. New York: McGraw-Hill, 1991.

Guggisberg, Charles A.W. *Man and Wildlife.* London: Evans, 1970.

Gürlt, Ernst F. *Thierische Missgeburten.* Berlin: Hirschwald, 1877.

Gurney, Gene. *Kingdoms of Europe.* New York: Crown, 1982.

Guthrie, R. Dale. *Frozen Fauna of the Mammoth Steppe.* Chicago: University of Chicago Press, 1990.

Gutsche, Thelma. *There Was a Man.* Cape Town: Timmins, 1979.

Habel, Robert E. "Anatomy: Past, present, future." *Cornell Vet.* 75 (1985): 27-55.

Habermehl, Gerhard. *Venomous Animals and Their Toxins.* Berlin: Springer-Verlag, 1981.

Haeckel, Ernest. *The Evolution of Man: vol. II The Evolution of the Species or Phylogeny.* New York: G.P. Putnam's Sons, 1910.

Haeckel, Ernest. *The History of Creation or the Development of the Earth and its Inhabitants by the Action of Natural Causes.* Fifth Edition translation revised by E. Ray Lankester. Vol. I of II vols. New York: D. Appleton Co., 1911.

Haldane, John B.S. *The Causes of Evolution.* Princeton: Princeton University Press, 1990.

Haldane, John B.S. "Disease and evolution." *La Ricerca Scientifica Suppl.* 19 (1949a): 68.

Haldane, John B.S. "The detection of antigens with an abnormal genetic determination." *Journal of Genet.* 54 (1956): 54.

Hall, Stephen J. *Two Hundred Years of British Livestock Farming.* London: British Museum (Natural History), 1989.

Hallgren, Willy. *Svensk Veterinärhistoria.* Malmo, Sweden: Allhem, 1960.

Hancock, Reginald. *Memoirs of a Veterinary Surgeon.* London: MacGibbon, 1952.

Hank, Davis and Balfour, Dianne, eds. *The Inevitable Bond: Examining Scientist-Animal Interactions.* Cambridge: Cambridge University Press, 1992.

Hanssen, Peter. *Geschichte der Epidemien bei Menschen und Tieren im Norden.* Glückstadt: Augustin, 1925.

Hardie, R.M. and Watson, J.M. "Mycobacterium bovis in England and Wales: past, present and future." *Epidemiol. Infect.* 109 (1992): 23-33.

Harris, Marvin. *Good to Eat.* New York: Simon & Schuster, 1985.

Harris, Marvin and Ross, Eric B., eds. *Food and Evolution.* Philadelphia: Temple University Press, 1987.

Hart, George. *Egyptian Myths.* London: British Museum, 1990.

Hart, Gerald D, ed. *Disease in Ancient Man.* Toronto: Clarke Irwin, 1983.

Hart, Susanne. *Too Short a Day.* New York: Taplinger, 1967.

Hartl, Daniel L. *Our Uncertain Heritage.* Philadelphia: Lippincott, 1977.

Hartman, H. "The evolution of natural selection: Darwin versus Wallace." *Pers. in Biol. and Med.* 34 (1990): 78-88.

Harvey, William. *On the Motion of the Heart and Blood in Animals.* Trans. Robert Willis. Buffalo: Prometheus, 1993.

Hatschbach, Percy I. "The teaching of veterinary medicine in Brazil: its origin and development. *A Hora Veterinária.* Ano 11 no.62 (July/Aug. 1991): 41-46.

Hausmann, W. *Monumenta Medicinae Veterinariae Historica.* Munich: Hans Marseille, 1980.

Hausmann, Walter and Joechle, Wolfgang. "The discovery of Chiron's Cave, a prehistoric school of medicine for animals and humans." *Canadian Vet. J.* 29 (1988): 857-860.

Hayes, John R., ed. *The Genius of Arab Civilization.* Cambridge: Massachusetts Institute of Technology Press, 1978.

Hayes, M. Horace. *Veterinary Notes for Horse Owners.* 6th ed. London: Hurst, 1903.

Hayter, Earl W. "Livestock doctors, 1850-1890." *The Veterinarian* 2 (1964): 65-74.

Hearne, Vicki. *Adam's Task.* New York: Vintage, 1987.

Heath, Agnew E. *A History of Hereford Cattle and their Breeders.* London: Duckworth, 1983.

Hendrickson, Robert. *More Cunning Than Man.* New York: Dorset, 1983.

Henning, Michiel W. *Animal Diseases in South Africa.* 1st ed. 1931, 2nd ed. Johannesburg: Central News Agency, 1949. 3rd ed. 1956.

Herman, Harry A. *Improving Cattle by the Millions.* Columbia, Missouri: University of Missouri Press, 1981.

Herms, William B. *Medical and Veterinary Entomology.* 2nd ed. New York: Macmillan, 1923.

Himmelfarb, Gertrude. *The Idea of Poverty.* New York: Vintage, 1985.

Highwater, Jamake. *Native Land.* Boston: Little, Brown, 1986.

A History of the Angus Breed. Rev. and repr. ed. St. Joseph, Mo: American Angus Association, 1981.

Hitches, Barbara. *Wool in Australia, 1788-1988.* Parkville, Victoria: Australian Wool Corporation, 1988.

Hitti, Philip K. *Makers of Arab History.* New York: Harper & Row, 1968.

Hoare, Cecil A. *The Trypanosomes of Mammals: A Zoological Monograph.* Oxford: Blackwell, 1972.

Hobson, William. *World Health and History.* Bristol, UK: Wright, 1963.

Hoff, H.E., Geddes, L.A. and McCrady, J.D. "The contributions of the horse to knowledge of the heart and circulation." 4 parts. *Connecticut Medicine,* vol. 29, (1965). 795 800 and 866 876; vol.30, (1966): 43 48 and 126-131.

Hollister, C. Warren. *Medieval Europe.* 3rd ed. New York: John Wiley, 1974.

Horhan, Dominique and Lorenz, Konrad. *Sa vie, son oevre, interet en medicine vétérinaire.* Thèse, Ecole Nationale Vétérinaire de Lyon, 1979.

Hosgood, Giselle. "The history of surgical drainage." *JAVMA* 196 (1990): 42-44.

Houck, U.G. *The Bureau of Animal Industry of the United States Department of Agriculture, Its Establishment, Achievements and Current Activities.* Washington: published by the author, 1924.

Houghton of Sowerby. *Dogs in the U.K.* London: Walter House for Joint Advisory Committee on Pets in Society, 1975.

Howard, Jonathan. *Darwin.* Oxford: Oxford University Press, 1982.

Howey, Mary Oldfield. *The Horse in Magic and Myth.* London: Rider, 1923.

Howey, Mary Oldfield. *The Encircled Serpent.* London: Rider, 1926.

Howey, Mary Oldfield. *The Cat in the Mysteries of Religion and Magic.* London: Rider, 1930.

Howey, Mary Oldfield. *The Cults of the Dog.* Ashington, Rochford, Essex: The C.W. Daniel Co., 1972.

Hoyt, Edwin. *A Short History of Science.* Vol. 1. New York: Day, 1965.

Huang, Kee Chang. *The Pharmacology of Chinese Herbs.* Boca Raton, Fla: CRC Press, 1993.

Hubbard, Clifford L.B. *Working Dogs of the World.* London: Sidgwick and Jackson, 1947.

Hufton, Olwen H. *Europe, Privilege and Protest 1730-1789.* Ithaca: Cornell University Press, 1980.

Hughes, Sally Smith. *The Virus: A History of the Concept.* New York: Science History, 1977.

Hull, David L. *Science as a Process.* Chicago: University of Chicago Press, 1988.

Hull, Denison B. *Hounds and Hunting in Ancient Greece.* Chicago: The University of Chicago Press, 1964.

Hunting, William. *Glanders: a Clinical Treatise.* London: H & W Brown, 1908.

Hutyra, Franz and Marek, Josef. *Special Pathology and Therapeutics of the Diseases of Domestic Animals.* Trans. John R. Mohler, et. al. 2nd American ed. Vol 1. Chicago: Eger, 1920.

Huxley, Julian. *Evolution in Action.* New York: Mentor, 1957.

Huxley, Thomas H. *Man's Place in Nature.* New York: Appleton, 1896.

Hyams, Edward. *Animals in the Service of Man.* Philadelphia: Lippincott, 1972.

Ingold, Tim. *Hunters, Pastoralists and Ranchers.* Cambridge: Cambridge University Press, 1980.

"In marks of ancient bit, clues to earliest riders." *New York Times,* June 26, 1990.

Innes, James Robert M. and Saunders, Leon Z. *Comparative Neuropathology.* New York: Academic Press, 1962.

International Conference on Biochemical Evolution. *Biochemical Evolution and the Origin of Life.* Amsterdam: North Holland, 1971.

Ions, Veronica. *Egyptian Mythology.* New rev. ed. New York: Newnes, 1982.

Isaac, Erich. "On the domestication of cattle." *Science* 137 (1962): 195-203.

Jackson, Jaime. *The Natural Horse.* Flagstaff, Ariz: Northland, 1992.

Jettmar, Karl. *Art of the Steppes.* Rev ed. New York: Greystone, 1967.

Jöchle, Wolfgang. "Samenübertragung, Besamung und ihre Bedeutung in der griechischen Mythologie." *Dtsch. Tierärztl. Wschr.* 94: 444-496.

Johnson, Andrew. *Factory Farming.* Oxford, UK and Cambridge, USA: Blackwell, 1991.

Jones, David M. "The veterinary surgeon in the zoo world." *Vet. Record* 111 (1982): 526-528.

Jordan, David S. *Evolution and Animal Life.* New York: Appleton, 1907.

July, Robert William. *Precolonial Africa.* New York: Scribner, 1975.

Kalechofsky, Roberta. *Autobiography of a Revolutionary: Essays on Animal and Human Rights.* Marblehead, Ma: Micah Publishing, 1991.

Kalra, S.K. "Possibilities of relating modern veterinary science literature to the growth of relevant knowledge in ancient India." *Indian J. Hist. Sci.* 22 (1987): 141-157.

Kaplan, M.M. and Bögel, K. "Historical perspective of the origins and development of international veterinary public health in the World Health Association." *Rev. sci. tech. Off. int. Epiz.* 10 (1991): 915-931.

Karasszon, Denes. *A Concise History of Veterinary Medicine.* Trans. E. Farkas. Budapest: Akadémiai Kiadó, 1988.

Karasszon, Denes. "History of the Budapest Veterinary School." *Acta Veterinaria Hungarica* 35 (1987): 9-48.

Karstad, Lars, Nestel, Barry and Graham, Michael. *Wildlife Disease Research and Economic Development.* Ottawa, Can: International Development Research Centre, 1981.

Katic, Ivan. *Dansk-russiske veterinaere forbindelser 1796-1976.* Copenhagen: n.p., 1982.

Keegan, John. *A History of Warfare.* New York: Alfred A Knopf, 1993.

Keen, Maurice. *Chivalry.* New Haven: Yale University Press, 1990.

Keith, Thomas B. *The Horse Interlude.* Ed. Clifton Anderson. Moscow: University of Idaho Press, 1976.

Kertesz, Peter. *A Color Atlas of Veterinary Dentistry and Oral Surgery.* Aylesbury, U.K.: Wolfe, 1993.

Kilgour, Ronald and Dalton, Clive. *Livestock Behavior.* Auckland, NZ: Methuen, 1984.

Kinder, Hermann and Hilgemann, Werner. *The Penguin Atlas of World History.* Trans. Ernest A. Menze. 2 vols. London: Penguin, 1978.

King, J.O.L. "The transport of animals." *UFAW Courier* 13 (1957): 7-15.

King, Lester S. *The Growth of Medical Thought.* Chicago: University of Chicago Press, 1963.

Kinross, Patrick B. *The Ottoman Centuries.* New York: William Morrow, 1979.

Kitasato, Shibasaburo. *Collected Papers of Shibasaburo Kitasato.* Tokyo: Kitasato Institute, 1977.

Ki-Zerbo, Joseph., ed. *Methodology and African Prehistory.* Abridged ed. London: Currey, 1990.

Kliks, M.M. "Helminths as heirlooms and souvenirs: A review of New World paleoparasitology." *Parasitology Today* 6 (1990): 93-100.

Klinkenborg, Verlyn. "If it weren't for the ox, we wouldn't be where we are." *Smithsonian* 24 (Sept. 1993): 82-93.

Kloster, Hans. *Svinets Historie.* Copenhagen: DSR Forlag, 1984.

Knappert, Jan. *Indian Mythology.* London: Aquarian-Harper Collins, 1991.

Knight, David. *Ordering the World.* London: Burnett, 1981.

Koch, Robert. *Essays of Robert Koch.* Trans. K. Codell Carter. New York: Greenwood, 1987.

Koebner, Linda. *Zoo Book: The Evolution of Wildlife Conservation Centers.* New York: Forge, 1994.

Koenigsberger, H.G. *Medieval Europe 400-1500.* Harlow, Essex: Longman, 1987.

Konczacki, Z.A. and J.M., eds. *An Economic History of Tropical Africa.* Vol 1. London: Cass, 1977.

Koolmees, Peter A. *Department of the Science of Food of Animal Origin: History and Bibliography, 1918-1993.* Utrecht: Faculty of Veterinary Medicine, Utrecht University, 1993.

Korea Oriental Medical Academy. "The diet as complementary element in acupuncture treatment." In *A Collection of Treatises: In Commemoration of One Century Research in East-West Medicine.* Seoul, Korea: Sung-Yen Han, 1975.

Korovkin, F. *A History of the Ancient World.* Trans. Sergei Sossinsky. Moscow: Progress, 1985.

Kosambi, Damodar D. *Ancient India, A History of Its Culture and Civilization.* New York: Pantheon, 1965.

Kraig, Bruce. "The formation of civilization." In *The Forum Series.* St. Louis: Forum, 1979.

Kuthan, V. "Some contributions of J.E. Purkinje to the visual physiology." *Physiologia Bohemoslovaca,* 36 (1987): 255-267.

Kutumbia, P. *Ancient Indian Medicine.* Bombay: Orient Longmans, 1962.

Kyle, Russell. *A Feast in the Wild.* Oxford: Kudu, 1987.

Laidlaw, Patrick P. *Virus Diseases and Viruses.* New York: Macmillan, 1939.

Lajoux, Jean-Dominique. *The Rock Paintings of Tassili.* Cleveland: World, 1965.

Lambrecht, Frank L. "Aspects of evolution and ecology of tsetse flies and trypanosomiasis in prehistoric African environment." Fage, J.D. and Oliver R.A. eds. *Papers in African Prehistory.* Cambridge: University Press, 1970.

Larousse Encyclopedia of Ancient and Medieval History. Trans. Delano Ames and Geoffrey Sainsbury. New York: Excalibur, 1981.

Law, James. *Textbook of Veterinary Medicine.* 5 vols, 1896,1900,1901, 1902,1903. Ithaca: Published by the author, 1896-1903.

Laycock, George. *The Hunters and the Hunted.* New York: Outdoor Life-Meredith, 1990.

Lechevalier, Hubert and Solotorovsky, Morris. *Three Centuries of Microbiology.* New York: McGraw-Hill, 1965.

Leclainche, Emmanuel. *Historie de la Medicine Vétérinaire.* Toulouse: Office du Livre, 1936.

Lee, Richard B. and DeVore, Irven. *Man the Hunter.* Chicago: Aldine, 1968.

Leffingwell, Albert. *The Vivisection Question.* New Haven: Tuttle, 1901.

Legg, Stuart. *The Barbarians of Asia.* New York: Dorset, 1970.

Leighton, Albert C. *Transport and Communication in Early Medieval Europe AD 500-1100.* New York: Barnes, 1972.

Lemonds, Leo L. *A Century of Veterinary Medicine in Nebraska.* Hastings, Neb: L.L. Lemonds, 1982.

Leonard, Ellis P. *A Cornell Heritage: Veterinary Medicine 1868-1908.* Ithaca: New York State College of Veterinary Medicine, 1979.

Leonard, Ellis P. *In the James Law Tradition 1908-1948.* Ithaca, NY: NYS College of Veterinary Medicine, 1982.

Leonard, Ellis P. *A Veterinary Centennial in New York State.* New York: State Veterinary Medical Society, 1989.

Leroi-Gourhan, André. *Treasures of Prehistoric Art.* New York: Abrams, 1967.

Leslie, Charles, ed. *Asian Medical Systems: A Comparative Study.* Berkeley: University of California Press, 1976.

Léveque, Pierre. *The Greek Adventure.* Trans. Miriam Kochan. Cleveland: World, 1968.

Libro commemorativo de Bicentenario de la Facultad de Veterinaria Universidad de Madrid 1793-1993.

Liedtke, Walter. *The Royal Horse and Rider.* New York: Metropolitan Museum of Art and Abaris, 1989.

Linberg, David C. *The Beginnings of Western Science.* Chicago: University of Chicago Press, 1992.

Linden, Eugene. *Apes, Men and Language.* Updated with a new afterword. London: Penguin, 1981.

Linton, Alan H. *Microbes, Man and Animals.* Chichester, UK: Wiley, 1982.

Linzey, Andrew. *Christianity and the Rights of Animals.* New York: Crossroad, 1987.

Livestock. In *Managing Global Genetic Resources* Series. Washington: National Academy, 1993.

Lizet, Bernadette. *Le Cheval.* Paris: Berger-Levrault, 1982.

Lloyd, G.E.R. *Early Greek Science: Thales to Aristotle.* New York: Norton, 1970.

Lodrick, Deryck O. *Sacred Cows, Sacred Places.* Berkeley: University of California Press, 1981.

Loew, Franklin M. and Wood, Edward H. *Vet in the Saddle.* Saskatoon, Can: Western Producer Prairie, 1978.

Loew, Franklin M. "Turning plowshares into Volvos: changing American attitudes toward livestock." *J. Agr. Envtl. Ethics,* 6 (suppl.1) (1993): 105-109.

Lommel, Andreas. *Prehistoric and Primitive Man.* New York: McGraw-Hill, 1966.

Long, Esmond R. *A History of Pathology.* New York: Dover, 1965.

Long, James. *The Book of the Pig.* London: Gill, 1886.

Longrigg, Roger. *The English Squire and His Sport.* London: Joseph, 1977.

Lonsdale, Steven. *Animals and the Origins of Dance.* London: Thames, 1981.

Lorenz, Konrad Z. *The Foundations of Ethology.* New York: Touchstone, Simon & Schuster, 1981.

Luce, Gay G. *Biological Rhythms in Human and Animal Physiology.* New York: Dover, 1976.

Lush, J.L. *Animal Breeding Plans.* Ames: Iowa State College Press,1937

Lush, J.L. "Family merit as bases for selection." *Am. Nat.* 81 (1947): 241.

Lyons, Albert S. and Petrucelli, R. Joseph, II. *Medicine, An Illustrated History.* New York: Abrams, 1978.

MacDonald, June F. *Animal Biotechnology.* Ithaca, NY: National Agricultural Biotechnology Council, 1992.

MacFadden, Bruce J. *Fossil Horses.* Cambridge: Cambridge University Press, 1992.

Machado, Manuel A., Jr. *Aftosa.* Albany: SUNY Press, 1969.

Mackay-Smith, Alexander, Druesedow, Jean R. and Ryder, Thomas. *Man and the Horse.* New York: Simon & Schuster, 1984.

MacQuitty, William. *Ramesses the Great.* New York: Crown, 1978.

Maehle, Andreas-Holger. "Literary responses to animal experimentation in seventeenth- and eighteenth-century Britain." *Med. Hist.* 34 (1990): 27-51.

Magner, Lois N. *A History of the Life Sciences.* 2nd ed. New York: Marcel Dekker, 1984.

Magrane, William G. *A History of Veterinary Ophthalmology.* Elkhart, Indiana: Franklin, 1988.

Majno, Guido. *The Healing Hand.* Cambridge: Harvard University Press, 1975.

Major, J. Kenneth. *Animal-Powered Machines.* Aylesbury, UK: Shire, 1985.

Malek, Jaromir. *The Cat in Ancient Egypt.* London: British Museum Press, 1993.

Malkin, Harold M. "Rudolf Virchow and the durability of cellular pathology." *Pers. in Biol. and Med.* 33 (1990): 431-443.

Malin, Donald F. *The Evolution of Breeds.* Des Moines, Ia: Wallace, 1923.

Manning, Aubrey and Serpell, James. eds. *Changing Perspectives.* London: New York: Routledge, 1994

Marek, Joseph. *Lehrbuch der Klinische Diagnostik der Inneren Krankheiten der Haustiere.* Jena: Verlag von Gustav Fischer, 1912.

Markham, Sidney D. *The Horse in Greek Art.* New York: Biblo, 1969.

Marquardt, Kathleen. *Animal Scam: The Beastly Abuse of Human Rights.* Washington, DC: Regnery Gateway Lanham MD: National Book Network, 1993.

Marshall, B.J., ed. *Sustainable Livestock Farming into the 21st Century.* Reading, UK: Centre for Agricultural Strategy, 1992.

Martin, Phyllis M. and O'Meara, Patrick, eds. *Africa.* Bloomington: Indiana University Press, 1977.

Maslow, Jonathan. *Sacred Horses.* New York: Random House, 1994.

Mason, Jim. and Singer, Peter. *Animal Factories.* New York: Crown, 1980

Mathijsen, August H.H.M. *Publication and Dissertations from the Veterinary College, later on the Faculty of Veterinary Medicine, in the Period 1921-1971.* Utrecht: University Library, Department of Veterinary Medicine, 1981.

Mathijsen, August H.H.M. "Recente publikaties van veterinair-historisch belang. *Argos* nr. 3 (1990): 79-82.

Maton, A., Daelemans, J., and Lambrecht, J. *Housing of Animals.* Amsterdam: Elsevier, 1985.

Maule, John P. *The Cattle of the Tropics.* Edinburgh: Edinburgh University Press, 1990.

Mayhew, Edward. *The Illustrated Horse Doctor.* 12th ed. London: W.H. Allen, 1881.

Mayhew, Edward. *The Horse's Mouth, Showing the Age by the Teeth.* 2nd ed. London: Messrs. Fores, n.d.

Mayhew, Edward. *Dogs, Their Management.* with revisions by Sewell, A.J. London: Routledge, 1901.

Mayr, Ernst. *The Growth of Biological Thought.* Cambridge: Belknap-Harvard University Press, 1982.

Mayr, Ernst. *One Long Argument.* Cambridge: Harvard University Press, 1991.

Mayr, Ernst and Provine, William B. *The Evolutionary Synthesis.* Cambridge: Harvard University Press, 1980.

McBride, Anne. *Rabbits and Hares.* London: Whittet Books, 1988

McDonald, Jerry N. *North American Bison.* Berkeley: University of California Press, 1981.

McDonald, John M. "Ramazzini's dissertation on rinderpest." *Bull. Hist. Med.* 12 (1942): 529-539.

McEvedy, Colin. *The Penguin Atlas of African History.* New York: Penguin, 1980.

McEvedy, Colin. *The Penguin Atlas of Ancient History.* New York: Penguin, 1967.

McFadyean, J. *The Anatomy of the Horse: A Dissection Guide.* New York: William R. Jenkins, 1884.

McGee, James O., et. al., eds. *Oxford Textbook of Pathology.* Oxford: Oxford University Press, 1992.

McGuire, J. Dennis. and Hansen, James E.II. *Chiron's Time.* Fort Collins, Colo: College of Veterinary Medicine and Biomedical Sciences, 1983.

McHugh, Tom. *The Time of the Buffalo.* New York: Alfred A. Knopf, 1972.

McKeown, Thomas. *The Role of Medicine.* Princeton: Princeton University Press, 1979.

McKinney, William T. *Models of Mental Disorders: A New Comparative Psychiatry.* New York: Plenum Medical, 1988

McLoughlin, John C. *The Canine Clan.* New York: The Viking Press, 1983.

McNeil, William H. *Plagues and Peoples.* New York: Anchor, 1976.

McSherry, Bernard J. and Valli, V.E.O. "Veterinary clinical pathology 1888-1988." *J. Comp. Path.* 99 (1988): 27-40.

Mead, Kate Campbell Hurd. *A History of Women in Medicine.* Haddam, Conn: Haddam Press, 1938.

Meadows, Jack. *The Great Scientists.* New York: Oxford University Press, 1987.

Merrilat, L.A. and Campbell, D.M. *Veterinary Military History of the United States.* 2 vols. Chicago: Veterinary Magazine Corp. 1935.

Mery, Fernand *The Life, History and Magic of the Cat.* New York: Grosset and Dunlop, 1968.

Mery, Fernand. *The Life, History and Magic of the Dog.* New York: Grosset, 1970.

Meyer, Karl F. *Medical Research and Public Health. An interview conducted by Edna Tartaul Daniel in 1961 and 1962.* Berkeley: Regents of the University of California, 1976.

Michell, A.R., ed. *The Advancement of Veterinary Science: The Bicentenary Symposium Series.* 4 vols. Wallingford: C.A.B. International, 1993.

Mickartz, G.V., Heer, A., Demmler, T., Rehder, H. and Seidler, M. "Tierschutz und tierseuchengerechtes Töten von Rindern, Schweinen und Schafen mit Hilfe einer transportablen Elektro-Anlage zur Schladtiertäubung (Schermer, Typ EC)." *Dtsch. tierärztl. Wschr.* 96 (1989): 85-156.

Miles, Gary B. *Virgils Georgics.* Berkeley: University of California Press, 1980.

Miller, Everett B. *United States Army Veterinary Service in World War II.* Washington: Office of the Surgeon General, Department of the Army, 1961.

Miller, William R. History of the Federal Meat and Poultry Inspection Program in Woods. George, T. ed. *Practice in Veterinary Public Health and Preventive Medicine in United States.* Ames, Ia: Iowa State University Press, 1986

Milner, Mordaunt. *The Godolphin Arabian.* London: J.A. Allen, 1990.

Ministry of Agriculture, Fisheries and Food, Great Britain. *Animal Health A Centenary 1865-1965.* London: HMSO, 1965.

Mitchell, Chas. A. "A note on the early history of veterinary science in Canada." *Can. J. Comp. Med.* (1938-1940): In several articles.

Mitchell, Timothy. *Blood Sport: A Social History of Spanish Bullfighting.* Philadelphia: University of Pennsylvania Press, 1991.

Mitra, Rajendalala. "Description of contents of five manuscripts treating of ancient Hindu veterinary art." *Proc. Asiatic Soc. of Bengal.* (July, 1885): 91-95.

Mizuno, Kogen. *The Beginnings of Buddhism.* Trans. Richard L. Gage. Tokyo: Kosei, 1980.

Moore, John A. "Science as a way of knowing IV—developmental biology." *Am. Zool.* 27 (1986): 1-159.

Moorehead, Alan. *Darwin and the Beagle.* London: Penguin, 1971.

Moorhouse, Geoffrey. *India Britannica.* London: Paladin, 1983.

More, Daisy and Bowman, John. *Aegean Rivals.* Boston: Boston, 1986.

Morgan, Thomas H., Sturtevant, A.H. Muller, H.J. and Bridges, C.B. *The Mechanisms of Mendelian Heredity.* New York: Henry Holt, 1915. 2nd ed. 1923.

Morgan, Thomas H. *A Critique of the Theories of Evolution: Lectures Delivered at Princeton University.* Princeton University Press: 1916.

Morris, Desmond. *Catlore.* New York: Crown, 1987.

Moss, Henry St.L.B. *The Birth of the Middle Ages 395-814.* New York: Galaxy-Oxford University Press, 1964.

Moulé, L. *Histoire de la Médicine Vétérinaire. Deuxieme Periode. Histoire de la Médicine Vétérinaire au Moyen Age (476-1500AD).* Bull. de la Société Centrale de Médicine Vétérinaire. Paris: Asselin et Houzeau, 1896.

Moulin, Raoul-Jean. *Prehistoric Painting.* Trans. Anthony Rhodes. New York: Funk & Wagnalls, 1969.

Müller, Georg, and Glass, Alexander. *Diseases of the Dog.* Chicago: Eger, 1926.

Muller, H.J. "Artificial transmutation of the gene." *Science,* 46 (1927): 84

Murdock, George P. *Africa: Its Peoples and Their Culture History.* New York: McGraw-Hill, 1959.

Murray, Jacqueline. *The First European Agriculture.* Edinburgh: Edinburgh University Press, 1970.

Myers, J. Arthur. *Captain of All These Men of Death.* St. Louis: Green, 1977.

Myers, Kathleen. *The Southdown.* Bellefonte, Penn: American Southdown Breeders' Association, 1982.

Nalbandov, Andrew V. "Puzzles of reproductive physiology." *J. Reprod. Fert.* 34 (1973): 1-8.

National Research Council. *Little-Known Asian Animals With a Promising Future.* Washington, DC: National Academy Press, 1983.

Netting, Robert M. *Cultural Ecology.* 2nd ed. Prospect Heights, Il: Waveland, 1986.

Neu, Harold C. *New Antibacterial Strategies.* Edinburgh; New York: Churchill Livingstone, 1990.

Neugebauer, Otto. *The Exact Sciences in Antiquity.* 2nd ed. New York: Dover, 1969.

New Larousse Encyclopedia of Mythology. Trans. Richard Aldington and Delano Ames. New ed. London: Hamlyn, 1968.

The New World Screwworm Eradication Program: North Africa, 1988-1992. Rome: Food and Agriculture Organization of the United Nations, 1992.

Nitecki, Matthew H., ed. *Extinctions.* Chicago: University of Chicago Press, 1984.

Nordenskiöld, Erik, *The History of Biology.* Trans. Leonard B. Eyre, New York: Tudor, 1949.

Nuland, Sherwin B. *Doctors, The Biography of Medicine,* New York: Alfred A. Knopf, 1988.

Oates, Joan. *Babylon.* Rev. ed. London: Thames, 1979.

Ochman, Howard and Wilson, Allan C. "Evolution in bacteria: Evidence for a universal substitution rate in cellular genomes." *J. Molecular Evolution.* 26 (1987): 74-86.

Oder, Eugen. *Apsyrtus: Lebensbild des Bedeutendsten Altgriechischen Veterinärs.* Leipzig: Verlag Walter Richter, 1926.

Office International des Epizooties. "Early methods of animal disease control." *OIE Sci. Tech. Review,* 13, No.2, (June 1994).

Olby, Robert C. *Origins of Mendelism.* New York: Schocken, 1966.

Oliver, Daniel T. *Animal Rights: The Inhumane Crusade.* Washington, DC: Capital Research Center, 1993.

Olivova, Vera. *Sports and Games in the Ancient World.* New York: St. Martin's Press, 1984.

O'Malley, Charles D., ed. *The History of Medical Education.* Berkeley: University of California Press, 1970.

Osler, William. *The Evolution of Modern Medicine.* New Haven Conn: Yale University Press, 1921.

Outteridge, Peter M. *Veterinary Immunology.* London: Academic, 1985.

Pääbo, Svante. "Ancient DNA." *Scientific American,* Nov. 1993: 86-92.

Packer, R. Allen. "Veterinarians challenge Dr. Robert Koch regarding bovine tuberculosis and public health." *JAVMA* 196 (1990): 574-575.

Pallottino, Massimo. *Etruscan Painting.* Geneva: Skira, 1952.

Parascandola, John. *The Development of American Pharmacology.* Baltimore: Johns Hopkins University Press, 1992.

Parliamentary Office of Science and Technology. *The Use of Animals in Research, Development and Testing.* London: P.O.S.T., 1992.

Parry, Herbert B. *Scrapie Disease in Sheep.* London: Academic, 1983.

Passmore, John. "The treatment of animals." *J. Hist. Ideas* 36 (1975): 195-218.

Pastoret, Paul P., Mees, G., and Mammerickx, M, eds. *De L'Art a la Science ou 150 ans De Médecine Vétérinaire à Cureghem.* Brussels, Belgium: Annales de Medicine Vétérinaire, 1986.

Patrick, Richard. *All Color Book of Greek Mythology.* London: Octopus, 1972.

Pattison, Iain. *A Great British Veterinarian Forgotten, James Beart Simonds.* 1990.

Pattison, Iain. *The British Veterinary Profession 1791-1948.* London: J.A. Allen, 1984.

Pattison, Iain. *John McFadyean.* London: J.A. Allen, 1981.

Pavlovsky, Evgeny N. *Natural Nidality of Transmissible Diseases.* Trans. Frederick K. Plous, Jr. Urbana: University of Illinois Press, 1966.

Pepin, Michael. *Historie des Veterinaires.* Montreal: Francois Lubrina, 1986.

Pericot, Garcia L. *Prehistoric and Primitive Art.* New York: Abrams, 1968.

Perkins, Dexter Jr. "Fauna of Catal Hüyük: Evidence of early cattle domestication in Anatolia." *Science* 164 (1969): 177-179.

Peters, A.R. and Ball, P.J.H. *Reproduction in Cattle.* London: Butterworths, 1987.

Pfeiffer, John E. *The Creative Explosion.* Ithaca: Cornell University Press, 1982.

Phillipson, Andrew T., Hall, L.W., and Pritchard, W.R. *Scientific Foundations of Veterinary Medicine.* London: Heinemann, 1980.

Phillipson, David W. *African Archaeology.* Cambridge: Cambridge University Press, 1985.

Porter, Roy, ed. *Man Masters Nature.* New York: Braziller, 1988.

Portsmouth, Gerald V.W. *British Farm Stock.* London: Collins, 1950.

Portugal, Franklin H. and Cohen, Jack S. *A Century of DNA.* Cambridge: Massachusetts Institute of Technology Press, 1977.

Postan, M.M. ed. *The Cambridge Economic History of Europe.* 2nd. Ed. vol.1. Cambridge: Cambridge University Press, 1966.

Pounds, N.J.G. *A Historical Geography of Europe.* Cambridge: Cambridge University Press, 1990.

Prideaux, Tom. *Cro-Magnon Man.* New York: Time-Life, 1973.

Pritchard, D.G. "A century of bovine tuberculosis 1888-1988: Conquest controversy." *J. Comp. Path.* 99 (1988):357-399.

Prusiner, Stanley, et. al., eds. *Prion Diseases of Humans and Animals.* New York: Ellis Horwood, 1992.

Pugh, L.P. *From Farriery to Veterinary Medicine: 1785-1795.* Cambridge: W. Heffer and Sons, 1962.

Rachels, James. *Created From Animals.* Oxford: Oxford University Press, 1990.

Railliet, Alcide and Moulé, L. *Historie de L'Ecole D'Alfort.* Paris: Asselin, 1908.

Rawson, Jessica. *Animals in Art.* London: British Museum, 1977.

Reader, John. *Man on Earth,* Austin: University of Texas Press, 1988.

Reed, Charles A. "Animal domestication in the prehistoric Near East." *Science* 130 (1959): 1629-1639.

Reed, Charles A. ed. *Origins of Agriculture.* The Hague: Mouton, 1977.

Regan, Tom, ed. *Animal Sacrifices.* Philadelphia: Temple University Press, 1986.

Reid, W. Malcolm. "History of avian medicine in the United States. Control of coccidiosis." *Avian Diseases* 34 (1990): 509-525.

Reinach, S. *Apollo.* Trans. Florence Simmonds. 3rd ed. New York: Scribner, 1924.

Reiser, Stanley J. *Medicine and the Reign of Technology.* Cambridge: Cambridge University Press, 1978.

"Remaking the wheel: Evolution of the chariot." *New York Times,* Feb 22, 1994: B5.

Renucci, Simon-Francois. *Thése Inaugurale sur la Découverte de L'Insecte qui Produit la Contagion de la Gale.* Paris: Didot le Jeune, 1855.

Rice, Tamara T. *Ancient Arts of Central Asia.* New York: Praeger, 1965.

Richards, Robert J. *Darwin and the Emergence of Evolutionary Theories of Mind and Behavior.* Chicago: University of Chicago Press, 1987.

Richards, Vincent. *The Landmarks of Snake Poison Literature.* Calcutta: Traill, 1885.

Richter, Gisela M.A. *Animals in Greek Sculpture.* New York: Oxford University Press, 1930.

Rieck, Wilhelm. "Die Entwicklung der veterinärhistorischen Forschung." *Veterinärhistorisches Jahrbuch,* jahrgang 7 (1935): 197-212.

Rindos, David. *The Origins of Agriculture.* Orlando: Academic, 1984.

Ritchie, Carson I.A. *Rock Art of Africa.* New York: Barnes, 1979.

Robinson, Michael H. and Tiger, Lionel. *Man and Beast Revisited.* Washington: Smithsonian Institution, 1991.

Roe, Frank G. *The Indian and the Horse.* Norman: University of Oklahoma Press, 1955.

Rogers, J.M. *Mughal Miniatures.* London: British Museum Press, 1993

Rogers, Leonard. *Happy Toil.* London: Muller, 1950.

Rolleston, Humphrey D. *The Cambridge Medical School.* Cambridge: Cambridge University Press, 1932.

Romanes, George J. *Mental Evolution in Animals: With a Posthumous Essay on Instinct by Charles Darwin.* New York: D. Appleton Co., 1884.

Romanes, George J. *Darwin, and After Darwin.* Chicago: The Open Court Publishing Co., 1896.

Ronan, Colin A. Science: *Its History and Development Among the World's Cultures.* New York: Facts on File, 1982.

Rosenberg, Charles E. and Golden, Janet. *Framing Disease: Studies in Cultural History.* New Brunswick, NJ: Rutgers University Press, 1992.

Rosenblum, Robert. *The Dog in Art: from Rococo to Post-Modernism.* London: John Murray, 1988.

Rosenkranz, Barbara G. "The Trouble With Bovine Tuberculosis." *Bull. Hist. Med.* 59 (1985): 155-175.

Ross, Ian C. *Memoirs and Papers.* Melbourne, Aust.: Oxford University Press, 1961.

Rothschild, Bruce M. and Martin, Larry D. *Paleopathology.* Boca Raton, Fla: CRC Press, 1993.

Rowan, Andrew N., ed. *Animals and People Sharing the World.* Hanover, NH: University Press of New England, 1988.

Ruckebusch, Y. *Evolution de la Therapeutique Vétérinaire.* Toulouse: Ecole Nationale Veterinaire, 1982.

Ruffié, Jacques. *The Population Alternative.* Trans. Laurence Garey. New York: Pantheon, 1986.

Rupke, Nicolaas A., ed. *Vivisection in Historical Perspective.* London: Routledge, 1990.

Ruse, Michael. *The Darwinian Paradigm*. London: Routledge, 1989.

Ruspoli, Mario. *The Cave of Lascaux*. New York: Abrams, 1986.

Russell, Howard S. *A Long Deep Furrow*. Abridged ed. Hanover, N.H.: University Press of New England, 1982.

Russell, Nicholas. *Like Engend'ring Like: Heredity and Animal Breeding in Early Modern England*. Cambridge: Cambridge University Press, 1986.

Ryder, Richard D. *Animal Revolution*. Oxford: Blackwell, 1989.

Sackmann, Werner. *Veterinary Literature of Seven Centuries (13th-19th)*. Basel Switzerland: University Library Basel, 1988.

Salisbury, Joyce E. *The Beast Within: Animals in the Middle Ages*. New York: Routledge, 1994.

Sandars, Nancy K. *Prehistoric Art in Europe*. 2nd ed. New York: Penguin, 1985.

Sanders, Alvin H. *Short-Horn Cattle*. Chicago: Sanders, 1918.

Sanders, Alvin H. *The Cattle of the World*. Washington: National Geographic Society, 1926.

Sanderson, Ivan T. *A History of Whaling*. (First published as "Follow the Whale.") New York: Barnes and Noble, 1993.

Sandvik, Olav and Naess, Bjorn. *Animal Health Standards in Norway*. Oslo: Esset Grafisk AS, 1992.

Sanford, James K. *A Century of Service: 1894-1994*. Salem, Va: Virginia Veterinary Medical Association, 1994.

Saunders, Leon Z. *Veterinary Pathology in Russia, 1860-1930*. Ithaca: Cornell University Press, 1980.

Saunders, Nick. "The civilizing influence of agriculture." *New Scientist* 106 (June 13, 1985): 16-18.

Sayce, Roger. *The History of the Royal Agricultural College Cirencester*. Wolfeboro Falls, NH: Sutton, 1992.

Schäffer, Johann. "Der Waffenschmied: ein Tierarzt als Opernfigur." *Historia Medizina Veterinaria* 9 (1) (1984): 14-24.

Schäffer, Johann. "Die Pferdeheilkunde in der Spätantike—zum Stand der Bearbeitung des *Corpus Hippiatricorum Graecorum*." *Pferdeheilkunde* 1 (1985): 75-94.

Schäffer, Johann. "Über die tierärztliche Hämatoskopie in der Spätantike." *Tierarztl. prax.* 13 (1985): 131-139.

Schäffer, Johann. "Zur Semiotik und Diagnostik in der Pferdeheilkunde der Spätantike." *Pferdeheilkunde* 2 (1986): 139-166.

Schäffer, Johann. "Wenn eine Stute Zwillinge wirft..." Mesopotamische Geburtsomina und ihre (Be-) Deutung." *Pferdeheilkunde* 5 (1989): 81-87.

Schäffer, Johann. "Blutdiagnostik vor 200 Jahren-Ein Beitrag Hämatoskopie in der Veterinärmedizin." *Berl. Munch. Tierarztl. Wschr.* 104. (1991): 403-408.

Schäffer, Johann. "Pull (sfh)-Cattle obstetrics in ancient Egypt." *Proc. 25th. Int. Cong. Hist. Vet. Med.* Ankara, Turkey. (1992): p.184.

Schirokauer, Conrad. *A Brief History of Chinese and Japanese Civilizations*. 2nd ed. San Diego: Harcourt Brace Jovanovich, 1989.

Schönherr, W. "History of veterinary public health in Europe in the 19th century." *Rev. sci. tech. Off. int. Epiz.* 10 (1991): 985-994.

Schwabe, Calvin W. *Cattle, Priests, and Progress in Medicine*. Minneapolis: University of Minnesota Press, 1978.

Schwabe, Calvin W. *Veterinary Medicine and Human Health*. 3rd ed. Baltimore: Williams & Wilkins, 1984.

Schwartz, H.J. and Dioli, M. editors: *The One-Humped Camel in Eastern Africa*. Weikershein: Margraf, 1992.

Secord, William. *Dog Painting 1840-1940: A Social History of the Dog Art*. Woodbridge, Suffolk: Antique Collector's Club, 1992.

Serpell, James. In the Company of Animals: *A Study of Human–Animal Relationships*. New York: B. Blackwell, 1986.

Seth-Smith, Michael, et. al. *The History of Steeplechasing*. London: Joseph, 1969.

Shafer, Byron E., ed. *Religion in Ancient Egypt*. Ithaca: Cornell University Press, 1991.

Sharma, R.D., Kumar, Rakesh and Sridhar. "Historical background and analysis of scientific content of ancient Indian literature on practices for the treatment of diseases in domestic animals." *Indian J. Hist. Sci.* 22 (1987): 158-163.

Sharp, Robert. *The Cruel Deception*. Wellingborough, UK: Thorsons, 1988.

Shepard, Paul. *Thinking Animals*. New York: Viking, 1978.

Sheppard, Philip M. *Natural Selection and Heredity*. 3rd ed. London: Hutchinson, 1967.

Sherer, John. *Rural Life Described and Illustrated, in the Management of Horses, Dogs, Cattle, Sheep, Pigs, Poultry etc., Their Treatment in Health and Disease, and a Complete System of Modern Veterinary Practice*. London: London Printing and Publishing Co., 1868.

Shesgreen, Sean. ed. *Engravings by Hogarth*. New York: Dover, 1973

Shoshan, Arieh. *Animals in the Jewish Literature*. Rehovot: Shoshanim, 1971.

Shryock, R.H. *The Development of Modern Medicine*. Madison: University of Wisconsin Press, 1979.

Siegel, Judith M. "Companion animals: In sickness and in health. *J. of Social Issues*. 49. (1993): 157-167.

Sieveking, Ann. *The Cave Artists*. London: Thames, 1979.

Sigerst, Henry E. *The Great Doctors*. New York: Dover, 1971.

Simonds, Jas. B. *A Biographical Sketch of Two Distinguished Promoters of Veterinary Science, Delabere P. Blaine—William Youatt*. London: Adlard, 1896.

Singer, Peter. *Animal Liberation*. New York: Avon, 1975.

Singh, Harbans. *Domestic Animals*. New Delhi: National Book Trust, 1966.

Siraisi, Nancy G. *Medieval and Early Renaissance Medicine*. Chicago: University of Chicago Press, 1990.

Sisson, Septimus. *Anatomy of the Domestic Animals*. 2nd Ed. Philadelphia: Saunders, 1914.

Skellet, Edward. *A Practical Treatise on the Parturition of the Cow, or the Extraction of the Calf: and Also on Diseases of the Neat Cattle in General*. London: 1807.

Skovenborg, Erik. *Danske dyrlaege—exlibris: Veterinary Bookplates*. Skovenborg, E., 1992.

Smith, Bradley. *Spain, A History in Art*. New York: Gemini-Smith, 1966.

Smith, Frederick. *The Early History of Veterinary Literature and its British Development*. 4 vols. Reprinted from The Veterinary Journal. London: J.A. Allen, 1976.

Smith, Frederick. "A veterinary history of the war in South Africa 1899-1902." *Supplement to the Veterinary Record,* (May 25th 1912): 1-320.

Smith, Frederick. *A History of the Royal Army Veterinary Corps 1796-1919*. London: Bailliere, 1927.

Smithcors, James F. *Evolution of the Veterinary Art*. Kansas City: Veterinary Medicine, 1957.

Smithcors. James F. "Medical men and the beginning of veterinary medicine in America." *Bull. Hist. Med.* 33 (1959): 330-341.

Smithcors, James F. *The American Veterinary Profession*. Ames: Iowa State University Press, 1963.

Smithcors, James F. *The Veterinarian in America 1625-1975*. Santa Barbara, Calif: American Veterinary, 1975.

Snead, Stella. *Animals in Four Worlds*. Chicago: University of Chicago Press, 1989.

Soave, Orland A. *An Introduction to Veterinary Law*. Philadelphia: WB Saunders, 1962.

Soma, Lawrence R. *Textbook of Veterinary Anesthesia*. Baltimore: Williams & Wilkins, 1971.

Sourkes, Theodore L. *Nobel Prize Winners in Medicine and Physiology 1901-1965*. London: Abelard, 1953.

Speedy, A.W. editor. *Progress on Sheep and Goat Research*. Wallingford, Oxon: CAB International, 1992.

Speiser, Werner. *The Art of China*. New York: Crown, 1960.

Spence, Wayman R. *Perez on Medicine*. Waco, Tex: WRS Publishing, 1993.

Spencer, A. Jeffery. *Death in Ancient Egypt*. Harmondsworth, UK: Penguin, 1982.

Spier, R.E. "Veterinary vaccines: From plagues to percentages." *J. Comp. Path.* 99 (1988): 121-131.

Stalheim, Ole H.V. *The Winning of Animal Health: 100 years of Veterinary Medicine*. Ames: Iowa State University Press, 1994.

Stange, C.H. *History of Veterinary Medicine at Iowa State College*. Ames, Ia: 1929.

Stanley, Steven M. *The New Evolutionary Timetable: Fossils, Genes, and the Origin of Species*. New York: Basic Books, 1981.

Stapeldon, Olaf. *Odd John and Sirius*. New York: Dover, 1972.

Steel, John H. *A Treatise on the Diseases of the Dog*. New ed. New York: John Wiley & Sons, 1894.

Steele, James H. "Veterinary public health in the United States, 1776 to 1976." *JAVMA* 169 (1976): 74-82.

Steele, James H. "A bookshelf on veterinary public health." *Am. J. Public Health,* 63 (1973): 291-311.

Steele, James H. "Veterinary Public Health: Early history and recent world developments." *JAVMA* 173 (1978): 1497-1504.

Steele, James H. "History of veterinary public health in the United States of America." *Rev. Sci. Tech. Off. int. Epiz.* 10 (1991): 951-983.

Stern, C. Sherwood. *The Origin of Genetics: A Mendel Source Book*. San Francisco: W.H. Freeman, 1966.

Stevens, Lewis. *Genetics and Evolution of the Domestic Fowl*. Cambridge: Cambridge University Press, 1991.

"Stonehenge" (being Walsh, J.H.) *The Greyhound*. London: Longman et al., 1853.

Striedter, Karl H., ed. *Rock Paintings from Zimbabwe*. Wiesbaden: Steiner, 1983.

Strouhal, Eugene. *Life of the Ancient Egyptians*. Norman: University of Oklahoma Press, 1992.

Struever, Stuart, ed. *Prehistoric Agriculture*. Garden City, NY: Natural History, 1971.

Struever, Stuart, and Holton, Felicia A. Koster: *Americans in Search of Their Prehistoric Past*. New York: Mentor, 1985.

Stubbe, Hans. *History of Genetics*. Cambridge: Massachusetts Institute of Technology Press, 1972.

Stubbs, George. *The Anatomy of the Horse*. The original 1766 edition and illustrations with a modern veterinary paraphrase by McCunn, J. and Ottaway, C.W.: (with 24 additional plates published for the first time). London: J.A. Allen, 1965.

Sturtevant, A.H. *A History of Genetics*. New York: Harper & Row, 1965.

Suares, Jean C. *The Indispensible Cat*. New York: Stewart, 1983.

Suffolk, Henry C.H. *Racing and Steeple-chasing*. London: Longmans, 1893.

Sullivan, Michael. *The Arts of China*. Rev. ed. Berkeley: University of California Press, 1967.

Sutcliffe, Antony J. *On the Track of Ice Age Mammals*. Cambridge: Harvard University Press, 1985.

Svinhufvud, Anne C. *A Late Middle English Treatise on Horses*. Stockholm, Swed: Almqvist, n.d.

Szabo, Kalman T. *Congenital Malformations in Laboratory and Farm Animals*. San Diego: Academic, 1989.

Talbot, Lee M. *The Meat Production Potential of Wild Animals in Africa*. Farnham Royal, UK: Commonwealth Agricultural Bureaux, 1965.

Talbott, John H. *A Biographical History of Medicine*. New York: Grune & Stratton, 1970.

Tang, Ho Yin. *The Enigma of Hog Cholera: Controversies, Cause and Control*. PhD Thesis at University of Minnesota, 1986.

Tannenbaum, Jerrold. "Veterinary medical ethics: A focus on conflicting interests." *J. of Social Issues*. 49 (1993): 143-156.

Taylor, J. "W.T. Kendall and his profession." in Australian Veterinary History-Special issue of the *Australian Veterinary Journal*, 69,(12) (December, 1992): 322-324.

Temple, Norman J and Burkitt, Denis P. *Western Diseases*. Totowa, NJ: Humane Press, 1994.

Temple, Robert. *The Genius of China*. New York: Simon & Schuster, 1986.

Tehver, J. "On the history of higher veterinary education at Tartu (1848-1973)." *Historia Medicinae Veterinariae* 1 (1976): 4-12.

Theodorides, Jean. *Des Miasmes Aux Virus: Histoire de Maladies Infectieuses*. Paris: Editions Louis Pariente, 1991.

Thèves, Georges. *Le Luxembourg et ses Vétérinaires 1790-1990*. Luxembourg: Arts et Livres, 1991.

Thompson, Larry. *Correcting the Code*. New York: Simon & Schuster, 1994.

Thompson, Ray. *The Good Doctors*. Fallston, Md: Maryland Veterinary Medical Association, 1986.

Thompson, Ruth D. *The Remarkable Gamgees*. Edinburgh: Ramsay Head, 1974.

Thorwald, Jurgen. *Science and Secrets of Early Medicine*. Trans. Richard and Clara Wilson. New York: Harcourt Brace Jovanovich, 1963.

Toft, Catherine A., Aeschilmann, Andre, and Bolis, Liana. *Parasite-Host Associations*. Oxford: Oxford University Press, 1991.

Townley, Johnson R. *Major Rock Paintings of Southern Africa*. Bloomington: Indiana University Press, 1979.

Toynbee, Arnold. ed. *Half the World*. New York: Holt Rinehart & Winston, 1973.

Toynbee, Arnold. *A Study of History*. New rev. and abridged ed. New York: Weathervane, 1979.

Toynbee, Jocelyn M.C. *Animals in Roman Life and Art*. London: Thames, 1973.

Travnickova, E. and Trojan, S. "Jan Evangelista Purkinye 1787-1869." *Physiologia Bohemoslovaca* 30 (1987): 181-189.

Travnickova. E. and Trojan, S. "Jan Evangelista Purkinye (Purkinje) 1787-1869" *NIPS* 2 (1987): 232-235.

Trew, Cecil G. *The Story of the Dog: and His Uses to Mankind*. London: Methuen, 1940.

Tringham, Ruth. *Hunters, Fishers and Farmers of Eastern Europe 6000-3000 BC*. London: Hutchinson University Library, 1971.

Trow-Smith, Robert. *English Husbandry*. London: Faber & Faber, 1951.

Trow-Smith, Robert. *A History of British Livestock Husbandry 1700-1900*. London: Routledge, 1959.

Trow-Smith, Robert. *Life From the Land*. London: Longmans, 1967.

Turek, V. Marek, J and Benes J. *Fossils of the World*. New York: Arch Cape Press, 1989.

Turk, Kenneth L. *Animal Husbandry at Cornell University*. Ithaca: Cornell Universityn Press, 1987.

Turner, Trevor and Lane, Dick. "One hundred years of small animal practice." *Vet. Record* 111 (1982): 519-523.

Tweddell, Colin E. and Kimball, Linda A. *Introduction to the Peoples and Cultures of Asia*. Englewood Cliffs, NJ: Prentice Hall, 1985.

Twigg, Graham. *The Black Death*. London: Batsford, 1984.

Tyler, John M. *The New Stone Age in Northern Europe*. New York: Scribner, 1921.

Ucko, Peter J. and Dimbleby, G.W., eds. *The Domestication and Exploitation of Plants and Animals*. Chicago: Aldine, 1969.

Ullmann, Manfred. *Islamic Medicine*. Edinburgh: Edinburgh University Press, 1978.

Underwood, E. Ashworth. *Boerhaave's Men*. Edinburgh: Edinburgh University Press, 1977.

United States Department of Agriculture: Bureau of Animal Industry. *Special Report on Diseases of the Horse*. Washington, DC: Government Printing Office, 1896.

United States Department of Agriculture: Bureau of Animal Industry: *Fourteenth Annual Report of the BAI for the Fiscal Year 1897*. Washington, DC: US Government Printing Office, 1898.

United States Department of Agriculture: Bureau of Animal Industry. *Special Report on Diseases of Cattle*. Washington, DC: Government Printing Office, rev. ed. 1923.

United States Department of Agriculture. *After a Hundred Years*. Washington, DC: Government Printing Office, 1962.

United States Department of Agriculture. *Hog Cholera and its Eradication*. Washington, DC: U.S. Dept. of Agriculture, 1981.

University of Pennsylvania School of Veterinary Medicine. *History of the School of Veterinary Medicine of the University of Pennsylvania 1884-1934*. Philadelphia: Veterinary Alumni Society, 1935.

Urquhart, Fred, ed. *The Book of Horses*. New York: William Morrow, 1981.

Van der Post, Laurens. *The Heart of the Hunter*. New York: William Morrow, 1961.

Van der Waerden, Bartel L. *Science Awakening*. Trans. Arnold Dresden, New York: Oxford University Press, 1961.

Van Doren, Charles. *A History of Knowledge*. New York: Ballantine, 1991.

Van Slyke, Lyman P. *Yangtze*. Reading, Mass: Addison-Wesley, 1988.

Varner, John G. and Varner, Jeannette J. *Dogs of the Conquest*. Norman: University of Oklahoma Press, 1983.

Velikovsky, Immanuel. *Ramses II and His Time*. Garden City, NY: Doubleday, 1978.

Veterinary Work in the Netherlands. Leidschendam, Netherlands: Veterinary Service Information Division, 1971.

Viborg, Erik. *Veiledning til Svinets Behandling som Huusdyr*. Copenhagen: Proft, 1804.

Villemin, Martial. *Les Vétérinaires Francais au XIX Siècle*. Maisons-Alfort: du Pont Vétérinaire, 1982.

Virchow, Robert. *Cellular Pathology*. Trans. Frank Chance. 2nd ed. New York: Dover, 1971.

Vogel, Colin. "From firing to phenylbutazone in equine practice." *Vet. Rec.* 111 (1982): 523-525.

Voipio, Paavo. "What did Mendel say about evolution?" *Hereditas* 107 (1987): 103-105.

Von der Königlichen Tierarzneischule zur Veterinärmedizinischen Facultätder Humboldt-Universität zu Berlin 1790-1990. München: Quintessenz-Verlag, 1990.

Walford-Lloyd, E. *The Southdown Sheep*. Chichester, UK: Willis, 1925.

Walker, R.E. "The veterinary papyrus of Kahun." *Vet. Record* 76 (1964): 198-200.

Walker, Stella A. *Sporting Art*. New York: Potter, 1972.

Wallace, Alfred R. and Bates, Henry W. *Wallace and Bates in the Tropics*. Ed. Barbara G. Beddall. London: Macmillan, 1969.

Walley, Thomas. *The Four Bovine Scourges*. Edinburgh: MacLachlan, 1879.

Waltner-Toews, David. "What is a healthy farm?" *J. Agr. Envth Ethics*. vol. 6. Special supplements 1 and 2. (1993): 199-201.

Walton, John, Beeson, Paul B., and Scott, Ronald B., eds. *The Oxford Companion to Medicine.* 2 vols. Oxford: Oxford University Press, 1986.

Wang, K.Chi-min and Wu, Lien-Teh. *History of Chinese Medicine.* Tientsin, China: The Tientsin Press, 1932.

Wang, Qinglan. Selections from texts and illustrations on ancient and traditional Chinese veterinary medicine. Vice-Dean Wang, Qinglan. Veterinary Medicine College, Beijing Agricultural University. 1993.

Ward, William E.F. *A History of Africa.* Nashville: Aurora, 1970.

Ware, Jean and Hunt, Hugh. *The Several Lives of a Victorian Vet.* London: Bachman, 1979.

Warren, Kenneth S. and Purcell, Elizabeth F., eds. *The Current Status and Future of Parasitology.* New York: Josiah Macy, Jr. Foundation, 1981.

Warren, Peter. *The Aegean Civilizations.* London: Elsevier-Phaidon, 1975.

Warwick, Everett J. *Breeding and Improvement of Farm Animals.* 7th ed. New York: McGraw-Hill, 1979.

Waterson, A.P. and Wilkinson, Lise. *An Introduction to the History of Virology.* Cambridge: Cambridge University Press, 1978.

Watson, William. *Ancient China.* New York: New York Graphic Society, 1974.

Wayne, R.K., Van Valkenburgh, B., Kat, P.W., Fuller, T.K., Johnson, W.E. and O'Brien, S.J. "Genetic and morphologic divergence among sympatric canids." *J. Heredity.* 80 (1989): 447-454.

Weatherford, Jack. *Indian Givers.* New York: Crown, 1988.

Weatherley, Lee. *Great Horses of Britain.* Hindhead, UK: Spur, 1978.

Wedgwood, Cicely V. *The Spoils of Time.* Garden City, NY: Doubleday, 1985.

Wester, J. *Die Physiologie und Pathologie der Vormägen beim Rinde.* Berlin: Verlag Richard Schoess, 1926.

White, Sheila, ed. *Electroacupuncture in Veterinary Medicine.* Trans. P.A. Herbert and Teressa Hwang. San Francisco: Chinese Materials Center, 1984.

Whitehouse, David and Ruth. *Archaeological Atlas of the World,* San Francisco: Freeman, 1975.

Whittick, William G. *Canine Orthopedics.* 2nd ed. Philadelphia: Lea & Febiger, 1990.

Wilkinson, J. Gardener. *The Ancient Egyptians.* 2 vols. New York: Crescent, 1988.

Wilkinson, Lise. *Animals and Disease.* Cambridge: Cambridge University Press, 1992.

Wilkinson, Richard H. *Symbol and Magic in Egyptian Art. New York:* Thames and Hudson, 1994.

Willet, Frank. *African Art: An Introduction.* New York: Praeger, 1971.

Williams, Eric I. *A History of the Oklahoma State University College of Veterinary Medicine.* Stillwater: Oklahoma State University, 1986.

Williams, Guy. *The Age of Agony.* London: Constable, 1975.

Williamson, G. and Payne, W.J.A. *An Introduction to Animal Husbandry in the Tropics.* 3rd ed. New York: Longman, 1978.

Williamson, Stanton. *50 Years of Educational Excellence and Practice Improvement.* Mishawaka, Indiana: The Association, 1983.

Wilson, Graham. "Veterinary microbiologists of the 19th century." *J. Comp. Path.* 98 (1988): 117-134.

Winslow, Charles-Edward A. *The Conquest of Epidemic Disease.* Madison: University of Wisconsin Press, 1943.

Wiseman, Julian. *A History of the British Pig.* London: Duckworth, 1986.

Wiser, Vivian, Mark, Larry, and Purchase, H. Graham, eds. *100 Years of Animal Health.* Beltsville, Md: Associates of the National Agricultural Library, 1987.

Wobeser, Gary A. *Investigation and Management of Disease in Wild Animals.* New York: Plenum, 1994.

Wobeser, Gary A. "Rumen overload and PEM: Diseases associated with consumption of grain by pronghorns." *Proc. Pronghorn Antelope Workshop* 11 (1984): 129.

Wolpert, Stanley. *A New History of India.* 3rd ed. New York: Oxford University Press, 1989.

Wolpert, Stanley. *India.* Berkeley: University of California Press, 1991.

Wrensch, Frank A. *Harness Horse Racing in the United States and Canada.* New York: Van Nostrand, 1948.

Wright, Sewall. "Principles of livestock breeding." *USDA Bull.* 905 (1920): 1.

Wright, Sewall. "Genetic principles governing rate of progress in livestock breeding." *Proc. Am. Soc. Amm. Prod.* (1939): 18.

Wright, Sewall. "Evolution in Mendelian populations." *Genetics,* 16 (1931): 97.

Wright, Sewall. "The physiology of the gene." Physiol. *Rev 21* (1941): 487-527.

Wu, Lien-Teh, et al. *National Quarantine Service Series III-1932: Cholera.* Shanghai, China: National Quarantine Service, 1933.

Wylder, Joseph. *Psychic Pets,* New York: Bonanza, 1978.Young, David. The Discovery of Evolution. London: Natural History Museum, 1992.

Xenophon, "On horsemanship"; "On hunting: a sportsman's manual or cynegeticus." In *The Works of Xenophon.* Translated by Dakyns, H.G. vol. III part II, pages 37-69 and 73-126. London: MacMillan, 1897.

Young, David. *The Discovery of Evolution.* London: Natural History Museum, 1992

Zeledón, Rodrigo. "Epidemiology, modes of transmission and reservoir hosts of Chagas' disease." *CIBA Foundation Symposium,* vol. 20 (1994): 51-73.

Zeuner, Frederick E. *A History of Domesticated Animals.* London: Hutchinson, 1963.

Zhao, Ji. *The Natural History of China.* New York: McGraw-Hill, 1990.

Zheng, Jingwen. *The Art of Wu Zuoren.* Beijing: Foreign Language, 1986.

Zhong, Lin, ed. *Pond Fisheries in China.* Oxford: International Academic, 1991.

Zimmerman, Leo M. and Veith, Ilza. *Great Ideas in the History of Surgery.* 2nd rev. ed. New York: Dover, 1967.

Zuckerman, Lord. *The Zoological Society of London 1826-1976 and Beyond.* London: Academic Press, 1976.

INDEX